Theory and practice of crown and fixed partial prosthodontics (bridge)

Theory and practice of crown and fixed partial prosthodontics (bridge)

Stanley D. Tylman

A.B. D.D.S., M.S., F.A.C.D.

Emeritus Professor of Prosthetic Dentistry, University of Illinois College of Dentistry, Chicago, Illinois; Professor Honoris Causa, Universities of Brazil, Argentina, Venezuela, and Bolivia; Certified State Board Specialist in Prosthodontics

Sixth edition

With 1,426 illustrations and 5 color plates

The C. V. Mosby Company

Saint Louis 1970

Sixth edition

Printed in the United States of America

Standard Book Number 8016-5165-4

Library of Congress Catalog Card Number 76-102405

Distributed in Great Britain by Henry Kimpton, London

Contributors

Claude R. Baker, M.S., D.D.S.

Professor of Dentistry, University of Missouri School of Dentistry, Kansas City, Missouri

R. C. Brumfield, C.E.

Formerly Associate Professor of Civil Engineering, Cooper Institute, New York, New York

Arthur E. Elfenbaum, D.D.S.

Professor Emeritus, Northwestern University School of Dentistry and University of Illinois School of Dentistry, Chicago, Illinois

Niles F. Guichet, D.D.S.

Instructor, University of California Postgraduate School of Dentistry, Anaheim, California

Parker E. Mahan, D.D.S., Ph.D., F.A.C.D.

Associate Professor of Dentistry, Emory University School of Dentistry, Atlanta, Georgia

John W. McLean, N.D.S., L.D.S., R.C.S.

London, England

George H. Moulton, D.D.S., F.A.C.D.

Professor and Chairman, Department of Crown and Bridge Dentistry; Dean, Emory University School of Dentistry, Atlanta, Georgia

Robert J. Pinkerton, B.S., D.D.S.

Anaheim, California

Lovingly dedicated to

Isabelle Hannam Tylman

Preface

Education and research are continuous processes. After many years of teaching and practice in crown and fixed partial prosthodontics, one appreciates that dentistry is not static and that new discoveries and concepts in related sciences and disciplines affect the progress, objectives, and procedures of dental education and practice.

Our efforts in the previous five editions have been to offer the student and practitioner those concepts and methods which were based on clinical experience and research of accepted leaders in biologic and related sciences. Fullest cooperation has always been given by dedicated teachers, research men, and manufacturers too numerous to thank individually at this time but gratefully acknowledged for posterity.

Likewise, we cannot sufficiently express gratitude to those pioneers in our field of restorative dentistry who have left us their heritage: Capon, LeGro, Taggart, Prothero, Dittmar, Goslee, Tinker, Thompson, Hollenback, McCollum, and many others.

I am also grateful to the following men, who have furnished either revisions or major new material for this edition: Drs. Claude R. Baker, Arthur E. Elfenbaum, Niles F. Guichet, Arthur C. Long, R. J. Pinkerton, Parker E. Mahan, John W. McLean, George H. Moulton, R. Vining, and Everitt Payne, and Professor R. C. Brumfield.

I am also thankful to those numerous dentists, journals, and dental manufacturers who so graciously cooperated in furnishing material and illustrations.

Stanley D. Tylman

Contents

Chapter 30

Construction of pontics for fixed partial dentures: indications, types, and materials, 650

Chapter 31

Gold alloys and soldering operations related to crown and fixed partial prosthodontics, 682

Chapter 32

Assembling retainers and pontics utilizing connectors (nonrigid and rigid), 699

Chapter 33

Installation, maintenance, and repair of crowns and fixed partial prostheses, 712

Chapter 34

History and development of metal-ceramic fixed partial dentures (bridges); early types to present-day restorations, 733

Chapter 35

Current dental restorations utilizing ceramics fired to gold-alloy castings (Thermalite, Micro-Bond, Ceramco porcelains), 757

Chapter 36

Alumina-reinforced ceramics, 780

Chapter 37

Gnathologic procedures utilizing the Denar Model D4-A and pantograph, 806

Color plates

Theory and practice of crown and fixed partial prosthodontics (bridge)

Chapter 1

History of crown and fixed partial prosthodontics (bridge)*

EARLY HISTORY

Man for many centuries has mutilated, decorated, and adorned his teeth.[1] This phase of expression, however, does not justifiably fit into the history of dental prosthesis. The literature on the subject is quite voluminous. In like fashion, teeth have always played an important part in the practice of magic. "Throughout prehistoric time, down through the centuries of written records, man has inflicted wounds and mutilations upon himself, inspired by vanity, fashion, generosity, mystical and religious ideas, and perversion of the senses."[1] The esthetic taste is indeed profound.

The histories of fixed and of removable partial prostheses go more or less hand in hand, and it is difficult at times to tell just where to draw the line between these types from the available data.

It seems apparent that the most ancient dental prosthetic appliances have been of the fixed bridgework type. These ancient relics of early civilization are artificial teeth, or detached natural teeth from one mouth adjusted to another by means of ligatures or similar contrivances to hold them in place. The ligatures employed for the maintenance of the interpolated teeth were threads of various materials, gold or silver wires, or gold ribbons, or connecting rings, which more or less provided for fixation (Figs. 1-1 and 1-2).

In one of the oldest tombs at Saida (ancient Sidon, dating between 300 and 400 B.C.) was found an extant Phoenician specimen consisting of gold wire fastened around six lower anterior teeth, two of the incisors being pontics (bridged-in teeth), natural teeth from which roots were removed with extra wires passing through holes in them and over the root ends, while another set of wires bound together the incisal edges. This relic now rests in the Louvre, Paris.[2]

Brown[3] stated: "There is no proof in extant relics or indubitable records that the ancient Egyptians practiced anything in the way of dental prosthesis or even ligated loose teeth; the only appliance for the latter purpose found in Egypt being the one described above, from a Roman grave of the first century A.D.

"But I was assured recently at the great Egyptian Museum in Cairo and elsewhere in Egypt that no specimen of ancient Egyptian prosthetic dentistry is known to modern Egyptologists."[3]

There are also some statements regarding artificial teeth in the mouths of mummies.[4] It is probable that the Phoenicians, and not the Egyptians, were the first to construct dental bridgework.

The ancient dental prosthetists attempted not only to replace the missing member but also to fix it to the adjacent

*Text by Claude Rowe Baker, M.S., D.D.S.; Professor of Dentistry, University of Missouri at Kansas City. Figures by the author (S.D.T.).

A 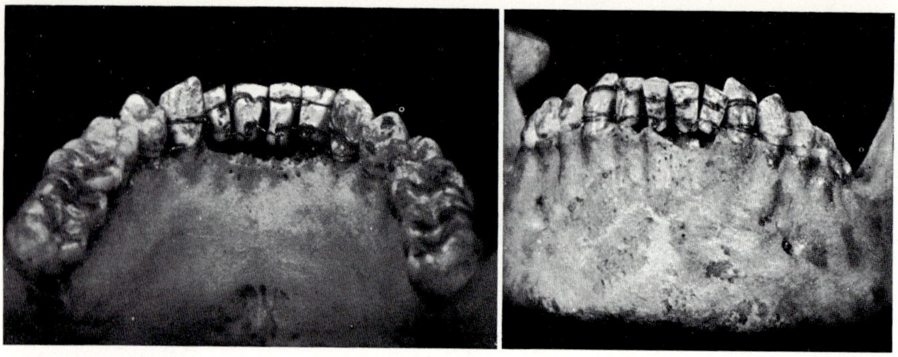 B

Fig. 1-1. A and **B,** Use of gold wires to fasten natural extracted teeth to remaining natural abutments.

A B C D 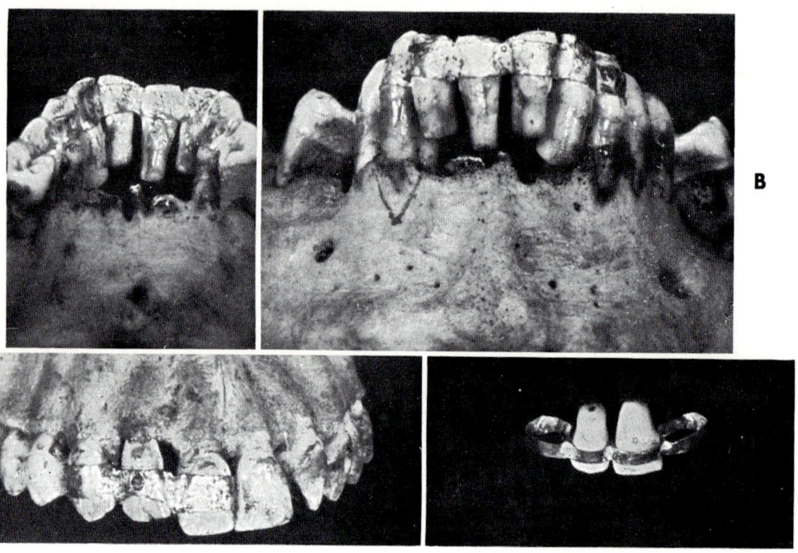

Fig. 1-2. A to **D,** Gold bands employed to attach extracted natural teeth to remaining natural teeth.

teeth. The fixation of weak teeth to adjacent stronger members was a very early practice. This principle, with modifications and variations, is employed by clinical dentists today. One of the earliest known appliances which employed this principle belongs to the sixth century B.C. It was found in an Etruscan necropolis and is now at the University of Ghent, Belgium. It was constructed for supporting loose teeth, and the condition of the sockets of the three wanting teeth evidences their existence until the end of the patient's life.[5]

As early as the middle of the first pre-Christian millennium are found artificial partial dentures, fixed and removable, made of soft gold and embracing natural or artificial pontics. One of the most interesting and earliest extant specimens of a carved block of teeth is an Etruscan dental bridge constructed before 500 B.C. It was made of a series of seven light gold rings soldered together, five of which embraced upper natural teeth, one holding an artificial left second bicuspid, the other retaining a block of two artificial central incisors riveted in place; it probably was carved from a single tooth of an ox or calf[6] (Fig. 1-2, *D*).

It is quite probable that the Etruscans introduced fixed dental bridgework to the Romans. Brown[3] stated that from his own examination of several types of Etruscan and Roman birdge dentures in Italy, he is convinced that most of them were removable, while some of them were permantly fixed. Artificial dentures of this type were employed by the Romans before Cicero's time, as Brown makes reference to them in speaking of the Roman Laws of Twelve Tables, 45 B.C.* Horace also makes reference to Roman dental prostheses, 35 B.C.†

Brown[7] believed it not improbable that dentures such as those described by Abulcasis (ca. 1100) were introduced to India in the twelfth century, and that artificial teeth were probably not known to the very early Hindus. Modi[8] was not of the same opinion.

In the *Chirurgia Magna* of the French surgeon, Guy de Chauliac (written in 1363 and first published in 1478), it is suggested that, when a person has lost some teeth, substitutes from another mouth or artificial teeth of ox bone may be tied in with fine ligatures.[3]

Marco Polo,[9] late in the thirteenth century, reported that men and women of southeast China covered their teeth with thin plates of gold. It would be impossible to determine, without more concrete evidence, whether this type of treatment supplanted lost teeth or was purely ornamental in purpose. It would probably be safer to select the latter since it was a rather widespread custom among those who could afford it.

Partial dentures carved from bone or ivory and ligated to the natural teeth were used in Spain in the middle of the sixteenth century. This information is obtained from the *Coloquio Breve* of Francisco Martinez. Martinez,[10] however, did not consider a full denture, either upper or lower, a possibility. Koch[11] made reference to Ambroise Paré, who stated that artificial teeth for the front of the mouth were carved from a single piece of bone or ivory or from the tooth of a rohart, and were ligated to the proximating teeth. Guerini[10] stated that rohart is an old French word meaning, perhaps, hippopotamus. Brown[3] considered rohart as meaning walrus.

Dental crowns, said to be cast of gold, or tooth caps, independent of supporting loops, were found in a tomb near Vitulenia in Italy.[12] Brown stated: "The first dentist who is known to have employed tooth caps of this type is C. Mouton, about 1740. He applied his *calottes d'or* to defective teeth, both anteriors and posteriors, and even had the former enameled to resemble the natural dental organs."[3]

During the seventeenth and eighteenth centuries references are made to dental prostheses in some of the works of well-known writers of the period. In Francis Bacon's *Sylvia Sylvarum,* 1627, he spoke of "the binding-in of artificial teeth where natural teeth have been stricken out."[13]

Samuel Pepys[1] in his *Diary,* dated March 11, 1660, recorded: "My wife came home, and she had got her teeth new done by LaRooche, and they are now pretty handsome."[14] He probably referred to an upper anterior fixed partial denture.

An interesting reference is found in Jonathan Swift's version of "A Beautiful Young Nymph Going to Bed" in 1730:

> Now dextrously her plumpers [she] draws,
> That serve to fill her hollow jaws [cheeks],
> Untwists a wire, and from her gums
> A set of teeth completely comes.*

*From Cicero: De Legibus, II, XXIV, 60.
†From Horace: Epode V.

*From Swift, Jonathan, 1730.

It is probable that partial dentures carved entirely of wood were used in Japan as early as the middle of the seventeenth century. Later they made complete dentures with loose plates of wood and teeth of ivory or marble.[15]

Kerr and Rogers[16] suggested that teeth of ivory or bone, secured by copper wire or catgut string, were used in China for ages before they were introduced to Europe.

There are numerous descriptions of prosthetic appliances used in the East Indies that seem to be similar to the ancient Roman and Jewish appliances. However, for the most part, the history during the seventeenth and eighteenth centuries deals with the use of gold and dyes for enhancing an individual esthetic taste, no particular technical advances being made. There seems to be little doubt that early East Indian artificial teeth of gold and other metals were of native origin. There is no concrete evidence that metal teeth were used in Europe or America until the middle of the nineteenth century. In short, there were no improvements over the early Etruscan appliances until the advent of Pierre Fouchard.

Pierre Fouchard[17] has often been referred to as the father of modern dental prosthesis. There may have been other clinical dental practitioners who practiced with the same excellence, but they did not record their work. His work, *Le Chirurgien Dentiste* (written in 1723, published in 1728 with forty plates, revised in 1746 and 1796 with forty-two plates), suggests that he made many improvements in dental prosthesis. He practiced in Paris. In the field of fixed partial prosthesis he was doubtlessly active, using appliances of this type, ranging from one tooth to nearly a whole set. He used what he called "tenons," which were in reality dowels or pivots screwed into the roots to retain some of his bridges; and it is possible that he may have been the first to attach dental bridges to tooth roots by this method. Brown illustrates a medal conferred upon John Allen by the American Society of Dental Surgeons for his "metallic bulbs." These were secured to the natural teeth by means of clasps or springs. They are described and illustrated in his United States patent, dated December 16, 1845.[18]

THE NINETEENTH CENTURY

Crown and fixed partial prosthesis was indeed in a crude state of development as late as 1850. Modern methods in this field had their inception after this date, and mechanical progress in all fields of restorative dentistry was well under way. The foundation laid down by the French during the latter part of the eighteenth century was ably built upon by the architects of this profession in the nineteenth century.[19]

The most popular method at the middle of the nineteenth century of restoring lost coronal surfaces was by placing a so-called pivot crown. A wooden pivot was adapted to the artificial tooth and to the canal of the root. This was thrust into position and held in place until the moisture of the mouth caused the wood to swell, thus affording sufficient anchorage. This frequently caused the root to split.

The first presentation of modern methods of supplying missing teeth by means of bridgework was by F. Maury in 1828 in a French work entitled *A Treatise on Dental Art,* which was translated into English by J. B. Savier in 1843.[20]

The following chronology relates important events applicable to the practice of fixed partial prosthesis.

1805 J. B. Gariot, of France, introduced the first dental articulator. It employed a hinge principle only.

1840 Daniel T. Evans, of Philadelphia, patented an articulator, the first to embody protrusive and lateral movements.

1856 Oxychloride of zinc cement was in general use.

1856 W. A. Divinelle suggested that which has

been termed the "progenitor of modern bridgework." It embraced a description of a method of adapting a coping to the end of a root, and attaching an artificial tooth to it. He stated: "A plate may be carried across the intervening space unoccupied by roots, and an unbroken row of teeth mounted upon it."[19]

1857 John Thom, of Lambeth, England, obtained a patent on an interchangable facing, similar to Steele's facing, antedating the latter's patent by forty-six years.

1858 W. G. A. Bonwill, of Philadelphia, evolved an articulator from his triangle hypothesis. He assumed that the distance between each condyle and the incisor point averaged 4 inches.

1866 F. H. Balkwell, of England, presented an articulator that provided for the downward movement and lateral shift of the condyles.

1871 B. J. Bing developed an artificial porcelain tooth to which a platinum bar extended from each lateral side. The ends of this bar were to be anchored in fillings in adjacent natural teeth.

1873 J. B. Beers patented a gold banded crown with swaged cusps ("gold shell crown").

1878 A. E. Matteson introduced the "openfaced" crown.

1886 Low-fusing porcelain, fused in a gold matrix, made its appearance.

1889 C. H. Land, of Detroit, introduced a method of constructing full pocelain veneer crowns. He also made high-fusing porcelain inlays, fused in a platinum matrix.

1896 William E. Walker, Pass Christian, Miss., studied mandibular movements with respect to dental prosthesis. He devised an adjustable articulator for individual mandibular movements, taking registrations of the inclination of individual condylar paths, extraorally.

1898 N. S. Jenkins, of Dresden, Germany, proclaimed a low-fusing porcelain perfected as to color and durability.

1900 High-fusing porcelain was generally employed. Its application was in somewhat of a slump until the full porcelain veneer crown was more widely used.

The dentists of this period were not aware of the pathology created at the root ends of the abutments that were devitalized mainly for the purpose of establishing greater mechanical retention by means of placing dowels into the root canals. Indeed, it was common practice to cut off the crown of a perfectly healthy, sound tooth and to place a porcelain-faced dowel crown (Richmond's crown) to serve as a retainer for a bridge. The following technics were the most popular among the practitioners: the retainers, for the most part, consisted of complete gold shell crowns, or similar dowel types, on the posterior teeth; porcelain-faced dowel crowns were used as retainers on the anterior teeth; the pontics for the bridges consisted of swaged occlusal surfaces soldered to porcelain facings; and the remaining contour was filled in with 22-carat solder. The materials used were porcelain, gold and platinum plate, gold and platinum wire, gold solder, and screw dowels and pivots of all varieties. These materials and the various individual technics were manipulated to produce the fixed partial prosthetic appliances of the time.

THE TWENTIETH CENTURY

Early developments

1901 Carl Christensen devised an intraoral method of securing positional relations of condylar paths.

1906 Carmichael introduced the partial veneer gold crown. Its construction consisted of a wire staple fitted into slots cut in the tooth, over a burnished gold plate, the two united and strengthened with solder.

1907 William H. Taggart announced his method of making gold castings, using a disappearing wax pattern. This application of an old method revolutionized the technical aspect of restorative dentistry. It made possible exceptional refinements in the construction of fixed partial prosthetic appliances.

1910 The casting method by this time was in quite general use. This method largely facilitated the development of the so-called three-quarter veneer gold crown that became popular as an anterior bridge retainer or wherever the display of gold on the labial or buccal surfaces of the teeth was undesirable. Technically, it was a refinement of the Carmichael crown. This restoration was largely developed by E.

T. Tinker, of the Crown and Bridge Staff at the University of Minnesota. The only recent technical alteration has been the elimination of the shoulder at the gingival border in favor of a beveled margin (chamfer).

1910 Forrest H. Orton developed a double-banded cast gold crown technic applicable to posterior abutments. He was largely responsible for the development of many technical advances in this field. His enthusiasm for a technical ideal still lives in the minds of those who knew him.

Up to this time the American dentists, independently from a basic biologic attitude, were developing and producing extensive dental restorations. Complicated crowns, supporting spans of any number of pontics, were adapted to hopelessly diseased and broken-down roots (Fig. 1-3).

William Hunter very loudly and very definitely denounced American dentistry. He said: "The worst cases of anemia, gastritis, . . . actual lesions of the cord, . . . chronic rheumatic affections of kidney disease are those which owe their origin to, or are gravely complicated by, the oral sepsis produced in private patients by those gold traps of sepsis [Fig. 1-4]. . . . Gold fillings, gold caps, gold bridges, gold crowns, fixed dentures, built in, on, and around diseased teeth, form a veritable mausoleum of gold over a mass of sepsis to which there is no parallel in the whole realm of medicine or surgery."[21]

The reaction was fairly prompt. The pendulum swung the other way under pressure of the medical practitioners. In a span of but a few years, the institution of fixed bridgework was held in ill repute.

The discussion which followed a paper pertinent to fixed bridgework, read by Alden J. Bush in Rochester, New York, on July 7, 1914, is rather interesting in that it portrays the status of fixed bridgework at this time. H. W. Gillett of New York City, stated: "I regard the day of fixed bridgework as having passed, and I believe the next decade will see the end of its use. It is time the colleges of the country stopped teaching it, because it has been most thoroughly discredited."[22] A similar reference is found in the discussion of a paper entitled *Properly Constructed Bridges and Their Hygienic Care,* read in 1916. It was largely one of protest against the use of fixed bridges by the "pillars"

A 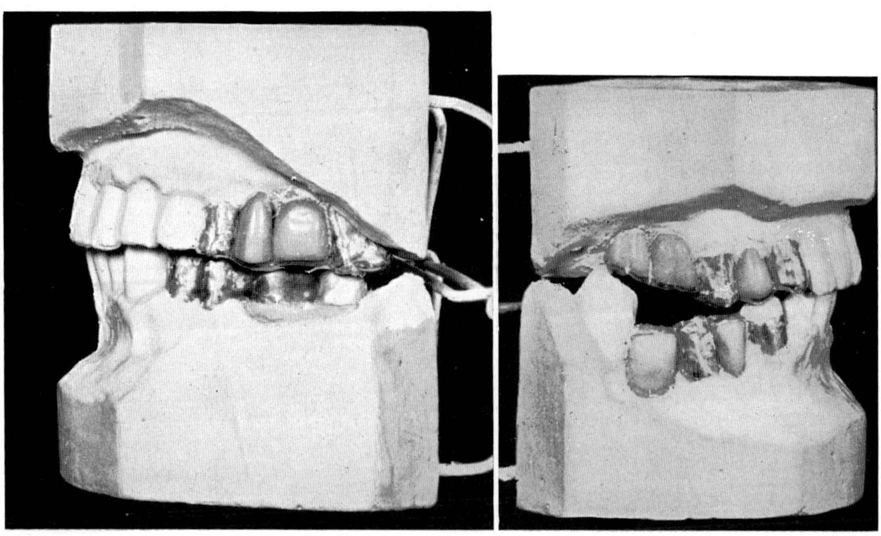 B

Fig. 1-3. Improperly constructed bridges: lack of contour and sanitation. **A,** Improperly constructed bridge on left side. **B,** Improperly constructed bridge on right side. Cantilever bridge is attached to two bicuspids.

of the dental profession. They contended that fixed bridgework was definitely becoming a thing of the past. To quote R. Ottolengui of New York City: ". . . it is my sincere hope that the time is not far distant when there will be so few fixed bridges in the mouth that no manufacturer could be tempted by the commercial profit to make a special brush to clean fixed bridgework."[23]

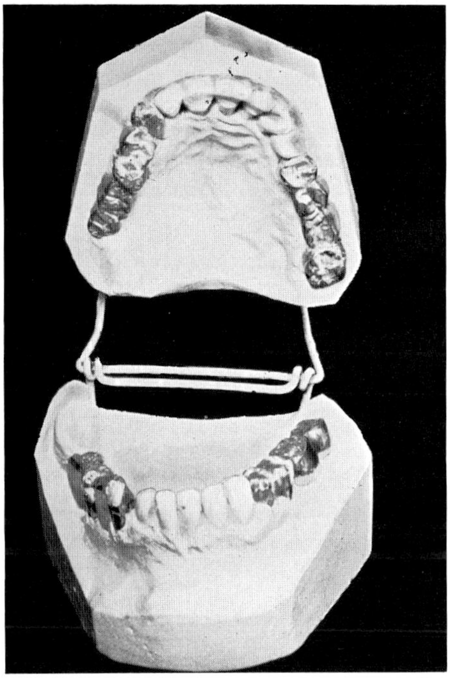

Fig. 1-4. Hunter's "gold traps of sepsis."

Forrest H. Orton,[24] in 1919, at the University of Minnesota, very logically placed before the dental profession the reason for the existence of many faults in this field of endeavor. He was one of the first to attempt the reformation of this type of treatment. He dealt with the importance of occlusion and anatomic form in the construction of this prosthesis[25] (Fig. 1-5).

Karl Knoche also heralded the revival of fixed bridge methods and suggested in 1918 that "crown and bridgework is the necessity of preserving the normal functions of the organ and of the individual teeth" and that its success "all points to a normal function"[26] (Fig. 1-6). In the same vein of thought, Bunting, in *Review of Dental Literature,* in 1920, quoted Mauk, who voiced the opinion "that the scathing criticisms which Hunter made of this branch of dentistry were not altogether fair or justifiable in that his deductions were drawn from examples of the poorest type rather than from those which were of the best or even average types."[27] Also, in 1919, Mauk[28] had enumerated the basic principles upon which this type of treatment should be constructed. These principles were, namely: physiologic tone of all supporting anatomic elements; adequate support in preparation to the work demanded; protection for soft tissues—correct anatomic contour; and normal articulation and normal occlusion (Fig. 1-7).

A

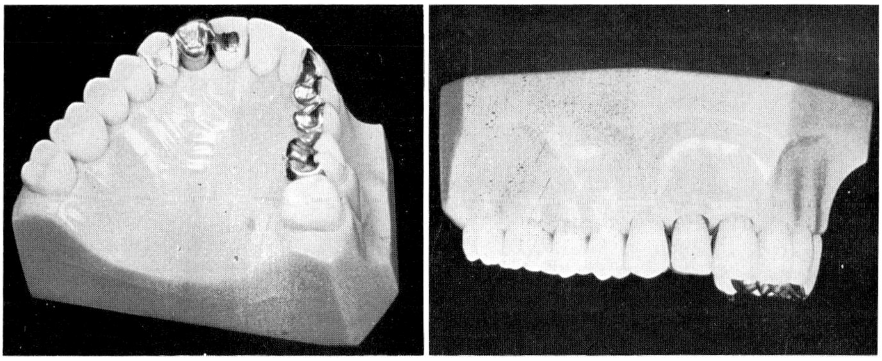

B

Fig. 1-5. A, Modern type of fixed bridge, lingual view. **B,** Labial view of bridge shown in **A.**

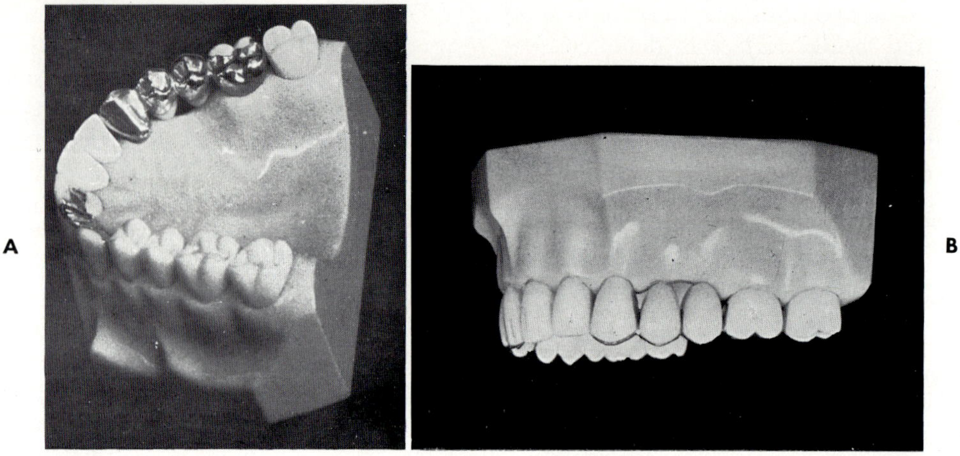

Fig. 1-6. A, Lingual view of upper posterior fixed bridge. **B,** Buccal view of bridge shown in **A.**

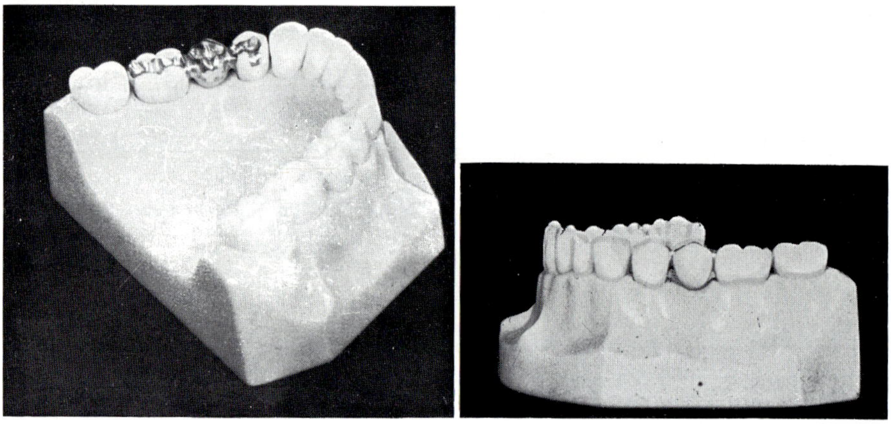

Fig. 1-7. Lingual and buccal views of lower semifixed bridge.

Following the year 1920, there is evidenced a decided change in attitude. This change, however, is manifest largely by prodigious strides in excellence of technic and attention to mechanical details. The complete intermarriage of a biologic attitude and mechanical application is absent. This is largely true today. Selberg[29] pointed out in 1936 that, fundamentally, the basic materials had changed but little in the past few years. These materials were gold or porcelain or a combination of the two. He summed up by saying that the restoration must meet the following requirements: protection, comfort, esthetics, durability, and utility. He stated that sources of irritation, as well as traumatic occlusion, must be avoided. It can be seen that there has been great advancement in this field of prosthesis, from a biomechanical aspect, in the last five decades.

Philosophically, man is a vain creature. The loss of a tooth, or teeth, particularly in the front part of the mouth, detracts from his appearance. It is then quite natural to suppose that the early attempts to replace these missing members had a

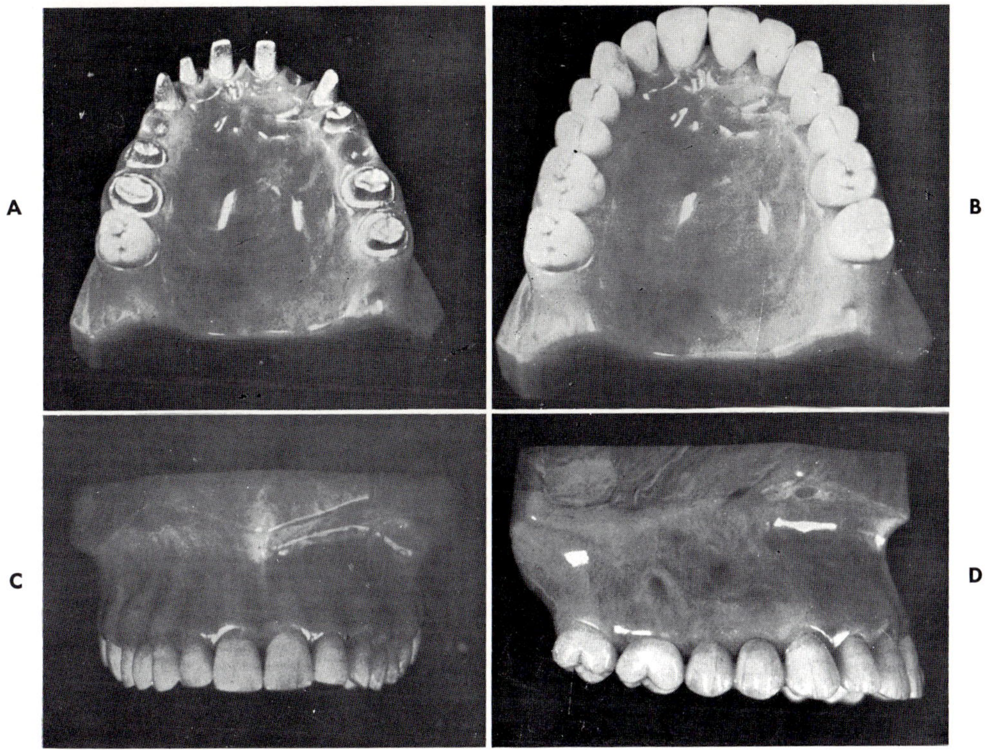

Fig. 1-8. A, Partially edentulous mouth having teeth prepared for porcelain veneer crowns and bridges. **B,** Lingual view of same mouth, showing all-porcelain restorations. **C,** Labial view of same mouth, showing porcelain veneer crowns and bridge restorations. **D,** Buccal view of same mouth, showing porcelain bridge extending from second bicuspid to cuspid.

primary purpose. If public opinion were to control this particular phase of treatment today, the esthetic factor quite likely would remain of paramount importance.

It is evident that some of the ancient dental prostheses, engaged in the restoration of charms ravaged by caries and the loss of teeth, were essentially the work of craftsmen. As the appreciation of the esthetic became even more manifest, fashioning of these prostheses tended to develop definitely toward a technical perfection. It was virtually a mechanical trade. There was, however, a dormant appreciation of a possibility of advancement along more scientific lines (Fig. 1-8).

In the decade following 1880, Miller, Black, and Williams committed dentistry to a course of development from a more scientific angle. This was met, inevitably, by a wave of protest, since it was assumed by a larger percentage of dental practitioners that the attempts would prove entirely impractical. Unfortunately, the same belief exists among some today. On the other hand, the trend, both educationally and professionally, is definitely biologic.[30] Various researches leading to our present-day knowledge of the bacteriopathology of the oral cavity and a suspected causal relation of mouth infection to systemic disease (?) have given to the science and art of dentistry a new birth and perspective.[31] The result will become primarily vital. The mechanical procedures employed in this particular phase of dentistry should be considered, not as ends in themselves, but rather as means to an end in relation to a biologic field. The dental pioneers have established profound and convincing evidence; i.e., that the dental profession must assume greater responsibility in rendering a health service. Esthetics was the cause of fixed partial prosthesis. Not to detract from its importance, it need not, and should not, be the result per se. Clinical restorative dentistry today accepts this type of treatment as a suitable substitute for lost segments of the dental arch.

Further developments*

1928 This year marked the beginning of a new era in dentistry. A publication by R. L. Coleman,[32] *Physical Properties of Dental Materials,* issued by the Bureau of Standards, was the first attempt to study scientifically the physical properties of materials used in dental practice. A second report was issued in 1942 by the Bureau under the heading, *Circular C433.*[33]

1932 to 1933 C. H. Scheu developed a technic employing hygroscopic expansion of investment to compensate for shrinkage of castings. He also determined that a difference existed in the percentage of shrinkage in different gold alloys.

1935 to 1940 This period marks the development of a technic based on scientific data to give accurately fitting cast inlays. The work of Volland,[34] Scheu,[35] and Hollenback[36] culminated in our present hygroscopic expansion technic employing the vacuum for mixing and investing the inlay.

1933 to 1950 H. Spiro[37] in 1933 presented the hydrocolloid impression technic for inlays, crowns, and fixed bridges. This was followed by further research by Sears,[38] Thompson,[39] Paffenbarger,[40] and Skinner, Cooper, and Beck[41] resulting in our present-day hydrocolloid indirect technics for crowns and fixed partial dentures. The synthetic resins were used for complete denture bases as early as 1936. It was not until 1940 that the synthetic resins were applied to restorative dentistry in the United States, particularly in the field of crowns and fixed partial dentures. In that year, W. E. Wilson presented his technic of casting plastic inlays and crowns. During the following five years, H. Vernon, L. W. Harris, F. Slack, A. Nelson, W. Skinner, C. Nelson and F. Peyton,[42] and members of the United States Bureau of Standards contributed further knowledge in the use of the synthetic resins in restorative dentistry.

1951 to 1964 The introduction of the rubber type (mercaptan) and silicone impression materials, and the development of carbide burs, ultrahigh-speed cord handpieces, and water and air rotor handpieces occurred. This period also saw further development of B. B. McCollum type of gnathographic articulators by E. Granger and C. Stuart and also of checkbite instruments by Hanau. A renaissance of the use of fired porcelain to cast metal crowns and fixed partial dentures (bridges) due to new alloys and porcelains occurred, along with the introduction and development of improved diamond stones and carbide burs accompanied by super high-speed cutting technics.

1965 to 1970

Refinement of methods for the pin type of retainers
Improvement in crystals of cast gold alloys
Development of high-temperature refractory die materials
Development of the aluminous porcelains employing alumina crystals
Improvement in vacuum-fired ceramics and furnaces
Improvement in gnathologic instruments and technics
Greater recognition of engineering principles involved in restorative dentistry

*Added by the author (S.D.T.).

DEFINITIONS RELATED TO CROWN AND FIXED PARTIAL PROSTHODONTICS*

Prosthesis—Replacement of an absent part of the human body by an artificial part

Dental prosthesis—Artificial replacement of one or more teeth and/or associated structures

Prosthodontics, prosthetic dentistry—Branch of dental art and science pertaining to the

*Definitions formulated by the Curriculum Committee on Partial Denture Prosthetics, Survey Committee, American Association of Dental Schools. A Course of Study in Dentistry, 1935; also, Glossary of Prosthetic Terms, ed. 3, by Nomenclature Committee of the Academy of Denture Prosthetics, J. Prosth. Dent. 1968.

restoration and maintenance of oral function by the replacement of missing teeth and associated structures by artificial devices

Dentition—Natural teeth in the dental arch considered collectively; may be deciduous, permanent, or mixed

Denture—Artificial substitute for missing natural teeth and adjacent tissues

Complete denture—Dental prosthesis that is a substitute for the lost natural dentition and associated structures of the maxillae or mandible

Partial denture—Dental prosthesis that replaces one or more of, but less than all of, the natural teeth and/or associated parts and that is supported by the teeth and/or the mucosa; may be removable or fixed

Fixed partial denture—Restoration of one or more of, but less than all of, the natural teeth, primarily supported by the teeth or roots; it is often designated as "Fixed bridge"

Pontic—Artificial tooth on a fixed partial denture; replaces the lost or missing natural tooth, restores its function, and usually occupies the space occupied by the natural crown

Abutment—Natural tooth or root used for the support or attachment of a fixed or removable prosthesis, either terminal or intermediate

Intermediate abutment (pier)—Natural tooth or root, without other natural teeth in proximal contact, which is used as an abutment, in addition to two terminal abutments

Retainer—That part of a fixed partial denture which attaches the prosthesis to the abutment; may be an inlay, partial-veneer crown, or a complete crown

Connector—Part of a fixed partial denture that unites its component parts, i.e., pontics and retainers; may be rigid or nonrigid

Crown—anatomic—Portion of a natural tooth that extends from its dentinoenamel junction to the occlusal surface or incisal edge

Crown—artificial—Fixed restoration of the major part or of the entire coronal part of a natural tooth; usually of gold, porcelain, synthetic resin, or their combinations

SELECTED REFERENCES

1. Magitot, E.: The history of the mutilation of teeth, D. Items Int. **15**:356, 1892.
2. Guerini, V.: History of dentistry, Philadelphia, 1909, Lea & Febiger.
3. Brown, L. P.: The antiquities of dental prostheses, D. Cosmos 76:830, 1934.
4. Blumenbach, J. F.: Gottinger Magazin **1**:110, 1780.
5. Sudhoff, K.: Geschichte der Zahnheilkunde, ed. 2, Leipzig, 1926, A. Lorentz.
6. Sudhoff, K.: Geschichte der Zahnheilkunde, ed. 2, Leipzig, 1926, A. Lorentz.
7. Brown, L. P.: Cosmic teeth, The Open Court **44**:77, 1930.
8. Modi, J. J.: Dentistry in ancient India, Indian D. J. **6**:1, 1931.
9. Marsden, W.: Translation of the travels of Marco Polo, New York, 1926, Boni and Liveright.
10. Guerini, V.: History of dentistry, Philadelphia, 1909, Lea & Febiger.
11. History of dental surgery, Fort Wayne, Ind., 1910, National Art Publishing Co.
12. Weinberger, B. W.: Ancient dentistry, Ann. Med. Hist. **6**:269, 1924.
13. Bacon, F.: Sylvia Sylvarum, VIII: 757, 1627.
14. Pepys, Samuel: Diary, March 11, 1660.
15. Chiwaki, N.: Dentistry in Japan, Tr. Fourth Dent. Cong. **3**:426, 1904.
16. Kerr, J. G., and Rogers, L. W.: Chinese dentistry, D. Cosmos **19**:382-385, 1877.
17. Kirk, E. C.: Pierre Fouchard, D. Cosmos **65**: 881, 1923.
18. New light on dental history, D. Cosmos **62**: 942, 1920.
19. Lufkin, A. W.: A history of dentistry, Philadelphia, 1938, Lea & Febiger.
20. Goslee, H. J.: Principles and practice of crown and bridgework, ed. 5, Brooklyn, 1928, Dental Items of Interest Publishing Co.
21. Hunter, W.: The role of sepsis and antisepsis in medicine, D. Brief **16**:852, 1911.
22. Bush, A. J.: Proposed classification of fixed bridge work and law governing its application, J. Nat. D. A. **2**:221, 1915.
23. Sarrazin, J. J.: Properly constructed bridges and their hygienic care, J. Nat. D. A. **3**:251, 1916.
24. Orton, F. H.: The general improvement in technic in crown and bridgework, J. Nat. D. A. **6**:91-109, 1919.
25. Orton, F. H.: The predicament of crown and bridgework, J. Nat. D. A. **4**:327, 1917.
26. Knoche, K.: Standardizing crown and bridgework, J. Nat. D. A. **5**:394, 1918.
27. Bunting, R. W.: Review of dental literature, April, 1919, to April, 1920, J. Nat. D. A. **7**:526, 1920.
28. Mauk, E. H.: Favorable and unfavorable conditions in bridgework, J. Nat. D. A. **6**: 487-497, 1919.
29. Selberg, A.: Modern fixed partial restorations, J.A.D.A. **23**:460, 1936.
30. Editorial: The passing of the dental cosmos, J.A.D.A. **26**:114, 1939.

31. Editorial: Dental internship, J.A.D.A. **25:** 1849, 1938.
32. Coleman, R. L.: Physical properties of dental materials, U.S. Government Printing Office, Washington, D. C., 1928.
33. Souder, W., and Paffenbarger, G. C.: Physical properties of dental materials, Circular C433, U. S. Government Printing Office, Washington, D. C.
34. Volland, R. H.: Wax patterns for cast gold inlays, J. Nat. D. A. **9:**569, 1922.
35. Scheu, C. H.: Precision casting utilizing the hygroscopic action of plaster investment in making expanded molds, J.A.D.A. **20:**1205, 1933.
36. Hollenback, G. M.: Precision gold inlays made by a simple technic, J.A.D.A. **30:**99, 1943.
37. Van Minden, F. A.: A new method of fixed bridge construction in two settings, Illinois D. J. **11:**457, 1933.
38. Sears, A. W.: Hydrocolloid technic for inlays and fixed bridges, D. Digest **43:**230, 1937.
39. Thompson, M. J.: Reversible hydrocolloid impression material: its treatment and use in operative and prosthetic dentistry, J.A.D.A. **39:**708, 1949.
40. Paffenbarger, G. C.: Hydrocolloid impression materials: physical properties and a specification, J.A.D.A. **27:**373, 1940.
41. Skinner, E. W., Cooper, E. N., and Beck, F. C.: Reversible and irreversible hydrocolloid impression materials, J.A.D.A. **40:**196, 1950.
42. Tylman, S. D., and Peyton, F.: Acrylics and other dental resins, Philadelphia, 1946, J. B. Lippincott Co.

GENERAL REFERENCES

Academy of Denture Prosthetics: Glossary of prosthetic terms, ed. 3, St. Louis, 1968, The C. V. Mosby Co.

Bassett, R. W., Ingraham, R., and Koser, J. R.: An atlas of cast gold procedures Buena Park, California, 1964, Uni-Tro Press.

Coelho, D. R., and Rieser, J. M.: A complete fixed bridge procedure, ed. 3., New York, 1963, New York University Press.

Council on Dental Materials and Devices: Certification program for dental materials: list of certified dental materials revised to January 1, 1968, J.A.D.A. **76**(2):366-372, 1968.

Ewing, J. E.: Fixed partial prosthesis, ed. 2, Philadelphia, 1959, Lea and Febiger.

Greider, A., and Cinotti, W. R.: Periodontal prosthesis, St. Louis, 1968, The C. V. Mosby Co.

Hollenback, G. M.: Science and technic of the cast restoration, St. Louis, 1964, The C. V. Mosby Co.

Huffman, R. W., Regenos, J. W., and Taylor, R. R.: Principles of occlusion, Columbus, Ohio, 1969, R and R Press.

Kornfeld, M.: Mouth rehabilitation—clinical and laboratory procedures, St. Louis, 1967, The C. V. Mosby Co.

Johnson, W. W.: History of prosthetic dentistry, J. Prosth. Dent. **9:**841, 1959.

Johnston, J. F., Phillips, R. W., and Dykema, R.: Modern practice in crown and bridge prosthodontics, Philadelphia, 1965, W. B. Saunders Co.

Lucia, V. O.: Modern gnathological concepts, St. Louis, 1961, The C. V. Mosby Co.

Myers, G. E.: Textbook of crown and bridge prosthodontics, St. Louis, 1969, The C. V. Mosby Co.

Peyton, F. A., editor: Restorative dental materials, ed. 3, St. Louis, 1968, The C. V. Mosby Co.

Posselt, U.: The physiology of occlusion and rehabilitation, Oxford, 1964, Blackwell Scientific Publications.

Rath, G.: History of prosthetic dentistry, I, D. Abst. **4:**50, 1959.

Rath, G.: History of prosthetic dentistry, II, D. Abst. **4:**8, 1959.

Schweitzer, J. M.: Oral rehabilitation problem cases—treatment and evaluation, St. Louis, 1964, The C. V. Mosby Co.

Sicher, H.: Orban's oral histology and embryology, ed. 6, St. Louis, 1966, The C. V. Mosby Co.

Skinner, E. W., and Phillips, R. W.: Science of dental materials, ed. 6, Philadelphia, 1967, W. B. Saunders Co.

Some interesting examples of early crown and bridge prosthesis, D. Mag. & Oral Topics **79:** 96, 1962.

Stallard, H.: The good mouth—a syllabus on oral rehabilitation and occlusion, San Francisco, 1968, University of California.

Stuart, C. E., and Stallard, H.: Syllabus on oral rehabilitation and occlusion, San Francisco, 1968, University of California.

Weinberg, L. A.: Atlas of crown and bridge prosthodontics, St. Louis, 1965, The C. V. Mosby Co.

Wilson, W. H., and Lang, R. L.: Practical crown and bridge prosthodontics, New York, 1962, McGraw-Hill Book Company.

Chapter 2

Factors relating to examination of patient requiring crowns and fixed partial prostheses

Before any preventive or restorative treatment can be intelligently applied, it must be preceded by a complete and thorough roentgenographic and clinical examination and evaluation of findings. To make such a diagnosis, it is imperative that the information and data be gathered by a definite and systematic method. This implies more than the mere recognition and location of cavities and edentulous areas. The ability to make a satisfactory examination is the result of careful study, thoroughness, and experience. The faculty of careful observation is very important, for the degree of its acuteness will determine the dentist's ability to recognize and distinguish between normal conditions and the first stages of pathologic conditions. The ability to interpret physical and laboratory findings of a specialized nature is also a desirable asset.

The examination of a patient should not be focused or limited to the immediate oral impairment of the patient. Except in those instances requiring emergency treatment for the relief of pain, the tendency should be toward a method of examination that will include a complete case history, a physical examination if necessary, an oral examination, and a careful recording of the data obtained from those examinations. This is particularly important with new patients, whether they be children or adults. Once such a complete record for a patient has been obtained, it is filed so that it may be readily accessible for reference upon subsequent visits of the patient for further health services.

Parents may be questioned about the general health and oral factors relative to their children. If the patient is an adult, little difficulty should be experienced in obtaining the desired data, once the patient understands the purpose of the examination. Most persons have a definite reason for visiting the dentist, and it is well to listen to their account of the symptoms and their reasons for the existing troubles. At times much valuable information may be obtained from the patient in this manner. It is said that a good diagnostician is always a good listener. Other facts are frequently disclosed during a conversation which will be of assistance to the dentist in making his general physical examination.

On the other hand, there are patients who have no specific, immediate disorder, but who desire a general examination and checkup. With such a patient our approach is slightly different. We may first suggest a thorough prophylactic treatment prior to the detailed examination of the teeth. Casual though pointed questions may be asked at intervals during the treatment, and in this way facts pertinent to the individual's condition may be obtained. During the recitation of the complaint by the patient, the astute operator often can make observations relative to his general health condition; these observations may relate to his physical, mental, and emotional states (Chapter 8).

The dentist should also be interested in the family history of the patient. Those patients having supernumerary or congenitally missing teeth, facial abnormalities, excessive caries, or known heart, kidney, and other disturbances can be questioned further and investigated. If there is the necessity to use anesthesia, it is well to ascertain from the patient what the effects were following previous administrations. It is routine procedure in all cases to obtain the patient's full name, address, telephone number, references, sex, age, occupation, and a complete record of the present complaint and its history (Fig. 33-1).

When a patient who has been under dental care returns for a periodic routine examination, it is well to study and review his record prior to seating him in the chair. All the previous roentgenographs and records of this patient should be examined. When the patient is seated, the dentist is able to examine all former restorations and to determine their present condition. A comparative study of previous roentgenographs will also enable him to recognize any changes taking place in the supporting structures (Fig. 33-2).

GENERAL EXAMINATION

A general examination of the patient is often the next consideration. The mouth should never be regarded as an entity isolated from the rest of the body; it is an essential and related structure of the human mechanism. Constitutional diseases and disturbances often manifest themselves first in the mouth and the teeth. The fact that a patient complains of heart trouble, headaches, rheumatism, or a general tired feeling frequently may indicate the presence of focal infection. It may be that certain laboratory tests are indicated, or possibly a general physical examination by the family physician. Blood and urine analyses are important in the differential diagnosis of certain gingival lesions. The dentist should recognize an unusual condition and take the necessary means to identify the cause. If surgery is undertaken in patients with leukemia or agranulocytosis, it may terminate fatally. Diabetes, nephritis, tuberculosis, and syphilis require more than dental service alone.

If questioning discloses the fact that the patient is under the care of his physician, it is well to arrange for a consultation with him to receive aid in the diagnosis and plan of treatment. Very often the dentist is the first one to make observations indicative of general systemic disorders, such as malignancies. In such circumstances the cooperation of the patient and his physician is essential in making a further study and diagnosis.

INDICATIONS

Although a fixed partial denture may be considered in most of the partially edentulous arches and for patients of every age, we find that this type of service is indicated primarily for the adult patient. A fixed partial denture is ordinarily contraindicated in children and young adolescents, because their teeth very often are not fully erupted, and pulp is unusually large and hence may be easily exposed or damaged during the preparation of the abutment. When placed in a child's mouth, a fixed appliance is primarily employed as a space maintainer following the loss of a tooth at an early age (Figs. 2-1 and 3-1). These space maintainers serve an intermediate function. They should be replaced by a permanent structure when the patient is older.

The tabulation of several thousand bridge patients shows that, in less than 10

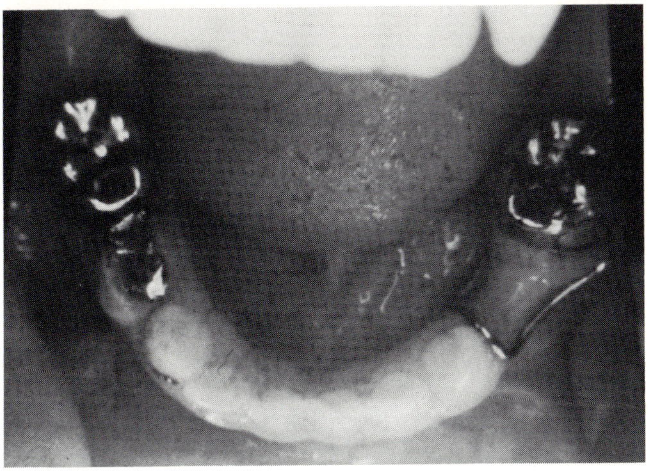

Fig. 2-1. Retainer placed on permanent molar to prevent it from tipping anteriorly.

percent, the restorations placed were for patients between the ages of 17 and 19 years. This period in life may well be considered the normal, minimum age limit for this type of service. It is true that fixed prostheses were placed for patients younger than 17 years of age, but they were of a more or less temporary nature. In studying this type of service for women, it was noted that less than 8 percent of the total number of patients requiring bridges are found in the 17- to 19-year age bracket. It is interesting to observe that, among the older patients, those 50 years of age or more, the percentage was less than 5 percent of the total requirements for all patients served (see Chapter 8).

The question may be raised whether it is practical or advisable to place extensive fixed restorations for very old patients, for many changes occur in the human body with aging. Likewise, at this period of life it is more difficult to determine and differentiate the normal and the abnormal. These facts should be considered in the diagnosis and plan of treatment (see Chapter 8). Tissues of young people, when subjected to unfavorable conditions, respond favorably more often than those of the aged. Hence, while the same condi-

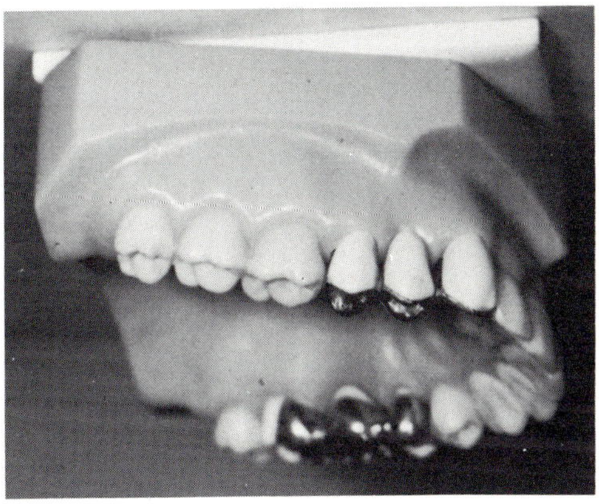

Fig. 2-2. Two upper posterior fixed partial dentures.

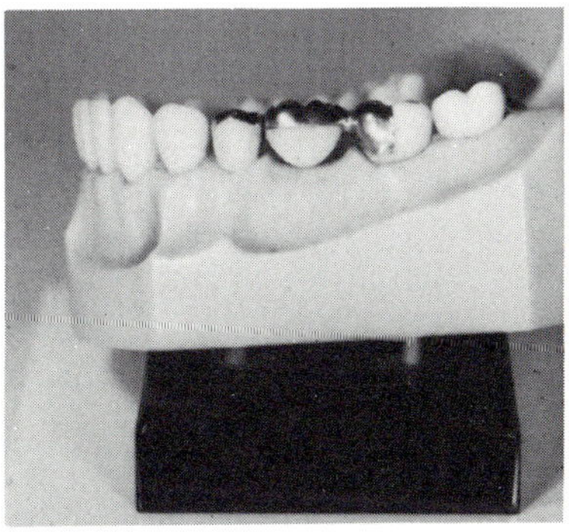

Fig. 2-3. Lower posterior restoration with mesial half-crown retainer on molar and intracoronal retainer on biscuspid.

tions may be present in a young patient as in an old one, it frequently happens that in the latter the tissue compensation may be deficient and may cause the appliance to fail.

Fixed partial denture service, therefore, is primarily intended for those patients between the ages of 20 and 55 years (Figs. 2-2 and 2-3). The greatest need for this service for men comes between the ages of 20 and 30 years, while for women it is between the ages of 30 and 39 years. When a fixed appliance must be placed in the mouth of a young patient, it is a good procedure to employ extracoronal instead of intracoronal retainers; i.e., the three-quarter partial veneer or the onlay types of retention, rather than the MOD types, are favored. In older patients it is quite safe to use the intracoronal types because of the completed formation of the coronal dentin and the gradual withdrawal of the pulp due to the presence of secondary dentin.

Generally, the fixed type of partial denture is indicated when one to three teeth are missing; it may prove a failure when it involves more. Many fixed bridges have failed because the length of the span between the abutments was too great for the forces imposed upon them. Other failures may be attributed to an insufficient vertical

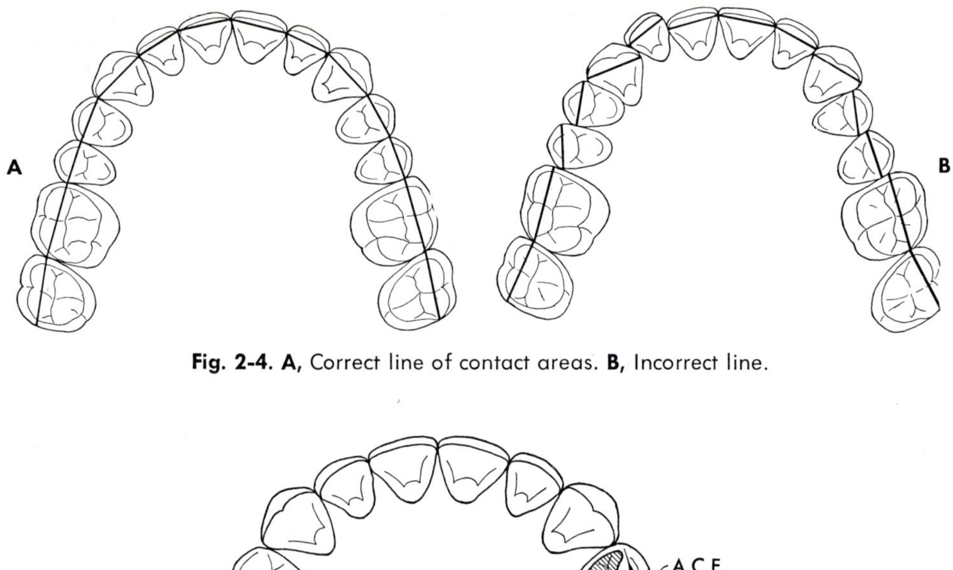

Fig. 2-4. A, Correct line of contact areas. **B,** Incorrect line.

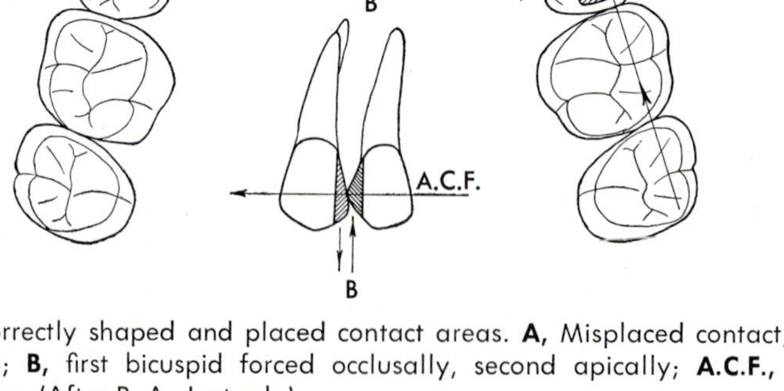

Fig. 2-5. Incorrectly shaped and placed contact areas. **A,** Misplaced contact, causing rotation of teeth; **B,** first bicuspid forced occlusally, second apically; **A.C.F.,** anterior component of force. (After R. A. Jentzsch.)

distance between the crest of the ridge and the opposing occlusal surfaces; such a condition does not allow the required amount of metal or the needed space for a cleansable pontic. In mouths that have been permitted to remain partially edentulous for a long time, the chewing habits of the patient are modified; the side having teeth is used to a greater degree than the partially edentulous one. Therefore the latter, because of partial disuse, undergoes physical, anatomic, and physiologic changes. Normal contacts are lost or modified, teeth move mesially or distally, and in some instances teeth gravitate or rise in their sockets (Figs. 2-4 and 2-5). Changes also occur in the periodontal membrane and in the bone supporting those teeth whose normal forces have been reduced or removed. It is unwise to use as abutments those teeth not having a normal bony support (Fig. 3-32).

The question is frequently raised whether pulpless teeth are useless as bridge abutments. Decision in this respect should be determined by the findings of the patient's complete case history, together with the roentgenographic evidence of previously treated teeth present in the mouth. Certain systemic disturbances also may contraindicate additional root treatments.

The dentist should take nothing for granted when he is making a diagnosis for a fixed restoration. A tooth that apparently exhibits favorable conditions for its use as a bridge abutment will sometimes disclose its weakness upon roentgenographic examination. This is especially true when the clinical crown of a tooth is sufficiently long, but upon roentgenographic examination it is found to have a root relatively short in proportion to the total length of the crown (Fig. 2-6). Such a root necessarily has a small area of periodontal membrane attachment, and the additional forces developed during the normal functional movements of a bridge might very quickly destroy the usefulness of such a tooth as a support. Where an edentulous area has existed for any length of time, particularly in the posterior region of the lower arch, we find almost without exception a mesial tipping and lingual inclination of the teeth posterior to the space (Fig. 9-1).

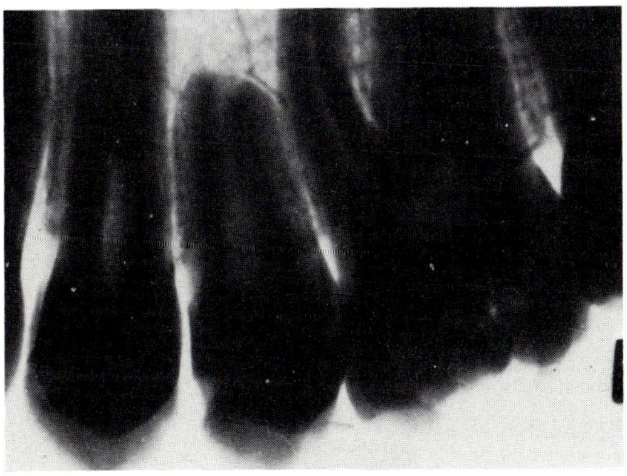

Fig. 2-6. Shortened root length of second bicuspid caused by absorption.

Those teeth tipped 24° from the vertical position as a rule should not be used for bridge abutments. If they are, the vertical forces on the bridge will not be transmitted in the direction of the long axis of the tooth. The result will be a periodontal membrane that is crushed, and a breaking down of the tissues on the mesial aspect of the tooth.

Another important factor in the consideration of a fixed prosthesis is the distribution and number of teeth present in relation to the number of teeth that are to be replaced with the restoration. The ideal condition exists when two abutment teeth are used to support one replaced tooth; however, two abutment teeth under certain conditions may carry very satisfactorily the pontics of two missing teeth (Fig. 2-7). This is true where a posterior bridge extends approximately in a straight line from abutment to abutment and where the teeth are similar functionally. There are occasions when three or four missing teeth may be replaced satisfactor-

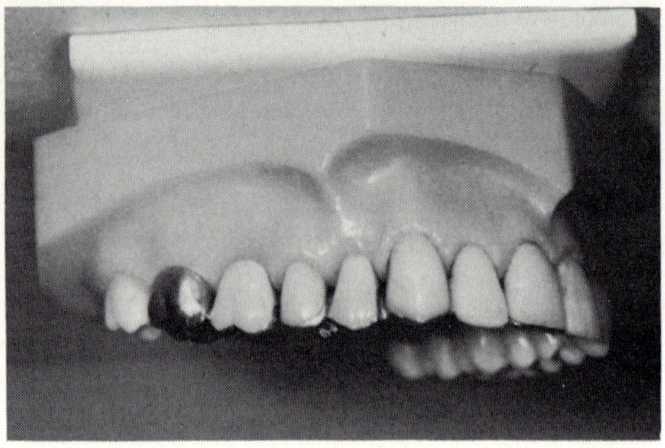

Fig. 2-7. Anterior restoration attached to cuspid and central incisor with lateral pontic; posterior restoration extends from first bicuspid to second molar, replacing first molar and second biscuspid.

ily with a fixed appliance. Such a condition is occasionally found in a bridge extending from a cuspid to a second molar, or sometimes even to the third molar if the opposing arch is a mucosa-borne artificial appliance. We find in these circumstances that the force which a patient can exert on the bridge will approximate only 20 percent of the normal poundage that could be exerted if the opposite natural teeth were present.

ORAL EXAMINATION

The examination of oral conditions may be made next. Many means are available to accomplish this, not the least of which is the direct visual examination of the mouth and the teeth. To be of most value this should be done thoroughly and in great detail. The fact must never be lost sight of that, although the examination is primarily of a dental and oral nature, the dentist constantly must be alert to the possible presence of oral lesions having a related systemic significance.

The prime requisite for an oral examination is good light, either natural or artificial. In addition there should be a mirror, an explorer, and a retractor available for use. An examination of this type should include a complete set of roentgenographs, as well as upper and lower study models of the mouth. A careful visual examination may disclose variations in tooth form and contour, the presence or lack of contact areas, or possibly improperly placed contact areas. Incipient caries may be located by the discoloration of the enamel, even though the caries may not be disclosed in the roentgenographs. Rotated, malposed, and displaced teeth in the arch are easily observed. The face and lips should be carefully inspected to see if any swelling or lesions are present. The inside of the mouth should also receive careful inspection to ascertain whether the cheeks, palate, tongue, and the sublingual regions are normal. The condition, contour, and relationship of the dental arches, both in centric relationship and in masticatory positions, should be noted. Very frequently abnormal forces and malocclusion manifest themselves by a breakdown of the gingival and periodontal structures. The presence of deposits or pus may also be determined. A discolored tooth very frequently indicates a dead pulp. These and many other conditions may be determined by visual observation.

If swelling is present, we note its qualities—whether it is soft, hard, elastic, or fluctuant. Lymphatic glands may also be felt and the state of induration determined by their softness or hardness. If vertical pressure applied to the crown of a tooth results in pain, there is a strong likelihood of an apical involvement; whereas pain resulting from a horizontal pressure from either the mesial, distal, or buccal direction indicates a probable periodontal infection or involvement.

Necessity for roentgenographs

Complete sets of roentgenographs are indispensable in making an examination. By means of these we can determine (1) the size, shape, and length of the root; (2) the size and position of the pulp chamber; (3) the condition of the supporting tissues; (4) the type and amount of supporting alveolar bone, i.e., whether it is dense or loosely trabeculated; and (5) the position of the root in its relationship to the crown of the tooth and to the mandible or maxilla. The roentgenographs may also disclose pathologic conditions such as bone destruction, odontomas, impactions of teeth, remnants of broken-off roots, and the presence of necrotic areas following the extraction of teeth. Roentgenographs may also help to reveal the presence of trauma and many other pathologic conditions. It is important to be able to recognize and interpret changes in the bone because of their practical significance in bridge restorations. When a roentgenograph reveals the destruction of bone on the mesial surface of a posterior tooth tilted mesially (if the destruction is not excessive), the further tilting may often be stopped by the placement of a fixed bridge. In similar cases, where the edentulous space is very narrow, a crown establishing contact anteriorly will also stop this movement. If, however, the roentgenograph discloses that such a tilting and excessive bone destruction have produced a deep, infected gingival pocket, and if, in addition to this, the examination discloses an involvement of the root bifurcation, such a tooth should not be used as a bridge abutment, for its life expectancy is short.

Roentgenographs further reveal the amount of periodontal membrane attachment and its relative thickness; the bite wing types are also valuable. Important as they are, roentgenographs were never intended to supplant the other forms of examination; they are merely a check upon other methods of examination. To be of full value, roentgenographs must be taken at the proper angles and in a sufficient number of views.

Transillumination may also be employed in making an oral examination. It is especially valuable for disclosing the pathologic involvement of the sinus.

Recording data

One of the most important and yet most frequently neglected factors in an examination is recording of important data and measurements. This applies to the young, to adults, and to older patients. When a patient is examined, his records should include the form and general shape of his arches at that time. This is best accomplished by constructing a set of articulated study casts. His record may also include the outline of his profile; this may be obtained either in lead wire or with a cutout pattern. Finally, his record should include the form and color of his teeth, both anterior and posterior. This information will prove very valuable should the patient require extensive partial or complete artificial dentures later in life. It is also well to obtain a record of the poundage the patient is capable of exerting on each of his natural teeth (Fig. 33-2). This may be obtained with any of the standard gnathodynamometers.

Pulp tests

An examination for the vitality of the pulp of each tooth should be routine procedure. These tests may be either electrical or thermal or both. Although the electrical test is valuable, it is not an infallible one; a sensation may be obtained in a tooth whose pulp is not normal. Occasionally we find a diseased pulp in which the nerves react as in a normal pulp. The response of a pulp to an electrical test varies in different teeth and in accordance with the amount of secondary dentin present. The thermal tests are generally more reliable than the electrical.

Although the examination of teeth with exploring instruments is perhaps the oldest method employed, it is still one of the best, if properly done. To do so, all the teeth first should be cleaned thoroughly and each tooth examined separately by taking one surface at a time. A sharp explorer, a good light, and a systematic procedure are still the recommended means of examining the teeth. Sometimes, when difficulty is experienced in examining the proximal surfaces of teeth, the application of a separator may allow better access to the proximal area. This, however, should be done rarely and with caution because of the possible damage to the periodontal membrane. Dental ligature passed through the contact area frequently discloses the presence of a carious lesion by its fraying.

At this time the periodontal tissues around each tooth should be investigated. The depth of the gingival crevices and pockets should be measured and recorded.

The examination discloses certain facts and information; these must be recorded on a suitable record chart. Whether the record is simple or extensive, it is important that it contain all the essential information. Many such charts have been developed and presented to the profession in the dental literature. Such records are kept as a permanent file for future reference. In addition to the written records, many dentists obtain photographs of the patient from anterior and profile views. These may prove extremely important, both to the dentist and the patient, if it is necessary to make complete dentures for the same patient 20 to 25 years later. Some dentists also recommend that plaster impressions be taken of the face and a permanent facial mask be made and filed. Additional data and information may be obtained by the use of head plate roentgenographs. All of the methods of recording that have been enumerated ultimately enable both the patient and the dentist to judge the degree of correction or success obtained in any individual undertaking.

Former oral health service

A patient requesting partial denture service has usually had dental restorations previously placed in his mouth. It is very important to check the oral health service formerly received by the patient. In our zeal to diagnose and determine a plan of treatment for the major needs of the mouth, let us not overlook the many small and apparently insignificant deficiencies that may also exist. Unless these are recognized and corrective steps are instituted, the entire scheme of restoration may fail (see Chapters 7 and 12). Such a complete check is made not only for the benefit of the patient, but also to ensure ourselves against failure that may result from the neglect of another operator. Hence, we should note the quality, the kind, and the duration of the service of all restorations, as well as their present condition.

Fillings

The fillings should be carefully checked for the integrity of cavity margins and to find if the margins of the preparation are extended into immune or cleansable areas, thus preventing the recurrence of caries. The presence or lack of contact areas and their proper placement are determined, and, finally, the occlusion in the restorations is noted to see whether any trauma is present. The roentgenograph is very useful in this phase of the examination, for it frequently discloses overhanging gingival margins that might escape visual and instrumental examination. The hygienic condition in which the mouth is kept may be an index to the probable future cleanliness the patient will maintain. If a patient has taken good care of his mouth in the past, the probability is that he will continue to do so in the future; but if he is neglectful and does not practice good mouth hygiene and if, as a result, the restorations are in a poor state of preservation, it is quite likely that the new restorations will encounter a similar fate. When making the examination, it is well to indicate on the record all the restorations present when the patient first applied for dental service. When a previous restoration that does not meet the correct specifications or that shows signs of disintegration is found, it should be called to the patient's attention. This should be done in a way not to deprecate the operator who placed it; to do so will not benefit anyone in particular. Such an attitude, however, does not justify one in hiding from the patient the existence of a dangerous condition. If a careful check of all restorations is not made and the patient is dismissed in the belief that his mouth is in a healthy state and a few months later a serious disorder develops, it might prove very embarrassing to explain such an oversight.

Crowns

The same diligence and thoroughness should be exercised when examining artificial crowns. The crown should be checked for its gingival fit; it must be determined whether there are any overhanging or deficient margins and whether any pieces of cement were overlooked when the crown was cemented to position. An examination of the crown will disclose the condition of its investing tissues. If there are signs of inflammation, suppuration, or pocket formation, the cause should be determined and removed, even though it requires the removal of the crown. It is well to look for minute openings worn through the occlusal surfaces of gold crowns. This condition is usually present when the crown is made of swaged gold only and occludes with a porcelain tooth. Very often these minute openings expose the underlying, enclosed natural tooth structure to caries, which goes unnoticed. Unless detected and corrected, the covered coronal portion of the natural tooth may be destroyed before the patient is aware of the condition.

The lack of proper contour, occlusion, or contact areas may also induce severe pathologic reactions, necessitating the removal of the tooth. In the anterior part of the mouth a recession of the gingival tissues may be found that leaves exposed a dark gingival region and destroys the esthetic values. There are other instances in which a single crown, due to its improper occlusal relationship with its antagonist, has thrown both arches out of harmony and equilibrium. Such restorations, if they cannot be properly corrected, should be removed and remade.

Fixed partial dentures

Since crowns are frequently used as bridge retainers, all such retainers should be examined for the same conditions that occur in the individual crowns. The presence of previously placed fixed bridges in the patient's mouth offers a more serious problem than that of a single crown. As is well known, the type and quality of fixed prostheses placed vary almost with the number of dentists who place them. At times, it is necessary to be cautious and diplomatic in explaining to the patient the conditions the examination discloses.

In examining bridges, not only is the question of mechanics and functional efficiency involved but also the biologic reactions of the tissues to the appliance must be recognized (Chapter 11). It is true that many poorly constructed bridges have given service for many years; yet this service was purely a mechanical one, since at the same time the presence of these bridges imposed a severe biologic handicap upon the entire body. Many patients are not aware of the close relationship between oral and systemic conditions; consequently, it may require a thorough presentation and explanation of the facts in order to make them understand the existing conditions. Although modern dental technic offers the dental profession the possibility of giving patients cleansable and sanitary fixed partial dentures, there are still many patients today who are receiving fixed restorations of a type prevalent 50 years ago.

We may find bridges, otherwise satisfactory, where the ridges have absorbed, leaving a considerable space between the crest of the ridge and the pontic. This open space proves annoying to the patient because it acts as a food trap. In such instances it may be advisable to fire additional porcelain to the pontics. Now and then we see a cantilever bridge where the pontic has been displaced and the entire abutment has been tilted. In such instances the periodontal membrane is frequently crushed on the mesial surface and a pocket is present. Such restorations should be removed and replaced with a prosthesis that is supported at each end. If, on the other hand, a cantilever bridge has given years of service and shows no tendency toward rotation or tilting and if the investing tissues are normal, it is quite likely that the environment is such that the bridge will continue to give satisfactory service for many years to come. Its removal is justified only as a precautionary measure.

There are times when we find an arch that is partially edentulous on one side, with the other side restored by a fixed partial denture. In such circumstances it is well to examine the existing bridge with the thought in mind of removing it to allow the placement of a bilateral removable partial denture. It is very disconcerting to place a fixed partial denture on one side, only to find that in a very short time the old restoration on the other side of the arch has failed because of an abscess or some other reason, and a bilateral removable partial denture is ultimately required.

Existing fixed restorations must be examined for occlusion, esthetics, and the recurrence of caries; the condition of the investing tissues must likewise be ascertained.

Removable partial denture

Where a removable partial denture is present, the individual retaining teeth are examined for caries, abrasion, and degree of firmness. Ocasionally it will be found that a clasp type of removable partial denture is causing discomfort to the patient because of the encroachment of the clasps upon the sensitive cementoenamel junction. This encroachment may frequently extend into the gingival tissues, causing a paradentosis. Clasps that are improperly designed or placed likewise may promote decalcification of the enamel. Where tissue resorption has occurred under the base of the denture, it may be necessary to rebase or to remake the appliance. The presence of a removable partial denture in the arch opposite the one in which a fixed partial denture is being considered may change or modify the type and design of the fixed partial denture.

Complete denture

If one of the arches contains a complete denture (Fig. 3-7), its presence may also modify the type of fixed restoration that is to be placed in the opposing arch, for we know that a mucosa-borne appliance is not capable of exerting the same degree of chewing force that the natural teeth do; consequently, the type of retainers used is sometimes determined by the existing reduced functional force.

Orthodontic treatment

Previous orthodontic treatment at times may be a factor closely related to fixed partial denture prosthesis. This is particularly true if the roots of the abutment teeth are shortened by resorption (Fig. 2-8). In these instances extreme caution must be exercised when contemplating the use of such teeth for supporting fixed partial dentures. The dentist is sometimes called upon to construct a fixed prosthesis to serve a dual purpose; first, restoring lost function to the edentulous area; and second, acting in the capacity of an orthodontic retainer. When the latter purpose is a major one, close cooperation with the orthodontist is essential. Similarly, when

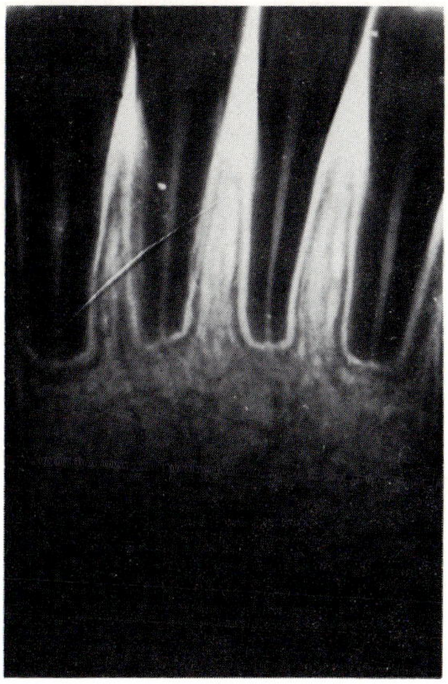

Fig. 2-8. Resorption of lower anterior root apices.

the use of a bite plane is indicated prior to undertaking restorative treatment, it is advisable to consult an orthodontist.

Surgery

Surgery to which the oral tissues have been subjected may be an important element in the problem of a fixed partial denture prosthesis. Generally, where a great deal of tissue has been removed surgically, it will be found that a removable partial denture is preferable to a fixed one. Where excessive destruction or removal of tissues has not occurred, it should be observed whether or not normal healing has taken place following surgical interference. If roots have been resected, the condition should be checked with roentgenographs to ascertain the success of the operation. The removal of cysts, tumors, and other pathologic conditions frequently may necessitate deferring the placement of a fixed appliance until the time when all possibility of recurrence has passed.

Frequently an examination of a mouth discloses at once the type of service the patient needs. The existing oral conditions may also disclose immediately the probable duration of any service that might be rendered.

From the standpoint of occlusion, it will be found that, all other factors being equal, in those cases where malocclusion exists, a fixed bridge is preferred to a removable one; the latter is more serviceable with an occlusion that is balanced. A fixed appliance makes it possible not only to replace lost teeth but also to restore the occlusion physiologically. In mouths that have been partially edentulous for a long time it is found that, almost without exception, there has been a drifting of teeth and a malalignment of occlusal relationships. Orthodontic procedures are usually first employed to correct the malrelations of such teeth.

Oral abnormalities

Oral abnormalities and deficiencies may play an important role in the diagnosis for fixed partial dentures. Such apparently unimportant items as supernumerary cusps and teeth must be taken into consideration, for these frequently modify or change the contemplated plan of treatment. At times tumors and bony prominences are present; these should be corrected by surgery. To place a fixed partial denture in the region of a tumor would be ill advised, for it is quite likely that later the bridge would be damaged or even removed during an operation for the removal of the growth. A bridge placed in the vicinity of a tumor might prove just the irritant needed to change a benign growth into a malignant one. Again, the recognition of a malignancy in its early stages may avoid placing the responsibility for its existence on the bridge.

There are times when the bony prominence of a ridge leaves only a short vertical space for pontics. If a fixed appliance is placed in these conditions, it usually fails because the pontic lacks sufficient bulk gingivoclusally. Surgical interference may be employed to remove enough tissue to give the needed space for a strong, hygienic type of pontic. Dental cysts are frequently found in the incisor and bicuspid regions. Unless corrected, they may nullify the usefulness of the abutment teeth involved. Benign tumors arising from precartilaginous connective tissue, such tissue as exostoses, chondromas, fibromas, and the like, have a slow process of growth; frequently, many years intervene before the symptoms are such that treatment is sought. If placing a fixed appliance in the vicinity of such conditions causes an irritation and inflammation of the overlying soft tissues, these may undergo a change into malignancy.

Alveolar bone. Change in the alveolar bone is another factor to be observed carefully. The alveolar process exists only by virtue of the presence and function of the tooth. When a tooth is extracted, the process is resorbed. The same condition prevails in modified form in those teeth that are out of normal function; here we see a partial atrophy of the bone. There is a question whether the loss of alveolar bone with teeth present may be due to the loss of their normal functions.

Cleft palate. There are other conditions that influence the use of a fixed partial prosthesis. A perforated or a cleft palate may require the modification of the fixed partial denture so that it may also help to retain an obturator placed in the cleft. In the case of an arch that is bilaterally partially edentulous, a removable partial denture with an obturator may be the restoration of choice.

Systemic disease. If a systemic disease such as tuberculosis, syphilis, diabetes, and pernicious anemia is present, it should be treated by a physician; such a disease has a direct bearing on the success of the prosthesis. All restorative services are dependent upon the health of the periodontal tissues, and since the health of these tissues depends upon the systemic condition of the patient, it is evident that a patient suffering from any of these general maladies does not possess the necessary stamina or resistance to receive and tolerate any additional loads that an appliance may impose. For his own protection, as well as that of his patient, the dentist should understand and be able to recognize the early manifestations of these various general disorders.

An examination should also take into consideration the local disturbances, particularly the so-called stomatitis. This usually accompanies some constitutional ailment or deficiencies of certain of the vitamins; metallic poisoning may also be a contributing factor. The presence of stomatitic conditions should cause us to question the possibility of systemic complications, which, if verified, must be eliminated before any prostheses are placed.

Devitalized teeth. Not many decades ago it was considered good practice to devitalize teeth prior to the placement of crown or bridge retainers. It is comparatively recently that the inlay and the extracoronal types of bridge retainers have supplanted the more generally used dowel crowns. It is now the unavoidable exception rather than the rule to remove pulps from abutment teeth routinely. The concept of a prosthesis as a health service assumes that every safeguard has been taken to conserve and protect the remaining tissues, that the appliance has been carefully designed and constructed, that it may be expected to last for a considerable length of time, and, finally, that its placement in the mouth will not result in any harm to the patient.

Research and study in the fields of dental pathology, histology, and bacteriology have definitely influenced the type of prosthetic appliances used today. The simplest appliance that is compatible with the needs of living tissues is far more

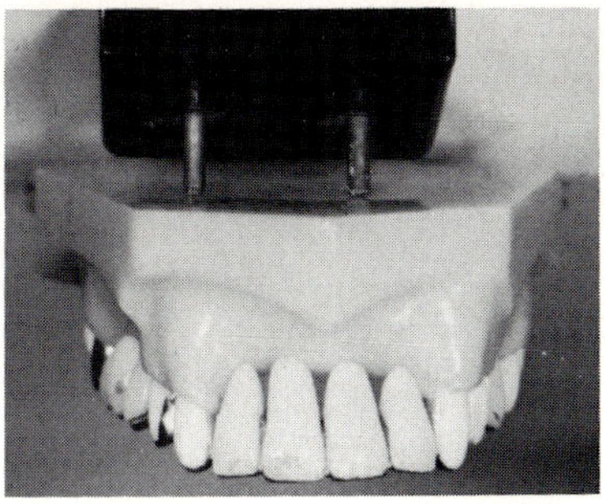

Fig. 2-9. Four upper incisors missing; ridge resorbed extensively. Removable partial denture normally indicated. Long pin facing used, with glazed porcelain root extensions touching crest of ridge.

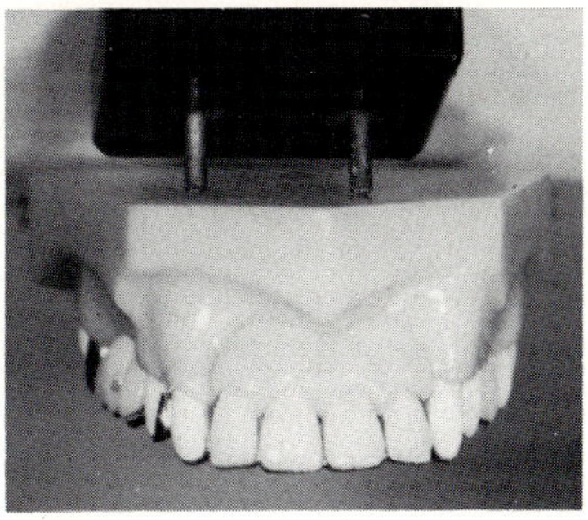

Fig. 2-10. Removable, gum-colored acrylic veneer, automatically held in position by lip; esthetic and hygienic, it prevents escape of air in playing wind instrument.

desirable and superior to an intricate and complex restoration that neglects these essentials.

Upper anterior restorations

For many years the placing of a bridge from cuspid to cuspid, employing only two abutment teeth, was common practice. A careful study of all bridges so placed during the last 50 years indicates that an appliance of this type will serve satisfactorily under certain favorable conditions. The success of such a bridge in the upper anterior region is problematic if the patient still retains his lower anterior teeth and is wearing a lower mucosa-borne appliance that restores the posterior teeth bilaterally. In this instance the major forces of mastication are borne by the anterior teeth. In a few years there may be a labial drift of the entire upper bridge that bodily moves the abutment teeth and the supporting tissues. Some of these appliances are known to have moved forward as much as 5 mm.

When such an edentulous space exists in the mouth and an anterior fixed bridge must be used—for example, for a wind instrument musician—it is recommended that at least the two first bicuspids be included as abutments in addition to the two cuspids (Figs. 2-9 to 2-11). These

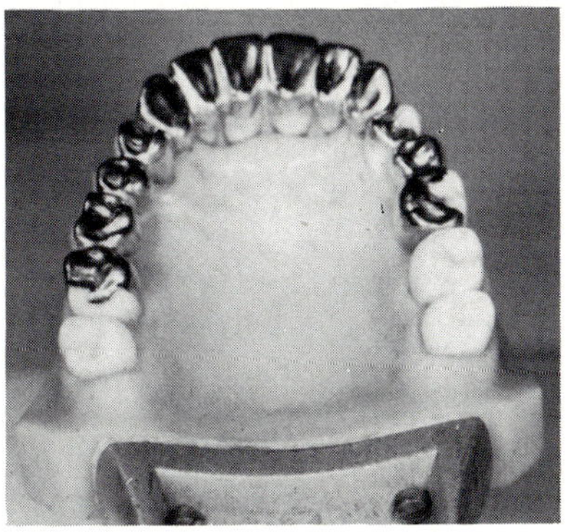

Fig. 2-11. Lingual view of veneer filling in cervical interproximal pontic spaces.

are then united with rigid connectors, giving a double terminal retention that will reduce the tendency toward labial drift.

Cantilever bridges are contraindicated in most conditions in the mouth. In the exceptional cases where a missing lateral incisor is supplied by suspending it from a cuspid retainer, it is a risky procedure. Many such restorations show that the lateral pontic gradually moves labially, rotating about the long axis of the cuspid unless supported also by the central.

Biologic aspects of foundation

Some teeth, because of their morphology, root length, and favorable amount and structure of bone, are more capable of accommodating the increases in force that accompany the placement of a bridge. The first molars, both maxillary and mandibular, are by far the strongest teeth available as bridge abutments. The cuspids, second molars, bicuspids, and upper central incisors are next in order of usefulness. The upper lateral incisors and the lower incisors are the weakest teeth available for this purpose (Tables 11-1 to 11-4). Even this classification is subject to certain qualifications. For example, if the cuspid is in an unfavorable position in the arch, if its root is short, or if the supporting tissues are deficient, it is evident that even a cuspid may be contraindicated as a fixed bridge abutment.

A careful study of the periodontal membrane frequently may be the determining factor in the success or failure of a fixed bridge. The periodontal membrane is so constructed that forces directed in the long axis of the tooth are received as in a hammock of suspending fibers. The occlusal pressure forces are then transmitted to the surrounding alveolar bone as tensile forces. It is a biologic characteristic of bone that, when subjected to a continuous slight pressure, it resorbs; however, it is stimulated by a pulling force or tension and responds to it by depositing bone. This pulling force, intermittently applied, maintains a healthy alveolar bone. When the position of a tooth is such that the forces directed upon it are not transmitted properly to the bone but result in a pressure area, resorption of the bone occurs. When a tooth is not in function, the periodontal membrane is usually very narrow or thin. Ordinarily, a thinner periodontal membrane gives a less mobile tooth. However, the fact that a tooth is firmer does not necessarily mean that its attachment is stronger. In a functioning tooth the periodontal membrane is wide and has strong, regularly oriented principal fibers that are capable of withstanding the forces of occlusion. When out of occlusion, the principal fibers are lost and only irregular interstitial strands of the fibers are present. Therefore, it is important to determine: first, whether the physical makeup of the periodontal membrane is such that it is capable of withstanding the additional forces of mastication which the bridge will impose upon it; and, second, whether the bridge can be so constructed that the stresses developed will be transmitted in line with the long axes of the abutments (Fig. 11-5).

The periodontal membrane, the alveolar process, and the other investing tissues form the real foundation for any restoration we may undertake; in order that the tissues may be acceptable and the foundation satisfactory, there must be no evidence of any existing pathologic lesion, either acute or chronic.

By the exercise of good judgment and the ability to discern the capacity of tissues to tolerate additional work we can render the best type of health service to the patient. If the restored function and service of a bridge are outweighed by the harm which the teeth and the supporting tissues might sustain, a bridge should not be placed. Sometimes there exists a disposition to divide the human body into many parts and to assign a specialist to the care of each part. There further exists the tendency for each of these specialists to subdivide and localize his interests, with the result that the body and its functions are no longer regarded and treated as a biologic unit. Such a dividing and subdividing is not a natural condition, nor is it regarded as such by nature, for we know that the violation of certain natural laws of health in one part of the body will react unfavorably in other parts. This excessive subdividing and focusing on minutiae very frequently lead to controversies that are not fundamental.

For example, we know that a tooth has movement in various directions, name-

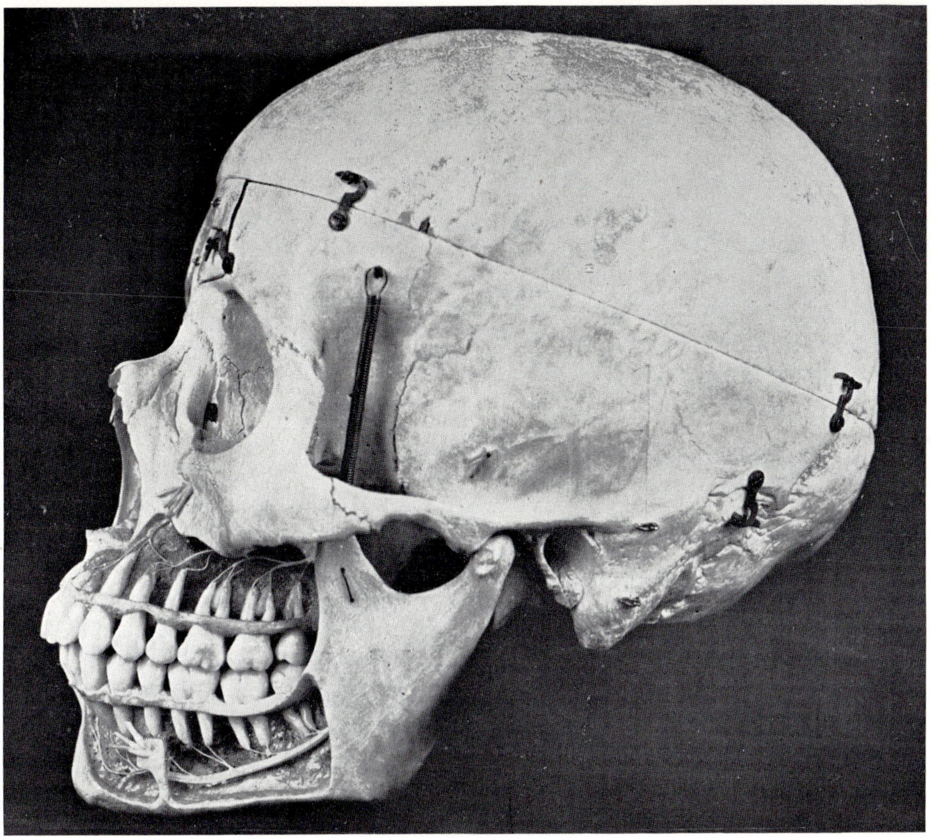

Fig. 2-12. Natural dentition; axes of upper and lower teeth meeting at angle directed anteriorly.

ly, buccolingually, mesiodistally, and apically. We know that the average thickness of the periodontal membrane is from 0.20 to 0.30 mm. and, consequently, the amount of movement a tooth undergoes is very limited. Nevertheless, it has been stated that even a slight inhibition of this small amount of movement is extremely injurious to the supporting teeth.

If it were true that the placement of a fixed restoration produced absolute fixation of the abutment teeth, a danger might exist. This, however, is not the case because of the arrangement, the position, and the structural form of the periodontal membrane. A study extending over 45 years to determine tissue reaction to fixed partial dentures has shown that those teeth supporting fixed bridges receive an amount of exercise and stimulation sufficient to maintain them in a state of health. It is found that nature very readily compensates for any slight inhibition that occurs in the movement of teeth. The entire arch, consisting of all the teeth, moves and functions in such a way that all the teeth perform as a unit in a functioning whole. Normal occlusion is found only when all the teeth meet their respective responsibilities and duties collectively (Fig. 2-12). It has been shown that it is not fixation but the occurrence of traumatic occlusion in a prosthesis which is the prime cause for the loss of abutment teeth.

It is difficult to obtain normal occlusion when (1) a tooth has tilted forward mesially or lingually to the point where half or more of its occlusal surface is out of function; (2) the tooth has either risen or gravitated in its socket beyond the occlusal plane of the adjacent teeth; and (3) the opposing teeth are not normal morphologically.

Although the essentials of fixed prostheses are sometimes limited to comfort, esthetics, and utility, they also restore function and help to promote the health of the patient. A fixed prosthesis is so constructed that it may be easily kept clean by the natural self-cleansing action of the mouth. It is not conducive to pathologic conditions of either the prepared tooth or the underlying tissues. It is so planned that its insertion does not produce inflammation or infection. By establishing the proper relationship between the pontics, retainers, and the underlying tissues, it is possible to obtain a constant stimulation of the gingival tissues and so to maintain a state of health in the mucosa. Finally, there are the very practical and essential considerations; namely, that fixed restorations, barring accident, should last throughout the greater part of the patient's life and that they should be simple and inexpensive to produce, so that a large proportion of the population may avail itself of this service.

Tooth form and function

The dental arches. Normal anatomic tooth form and relationship in the dental arch occupy an important place in crown and bridge practice. The dental arch encompasses more than a curved structure. The Dental Glossary defines the arch as "a composite structure of natural dentition and the alveolar ridge or the remains thereof after the loss of some or all of the natural teeth." As envisioned by the engineer, the teeth follow a curved line that passes through the center of gravity of the cross section of each tooth; the section also contains the center points of the ideal interproximal contact areas on either side of the tooth.

If the correct form of a tooth has been restored, it will be found that its function is usually regained. Restoring the correct form of the tooth is not synonymous with prominent cusps, deep sulci, and sharp marginal ridges. By reestablishing correct form is meant that the restoration is in harmony with the conditions that exist in the mouth at the time the restoration is placed. Missing teeth must be replaced correctly not only with reference to their anatomy, but also in their proper relationship to other teeth and investing tissues. We find in young patients that, although the cusps and ridges are sharp and unworn, the hinge movement of the mandible also predominates, resulting in little lateral movement. As the patient grows older, the occlusal forms of the teeth change due to the wearing down and flattening of the ridges and cusps; this is coincidental with the development of a greater functional range of the mandible. This process of cuspal coordination is a gradual one and continues until an optimum condition is attained. When the wear of teeth reaches a stage where their multiple shearing action is largely replaced by a crushing and mashing action, greater force is required in the mastication of food, and the periodontal membrane and the supporting bone are called upon to endure excessive loads.

Occlusal wear. An excessive wear of the occlusal surfaces of teeth very frequently results in the loss of a coordination of the occlusal and incisal surfaces. To maintain healthy teeth and investing tissues and to ensure a nondestructive function, the essential anatomic factors must be maintained. The shape of the teeth and their position in the arch are very important to the oral health of the patient. To protect the gum margins and to divert the food over them harmlessly, due regard must be paid not only to the occlusal anatomy of the teeth but also to their axial convexities and concavities, contact areas, and the curvatures in the gingival regions. Many crowns and bridges fail, in spite of their mechanical efficiency, because the restoration disregards the protection that is so essential to the soft tissues. If the convexities, sulci, and cusps characteristic of teeth were not essential to the well-being of human beings, nature by the process of evolution long ago would have eliminated them and given men teeth with flat surfaces throughout. It is certain that these contours have a very definite purpose.

Contact areas and facets. Occasionally we find a crown that meets all the requirements of correct anatomy and occlusion with one exception, that of proximal contact relationship. True, a tooth may be contacting its neighbor, but this alone is not sufficient. The form of the contact areas and the area where it is placed, both buccolingually and gingivoclusally, is extremely important. If it is placed too far buccally, the tendency will be to drive the tooth in the buccal direction; on the other hand, if the contact is placed too high occlusally, it will have a tendency to exert a lifting force on the tooth (Fig. 2-5). It is only when this area is correctly established and preserved that we may expect a perfectly equalized arch. An unnatural contact relationship is one reason why rotated teeth usually result in an unbalanced denture. Clinical observation discloses the fact that the most frequent failure of the arches resulting from improper contacts is found in the region of the cuspid and lateral. This is most common in the lower arch, and, when it occurs, the molar and bicuspid move anteriorly, pushing the cuspid past the lateral incisor. A proper contact relationship also protects the tissues from food that may otherwise be forced onto the interproximal gum tissues.

As patients grow older, it is found that the interproximal contacting surfaces lose their original convexities and develop flat facets. These result from the movement of the teeth against each other during function. In older patients there is likely to be a concomitant loss of alveolar bone and gum recession. Such flattened interproximal contacts give the teeth added support against the forces of mastication.

Therefore, in restorations for older patients, the contacts are usually less convex or slightly flatter than for younger patients.

Correct contour. The concept sometimes prevails that, if a crown is made with convex axial surfaces from the occlusal to the gingival, it meets the requirements of correct morphology. While a convexity may be desirable and beneficial in the indicated areas, it may prove definitely detrimental if used in the wrong areas.

Wheeler[12] has called our attention to the importance of correct contour in the cervical third region of human teeth. He has shown that, while the correct convexities assist in maintaining and protecting the health of the gingivae, an excessive contour in this area causes the investing tissues to lose their tone and also results in the formation of a debris pocket, causing a chronic inflammation of the gum tissues.

These convexities of the gingival third areas are fairly consistent in the arc they describe in each locality of the mouth. So important and so essential are these considered to the well-being of the investing tissues that their loss or exaggeration is discouraged in the placement of prosthetic restorations.

Wheeler further found that the contours of the cervical third of the upper teeth are quite similar on the labial, buccal, and lingual surfaces. Similar curvatures exist on the buccal surface of the lower posterior teeth to those on the upper, except that on the lower lingual surfaces the highest point of the contour lies midway between the cementoenamel junction and the tip of the cusps. In the lower anterior teeth he found that the contour of the cervical third was less than that in the upper anterior teeth.

Tooth form. While the dentist is primarily interested in the six anterior teeth when harmonizing tooth form with the shape of the arches and the face, it is important for him to recognize that the square, tapering, and ovoid characteristics of the anterior teeth are usually inherent in the posterior teeth. Those patients with long, tapering anterior teeth usually have long bicuspids and molars in proportion to their diameter. Such patients also tend toward a vertical mandibular movement rather than a lateral one. This is due primarily to the fact that their posterior teeth have high cusps and definitely inclined steep planes.

On the other hand, in the broad, square type of face, which has the characteristic square type of tooth, it is found that the anterior teeth are not as long; they are more square and the bicuspids and molars have shorter cusps and comparatively flat inclined planes. This condition is conducive to a more lateral function of the mandible. The difference in the type of function not only is related to the shape of the teeth but also is reflected in the shape of the head of the person; those patients with vertical mandibular movements usually tend toward the long, tapering types of face, while the lateral functioning types result in broad, wide faces.

So definitely does facial form respond to the existing type of function that the Eskimo, who normally belongs to the tapering type, acquires the broad, wide facial type at maturity. He uses his teeth so vigorously because of his native diet of frozen fish and blubber that he completely wears down all cuspal interference, which then allows him free and extensive lateral movements, resulting in the lateral development of his face.

When placing crowns or bridges, it is essential that the characteristic tooth form be reproduced so that it harmonizes with the cusp height and plane inclination of the remaining teeth.

Root anatomy

When the teeth of one arch are brought in contact with those of the other, certain forces and relationships are established. Our knowledge of dental anatomy tells us that the roots of the molars, both upper and lower, are not at right angles to the planes of their occlusal surfaces (Fig. 2-12). We find that in both the upper and lower molars, roots incline and slope distally. A line drawn through the long axis of the upper root and another line drawn through the long axis of the lower root will meet to form an acute angle directed anteriorly (Fig. 11-5). The axis of the tooth has been defined by Brumfield as "that line which connects the center of rotation of the tooth in its structure with the center of gravity of the tooth cross-section above, which also contains the centers of interproximal contact areas." Consequently, during the act of mastication or closure of the jaw, when the upper and lower teeth meet, the tendency is to drive the teeth anteriorly. This so-called anterior component of force must be taken into consideration when constructing partial prostheses. This may also help explain the lower cuspid migration anteriorly and labially. The normal anatomy of a tooth may be modified to reduce occlusal stresses and to enhance their self-cleansing qualities when pontics are used; frequently, natural grooves are deepened and supplementary ones placed through the marginal ridges. Such modifications facilitate the self-cleansing action of the restoration and also permit the escape of food into the oral cavity once it has been crushed.

Forces and stresses

Many fixed bridges fail because of the periodontal lesions that result from a disharmony of the occlusion. The stresses that result from tortioned abutment teeth, interfering cusps, and improper occlusal contacts and relationships very frequently result in a biologic handicap which the tissues cannot overcome. When such conditions are encountered, they should be corrected prior to the construction and placement of a fixed partial denture.

During function most teeth are subjected not only to vertical forces, but also to varying degrees of lateral and anteroposterior forces. Where vertical forces are proportionately greater than the lateral or anteroposterior forces, we may expect a healthy condition of the investing tissues and a long life of the teeth.

When the occlusion is not well balanced in either the lateral or forward movements of the mandible, it will lack an equitable distribution of forces on all the teeth. In such circumstances one or only a few of the teeth bear the brunt of the work, and in a short time they become tender and accompanied by inflammatory processes of the periodontal membranes; this frequently is followed by the loss of the tooth. Although the vital powers of a tooth are capable of compensating for slight unnatural forces, experience has shown that, unless points of excessive interference are reduced, the tooth becomes loosened and is lost. On the other hand, when the occlusion and the arrangement of teeth are harmonious during the lateral excursions of the mandible, the periodontal membrane and other supporting tissues are capable of withstanding the normal forces of mastication without any harmful effects.

Areas of interception existing in either a crown or bridge should be corrected immediately. Formerly, when softer golds were used for prostheses, the high areas in gold were worn down before a definite breakdown of the tissues occurred. Today, when the harder types of gold alloys are used, a harmful reaction takes place in the tissues.

Concepts of occlusion

Normal occlusion has been considered as an innocuous distribution of forces on the teeth in their various contacts. Traumatic occlusion, therefore, is an abnormal and injurious distribution of forces on teeth experienced during the various phases of functional occlusion that will result in the impairment of the tooth and its supporting tissues. Normal occlusion implies, therefore, not only the closure maintained in centric relationship but also the full range of relationships in the various positions and movements of the mandible against the maxillae. (A more inclusive definition of occlusion in its varied applications may be found in *Glossary of Prosthodontic Terms.**) For a comprehensive, well-illustrated, and understandable presentation of the principles of occlusion based on present-day concepts, the recent work of Huffman, Regenos, and Taylor is recommended.[11]

In partial denture prosthesis every effort should be made to maintain a normal physiologic occlusion. This objective is difficult to attain if we attempt to use abutments that are tipped to such an extent that occlusal relationships cannot be restored, or if we attempt to place restorations in edentulous areas which oppose teeth that are extruded beyond the occlusal plane of the opposing arch without first having brought these to their proper occlusal relationship. Neither can be secure normal occlusion in restorations if we fail to restore the correct tooth anatomy.

To distinguish between normal and abnormal occlusion, a distinction should be made between a functional centric relation occlusion and a pseudocentric occlusion.[2] This can best be done by mount-

*Nomenclature Committee, The Academy of Denture Prosthetics: Glossary of prosthodontic terms, ed. 3, St. Louis, 1968, The Journal of Prosthetic Dentistry, The C. V. Mosby Co.

ing the upper and lower casts in an adjustable articulator with a hinge axis face-bow registration that has been adjusted to the correct centric, protrusive, and lateral positions of the mandible in the glenoid fossae (Chapters 29 and 37).

While the perfect coordination of all natural teeth in both arches is a rarity in nature, the dentist should make every effort to detect uneven distribution of forces and to take the necessary corrective steps to remedy them. He should likewise make every effort to equalize forces by eliminating all points of interception between the various movements and positions of the mandible and the maxillae.

GENERAL CONSIDERATIONS OF PATIENT

The general information concerning the patient should now be examined as it relates to his fixed partial prostheses. Those factors that may influence the decision will be age, sex, and possibly the habits of personal hygiene. As stated previously, fixed partial denture service is most frequently indicated and rendered to patients between the ages of 20 and 55 years. When partially edentulous conditions exist in patients younger or older than this, serious consideration should be given to some type of restoration other than fixed. Since in fixed appliances it is necessary to cut into teeth, there is danger, in the case of young patients, of encroaching upon or exposing the pulp, unless the tooth and pulp chamber are fully formed. In senescence there are also characteristic dangers. It has been found that in patients beyond the age of 55 years the teeth are not as strong as in youth, nor are they able to withstand as well the forces to which abutment teeth are subjected. The vitality of the supporting and investing tissues apparently decreases with age. For this reason some other type of restoration for the older patients is frequently preferred. The question of age is an important one in certain patients (Chapter 8).

Type of patient

Generally the teeth of a powerfully built man are stronger than those of a dainty, frail woman. Likewise, the tissue vitality, on the average, is better in the robust type of patient than in the frail. Although the quality of esthetics is a desirable one in every fixed partial denture, it is more desirable when the appliance is placed for a woman, particularly in the anterior part of the mouth. The fact that the appliance is for a woman will sometimes indicate the placement of a fixed rather than a removable restoration because of the apparent aversion of women to removable prostheses (Figs. 3-37 to 3-42).

Personal hygiene. The personal hygiene of a patient often determines the type of prosthesis to be employed. Unless mouth hygiene is rigidly pursued, the most perfectly constructed and sanitary type of fixed partial denture will soon fail. A removable prosthesis, since it can be cleaned more quickly and more readily, is preferred for those patients who, the dentist suspects, will not be diligent and careful in maintaining oral cleanliness. Studies (see Chapter 11) have definitely shown that men exert a greater force in chewing than women; hence, men usually require a sturdier type of restoration.

General health. The general health factor of the patient should not be overlooked. Although most of the patients who seek dental service are in good health, a certain percentage of these are either sick or in questionable physical condition. The alert operator should be able to recognize the different types. In children we occasionally see a retardation of the eruption of teeth or the persistence of the deciduous teeth. This may be associated with a hypopituitary condition. Frequently the type of edentulous areas and the degree of deposits on teeth may raise the suspicion of a diabetic condition in a patient beyond the age of 50 years. Cyanosis of the lips and mucous membrane may indicate a serious heart disease. Systemic disturbances may also manifest themselves through bleeding gums, which may be a sign of a more serious type of deficiency disease. We observe at times a discoloration of the gingival margins due to a metallic intake. Lead and bismuth are the two metals most commonly involved. Pigmentation sometimes occurs in Addison's disease.

Occupation of patient. The vocation or occupation of a patient is a factor to be considered, particularly when the appliance is planned for a patient who depends largely upon his personal appearance as a means of earning his livelihood. This is more important if the restoration is in the anterior part of the mouth. If the factor of occupation is of prime importance, it may be necessary to modify the design of the appliance in such a manner that the mechanical and physiologic requirements of the restoration are subserved in order to enhance those of the esthetic. For those patients whose clarity of speech or voice is a prime consideration, the appliance must be designed to meet these specifications. There are instances in which extreme compromises must be made; singers and musicians using wind instruments are often in this category (Figs. 2-9 to 2-11). Although removable partial dentures may be indicated on the basis of the factors disclosed during the oral examination, fixed appliances are sometimes constructed because of the utilitarian requirements. In those cases in which a radical departure from the essential physiologic and mechanical principles has been made, the patient should recognize and accept his share of the responsibility and should be appraised of the future prespects of the appliance. The qualities of function, mechanical strength, and esthetics are desirable in every restoration, but when the values of one must be sacrificed to enhance those of the others, it should be done only with the full understanding and *written* consent of the patient.

The financial status of the patient has sometimes been indicated as a possible factor to be considered. This should be left to the discretion and good judgment of the dentist and his patient.

DENTAL ANALYSIS

Number and location of teeth

Since the fixed partial denture is a tooth-borne appliance, the teeth should next receive attention. The loss of one or more of the natural teeth generally creates abnormal physical changes with accompanying abnormal functions and forces. An increased load is placed on some teeth, while others suffer through a loss or diminution of function. The deleterious change from normality, while slow, is continuous and may become progressively worse with the lapse of time. The chewing habits of the patient are frequently modified, and further abnormalities may develop to the degree that the entire dental mechanism is thrown out of equilibrium and effective use. Hence the number of teeth present and their location are important considerations. It is an accepted axiom that the ideal fixed partial denture consists of two abutment teeth supporting one pontic. There are times, however, when two abutments may safely support two pontics. It has been observed that bridges confined to one area or quadrant of the mouth, where the teeth have similar functions, render the best service to the patient. Each tooth to be used as an abutment should have its pulp vitally determined. Although teeth with vital, normal pulps are normally utilized, those that have been properly treated and filled may be safely used as abutments if they are satisfactory clinically and roentgenographically (Tables 9-1 to 9-12).

Form, position, size of teeth

The characteristic form, size, position, and color of teeth should be observed and noted. A tooth that is small, malformed, or excessively thin labiolingually, or one whose crown is short gingivoclusally, may not be safely used as a bridge abutment. If such a tooth must be employed, the type of retainer placed on it must be modified to meet the prevailing conditions.

The position of a tooth or root in the arch may be studied more easily with the study cast and the roentgenographs. Very often the malposition of a tooth in the arch not only contraindicates its use as an abutment but also changes the type of prosthesis indicated. In other words, instead of restoring the edentulous area with a fixed appliance, a removable one is used. Occasions arise where the MOD and simpler types of retainers are supplanted by complete crowns because of their greater mechanical strength and retention.

The size and shape of the root are also very important. If the root is disproportionately short to the length of the crown, it may be ruled out as an abutment. If the position of the tooth is such that the root will not receive forces in line with its long axis, this also may exclude its use as a bridge abutment. It is frequently found that secondary dentin has practically obliterated the root canal of teeth of very old patients or teeth that have been subjected to trauma. If it is necessary to treat and fill such a root, the existing physical handicap may preclude the possibility of a successful root canal treatment; therefore, such a tooth is questionable.

Analysis of occlusion

A careful analysis should be made of the occlusion of each partially edentulous mouth. If corrective means are immediately employed after teeth are lost, little if any deviation from normal will take place. There is clinical evidence to indicate that, even in those patients in whom a partial impairment due to missing teeth has been sustained, the mechanical and biologic factors can be favorably restored by correct crown and bridge prostheses. Nature adapts herself readily to a new environment if the restoration is properly designed, constructed, and maintained. Hence, even in those mouths in which normal occlusion is lacking, the patient can be helped by proper corrective grinding or restorative procedures.

Much has been said and written on the importance of normal occlusion. Suffice it to say that, if the examination shows that the placement of a fixed partial denture will restore, even to a limited degree, the normal, physiologic functions of the oral mechanism and prevent any further pathologic changes, such a restoration should be placed, even though an ideal occlusion is not attainable. It should be noted also whether the existing type of occlusion has produced a breakdown of the supporting and investing tissues; if not, it is evident that the impaired conditions are not beyond the compensatory powers of nature, and therefore the prognosis is favorable for a fixed partial denture.

Dental abnormalities

Since dental caries is the most extensive pathologic condition that involves teeth, it is well to determine its extent and the patient's degree of active susceptibility. Other teeth may show signs of dystrophy, erosion, or opalescent dentin, or may be otherwise abnormal. Although attrition and fractures may not be classified as pathologic conditions, they present a problem in partial denture prosthodontics. The extreme manifestitation of any of these can and does modify the type of bridge-retainer placed on the abutment tooth, and it also may change even the type of prosthesis employed. Discoloration, hypoplasia, and torsion are other factors to be considered.

Although teeth normally exhibit a slight mobility in their sockets, excessive movement should excite our curiosity sufficiently to determine its cause. A bridge should not be considered or placed unless all oral pathologic conditions have been corrected and the remaining natural teeth restored to a healthy state. The eradication of all foci of infection is a distinct prerequisite to the placement of any type of bridge. If abutment teeth are so situated in the arch as to be in traumatic occlusion, the placing of a fixed partial denture on them will inevitably result in the loss not only of the prosthesis, but also of the abutment teeth.

Extraction

The extraction of teeth is an item of major importance. Those teeth that are physically beyond the realm of usefulness should be removed as well as those that show hopeless, pathologic, periapical involvements. Teeth that do not have proper supporting or investing tissues to enable them to serve satisfactorily as bridge abutments should be removed. When it is impossible or impracticable to move a malpositioned abutment to normal alignment by orthodontic means, it may be necessary to remove such a tooth and not use it as an abutment. Another consideration arises relative to the extraction of teeth; namely, when should the extraction be made? Those teeth designated for extraction are usually removed as soon as possible to allow the ridges to heal prior to the placement of the fixed partial denture. There are other times, however, when the so-called immediate replacement type of fixed partial denture is employed, in which event the teeth are not extracted until the fixed appliance is constructed and ready for insertion at the time the teeth are removed.

Periodontal membrane (ligament)

The periodontal membrane very often has been neglected among the factors to be considered prior to the placement of a fixed partial denture. The type of the periodontal membrane should be noted to see whether it is thick or thin. This can best be done with the aid of roentgenographs. The determination of this fact may indicate whether the tooth is in function or not. Occasionally the relative thickness of the periodontal membrane may disclose a localized traumatic condition. We know that a functioning tooth has a thicker periodontal membrane, while one out of function has a thinner one. To use a tooth safely as an abutment for a fixed partial denture, the length of its periodontal membrane attachment should be at least one-half to two-thirds that of its normal root attachment. Those teeth having less than half the normal length of periodontal attachment have not proved satisfactory as abutments in the past (Chapter 4).

The ability of the periodontal membrane to withstand the additional load incident to placing a fixed partial denture is often predetermined by its previous degree of function; i.e., a tooth in function usually has a periodontal membrane of normal thickness, and it also has an alveolar process of normal structure. Those teeth, however, that have been out of function have a thin periodontal membrane and an alveolar process and supporting bone containing large marrow spaces. Since the reestablishment of function in teeth out of function places them under an immediate, additional load, extreme care and judgment must be exercised when utilizing them for bridge supports. It is true that in time the new functions will reestablish normal conditions in both the membrane and the supporting bone. The possible pathologic conditions of the periodontal membrane are also to be considered. If any infection of the membrane is present, it must be removed before such a tooth may be safely considered for an abutment; likewise, if the membrane is injured either mechanically or chemically, it must be brought back to a normal state. Occasionally we encounter in the periodontal membrane the effects of systemic disturbances. If such conditions are disclosed, the cause should be removed; if this is impossible, a different type of restoration may be indicated.

The pulp

The pulp, its size, and its location have a very practical significance in a fixed partial denture prosthesis. Although the pulp is the dentin builder and the dental sensory organ, it is very responsive to thermal changes and trauma. The size and position of the pulp are relatively constant with reference to any individual tooth, yet it is necessary to be on the alert for abnormalities. Many pulp exposures have resulted because residual strands of pulpal horns extended high up into the cusps; on rare occasions pulps have been exposed because vascular inclusions and other structural imperfections were encountered in unlooked-for locations. The roentgenograph may serve as an index to the general size and location of the pulp. As aging progresses there is an increase in the amount of secondary dentin formed; a similar reaction occurs in teeth whose dentin is exposed. These facts have a direct bearing on cavity preparation. In youth, the presence of large pulp chambers and the lack of secondary dentin may cause cavity preparations to encroach closely upon the pulp. Temperature changes to which the pulp is subjected when relatively large masses of metal are placed in close proximity to it may also be etiologic factors in pulp degeneration. In the young patient, therefore, the position and size of the pulp frequently determine whether a fixed or a removable partial denture is to be placed. Intermediate appliances are often made until the pulp has receded sufficiently. The presence of pulpstones or bone-like tissue within the pulp also raises the question of using such teeth for bridge abutments.

Treated teeth

The problem of treated teeth is an important one. A tooth with a normal, vital pulp is the ideal abutment. However, one that has been properly treated and filled may also be used, provided that the patient is healthy and not suffering from systemic disturbances and that the teeth previously treated for the patient disclose reactions that are satisfactory both roentgenographically and clinically.

When it is necessary to resort to pulp canal therapy for intended abutments, it is good procedure to wait a reasonable length of time after filling the root canal before placing a prosthesis. Many fixed partial dentures, otherwise satisfactory in every respect, have failed because the treated tooth was unable to adjust itself to the added load immediately after undergoing the trauma incident to pulp extirpation and root canal filling. The question is sometimes raised whether a crown should be placed on a tooth before or after an apicoectomy. It is the experience and general practice of many to place the restoration on the tooth first, and then to resect the root end. The life and usefulness of teeth so treated, however, are uncertain.

Dental fractures and tissue dyscrasias

The loss or absence of tooth structure may be due to one of or a combination of any of the following causes: (1) caries, (2) internal and external root resorption, (3) erosion, (4) hypoplasia, (5) effects of abnormal habits, (6) abrasion, (7) attrition, or (8) the results of failures of operative restorations. Without doubt, the largest percentage of teeth requiring operative or prosthetic restorations are those affected by caries.

Caries

Dental caries is generally considered a bacterial disease of the hard tissues of teeth with a resultant loss of tooth structure. So prevalent is it that 95 percent of the population is affected by it; people are most susceptible during the first 20 years of life.

While the cause of dental caries has not been definitely established, it is generally agreed that it is essentially bacteriologic in character and that its progress is associated with many other contributing factors. The bacteria involved in this degenerative process are primarily the acidogenic and proteolytic types. In order for them to function effectively, the bacteria must find a protected location; lacking this, they seek the assistance of other bacteria to develop the means of confining and protecting the acid produced. The so-called protective bacterial plaques are generally associated with the *Leptothrix* organisms.

In addition to bacteria, there are other factors involved in the mechanism of caries. Among these is the decalcification of enamel and dentin. As is well known, there are on teeth certain areas of relative susceptibility and of immunity. With certain exceptions it has been found that the occlusal and incisal surfaces, also the buccal, labial, and lingual surfaces, are comparatively immune. These surfaces are exposed to the natural cleansing and scouring action of the food, cheeks, and tongue, which prevents the formation of bacterial plaques so necessary for the beginning of dental caries. The presence of pits and deep fissures, however, will predispose even these surfaces to decay.

The proximal surfaces, particularly the area lying cervically from the contact area, are similarly susceptible, especially if the interproximal tissue has receded. It has been estimated that over 80 percent of cavities start either in a pit or fissure. Cavities beginning on smooth surfaces very rarely extend beyond the line angle into other surfaces. The point to remember clinically is that, when a margin of a filling or a partial crown does terminate on a smooth surface, it must be placed in a position where it automatically will be kept clean by the excursion of food or where the patient can keep it so by the use of a toothbrush.

The shape and position of the interproximal space assume importance in fixed partial denture prosthesis. An effort is made in the construction of a partial prosthesis to make wide embrasures between the pontics and the retainers to develop the self-cleansing or cleansable characteristics so necessary to prevent recurrence of decay along the gingival or proximal margins.

By studying ground sections of a carious tooth, the course which dental caries follows may be seen (Fig. 2-13). It will be observed that in pit and fissure cavities the decay assumes the form of a wedge, with its base directed toward the dentinoenamel junction, while the apex is pointed toward the occlusal opening. In the surface types of decay caries also progresses as a wedge, but its base is on the outer surface of the enamel with its apex directed toward the dentinoenamel junction. It is characteristic that caries is very rapid and appears in its most intense form in the pit and fissure types of decay.

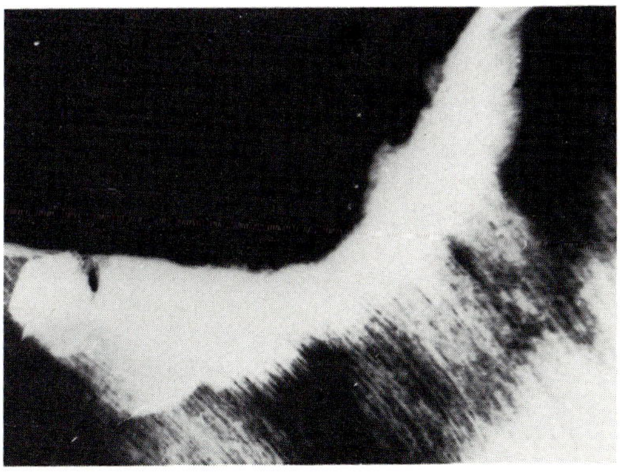

Fig. 2-13. Penetration of caries into dentin.

Once decalcification and decay have reached the dentinoenamel junction, they spread laterally along the dentinoenamel plane. From this area the decay then progresses through the dentin in the form of a wedge with its apex directed toward the pulp.

It must be remembered that decay of dentin can progress even though it is covered by the remnants of decalcified enamel. The acid formed by the bacteria on the surface of the decalcified enamel permeates through it and affects the dentin, even though the bacteria are not in direct contact with it. Once the enamel rods have fallen out and the bacteria come in contact with the surface of the dentin, the organisms then invade the dentin; authorities[1, 2] are not agreed whether this invasion occurs before or after its inorganic constituents have been decalcified. The remaining organic matrix of the dentin then acts as the food for the growth of the bacteria. For this reason, in the preparation of cavities it is absolutely essential to remove all carious dentin, even that which seems to be affected only by the acid end products of bacteria, although not actually invaded by the organisms. When dentin is affected by caries or other irritants, it is capable of a limited self-defense by depositing secondary dentin or by changing the nature of its structure into the sclerotic type (Fig. 2-14).

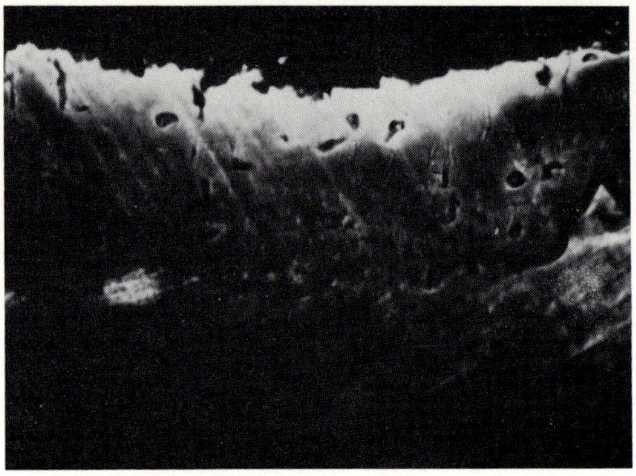

Fig. 2-14. Sclerotic dentin.

While definite proof has not been presented that diet can either prevent or stop dental caries, it has been shown that diet rich in sugars tends to make individuals more susceptible to caries; likewise, other diets help to check the progress of caries noticeably. The physical characteristics and qualities of the food used are also contributing factors, since rough fibrous foods exert cleansing and scouring actions that are lacking in the softer types. The fact that one or the other type of food is characteristic of certain races is clinically important because the cavity margins are extended for prevention in proportion to the carbohydrate and sugar diet of the individual. It is doubtful whether heredity plays an important part as a direct factor in dental caries.

Individuals are occasionally found whose susceptibility to caries and loss of tooth structure cannot be explained, except by the possible presence of structural microscopic defects in the enamel of the tooth or by the poor mineralization of tooth structure. Such reasoning, however, is purely hypothetical.

Fractures of teeth: resorption and repair

The loss of tooth structure may also result from fractures. Because of their position in the arches, anterior teeth are the ones most frequently involved, particularly in accidents. Adolescents are by far the largest group suffering from such loss of tooth structure.

Fractures may be coronal or radicular, i.e., they may involve either the crown or root portions of the tooth. When a part of the crown is fractured, it usually involves one of the incisal angles; the line of fracture is diagonal from the incisal angle gingivally (Fig. 3-9). In these situations the first consideration from a restorative standpoint is to determine whether or not the pulp is involved. If there is no pulp exposure, then its condition and vitality should be determined. The blow causing

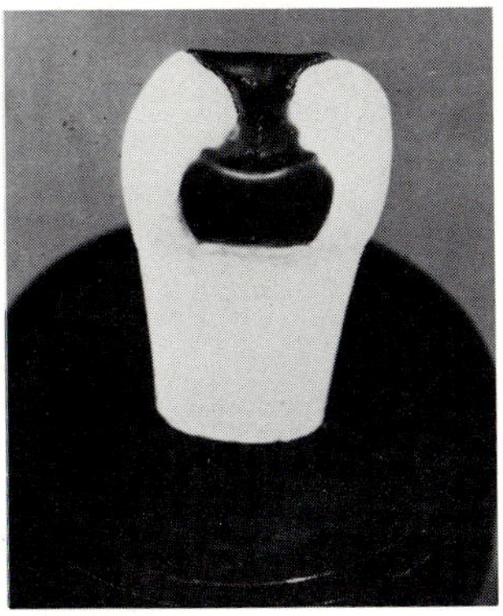

Fig. 2-15. Unprotected lingual cusp on devitalized bicuspid.

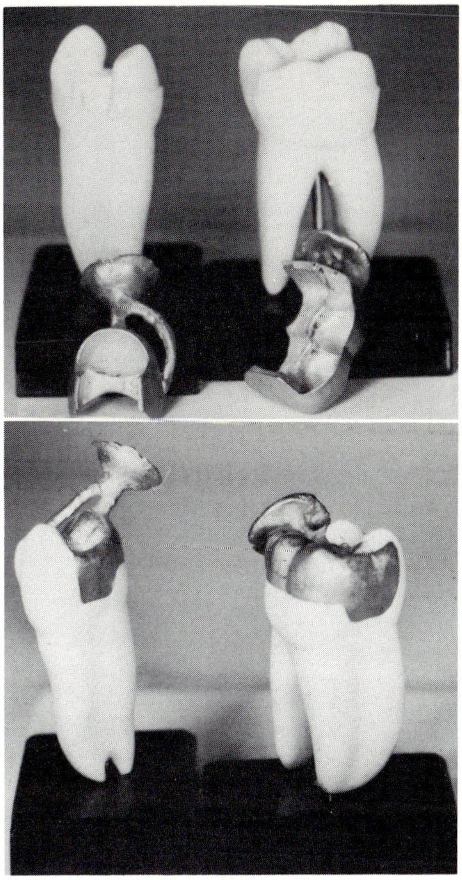

Fig. 2-16. A, Protected lingual cusp preparation on devitalized upper bicuspid and protected buccal cusp preparation on devitalized lower first molar. **B,** Castings for teeth in **A.**

the fracture will usually produce an inflamed periodontal membrane. If this occurs, it may be necessary to relieve occlusal or lingual contacts by grinding to afford relief from pressure. The dentin exposed by such fracture should be protected by some temporary means, and the tooth should be kept under observation for a length of time sufficient to ensure the reestablishment of normal conditions in the pulp and in the investing tissues. If this occurs when the patient is young, the method employed is primarily temporary in character, and the restoration will so function until such a time as the patient's age and circumstances permit a more permanent type of service.

If a partial coronal fracture has exposed the pulp, it should be removed under aseptic conditions and the root canal treated and suitably filled. This procedure is preferable to the questionable pulp capping so frequently used. Then, again, a partial fracture may come so close to the pulp and the shock of it may be so great that it gradually degenerates and its death ensues. If after a fracture the soreness and tenderness persist with a gradually increasing pain, which stops suddenly, it usually is evidence that the pulp has died, and steps should be taken immediately to remove it before the infection spreads.

Patients do not always seek dental advice or service immediately following such accidents. In fact, many of them permit the tenderness to subside and give no further thought to it until a discoloration calls their attention to the fact that all is not well with the tooth. By that time the pulp has died and very often a periapical involvement necessitates the extraction of the tooth.

Fractures of teeth also occur in the posterior regions, particularly in the bicuspids. This sometimes occurs when a mesiodistoclusal inlay is placed in a tooth that has been extensively undermined by decay and that has not been sufficiently protected by having the cusps covered with metal (Figs. 2-15 and 2-16). There are times when the lingual cusp of an upper biscuspid is fractured and still the pulp is not exposed. In such a situation the exposed dentin should be protected by a temporary covering until such time as the pulp can form secondary dentin; meanwhile, the tooth must be observed. Permanent restorations may be placed on these teeth if no harmful changes have taken place after 6 to 12 months' observation.

There are instances in which a fracture extends below the cementoenamel junction and involves a part of the root; even such teeth may be saved if the fracture does not extend too far apically.

Radicular fractures sometimes occur without the patient being aware of their existence. When a fractured root exists, its presence is usually disclosed by roentgenograms (Fig. 2-17). This condition is found most frequently in the anterior teeth. Such a fracture does not always necessitate the extraction of the tooth. The nearer to the apex of the root that a fracture occurs, the more favorable is the prognosis for the retention of such a tooth. Fractures occurring near the cervical line cause the remaining coronal portion of the tooth and root to move about freely, thus setting up inflammatory reactions.

Root fractures not exposed to saliva are capable of being immobilized and will heal and function as any other tooth. In addition to immobilization and lack of infection, its is also necessary that the two parts be in close apposition to heal properly. In teeth that have healed in this manner, it will be found roentgenographically that the portion of the pulp extending toward the crown has been altered or replaced and the space filled in with a bone-like structure. Fig. 2-18 shows the typical tissues found in this part of the pulp chamber and canal. The apical portion of the root contains a normal and vital pulp tissue. Fig. 2-17 shows roentgenograms of a tooth used as an abutment for an anterior restoration that gave satisfactory service for many years. This, of course, was an extreme use of a repaired

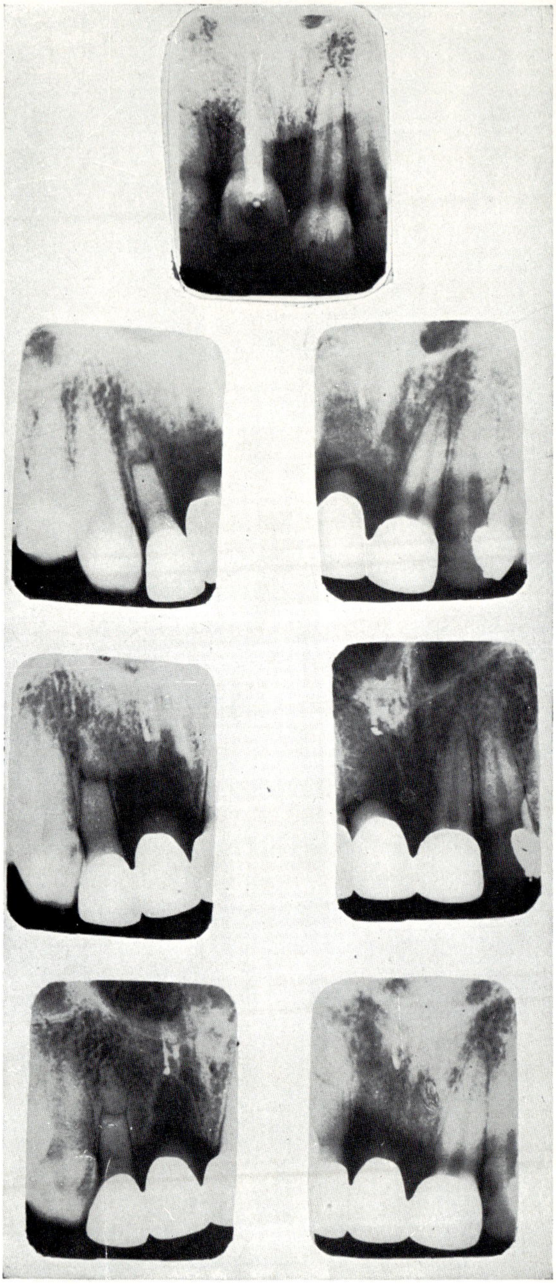

Fig. 2-17. Fractured root of vital tooth used as abutment for fixed partial denture.

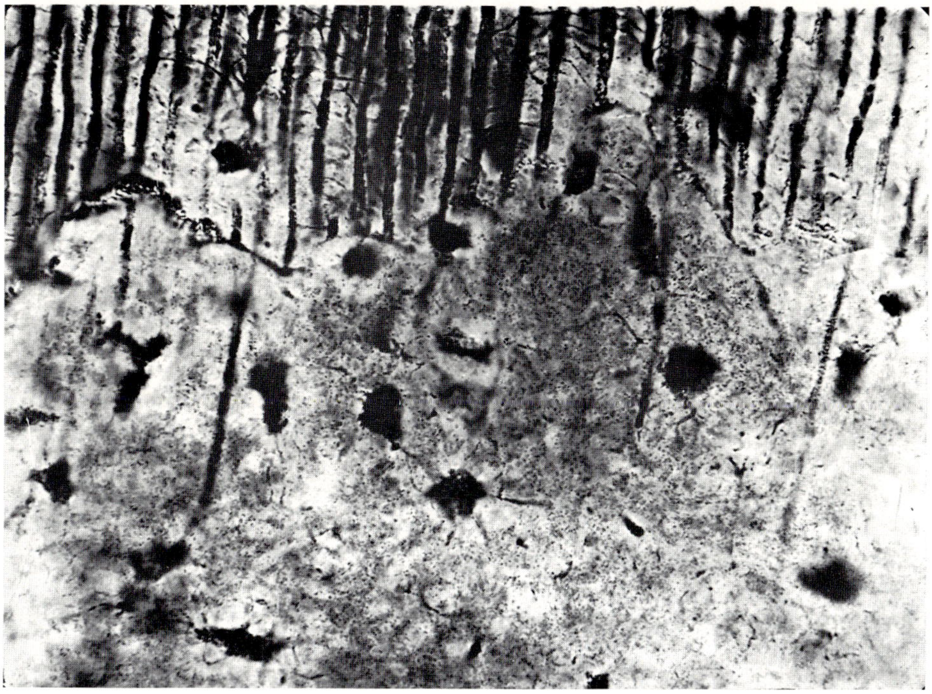

Fig. 2-18. Magnified view of absorption of dentin and deposition of bone-like tissue enclosing dentinal fibrils.

tooth, but it indicates what may occur under favorable circumstances.

Internal and external resorption

In considering this type of dyscrasia, Mahan makes the following observations:

Both the crowns and roots of teeth are subject to resorption from the pulpal side of the dentin. This internal resorption may be a slow, intermittent, progressive process or it may develop rapidly and perforate the tooth within a matter of months. In its advanced stage the color of the pulp shows through the thin plate of remaining enamel and the condition has been called "pink spot."

In internal resorption the dentin and enamel seem to be destroyed by macrophages and multinucleated giant cells that resemble osteoclasts. The resorbed dentin may be replaced by chronic inflammatory tissue or by a cancellous bone-like substance with fibrous or fatty marrow spaces. Any tooth may be involved but the most common sites are the upper anterior teeth.

Internal resorption may follow traumatic injury to the teeth. A small amount of resorption often occurs in teeth with pulpitis and it has been reported in the abutment teeth of fixed partial dentures. A possible familial tendency for internal resorption has been reported.

If the resorptive process has not advanced sufficiently to perforate the root, endodontic therapy will prevent further destruction of the tooth.

A process of root resorption may begin in the periodontal connective tissue. This external resorption of the cementum and dentin also resembles osteoclastic resorption. Once the pulp is entered, a pulpal pathosis follows and it becomes difficult to distinguish whether the process is internal or external resorption. Comparison of several radiographs taken at different angles will usually help distinguish between the two. If the resorbed area on the root surface is concave, one should suspect the process to be external resorption.

A resorption of root tips of anterior teeth is not infrequently observed in postorthodontic patients wearing retainers with labial arch wires It is also seen in abutment teeth on long span, fixed partial dentures. This type of external resorption seems to result from traumatic occlusion involving a "jiggling" action of the teeth.

External resorption of the gingival third of the root may be treated by making a flap and restoring the resorbed cavity with amalgam. If the area is too large to restore, the tooth can only be extracted. Endodontic procedures will not prevent the further progress of external resorption.*

Erosion

Another cause of tooth loss is erosion. Two general types are recognized, the saucer and the wedge shapes. While this process of disintegration of tooth structure is a slow one, it should be kept under constant observation, especially the wedge type. If permitted to progress to far, so much of the tooth will be destroyed that the amount remaining will not be sufficient to support a crown. Although operative procedures are usually resorted to, these are mostly of a temporary character, since the erosion will continue beyond the margins of a filling. The best known method of preserving such teeth in serviceable condition is to restore them with complete veneer procelain crowns. This, however, must be done before the tooth is excessively eroded.

*Mahan, P. E.: Personal Communication.

Enamel hypoplasia

While enamel hypoplasia is not, in the strict sense, a loss of tooth structure, but is rather a lack of normal enamel, it properly may be considered at this time (Fig. 2-19). When the structural disturbances in the enamel are of such magnitude that the quality of esthetics is destroyed or when an environment of lowered resistance to caries is established, the condition may be corrected by covering the entire coronal portion of the tooth with a restoration such as the porcelain veneer crown. This restores not only the function but also the form and esthetics of the natural tooth.

A

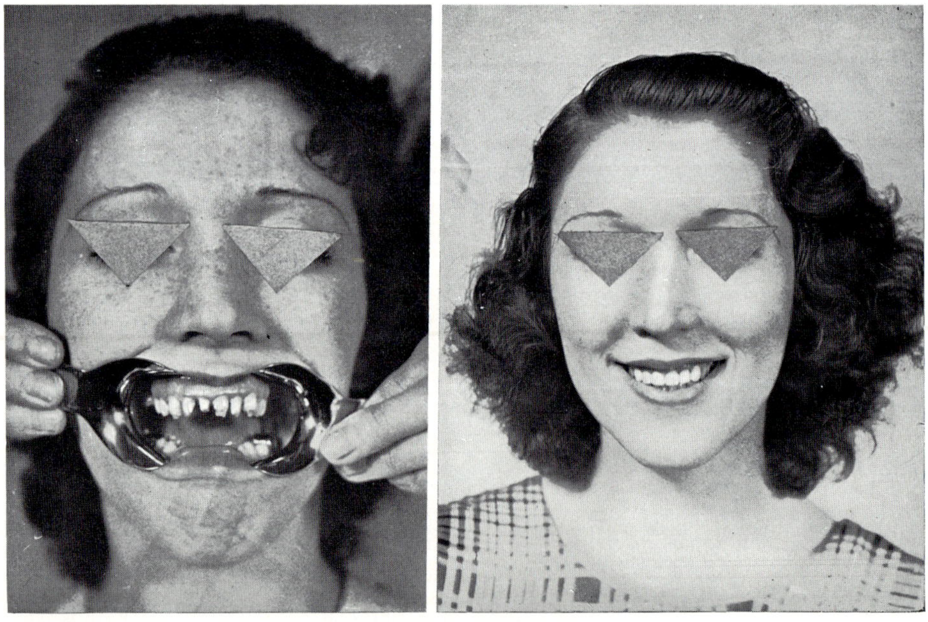

B

Fig. 2-19. Patient with enamel hypoplasia. **A,** Before, and **B,** after placement of complete veneer porcelain crowns.

Abrasion and attrition

Sometimes a wearing down of the natural teeth occurs because of certain abnormal habits that patients possess. These conditions are manifest in such individuals as traffic policemen who constantly keep a whistle between the anterior teeth, pipe smokers who habitually hold the stem of the pipe in one position (this is more marked if the pipe stem is made of clay), seamstresses who have been known to develop deep grooves in their anterior teeth caused by biting off thread. Many other similar examples could be cited. Usually such defects can be corrected by the placement of complete or partial veneer crowns.

Abrasion and attrition are two conditions which, in many instances, result in loss of tooth structure. While the end result is the same in both, the causes producing one differ from those responsible for the other. While abrasion is an unnatural and rapid wearing away of the teeth resulting from the friction of foreign materials, attrition is a normal, functional process involving the normal wear of tooth structure incidental to mastication. Two methods of procedure may be followed in dealing with these conditions.

If the degree of tooth loss has not reached a point necessitating prosthetic procedures, the cause should be determined and the patient instructed in methods of preventing further damage. If the amount of lost tooth structure has reached the stage that necessitates rebuilding the teeth to new relationships, both vertically and horizontally, this can best be done by the use of complete crowns or by combining crowns with some form of a partial denture prosthesis.

Prosthetic service is indicated in those teeth in which the loss of structure accompanies failures of previous operative restorations. It is not uncommon to find fillings placed in teeth whose enamel walls are entirely unsupported or are supported by carious dentin. Such restorations are not permanent, for very shortly the enamel walls and even entire cusps fracture under the forces of mastication. Such teeth usually necessitate removal of the previous restoration before the placing of a complete crown; before doing so, the vitality of the pulp should be ascertained.

Opalescent dentin or dentinogenesis imperfecta

There is another condition that is unusual but of sufficient occurrence to merit attention; it is found in patients with hereditary opalescent dentin. Those afflicted with this condition manifest certain phenomena, for, while they are comparatively immune to caries, it is found that the crowns of both arches are usually worn down to the gum line if left as they are (Fig. 2-20). In spite of this extraordinary destruction of tooth structure, there is rarely a pulp exposure. It is characteristic of these teeth that, even before they are worn down, their pulp chambers are small and the pulp is remotely receded from the outer surfaces of the tooth. The structural form of dentin in this type of tooth differs from that found in a normal tooth. There is no regularity of arrangement of the dentinal tubules; instead we find a promiscuous and indefinite arrangement of tubules in the dentin

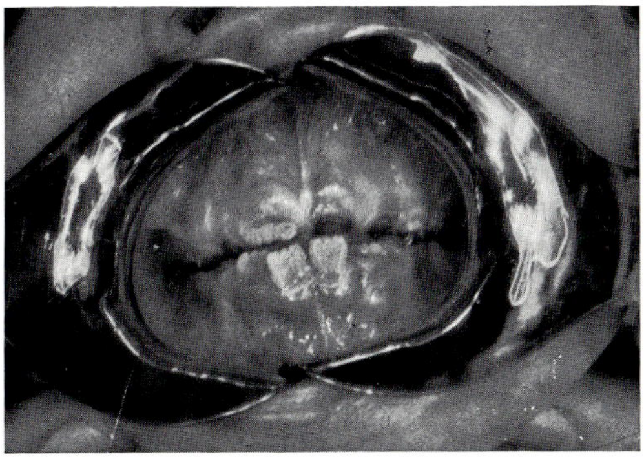

Fig. 2-20. Opalescent dentin, upper deciduous teeth worn down (see Plate 1).

(Fig. 4-3). A characteristic of this type of dentition is that its rate of eruption is much more advanced than the eruption of normal teeth.

Plate 1 shows a patient with opalescent teeth. Because of the close vertical relationship of the mandible and maxillae on account of the worn teeth, it was necessary to reestablish a correct vertical distance to enable the normal, active eruption of the permanent teeth. To accomplish this, crowns were placed on the permanent first molars, which established and maintained the correct functional distance and thus permitted the anterior teeth to come into their proper relationships. Plate 1 shows the mouth 7 months after the crowns were placed on the molars. What the value might be of such teeth from the standpoint of permanent restorations was problematic. This particular reconstruction lasted for over 24 years. It is interesting to note that the condition is definitely a hereditary one, as indicated by the chart shown in Fig. 2-21.

Porphyria erythropoietica

Porphyria erythropoietica is a rare disease resulting from an imbalance of porphyrin metabolism. It appears in infancy or childhood and is charactertized by a vesicular skin eruption, sensitivity to sunlight, and severe scarring of exposed skin areas. Increased hemolysis and splenomegaly are found in these patients. The patient seen in Plate 2 was first seen at 11 years of age at the University Clinic. The teeth were reddish purple and the skin surfaces of her face and body were scarred. After a splenectomy she improved from a dermatologic standpoint. She was again seen at 16 years of age; she was mentally alert and in good physical condition, but socially withdrawn for obvious reasons. Her oral hygiene was good. She had a full complement of teeth, all showing a dark red discoloration evenly distributed. The gingiva was normal but also discolored. Fissures and canker sores were present on her lips and corners of her mouth. Her mouth was small with tense

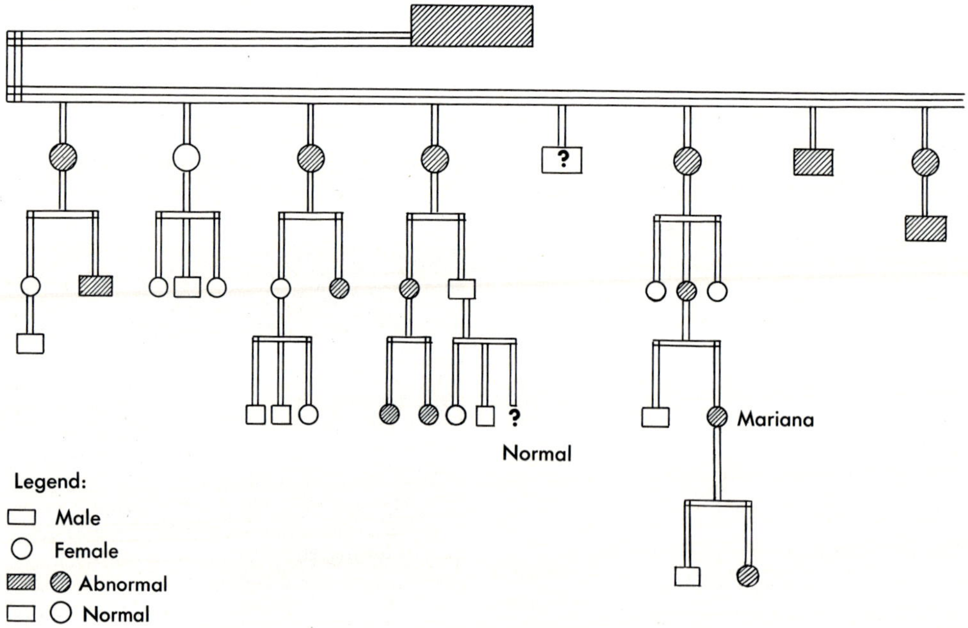

Fig. 2-21. Five generations of opalescent dentin.

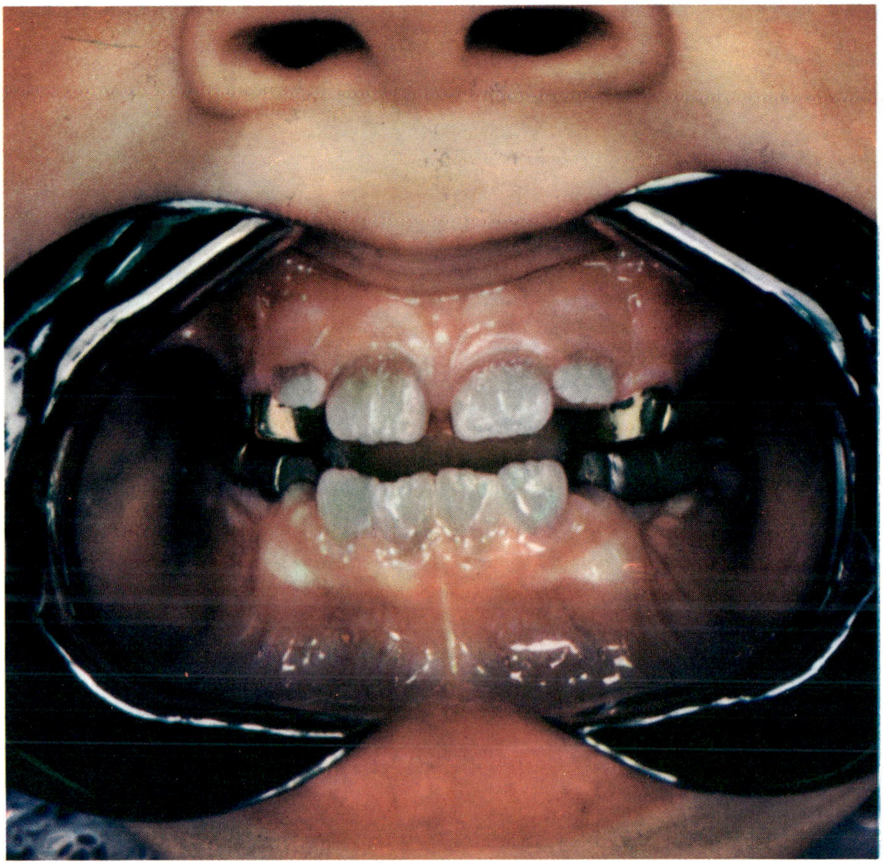

Plate 1. Opalescent dentin, or dentinogenesis imperfecta; same patient as in Fig. 2-20. (Photograph by E. Anderson.)

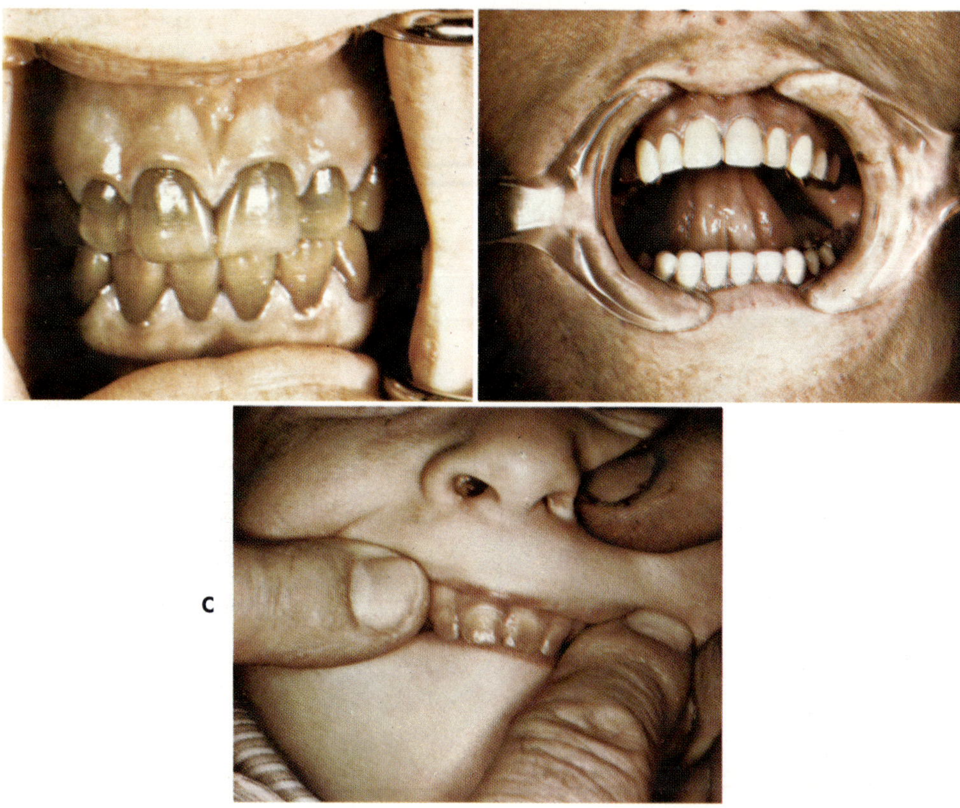

A B C

Plate 2. A, Appearance of teeth characteristic of patients with porphyria erythropoietica; **B,** restoration with individual veneer crowns; **C,** deciduous teeth of patient's first child.

circumoral musculature. There was no temporomandibular disorder. The pulps appeared well formed, as did the trabecular bone. Laminographs disclosed a slight subluxation due to a poorly formed articular eminence.

Basically, the patient's desire for dental service was to eliminate the displeasing color of her natural teeth caused by her congenital disorder. Examination of the roentgenograms revealed the pulps to be too large to prepare the teeth for conventional porcelain veneer crowns. It was decided that processed acrylic veneers be constructed for the six upper anteriors; for the upper first and second bicuspids, modified chamfer-shoulder preparations with porcelain-fused-to-metal crowns were constructed. The lower six anterior teeth together with the first and second bicuspids bilaterally were likewise crowns of the porcelain-fused-to-metal castings. Plate 2 shows the teeth seven years later when the patient presented at the clinic again. At this time she was already married and at our request she brought her first child along with her for our examination. The deciduous teeth of the child showed a slight discoloration of the enamel but he exhibited none of the systemic disorders of the mother's porphyria erythropoietica. The consulting physician expressed the opinion that, when the child's permanent teeth erupted later, he expected them to be of normal texture and color.[13] This we shall await with interest. The roentgenograms which we took of the child show a normal pulpal condition.

SELECTED REFERENCES

1. Miller, W. D.: A study of some dental anomalies with reference to eburnitis, Dent. Cosmos **43**:845, 1901.
2. Aisenberg, M. S.: Bone in pulp chamber, J. Dent. Res. **17**:371, 1938.
3. Warner, G. R., and others: Internal resorption of teeth: interpretation of histologic findings, J.A.D.A. **34**:468, 1947.
4. Goldman, H. M.: Spontaneous intermittent resorption of teeth, J.A.D.A. **49**:522, 1954.
5. Sullivan, H. R., and Jolly, M.: Idiopathic resorption, Australian Dent. J. **2**:193, 1957.
6. Deeb, E.: Idiopathic resorption of permanant teeth, J. S. California Dent. Assn. **28**: 210, 1960.
7. Rowe, W. H.: Peripheral granuloma of internal resorption, J. Canadian D. A. **26**:267, 1960.
8. Simpson, H. E.: Internal resorption, J. Canadian D. A. **30**:355, 1964.
9. Manson-Hing, L. R.: Familial internal resorption, Oral Surg. **13**:201, 1960.
10. Ramfjord, S. P., and Ash, M. M.: Occlusion, Philadelphia, 1966, W. B. Saunders Co.
11. Huffman, R. W., Regenos, J. W., and Taylor, R. R.: Principles of occlusion, Columbus, Ohio, 1969, H. and R. Press.
12. Wheeler, R. C.: Textbook of dental anatomy and physiology, Philadelphia, 1968, W. B. Saunders Co.
13. Rosenthal, I. M., Lipton, E. L., and Asrow, G.: Effect of splenectomy on porphyria erythropoietica, Pediatrics **15**:663, 1955.

GENERAL REFERENCES

Adams, J. D.: Planning posterior bridges, J.A.D.A. **53**:647, 1956.

Alldritt, W. A.: Occlusal disharmony, Brit. Dent. J. **119**:406-408, 1965.

Asling, C. W.: Recent developments in biologic studies on the osseous system, Amer. J. Orthodont. **47**:830, 1961.

Atkinson, H. F., and Harcourt, J. K.: Some observations on the peritubular translucent zones in human dentine, Australian D. J. **6**:194, 1961.

Avery, J. K., and Meyers, R. A.: Studies of internal and external resorption of root dentine, I.A.D.R. **40**:10, 1962.

Awazawa, Y.: Electron microscopic images of carious dentin—with particular reference to aspects of carious dentin with cross-sectioned dentinal tubules, J. Nihon Univ. School Dent. **4**:59, 1961.

Baker, C. R.: Why fixed partial denture prosthesis? J. Canadian D. A. **16**:565, 1950.

Barber, T. K.: The concept of preventive orthodontics, J. Dent. Child. **33**:75-86, 1966.

Bartels, J. C.: Oral diagnosis and restorative treatment, J. S. California D. A. **26**:308, 1958.

Bates, J. F., and Murphy, W. M.: A survey of edentulous population, Brit. Dent. J. **124**:116-121, 1968.

Beaudreau, D. E.: Objectives of fixed partial dentures, J. Tennessee Dent. Assn. **47**(1):7-10, 1967.

Besic, F. C.: Fate of bacteria sealed in dental cavities, J. Dent. Res. **22**:349, 1943.

Best, E. S., and Waldron, C. W.: Oral diagnosis: cleaning up a diseased mouth, J. Nat. D. A. **9**:134, 1922.

Bhaskar, S. N.: Cancer and the dentist, J. Dist. Columbia D. Soc. **36**:16, 1961; Massachusetts D. Soc. J. **10**:23, 1961.

Bhaskar, S. N.: New approach to oral diagnosis, J. Maryland D. A. **4**:81, 1961.

Black, A. D.: Examination and diagnosis by the dentist, J.A.D.A. **18**:62, 1931.

Bowen, R. L., and Rodriguez, M. S.: Tensile strength and modulus of elasticity of tooth structure and several restorative materials, J.A.D.A. **64**:378, 1962.

Boyne, P. J., and Kruger, G. O.: Fluorescence microscopy of alveolar bone repair, Oral Surg. **15**:265-281, 1962.

Brecker, S. C.: Management of abnormal conditions in crown and bridge prosthesis, J. California D. A. **37**:21, 36, 1961.

Bregstein, S. J.: Diagnosis and treatment planning: a philosophy, Ann. Dent. **21**:37, 1962.

Brescia, N. J.: Roentgenographic study of the trabecular pattern of the alveolar processes of the human maxilla and mandible, J. Dent. Res. **39**:730, 1960.

Bricker, J. S.: The re-establishment of fixed bridge work, J. Canadian D. A. **2**:154, 1936.

Brill, N.: Gingival conditions related to flow of tissue fluid into gingival pockets, Acta Odont. Scand. **18**:421, 1960.

Brill, N., Hedegard, B., and Osborne, J.: Dental prosthetics, Norske Tannlaegoforen Tid. **77** (5):277-292, 1967.

Brooks, E. C.: A practical approach for crown and bridge construction. Paper read before Kentucky State Dental Association, Louisville, April, 1955.

Buonocore, M. G.: Principles of adhesive retention and adhesive restorative materials, J.A.D.A. **67**:382, 1963.

Burman, L. R., and Tang, C.: The abutment tooth, J. Dent. Med. **18**:83-91, 1963.

Bush, J. B.: Effective communication to the patient of the meaning of the proposed treatment plan, Dent. Clin. N. Amer., pp. 67-72, March, 1961.

Cacciatore, A. C.: Modern principles of periodontics related to prosthodontics, Dent. Clin. N. Amer., Nov. 1962, pp. 787-798.

Campbell, J. F.: Electrogalvanic action in the mouth, Texas D. J. **60**:221, 1942.

Castagnola, L.: The advantages of removable-fixed bridges over fixed bridges, Int. Dent. J. **18**:276, 1968.

Cavanagh, W. D.: Simplified crown and bridge treatment for the general practitioner, J. Canadian D. A. **25**:294, 1959.

Chayes, H. E.: Crown and bridge work on a physiologic basis, Summary **36**:1063, 1916.

Chirnside, I. M.: Bacterial invasion of non-vital dentin, J. Dent. Res. **40**:134, 1961.

Coelho, D. H.: Criteria for the use of fixed prosthesis, Dent. Clin. N. Amer., p. 299, March, 1957.

Coelho, D. H.: Present day rationale of fixed restorations, J. Dent. Med. **7**:31, 1952.

Coleman, R. L.: Physical properties of dental materials, National Bureau of Standards Research Paper No. 32, Washington, D. C., 1928, U. S. Government Printing Office.

Craig, R. G., and others: Compressive properties of enamel, dental cements, and gold, J. Dent. Res. **40**:936, 1961.

Dalmau, L. B.: Use of non-vital teeth in crown and bridge-work, J. Puerto Rico D. A. **1**:21, 1961.

Dubner, R., and Stanley, H. R.: Reaction of the human dental pulp to temporary filling materials, Oral Surg. **15**:1009, 1962.

Dykema, R. W.: Fixed partial prosthodontics, J. Tennessee D. A. **42**:309, 1962.

Edison, R. L.: A rationale for the changing concepts in restorative procedures, J. S. California Dent. Ass. **34**:334-336, 1966.

Elfenbaum, A. E.: Color changes in the oral mucosa, Oral Hyg. **51**:52, 1961.

Elfenbaum, A. E.: Diagnostic procedure in dental practice, Illinois D. J. **30**:12, 1961.

Elfenbaum, A. E.: Practical application of diagnosis in the dental office, J. Canadian D. A. **27**:780, 1961.

Ericson, S., Hedegard, B., and Wennstrom, A.: Roentgenographic study of vital abutment teeth, J. Prosth. Dent. **16**(5):981, 1966.

Ericsson, S. G., and Marken, K.: Effect of fixed partial dentures on surrounding tissues, J. Prosth. Dent. **20**(6): 517, 1968.

Ewing, J. E.: Fixed partial prosthesis, ed. 2, Philadelphia, 1959, Lea & Febiger.

Ferranti, P.: Simple technique for treatment of hypersensitive exposed dentin, D. Digest **68**: 14, 1962.

Fox, L.: Control of pain and apprehension and use of local anesthesia in periodontics, Dent. Clin. N. Amer., July, 1961, pp. 329-340.

Friedman, Samuel: Effective use of diagnostic data, J. Prosth. Dent. **9**:729, 1959.

Friend, George: Bridge work as a routine treatment in dental practice, Brit. D. J. **111**:394, 1961.

Fusayama, T., and others: Corrosion of gold alloy by contact with amalgam fillings, J. Dent. Res. **41**:734, 1962.

Gardner, A. F.: Trauma and fractures of teeth, S. Carolina D. J. **20**:8, 1962.

Georgiade, N. G.: Temporomandibular joint dysfunction and facial pain, J. North Carolina D. Soc. **44**:110, 1961.

Gerson, S. J., and Meyer, J.: Metaplastic keratinization in the human buccal mucosa, J. Dent. Res. **43**:536-547, 1964.

Gralnick, I. J.: Periodontal aspect of fixed bridge diagnosis and construction, J. Second Dist. D. Soc. (N. Y.) **32**:172, 1946.

Granger, E. R.: Practical procedures in oral rehabilitation, ed. 1, Philadelphia, 1962, J. B. Lippincott Co.

Grant, A. W.: Responsibility of the general practitioner in oral diagnosis, Bull. Acad. Gen. Dent., pp. 36-44, Sept. 1962.

Gratzinger, M.: Use of plate appliances in the treatment of periodontal trauma, D. Pract. **8**: 12, 1957.

Greene, J. C.: Oral hygiene and periodontal disease, Amer. J. Public Health **53**:913-922, 1963.

Gorman, W. J.: Prevalence and etiology of gingival recession, J. Periodont. **38**:316-322, 1967.

Hagerman, D. A., and Arnim, S. S.: The relation of new knowledge of the gingiva to crown and bridge procedures, J. Prosth. Dent. **5**:538, 1955.

Hayes, R. L.: Idiopathic internal resorption of teeth, Oral Surg. **13**:723, 1960.

Held, H. W.: Hereditary dentinogenesis imperfecta, D. Radiog. **35**:3-6, 1962.

Henschel, C. J.: Heat impact of revolving instruments on vital dentin tubules, J. Dent. Res. **22**:323, 1943.

Hildebrand, G. Y.: Studies in dental prosthetics, Stockholm, 1937, A. B. Fahlcrantz' Boktryckeri.

Hillman, S. H.: Emotional problems involved in the practice of dentistry, Brit. D. J. **113**:295, 1962.

Jarabak, J. R.: Orthodontic treatment preparatory to fixed partial denture prosthesis, Dent. Clin. N. Amer., p. 31, 1959.

Jarby, S.: Response of the dental pulp to heated filling materials, Odont. Tskr. **70**:5, 1962.

Johnston, J. F., Phillips, R. W., and Dykema, R. W.: Modern practice in crown and bridge prosthodontics, ed., 2, Philadelphia, 1965, W. B. Saunders Co.

Kabnick, H. H.: Divergent biomechanical and physiological concepts in case planning and treatment, Fort. Rev. Chicago D. Soc. **44**:11, 29, 1962.

Karlsen, K.: Fixed bridgework as opposed to fixed-removable appliances, Int. Dent. J. **18**: 269, 1968.

Kerr, D. A.: The cementum: its role in periodontal health and disease, J. Periodont. **32**: 183, 1961.

Kerr, K. M.: Prosthodontic practice in dentistry, J. Canadian D. A. **27**:217, 1961.

Klaffenbach, A. O.: Analytic study of modern abutments, J.A.D.A. **23**:2275, 1936.

Klaffenbach, A. O.: The role of crown and bridge prosthesis in the Field of restorative dentistry, J.A.D.A. **25**:536, 1938.

Klaffenbach, A. O.: Some important aspects of fixed bridge restorations, J.A.D.A. **27**:738, 1940.

Klavan, B.: Occlusal trauma and periodontal disease, D. Progress **2**:160, 1962.

Klecinic, E. P., and Fedi, P. F.: Periodontal preparation for fixed partial dentures, J. Prosth. Dent. **20**(6):511, 1968.

Klenda, H. M.: Consultation examination and treatment planning, J.A.D.A. **58**:86, 1959.

Kossoff, G., and Sharpe, C. J.: Examination of the contents of the pulp cavity in teeth, Ultrasonics **4**:77-83, 1966.

Kramer, I. R. H.: Alveolar bone in health and disease with special reference to local factors, D. Pract. **12**:327, 1962.

Kurahashi, Y., and Takauma, S.: Electron microscopy of human gingival epithelium, Bull. Tokyo D. Col. 3:29, 1962.

Kustaloglu, O.: Hereditary dentinogenesis imperfecta, D. Radiog. **35**:7-10, 1962.

Lain, E. S., and Coughron, G. S.: Electrogalvanic phenomena of the oral cavity caused by dissimilar metallic restorations, J.A.D.A. **23**:1641, 1936.

Lakermance, J., and Laudenbach, P.: Indications and contraindications for fixed prostheses, Rev. Stomat. **63**:46, 1962.

Langeland, K.: Effect of various procedures on the human dental pulp: pulp reactions to cavity preparation and gutta-percha, Oral Surg. **14**:210, 1961.

Lefkowitz, W.: Pulp and operative dentistry, J. D. Med. **17**:129, 1962.

Lehman, M. L.: Tensile strength of human dentin, J. Dent. Res. **46**(1):197, 1967.

Listgarten, M. A.: The ultrastructure of human gingival epithelium, Amer. J. Anat. **114**:49-69, 1964.

Lucia, V. O.: Modern gnathological concepts, ed. 1, St. Louis, 1961, The C. V. Mosby Co.

MacBoyle, R. E.: Modern fixed bridgework, Oral Health **22**:532, 1932.

McCracken, W. L.: Differential diagnosis: fixed or removable partial dentures, J.A.D.A. **63**:767, 1961.

McHugh, W. D.: The keratinization of gingival epithelium, J. Periodont. **35**:338-348, 1964.

McKenzie, R. Tait: Human facial types—facial expressions, D. Cosmos **77**:639, 1935.

Marshack, M.: Four aspects of fixed prosthesis, Bull. Acad. Gen. Dent., pp. 12-18, Dec., 1962.

Maves, H. A.: A plea for healthier environment tissues in crown, bridge, and partial denture construction, D. Cosmos **74**:277, 1932.

Maves, T. W.: Fixed bridgework, Dom. D. J. **42**:287, 1930.

Millard, H. D.: Oral diagnosis procedures, J. Michigan D. A. **42**:156, 1960.

Miller, S. C., and Rosof, I. L.: The use of dental restorations in improving function and facial contour, D. Digest **41**:364, 367, 1935.

Mitchell, L. D., Jr.: Panoramic roentgenography—a clinical evaluation, J.A.D.A. **66**:776, 1963.

Mjor, I. A.: Effect of zinc oxide and eugenol on dentine evaluated by micro-hardness testing, Arch. Oral Biol. **7**:333, 1962.

Mohammed, Y. R., Van Huysen, G., and Boyd, D. A.: Filling base materials and the unexposed and exposed tooth pulp, J. Prosth. Dent. **11**: 503, 1961.

Moorehead, F. B.: The prevalence of chronic mouth infections and their management, J.A.M.A. **67**:845, 1916.

Moses, C. H.: Biologic emphasis in prosthodontics, J. Prosth. Dent. **12**:695, 1962.

Moulton, G. M.: Esthetics in anterior fixed bridge prosthodontics, J.A.D.A. **52**:36, 1956.

Moulton, G. H.: Importance of centric occlusion in diagnosis and treatment planning, J. Prosth. Dent. **10**:921, 1960.

Mylin, W. K., and others: Internal resorption of the dentine with extensive osseous metaplasia of the pulp: report of a case, Oral Surg. **21**: 75-82, 1966.

Nagai, K., and Imazeki, T.: Correlational study between metallographical findings of metals and their tissue reactions in vital body, J. Nihon Univ. School Dent. **2**:66, 1959.

Nagai, K.: Behavior of metals in oral cavity, J. Nihon Univ. School Dent. **1**:203, 1959.

Nelson, E. A.: Significant factors in occlusal restoration by means of crown and bridge prosthesis, Pennsylvania D. J. **16**:3, 1949.

Nelsen, R. J., and Nelsen, A. E.: Patient, the tooth and the dentist; a modern perspective of tooth preparation, J.A.D.A. **58**:1, 1959.

Niswonger, M. E.: The rest position of the mandible and centric relation, J.A.D.A. **21**:1572, 1934.

Norman, R. D., and others: Additional studies on the solubility of certain dental materials, J. Dent. Res. **38**:1028, 1959.

Nuttall, E. B.: Clinical and technical aspects of crown and bridge prosthesis, Bull. Philadelphia Co. D. Soc. **14**:128, 1950.

Nuttall, E. B.: Diagnosis and correction of occlusal disharmonies in preparation for fixed restorations, J.A.D.A. **44**:399, 1952.

Oliver, R. T.: Patient management and treatment planning, Dent. Clin. N. Amer., pp. 31-41, March, 1961.

Owen, E. B., and Bruening, E. H.: A study of facial form and complexion colors, J.A.D.A. **13**: 1564, 1926.

Parfitt, G. J.: Investigation of the normal variations in alveolar bone trabeculation, Oral Surg. **15**:1453, 1962.

Peyton, F. A., Mahler, D. B., and Hershenov, B.: Physical properties of dentin, J. Dent. Res. **31**: 366, 1952.

Philippas, G. G.: Influence of occlusal wear and age on formation of dentin and size of pulp chamber, J. Dent. Res. **40**:1186, 1961.

Phillips, R. W.: Certain biological considerations in the use of restorative materials, New York D. J. **282**:397, 1962.

Phillips, R. W., and Ryge, G.: Adhesive restorative dental materials, J.A.D.A. **66**:627, 1963.

Pietrokovski, J.: Extraction wound healing after tooth fracture in rats, J. Dent. Res. **46**(1):232, 1967.

Pini, C. E.: Co-report: hygienic considerations in crown and bridge prosthesis, Int. Dent. J. **8**:357, 1958.

Plainfield, S.: Psychological considerations in prosthetic dentistry, Dent. Clin. N. Amer. pp. 669-681, Nov., 1962.

Potter, H. R.: Does modern fixed bridge construction fulfill contemporary scientific specifications? Pacific D. Gaz. **39**:325, 1931.

Prothero, J. H.: Prosthetic dentistry, ed. 4, Chicago, 1928, Medico-Dental Publishing Co.

Pruden, K. C.: Abutments and attachments in fixed partial dentures, J. Prosth. Dent. **7**:502, 1957.

Pruden, W. H.: Role of study casts in diagnosis and treatment planning, J. Prosth. Dent. **10**: 707, 1960.

Pruden, W. H., II: Today's approach to fixed partial denture prosthesis, J. New Jersey D. Soc. 32:11, 1960.

Pulver, F.: An atypical form of dentinogenesis imperfecta, J. Dent. Child. **29**:123, 1962.

Ramfjord, S. P.: Bruxism, a clinical and electromyographic study, J.A.D.A. **62**:21, 1961.

Reinhard, M. C., Goodale, H. I., and Soloman, H. A.: The possibility of precancerous oral lesions from electrical causes, D. Digest **39**: 142, 1933.

Reynolds, R. L.: The determination of pulp vitality by means of thermal and electrical stimuli, Oral Surg. **22**(2):231-240, 1966.

Riley, W. J.: Dentist-patient relationship, J. Ontario D. A. **39**:9, 1962.

Schweiger, J. W.: Prosthetic considerations for the aging, J. Prosth. Dent. **9**:555, 1959.

Rinehart, R. J.: Indications for fixed bridgework and construction of abutment pieces, J.A.D.A. **21**:296, 1934.

Ritchie, G. M.: Repair of coronal fractures in upper incisor teeth, Brit. D. J. **112**:459, 1962.

Rivault, M. A.: Functional re-establishment of mastication by means of fixed prostheses, Int. Dent. J. **16**:413-422, 1966.

Robinson, H. B. G.: Oral diagnosis as a key to practice administration and patient care, J. Tennessee D. A. **41**:208, 1961.

Robinson, H. B. G., and Lefkowitz, W.: Operative dentistry and the pulp, J. Prosth. Dent. **12**:985-1001, 1962.

Rosenow, E. C.: Mouth infection as a source of systemic disease, J.A.M.A. **63**:2021, 1914.

Schouboe, T., and Macdonald, J. B.: Prolonged viability of organisms sealed in dentinal caries, Arch. Oral Biol. **7**:525, 1962.

Schriever, W., and Diamond, L. E.: Electromotive forces and electric currents caused by metallic dental fillings, J. Dent. Res. **31**:205-229, 1952.

Selberg, A.: Modern fixed partial restorations, J.A.D.A. **23**:460, 1936.

Seniff, R. W.: Change in enamel surface caused by oxyphosphate cement, J. Dent. Res. **40**:642, 1961 (abst.).

Simpson, D. H.: Considerations for abutments, J. Prosth. Dent. **5**:375, 1955.

Smith, Donald E.: Twenty-five years of fixed bridge work, J. S. California D. A. **3**:794, 1936.

Smith, G. P.: Objectives of a fixed partial denture, J. Prosth. Dent. **11**:463, 1961.

Soni, N. N., and others: Polarized light and microradiographic study of dental tissues in dentinogenesis imperfecta, J. Dent. Res. **46**(2): 434, 1967.

Stanford, J. W., and others: Compressive properties of hard tooth tissues and some restorative materials, J.A.D.A. **60**:746, 1960.

Stone, E.: Consultation and treatment planning in occlusal rehabilitation, J. Prosth. Dent. **12**: 326, 1962.

Stuart, C. E.: Divergent concepts in case planning and treatment, Fort. Rev. Chicago D. Soc. **44**:12, 61, 1962.

Swartz, M. L., Phillips, R. W., Norman, R. D., and Oldham, D. F.: Strength, hardness and abrasion characteristics of dental cements, J.A.D.A. **67**:367, 1963.

Thomas, G. A.: Approach to the new patient, J. Tennessee D. A. **42**:190, 1962.

Thompson, J. R.: The rest position of the mandible and its significance to dental science, J.A.D.A. **33**:151, 1946.

Tinker, E. T.: Fixed bridgework, D. Summary **40**:175, 1920.

Tinker, E. T.: Some of the fundamentals in the construction and application of crown and bridge restorations, J.A.D.A. **12**:1347, 1925.

Tyldesley, W. R.: The mechanical properties of human enamel and dentine, Brit. Dent. J. **106**: 269-278, 1959.

Tylman, S. D.: Some factors essential to a correct crown and bridge practice, D. Cosmos **72**: 50, 1930.

Tylman, S. D.: To what degree can the partially edentulous patient be rehabilitated biologically and mechanically by means of crowns and fixed bridges? J. Ontario D. A. **30**:255, 314, 1953.

Tylman, S. D.: Fixed partial denture prosthodontics, Int. Dent. J. **10**:58, 1960.

Tylman, S. D.: Discussion of crown and fixed bridge prosthesis, J. Ninth Internat. D. Cong. **7**:408, 1936.

Tylman, S. D.: Biologic concepts of fixed partial dentures, New York J. Dent. **18**:386, 1948.

Tylman, S. D.: Crown and fixed bridge prosthesis: a phase of restorative dentistry, Int. Dent. J. **4**:457, 1952.

Van Huysen, G.: Microstructure of normal and sclerosed dentine, J. Prosth. Dent. **10**:976, 1960.

Van Huysen, G.: Historadiographic study of dentin sclerosis, Alum. Bull. Indiana Univ. School Dent., pp. 4-5, 50, March, 1961.

Vedder, F. B.: Some important changes in the practice of bridgework, J.A.D.A. **14**:608, 1927.

Vedder, F. B.: Some indications for fixed and removable bridgework, D. Cosmos **72**:1266, 1930.

Vermeersch, A. G.: Recent advances in crowns and bridges, Int. Dent. J. **7**:238, 1957.

Wasser, V. E.: Harmonious occlusion in fixed partial dentures, J. Prosth. Dent. **7**:500, 1957.

Williams, P. E.: Humane approach to the patient, Dent. Clin. N. Amer., pp. 791-794, Nov., 1959.

Wilson, W. H.: Practical application of oral physiology, J. Prosth. Dent. **6**:53, 1956.

Wilson, W. H., and Lang, R. L.: Practical crown and bridge prosthodontics, New York, 1962, McGraw-Hill Book Company.

Yock, D. H.: Fixed crown and bridge work, J. Tennessee D. A. **32**:265, 1952.

Yurkstas, A. A.: The effect of missing teeth on masticatory performance and efficiency, J. Prosth. Dent. **4**:120, 1954.

Chapter 3

Types of restorations utilized in crown and fixed partial prosthodontics

Prior to starting tooth preparation and construction of a dental restoration for a patient, it is necessary for the dentist to first make a complete and thorough examination of the mouth and to obtain a complete physical appraisal when it is deemed advisable. This information will serve as the basis for making a meaningful diagnosis of the available information and design a dental restoration that will be compatible with engineering principles and biologic acceptance.

Diagnosis may be considered as the determination of the nature, causes, and location of a disease. It includes an evaluation of the normal, vital, physiologic processes as well as the functional and structural changes caused by disease. Oral diagnosis includes not only the determination of the nature, causes, and location of a disease, but also any deviations from the normal function or form of the masticatory organ. Such changes from normality may be due to systemic disturbances, loss of tooth, or improper functioning of the teeth due to malocclusion.

An analysis should be made of the data obtained during the examination. The information in the case history obtained in questioning the patient and others and in the records of former restorations and previous examinations may disclose the causes of existing conditions. A study of laboratory reports, together with those of the physician concerned with the general health of the patient, may also help. The information obtained by visual, roentgenographic, exploratory, and dynamic tests, as well as those gained by palpation, percussion, transillumination, and pulp tests, should be scrutinized for the probable causes of the disorder.

The analysis of the case should include a careful study of the patient's photographs, study models, and roentgenographs. A critical breakdown of these data should determine the conditions, both physical and functional, that are present; namely, the general health factors of the patient; the teeth, periodontal membrane, and pulps and pulp cavities; former oral health services; oral abnormalities and deficiencies, diseases, and facial factors; the condition of the maxillae, the mandible, the mucous membrane, the soft palate, the tongue, and the mucous and salivary glands; and the movements and relationships of the mandible to the maxillae.

The diagnosis having been made, the patient should be informed of the existing conditions and of service necessary to correct them. During such a conference with the patient, the availability of study models, roentgenographs, and the complete examination records will simplify for the dentist the task of explaining the present, existing deficiencies or abnormalities, the proposed method of restoration, and the prognosis of the proposed plan of treatment.

IMMEDIATE FIXED PARTIAL DENTURE SERVICE

Normally, fixed partial dentures are employed to replace teeth that were extracted long ago and that now have healed ridges. Immediate partial denture service differs from this in that the fixed partial prosthesis is constructed prior to the removal of the teeth and is placed in position immediately after the teeth are extracted; this is usually done at the same sitting. Although it is preferable to let the ridges heal before the placement of a fixed partial denture, certain conditions indicate the immediate replacement type of service.

It is a tragedy to most patients when it becomes necessary to lose one or more of their natural teeth. This feeling is intensified if the tooth happens to be in the anterior region of the mouth. Patients will undergo much discomfort and inconvenience in order to avoid this toothless plight; therefore, any technic or method that will enable them to continue their daily and social activities without interruption will be tolerated. This attitude constitutes one of the main reasons why such immediate dental service is frequently rendered. (See Chapter 33.)

In this method the abutment teeth are prepared first for retainers before extraction. After being cast, the retainers are placed in position, the impressions, registration, and shade are taken, and the working models are constructed. The tooth or teeth to be extracted are cut from the working model, and the pontic is properly fitted in its place and united with the retainers. Upon the completion of the prosthesis, the patient is recalled and the natural tooth or teeth are removed; the finished restoration is then immediately inserted. Such a bridge is usually set with temporary cement. Following a period of observation, if the condition of the tissues is compatible with the appliance so that a normal healing process takes place and if no changes in the pontic are needed, it is removed and prepared for permanent cementation.

In addition to overcoming social handicaps, there are other advantages to the immediate type of restoration. It has been stated that, with artificial complete dentures, the immediate replacement of complete dentures helps to conserve the alveolar process and promotes the condensation of the bone. It was observed that in such instances the healing process was more satisfactory and materialized quicker and that less irritation and infection followed such a method of treatment. It was further noted that immediate replacement controlled excessive bleeding by assisting in the formation and protection of the blood clots following the extraction of the teeth. It is probable that the same advantages are inherent to a modified degree in the immediate replacement type of fixed partial dentures.

Whenever a tooth is extracted, the resulting space often proves very annoying to the patient, who unconsciously seeks the edentulous area with his tongue. Later, when a fixed partial denture is inserted, the patient again experiences a foreign environment, for by that time his tongue has become accustomed to the open space. Since a patient quickly becomes adjusted to the new structure, this is a minor objection; still, it is a readjustment that is avoided when the immediate replacement type of prosthesis is employed.

It is not uncommon to find patients carrying infected teeth in the anterior region of the mouth for many years because they dread being edentulous even for a short time. The immediate replacement type of service permits the patient to elim-

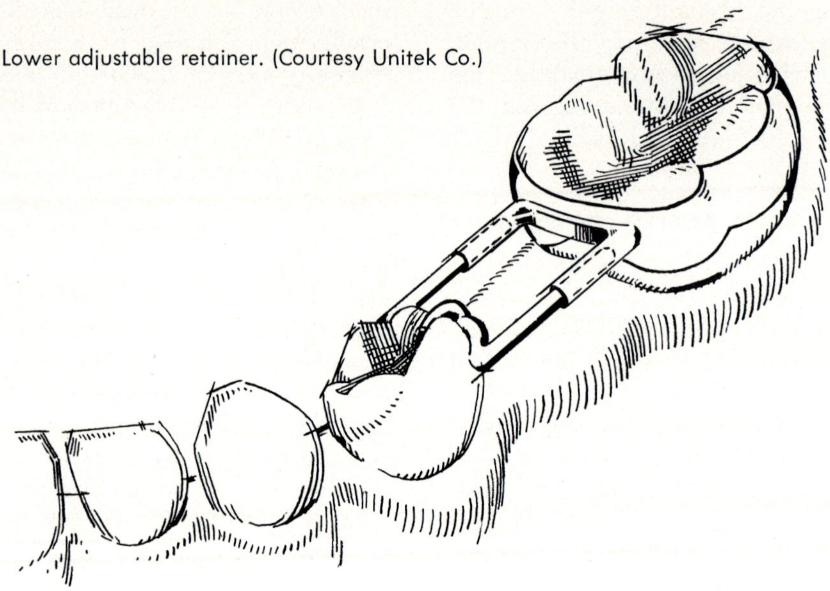

Fig. 3-1. Lower adjustable retainer. (Courtesy Unitek Co.)

inate the focus of infection in his mouth and still be presentable at all times.

In those younger patients who still have a mixed dentition, it is frequently necessary to place an appliance that serves the dual purpose of function and space maintenance (Fig. 3-1). For such, the prosthesis may also be previously constructed and placed immediately following the extraction of the deciduous teeth.

Prerequisites

There are certain prerequisites for succeeding with the immediate replacement type of restoration for adults. First, it must be certain that there is no danger of secondary infection following the removal of the tooth. A disregard of this precaution will cause the appliance to fail within a very short time. The type and the amount of alveolar bone present must be ascertained to assure a degree of permanency and to maintain the relative position of the investing tissues and the pontics. Ultimate success with this type of restoration depends also upon the presence of a sufficient and a normal alveolar process before and after the extraction of the tooth. If the labial plate of bone is lacking or destroyed during extraction, the immediate replacement type of fixed denture is contraindicated.

Finally, the success of this type of service is contingent upon the proper execution of the technical steps involved in its construction. This will be discussed fully when the various types of pontics are considered in Chapter 30. However, it can be stated now that this type of service is usually limited to the anterior part of the mouth; it restores one or two teeth at the most and tolerates no pressure between the pontic and the surrounding tissues, especially the bone.

Since the degree of tissue resorption that occurs following an extraction is not predictable, it is suggested that, in setting these bridges, the porcelain member of the pontic be attached to the bridge proper with temporary cement. In the event that excessive resorption occurs while the bridge is still under observation, additional porcelain may be added to the pontic at a later period without destroying or remaking the entire bridge. After a patient has worn the appliance for one week, it

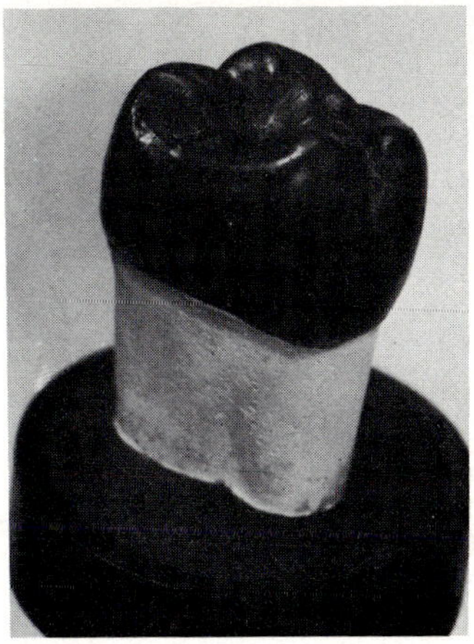

Fig. 3-2. Upper first molar cast gold crown.

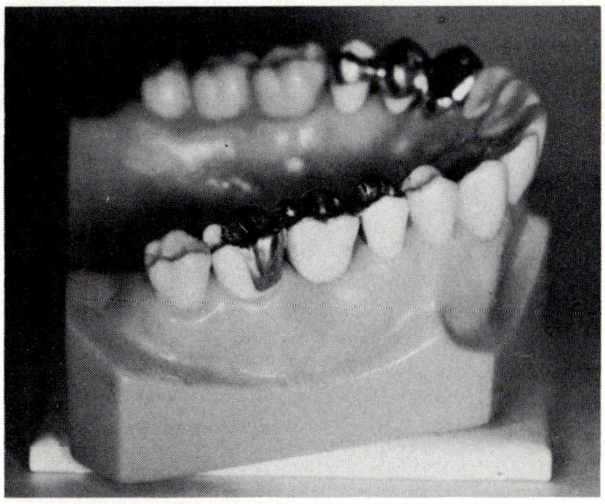

Fig. 3-3. Two upper fixed partial prostheses with intracoronal and extracoronal retainers.

should be removed and the underlying tissues should be examined carefully. If the healing process has progressed normally, it is suggested that the bridge again be set with temporary cement and kept under observation for another 2 weeks. The bridge may be cemented permanently if, following this second period of observation, it discloses an alveolar fundus with normal, soft tissues surrounding the surface of the porcelain pontic. There may be instances, however, in which it will be advisable to keep such temporarily set appliances under observation for as long as 6 months. Unusual developments may require the construction of an entirely new bridge, in which event the first one may be worn during the interval that the second is being constructed.

When more than one tooth is replaced in a restoration, the alternative and sometimes preferable method consists in giving the patient a small removable partial denture that may be worn until the ridges heal. Such an appliance may be worn by the patient from the time of the extraction until the fixed restoration is finished and ready to cement.

After having considered the factors disclosed in the examination and evaluation of the data, it is important that a suitable plan be developed before any restorative work is undertaken. This is necessary in order to coordinate and harmonize all restorations with each other and to reestablish a well-functioning oral organ both physiologically and mechanically.

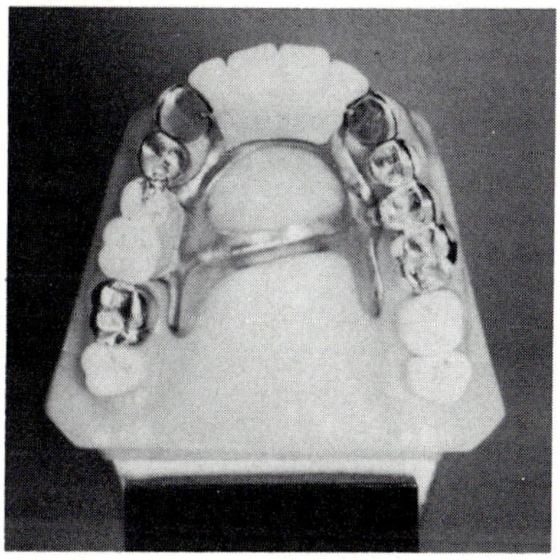

Fig. 3-4. Upper removable precision partial denture and fixed restoration from left cuspid to first molar utilizing nonrigid precision connector in second bicuspid pontic of fixed partial denture.

The restorations entering into the consideration of such a plan of prosthetic treatment are classified as follows: (a) individual crowns (Fig. 3-2); (b) fixed partial dentures (Fig. 3-3); (c) a fixed partial denture in combination with a removable partial denture or complete denture (Fig. 3-4); (d) a removable partial

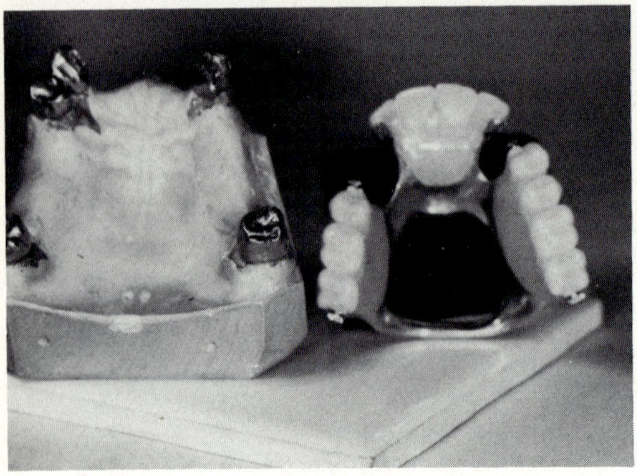

Fig. 3-5. Upper removable precision partial denture restoring four anterior teeth and posterior teeth bilaterally.

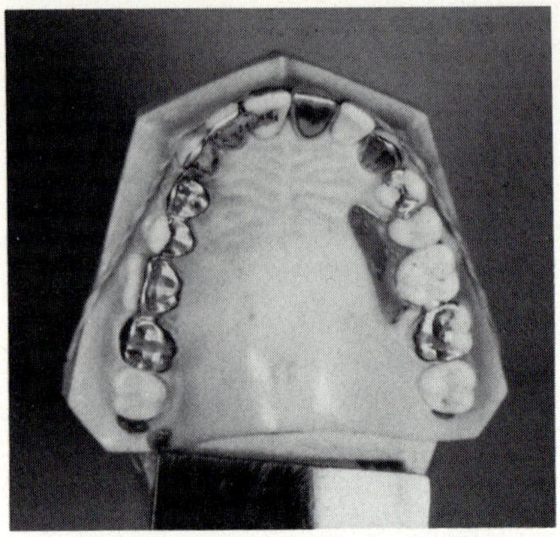

Fig. 3-8. Anterior and posterior fixed restorations on patient's right side; removable precision partial denture on opposite side.

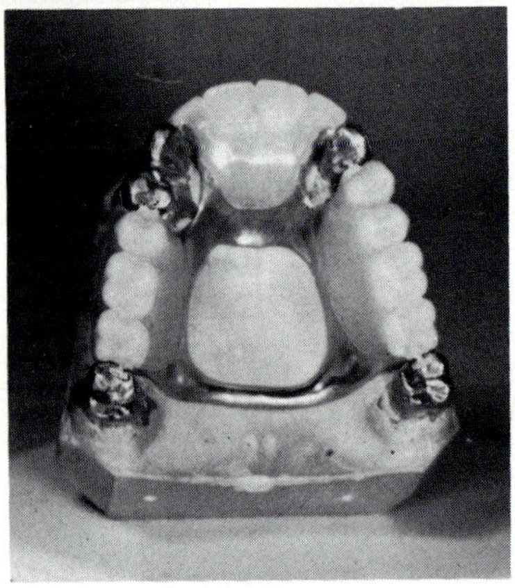

Fig. 3-6. Upper partial denture shown in Fig. 3-5, in position on abutment teeth.

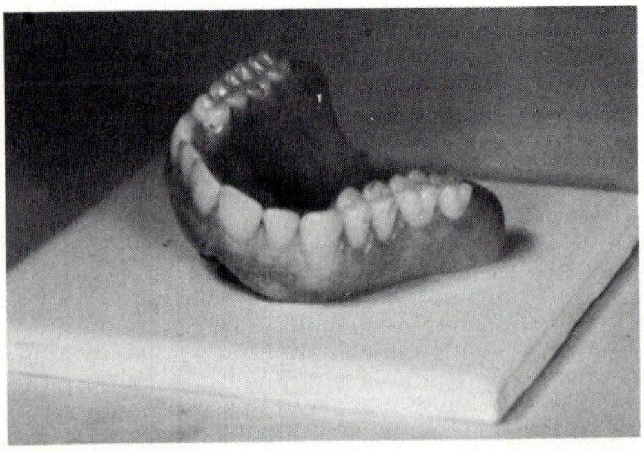

Fig. 3-7. Complete upper denture with complete porcelain fired base.

denture (Figs. 3-5 and 3-6); (e) a complete upper denture (Fig. 3-7); (f) a combination of an anterior and a posterior fixed prosthesis and a removable partial denture (Fig. 3-8); and, finally, (g) any combination of these employed in planning a reconstruction.

The crown may be considered the single unit of partial denture prosthesis and is usually indicated in teeth that cannot be restored to proper function or form by operative procedures. Crowns are also used as retainers for fixed and removable partial dentures.

Types of crowns

When crowns are the restorations under consideration, the plan may indicate the use of partial veneer crowns or complete crowns—either without a dowel or with a dowel.

Partial veneer crowns. Although the partial veneer crown is used mostly as a bridge retainer, it may be employed as an individual restoration when it is desirable or necessary to restore the two proximal surfaces and part or all of the lingual and occlusal surfaces of a tooth. This type of restoration may be placed on either anterior or posterior teeth (see Chapters 17

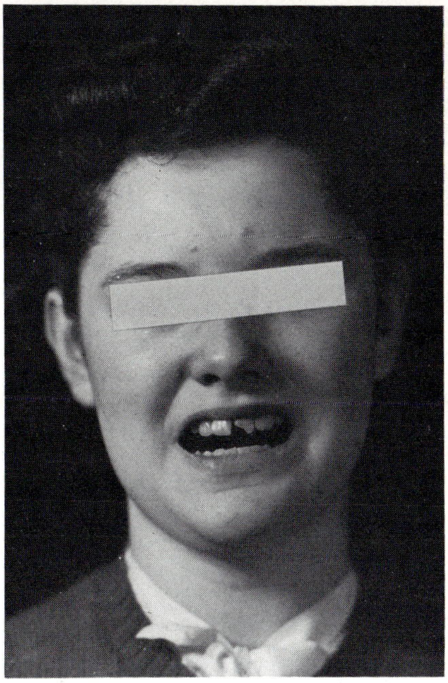

Fig. 3-9. Patient with diastema and fractured incisor.

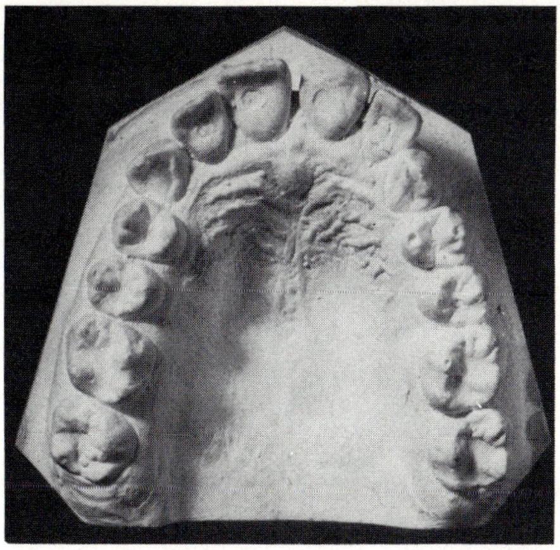

Fig. 3-10. Study casts of patient shown in Fig. 3-9 after endodontic treatment of four incisors.

and 18); it is useful on either a vital or a pulpless tooth. The plan of restoration may include an anterior partial veneer crown with (1) incisal and proximal axial grooves (Fig. 17-1), (2) proximal axial grooves without the incisal groove (Fig. 17-20), (3) proximal axial boxings without involving the incisal surface (Fig. 19-11), and (4) modifications and special types (Fig. 19-10). The first type with the incisal and axial grooves is considered only in those cases of unusual occlusal force and where the esthetic consideration is not of prime importance. Types 2, 3, and 4 are preferred to Type 1 because there is no display of gold or discoloration at the incisal edge. In Type 3 only the gingival two-thirds of the lingual and the two proximal surfaces are involved; this latter type leaves the incisal plane uncut and not covered by metal.

When teeth are rotated or otherwise malpositioned, the partial veneer also may be used on the distal or mesial halves of the coronal part of a tooth.

Partial veneer restorations are also indicated in posterior teeth whose occlusal surface and three or more axial surfaces are involved. When these restorations are used on upper bicuspids or molars, the mesial, distal, occlusal, and lingual surfaces are involved (Fig. 18-6). When they are placed on the lower molar teeth, then the mesial, distal, occlusal, and buccal surfaces are involved (Fig. 18-3). In the lower bicuspids the mesial, distal, lingual, occlusal, and very frequently a part of the buccal surfaces are included (Fig. 18-8). The modifications of the partial veneer crown for posterior teeth include the MacBoyle and other similar crowns (Fig. 19-13). There is also the so-called veneer one-half crown, which restores a part of the occlusal surface, one of the proximal surfaces, and those halves of the buccal and lingual surfaces lying adjacent to the involved edentulous space (Fig. 18-32).

The partial veneer crowns for posterior teeth are indicated: (1) when extensive caries involves the surfaces normally included in such a preparation; and (2) to reestablish normal occlusal and proximal relationships on sound but malposed teeth.

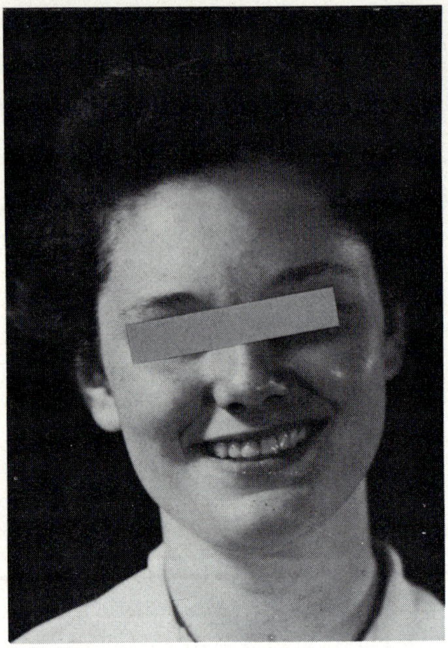

Fig. 3-11. Two central incisors restored with porcelain veneer crowns.

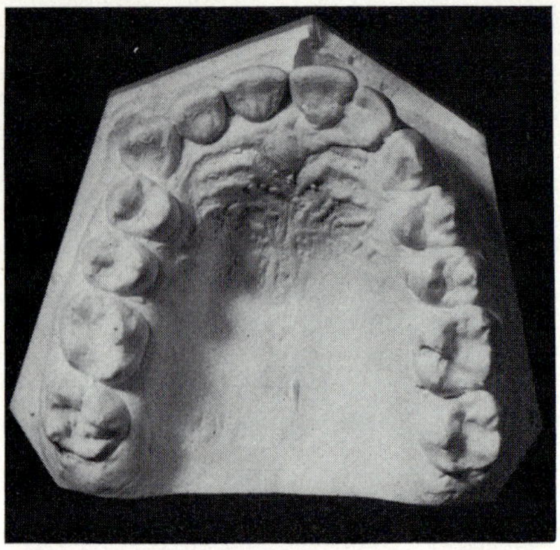

Fig. 3-12. Palatal view of cast showing completed crowns closing diastema.

In the presence of caries cautious planning may indicate complete, rather than the three-quarter or one-half partial, veneer restorations.

When either a partial veneer or a complete veneer porcelain (jacket) crown is a possible restoration for anterior teeth, it will be found in some situations that the complete veneer porcelain crown is preferred from the standpoint of esthetics (Figs. 3-9 to 3-12).

Complete crowns. In selecting complete crowns as individual restorations, there are many types from which to choose. There are two general classes: the complete crown without a dowel and the complete crown with a dowel. The first type may be placed on vital or pulpless teeth, while the second is employed only on pulpless teeth.

Complete crowns without dowels. Crowns without dowels may be of two general types—the shoulder type and the shoulderless type. Modifications of these with their special types may also be used.

A complete crown is planned for a tooth only when it cannot be restored by operative measures. Every effort should be made to maintain a vital, normal pulp in a healthy state. If the pulp is not exposed following the removal of decay, an effort should be made to maintain its vitality. If the condition of the pulp is questionable, it should be protected and kept under observation for a length of time sufficient to give assurance of its continued healthy condition. The shoulder type of crown may be placed either in the anterior or the posterior regions of the mouth. The complete veneer porcelain or so-called porcelain jacket crown is an example of this type of restoration (Fig. 26-3). The shoulder type of crown is equally useful in the posterior teeth; it may be constructed either of porcelain or of metal (Fig. 23-45). This type of crown requires the removal of a greater amount of tooth structure than does the shoulderless type. When used posteriorly, it is placed on teeth having sufficient tooth structure left after being prepared to withstand the forces to which they might be subjected.

The shoulderless type of complete crown without a dowel is used mainly in the bicuspid and molar regions. Because its preparation requires less cutting of tooth structure than the shoulder type, it may be successfully used on smaller teeth or those with little tooth structure remaining. Although the shoulder type of crown may be made of porcelain, the shoulderless type is usually constructed of metal or metal in combination with porcelain. The latter modification is applicable to either the shoulder or shoulderless type and is employed either anteriorly or posteriorly.

Complete crowns with dowels. The complete crown with a dowel is placed on pulpless teeth. A restorative plan may use it in either the anterior or the posterior regions of the mouth; it may be constructed with or without a metal base. If the remaining root or tooth is badly broken down, a metal base, usually cast, is indicated (Figs. 27-2 and 27-4). Metal pins locked in dentin are sometimes used to restore, with amalgam, that portion of the crown lost by caries. This is preferable to using cement alone for this purpose. The superstructure of a crown with a metal base may be made entirely of porcelain, gold, or gold and procelain combined (Figs. 24-42 and 24-43).

When a posterior tooth is badly broken down, the restorative plan may indicate a type of gold crown that receives its support and retention from a dowel extended into one or more of the treated and filled root canals (Fig. 23-1).

In those instances in which a sufficient amount of tooth structure remains, a complete porcelain crown with a dowel may be fitted to the root without any metal intervening.

One of the determining factors in the plan of treatment is whether sufficient tooth structure remains to afford the necessary retention and fit of the crown.

Many modifications of these two types will suggest themselves, and their success or failure will depend entirely on the manner in which they fulfill the functional requirements of their individual restoration.

In planning crowns it is necessary to decide the type of construction that is to be employed. Those crowns limited as to space, but exposed to excessive forces of mastication, must necessarily be constructed of the strongest materials available. Those having sufficient space and a normal or weak bite may use the weaker but the more esthetic types of materials.

TYPES AND COMPONENTS OF FIXED PARTIAL DENTURES: ANTERIOR AND POSTERIOR

Having determined the individual crown restorations, attention is next focused on those edentulous areas requiring partial dentures. This type of prosthesis is divided into two general groups—the fixed partial denture and the removable partial denture. The fixed partial denture may be placed in either the anterior or the posterior region of the mouth. As stated previously, an ideal or exemplary fixed bridge consists of three units, namely, two retainers and one pontic. There are rare instances in which a two-unit cantilever bridge may be placed in the anterior part of the mouth. Anterior bridges are divided into unilateral and bilateral types. The unilateral anterior bridge is the two- and three-tooth fixed prosthesis that does not cross the median line (Figs. 3-13 to 3-15). The bilateral anterior restoration may be a three-, four-, five-, or six-tooth fixed partial denture and may involve teeth on both sides of the median line (Figs. 3-16 to 3-19). In the unilateral bridge the central and lateral incisors and the cuspid of one quadrant may be involved; in the bilateral the two central incisors, the two lateral incisors, and the two cuspids may be involved in the prosthesis.

The design for a fixed partial denture is usually determined by the length of the span, the condition of the abutment teeth, the type of existing functional occlusion, the distribution, length, and number of abutment teeth, the general health of the patient, and the habitual care the patient gives his mouth. In the anterior part of the mouth the esthetic factors also play an important part in determining the type of restoration to use.

For convenience in planning the design of the unilateral restoration, it is considered according to its location in the arch and the physical and biologic characteristics of the available abutment teeth. In the anterior area the cuspid may be used as an abutment with a central incisor. In unusual situations the cuspid may also be utilized by itself to support a cantilever pontic.

The mediate area posteriorly usually in-

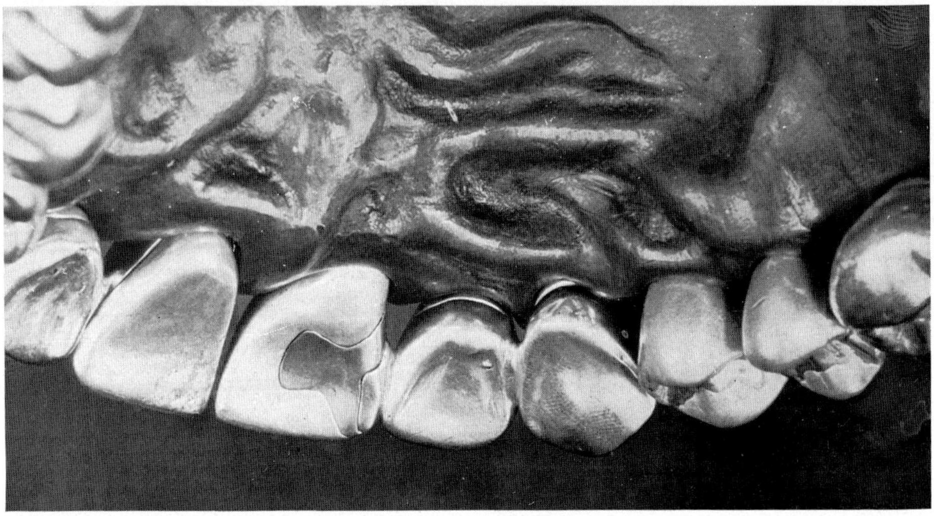

Fig. 3-13. Lingual view of fixed partial denture. Note broken-stress type of connector between lateral pontic and central retainer.

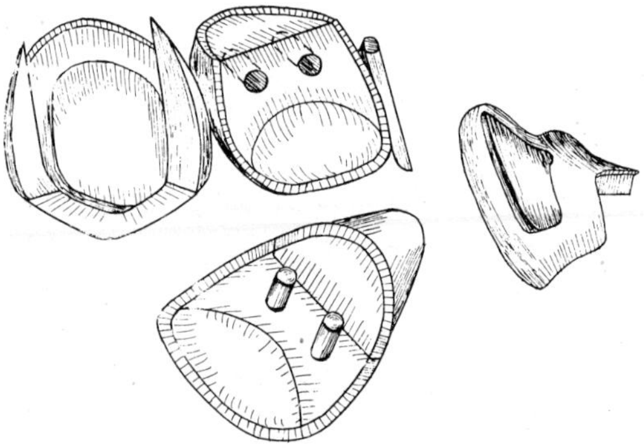

Fig. 3-14. Parts of restoration shown in Fig. 3-13. Shown are typical key and keyway nonrigid indirect retainer in lateral incisor, cuspid three-quarter crown acting as direct terminal retainer, and rigid soldered connector between three-quarter crown and lateral incisor pontic.

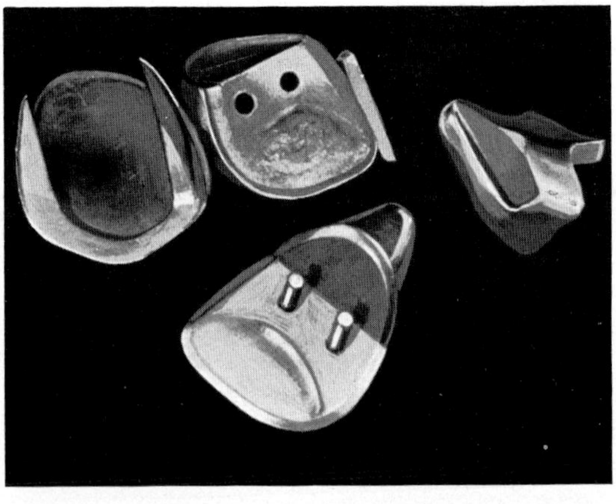

Fig. 3-15. Component parts of restoration shown in Figs. 3-13 and 3-14. Note near parallelism of proximal grooves in cuspid retainer; also hollow grinding of lateral pontic, incisal third.

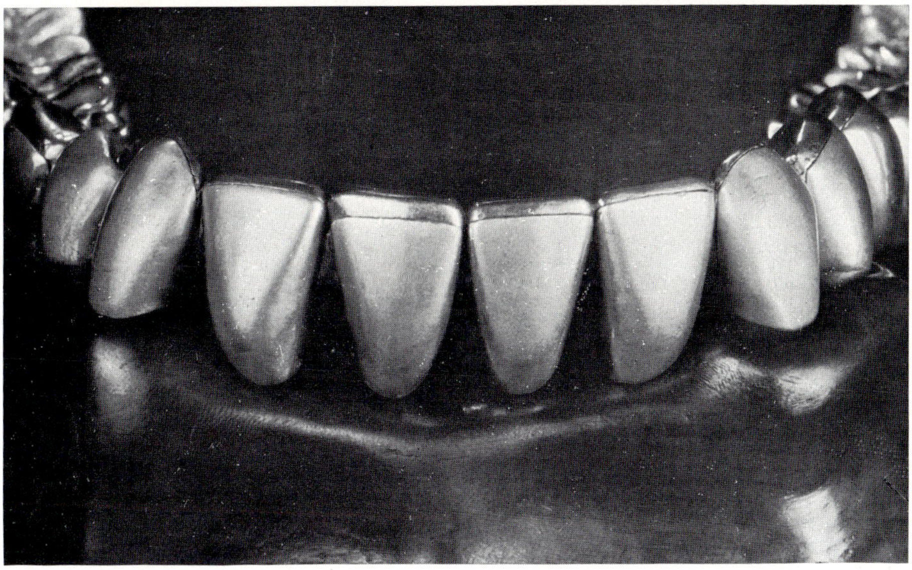

Fig. 3-16. Six-tooth fixed partial denture bilaterally replacing four incisors. Because gingival portion of lower anterior teeth is not ordinarily visible, embrasures may be made relatively wider. Pontics touch crest of ridge.

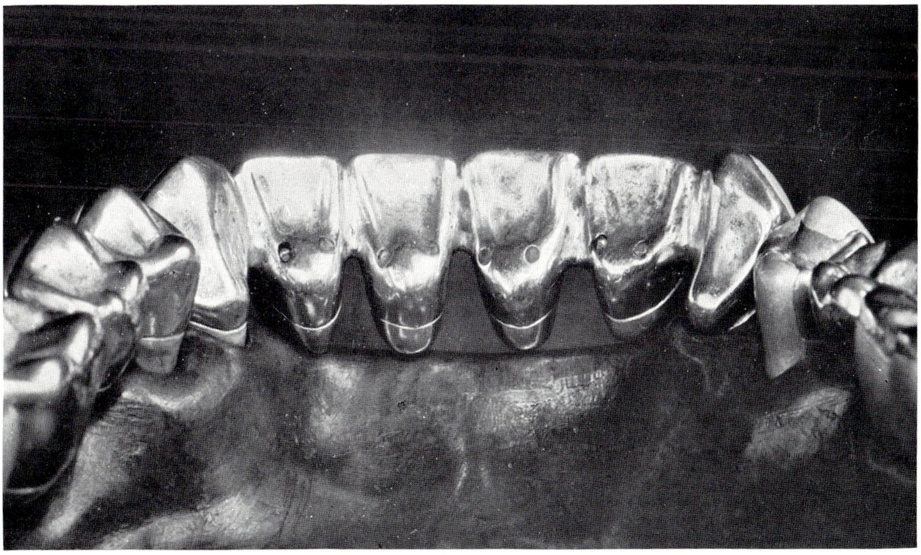

Fig. 3-17. Lingual view of fixed partial denture shown in Fig. 3-16. Note wide lingual embrasures, lingual contour, position and shape of soldered connectors, and porcelain portion of pontics in contact with crest mucosa. Platinum pins are riveted to gold portion of pontics, in addition to cementation.

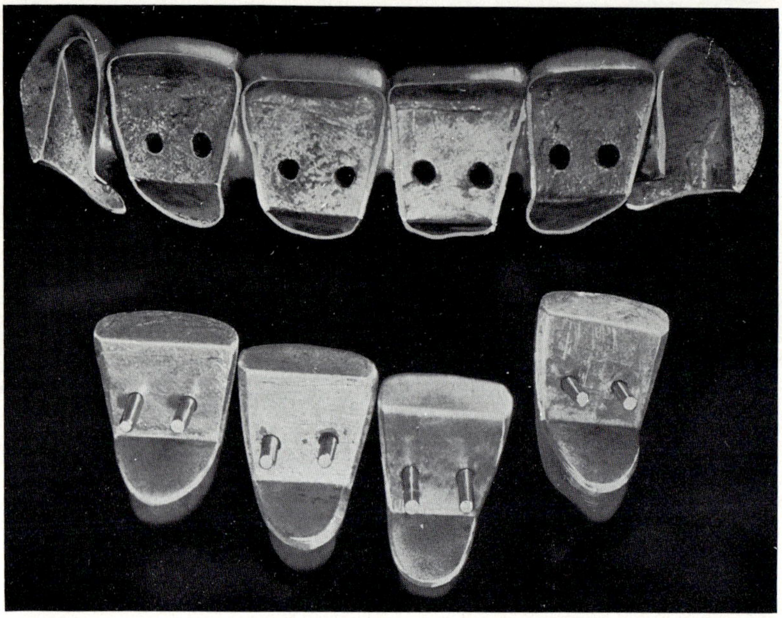

Fig. 3-18. Parts of fixed partial denture shown in Figs. 3-16 and 3-17. Occasionally incisal portion of porcelain facing is restored in porcelain instead of gold.

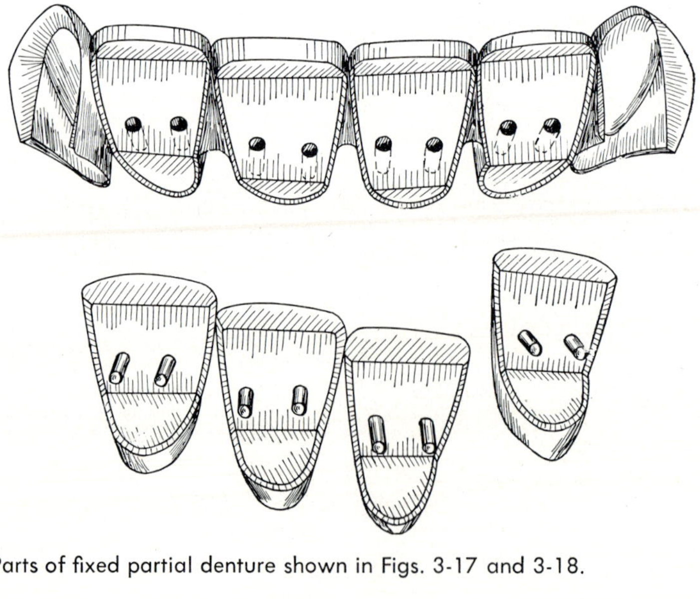

Fig. 3-19. Parts of fixed partial denture shown in Figs. 3-17 and 3-18.

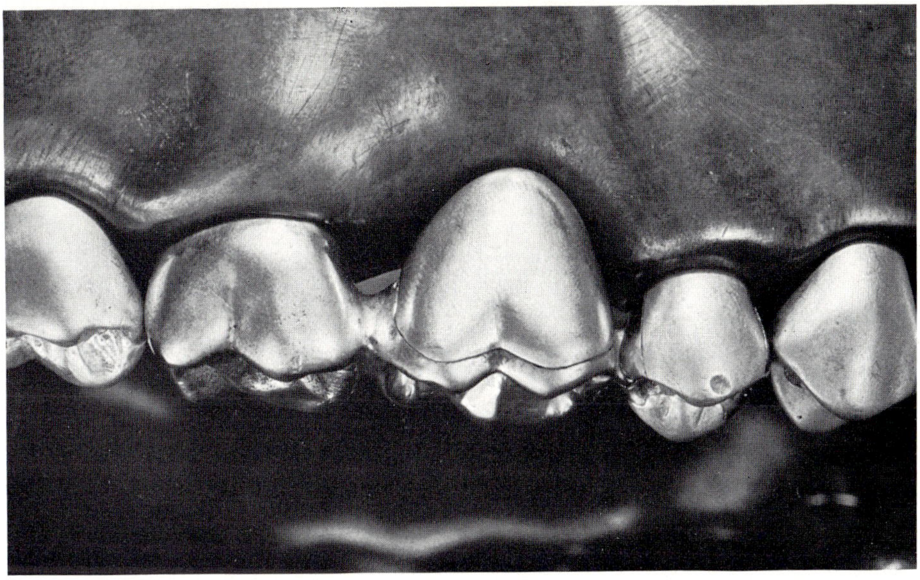

Fig. 3-20. Buccal view of fixed partial denture with rigid connector between first and second molars; broken-stress connector used between pontic and second bicuspid.

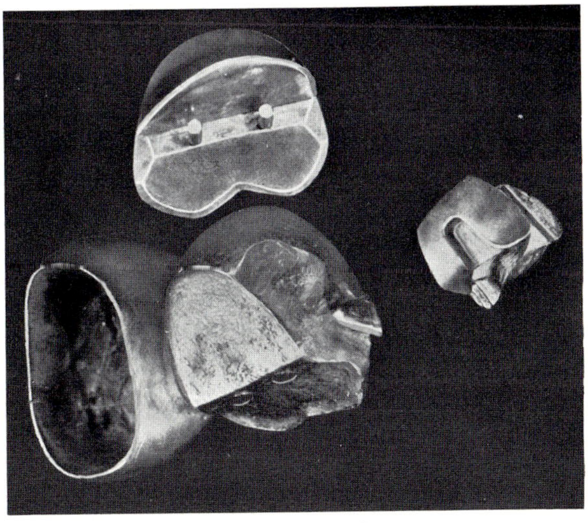

Fig. 3-21. Component parts of fixed partial denture shown in Fig. 3-20.

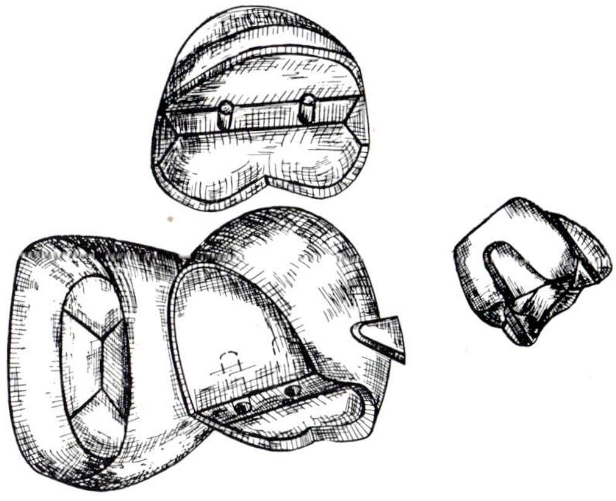

Fig. 3-22. Parts of restoration shown in Fig. 3-21.

volves the bicuspids and their adjoining cuspid or molar (Figs. 3-20 to 3-22). The restoration may restore both of the missing bicuspids, whereupon the cuspid and first molar are utilized as abutments. If the first bicuspid is to be restored, the cuspid and the second bicuspid are usually used for abutments; if the second bicusipd is missing, then the first molar and first bicuspid become the abutments for the restoration. The connectors may be nonrigid, or soldered types; the latter type is usually preferred.

The third type of unilateral restoration involves the posterior area and utilizes two or more of the molar teeth (Figs. 3-23 to 3-25).

Infrequent situations arise unilaterally which encompass the anterior, the mediate, and the posterior areas from central incisor to molars. Figs. 3-26 to 3-28 illustrate the possibility of constructing such a restoration with a broken-stress, nonrigid connector between the anterior area and the anteroposterior regions. In this instance, however, it would be advisable to utilize a complete cast crown on the cuspid instead of the MLD retainer and to have soldered rigid connectors throughout the structure. If a broken-stress connector was deemed necessary, a Stern or Chayes precision connector would be utilized in the cuspid cast crown. Such extensive restorations under normal circumstances rarely render the service which is expected from a well-planned and well-constructed prosthesis.

Removable partial dentures. No discussion of the removable partial dentures is considered here, other than to say that they are also classified into anterior and posterior types. The anterior may be unilateral and so constructed that it is tooth-borne or mucosa-borne; or it may extend bilaterally and also be tooth-borne or mucosa-borne. Of the posterior types of removable partial dentures, there are the unilateral and the bilateral. The former may be entirely or partially tooth-borne; whereas the bilateral may be entirely or partially tooth-borne, entirely mucosa-borne, or a combination of both. The den-

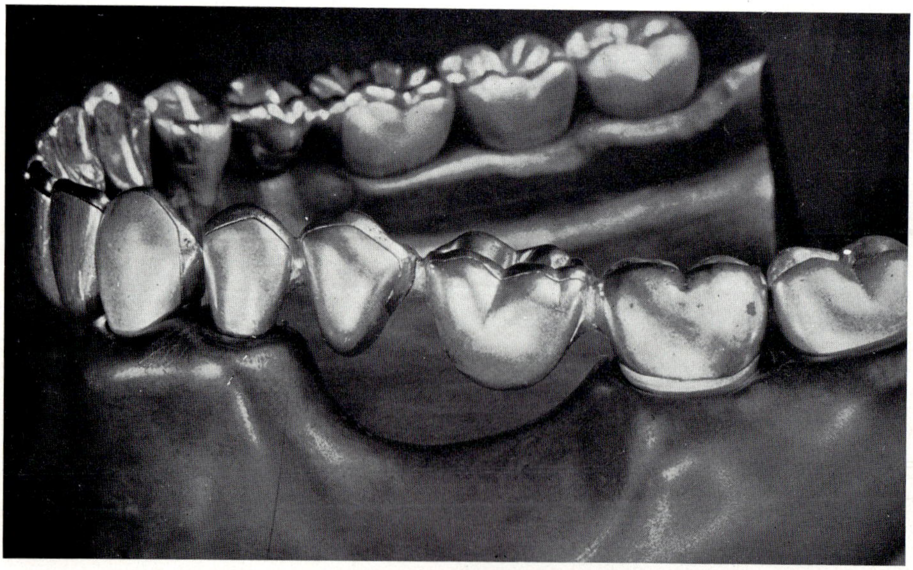

Fig. 3-23. Second bicuspid and first molar restored with fixed partial denture rigidly soldered to both retainers. Because of excessive ridge resorption, space is left between tips of pontics and ridge crest.

tist, after a careful analysis of the examination data, should be in a position to select the type of restoration best suited to the particular requirements of the patient. Having determined the type of prosthesis best suited to the existing conditions, one is in a better position to consider the elements involved in the fixed partial denture.

Elements of a fixed partial denture. The first and most important element to be considered is the abutment tooth. It is necessary to decide which teeth are to be used for the direct retention of the bridge and which teeth are to be used only for support or indirect retention (Fig. 3-29). Likewise, it must be determined whether the simple or the compound type of retention is to be employed and whether the teeth available are suitable for the type of retention selected.

The second element of a fixed partial denture is the retainer. Retainers may be direct or indirect (broken-stress); of the direct type we have the two- and the three-surface inlays, the three-quarter crowns, and the complete crowns (Chapters 15 to 18). These are the simple types of direct retainers.

There are two types of indirect retainers, the simple and the compound. The simple type of indirect retention is exem-

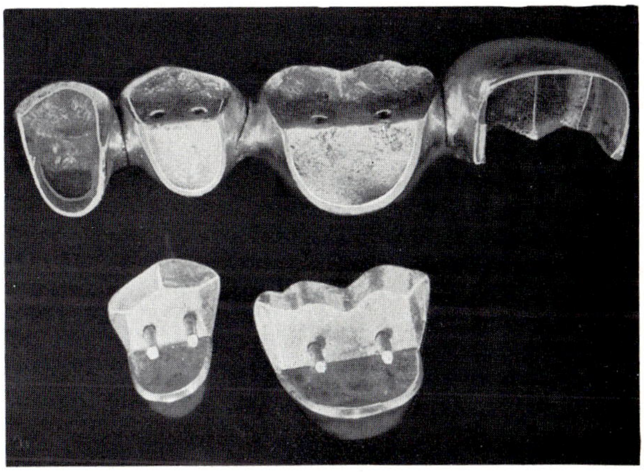

Fig. 3-24. Parts of restoration shown in Fig. 3-23.

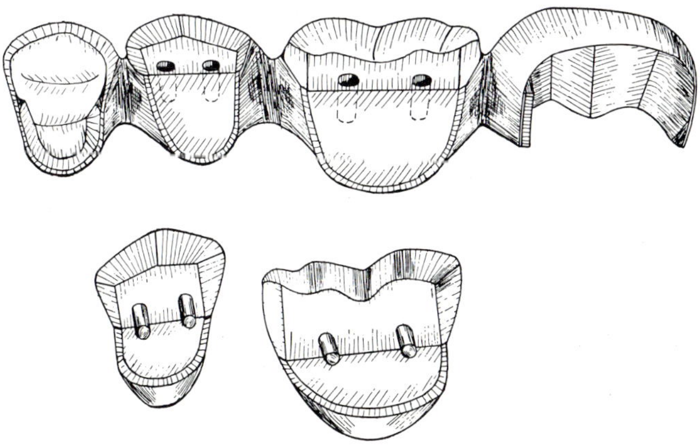

Fig. 3-25. Parts of restoration shown in Fig. 3-24.

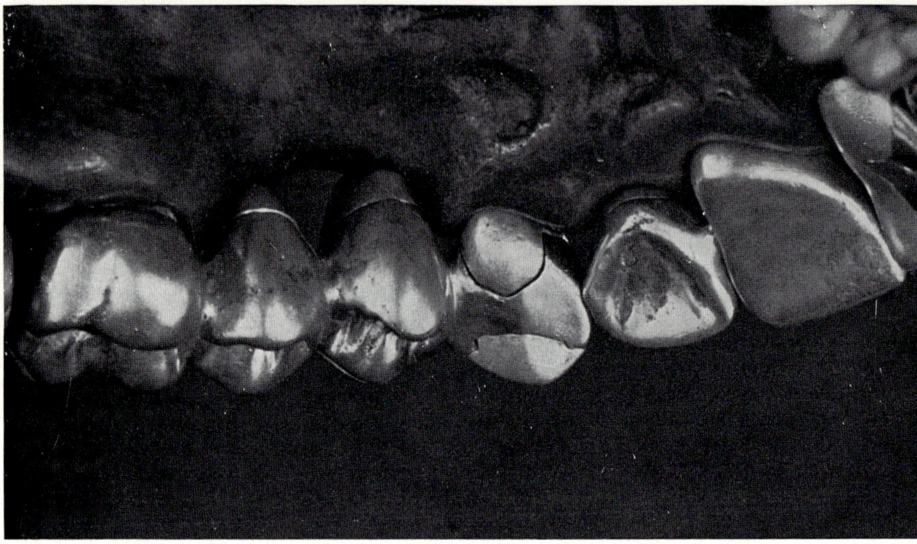

Fig. 3-26. Lingual view of multiple area restoration. Three fixed soldered connectors and one broken-stress type between the cuspid and lateral pontic are utilized. (See text for variation.)

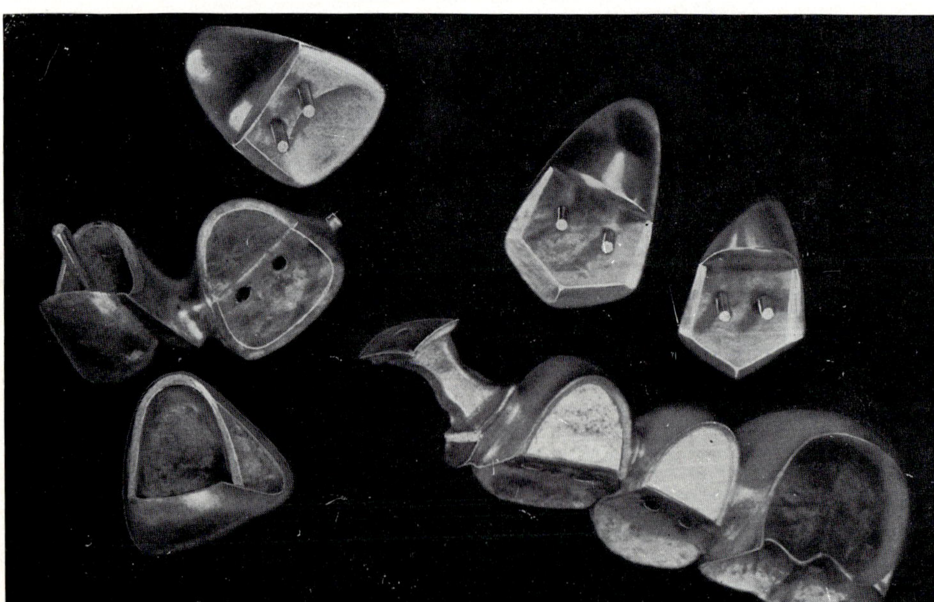

Fig. 3-27. Parts of restoration shown in Fig. 3-26. Note proximal wing extension on distal surface of central cast core.

plified by the surface rest, while the compound consists of the recessed tapered key and keyway, also called the broken-stress. Because of the additional retentive strength obtained from the precision compound types of recessed key and keyway, they are used more extensively in present-day prostheses and are exemplified by the Chayes and the Sterns attachments.

There are many modifications of these types of retainers. The type of retention employed is determined entirely by the physical and functional factors disclosed in the oral examination.

In planning restorations, it is essential that careful attention be given to the pontic element (Chapter 30). We must determine whether the pontics are to be of metal, porcelain, or a combination of the metal and porcelain types. The all-metal type of pontic is rarely used today, except in the posterior part of the mouth where the edentulous space is extremely short vertically.

The all-porcelain type of pontic is employed mainly in porcelain restorations. If the plan of reconstruction calls for a porcelain type, the pontics used may be prefabricated porcelain crowns or replaceable Steele's or long-pin facings, which are fired to the metal truss of the bridge with porcelain. Finally, pontics may possibly be built entirely of fired porcelain. A strong and esthetic porcelain restoration is obtained when the pontics are fired on a metal truss made an integral part of the restoration.

The third type of pontic uses the combination of cast metal and a prefired porcelain facing and is used extensively. It may be cast, soldered, or the combination dowel type; of these, the cast type is used most frequently.

Many modifications of pontics have been developed and reported in the literature describing the indications for the use of each type. The determining factors in selecting and planning the pontic depend entirely uopn the length of the bridge span, the vertical space available, and the requirements of esthetics and strength.

The connector is the fourth and final

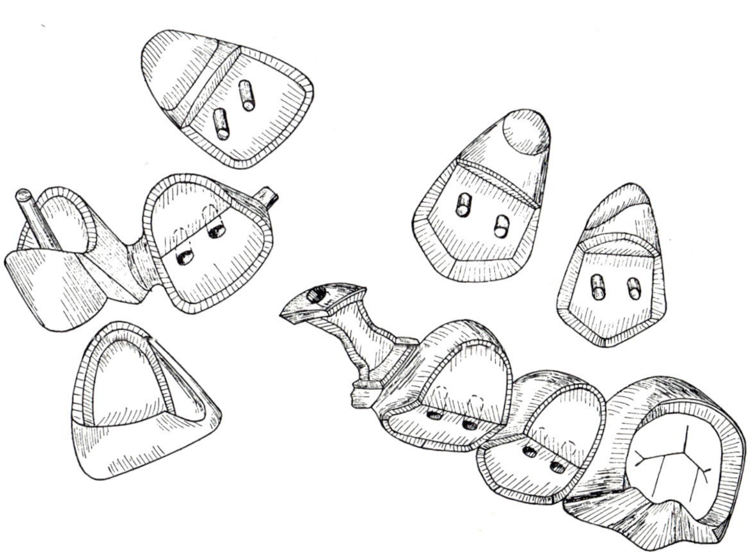

Fig. 3-28. Parts of restoration shown in Fig. 3-27. Note weakest design of subocclusal broken-stress connector placed in cuspid retainer. See text for correct alternative retainer and connector.

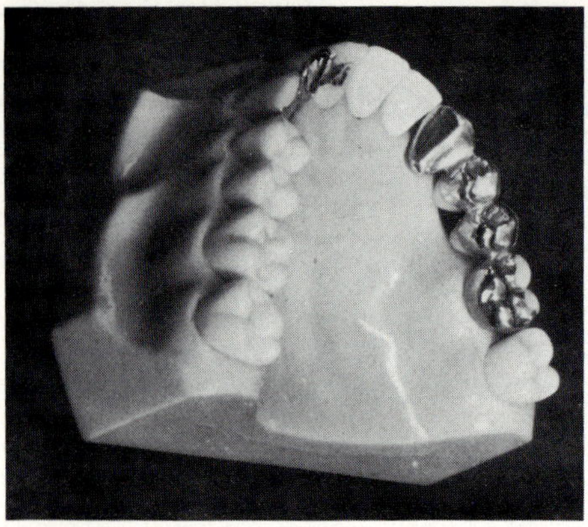

Fig. 3-29. Upper left quadrant restoration with three-quarter direct (primary) retainers on cuspid and first molar; opposite anterior area has indirect broken-stress retention in lateral pontic, key resting in keyway of central incisor inlay.

element to be considered in planning fixed partial dentures. There are two general types of connectors, the major, used in removable partial dentures, and the minor, used in fixed partial prostheses. The major connector is not of immediate interest at present, since it is employed primarily in the removable types of partial dentures. The palatal and the lingual bars are examples of the major connectors (Figs. 3-4 to 3-6). These may be made of either synthetic resin or metal.

The minor connectors used in fixed prostheses are of two general types, the rigid and the nonrigid. The rigid may consist of the porcelain or metal types; the latter may be either soldered or cast. Nonrigid connectors are of two types, the simple and the compound, the simple being a wire rest and the compound type embodying a mechanical key and keyway. It is recalled that a connector is that part of a fixed dental restoration which unites the pontic or body of the bridge to a retainer.

After the prosthetic needs of the patient have been determined, it is advisable to sketch the proposed restorative plan on the dental chart and sometimes on the study models also. The chart should summarize the reasons for the selection of the individual parts of the prosthesis, as well as the materials which are to be used in each.

Some dentists have found it helpful to make duplicate study models and on these to cut the prepartions of the various abutment teeth. This prepared model is later used as a reference model at the time cavities are being prepared. This method is especially valuable to those who have difficulty in paralleling the walls of a preparation in one tooth with those in another. Such models are also helpful when preparing teeth that are severely rotated or protruded, or whose long axes are malrelated; they may assist the operator in avoiding pulp exposures.

A thorough and precise method of planning should not be regarded as superfluous if it will safeguard the health of the patient and at the same time facilitate the operative procedures.

Many dentists who otherwise are good operators and excellent technicians may fail because they neglect to make a comprehensive examination of each patient. The reader is referred to Chapters 39 and 40.

PULPLESS TEETH

The problem of root canal therapy is one that must be approached cautiously. It is necessary at times to decide whether a pulpless tooth is to be retained or extracted, and, if retained, what the possibilities are of its giving satisfactory service. Although it is unquestionably true that a tooth with a vital pulp is better than one without it, in an analysis of many case histories it was found that pulpless teeth serve satisfactorily as bridge abutments if the tooth is carefully treated, filled, and kept under periodic radiographic surveillance. Our decision should be influenced by the condition and service rendered by previously treated teeth. If roentgenographic evidence indicates an unfavorable biologic tissue reaction to treated teeth, it is unwise to employ additional teeth for bridge supports. If an examination of the patient's record indicates that the prognosis for root treatment is favorable, one should not hesitate to use such teeth when it is necessary to do so.

ORTHODONTIC PROCEDURES: ROTATED AND TILTED TEETH

Many patients requiring fixed partial denture service have teeth which have moved out of their normal position and relationship (Fig. 3-30). What sometimes appears to be an extremely difficult restorative procedure may be simplified if orthodontic aid is utilized prior to the construction of the bridge. This is especially true of rotated or tilted teeth. Such conditions are encountered most frequently in the lower molar regions. Figs. 3-1 and 3-2 show how simple appliances may prevent, or reposition tilted teeth and close open spaces. The extraction of a lower first molar, if a prosthetic appliance is not immediately employed, will result in a drifting and tipping anteriorly of the second molar. This condition becomes progressively worse until only the distal cusps of the lower molars are in occlusal contact with the upper teeth. To place a fixed appliance on a tooth having such an angle of inclination subjects it to unusual stresses since the forces of mastication will not be transmitted to the normal axis of the tooth. It is sound procedure, therefore, to restore such teeth to their correct, vertical relationships by orthopedic procedures.

ARROWHEAD BITE PLANE

If there is an overclosure of the vertical dimension with accompanying local dental tissue involvement and temporomandibular disturbances, we must decide whether to establish an increased vertical height immediately with restorations or whether to resort to orthopedic treatment —if the latter, then the bite plane can be utilized (Fig. 3-31).

The use of the bite plane in not new.[1] It has been used in orthodontic and later in periodontic practice. Its adaptation as an ancillary method in the treatment of the partially edentulous prosthetic patient is comparatively recent.[2]

We are aware that when a tooth becomes functionless due to the loss of its occluding opposing tooth, it egresses from its former plane of occlusion (Fig. 3-32). This movement, up or down, depending on whether the tooth is a lower or upper one, is accompanied by the movement of the entire periodontium, the gingivae, the

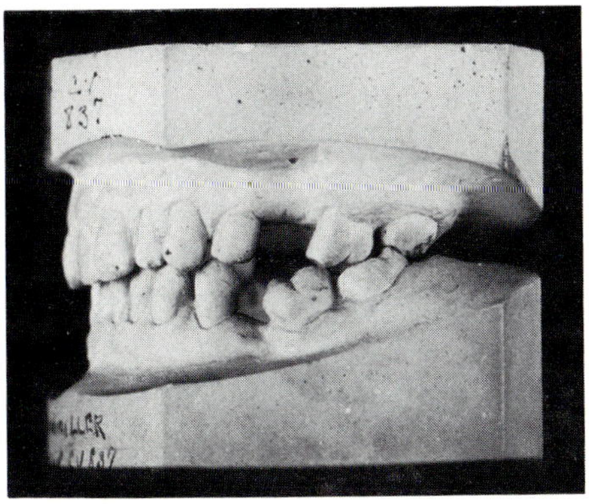

Fig. 3-30. Upper and lower casts of rotated, egressed, and tilted teeth.

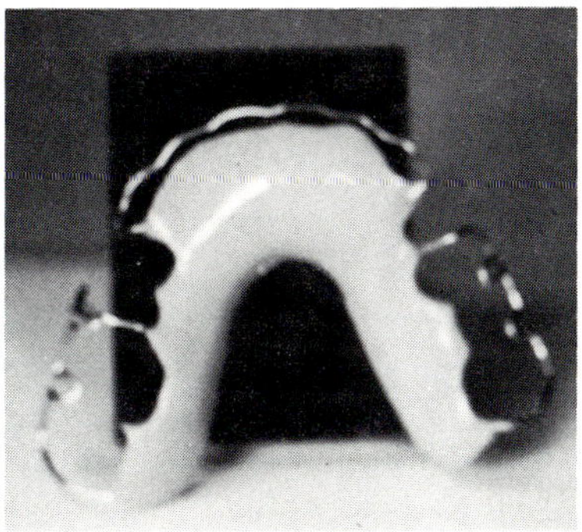

Fig. 3-31. Functional gnatho-orthopedic Andersen bite plane.

A 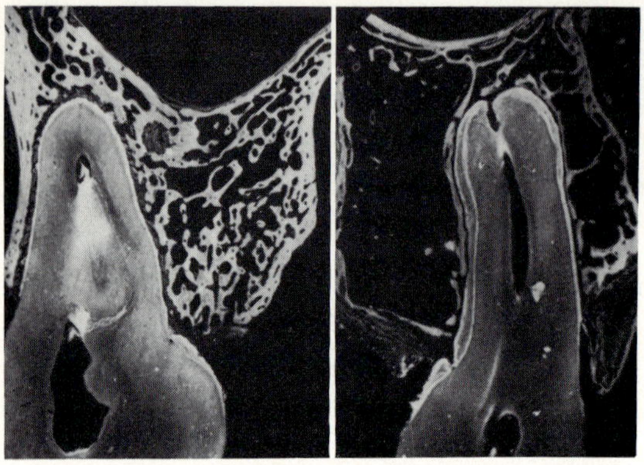

Fig. 3-32. A, Normal tooth. B, Functionless tooth. (Courtesy B. Orban.)

B 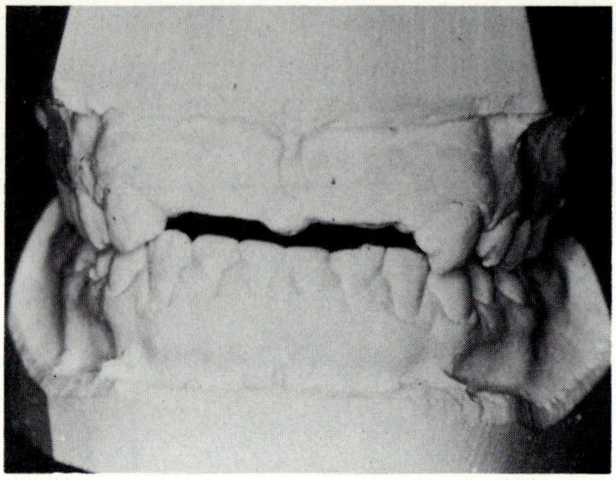

Fig. 3-33. Casts of patient with limited vertical dimension prior to wearing bite plane. (Courtesy E. C. Brooks.)

periodontal membrane, and the lamina dura; a change also takes place in the supporting bone trabeculae. This mass movement continues until the tooth meets an opposing stop, usually an opposing tilted or rotated tooth. If no opposition is encountered the tooth may egress to the extent that it touches the mucosa of the opposing edentulous ridge. Recognizing this unique biologic phenomenon of nature in egressing functionless teeth, the bite plane is often utilized to assist biologically in the establishment of a desired increased vertical height.

The use of the bite plane in general practice will mitigate some of the mechanical and biological problems that confront the dentist.

Due to the excessive overclosure, relatively young age, and sex of the patient seen in Fig. 3-33, a fixed bilateral restoration was planned for this patient instead of a removable appliance. She was given a bite plane to increase her vertical dimension in order to accomodate a fixed partial denture (Figs. 3-34 and 3-35).

On the other hand, we must keep in mind that taking teeth out of function *permanently* would not only cause them to egress, but would cause harmful changes to take place in their supporting and contiguous tissues; namely, (1) the

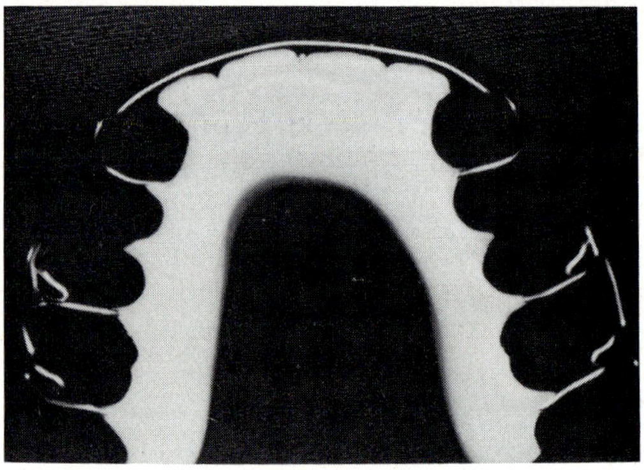

Fig. 3-34. Orthopedic bite plane with arrowhead clasps and anterior retaining labial wire; worn by patient. (Courtesy E. C. Brooks.)

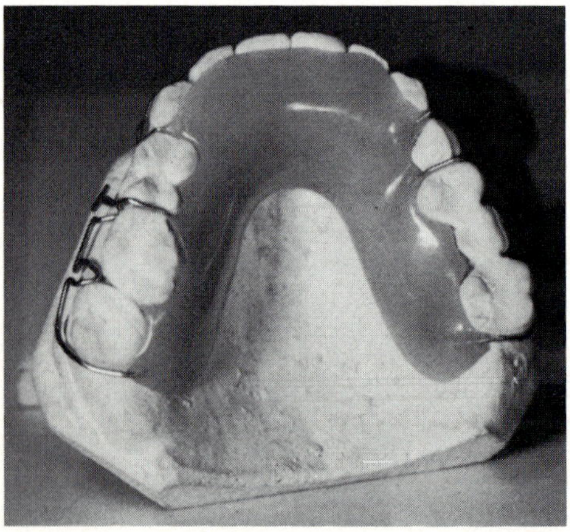

Fig. 3-35. Completed bite plane with four anterior teeth on model. (Courtesy E. C. Brooks.)

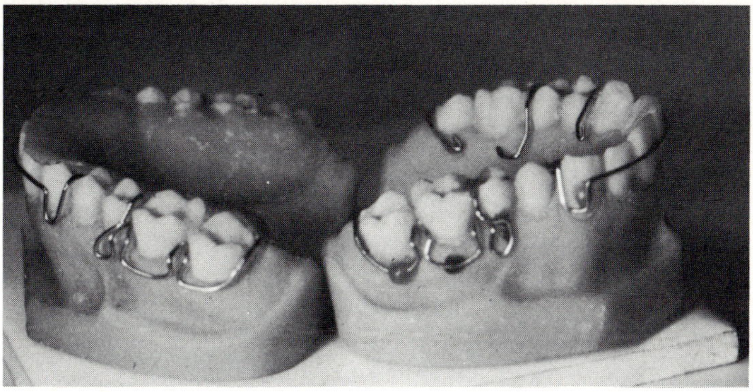

Fig. 3-36. Left, Design, placement, and means of retaining clasps and labial wire in acrylic base. **Right,** Remaining components prior to embedding in acrylic base. (Courtesy F. Milford.)

width of the periodontal membrane would decrease, and (2) the supporting alveolar bone would gradually be diminished in form and size, causing an increase in the size of the marrow spaces. This is not desirable, and consequently it is recommended that the patient should wear the appliance continuously but that he remove it at mealtime and then replace it.

The stimulation the teeth receive during these three functioning periods prevents the deleterious tissue changes in the periodontium, even though the entire mass is moving occlusally.

Later, when final rehabilitation is accomplished, a new bite plane is made for the patient, which is worn only at night. The length of time it is worn varies with different individuals. The bite plane is a relatively simple appliance made of acrylic resin and sometimes with retentive clasps (Fig. 3-36). It is horseshoe shaped and leaves most of the palate area uncovered. An anterior wire extends from cuspid to cuspid to secure the stability of the anterior teeth (Fig. 3-35). The clasps are the arrow type and are placed in the bicuspid and molar interdental, buccal embrasures, near the cervical region (Fig. 3-36). This type of retainer does not restrain the occlusal movement of the bicuspids and molars.

On the anterior palatal surfaces of the bite plane a flat bite-wall is made, extending from cuspid to cuspid (Fig. 3-35). This flat plane meets the incisal edges of the lower six anterior teeth at an exact angle of 90° so that only a vertical force is exerted on the teeth. It is usually necessary to level their incisal edges so that uniform contact is made against the bite plane of the appliance. There should be no depressions in the flat plane. This would prevent the free positioning of the mandible to its true centric relation. The height of the bite plane should allow the patient 1.5 to 2.0 mm. of freeway space.

Because of the smooth, flat incisal plane and a sufficient freeway space, the patient will be able to maintain physiologic rest and centric positions, the condyles will be relieved of any strain, and consequently the correct neuromuscular pattern will gradually condition the patient into a correct centric relationship closure. This will be a great help when the various jaw registrations for mounting the casts are taken.

The patient wears the bite plane from 3 to 6 months, sometimes longer if orthodontic treatment is also included. Since an increased interocclusal space is created between the opposing bicuspids and molars by the anteror bite plane of the ap-

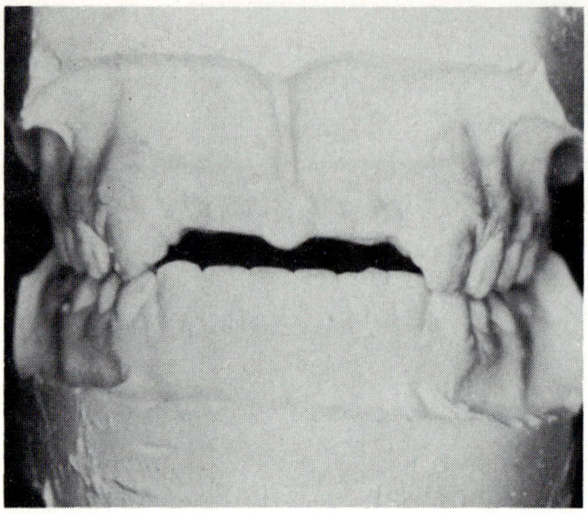

Fig. 3-37. Desired increase in vertical dimension obtained after 8 months of therapy. (Courtesy E. C. Brooks.)

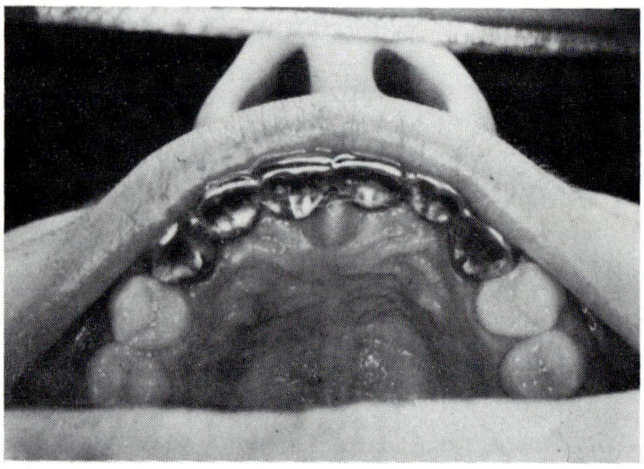

Fig. 3-38. Fixed bilateral partial denture cemented in patient's mouth.

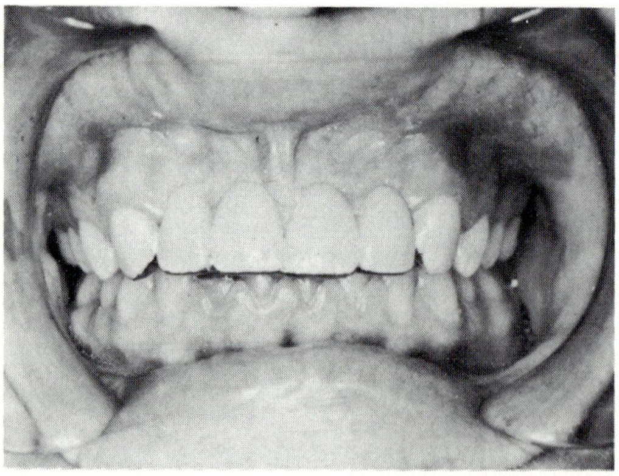

Fig. 3-39. Labial view of restoration cemented on abutments. Note vertical increase. (Courtesy E. C. Brooks.)

pliance, the upper and lower posterior teeth gradually egress until they contact each other (Fig. 3-37). The question as to how much the teeth should be allowed to egress is important. This can be determined by checking the position of the lower incisal edges in a position of closure, also the cuspid clearance in eccentric occlusions; this may be done in the mouth or on the casts mounted on the articulator in their correct hinge axis relationship.

When normal masticatory movements can be made without premature, injurious contact of the anterior teeth, the proper posterior opening has been attained and the permanent reconstruction may be initiated and completed (Figs. 3-38 and 3-39).

SURGICAL TREATMENT

It is not always possible to initiate the restorative program immediately after the completion of the examination and diagnosis. It is frequently necessary to seek surgical treatment prior to the construction of fixed partial dentures. The one most frequently required is the extraction of roots or teeth. The dentist must decide whether the extraction is to be done as soon as possible to permit the ridges to heal before constructing the bridge or whether an immediate replacement type is to be constructed prior to the extraction of the tooth; the latter is especially important in the anterior region of the mouth. It may also be necessary to decide on the time for the removal of residual areas of infection. Almost without exception the removal of all such areas is a prerequisite to the placement of fixed dental prostheses.

If a cyst is present, its extent and location will determine whether the restorative work is to be done before or after its removal. If the cyst involves any of the abutment teeth, sound procedure suggests surgical service prior to the prosthetic service.

Alveolotomy is less required in partial than in complete denture prosthesis. When resorted to in fixed prosthesis, it is localized and is generally limited to the removal of sharp spicules of bone and a rounding off of the process, so that the healed ridge will be well formed.

The reduction of part of the ridge is sometimes suggested in order to increase the vertical space to be occupied by the pontics. Ordinarily, a short vertical space contraindicates a fixed type of restoration; a removable one is preferred. When this condition is encountered, it is a simple matter to reduce the bone to any desired height at the time of the extraction. If a ridge is healed and is of long standing, one should resort to surgical reduction only after other methods of reconstruction are contraindicated.

Another condition may be present, namely, that of localized areas covered with hypertrophied mucous membrane. If the hypertrophy is excessive, the tissue should be removed and a firm, well-rounded ridge established prior to undertaking fixed prosthesis. Likewise, localized bony eminences should be smoothed and rounded off.

The excision of muscular attachments is indicated more frequently when complete rather than partial dentures are reconstructed. When such excision is performed, it is done almost exclusively because of the presence of cicatricial tissue.

Cleft palate

The dentist is occasionally called upon to make restorations for a patient with either a cleft or a perforated palate. The retention of an obturator may have a direct dependence upon the prosthesis that is to be placed. If a perforation in the hard palate is remote to the region of the fixed partial prosthesis, it may be closed either surgically or with a self-retaining mechanical appliance before or after the placement of the prosthesis. If, however, the perforation, such as an opening into the maxillary sinus, is located in the immediate region of the prosthesis, it should be corrected prior to placing the bridge restoration.

Oral disorders

Of prime consideration is the treatment of existing inflammatory gum conditions or other oral diseases. Until such disorders are corrected, no crowns or bridges should be undertaken. Oral diseases, whether they be acute or chronic, benign, malignant, or infectious, if they persist, may alter the entire plan of prosthetic procedure.

The treatment for tissue tone prior to taking impressions is sometimes instituted prior to the construtcion of partial dentures. The purpose of such procedures is to shrink pendulous mucosa overlying the bone structure so that an impression may be obtained of it in this reduced condition. The model resulting from such an impression is reduced slightly in size. Pontics fitted accurately to such a model and later coming into contact with the normal, relaxed mucosa, will establish a glazed-surface contact sufficient to establish a physiologic stimulation in the contacting mucosa (see Chapter 30). This has been accepted as a physiologic relationship between the prosthesis and the tissues. It eliminates the guesswork that accompanies the "scraping" of a cast. The application of an astringent to the edentulous area for several minutes has also been employed; likewise, the use of ice-cold water has been recommended for this purpose.

Every patient seeking dental service of any nature should first receive a thorough prophylaxis. Correct dental practice does not approve the placement of any type of restoration prior to this service.

The dentist should also decide on the order of procedure for operative restorations, root canal therapy, or other services prior to placing fixed partial dentures. If operative restorations are needed, these may often be included as a part of the fixed partial denture.

MATERIALS USED

In the construction of a fixed partial denture the mechanical aspects of replacing teeth are sometimes overemphasized, and a full appreciation of the mutual relations between the appliance and the oral tissues is lacking. Unless the environment in which the appliance functions is favorable to the tissues and can be kept so permanently without injury to them, the restoration will not last very long. One of the most exacting demands of any prosthesis is that it be kept clean. This naturally implies that it is cleansable and that it is constructed of such material and is of such design that the patient can keep it in a sanitary condition with an average amount of care.

An acceptable material must be used in fabricating fixed partial denture prostheses so that it be nonirritating to the soft tissues. This implies a substance that is dense, strong, and smooth, that maintains its form, and that will not react with the fluids of the mouth to give off either unpleasant odors or a disagreeable taste. Although gold, porcelain, and synthetic resins are the materials principally used by the partial denture prosthodontist, unless manipulated and finished properly, they too may become irritating to the tissues.

The surface of any gold restoration placed in the mouth must be so polished that there are no scratches or nodules capable of acting as irritants to the soft tissues. Rough areas allow the accumulation and retention of debris particles, which later undergo putrefaction and are accompanied by disagreeable odors and unfavorable tissue reactions. Poor castings should be discarded because of their inherent mechanical weakness and also because they are a hygienic liability.

Although glazed porcelain has proved highly acceptable to the soft tissues of the mouth, its improper manipulation may also result in serious sequelae. To be compatible with the tissues, a porcelain surface must be smooth and absolutely impervious to moisture. This implies that it has been carried to a sufficiently high temperature during the process of vitrification and that all the surface pores have been sealed and eliminated. Such a surface prevents the retention and accumulation of food debris and stimulates and maintains the adjacent soft tissues in a healthy state. Rarely do we find pathologic symptoms associated with properly designed, glazed, and contoured porcelain restorations correctly related to tissues.

It is when porcelain has been ground and not reglazed that irritation and inflammation ensue. Bridge facings formerly were ground to fit the ridge and then placed against soft tissues without reglazing the ground surfaces. Such a technic of pontic construction not only creates shelves that catch and retain food but also places a rough, porous, sharp-edged surface in intimate contact with the delicate mucosa. The slight movement of the bridge normally present during mastication, plus any retained putrefying debris, is sufficient to cause a chronic inflammation of the soft tissues. Modern procedures and technics eliminate the excuse for such practices today.

The synthetic resins have come into extensive use. If properly manipulated and processed, they are compatible with the tissues of the mouth. If not properly used, they also are likely to be porous and irritating to the tissues.

Use of dissimilar metals

The question is sometimes raised relative to the possible harmful effects resulting from the use of dissimilar metallic restorations in the same mouth. It is reported that such a condition results in the creation of galvanic currents. Some men have associated these electrical currents with the etiology of oral malignancies. Although evidence has been submitted to prove the existence of such currents in the mouth, the proof that these currents are responsible for such lesions has not yet been definitely established. The metallic taste which patients sometimes experience has likewise been attribtued to the presence of dissimilar metals in the mouth. Although no definite correlation has been established between these findings, whenever possible we should confine the metals used to one group of alloys.

When unfavorable symptoms develop from the wearing of fixed partial dentures, it is well to investigate the materials and their surface texture and to determine if the material has been properly manipulated to restore the correct form and function of the missing teeth. A bridge retainer or pontic of gold alloy may be highly polished, yet if its contour is improper and its anatomy violates the laws of occlusion, or if the shape and position of the axial surfaces fail to protect the soft investing tissues from impingement and harmful excursions of food, the hygienic benefits of the material itself will be nullified. On the other hand, it is possible for a highly glazed and properly contoured porcelain pontic to be the source of irritation and the cause of an unhygienic condition if the pontic, correct in every other respect, exerts excessive pressure on the ridge. It may cut off the circulation of the blood in the contacting area with a resultant resorption or development of a hypertrophied and inflamed tissue. When either condition develops, it is impossible for the patient to maintain a healthy mouth hygiene.

Preventive measures

Fixed partial dentures must be so constructed that they are largely self-cleansing (see Chapter 30). Their form and relationship to the soft tissues must be such that the patient can keep the appliance in a sanitary condition by the judicious use of the toothbrush and ligature. There are times when this care may be supplemented by the use of mechanical water syringes. No prosthetic service may be considered complete until the dentist has given the patient full instructions and training in the proper method of maintaining a hygienic oral condition. It is the duty of the dentist also to check periodically to see whether the patient is following these instructions properly; if not, he should be helped to secure the desired oral hygiene.

Many a well-restored mouth has failed either because the dentist neglected to instruct his patient in its proper care or because the patient failed to comply with the instructions given him by the dentist. Too much emphasis, therefore, cannot be placed in stressing these facts to the patient.

Dental caries, the most prevalent of human diseases, is not yet fully understood. Two facts, however, have been established: first, it is more likely to occur before maturity, although this does not imply that older persons are immune to it; and second, research has disclosed the fact that diet in some undetermined way is also a factor. The main thought and energies of the profession today are directed toward the prevention of dental caries. It is to be hoped that some day its cause will be understood and eliminated.

While preventive measures are constantly employed, when they still fail, the next best resort is restorative dentistry. If caries is checked in its early stages by suitable operative procedures, the smallest amount of tooth structure is then involved and rarely is prosthetic service necessary, except in those cases involving accidents. A restorative procedure, whether it be operative or prosthetic, must be such that it not only rebuilds and restores lost form and function, but also prevents future recurrence of caries in the same region. Complete crowns are placed to preserve what remains of the natural tooth and to safeguard it against future destruction by caries. Where a carious tooth is involved to the point that its restoration requires a partial crown or inlay, the margins must be carried into self-cleansing or naturally immune areas.

In observing the principles of extension for prevention, care should be exercised not to overextend the margins of the preparation.

If the patient is susceptible to caries, a removable partial denture on natural teeth to support retaining clasps will result in the loss of the abutment teeth. To avoid such a mishap, place complete crowns on the retaining teeth that carry clasps. This will ensure them against decay and give years of additional service.

SELECTED REFERENCE

1. Andresen, V.: Functional gnatho-orthopedics, Acta Gnathology **4**:11, 1930.
2. Tylman, S. D.: The use of the bite plate as a pre-restorative measure, J. Canadian D. A. **33**:134-140, 1957.

GENERAL REFERENCES

Ante, I. H.: The fundamental principles, design and construction of crown and bridge prosthesis, D. Items of Interest **50**:215, 1928.

Ante, I. H.: The fundamental principles, design and construction of fixed and partial prosthesis, J. Michigan State D. Soc. **17**:187, 1935.

Ante, I. H.: The fundamental principles, design and construction of bridge prosthesis, J. Canadian D. A. **10**:1, 1938.

Beaver, H. A., and Kopel, H. M.: A new appliance for space maintenance, J. Michigan Dent. Ass. **49**(10):299-300, 1967.

Berman, H., and Lustig, L. P.: Primary substructures and removable telescopic superstructures in dental reconstruction, J. Prosth. Dent. **10**:724, 1960.

Boos, R. H.: Preliminary treatment of prosthetic patients, J. Prosth. Dent. **15**:1002-1009, 1965.

Bowman, J. F., and others: Operative dentistry as related to removable partial dentures, Pennsylvania Dent. J. **33**:83-88, 1966.

Braly, B. V.: A preliminary wax up as a diagnostic aid in occlusal rehabilitation, J. Prosth. Dent. **16**:728-730, 1966.

Brenman, H. S., Weiss, R. C., and Black, M.: Sound as a diagnostic aid in the detection of occlusal discrepancies, Pennsylvania Dent. J. **69**:33-39, 1966.

Buonocore, M. G.: New anterior restorative materials, Int. Dent. J. **18**(2):406-420, 1968.

Bush, A. J.: Proposed classification of fixed bridgework and law governing its application, J. Nat. D. A. **2**:221, 1915.

Castagnola, L.: The advantages of removable-fixed bridges over fixed bridges, Int. Dent. J. **18**(2):276-278, 1968.

Cohen, D. W., and Chacker, F. M.: Criteria for selection of one treatment plan over another, Dent. Clin. N. Amer. pp. 3-22, March, 1964.

Cohn, L. A.: Physiologic basis for tooth fixation in precision-attached partial dentures, J. Prosth. Dent. **6**:220, 1956.

De Boer, J. G.: Prerestorative operations, Nederl. T. Tandheelk **72**(12):864-868, 1965.

Dietz, W. H.: Means of saving mutilated teeth, J. Prosth. Dent. **11**:967-972, 1961.

Dixon, C. M., and Rickert, U. G.: Tissue tolerance to foreign material, J.A.D.A. **20**:1458-1472, 1933.

Gordon, T.: Telescopic reconstruction: an approach to oral rehabilitation, J.A.D.A. **72**:97-105, 1966.

Gratzinger, Max: Use of removable orthodontic plate appliances in the management of chronic periodontal disease, Dent. Clin. N. Amer., pp. 403-417, July, 1959.

Greeley, J. H.: Planning for fixed prosthesis. J. Prosth. Dent. **20**(5):412-416, 1968.

Griffiths, N. H.: Mouth preparation and management of abutment teeth for the removable partial denture, New York J. Dent. **35**:130-135, 1965.

Harrison, J. D.: Crown and bridge preparation, design, and use, Dent. Clin. N. Amer. pp. 185-193, March, 1966.

Helmers, G. B., and others: Treatment of dentitions affected by hereditary amelogenesis and dentinogenesis imperfecta, Dent. Clin. N. Amer. pp. 437-447, July, 1966.

Holmes, J. B.: Preparation of abutment teeth for removable partial dentures, J. Prosth. Dent. **20**:396, 1968.

Johnston, J. F.: Preparation of mouths for fixed and removable partial dentures, Alum. Bull. Indiana Univ. School Dent., pp. 4-7, 34-35, Sept., 1960; J. Prosth. Dent. **11**:456, 1961.

Kabnick, H. H.: Divergent biomechanical and physiological concepts in case planning and treatment, Fort. Rev. Chicago D. Soc. **44**:11, 29, 1962.

Kahn, A. E.: Considerations in the use of partial

and full coverage in periodontal prosthesis, J. Prosth. Dent. **15**:83-99, 1965.

Kahn, A. E.: Partial versus full coverage, J. Prosth. Dent. **10**:167-178, 1960.

Kantorowicz, A.: Klinische Zahnheilkunde, Berlin, 1932, Hermann Meusser, Part IV. Salamon, H.: Dental bridgework systematized, D. Cosmos **66**:1303, 1924.

Karlsen, K.: Fixed bridgework as opposed to fixed-removable appliances, Int. Dent. J. **18** (2):269-274, 1968.

Karlstrom, S.: Efterkontroll av brofall framstallda enlight den s. k. pontostruktormetodiken (Follow-up examination of bridges prepared by the Pontostructor method), Svensk tandl. Tidskr. **53**:957-972, 1960.

Katz, Benjamin: Orthodontics as an adjunct to oral prosthesis in adults, New York D. J. **27**: 30, 1961.

Knowles, L. E.: Biomechanics of removable partial dentures and its relationship to fixed prosthesis, J. Prosth. Dent. **8**:426, 1958.

Linkow, L. I.: Mesially tipped mandibular molars, J. Prosth. Dent. **12**:554-558, 1962.

Lorey, R. E., and Myers, G. E.: The retentive qualities of bridge retainers, J.A.D.A. **76**(3): 568-572, 1968.

McCracken, W. L.: Mouth preparations for partial dentures, J. Prosth. Dent. **6**:39-52, 1956.

Malone, W., and others: Early treatment of amelogenesis imperfecta, J. Prosth. Dent. **16**:540-544, 1966.

Mark, F.: Preparation of the ridge for fixed and removable restorations, J.A.D.A. **25**:21, 1938.

Massler, M.: Biologic considerations in the selection and use of restorative materials, Dent. Clin. N. Amer. p. 131, 1965.

Norton, L. A., and Proffit, W. R.: Molar uprighting as an adjunct to fixed prostheses, J.A.D.A. **76**:312, 1968.

Nuttall, E. B.: Diagnosis and correction of occlusal disharmonies in preparation for fixed restorations, J.A.D.A. **44**:399, 1952.

Paris, L.: A change in dental lamina dura terms for the clinician, J. Maine. Med. Ass. **57**:134, 1966.

Peterson, E. A., Phillips, R. W., and Swartz, M. L.: A comparison of the physical properties of four restorative resins, J.A.D.A. **73**:1324, 1966.

Pietrokovski, J., and Massler, M.: Ridge remodeling after tooth extraction in the rat, J. Dent. Res. **46**:222-231, 1967.

Porter, M.: Dental problems in wind instrument players, Chir. Dent. France **38**(18):23-40, 1968.

Pruden, W. H., II: Partial coverage retainers: a critical evaluation, J. Prosth. Dent. **16**:545-548, 1966.

Ravinett, S.: Factors influencing fixed partial dentures for adolescents, J. Prosth. Dent. **15**:880-888, 1965.

Reynolds, J. M.: Abutment selection for fixed prosthodontics, J. Prosth. Dent. **19**:483, 1968.

Roberts, D. H.: The use of the three-quarter crown in standard and modified form in bridge work, Brit. Dent. J. **112**(10):430-434, 1967.

Rudd, K. D., and others: Stabilizing periodontally weakened teeth by using guide plane removable partial dentures: a preliminary report, J. Prosth. Dent. **16**:721-727, 1966.

Sassouni, V.: The prevention and control of malocclusions, Dent. Clin. N. Amer. pp. 41-49, March, 1966.

Sauser, C. W.: Pretreatment evaluation of partially edentulous patients, J. Prosth. Dent. **11**: 886, 1961.

Schachter, Joseph J.: Adjustable space maintainer for the general practitioner, J.A.D.A. **66**:817, 1963.

Schulke, M. D.: A fixed bridge that is removable, J.A.D.A. **74**:403, 1967.

Schwarz, A. M., and Gratzinger, M.: Removable orthodontic appliances, Philadelphia, 1966, W. B. Saunders Co.

Schweitzer, J. M.: Discussion of "crown and sleeve-coping retainers for removable partial prostheses," J. Prosth. Dent. **16**:1086, 1966.

Shearer, W. L.: Cleft palate and cleft lip, J.A.D.A. **21**:1447, 1934.

Shelby, D. S.: Tooth and tissue supported fixed partial dentures, J. Prosth. Dent. **17**:590, 1967.

Shell, J. S., Hollenback, G. M., and Villanyi, A. A.: Comparative abrasion rates on restorative materials, J. California Dent. Ass. **42**:6, 1966.

Slater, L. M.: A practical technique for restoration of an overlapping anterior tooth, Dent. Dig. **72**:314-315, 1966.

Smith, D. E.: The immediate restoration, Pacific D. Gaz. **40**:82, 467, 519, 1932.

Smith, R. A.: Cooperation between prosthodontist and oral surgeon, J. Philippine D. A. **13**:25, 1960.

Tuccillo, J. J.: Tele-seal pontic-seal bridgework, Thermotrol Technician **21**:3, 1967.

Tylman, S. D.: Co-report: problems in the construction of crowns and bridges, Int. Dent. J. **8**:353, 1958.

Tylman, S. D.: Biologic factors involved in fixed prostheses, J. Canadian Dent. Ass. **33**:67, 1957.

Willey, R.: Why do bridges fail? J. Florida D. Soc. **31**:18-22, 1960.

Wilson, W. H., and Lang, R. L.: Practical crown and bridge prosthodontics, ed. 1, New York, 1962, McGraw-Hill Book Company.

Chapter 4

Histologic structure of teeth and supporting tissues in relation to crown and fixed partial prosthodontics

The subject of dental histology in recent years has assumed its rightful place in the minds of dental students and dentists. It is more manifest daily that, in order to comprehend diseased conditions, one must necessarily understand the structure of healthy tissues; otherwise, how can one differentiate between normal and abnormal conditions? Certainly it is not unreasonable to expect those who are undertaking to make a comprehensive examination and accurate diagnosis and to execute a plan of treatment for the restoration of lost form and function by means of prosthetic procedures to have a working knowledge of the dental tissues involved.

Standard texts on histology cover the subject in detail; here we are interested mainly in the application and relationship existing between histologic knowledge and fixed partial denture prosthodontics.

Dental tissues may be grouped into two general divisions—the calcified and the noncalcified. In the first group are included enamel, dentin, cementum, and the alveolar process; the second group embraces the pulp, the periodontal membrane, and the soft tissues, including the gingivae (Plate 3).

CALCIFIED DENTAL TISSUES

The enamel

The tissue with which the dentist is most engaged and on which the success or failure of his work largely depends is the enamel. Enamel is generally defined as the material that covers the anatomic crown of a tooth. The anatomic crown extends to the cementoenamel junction and is distinguished from the clinical crown, which consists of the coronal portion of a tooth extending into the mouth from the bottom of its gingival crevice. This distinction is important from a prosthetic point of view since a clinical crown may be shorter or longer than the anatomic crown.

Because of the type of work enamel is called upon to do, nature has made it one of the hardest of animal tissues and one that is very resistant to wear. It is not equally distributed in thickness over the coronal portion of a tooth; it is thicker in the occlusal or incisal third and it gradually diminishes in thickness until it ends in a thin line at the cementoenamel junction. The inner surface of the enamel cap is not a smooth surface; instead, it meets the underlying dentin in a series of pointed

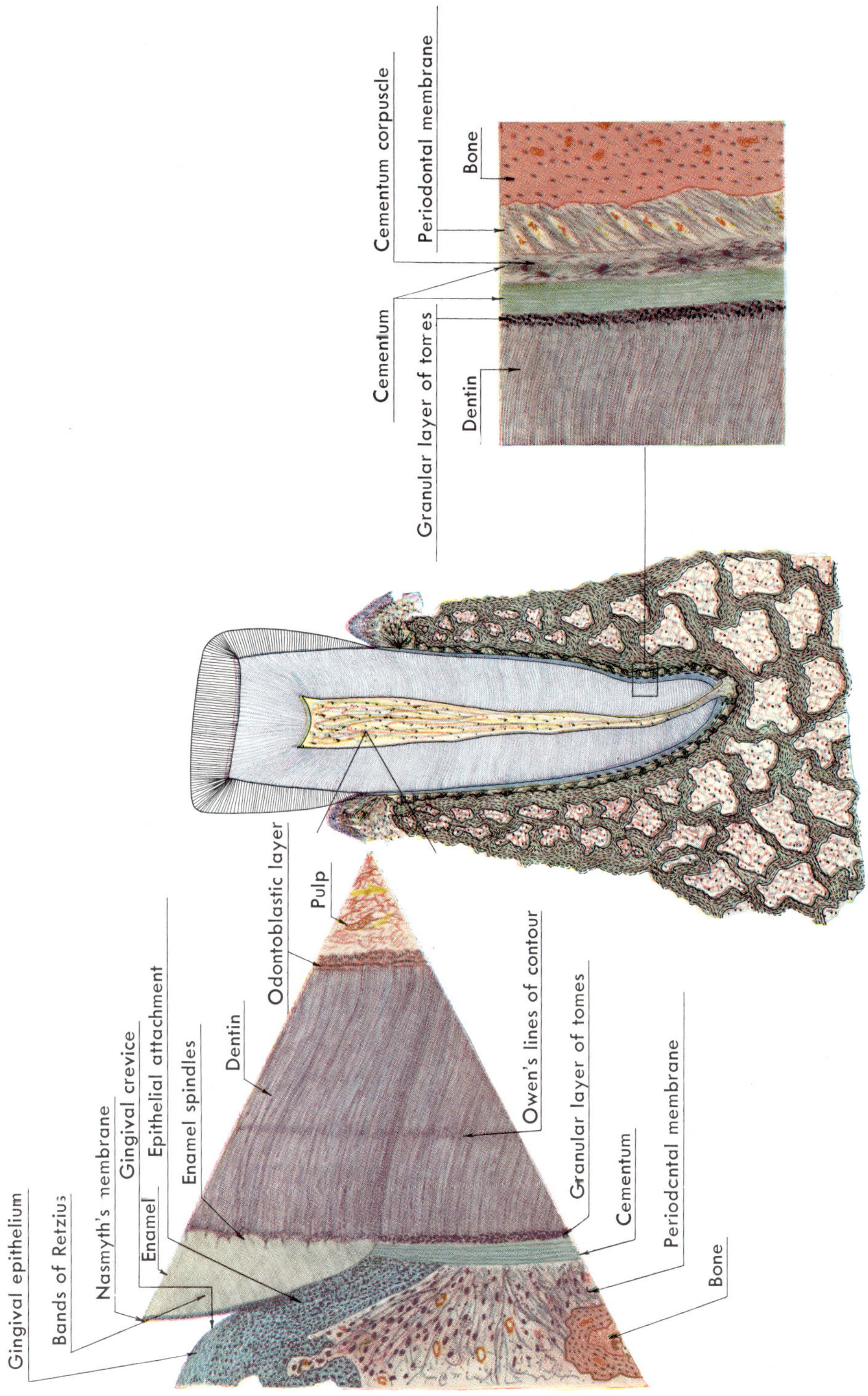

Plate 3. Dental tissues. (Drawing by E. H. Ragan.)

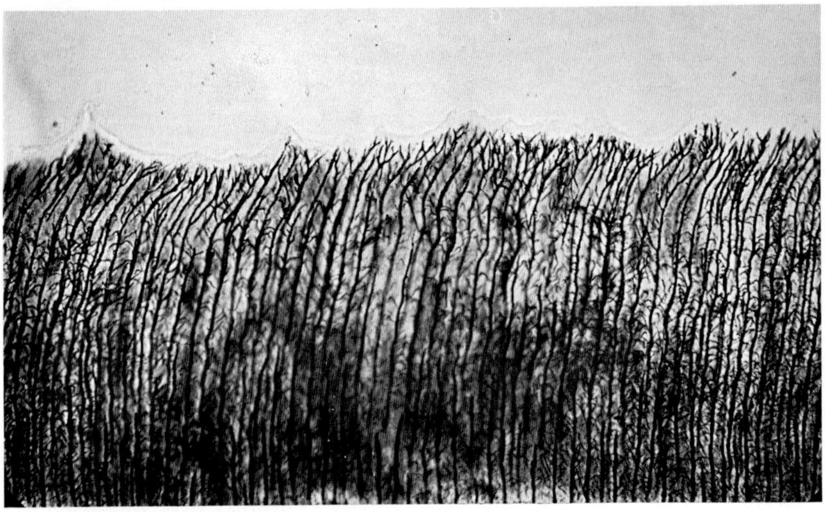

Fig. 4-1. Scalloped type of union between dentin and enamel.

dentin processes.[1] In a microscopic cross section of this area a scalloped effect is obtained (Fig. 4-1). The clinical significance of this arrangement is realized when an attempt is made to remove the enamel from a tooth that is being prepared to receive a porcelain (jacket) veneer crown. This helps to explain the difficulty experienced when denuding the coronal portion of a tooth of its enamel.

As is well known, enamel consists of globulated rods and interprismatic substance. These rods on most of the axial surfaces are usually of a uniform diameter throughout their length and generally are in a straight line from the dentinoenamel junction to the surface. In the posterior teeth, however, these rods lose their parallelism a short distance from the surface and assume a gnarled and twisted shape as they approach the dentinoenamel junction.[3] These facts are of particular significance in the cutting of enamel and in the finishing of its margins. The enamel rods are united and held together by an interprismatic substance that is more soluble than the rods and is not as strong. When pressure with a cutting instrument is applied along cleavage lines on the surface of the enamel, the rods separate quite readily, especially if the enamel is unsupported by sound dentin. While this cleavage is definite and usually extends from the surface to the dentinoenamel junction on the axial surfaces, the same conditions do not prevail in the cusp areas of bicuspids and molars; here the enamel rods are parallel for a short distance, then change into the gnarled and twisted types. These latter do not cleave easily, nor do they cut readily with a steel bur.

It is usually accepted that, once the enamel has been completely formed, it is not modified further by subjective biologic reactions; but it does respond to external chemical and physical influences.

The strength of enamel is not inherent; it is contingent upon the support received from sound dentin. Therefore, the types and designs of tooth preparations are determined not only by the direction of the enamel rods, but also by the assurance that the enamel walls rest upon sound dentin. Clinically, whenever unsupported enamel is found while preparing a tooth for a bridge retainer, the enamel is either removed or included within the metallic casting, so that it will not fracture under the forces of mastication.

Unsupported and unprotected enamel

rods are likely to break down when a cavity for a filling or a bridge retainer is filled temporarily until the permanent restoration is set. While gutta-percha and similar plastic materials have been generally advocated and used for this purpose, they do not afford the same degree of protection that is obtained from a temporary metallic casting or from a temporary metallic covering.

Unless the operator knows the general direction of the enamel rods at a cavity margin, there is some danger of breaking or injuring these rods during the fitting and burnishing processes incident to the construction of crowns or bridges.

The danger of leaving unsupported enamel rods at the margin can be avoided if the operator has an accurate knowledge of the direction of enamel rods so that the correct angle of the wall may be established and the proper bevel given to the margin (see Figs. 13-29 and 13-30).

It has been found in studying a large number of teeth, regardless of the age of the patient, that in 60 to 65 percent of all the teeth examined the cementum overlapped the margin of the enamel, in 30 percent of the teeth the margins of the enamel and cementum met, and in the remaining 5 to 10 percent there remained a slight space between the cementum and enamel. These facts are of special interest to the prosthetist planning the construction of a complete veneer crown, which may require the removal of the tooth enamel. This relates particularly to the preparation of teeth for complete veneer porcelain crowns, the so-called jacket crowns.

One group of operators recommends removing all the enamel, because it enables them to cut an accurate shoulder more easily at the correct cervical plane, to which the crown may then be accurately fitted.

Another group of operators claims that the removal of all the enamel is neither necessary nor desirable because: first, an accurate shoulder in the enamel may be made against which to finish the crown without leaving any unsupported enamel rods; second, to remove all the enamel results in injury to the soft investing tissues; third, its removal destroys more tooth structure, since the gingival margin is placed farther down on a tapering root; and finally, once all the enamel is removed, it is difficult, if not impossible, to restore the correct anatomy. The niceties of contour whose landmarks are left if some of the gingival enamel remains are said to serve as a guide in rebuilding the crown. The claims and merits of each group will be more fully appreciated when the gingival crevice and tissues are discussed.

It is to be remembered that generally the direction of the enamel rods may slope from a horizontal plane to 6 to 12° apically.

In view of the structural form of enamel its removal from the tooth may be approached clinically in three ways: first, if the enamel is undermined, by the application of a cutting instrument along the cleavage lines of the interprismatic substance; second, if the enamel is not undermined but is supported by sound dentin, by first removing the supporting dentin with burs, following which the undermined enamel is chipped off with cutting instruments; third, if the access for undermining enamel is not available and it must be obtained through cutting away its outer surface, the best means for doing so is by the use of diamond stones with high speeds in conjunction with cocoa butter and a stream of lukewarm water. Once the stone has penetrated the enamel and exposed the dentin, the cutting may be continued with carbide burs until the desired outline and preparation of the cavity are completed.

In those preparations where it is not necessary to remove the enamel entirely, the major cutting of the outer surfaces of enamel is best done by means of diamond stones properly lubricated and bathed in lukewarm water. With the advent of high-speed technics, enamel is frequently reduced using only carbide burs and a stream of water.

The dentin

A thorough understanding of the nature and distribution of dentin is likewise important to the rendering of a correct prosthetic service. As is well known, dentin is a strong connective tissue substance that is calcified, but in contradistinction to enamel the type and degree of its calcification do not leave it brittle; instead, it is a comparatively elastic substance. The body of the dentin usually determines the general form of the tooth. Dentin is penetrated by minute canals containing protoplasmic fibers that are extensions of the odontoblasts. In young dentin these minute canals are filled with a very vital and responsive protoplasmic material; whereas in old teeth, due to the process of continued calcification, these projections are calcified and very frequently obliterated entirely. The clinical significance of this lies in the fact that in the former type of dentin greater sensitiveness is experienced during operative procedures than in the latter or older types. One other factor should be remembered in connection with the distribution of the dentinal tubules: it has been shown that there are four times more tubules per square millimeter in the dentin near the pulp than there are near the peripheral surface that approximates the dentinoenamel plane. This fact may help to explain why cavities are more sensitive in proportion to the depth to which the dentin is cut and the proximity of the cavity wall to the pulp.

Not only is dentin one of the most highly specialized connective tissues in the human body, but it is also one of the most sensitive in its response to irritation. When affected by thermal, mechanical, or other stimuli, dentin has the power of laying down a secondary tissue known as secondary dentin. This is a biologic protection that dentin employs to safeguard the vitality of the pulp and to prevent its exposure.[2]

As the dentinal tubules approach the dentinoenamel region, there are extensive branchings and anastromoses[1] (Fig. 4-2). Cutting into this area containing the complex network of sensitive fibrils causes the extreme sensitiveness sometimes experienced during the preparation of teeth for retainers and crowns.

The dentinal fibrils are also affected by the exposure of dentin through decay, attrition, or abrasion reaching the dentinoenamel junction, and by the exposure of sound dentin through operative procedures.

While dentinal fibrils and their odontoblasts are irritated by the processes of abrasion or decay, this irritation is usually gradual and enables the odontoblasts and their protoplasmic extensions to react biologically to protect themselves by the simple expedient of laying down secondary dentin. On the other hand, when sound dentin is exposed during abutment preparations for inlays, partial veneer crowns, or complete veneer crowns, the exposure of dentin with its associated irritation is so sudden and intense that, before the odontoblasts have time to react by laying down protective layers of secondary dentin, the pulp may become involved and is sometimes lost.

The concept that we are dealing with a vital tissue susceptible to infection is occasionally disregarded by operators cutting and exposing sound, healthy dentin. If it is kept in mind that the exposure of the fibrils in sound dentin to the organisms of the mouth may result in infection of the pulp, greater care will be exercised to maintain surgical precautions during operative procedures.[3, 4]

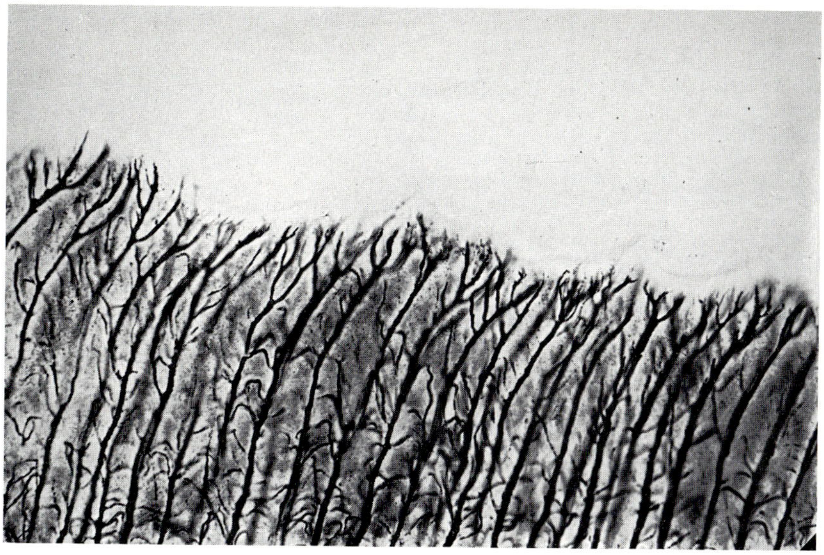

Fig. 4-2. Magnification of dentinoenamel junction showing branchings and anastomoses of dentinal tubules.

When pulps sometimes die under fillings or crowns for apparently no valid reason, the cause may be due to unprotected dentin left exposed prior to the placement of the finished restoration.

Whenever the possibility exists of involving the dentin through the presence of infection in the gingival region of a tooth, every precaution should be taken not to expose the dentin in this area. If the nature of the preparation is such that a considerable amount of dentin must be cut and exposed, the precaution of using a rubber dam should be resorted to at all times. The use of a rubber dam in the preparation of extensive carious cavities serves another purpose; during the removal of carious and infected tooth tissue, there is ample opportunity for chips and particles of infected debris to be carried back in the throat and sometimes into the air passages of the patient and the dentist with subsequent serious results. The use of a rubber dam avoids this danger.

When preparing teeth for bridge retainers or crowns, occasionally the alternative exists of leaving a small amount of carious dentin in the cavity to prevent exposure of the pulp or of removing it and thus exposing the pulp. If the latter is decided upon, the rubber dam should be applied and the pulp should be exposed and treated. It is much better to do this before the restoration is placed than sometime later, following its cementation.

Dentin should be protected, therefore, from saliva and bacterial invasions during the time that the tooth is being prepared and before the restoration is cemented. If such protection is not given the dentin, another disagreeable reaction may result; namely, the tooth becomes hypersensitive because of osmotic pressure and change in the surface tension of the cytoplasm within the tubuli. If dentin surfaces are not kept dry during the preparation of the cavity, they should be washed with 3 percent hydrogen peroxide, dried, and protected between visits of the patient. Temporary fillings or crowns cemented with zinc-oxide–eugenol cement may be employed for this purpose. If other drugs are used, only those which will not be irritating to the pulp or cause discoloration of the tooth should be employed.

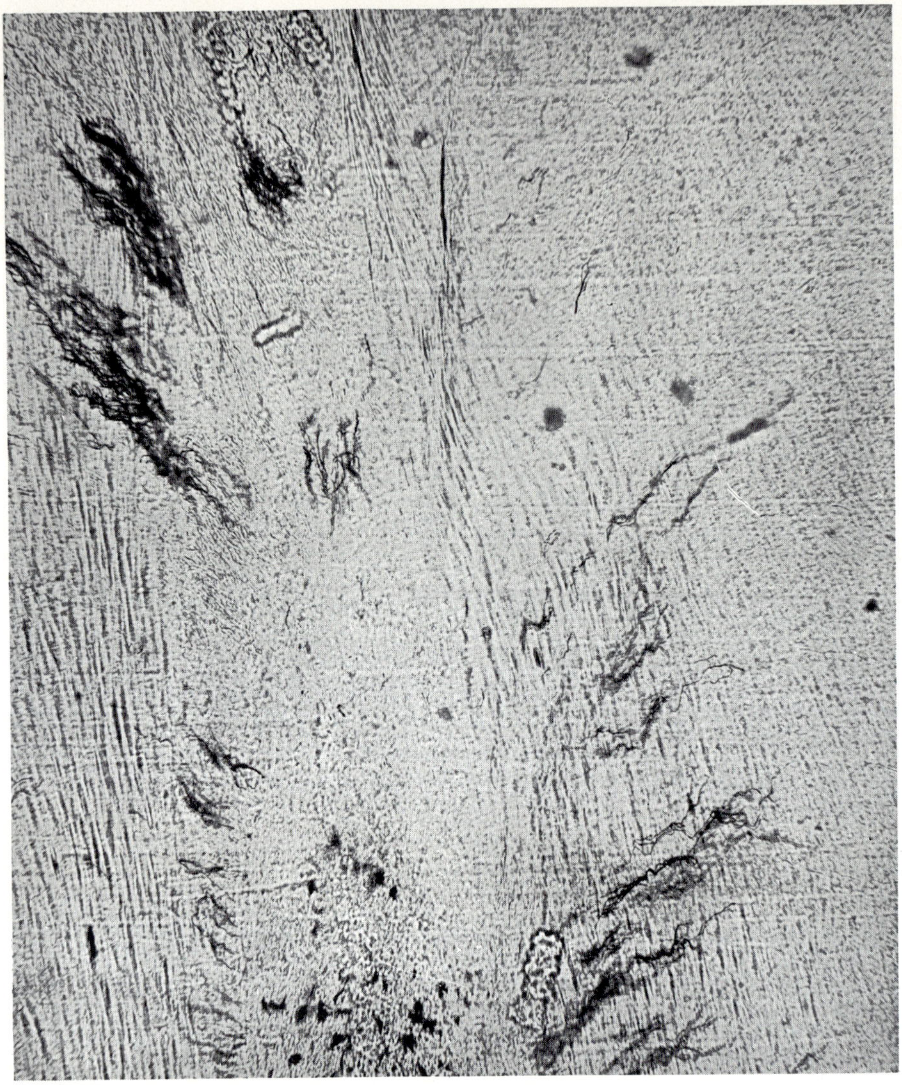

Fig. 4-3. Promiscuous distribution of dentinal tubules in opalescent dentin. (Courtesy E. Falkenstein.)

If the extent of the decay or the depth of the cavity approaches the pulp very closely, the remaining thin layer of sound dentin should be protected with a cavity lining and a thin layer of calcium hydroxide paste; over this a layer of zinc phosphate cement is flowed without pressure. This helps to seal the dentinal tubuli and helps insulate the pulp against thermal shocks caused by the metallic restoration. Zinc-oxide–eugenol paste is often used in place of calcium hydroxide.

Finally, after the tooth has been prepared, every preparation involving the dentin must have a bulk of dentin remaining of sufficient amount to withstand the forces of mastication.

It has been observed clinically that the dentin of teeth from which the pulp has been removed becomes very brittle and less elastic. Such a condition demands that certain precautions be taken in the preparation of a cavity to prevent the splitting or fracturing of the cusps. This is especially important in the posterior regions where bicuspids and molars are used as abutments for mesioclusodistal retainers. In all instances of devitalized teeth used for this type of retainer, the entire occlusal surface should be reinforced by including the buccal and lingual cusps in the casting; this additional protection will prevent fractures (see Figs. 16-15 to 16-18).

Opalescent dentin or dentinogenesis imperfecta. An unusual type of dentin is encountered on rare occasions and should be recognized when seen; it is the so-called opalescent dentin. Patients with this type of dentin have teeth that are easily recognized by their more or less translucent, bluish-gray opalescence (Plate 1). The dentin of such teeth does not possess the regularly arranged tubules found in normal dentin; instead, a microscopic section of such a tooth will reveal a promiscuous distribution of tubules throughout the mass of dentin (Fig. 4-3). It has been observed clinically that such patients are comparatively immune to caries and that there is a pronounced recession of the pulps; in addition, the teeth are worn down rapidly to the very gum line.

The cementum

Cementum retains a tooth in position by attaching the periodontal membrane fibers to its root. Cementum may be deposited on a treated tooth or on one having a vital pulp; hence, its existence and nourishment depend not on the pulp but upon the periodontal membrane. Cementum, like bone, is highly responsive to the forces and conditions of its environment; in order to meet the changing conditions, periodontal fibers are being constantly detached and new ones formed with a simultaneous laying down of new cementum that reattaches the new fibers. A characteristic of cementum is that the number of its layers is constant and that the difference in thickness of cementum in the different areas is due primarily to the varying thickness of each layer and not to the increased number of layers. As previously stated, cementum sometimes overlaps and covers the enamel at the cementoenamel junction. Primarily, the cementum covers the dentin of the root; it also extends a short distance into the apical opening. The cementum not only serves the capacity of retaining the tooth in position but also protects the dentin of the root when the latter is exposed by the recession of the investing tissues. In such cases, however, should the cementum be absent or destroyed, an area of extreme sensitivity develops.

Kronfeld[5] has made the following observations relative to cementum:

> The distribution of cementum throughout the animal kingdom varies greatly among the various species. Generally, the herbivores have thick cementum and the carnivores, thin cementum. Man occupies an intermediate position.
>
> The basic biologic difference between cementum and bone is that cementum is normally deposited continuously without resorption; whereas in bone, deposition and resorption occur simultaneously throughout life.
>
> Teeth in occlusion usually have thinner cementum than teeth without antagonists and imbedded teeth. Occasionally, cementum is distributed on the root surface in accordance with prevailing functional stress.
>
> Cementum deposition upon the enamel (coronal cementum) is frequently found in imbedded teeth. Sometimes it also occurs in the occlusal fissures of normal, unerupted teeth of children.
>
> Resorptive processes on the root surface are usually offset by cementum deposition. Such resorption may be caused by trauma, pressure, inclination or systemic disturbances.
>
> On rare occasions, a bony union (ankylosis) between alveolar process and root develops during formation of the reparative cementum following root resorption.*

The clinical significance of cementum is obvious when we remember that, if functional forces or other irritants are beyond the compensatory powers of cemen-

*From Kronfeld, R.: The biology of cementum, J.A.D.A. **25**:1451, 1938.

tum, a resorption and loosening of teeth result; on the other hand, if such irritants are not excessive, a readjustment to the new conditions is made by the deposition of secondary cementum.

The alveolar process

A thorough understanding of the character and function of the alveolar process is extremely important to successful partial denture prosthesis. These processes, supporting teeth in the mandible and the maxillae, completely surround the root and normally extend to within 2 or 3 mm. of the cementoenamel junction. For purposes of fixed partial denture retention, it is essential that abutment teeth have a normal amount and distribution of alveolar bone. Few teeth whose alveolar processes have been resorbed or reduced more than half their original heights are suitable for bridge abutments. While the cribriform and the cortical plates of the alveolar process are comparatively constant, the supporting bone or that portion of the alveolar process lying between the cribriform and cortical plates varies considerably. In normal cases favorable for fixed partial denture service the trabeculae of the cancellous bone between the cortical and cribriform plates are uniform, both in their size and distribution, and thus can absorb the forces of occlusion. In teeth out of function it will be found that the supporting bone is very sparse with arrangement of the trabeculae irregular and comparatively thin; also, the marrow spaces are enlarged. The clinical significance of the two types of alveolar process becomes apparent when it is remembered that the placing of a fixed partial denture on teeth that have been out of function for many years submits such abutments to an increased load, which may be far beyond the capacity of their endurance. When the roentgenographs and case history reveal the existence of such an impaired alveolar structural arrangement, a temporary type of fixed partial denture should be utilized to fulfill partially the functional requirements, thus subjecting the abutment teeth to a partial load only. The stimulation resulting from such a partial function will tend to develop new trabeculae oriented to meet the new forces; it will be found that the size of existing trabeculae will also increase. The very large marrow spaces underlying nonfunctioning teeth will gradually diminish until eventually the supporting bone is so rebuilt that it can conveniently withstand and transmit normal masticatory forces to the cortical plate. Concomitant with this change in the supporting bone from a nonfunctioning to a functioning tooth will be observed the changes that occur in the periodontal membrane. As later discussed, the nonfunctioning tooth has a typical narrow periodontal membrane, while a tooth in function has one that is normal and wider.

All other things being equal, it is found that the closer the crest of the alveolar process approaches the cementoenamel junction of the crown, the greater the likelihood of having a firmer and sounder abutment for a bridge.

Alveolar bone responds characteristically to different types of forces. It is known that bone reacts to undue pressure by resorption and that the response to tension is the building of new bone. When the compression is within physiologic limits, newly formed bone is of the cancellous type; when the physiologic forces are of the bending and twisting types, compact bone will be the result.

The function of bone is not only to give support to the tooth, but also to resist and counteract the transmitted forces of occlusion. The structure of the alveolar process is in harmony with its functional forces, for it is found that the cortical plate is composed of both subperiosteal and the haversian system bone. Although the cribriform plate, the so-called lamina dura, is pierced by many openings to accommodate the blood vessels, it has the characteristics of cortical bone and can be distinctly recognized in roentgenographs as a denser bone. This cribriform plate is subjected to the tensile and twisting actions of the functioning tooth in its socket; hence, it reacts with its characteristic type of bone. The supporting intervening bone, the so-called spongiosa, is the typical cancellated type that receives the pressure transferred from the cribriform to the cortical plates of bone.

Alveolar bone is extremely sensitive to any changes in the magnitude or direction of transmitted forces. When teeth are to be subjected to new forces (for example, when a bridge is placed), it must be definitely established that the character of the supporting bone is such that it will be able to withstand and counteract the newly imposed forces. If not, the restoration will fail with the failure of the abutment.

It is recalled that pressure is exerted against the buccal and the labial cortical plates in the upper arch, while tension is exerted on the lingual. Hence, the response to tension results in a larger bulk of bone on the lingual aspect of the upper teeth. Finally, it must be remembered that the vitality and the ability of bone to respond to new stimuli decrease with age, and consequently the biologic efficiency is likely to decrease in its ability to meet the mechanical requirements of fixed bridges in older patients.

NONCALCIFIED DENTAL TISSUE

The pulp

A most important consideration in placing prosthetic restorations on vital teeth is to preserve the normal condition of the pulp. Any procedure or technic that jeopardizes the health of the pulp should not be employed. Since the pulp is located centrally within the body of the tooth, it cannot expand beyond the limiting walls of dentin. The fact that the nerves, arteries, and veins of the pulp enter through a small apical foramen exposes the pulp to certain dangers. Since the primary sensation of the pulp is sensory, it responds very definitely to sudden temperature changes. This range of temperature response extends from 68° F. and below to 122° F. and above. If a pathologic pulp condition exists, the response is more acute. This response to temperature change is utilized in testing pulp conditions.

When an irritant, be it thermal, chemical, or otherwise, is applied to the pulp, the arteries dilate and an increased amount of blood enters the pulp. So long as the veins are capable of carrying off this excess supply of blood from the pulp chamber, no harm results; but, if the pressure becomes so great that the lumina of the veins at the root end become constricted to the extent that the outflow of the venous blood is prevented, congestion, degeneration, and necrosis of the pulp may ensue. Serious damage rarely results from an occasional mild, hyperemic reaction of the pulp; however, danger exists with a sudden, intense irritation or a chronic condition, which results in a lowered tone of the tissues and the inability of the blood vessels to resume their normal functions even after the irritation has subsided.

Irritants to pulp. Hildebrand[6] has pointed out four possible irritants that might definitely affect the pulp: (1) the mechanical, which is incidental to the grinding of tooth structure; (2) the thermal, which may be produced by the heat generated during the grinding and preparation of teeth or by contacting liquids of extremely high or low temperatures; (3) the chemical irritation produced by drugs, saliva, and various ingredients in food; and (4) the bacteria that may affect the pulp by invading the dentinal tubuli exposed by caries or by dental operations. He also includes in this group the effect of anesthetics on the vessels of the pulp, and the continuous thermal shocks caused by large metallic fillings placed too close to the pulp. Degenerative changes in the pulp are attributable in a large number of cases to this particular factor.

The normality of the pulp or the degree of its deviation from the normal should be established before undertaking restorative treatment for a patient. A pulp is usually normal clinically if it exhibits no signs of pain and is covered by sound tooth structure. It should give a definite response to electrical and thermal tests and should not disclose any pathologic condition roentgenographically. Three varieties of the abnormal pulp are possible; namely, the hyperemic, the inflamed, and the necrotic.

Serious injury from mechanical trauma may result to the pulp if a filling, crown, or bridge is not in correct occlusal relationship with its opposing teeth. If such a condition is permitted to continue, there will be a breakdown of the periodontal membrane and very frequently the pulp will become involved, necessitating its removal. Therefore, all restorations, whether of the individual or the multiple unit types, should be checked not only in centric relationship, but also in all the lateral movements of the mandible. This can be done either by the use of carbon ribbon or by casts properly oriented on an adjustable articulator. The high points will be disclosed as carbon marks or as perforations in the wax bite, indicating premature initial occlusal contacting areas.

The shock that a pulp undergoes from mechanical irritation during the cutting of tooth tissue and the severity of the pulpal reaction have not been definitely determined as yet. However, we do know that changes occur in both the dentin and the pulp whenever dentin is exposed to saliva either by the process of attrition or by cutting it with stones and burs. Pulpal reaction may be less severe in older patients than in younger ones, due to the presence of secondary dentin in the former. Therefore, in preparing teeth for crowns or bridge retainers, extreme care should be exercised not to cut deeply or to cut more tooth structure than is necessary to secure sufficient mechanical retention. Irritation of this type can be largely alleviated by the use of sharp cutting instruments and stones that are true. This is more fully discussed in Chapter 15.

Pulp protection. After the tooth preparation is completed, the exposed dentin surfaces should be dried and a eugenol dressing applied for a few seconds. The oil is then volatilized, the cavity is again dried, and the dentin portion of the cavity is given an application of a thin solution of cavity varnish. Only a sufficient amount should be used to seal the dentinal tubules against the ingress of saliva and bacteria. If the cavity has not been kept dry during its preparation, it must be mechanically cleaned with pumice and brush, washed with hydrogen peroxide and normal saline solution, and dried with cotton prior to the application of the varnish. Many methods of sterilization are advocated; some suggest the use of phenol followed by alcohol; others advocate the use of silver nitrate precipitated with eugenol on posterior teeth. Many feel that wiping the dry cavity with eugenol followed by cavity varnish is sufficient. Evidence from all studies and research to date indicates there is no proved method of dentin sterilization other than the superficial layer. If all carious dentin is removed to sound, calcified dentin, bacteria still in the dentinal tubuli lie dormant or die when the filling is cemented in the tooth.

Sometimes extreme sensitiveness develops after cementing a large filling or a crown on a tooth with a vital pulp. To alleviate such a condition the precaution may be taken of adding one drop of eugenol to the cement liquid prior to mixing with the powder. In most occurrences of mild hyperemia such conditions will subside and the patient again will be able to use the restoration in comfort and with no danger to the health of the pulp. Harm may also result in the final step of the service; therefore, care must be exercised while using finishing strips and disks not to develop frictional heat to the point of irritating the pulp; a stream of air or water will mitigate this condition.

A safe rule to follow is to so plan one's work that once a tooth is cut into, the preparation is completed during the same sitting. When a partially prepared tooth is worked on several times before being completed, it will be found that with each succeeding visit the tooth becomes more sensitive. This condition develops even if a temporary filling is carefully sealed in the cavity, because the pressure of a semi-plastic filling material in the cavity presses against the terminal endings of the dentinal fibrils and sets up an irritating reaction in the odontoblasts and the pulp.

Pulp reactions to irritants. When a pulp is subjected to severe shock, the possibility exists that this may be the beginning of its subsequent degeneration, inflammation, and death, even if at the time of cementation it apparently recovers its normal condition.

With all precautions taken during the preparation of a tooth to eliminate the possibility of either mechanical or thermal irritations, the danger still remains of irritating the pulp chemically Van Huysen and Gurley[9] have shown that, if only half the normal thickness of healthy dentin is removed and the surfaces are exposed to the fluids of the mouth for a short time, a cellular infiltration of the pulp periphery occurs. Their experiments indicate that not only are the dentin and odontoblastic layers disturbed, but there is also an increase in the cell contents of the pulp. They also observed that the closer the cavity approached the pulp, the more severe was the reaction following exposure to saliva.

The chemical irritant to which the pulp is exposed most frequently results from the improper mixing and use of cement. This occurs either in cementing the restoration or in placing a protective base over the pulpal wall, as in the case of deep caries. In order to minimize pulpal reaction to cement, the prepared tooth or cavity should never be dehydrated prior to cementing a restoration. The use of choloroform or alcohol for the drying of cavities is contraindicated. When alcohol is used, in addition to the irritation caused by dehydration of the dentin and the dentinal fibrils, a spongelike cavity surface that absorbs the excess cement liquid is left; thus the pulp is exposed to a double irritation.

The cavity should not be dehydrated, but only dried with cotton pellets and gentle puffs of warm air very briefly. The cement should be so mixed that there is a correct proportion of powder and the cement liquid; it should be mixed slowly and thoroughly on a slab that has been chilled in order to dissipate the heat generated during the mixing process. Many a pulp has been injured not only by the excess liquid in the cement but also by the intense heat resulting from an excessively rapid mixing technic. If excess liquid is left in the cement, that amount remaining after crystallization has taken place will be absorbed by the cytoplasm of the dentinal fibrils; this results in their degeneration and eventually in the impairment of the odontoblasts. In those cases, therefore, in which a cavity extends deeply and closely to the pulp, it is well to treat the dentin before cementation, either by painting the cavity with some enduring varnish or with a solution of chloroform and rosin. For further protection a layer of thick thymolized calcium phosphate paste made with eugenol is sometimes placed. This not only acts as an obtundant and insulator, but it also helps to seal the ends of the dentinal tubules.

A pulp may be exposed to chemical irritation even though the tooth structure has not been cut. Such a condition exists in the presence of excessive gingival recession that exposes the cementum of the tooth. In all such areas where the cementum is very thin or lacking, the exposed dentin may result in a severe pulp reaction when it is exposed to the chemical agents found in some foods.

The fourth possibility of pulp irritation results from exposure to bacteria. Authorities do not entirely agree on (1) whether bacteria invade the dentinal tubules when the dentin is exposed to the saliva or (2) whether they are present only superficially on the surface. It is claimed that bacteria do not penetrate dentin unless the tooth structure is decalcified in advance. In either case the danger of infection is present and, since the danger exists in the proportion that the number of bacteria are present as compared to the relative resistance of the patient, it is good policy to eliminate, or at least to reduce, the number of bacteria present on the surface of a cavity prior to setting an inlay or a crown. On the posterior teeth, where a possible discoloration of tooth structure would not be so objectionable, some recommended the use of silver nitrate precipitated with eugenol; others recommend the use of 30 percent H_2O_2 or liquefied phenol followed by an alcohol wash. It is claimed that these are self-limiting and therefore involve only the protoplasmic ends of the dentinal fibrils. When possible, the best method is to operate in such a way as not to infect the exposed dentin with saliva. In any event, either after sterilization or when clean surfaces are present, it is best to paint all exposed dentinal surfaces with a thin cavity varnish. This seals the tubules against the possible ingress of bacteria.

Whenever the preparation involves a cusp or the incisal edge of a tooth, a certain danger to the pulp also exists. We find that in younger patients the pulpal horns extend occlusally and incisally to a higher level than in similar teeth in older people. In the latter, secondary dentin causes the recession of the pulpal horns, and consequently there is less danger of accidentally exposing them during operative procedures. The age of the patient and the radiographs may serve as guides in guarding the pulp against accidental exposures.

The periodontal membrane (ligament)

The function of the peridontal membrane is such that it has been called the foundation of all restorative dentistry. In order to evaluate its importance, it is necessary only to recognize its sensory, vital, and physical functions. As is well known, the periodontal membrane is the tissue located between the alveolar socket wall and root of the tooth; it also extends coronally into the area of the gingivae. While each of its structural elements is important, the arrangement and functions of the periodontal fibers are of more immediate concern.

The mistaken notion sometimes exists that, because the tooth is capable of movement in its socket, it is suspended by elastic fibers. This "give" in the periodontal membrane is not due to the elasticity of fibers, but to the straightening out of the wavy, inelastic fibers when force is applied to them. When the force is removed, these fibers recoil to their original shape and length due to the resultant stresses developed within them by the applied force.

One of the important groups of principal fibers to the prosthetist is the free gingival group. It is this group of fibers that keeps the gingivae in close apposition to the crown or bridge; it is important, therefore, not to injure or sever these fibers during the preparation of a tooth.

It is a fact that periodontal membrane

fibers possess their characteristic arrangement as the result of functional forces rather than in anticipation of any unusual forces; when the direction or degree of force is changed, the periodontal fibers readjust themselves to meet the changed conditions.

Attaching the root to the alveolar bone is only one function of the periodontal membrane; another and equally important one is to sustain and dissipate the stresses that result from the forces of mastication. The oblique group of fibers offers the main resistance to these forces. These fibers are capable of withstanding excessive pound pressure per square inch, provided the pressure is directed in the direction of the vertical axis of the tooth, resulting in a tensile and not in a crushing force on the peridontal fibers. Horizontal or lateral forces exceeding physiologic limits produce compression and crushing of the soft tissues between the tooth and the bone with subsequent resorption of bone and necrosis of soft tissues. If the damage sustained is not excessive or recurrent, nature usually repairs the harm done by rebuilding and reattaching new tissues so that normal functions may continue.

Obviously, if all the groups of periodontal fibers are intact and function properly, the tooth is held more firmly in its position, yet a wire-spoke wheel based on a similar principle of torque distribution functions with only a slight impairment when several wire spokes are missing; on the other hand, misapplied lateral forces have ruined perfectly good wheels.

The width or the thickness of the periodontal membrane is relatively wide or narrow depending upon the use or disuse of the tooth. It has been found that in a tooth subjected to normal function the thickness of the periodontal membrane varies from 0.20 to 0.25 mm. in thickness. In those instances in which the occlusion is unusually strong, the thickness may increase to 0.35 mm. On the other hand, when a tooth is out of occlusion and not in function, the periodontal membrane is reduced to half the width of a normal one, sometimes reaching a thickness of only 0.10 mm. These changes in the periodontal membrane are usually concurrent with the changes in the alveolar bone previously described in this chapter. This reduction in the width of the periodontal membrane in nonfunctioning teeth is accomplished by additions of new cementum layers on the root surface.

When a nonfunctioning tooth with a narrow membrance is restored and placed back into function, it is found, after a period of use, that the normal, physiologic width of the periodontal membrane is restored. From the clinical standpoint, care should be taken in placing a large restoration, such as a fixed bridge, to make certain that too great a load is not suddenly imposed upon the periodontal membrane. Should excessive force or unusual lateral force be exerted upon such a tooth, the danger exists of crushing the membrane between the root and the alveolar bone, thus defeating the purpose of the restoration.

Another item of clinical importance relates to the width of the periodontal membrane at different root levels. The center of rotation of a single-rooted tooth in function is located apically from the middle portion of the root; an examination of a histologic section of this tissue will show that the periodontal space is narrower in this area, while the greatest widths of the membrane are located in the regions of the alveolar margin and the root end. Occasions arise in both operative and prosthetic operations to separate teeth in order to gain access to the proximal surfaces. If mechanical separation is obtained by the use of separators, extreme care must be exercised. In separating the contact areas of anterior teeth beyond 0.30 mm., there is great danger of crushing the periodontal membrane in the apical and gingival third regions; the width of the membrane in a normally functioning tooth rarely exceeds 0.20 to 0.30 mm. For this reason we believe that a method of slow separation is preferable to the rapid mechanical one.

The correct concept of the function of the periodontal membrane is not that of a cushion interposed between the root and the alveolar process to receive and distribute pressure forces; rather, it is the concept of the root being suspended in a limitless number of expansive, bellow-like springs oriented in different groups and in different locations. These receive pressure forces from the tooth and convert them into those of tension on the alveolar bone. It is this tension that acts as the stimulating factor in maintaining and building a healthy new alveolar process. While individual fiber bundles may extend from the cementum to the lamina dura, a more recent concept suggests that fibers extend toward each other from each side, meeting midway to form a plexus bundle in the membrane.

In its adaptation to functional changes the periodontal membrane, like all other tissues, responds more readily and more favorably in young patients than in older ones; this is an important consideration when planning fixed partial dentures for elderly patients. What might be a favorable indication for prosthesis in the mouth of a young person would be contraindicated in an older one.

The gums and gingivae

The gums and gingivae are closely related to the success or failure of any prosthesis. Although the chief function of these tissues is the protection of the underlying tissues, they have other characteristics that must be recognized and properly related. Without going into the histologic structure of gum tissue covering an edentulous ridge, it is recognized that two general types exist: (1) the thin, tightly drawn, unyielding type of mucosa, and (2) the thick, yielding, softer type. These distinctions should be carefully determined, because the technic employed when constructing pontics differs for each type. (See Chapter 30.)

Occasions arise when the type of tissue covering a ridge is modified by surgical means.

The location where the firm and comparatively immovable gum tissue blends into the movable oral mucosa of the cheeks and lips should be determined. This area indicates the position of the gingival limit of the pontics.

It is generally recognized that the soft tissues of the mouth heal very readily when subjected to traumatic injury; this is due to their high vascularity.

The gum tissues, in the presence of teeth, assume a specialized form around the cervices of the teeth; these are the so-called gingivae.[11] The gingivae, by their position, not only serve to protect the teeth against infection, but also help to maintain them in their proper position in the arch.

Epithelial attachment. The structure and relationship of the gingivae and their related parts have been the subject of much discusion in recent years. While formerly it was generally believed that the epithelium of the gingivae was attached to the tooth around the cementoenamel junction, the more recent and accepted concept indicates that the epithelium is attached to the enamel and extends to the cementoenamel junction at the time the tooth erupts. Instead of a space existing from the crest of the gingiva to the cementoenamel junction, an epithelial band is present that is attached to the enamel from its cementoenamel junction to a point incisally near the crest of the gingivae. This so-called epithelial attachment is in contact with the enamel. Whether this is an organic union or merely an intimate apposition is still being investigated (Plate 2).

Passive and active eruption. As is generally accepted, when the tooth germ perforates the mucous membrane of the oral cavity, the enamel epithelium and the oral epithelium unite while the tooth enters the oral cavity. The marginal epithelium is therefore of a dual origin. As the tooth continues to erupt into the oral cavity, more and more of the enamel epithelium separates from the enamel surface. This growth or so-called passive eruption of the tooth into the oral cavity is comparatively rapid until such time as it meets an opposing tooth. When this occurs, its eruption is slowed down. This increased lengthening of the crown of a tooth into the oral cavity by the progressive detachment of epithelium from the enamel is generally designated as the passive eruption of a tooth. There also exists the so-called active eruption of a tooth; this consists of a definite, bodily movement of the tooth in the direction of occlusion.

In the early stages of passive eruption the epithelial attachment is wide gingivo-incisally, but this gradually decreases in width as the eruption continues. When the detachment of the epithelium approaches the cementoenamel junction, there is a proliferation of the epithelial cells that grow apically along the cementum. The detachment of the epithelium from the enamel surface is concurrent with the downward growth of the epithelium along the tooth apically. From a prosthetic standpoint, it is well to remember that the detachment occurs at different levels in different areas around the circumference of a tooth.

Gingival crevice. Orban has defined the gingival crevice as "the space limited on one side by the enamel or enamel cuticle, and on the other by the epithelium."[12] The bottom, therefore, is the lowest point in the separation of these two tissues. Since the depth of the crevice may vary in its different locations, it is possible for the epithelial attachment to be in contact with the enamel in one area and with the cementum in another. Clinically, it is important to know that the height of the gingival tissues depends largely upon the height of the epithelial attachment.

Epithelial detachment. If the passive eruption of a tooth is normal, the depth of the gingival crevice should be very small or practically zero. If eruption is slow, it is generally regarded as a normal, physiologic process; whereas if the eruption is unduly rapid, it may be a pathologic one. The studies of Gottlieb and of Orban[12, 13] indicate that there are at least four stages in the passive eruption of a tooth. These correspond roughly to certain age groups. The first stage exists where the epithelium is in contact with the enamel and extends to the cementoenamel junction; we find this condition in young patients and frequently in those up to the age of 25 years. The second group, including individuals from 25 to 35 years of age, still has some epithelial attachment to the enamel, but a proliferation of the epithelium has also extended apically along the root on the cementum. The third group, which is rather rare, has the epithelium entirely detached from the enamel to the cementoenamel line, and the epithelium extends from this line apically along the cementum of the root. In those patients from 35 to 40 years of age and older a fourth stage exists in which a space exists between the cementoenamel junction and the attachment of the epithelium to the root. In the latter stage the cementum of the root is exposed to the oral fluids.

The figures given for the different age groups are approximate ones, for very frequently the fourth state of epithelial detachment may be found in patients 20 years of age or younger; then again, patients of 45 and 50 years of age exhibit types 1 and 2 of epithelial attachments. There are no definite data or figures for the rate of epithelial detachment from the tooth surface. Apparently, the maintenance of dental health and function depends upon gradual rather than rapid exposure of tooth surface; the slower this process occurs, the more favorable is the condition of the tooth.

While the average amount of detachment has been determined for the various age groups, it would be valuable to the prosthodontist to know the speed and amount of detachment that occurs from the time a tooth comes into occlusion to the ages of 45 or 50 years. Accepting the passive eruption theory in its entirety without knowing the rate of eruption, the circumstances, and the environment influencing this rate of eruption has its serious aspects. The impression is sometimes gained by students and dentists that, irrespective of the varying conditions found in different mouths, the rate of eruption is so rapid and so alterable that the exposure of gingival margins in all restorations is inevitable within a short time. As a matter of record and observation, passive eruption and its clinical evidences are practically nil in most mouths.

Position of gingival margin. The question is often asked: "Where should the gingival margin of an inlay or a crown be placed with reference to the adjacent soft tissues?" One group advocates a position slightly above the crest of the gingivae; another, at the crest; while still another suggests that it be carried below the crest of the gum tissue. Furthermore, the last group questions: "Just how far below?"

It is claimed that the placing of the margin below the crest of the gum tissue in young patients will result in the detachment of the epithelial attachment, which may result in the damage and infection of these tissues. On the other hand, it is pointed out that teeth erupt continuously and that eventually every submerged margin becomes exposed. It is said that the eruption of teeth does not stop during any period of life, but that it is only slowed down when the teeth come into occlusion. These facts place the dentist more or less in a dilemma. First, in order to obtain esthetic results, it is necessary to place the margins of crowns beneath the crest of the gum tissue; second, even though the margins are placed beneath the crest, because of the continuous eruption of teeth, the margins soon become exposed and consequently ruin the esthetic effect originally developed.

Nevertheless, numerous clinicians and dentists who have practiced for many years can produce clinical evidence that the margin of a filling or crown previously placed beneath the crest of the gum tissue 20 to 45 years ago maintains the same relationship today. If the eruption of the teeth is as irresistible and as constant as is sometimes implied, these margins should have become exposed in almost every instance; but this they have not done.

It is recommended, therefore, in those patients past the age of 25 years that the gingival margins of restorations be placed beneath the crest of the gum tissue. The level at which this line lies is *midway* between the crest of the gingivae and the deepest portion of its gingival crevice. If, however, the occasion does arise that a fixed bridge must be placed for a young patient having an epithelial attachment on the enamel, and if the exposed portion of the crown is sufficiently long to afford enough retention without carrying the preparation below the crest of the gum tissue, the margin of the crown is placed *at or slightly above* the gingival crest. If, however, the alternative exists either of detaching the epithelium or of not being able to obtain sufficient mechanical retention, we may be forced, of necessity, to extend the margin to a depth where sufficient retention can be obtained, even if in doing so the epithelium attachment is slightly detached. This, however, will occur rarely and should be avoided if possible.

The gingival crevice has been largely overemphasized from the standpoint of prosthetic restorative service. First, we find that fixed partial denture service is indicated mainly for patients between the ages of 20 and 55 years, and in most of these the epithelial detachment extends apically beyond the cementoenamel junction. Second, Orban[12] has found that in over 55 percent of all patients the depth of the crevice is 0.50 mm. or more, and the average depth of the gingival crevice is 0.80 mm.

Some have suggested placing the gingival margins of all restorations, fillings, or crowns above the crest of the gingivae for the following reasons: first, there is no danger of detaching the epithelial attachment; second, the subgingival space or crevice is not an immune area; and third, even if the margin is placed beneath the crest of the gingivae, the passive eruption of the tooth in a short time will again expose the margin.

Let us consider these points in their respective order. It is granted that in patients 20 years of age or younger it is normally inadvisable to extend the gingival margins apically. Prosthetic restorations for a young patient are usually of a temporary character and will be replaced at maturity. Excluding the esthetic factors, the reason for staying above the gingival crest is not so much the fear of epithelial detachment as it is the desire to avoid extensive cutting of the tooth and the possible involvement of the pulp. In adult patients, in whom the average gingival crevice is almost 1 mm. in depth, by employing a careful technic to depress the gingival tissues prior to tooth preparation and the placement of a crown, it is found that the gingival tissues again will resume and maintain their former position, leaving the margins of the restoration beneath the crest of the gingivae.

A carefully developed technic will enable the dentist to place his margins very safely from 0.50 to 0.60 mm. beneath the crest of the gingivae.

Research data have indicated and clinical evidence has verified the fact that the passive eruption of the tooth is very slow after the teeth have come into occlusion. Since the large percentage of patients requiring partial denture service is in the group whose epithelial attachment has gone beyond the cementoenamel junction, it is apparent that little, if any, danger exists of gingival injury in the average normal mouth.

Furthermore, the gingival margins of fillings and crowns are placed below the crest of the gingivae not because of any possible immunity associated with this area, but because the area immediately at the gingival crest is likely to be much more susceptible to caries. The subgingival crest margins of restorations properly contoured and finished have maintained a normal tissue relationship for many years without any apparent injurious effects. Moreover, the placing of the margin of a restoration above the crest of the gingivae may afford a margin or shoulder where food debris is caught. Hence, it is advisable to terminate the restoration approximately halfway between the crest of the gingivae and the bottom of the crevice, except in those restorations in which a margin is carried occlusally into an area of immunity.

Granting that a submerged margin may be exposed eventually, there are instances in which esthetic factors demand the placing of the margin in an invisible location. In these circumstances, even in younger patients, we have no alternative except to extend the margins below the crest of the gingivae. The exposure of the gingival margin of a restoration and the speed with which it occurs depend on the contour of the restoration, the relationship established between it and its neighbor, the finish of its margins, and the occlusal relationship established with its opposing teeth. If, then, after many years of satisfactory service, it is necessary to remake a restoration because the gingival margin is exposed, it is still possible to do so without any harm to the tooth.

SELECTED REFERENCES

1. Tylman, S. D.: The dentino-enamel junction, J. Dent. Res. **8**:615, 1928.
2. Diamond, D. D., Stanley, H. R., and Swerdlow, H.: Reparative dentin formation resulting from cavity preparation, J. Prosth. Dent. **16**:1127-1134, 1966.
3. Bender, I. B., Selzer, S., and Kaufman, I. J.: Infectibility of the dental pulp by way of dental tubules, J.A.D.A. **59**:466, 1959.
4. Fusayama, T., Higaki, T., and Uehara, C.: The directions of the enamel rods in central longitudinal sections throughout all kinds of permanent teeth, Bull. Tokyo Medical and Dental University **3**:43, 1956.
5. Kronfeld, R.: The biology of cementum, J.A.D.A. **25**:1451, 1938.
6. Hildebrand, G. Y.: Studies in dental prosthetics, Stockholm, 1937, Aktiebolaget Fahlcrantz' Boktryckeri, vol. 1.
7. Kesel, R. G., and Stephan, R. M.: Pathology and protection of the dental pulp in partial denture construction, J.A.D.A. **21**:1022, 1934.
8. Henschel, C. J.: Pain control by cold control, D. Digest **47**:444, 1941.
9. Van Huysen, G., and Gurley, W. B.: Histologic changes in the teeth of dogs following preparation of cavities of various depths and their exposure to oral fluids, J.A.D.A. **26**:87, 1939.
10. Wheeler, R. C.: A comparison of periodontal attachment levels: antero-posteriorly, D. Digest **41**:261, 1935.
11. Hagerman, D. A., and Arnim, S. S.: The relation of new knowledge of the gingiva to crown and bridge procedures, J. Prosth. Dent. **5**:538, 1955.
12. Orban, B.: Dental histology and embryology, Chicago, 1928, Rogers Printing Co.
13. Gottlieb, B., and Orban, B.: Biology and pathology of the tooth and supporting mechanism, New York, 1938, The Macmillan Company.

GENERAL REFERENCES

Boyne, P. J.: Osseous repair of the postextraction alveolus in man, Oral Surg. **21**:805-813, 1966.

Brannstrom, M.: Sensitivity of dentine, Oral Surg. **21**:517-526, 1966.

Cran, J. A.: Development of the gingival sulcus, Aust. Dent. J. **11**(5):322-328, 1966.

Frithiof, L., and Wersall, J.: A highly ordered structure in keratinizing human oral epithelium, J. Ultrastruct. Res. **12**:371-379, 1965.

Hashimoto, K., DiBella, R. J., and Shklar, G.: Electronmicroscopic studies of the normal human buccal epithelium, J. Invest. Derm. **47**:512-525, 1966.

Innes, P. B., and Shroff, F. R.: Orientation of the crystallites in the surface layer of human enamel, J. Dent. Res. **47**:1029, 1968.

Meyer, J., and Gerson, S. J.: A comparison of human palatal and buccal mucosa, Periodontics **2**:284-291, 1964.

Osborn, J. W.: Directions and interrelationship of prisms in cuspal and cervical enamel of human teeth, J. Dent. Res. **47**(3):395, 1968.

Osborn, J. W.: Three-dimensional reconstructions of enamel prisms, J. Dent. Res. **46**:1412-1420, 1967.

Richardson, E. R.: Comparative thickness of the human periodontal membrane of functioning versus nonfunctioning teeth, J. Oral Med. **22**:120-126, 1967.

Rivault, M. A., and Tabet, G.: Comparison between fixed and removable-fixed prostheses, Int. Dent. J. **18**:251, 1968.

Roucoules, L.: Biology and prosthetics, IV: biophysiologic principles; V: practical applications, Inform. Dent. **48**(46):4541-4555, 1966.

Schultz-Haudt, S. D.: The dento-gingival junction: a review, Mechanisms Tooth Support (Symp.) (Bristol) 33-37, 1967.

Selvig, K. A.: The fine structure of human cementum, Acta Odont. Scand. **23**:423-441, 1965.

Sicher, H.: Orban's oral histology and embryology, ed. 6, St. Louis, 1966, The C. V. Mosby Co.

Silverman, S.: Ultrastructure studies of oral mucosa, I: comparison of normal and hyperkeratotic human buccal epithelium, J. Dent. Res. **46**(6):1804-1809, 1967.

Soni, N. N., Van Huysen, G., and Swenson, H. M.: A microradiographic and x-ray densitometric study of cementum, J. Periodont. **33**:372-378, 1962.

Turck, D.: A histologic comparison of the edentulous denture and non-denture bearing tissues, J. Prosth. Dent. **15**:419-434, 1965.

Zwarych, P. D.: The adaptation of the microstructure of dental tissues to occlusal stress, Penn. Dent. J. (Phila.) **69**:10-14, 1965.

Chapter 5

Anatomy of the stomatognathic system related to crown and fixed partial prosthodontic therapy*

The stomatognathic system may be defined as the combined structures of the mouth and jaws. It includes the upper and lower teeth, hard and soft palate, tongue, cheeks, maxillae, mandible, temporomandibular joint, and the muscles that move the mandible. All of these structures are either directly or indirectly involved in the diagnosis of occlusal and dental restorative problems. The dentist must have an understanding of the detailed anatomy and function of the stomatognathic system if he is to maximize his success in dental diagnosis and treatment planning. In this chapter, emphasis will be placed on stomatognathic anatomy.

The temporomandibular joint demonstrates the correlation of structure and function in a manner that cannot be exceeded by any other joint in the body. These paired joints allow a remarkable freedom of motion of the mandible and still serve to guide and, in some positions, to limit its movement. When one is studying functional positions of the mandible he must consider the fact that the medial structures of one joint are reinforced by the lateral structures of the opposite joint, and vice versa. The temporomandibular joint does not function as a ball and socket joint but it articulates as a ball on a hill. The condyle most closely approximates and functions against the posterior incline, the crest, and, in some patients, the anterior incline of the articular eminence. It does not function against the depth or posterior incline of the glenoid fossa. As shown in Fig. 5-1, the articular surface of the glenoid fossa extends from a point anterior to the crest of the eminence to the squamotympanic fissure. This articular surface is not cartilage but is comprised of a fibrous protein, collagen. The collagen fibers in the articular surface are specifically arranged so that they exit from the bony surface perpendicular to

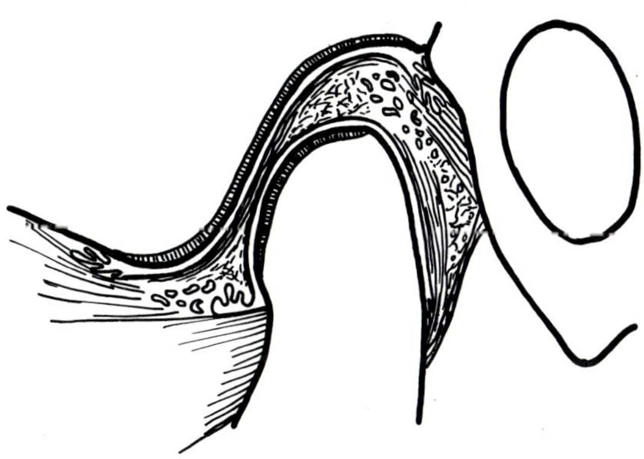

Fig. 5-1. Sagittal section through medial half of human temporomandibular joint.

*Text by Parker E. Mahan, D.D.S., Ph.D., F.A.C.D.; Associate Professor of Dentistry, Emory University School of Dentistry, Atlanta, Georgia.

that surface and then turn 90 degrees to run parallel to the surface. This arrangement of fibers is admirably suited to withstand forces of friction during translation of the condyle. It has been demonstrated that, in the healthy temporomandibular joint, the meniscus is tightly attached to the condyle at its medial and lateral poles and that translation occurs in the superior cavity of the joint.[1] The superior surface of the meniscus therefore glides across the articular surface of the eminence and glenoid fossa.

The superior cavity is lined at its periphery by a synovial membrane, which secretes the small amount of synovial fluid that lubricates the cavity. In the anterior and posterior of the cavity the synovial villi are arranged in long folds extending from medial to lateral. When the condyle translates down onto the eminence the villi in the posterior of the cavity unfold to allow the meniscus to translate with the condyle. Lymphatic capillaries are associated with the synovial villi and function to provide the aqueous phase of the synovial fluid.

The meniscus of the healthy temporomandibular joint does not contain cartilage but is comprised of collagen. The collagen fibers of the meniscus are oriented anteroposteriorly in the superior surface and anterior portion but run in all three directions in space and are enmeshed together so as to provide a flexible and yet very strong pad in the posterior portion just above the condyle.[2] The medial half of the anterior border of the meniscus is attached to the superior belly of the lateral pterygoid muscle. When sectioned in the sagittal plane the anterior portion of the meniscus is shaped like a foot with a heel, as shown in Fig. 5-1. The foot portion contains many blood vessels and Golgi tendon organs. Batson[3] has described a venous plexus that surrounds the periphery of the meniscus in which blood can be shunted back and forth during function to partially compensate for the volume vacated by the condyle. The central part of the meniscus lying between the posterior slope of the eminence and the condyle and that part over the medial pole of the condyle are very thin. Zola[4] has found the thickness in these areas to be only 0.4 to 0.2 mm., depending on the force applied to the vernier gauge. This indicates that the medial pole and anterior slope of the condyle may approximate the temporal bone very closely during function. The portion of the meniscus located just superior to the condyle is thicker than the central portion and, in the adult, is avascular. Just posterior to this region the meniscus bends down posteriorly over the condyle and contains a very rich vascular network. Griffin and Sharpe[5] have demonstrated that this vascular knee contains glomus cell anastamoses connecting the small arteries and veins. At the vascular knee the meniscus forms two distinct strata of connective tissue fibers separated by loose areolar tissue. The superior stratum of this bilaminar zone is very rich in elastin and is attached to the tympanic plate of the temporal bone. The protein, elastin, is a truely elastic fiber that will assume its initial length when applied tension is released. It is, in fact, essential that the attachment of the meniscus to the tympanic plate be loose or elastic if the meniscus translates forward with the condyle. The inferior stratum of the bilaminar zone is comprised mainly of collagen and it attaches to the posterior aspect of the neck of the condylar process. Since the mensicus in the healthy joint moves with the condyle there is no need for elasticity or laxity in this attachment of the meniscus. The collagen capsule of the joint extends from the condylar attachment of the inferior stratum to the tympanic plate of the temporal bone to complete the posterior aspect of the joint.

The inferior cavity of the joint lies between the meniscus and the condyle and is also surrounded at its periphery by synovial membrane. The synovial tissues are confined to the periphery of the cavities and do not extend over the superior and inferior surfaces of the meniscus. The attachment of the heel of the meniscus foot to the condyle is often higher than the attachment of the inferior stratum of the bilaminar zone in the posterior. The inferior belly of the lateral pterygoid muscle attaches to the condyle neck in a fovea just inferior to the articular surface and makes this anterior high attachment necessary.

The articular surface of the condyle is very small when compared with that of the glenoid fossa and articular eminence. In the saggital projection it extends from the pterygoid fovea only to the superior crest of the condyle (Fig. 5-1). This surface is also collagen, not cartilage as seen in other joints of the body. Its fibers are arranged parallel to the surface of the condyle. The secondary cartilage of the condylar process lies just beneath this layer of collagen. The presence of fibroblasts in the articular surface makes growth of the condyle by apposition possible. The fibroblasts may differentiate into chondroblasts to form new cartilage by appositional growth and the chondrocytes of the condylar cartilage can also undergo mitosis to provide new cartilage by interstitial growth. The persistence of the condylar cartilage accounts for the renewed growth of the mandible resulting in a class III or prognathic jaw relationship commonly seen in acromegalics.

The capsule of the temporomandibular joint is not as well defined and organized as the capsules of the larger joints of the body. Its lateral aspect is reinforced by the band of collagen fibers known as the temporomandibular ligament. This ligament extends from the zygomatic arch, down and posteriorly to the lateral aspect of the neck of the condylar process. Since it attaches in such a manner it allows translation of the condyle down and forward without need for increasing its length because it functions much like the arm on a pendulum as the condyle moves forward. The remainder of the lateral wall of the capsule and the lateral half of its anterior wall are remarkably flimsy and poorly organized. The anterior wall becomes a loose meshwork of fibers in the lateral half and is deficient completely in the medial half where the superior belly of the lateral pterygoid attaches to the meniscus. The medial and posterior walls are complete but are also loosely organized. The medial, posterior, and lateral walls of the capsule are innervated by a large branch from the auriculotemporal nerve, which extends superiorly from the nerve as it crosses posterior to the condyle neck.[6] The posterior deep temporal nerves supply a small portion of the lateral and anterior walls of the capsule and the masseteric nerves supply the remainder of the anterior wall and a small portion of the medial wall. The pressures created in the bilaminar zone of the joint meniscus have been shown to become negative when the condyle translates forward out of the fossa and to become positive when the condyle moves back into the fossa.[7] The maximum pressure measure was + 16 mm. of mercury with the usual range being about + 1 or − 1 mm. of mercury. These are not remarkably high pressures when one considers that the pressure in the alveoli of the lungs varies from + 3 to − 3 mm. of mercury during normal breathing. Several studies have shown that 60 to 70 percent of subjects studied translate their condyles anterior to the crest of the articular eminence on wide opening of the jaws.[8, 9] These are subjects who have not experienced temporomandibular joint pain syndrome or subluxation of the condyle with locking in the forward position. The concept that such extreme mobility of the condyle indicates joint dysfunction has not been validated by these studies. McLeran[9]

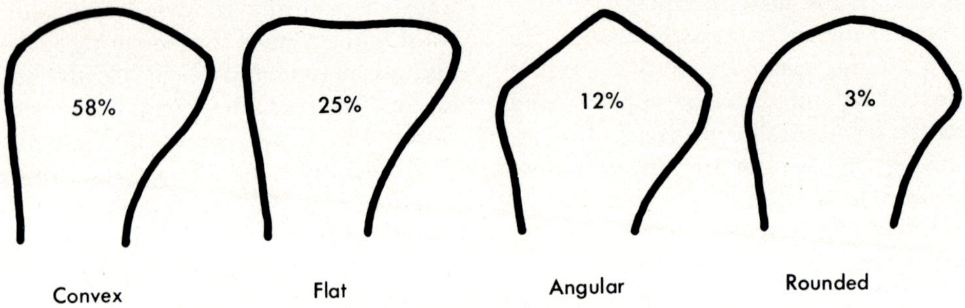

Fig. 5-2. Four shapes of human condyles viewed in frontal plane with their incidence reported by Yale. (Yale, S., and others: Oral Surg. **21**:169, 1966.)

has also demonstrated that many subjects with asymptomatic joints show considerable asynchrony of movement of the condyles during jaw function. The condyles in his subjects were shown to "hunt" toward and away from the articular eminence in a bizarre fashion as they translated out of the fossa. In some subjects one condyle would move forward at the first increment of opening while the opposite condyle would drop down and back. The concept that the condyle glides down and over the eminence smoothly along its surface seems to be in error in many cases.

The shapes of the frontal projection of thousands of mandibular condyles have been studied,[10] and their analysis has shown that there are four shapes to be considered (Fig. 5-2). The majority of human condyles (58 percent) are slightly convex superiorly with a radius of curvature greater than the distance from the medial to lateral poles. The next largest proportion (25 percent) of condyles are flat superiorly. Approximately 12 percent are pointed or angular in shape, and approximately 3 percent are bulbous or rounded in shape with a radius of curvature less than the distance from the lateral to medial pole. The surface of the articular eminence that most closely approximates the condyle is consistently congruent with the surface of the condyle.[11] The two condyles of a patient may be asymmetric; a combination of flat condyle on one side with a convex condyle on the other is most common. One never finds a rounded or bulbous condyle on one side associated with any other shape condyle in the absence of bony pathology.[11] The shape of the condyle would directly affect the nature of the Bennett shift of the mandible. A subject with an angular condyle functioning in an angular fossa would move his mandible inferiorly to a marked degree when making a lateral side shift, while a person with a flat condyle would not necessarily drop inferiorly at all during the lateral side shift. The patient with an angular condyle would be able to function with very steep cusps since a downward deflection of a condyle in the Bennett shift moves the teeth apart, especially on the working side.

It has been shown (Fig. 5-3) that the temporomandibular joint meniscus is tightly bound to the lateral and medial poles of the condyle independently of the capsule.[1] The capsule attaches below the meniscus at both sites and is not tightly bound between temporal bone and condyle poles. If the medial and lateral attachments of the meniscus to the condyle have not been damaged, it follows that the meniscus is placed on stretch from the condyle poles to the tympanic plate by elastin fibers and unfolded synovial membrane during wide opening of the mouth. Excessive tension will damage these fibers, especially in frail, small women. The den-

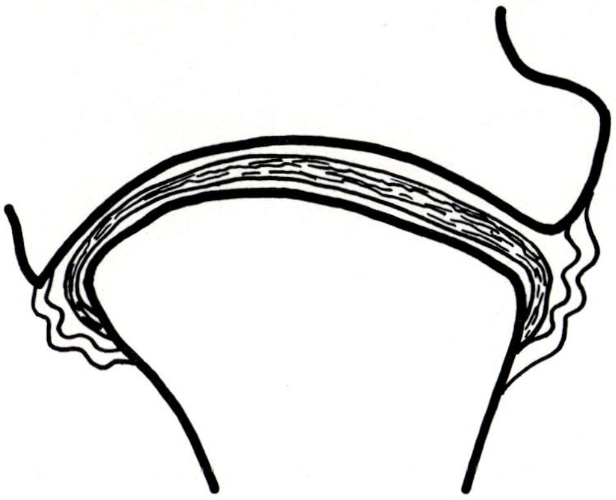

Fig. 5-3. Frontal section through human temporomandibular joint showing independent attachments of meniscus and capsule at condylar poles.

tist should keep these points in mind when applying great forces to seat crowns and bridges, during extraction of lower molars, when working with a rubber dam for extended periods of time, and when placing and removing impression trays. A significant percentage of temporomandibular joint pain syndromes have been shown to be initiated by dental treatment.[12]

The sphenomandibular and stylomandibular ligaments span the temporomandibular joint and are richly innervated by Golgi tendon organs. The sphenomandibular ligament extends from the spine of the sphenoid bone to the lingula on the mandibular foramen in the medial wall of the ramus. It represents the remnant of Meckel's cartilage, the primary cartilage of the mandibular arch. The stylomandibular ligament extends from the styloid process to the posterior border of the ramus near the angle. These ligaments are now considered to function by limiting jaw movement at maximum opening positions and to provide proprioceptive input to the central nervous system via their Golgi tendon organs.

Many muscles of the head and neck have an influence on the movement and position of the mandible. The masseter, temporalis, medial (internal) pterygoid, and lateral (external) pterygoid are described as the muscles of mastication. Of these, the masseter, temporalis, and medial pterygoid serve to elevate the mandible when they shorten. The lateral pterygoid, however, when shortening in conjunction with other muscles, including the opposite lateral pterygoid, serves to depress, protrude, or shift the mandible laterally.

The masseter extends from the zygomatic arch to the lateral surface of the mandibular ramus with its fibers generally directed downward and backward (Fig. 5-4). The posterior part of the muscle is divided into a superficial and a deep portion. The superior part contains many tendinous strands and one therefore observes bulging of the masseter on forceful jaw closure, mainly in the lower half of the muscle. The fibers of the masseter are arranged at an angle to the long axis of the muscle between layers of tendon. This arrangement of numerous, short fibers between layers of connective tissue affords the masseter great power of contraction.

The temporalis muscle takes origin from the temporal fossa on the side of the skull and from the inner surface of the temporal fascia. (Fig. 5-4). Its anterior fibers are directed vertically running deep to the zygomatic arch to attach to the anterior border, apex, and deep surface of the mandibular coronoid process. The fibers covering the anterior margin of the ramus extend almost to the level of the occlusal plane and are extremely sensitive to pressure. Impingement of a thick denture flange against the anteromedial aspect of the mandibular ramus will elicit excruciating pain in the temporalis fibers. The deep portion of the anterior temporalis fibers often attaches by a separate tendon to the interal oblique line on the medial aspect of the ramus low enough to affect insertion of the needle for mandibular

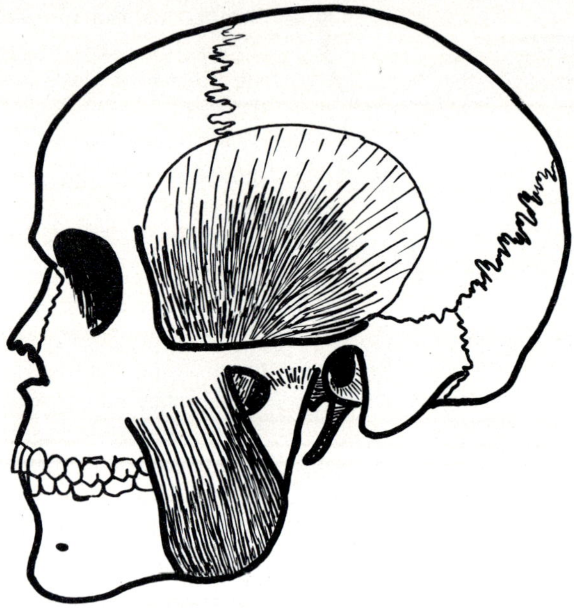

Fig. 5-4. Human skull showing only masseter and temporalis muscles.

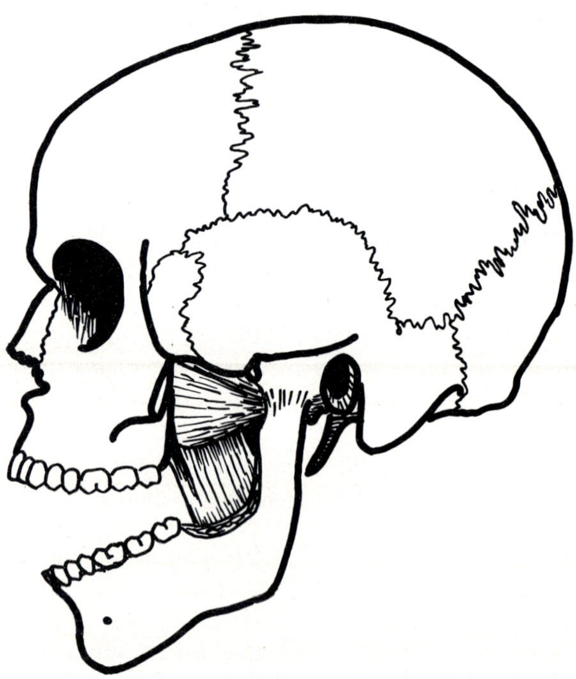

Fig. 5-5. Human skull showing relationship of lateral pterygoid muscle to medial pterygoid muscle.

block anesthesia. The middle and posterior fibers of the temporalis become increasingly oblique so that the most posterior fibers run forward horizontally and bend downward in front of the articular eminence. They attach to the coronoid process as far down as the depth of the mandibular notch. The fibers of the temporalis muscle are divided by tendinous plates as in the masseter but are much longer than those of the masseter. The temporalis muscle serves mainly as an elevator of the mandible. Its most posterior fibers, functioning around the root of the zygomatic process, serve to retrude the mandible to some extent.

The medial pterygoid muscle is located deep to the mandibular ramus and functions as a counterpart of the masseter (Fig. 5-5). It takes origin in the pterygoid fossa and on the medial surface of the lateral pterygoid plate of the sphenoid bone. It extends downward, backward, and outward to insert on the medial aspect of the angle of the mandible. The most anterior fibers of the medial pterygoid muscle often extend down onto the pyramidal process of the palatine bone and maxillary tuberosity so as to produce a definite facet in the posterior border of an upper arch impression. These fibers, when present, will often displace denture flanges during functional movements of the mandible. The fibers of the medial pterygoid are arranged internally the same as those of the masseter, but the medial pterygoid is not as powerful as the masseter.

The lateral pterygoid muscle is more intimately related to the temporomandibular joint than the other muscles of mastication (Fig. 5-5). Its large, inferior head takes origin on the lateral surface of the lateral pterygoid plate and extends upward, outward, and backward to insert in the pterygoid fovea on the neck of the condyle. The small, superior head takes origin from the horizontal portion of the greater wing of the sphenoid, medial to the infratemporal crest. It extends horizontally backward and outward to attach to the anteromedial corner of the temporomandibular joint meniscus and the pterygoid fovea. When both lateral pterygoids shorten simultaneously they either depress or protrude the mandible. If the mandibular elevators are only partially relaxed, the mandible is protruded. If the elevators are relaxed and the digastrics are contracted with a fixed hyoid bone, the mandible is depressed. If only one lateral pterygoid is contracted, it serves to move the mandible laterally to the opposite side. It is believed that the superior head of the lateral pterygoid serves to stabilize the temporomandibular joint meniscus on the condyle as it translates forward on the articular eminence. It therefore serves to assist the meniscus attachments at the medial and lateral poles of the condyle in holding the meniscus between the condyle and temporal bone in all forward excursions of the mandible.

The suprahyoid muscles extending from the skull and mandible to the hyoid bone serve to elevate the hyoid bone or to depress the mandible. They include the digastric, geniohyoid, mylohyoid, and stylohyoid. If the infrahyoid muscles are contracted so as to immobolize the hyoid bone, contraction of the suprahyoids depresses and retracts the mandible. If the mandible is fixed by contraction of the elevators, the suprahyoids elevate the hyoid bone and the larynx.

The muscles of facial expression are normally very thin, weak muscles that serve to move only the soft tissues of the face. Some of these muscles indirectly extend from the bones of the upper face to the mandible but under normal circumstances are not important in moving or positioning the lower jaw.

• • •

The temporomandibular joint in man

functions in a manner that resembles a ball on an inverted hill rather than a ball in a socket. The mandibular condyle moves anterior to the articular eminence during wide opening of the jaws in most individuals. It also moves away from and toward the surface of the eminence during functional movement of the mandible with a considerable degree of freedom. The meniscus is tightly attached to the medial and lateral poles of the condyle in the healthy temporomandibular joint, and its attachment to the tympanic plate is made up of elastic tissue. This anatomic arrangement allows the meniscus to translate with the condyle while being attached to the temporal bone posteriorly.

The central part of the meniscus is avascular in the adult but its periphery is richly supplied with blood vessels. Boyer and others[13] have demonstrated a great complexity and quantiy of blood vessels in the periphery of the meniscus in the monkey, which is very similar to that of man. Glomus cell arteriovenous anastomoses have been demonstrated in this vascular area of the human meniscus.

The major nerve innervating the temporomandibular joint capsule is a large branch from the auriculotemporal nerve, which approaches the joint from the posterior aspect of the neck of the condyle. The posterior deep temporal and masseteric nerves also supply the capsule.

The two condyles of a patient are often asymmetric, but one never finds a rounded or bulbous condyle on one side associated with a flat, oval, or angular condyle on the opposite side in the absence of pathology of the condyle.

The upper portion of the masseter muscle is comprised of a large proportion of tendinous strands, while the lower part is mainly made up of muscle fibers. This explains the fact that bulging of the masseter usually occurs in the lower half of the muscle when it is forcefully contracted in jaw closure. The anterior fibers of the temporalis, located just buccal to the maxillary tuberosity, are extremely sensitive to pressure and any impingement of denture flanges against these fibers will cause extreme pain in the muscle. The deep part of the anterior temporalis attaches by a separate tendon on the medial aspect of the ramus low enough to obstruct the path of insertion of the needle in a mandibular block injection. Piercing this muscle and tendon may divert the needle from the region of the lingula and inferior alveolar nerve, causing failure of the anesthesia. The posterior fibers of the temporalis are directed horizontally and serve to retrude the mandible to some extent. The anterior fibers of the medial pterygoid muscle often extend down onto the maxillary tuberosity so as to produce definite facets in the posterior border of upper arch impressions and to displace denture flanges during wide opening of the jaws. The lateral pterygoid muscle attaches to the medial, anterior corner of the temporomandibular joint meniscus and exerts an anterior pull on the meniscus during jaw opening, thus helping to stabilize the meniscus on the condyle as it translates forward. The muscles of facial expression indirectly extend from the bones of the upper face to the mandible but under normal circumstances are not important in elevating the lower jaw.

SELECTED REFERENCES

1. Choukas, N. C., and Sicher, H.: The structure of the temporomandibular joint, Oral Surg. **13**:1203, 1960.
2. Thilander, B.: The structure of the collagen of the temporo-mandibular disc in man, Acta Odont. Scand. **22**:135, 1964.
3. Batson, O. B.: The anatomist looks at the temporomandibular joint, Amer. Acad. Ophthal. Otolaryng. May: 413, 1956.
4. Zola, A.: Morphologic limiting factors in the temporomandibular joint, J. Prosth. Dent. **13**: 732, 1963.
5. Griffin, C. J., and Sharpe, C. J.: The structure of the adult human temporomandibular meniscus, Aust. Dent. J. **5**:190, 1960.
6. Thilander, B.: Innervation of the temporo-

mandibular joint capsule in man, Trans. Roy. Schools Stockh. Umea No. 7, 1961.
7. Findlay, I. A.: Mandibular joint pressures, J. Dent. Res. **43**:140, 1964.
8. Frommer, H., and Parker, L. A.: Roentgenographic temporomandibular joint survey, Oral Diag. & Path. **16**:1326, 1963.
9. McLeran, J. H., and others: A cinefluorographic analysis of the temporomandibular joint, J.A.D.A. **75**:1394, 1967.
10. Yale, S. H., and others: An epidemiological assessment of mandibular condyle morphology, Oral Surg. **21**:169, 1966.
11. Emmering, T. E.: A new approach to the analysis of the functional surfaces of the temporomandibular joint, Oral Surg. **23**:603, 1967.
12. Moulton, R.: Oral and dental manifestations of anxiety, Psychiatry **18**:261, 1955.
13. Boyer, C. C., and others: Blood supply of the temporomandibular joint, J. Dent. Res. **43**:223, 1964.

GENERAL REFERENCES

Boucher, L. J.: Anatomy of the temporomandibular joint as it pertains to centric relation, J. Prosth. Dent. **12**:464-472, 1962.

Brodie, A. G.: Occlusion from the standpoint of the fundamental sciences, Illinois D. J. **6**:6, 1937.

Fagerstom, K. G., and Brodie, A. G.: Cranial and facial growth in the pig as revealed by metallic implants and serial roentgenology, I.A.D.R. Preprinted Abstracts, No. 250, 1963.

Gasser, R. F.: The development of the facial muscles in man, Amer. J. Anat. **120**:357, 1967.

Hase, R. R.: Anatomical carving in crown and bridge prosthodontia, J. Philippine D. A. **15**: 17, 1961.

Hockstein, I.: Arch form—a study of various dimensions and relationships in the maxillary arch, Am. J. Orthodontics **48**:554, 1962 (abst.)

Lauritzen, A. G.: Function, prime object of restorative dentistry; a definite procedure to obtain it, J.A.D.A. **42**:503, 1951.

Lindblom, G.: Balanced occlusion with partial reconstructions, Internat. D. J. **1**:84, 1951.

Meyer, F. S.: Bridges cast to functional occlusion, Minneapolis Dist. D. J. **15**:9, 1932.

Meyer, F. S.: Cast bridgework in functional occlusion, J.A.D.A. **20**:1015, 1933.

Monson, G. S.: Occlusion as applied to crown and bridgework, J. Nat. D. A. **7**:399, 1920.

Morris, M. L.: Artificial crown contours and gingival health, J. Prosth. Dent. **12**:1146, 1962.

Moulton, G. M.: Esthetics in fixed bridge prosthodontics, J.A.D.A. **52**:36, 1956.

Piatowska, D.: Anatomical structure of the gingiva, Czas Stomat. **21**(10):1169-1173, 1968.

Pound, E.: Applying harmony in selecting and arranging teeth, Dent. Clin. N. Amer. pp. 241-258, March, 1962.

Sicher, H.: Oral anatomy, Saint Louis, 1965, The C. V. Mosby Co.

Thilander, B.: Innervation of the temporo-mandibular disc in man, Acta Odont. scand. **22**: 151, 1964.

Tinker, E. T.: Predetermination of occlusal surfaces of teeth, J.A.D.A. **18**:1046, 1931.

Tylman, S. D.: Discussion of the biologic factors involved in the fixed partial denture, J. Canad. D. A. **23**:67-75, 1957.

Wilson, W. H., and Lang, R. L.: Practical crown and bridge prosthodontics, ed. 1, New York, 1962, McGraw-Hill Book Co., Inc.

Chapter 6

The maxillae—mandible and related factors

If any degree of success is to be attained in partial denture prosthodontics, it is important to maintain the underlying bone in a healthy condition. The bones with which we are mostly concerned are the maxillae in the upper and the mandible in the lower part of the face. It is not necessary to review here the anatomy of the maxillary bones, since the complete anatomic descriptions are contained in standard texts on the subject. It is well, however, to remember the general outline and formation of the maxillary bones. The maxillary teeth are the anvils against which the muscles drive the lower jaw, and nature has so distributed and arranged the root system and the supporting bone that the blow is pneumatized in the posterior regions of the maxillae by large sinuses immediately overlying the root system. It is essential to determine the type and the extent of the maxillary sinus in the event that any teeth have been removed from this area. We must be certain that there are no postoperative openings into the sinus or infections present in this cavity. It would be dangerous for the patient if a fixed appliance were placed over such an edentulous area. The fact, however, that the apices of either the bicuspids or molars approach and sometimes extend into the floor of the sinus does not necessarily contraindicate the use of such teeth as abutments.

THE MAXILLAE: RIDGE AND ARCH FORM

There are two factors with reference to the maxillae that are of special interest to the dentist: first, the ridge, and second, the arch form (Fig. 6-1). As is well known, the maxillary ridge increases in width buccolingually as it extends posteriorly, ending in rounded tuberosities. We very frequently find undercuts on the labial and on the buccal surfaces. If removable partial dentures are contemplated, it is frequently necessary to remove these undercuts; this is not so essential if fixed appliances are placed. Two aspects of the size of the ridge are quite important in fixed partial prosthodontics: first, its vertical height; and second, its labiolingual or buccolingual width. From the standpoint of vertical height, if the ridge is too high there will not be enough room gingivocclusally for a sufficient bulk, and therefore strength, of the pontic. In these circumstances it is very difficult to construct a pontic that will be cleansable and sanitary. When the treatment plan calls for placing a fixed appliance, it must be decided whether a sufficient space will exist vertically for a pontic after ridge resorption has taken place. If not, then it may be necessary to resort to surgical procedures in order to establish the necessary vertical space.

There is another condition to consider in examining the ridge of an edentulous

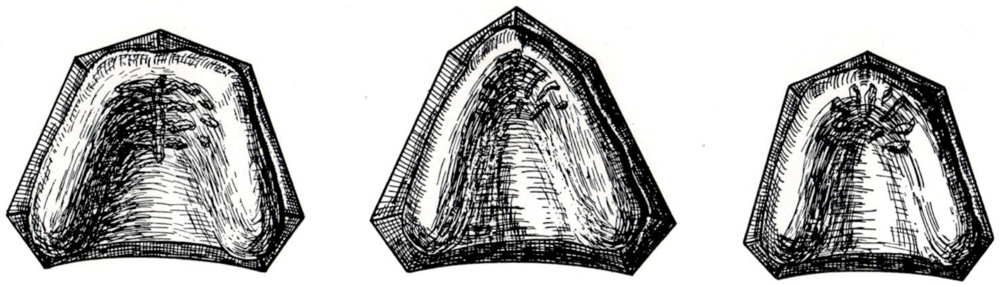

Fig. 6-1. Three types of arches: square, tapering, and ovoid.

area. If the spicules of alveolar bone are neither removed nor rounded off following the extraction of teeth, the ridge will heal with a very irregular surface continuity. It is difficult to construct a fixed bridge for this type of ridge so that it will maintain its self-cleansing qualities. Very frequently patients are seen following extractions whose ridges apparently refuse to heal and persist in remaining very tender and sore. An examination may disclose pieces of fractured bone or alveolar process that were sprung out of position or even detached during extraction. Unless they are removed, healing will not take place until nature absorbs or exfoliates them. If the dentist who constructs the fixed partial denture has the opportunity to see the patient prior to the extraction of teeth, he should decide on the amount and extent of alveolar process to be removed; this amount should be sufficient to allow the placement of a sanitary pontic. Less resorption of the ridge will take place if all irregular projections of alveolar process are removed at the time of extraction than if these are allowed to resorb completely by themselves.

Occasionally an excessive resorption of the ridge occurs (Fig. 30-21). This condition in the anterior part of the mouth may contraindicate a fixed appliance and specify a removable partial denture in order that the necessary esthetic effect can be obtained.

The ridge contour varies according to its position in the arch. Generally it will be found that the ridge is narrower labiolingually in the anterior region (Fig. 30-9, *B*) than in the posterior region (Fig. 30-13, *B*). The examination should disclose the approximate state of resorption that exists, as this will enable the dentist to place the gingival portion of the pontic in its proper relationship to the ridge.

There are times when nodules or exostoses, varying in size, appear on the ridges of the maxillae or the mandible. If these are likely to interfere with the proper placement of a fixed bridge or if there is a possibility of subsequent irritation, they should be removed prior to the construction of the appliance.

In focusing attention on the ridge, the aim should be to leave it in such shape and condition that (1) the fixed partial denture may be placed in the shortest possible time following the extraction of the teeth, (2) one can more easily arrange the pontics in a correct position, and (3) once the appliance is in place, it will be comfortable and sanitary in its relationship to the ridge.

The arch forms of both the maxillae and the mandible ordinarily correspond to the form of the face. Although there are the three typical types—square, tapering, and ovoid—many variations and combinations exist. The determination of the arch type and ridge form may help to select the type of teeth that are to be used in the restoration.

Alveolar process

The alveolar process is a part of the bony ridges (Figs. 11-1 and 11-2) and depends upon the presence of teeth for its existence. There is no alveolar process before the eruption of teeth, nor any after all the teeth have been lost. The alveolar process is the tooth-supporting portion of the arches. The amount and distribution of the alveolar process not only vary in different teeth and individuals, but also differ in each of the arches. In the upper arch, the forces to which teeth are subjected cause them to be moved buccally and labially, producing a tension on the lingual processes of the maxilla. It is known that bone resorbs when subjected to pressure but that it is stimulated to growth by physiologic tension; therefore, in the upper arch the greater amount of alveolar bone is laid down on the lingual aspect, while the labial plates are relatively thin. Since the type of alveolar bone is more or less contingent upon its functional activity, bone is formed where the forces of mastication are transferred to it by means of tension in the periodontal membrane. On the other hand, when a tooth does not receive normal functional forces, resorption of the alveolar bone takes place; a diffuse atrophy or pocket formation may even occur.

It is quite essential, therefore, to determine the condition of the alveolar bone around teeth, particularly around those to be used as bridge abutments. By grasping the coronal portion of a tooth between the thumb and finger of one hand and placing the tip of the index finger of the other hand above the apical region, and then by moving the tooth labiolingually or buccolingually, the dentist may ascertain the type and degree of periodontal membrane attachment, as well as the character of the bone in that region.

Changes following extraction

Certain changes take place in the tissues when a tooth is extracted. Ordinarily it takes from 4 to 8 weeks for the gum tissues to heal sufficiently to allow the cementation of a fixed restoration. One of the principal changes that occurs in the alveolar process is the marginal resorption of the sockets. Concurrent with this process there is a loss of contour and a general rounding off of the ridge, but at a lower level. It is significant that the alveolar resorption in the upper arch differs from that in the lower. In the maxillae the labial and buccal alveolar plates, as well as the crest of the alveolar processes, resorb much faster than do the lingual plates. This result is more noticeable in a completely edentulous mouth than in one that is partially so. The same relative and quantitative resorption also takes place in short edentulous spans. It will be found, in fitting pontics for the anterior or posterior regions of the mouth, that the labial or buccal gingival portion of the pontics usually rises rootwise above the lingual margin (Figs. 30-9, *B*, and 30-11). It will be noted in a completely edentulous mouth that, after complete resorption of the process has taken place, the size of the upper arch is reduced and the maxillary ridge lies wholly within the arch of the lower jaw. Later we shall see that the method and speed of alveolar resorption of the mandible differs from those of the maxillae.

Because resorption is progressive, it is necessary to ascertain whether an edentulous area is of recent extraction or of long duration. If the extraction is quite recent, allowance for this anticipated resorption within the near future must be made in fitting the pontic to the ridge. In cases of long duration the alveolar process is resorbed and the bone is regenerated; consequently, there is less likelihood of further resorption in the immediate future.

A determination should be made of the degree of healing of the alveolar process or ridge. Although the ideal condition for the placement of a fixed partial denture is that in which the ridge is entirely healed, there are occasions when the so-called immediate replacement type of prosthesis is employed (Fig. 30-16). This type of upper anterior prosthesis is employed only when there is a sufficient amount of normal alveolar process present prior to and after the extraction of the tooth. (See Chapter 30.)

In placing a pontic into the alveolar socket, it is well to remember that the upper labial process of bone resorbs more quickly than the lingual. Consequently, the pontic should be shaped with its labial gingival third curving toward the ridge, while the lingual surface of the pontic, in its gingival third, may follow the general axis direction of the alveolar socket. Some authorities, however, believe that the labial surface should be given its full contour.

The alveolar bone is one of the most responsive of the tissues in the human body. It appears and disappears in response to function, and during its life and existence it is one of the most active and versatile of the tissues. Pressure or tension will alternately produce resorption or deposition of bone in order to keep the tooth within its physiologic limits. Roentgenographically, it will be observed that the trabeculation of alveolar bone varies in thickness and architecture in proportion to the degree of functional force imposed upon it.

THE PALATES

While the palates, both hard and soft, do not enter directly into the consideration of a fixed partial denture prosthesis, it is always well to examine them. Not only should the form be verified to see that it coincides with the form of the face and the arch, but the presence or absence of any pathologic lesions should be determined. If a record is made with the view of using the data subsequently, possibly 20 to 25 years later, it might be well to note the extent of the hard and the soft palates. Although the rugae are regular and symmetric in most mouths, there are instances in which the variation from normal is such as to interfere with successful prosthetic restorations. The presence, location, size, and shape of a torus palatinus may influence the design of the pontic used in the restoration.

THE MANDIBLE

While the mandible shares certain characteristics of the maxillae, it differs markedly from the latter in other respects. The similarity lies in the fact that the alveolar process is developed and resorbed in response to the same stimuli as those in the maxillae. The vertical height of the mandible increases due to the development of the alveolar process and the upward growth of the condyle, which brings the mandible downward. This was shown by Thompson and Brodie[1] in their studies relating to the position of the mandible during growth. A similar development takes place concurrently in the upper arch.

Formerly, it was generally accepted that the mandible changed its form during the various periods of life, starting with an apparently flat mandible with an obtuse angle and gradually developing into one with a more acute angle during maturity. The latter was thought to change again into an obtuse angle during the edentulous stage of senescence.

The same investigators have presented evidence to indicate that the angular pattern of an individual persists throughout life. It was further stated that the proportions of a face are constant, as far as vertical height is concerned, when the jaw is in rest position. Hence it is important in an extensive program of mouth rehabilitation to recognize and register the various positions of the mandible. A further discussion of this phase of dentistry is found in Chapters 29 and 36.

These observations should be kept in mind when examining a patient, so that the type of occlusion, the strength of the bite, and the amount of wear of the natural teeth may be ascertained. Any prosthesis placed in a mouth should conform to the existing functional, physiologic tooth form. Natural teeth with worn cusps require a corresponding type of occlusal anatomy in the prosthesis; if it is markedly different, there will be a disharmony of function, resulting ultimately in the loss of the restoration.

Ridge and arch form

The ridge of the mandible ordinarily is not as large or as prominent as that of the maxillae. Not only is it reduced in height, it is also thinner labiolingually and buccolingually. Although the contour of the ridge is generally well rounded, its general shape should be noted, i.e., whether its walls are parallel, converging, or undercut. It is of great importance to the partial denture prosthesis whether the ridge has been excessively resorbed. When the placement of a fixed partial restoration is contemplated in the lower arch, this condition is not quite the handicap that it is in the upper. The factor of esthetics often rules out a fixed upper restoration, while in the lower arch it does not offer serious objections because the gingival regions are hidden by the cheeks and lip. In fact, a resorbed ridge in the lower arch very frequently helps to maintain the self-cleansing features of the fixed appliance.

Following the extraction of teeth in the mandible, the alveolar process is resorbed, the same as it is in the upper arch. There are certain points of difference, however, which are to be kept in mind. In the upper arch the forces of mastication move the teeth buccally and labially, exerting a tension on the lingual bone but a pressure on the labial and buccal plates. As a result, the labial and buccal plates of bone are very thin, and these, following extraction, resorb to a greater degree than does the lingual plate.

The forces exerted on the lower teeth are in a lingual direction; yet, because the mandibular teeth are arranged in the form of a closed arch, the amounts of bone on the lingual and on the labial surfaces are approximately the same. Because of this, it is generally true that the resorption of the alveolar processes of the mandible takes place at approximately the same rate in both the labial and lingual plates. This results in a symmetric reduction in height of a rounded ridge; the size of the arch is maintained, but it is at a lower level. This method of healing in the mandible as compared to that in the maxillae presents certain difficulties in complete artificial denture construction.

The healed ridge of the mandible may be well rounded or may assume a thin, knife-edged shape. Because the factor of esthetics is not limited in the lower as much as in the upper arch, it will be found that in most mandibular restorations a conical or spheroidal type of pontic may be used, contacting the ridge at its center or slightly buccally. It should be noticed whether the extraction is of recent date or is of long standing; it is known that the lower arch has a faster rate of resorption than the upper, and this should be taken into consideration when selecting the type of pontic that is to be used.

Mylohyoid ridge

While the mylohyoid ridge may not be regarded as of sufficient importance in the consideration of fixed partial dentures, it sometimes happens that the fibers of attachment of the mylohyoid muscles extend up over the mandible above the mylohyoid line for several millimeters. In such event this may be a factor in the establishment of the correct position and clearance of the pontics and the ridge. The head of the condyle should be located and its action observed, particularly when very extensive fixed restorations are to be employed in the establishment of new occlusal relationships. Changes in the relationship of the condyle head and the glenoid fossa may result from excessive tooth destruction or from malocclusion.

Mental foramen

The mental foramen is an important landmark when block anesthesia is used during cavity preparation. Its position should be located when a fixed partial denture is used to restore the lower first and second bicuspids. In the presence of excessive resorption of the process and ridge, it happens on rare occasions that the foramen is very close to the crest of the alveolar ridge. Its location should be definitely established in order not to impinge a pontic upon it. Should this happen, extreme discomfort and pain will result.

OTHER ORAL FACTORS: MUCOUS MEMBRANE

In examining the mucous membrane of the mouth, one should distinguish between the tissue that covers the ridge (usually designated as ridge mucosa) and that which is confluent with the cheeks and the tongue. The mucosa over a ridge is normally firm and unyielding; it is attached to the underlying bone by a dense and firm fibrous tissue. Ordinarily, this mucosa is not very sensitive to pain, its color is normally of a pinkish tint, and it is slightly yielding. An examination might disclose a mucosa of similar physical characteristics but of a slightly anemic color, which may be due to some impaired physical condition; it appears to be stretched tightly over the underlying bony support. There is also the type of mucosa that is flabby and pendulous (displaceable). This is quite sensitive and frequently demands surgical interference in order to reduce the ridges to a normal, firm condition. During the examination the dentist should distinguish between the three types, for the type of mucosa will determine the shape of the pontic and the amount and area of contact to be established between the pontic and the ridge.

While the mucosa over the ridge is relatively immovable, that of the border tissues is very mobile. The examination should disclose the plane or line at which this tissue connects with the immovable ridge tissue and whether this line is in a high, medium, or low position. It is well to note whether this border tissue is loosely or tightly attached. As shown in Chapter 30, the significance of this observation lies in the fact that, in fixed partial dentures, the pontic always terminates within the area of the immovable mucosa of the ridge. Whenever the gingival outline of the pontic extends beyond and into the movable border tissues, irritation and inflammation ensue.

The examination should also include the mucous membrane of the cheeks and the lips. Sometimes it is found that patients bite their inner cheeks because of faulty occlusion or shape of the teeth. This condition sometimes may be rectified by a judicious recontouring of the teeth. It is well known that many of the early malignant conditions of the oral cavity are recognizable long before the patient is aware of their existence. For this reason it is of utmost importance that the dentist carefully examine the cheeks, lips, and tongue for any signs of unusual growths or configurations of tissue.

The same is true of the mucous membrane of the soft palate. While a recognition of the physical conditions of this tissue is more important to the complete than to the partial denture prosthodontist, the latter should make careful study of this area to determine the presence of any abnormalities.

THE TONGUE

The tissues of the tongue are usually examined with those of the mucous membrane to detect any pathologic conditions. The size of the tongue varies in different patients. If abnormal in size, as in the case of macroglossia, there is the possibility of excessive force being exerted by the tongue against the teeth. If this horizontal force involves a bridge, it may cause the abutment teeth to shift either labially or buccally, and eventually the appliance may fail. If a bridge is placed under these circumstances, provision should be made to counteract the unnatural forces that might be present.

In examining partially edentulous mouths of long duration, it is frequently noted that the tongue becomes hypertrophied into an edentulous space. Later, following the placement of a fixed appliance, the patient may experience discomfort and may even bite his tongue. The patient should be informed of this tendency, and provision should be made to minimize this danger by properly contouring the lingual surfaces of the pontic and the bridge retainers.

GLANDS OF THE MOUTH

The glands of the mouth are divided primarily into their location and type of secretion. While the buccal and labial glands open into the vestibule, some maxillary and lingual glands empty directly into the inner oral cavity. The direct examination of the glands normally will be incident to some complaint on the part of the patient; the most common is that of a stone forming in the duct, preventing the normal flow of saliva. A determination of the type and the amount of saliva should be made. It should be established whether the saliva is primarily serous or mucous in character, for this finding may be related to the fact that the patient is or is not actively susceptible to caries. It is an established fact that a serous type of saliva aids in the mechanical cleansing of a restoration, while a mucous type tends to adhere to the teeth and restorations and helps in the formation of bacterial plaques. If, therefore, a patient is predisposed to caries and has a characteristic mucous secretion, it will influence the decision with respect to the type of prosthesis and the type and design of cavity preparation that should be employed. When the flow of saliva is exceptionally copious, the fact should be recorded and the necessary operative or medicinal treatment instituted to keep this condition under control, at least during the time that abutments are being prepared. The use of atropine is sometimes indicated in such instances.

If the glands are abnormal in size, it is well to investigate the possibility of infection.

MASTICATORY FORCE

It is known that different patients are capable of exerting a masticatory force varying from 20 to 50 pounds up to 250 to 300 pounds (Tables 11-1 to 11-3). This force, together with the condition of the muscles of mastication, is usually related to the physical status of the patient. Robust persons normally possess a strong musculature. It is also known that the greatest crushing power a patient is capable of exerting lies in the area of the first molars. In examining a partially edentulous mouth for fixed prosthesis, it is apparent that the location of the edentulous space and the type and the development of the muscles of mastication have an important bearing on the decision. Those prostheses that will be subjected to the greatest forces must of necessity be so designed and constructed as to possess maximum strength. This precaution still holds in spite of the fact that the limit of force a tooth can safely endure is not determined by the ultimate power that the muscles of mastication exert, but by the amount of force tolerated by the periodontal membrane. (See Chapter 9.)

FACIAL FACTORS

When teeth are lost, the face undergoes certain changes. The amount of change is usually in proportion to the number of teeth lost and the length of time following extraction. These changes are usually discernible in the lower half of the face. Teeth, therefore, are essential not only to the well-being of the patient but also to the maintenance of a normal facial contour. Patients may not wish to admit it, but the primary motivating factor in a large percentage of those seeking dental service is the desire to maintain the esthetic factors. Therefore, it is the function and duty of the dentist to correct not only any disturbed oral functions but also the impaired esthetic values. When a mouth is partially edentulous, these corrections are usually made in harmony with the remaining natural teeth; however, in those cases in which all the teeth are missing, it is necessary to restore the dental mechanism with reference to the facial contour of the patient.

At first it would seem that a study of the facial factors is an entirely unnecessary procedure in fixed partial denture prosthesis, since a fixed bridge ordinarily replaces only one or two missing teeth. Some might feel that an extensive study of the facial factors is not required, since the remaining natural teeth are the criteria for color, mold, position, and size. When extensive fixed restorations are involved, such as a cuspid-to-cuspid bridge or extensive porcelain veneer crown restorations in the anterior part of the mouth, the facial factors assume their maximum importance.

Although it is less difficult to meet the requirements of proper form and color of teeth in partial denture prostheses than in complete artificial dentures, still a knowledge and an understanding of the basic principles that guide these selections of correct color and tooth form enable one more easily to accomplish the desired results and to explain to the patient what is being done and why. While complete dental roentgenographs and mounted study model records of partially edentulous mouths are generally taken, it is also suggested that a record be kept of the type and color of the teeth still present. It is also well to obtain the profile outline of the patient either by a cutout form or by the use of a 12-gauge lead wire, which is bent to the facial contour; this outline is then transferred to the patient's record. Some dentists have developed a photographic technic that accomplishes the same purpose. These records should be taken with the jaw in a rest position.

Form and color harmony

The dentist who desires to render to his patients the most artistic as well as the most serviceable form of prosthesis must recognize in the human face certain factors of harmony and proportion, particularly those of form and color. Since these elements are existent and related in the human face, any appliance that the dentist makes for the patient must conform to identical standards in order to preserve the harmonious effect. A dental prosthesis may be ever so beautiful on a plaster cast, but if its form and color do not harmonize with the form and color of the patient's face, it will be a monstrosity when placed in the mouth. This is one of the reasons why the entire responsibility of designing and constructing an appliance cannot be left to a dental technician, for he does not have the opportunity of relating his technical skills to the esthetic requirements of the patient. The construction of an artistic as well as a useful appliance lies only in the domain of the trained dentist.

Facial form

Although no two patients are exactly alike in appearance or proportion, the large majority present a harmonious appearance. No doubt the harmony of the dental apparatus is the same as that found in any other smoothly functioning machine. Since a broad, well-developed face usually contains strong, wide teeth, and a delicate face has smaller, more delicate teeth, it is quite evident that there must be a balanced relationship existing between the forces that are produced, then transferred, and finally active in that machine. Without considering any hereditary factors that may be invloved, let us consider those that are purely functional. The process of molding and shaping the outline of the face, including the bones and muscles, is continuous until about 18 to 21 years of age. Since in a normal denture all the teeth, excluding the third molars, are formed and functioning by the twelfth to fourteenth year, it is evident that between the ages of 14 and 21 years the dental mechanism or the functional part of the mechanism is a determining factor in the development of the bones. This is one reason why it is so important to render proper dental service to the adolescent. The use of fillings that correct occlusal relationships, contacts, and contours, as well as space maintainers when teeth are lost, is extremely important during this formative period of facial contour.

Classification of facial form. The theory of face form that is usually used and accepted today is the typal. The original classification by Madame Schimmelpennick divided face forms into square, parallelogram, ovoid, circle, and triangle. From this basis Dr. J. Leon Williams reclassified faces into three general groups: square, tapering, and ovoid. Williams showed that the outline form of the face is closely related to the outline form of the upper central incisors. There is, however, a more fundamental relationship between outline form, function, and facial form. It has been shown that tooth form, type of occlusion, and facial form are closely related. In the square type of face the teeth generally have a square, flat contact area and cusps with shallow inclined planes; the tapering type of teeth have a narrow contact area with longer and relatively steeper inclined planes; the ovoid type presents a compromise between the tapering and the square. It is thought by some that the masticatory musculature is dependent upon the inherent growth pattern and, therefore, the facial form of the individual.

It might be asked what relationship exists between these facts and the construction of fixed partial dentures. In the practice of fixed partial prosthodontics it is very important to recognize the type of face with which we are dealing, so that the contour, cusp height, and occlusal plane inclination of the restoration may be reconstructed to harmonize with the remaining natural teeth and occlusion. The same is true in the reconstruction of entire arches. The extreme importance of correct typal recognition manifests itself when it is necessary to restore the upper six anterior teeth with complete porcelain veneer crowns. Such restorations are less noticeable and less objectionable if there is a slight deviation in their color, but if the true type form is not reproduced there is a clash with the general harmony of facial contour that immediately proclaims the artificiality of the restorations. Furthermore, if we fail to harmonize our restorations with the conditions found in the mouth, it will be found that an appliance, even though comfortable in centric relationship, will prove uncomfortable when subjected to functional movements. Malocclusion will usually result if the correct type of occlusion and contour of tooth are not employed; many bridges have failed because they lacked these important requirements. There are many variations of the three typal forms; hence, it is essential that the dentist be able to recognize and understand the features distinguishing one from the other. If the tooth form of the restoration harmonizes with the natural teeth, the harmony of function and the harmony of esthetics will be present.

Profile form

Usually the consideration of the profile form is not as important in the construction of a partial prosthesis as it is in a complete denture prosthesis. In the former a sufficient number of natural teeth is present to indicate the correct occlusion. When teeth are present, a knowledge of the correct facial proportions is essential in the event that a change is contemplated in the occlusal relationship of the two arches. Thompson[1] has pointed out that the correct height of the face, either in an edentulous patient or in one with teeth, is determined by the position of the mandible at rest. He stated further that "the difference between the height of the face when the mandible is at rest and when the teeth are in occlusion is determined by the amount of space between the upper and lower teeth when the mandible is at rest. This, which is called the freeway space, averages 2 to 3 mm. in a normal dentition. In abnormal, it may be 10 mm. or more". Niswonger,[2] more than a decade previously, had called attention to this same fact. Although profiles are generally classified as convex, straight, and concave, the typal form can be modified only to the extent of the changes that result from changing the vertical dimension of the face.

Color harmony

Just as tooth form harmonizes with that of the face and the arch, so also is the color of the tooth in harmony with that of the face. As a rule, a person with a dark complexion, dark eyes, and black hair has teeth that are relatively dark, i.e., the teeth tend toward the orange hues. On the other hand, a person with a blonde complexion having fair hair and light-colored eyes has teeth that are correspondingly light, i.e., they are lightly tinged with yellow or blue. A dark tooth for a blonde patient or a light tooth for a brunette would be a distinct shock to the sense of harmony.

However, teeth darken with age; it will be noticed that the complexion undergoes a concurrent change. In youth the skin is fair, pink, and of a light color, while in old age it changes to a sallow gray or even to a yellow color. Here again Nature shows her handicraft in maintaining color harmony. There are several reasons why the color of teeth may change; if the incisal edge or occlusal surfaces have been worn through the enamel, exposing the dentin, stains may penetrate through the dentinal tubules and alter the color effect considerably.

There are certain biologic changes that take place, such as the formation of secondary dentin in the pulp chamber with a resultant recession of the pulp. It is the redness of the pulp tissue that gives the live and vital orange tint to teeth in youth. When this disappears or is reduced in intensity, the yellow color of the dentin predominates, giving a dull yellow color to old teeth. Many classifications of patients as to color of teeth have been made. These range from yellow through red, gray, and brown. The sense of color harmony is one that has to be developed and acquired through study and long experience. The simplest method in determining these factors is to select two predominating colors. By placing both of these in the mouth alternately, the one that harmonizes most closely with the color of the face, hair, and eyes can be easily discerned. A more complete discussion of this subject will be found in Chapter 25.

Lips

The lips play a prominent part in the study of the face. Unless the lips are in harmony with the teeth, the character and expression of the patient will be lost. When rendering partial denture service in the anterior part of the mouth, it is noted that small teeth usually do not coincide with large, pendulous lips, nor do large teeth harmonize with thin, narrow lips.

In making the examination of the patient, it should be observed whether the color of the lips is pink, red, purple, or of a grayish tint. These colors usually accompany varying degrees of health, age, and vitality of the patient. Moreover, the position of the lips should be observed when they are at rest as well as during function, at which time the high and low lip lines may be noted and recorded on the study models. Some claim that the contour of the lips harmonizes with the head at the brow line. The lip line is used as a guide to determine the position of the incisal edge of the anterior teeth and is also helpful in locating the median line of the face and in the positioning of the cuspids with reference to the angles of the mouth. When restoring the mouth with extensive anterior restorations, care must be exercised that the philtrum is not eradicated. In those patients who are completely edentulous or who have worn down their natural teeth extensively, it will be observed that the lower lip has driven the upper lip upward, and in some instances a definite shortening of the upper lip has taken place. This results in the lip line being too high and practically eliminates the entire vermilion border. When making an extensive restoration for a patient of this type, one cannot be guided entirely by the position of the lip line, for it has been found that, after the vertical dimension has been increased to normal, the upper lip, in the course of 6 months to a year, lengthens to meet the new functional requirements.

It is important to check the positions that the lip assumes during speech, laughter, and repose. If the upper lip line is low, the pontics of an upper fixed bridge may be narrowed in the gingival area for hygienic purposes. If, however, the lip line is high and exposes the gingival line of the pontics during function, it will necessitate the construction of a different shape of pontic.

Facial landmarks

When a partial denture restores most of the anterior teeth, one cannot be guided entirely by the lip in locating the median line of the face. Sometimes the median line of the lip deviates to the right or the left, in which case the central incisors are placed in a position that will harmonize best with the average relationship of the eyes, nose, and chin.

There are other facial landmarks that need to be observed; these are the temporomandibular joint, the eyes, angles of the mouth, alae of the nose, median line of the face, and chin. The temporomandibular articulation should be studied carefully, particularly in those patients who require extensive dental service as the result of excessive wear and closure of the bite. If a patient complains of pain or other disturbances related to this region, an effort should be made to determine the cause and to remove it. In most patients requiring a one-tooth or two-tooth bridge, the temporomandibular joint is not seriously involved. The eyes should be noted, since the color of the eyes is often related to that of the teeth. The eyes may reveal the presence of certain systemic diseases. The color pigment of eyes may have a different color effect in a severe case of jaundice. The pupils may be abnormal in their relative position and function, as in tabes dorsalis. Sometimes the eye is used as a reference point from which measurements are made to establish the parallelism of the plane of occlusion.

It is very often possible to tell by the position of the angles of the mouth and the alae of the nose whether a patient has lost his normal facial expression. When his bite is closed, it will be observed that the angles of the mouth are stretched laterally, the lips are turned in, and the mouth appears as a narrow slit. It is natural in older people to have a nasolabial groove extending from the alae of the nose to the lip line, and not too much effort should be made in older patients to eradicate these grooves completely.

In edentulous patients or in those for whom we are establishing a new occlusal relationship, great care must be exercised to position the chin properly when taking the bite so that each condyle is seated in its glenoid fossa. The tendency for patients to protrude the jaw when registering the bite is well known.

When examining a patient for all the facial factors previously enumerated, it is well to stand back and try to visualize the patient as he was 20 years previously. If possible, obtain photographs of the patient taken earlier in life; these will aid in restoring the esthetic factors.

SELECTED REFERENCES

1. Thompson, J. R.: The rest position of the mandible and its significance to dental science, J.A.D.A. **33**:151, 1946.
2. Niswonger, M. E.: The rest position of the mandible and centric relation, J.A.D.A. **21**: 1572, 1934.

GENERAL REFERENCES

Lam, R. V.: Contour changes of the alveolar processes following extractions, J. Prosth. Dent. **10**:25, 1960.

Pendleton, E. C.: Anatomy of the maxilla and its relation to the problem of full denture retention, J.A.D.A. **19**: 543, 1932.

Schram, W. R.: Healing of tooth sockets following extraction by forceps and surgical methods, Bull. Northwestern Univ. **30**:1, 1930.

Tylman, S. D.: Relationship of the structural design of dental bridges to their supporting tissues, Int. Dent. J. **13**:303, 1963.

Chapter 7

Stomatognathic physiology related to crown and fixed partial prosthodontic therapy*

Posselt[1, 2] studied the limits of motion of the human mandible at many increments of jaw opening from tooth occlusion to maximum opening. He recorded these limits with intraoral needle point tracings at the different vertical openings, one above the other, to produce a solid form that demonstrated the movement space of the mandible. A midsagittal section through a typical movement space is shown in Fig. 7-1. It has been found that an arc, *BC*, exists for the mandible in which it rotates about an axis running through or near the condyles when they are seated up in the glenoid fossae. This arc is known as the centric relation closure arc and can be demonstrated on most patients using a hinge axis face bow procedure. The center of this arc is the terminal hinge axis or kinematic point. When a patient has opened to point *C* in the centric relation closure arc the condyles can no longer remain up in the glenoid fossae but must translate down and forward. The mandibular reference point will therefore be deflected at point *C*; the arc *CD* represents a combination of translation and rotation of the condyles. This movement, then, has a constantly changing center of rotation. At point *D* the mandible has reached maximum opening. The curve *DE* represents the maximum, protruded closure arc. The condyles are located forward, in many cases, anterior to the eminence during this closure. The irregular path from *E* to *A* represents the movement of the mandible from the maximum protruded occlusal position back to maximum intercuspation of the teeth. The irregular path is produced by the deflection

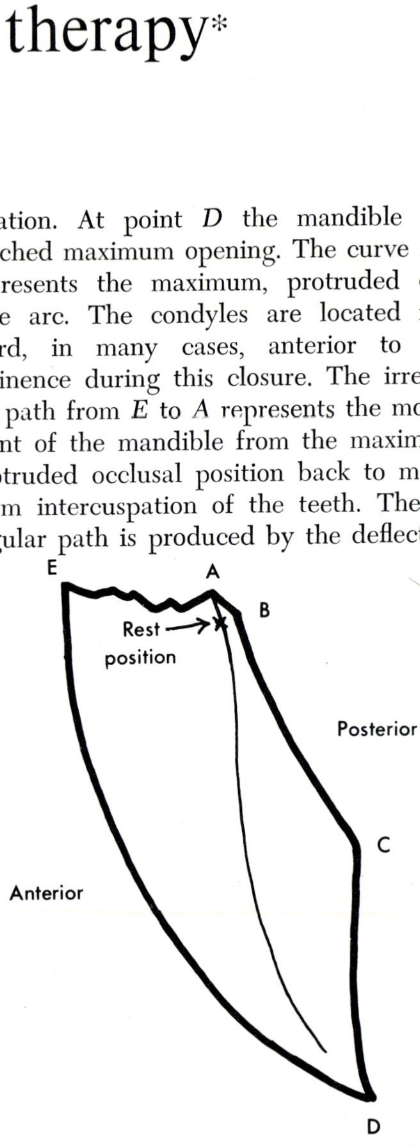

Fig. 7-1. Midsagittal section through mandibular movement space as described by Posselt. (Posselt, U.: Acta Odont. Scand. **10**:10, 1952.)

*Text by Parker E. Mahan, D.D.S., Ph.D., F.A.C.D.; Associate Professor of Dentistry, Emory University School of Dentistry, Atlanta, Georgia.

of the mandible by opposing inclines of the teeth as they move over each other.

SLIDE FROM RETRUDED CONTACT TO MAXIMUM INTERCUSPATION

Posselt found that 88 percent of the subjects in his study, when closing in the centric relation closure arc, first occluded their teeth at a retruded contact position (*B*); the mandible was then deflected up and forward to maximum intercuspation of the teeth at point *A*. He found that this slide from retruded contact to maximum intercuspation had a horizontal component of 1.25 ± 1.0 mm. and a vertical component of 0.9 ± 0.75 mm. relative to the sella-nasion line measured at the lower incisors. Many other investigators have studied the magnitude and direction of the slide. Beyron[3] found that 90 percent of forty-six adult aborigines had a slide that averaged approximately 1 mm.; Kydd and Sander[4] found that all fourteen of their subjects had a slide. Hodge[5] studied 101 young male adults and found that only 57 percent of them had a slide. These men had at least twenty-eight natural teeth and most of them had no dental restorations. Hodge measured the horizontal, vertical, and lateral component of the slide and found that although 57 percent of the subjects had an anteroposterior component to their slide, only 15 percent had a measurable lateral component. Lateral deviation in the slide is often associated with temporomandibular joint pain syndrome.[6-9]

The lower incisor teeth close up and forward at an angle of approximately 38 degrees to a perpendicular from the Frankfort plane during the last millimeter of closure.[10] This natural angle of closure serves to move the lower anterior teeth forward a distance almost equal to their vertical movement in the last millimeter of jaw closure. Therefore, adjusting the occlusion in a patient with a long anteroposterior slide may require very little removal of tooth structure on the opposing cuspal inclines. The distal inclines of lower teeth occlude against the mesial inclines of uppers in the slide. Since the lower teeth are moving forward in this final increment of jaw closure, tending to move these occluding inclines apart, interfering tooth substances that actually deflects the mandible is greatly minimized. When a jaw registration in the maximum intercuspation position is transferred to most adjustable articulators, there is one movement that the patient can make which the instrument cannot duplicate or simulate. That movement is the slide from retruded contact to maximum intercuspation. A dental patient will often close into the maximum intercuspation position when he is not guided or trained by the dentist.[11] When many occlusal surfaces are to be restored in an arch, the cuspal inclines that occlude in the slide may need excessive adjustment in the mouth after the restorations are seated when maximum intercuspation registration was established on the articulator so that the slide could not be simulated.

When the anterior teeth of a patient who has a slide are being restored on a nonadjustable instrument or simple hinge device, the maximum intercuspation registration will introduce less error than the retruded contact registration. This is true because the lower anterior teeth usually move up and forward to contact the lingual surface of the uppers at the end of the slide. When a retruded contact registration has been established on an adjustable instrument, the anterior teeth can be waxed so as to establish contact along the slide in the cingulum area of the upper incisors and cuspids.

Several studies using radio transmitters in fixed bridge pontics so that the keying contacts are closed by metal restorations in opposing teeth when the jaws are closed in specific occlusal positions have produced interesting results. It has been shown in one study[12] that four out of five subjects closed into retruded contact position when swallowing and cleansing the mouth. All five of the subjects closed into maximum intercuspation position while chewing peanuts and rye bread and when swallowing and cleansing the mouth. The movement back to retruded contact has also been observed in subjects when swallowing a bolus of food they have masticated while wearing extraoral needle point tracing devices.[13] Interferences in the slide are very often associated with temporomandibular joint pain syndrome.[6-9] The fact that retruded contact position is rarely used in normal function does not prevent interferences in this position from playing a role in temporomandibular joint dysfunction.

When attempting to adjust a patient's occlusion prior to extensive crown and bridge restoration one may observe that in one patient this adjustment will create an increased horizontal overlap of anterior teeth while the next adjustment will not alter this measurement.[10] This observation can be explained as shown in Fig. 7-2. In Fig. 7-2, *A*, the lower second bicuspid closes along the centric relation closure arc (arrow) until it contacts the upper second bicuspid at its cusp tip. It then slides up and forward to the cross (+) over the marginal ridges of the upper bicuspids. When the mesial incline of the upper bicuspid is adjusted by removing the stippled area, the jaws can then close so that the lower bicuspid moves to the cross on the centric relation closure arc. In this case the horizontal overlap of the incisors has been increased by the distance between the crosses. In Fig. 7-2, *B*, the lower bicuspid closes along the centric relation closure arc until it contacts the distal aspect of the upper second bicuspid cusp tip. It then trips over this cuspal incline and moves to the cross (+) over the marginal ridges of the upper bicuspids. When the upper bicuspid has been adjusted to eliminate the slide in this case the lower bicuspid moves to the same occlusal position it had before the adjustment, and the horizontal overlap of the anterior teeth is not altered.

It has been shown that the slide from retruded contact to maximum intercuspation in children is quite similar to that found in the adult.[14, 15] Ingervall[14] has demonstrated that the only statistical difference between the slide in 10-year-old girls and that in 20-year-old women is a larger lateral component in the girls. These data indicate that during the mixed dentition stage when the permanent teeth are erupting into position in the dental arch, lateral interferences are created that tend to be corrected with time alone.

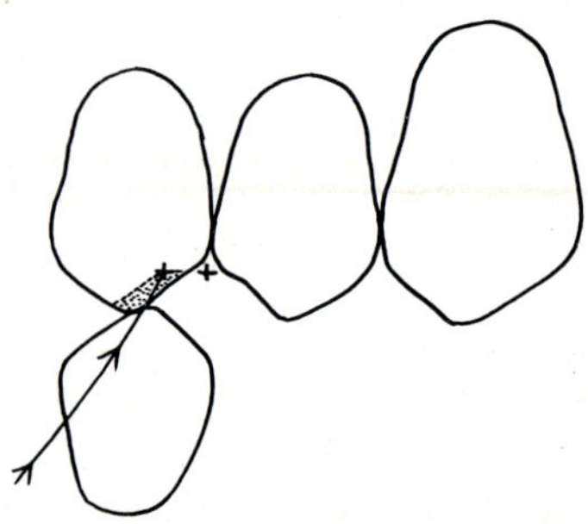

A

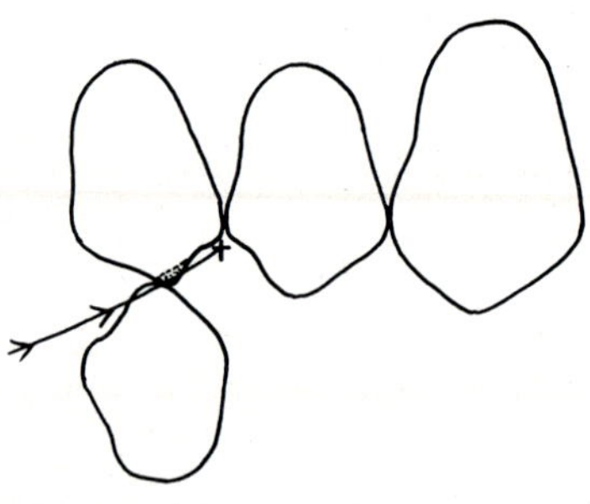

B

Fig. 7-2. Upper cuspid, first and second bicuspid with centric relation closure arc of lower second bicuspid indicated. **A,** Relationship that increases anterior horizontal overlap with occlusal adjustment. **B,** Relationship that does not alter anterior horizontal overlap with occlusal adjustment.

INTEROCCLUSAL DISTANCE AND MOVEMENT FROM REST POSITION TO MAXIMUM INTERCUSPATION

In 1908 Sir Norman Bennett[16] demonstrated that the center of rotation of his mandible from maximum intercuspation to rest position was located in the region of his mastoid process. In 1956 Nevakari[17] studied this movement in seventy-five dental students. He was interested in finding out whether or not this movement was a pure hinge movement with its center in or near the condyle. He found the average location of the center of rotation of this movement in his subjects to be also in the region of the mastoid process. His study further demonstrated that the condyle moves up and back approximately 1 mm. during this movement so that both translation and rotation occur simultaneously. He found that the lower cuspids move up and forward at an average angle of 11 degrees to a perpendicular to the Frankfort plane in the movement from rest to maximum intercuspation. Posselt demonstrated (Fig. 7-1) that the rest position in the average patient is not a border movement but lies within the movement space on the free opening-closing path. These data indicate that the mandible is not back in the centric relation closure arc when it is in rest position in most patients.

A number of electromyographic studies of interocclusal distance have been reported. Garnick and Ramfjord[18] found that the posterior temporalis muscle usually demonstrates electrical activity when the mandible is in the clinically determined rest position. They considered the distance between the teeth when the first elevator muscle came into electrical activity on jaw closure to be the electromyographic (EMG) interocclusal distance. In their study of twenty subjects this distance averaged 3.3 mm., while their clinically determined interocclusal distance averaged 1.7 mm. on the same subjects. They found an EMG resting range of 11.1 mm. in their subjects instead of a specific rest position. Prieskel[19] studied the variations in interocclusal distance with different head positions. He found that when the head was turned down 35 degrees from the horizontal orientation, the interocclusal distance decreased; when the head was turned up 35 degrees it increased. In each instance he found that the EMG interocclusal distance was greater than the clinically determined distance. It has not been practical to place electrodes on all of the mandibular muscles in these studies but it has been shown, on the muscles that are accessible for recording, that the concept that the mandibular muscles are at minimal activity at the rest position is probably not true. It seems that at least the posterior temporalis is active, counteracting the pull of gravity on the lower jaw at our clinically determined rest position. It will be interesting to see, with the advent of space travel in the future, what effect weightlessness will have on the interocclusal distance.

The rest position in children with class II, division 1 malocclusions is different from that in children with normal jaw relationships. Ingervall[20] located the average rest position in thirty-two class II, division 1 girls and found it to be down and forward of the maximum intercuspation position. It is located down and backward from the maximum intercuspation position in normal subjects. The class II patient may hold his jaw forward for esthetic reasons or to allow the muscles of the lips and chin to function properly.

The addition of an acrylic palatal base plate to a patient's mouth will increase the resting height of the face.[21] A study of rest position in thirteen dental students has demonstrated a statistical increase in rest face height and greater variation in rest position of the mandible when the subjects wore a palatal piece 2.5 mm.

thick. These subjects all had nearly full complements of natural teeth.

It is interesting that the interocclusal distance was reduced to zero over a 12-year period in a patient with a paralyzed right lateral pterygoid.[22] In this instance an imbalance between the elevators and depressors of the mandible in favor of the elevators established a new rest position at the occlusal vertical dimension. One of the generalizations in physiology that can be demonstrated repeatedly is that the organs of the living mammal function in a state of dynamic balance. In this state, opposing forces that may vary in magnitude from time to time balance each other in establishing the functions of life. The occlusal vertical dimension and the rest position are established in any given patient by a dynamic balance between various factors that tend to close the jaws and those that open them. It is a common observation that in some patients the teeth, when taken out of occlusion by the occlusal reduction of a full crown preparation, will rapidly extrude into occlusion if very accurate temporary crowns are not placed on them. In other patients the teeth that have been taken out of occlusion do not seem to extrude at all. When one is deciding whether or not to change the occlusal vertical dimension of a patient he should study the factors that have balanced to produce the vertical dimension and interocclusal distance in that patient. If it seems possible to alter these factors in favor of an increased vertical dimension then perhaps the bite can be successfully opened. One should always examine the interocclusal distance when he is contemplating increasing the occlusal vertical dimension in a patient. It has been found that increasing the vertical dimension in patients with small interocclusal distance is rarely successful.[23] Increasing the occlusal vertical dimension with case restorations or removable applicances may not alter the opposing forces that establish the dimension so that the teeth may intrude into the alveolar process and/or the condyle-fossa relationship of the temporomandibular joint may be changed. These changes may or may not be accompanied by pain dysfunction syndrome. It has been observed that opening the bite in some patients with temporomandibular joint pain syndrome will relieve the pain.[24] This relief is not uncommonly temporary and in those cases in which it recurs after the teeth have been intruded, the dentist is confronted with a most difficult problem. One should always carefully examine for temporomandibular joint pathology, muscle abnormality, interferences in the slide, balancing interferences, lateral deviations in the slide, and open or heavy centric stops at the patient's occlusal vertical dimension before considering opening a patient's bite.

CENTRIC RELATION CLOSURE ARC AND TERMINAL HINGE POSITION

Zola[25] has demonstrated a shiny facet in a depression in the medial wall of the glenoid fossa of an unspecified number of skulls. He has also demonstrated that the meniscus may be only 0.2 mm. thick over the medial pole of the condyle as it is positioned in these depressions. The seating of the right and left condylar medial poles in these depressions will establish a bony support for the mandible in its superior, posterior position and establish an axis about which it may rotate. It is reasonable that this anatomic relationship would establish a terminal hinge axis with a kinematic point on the face where this axis emerges from the head. This definite depression in the medial wall of the glenoid fossa cannot be demonstrated on many human skulls so these findings will not explain the presence of a terminal hinge axis in all patients. McCollum and Stuart[26] reported that the terminal hinge axis has remained constant in a few patients for as long as 9 years. The significance of the terminal hinge axis to jaw registration for occlusal restoration was pointed out by Moulton[27] in 1960.

Beck[28] located the terminal hinge axis on twelve subjects and studied its location relative to the image of the condyle on lateral cephalometric radiographs. Disregarding the complicated distortion of the cephalometric radiograph it can be seen from his study that the terminal hinge axis fell within the condyle in seven of his twelve subjects. In the other five subjects it was located posterior to, anterior to, or within the neck of the condylar process. Schallhourn[29] located the terminal hinge axis in seventy dental students and then marked the arbitrary axis point 13 mm. anterior to the tragus on a line to the outer canthus of the eye. He found the average discrepancy between these two points to be 1.7 mm. Ninety-seven percent of the arbitrary axis points fell within 5 mm. of the hinge axis points. The hinge axis points tended to lie slightly posterior to the arbitrary point. Fox[30] has estimated that cementation of crowns produces occlusal errors of 0.05 to 0.08 mm. He then calculated that an error of 1 mm. in locating the terminal hinge axis is acceptable because it will not result in greater occlusal discrepancy than 0.08 mm.

TYPES OF OCCLUSAL FUNCTION

Before one can properly diagnose and plan treatment for the occlusal restoration of a patient, he must know how the patient's teeth occlude during function. There are three general types of occlusal function found in the human dentition. These are balanced occlusion, working side occlusion, and cuspid rise or cuspid protected occlusion. All three are based on the assumption that opposing teeth are in contact in a centric stop position when the jaws are closed in maximum intercuspation position. The type of occlusal function in a specific patient may not be bilateral. It is not uncommon, for example, to find cuspid protected occlusion on one side and working side occlusion on the other in young patients.

Balanced occlusion is that relationship of the teeth in which they are in contact on the right and left sides and in the anterior and posterior simultaneously when the jaws are closed within the functional range of opposing occlusal surfaces. In this type of occlusion there is a buccal-to-buccal contact on the working side of the mouth and at least one contact of an upper lingual cusp against a lower buccal cusp on the balancing side. This type of occlusion is considered ideal in complete denture construction because three-point contact provides stability of the denture bases against the alveolar mucosa during occlusal function.

Working side occlusion is that type of occlusal function in which the cuspids and one or more posterior teeth are in contact, buccal-to-buccal, on the working side but there is no tooth contact on the balancing side. Weinberg[31] has reported that 65 per cent of one hundred patients having at least twenty-eight natural teeth had this type of occlusion. Working side occlusion is found in the Australian aborigines who abrade their teeth excessively throughout life. One explanation for the high incidence of working side occlusion (no tooth contact on the balancing side) in the human dentition can be found in the data of Conant.[32] In this study a sound transmission method was used to measure the forces exerted between the teeth in the chewing cycle in an unspecified number of subjects. The relationship of force exerted between the teeth to the amount of filtered and amplified 1,000 cycle/second sound transmitted from the forehead to the chin was determined on one subject. On the basis of this calibration of the system it was found that when subjects chew a soft bolus of food like chewing gum they exert maximum force between the teeth in the maximum intercuspation position at the top of the chewing cycle. When, however, they are chewing a tough bolus of food like raisins, the teeth move through maximum intercuspation into a balancing relationship on the bolus side and exert maximum closing force in this position. It therefore seems reasonable that the balancing inclines of the teeth would abrade away slightly ahead of the working inclines since more force is applied in this tooth position against tough and abrasive foods. It has been observed that balancing interferences are often associated with temporomandibular joint pain syndrome.[9, 33] These interferences are not infrequently found in mouths with missing lower molars and mesial tipping of the more distal molar. They are also found in postorthodontic patients when occlusal adjustment has not been accomplished after the teeth have closed up the band spaces interproximally and tightened up in the alveolar process.[34]

Cuspid protected occlusion is that type of occlusal function in which there are even centric stops around the arch in the maximum intercuspation position but any lateral or protrusive movement of the mandible immediately discludes the posterior teeth, with the lower cuspid occluding against the lingual surface of the upper cuspid.

D'Amico[35] pointed out the significance of this type of occlusal function when he noted that ancient California Indian skulls showed abraded cuspids and incisors with an occlusal function resembling that of the aborigine, while the modern California Indian (eating a soft diet) has cuspid protected occlusion. Weinberg[31] reported that only 19 percent of one hundred patients with twenty-eight natural teeth in his study had cuspid protected occlusion. This type of occlusal function would tend to put very heavy forces on single teeth, the cuspids, in eccentric occlusal positions. It has been noted in the cat[36, 37] that the periodontal membranes of the teeth, especially the anterior teeth, are richly innervated with nerve receptors whose primary cell bodies lie in the mesencephalic nucleus of the trigeminal nerve. These receptors are directionally oriented around the tooth roots so that slight displacement of

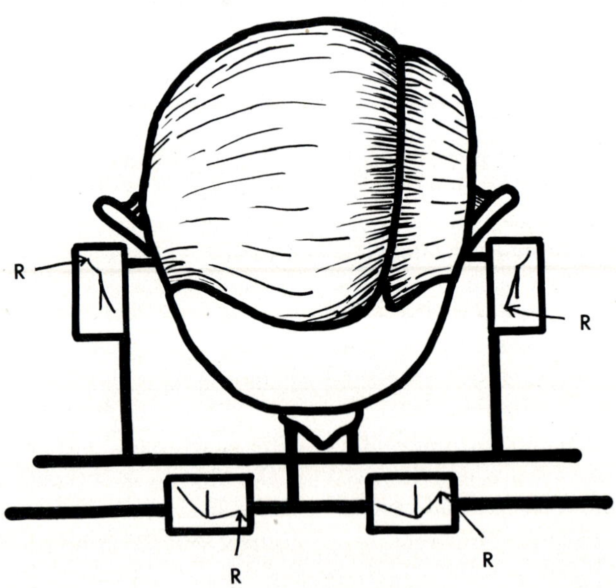

Fig. 7-3. The Bennett path and gothic arch tracings of a pantographic tracing.

the cuspid inhibits the motor output to the jaw-elevating muscles and stimulates the anterior belly of the digastric muscle. These neurons with specialized receptors, then, constitute the sensory side of a jaw-opening reflex. This type of proprioceptive mechanism may function in patients with cuspid protected occlusion to prevent traumatic occlusion and destruction of the cuspid periodontium. There is no agreement today among the men most experienced in occlusal restoration as to whether or not cuspid protected occlusion is a healthy and desirable occlusal function. Some feel that the lateral forces of occlusion should be distributed to as many teeth as possible,[33] while others think that the cuspids can withstand these forces and the posterior teeth may show premature periodontal deterioration when subjected to the lateral forces of balanced occlusion.[38] Only 16 percent of the patients in Weinberg's study had balanced occlusion of their natural teeth.

One can best visualize the movement of the mandible relative to the maxilla in both functional and nonfunctional positions by studying a typical pantographic tracing of a patient. Fig. 7-3 diagrammatically demonstrates four of the six tracings of a pantographic recording. The writing styli are not pictured so that the Bennett path and Gothic arch tracings may be viewed without obstruction. It should be noted that the Bennett path tracing tables are fixed to the maxilla and their writing styli are fixed to the mandible. The Gothic arch tracing tables, on the other hand, are fixed to the mandibular face bow and the styli are fixed to the maxilla. The simultaneous locations of the writing styli for a subject in the extreme right lateral position of the mandible are indicated by the letter *R* in Fig. 7-3. A typical pantographic Bennett path tracing is described in Fig. 7-4. It must be remembered that the stylus is lateral to the condyle so the Bennett tracing does not duplicate the movement of the condyle in any plane in space. The curved line from the centric occlusion point marked "working condyle path" represents the combination of rotation and lateral shift of the working condyle. The extent of straight lateral displacement of this curve from the centric occlusion point would approximate the actual amount of side shift of the mandible. The angle formed between the "working condyle path" and the sagittal plane is reported to range between 0 and 35 degrees.[39] An angle of 0 degrees would indicate no lateral shift of the mandible. Several studies[39, 40] have reported that all patients examined (seventy-six patients) showed Bennett shift of at least one condyle. The tracing marked "balancing condyle path" anterior to the centric occlusion point represents the movement of the condyle as it translates down and medially on the articular eminence when the mandible is moved to the opposite lateral position.

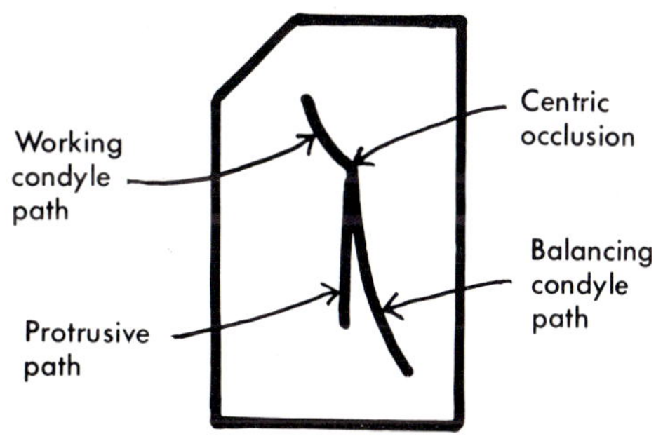

Fig. 7-4. Typical pantographic Bennett path tracing.

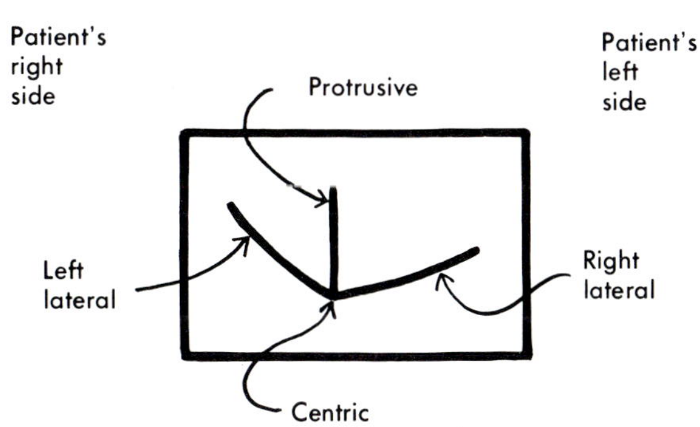

Fig. 7-5. Typical pantographic gothic arch tracing.

The third tracing represents the path of the mandibular stylus when the patient protrudes the jaw straight forward.

A typical pantographic Gothic arch tracing is shown in Fig. 7-5. The apex of the three tracing lines represents centric occlusion or retruded contact position. The patient's movement from retruded contact to maximum, straight protrusive would produce the tracing so labeled. When the jaw is moved to a right lateral position the tracing would actually move toward the patient's left, as indicated, because the stylus is fixed to the maxilla and the tracing table moves with the mandible. When the jaw is moved to a left lateral position the tracing would run from the centric occlusion point to the patient's right, as indicated.

A typical pantographic condyle path tracing is shown diagrammatically in Fig. 7-6. The mandibular side arm with its vertical and horizontal writing styli is not shown. It will be noted that the centric occlusion point is not located at the posterior end of the tracing. The portion of the tracing posterior to the centric point is traced when the jaw is moved laterally to the side of the tracing table. The condyle tracing table is fixed to the maxilla and is several centimeters lateral to the condyle. The writing stylus is fixed to the mandibular face bow and when the condyle rotates the stylus is moved posterior to its centric occlusion location. When the patient moves into straight protrusive the condyle usually does not drop as far inferiorly as it does when the jaw is moved to the opposite lateral position, as indicated. Only a small portion of the protrusive condyle path is traced before the lower anterior teeth have protruded beyond the upper anteriors. The length of the condyle path utilized in functional occlusal positions depends on the amount of horizontal and vertical overlap of the anterior teeth.

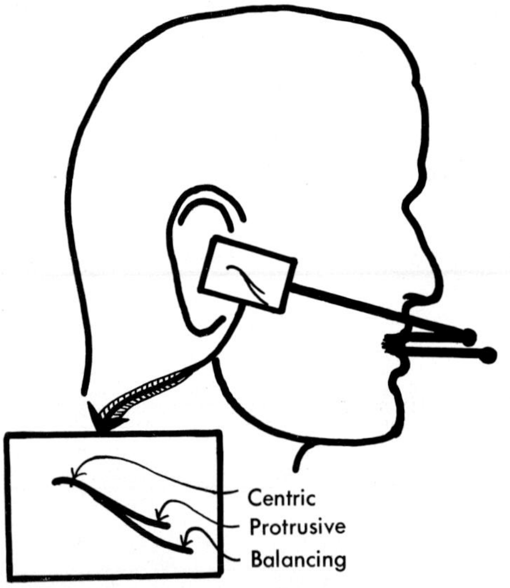

Fig. 7-6. Typical pantographic condyle path tracing.

There are many variations in pantographic tracings observed in patients, but the examples described demonstrate a fairly common set of tracings. Isaacson[39] has beautifully demonstrated the variability found in the Bennett path tracings in nine patients.

PROPRIOCEPTION IN THE STOMATOGNATHIC SYSTEM

The major receptors that subserve the function of proprioception are the muscle spindles and Golgi tendon organs. The muscle spindles are very complicated structures usually found in the central parts of the muscles.[41] There are two types of muscle fibers within the spindles that do not produce tension when they contract. These fibers have separate motor innervations and function only to alter the firing rate of the primary and secondary endings of the proprioceptive nerves. The muscle spindles, then, have a double motor and double sensory innervation and they provide the central nervous system with information on the instantaneous length and the rate of change of length of the muscle in which they are located. They help ensure that muscle tension will be proportional to stretch and they allow smooth coordination of phasic (intentional) movement with posture. The Golgi tendon organs are located in the ligaments and tendons of the muscles and are also constantly firing into the central nervous system.[42] The tendon organs have sufficiently low thresholds to tension to play a part in the moment-to-moment control of muscular contraction.

There are several unique features in the proprioceptive mechanism of the stomatognathic system. The cell bodies of the proprioceptive nerves in the muscles that elevate the mandible are found within the central nervous system in the mesencephalic nucleus of the trigeminal nerve.[43, 44] One would expect these primary sensory neuron cell bodies to lie in the semilunar ganglion since all the other proprioceptive cell bodies are located outside the central nervous system in the dorsal root ganglia. Secondly, there are no muscle spindles in the lateral pterygoid muscles and probably none in the anterior belly of the digastric.[45, 46] Anatomists have examined the lateral pterygoids of man, rat, goat, and cat, and none of these mammals have muscle spindles in the lateral pterygoids. The typical reciprocal activity of antagonistic muscles has been demonstrated by Kawamura and others[47] in the mandibular muscles. When they freed the mandibular muscles from their insertion in the cat and stretched one of them while recording in the motor nucleus they found that electrical activity in the antagonistic muscle was inhibited. This type of muscle function is typically attributed to the reciprocal activity of muscle spindles located in the antagonistic muscles. Since there are no muscle spindles in the depressor muscles of the mandible, one must find another explanation for these observations in the stomatognathic system. It has been shown that the capsule of the temporomandibular joint is richly innervated with proprioceptive nerve endings.[48] Griffin[49] has demonstrated recently that the meniscus of the temporomandibular joint is richly innervated by Golgi tendon organs in the area of attachment of the superior belly of the lateral pterygoid muscle. Jerge[36] has recently demonstrated in the cat that the periodontal membranes of the teeth, especially the anterior teeth, are innervated by complicated nerve receptors whose cell bodies lie in the mesencephalic nucleus of the trigeminal nerve. He has shown that these nerves may innervate single tooth periodontal membranes or two or more adjacent teeth and the adjacent gingival tissue. These receptors in the periodontal membranes are directionally oriented; pressure applied to the teeth is followed by jaw-opening movements. It therefore seems that the organs that need protection from jaw-closing action, the teeth, provide a large part of the sensory side of a jaw-opening reflex. The depressor muscles are protected by the Golgi tendon organs in their attachments and by the tendon organs in the temporomandibular joint.

It follows, then, that any time a dentist alters or restores the occlusal surface of a tooth having occlusal function, he is dealing directly with the proprioceptive innervation of the muscles. It has been shown[34] that muscle spasms rapidly disappear in the temporal muscles when occlusal interferences have been removed, as evidenced by electromyographic recording from the muscles. In cases where occlusal interferences were corrected with splints, the muscle spasms recurred almost immediately upon removal of the splint. These observations seem to indicate that the proprioceptive nerves from the periodontal membranes, the muscles ligaments, and joints of the stomatognathic system are extremely sensitive to the occlusion of the teeth. It also seems evident that an altered proprioceptive input due to occlusal interferences will lead to muscle pain and spasm in many patients.

Leff[50] has demonstrated that very slight changes in occlusal position of the teeth greatly alter the maximum closing pressure of the mandibular elevators. He first measured the amount of closure of the subjects' teeth into a soft acrylic resin interocclusal record. Then he placed casts of the subjects' arches in the acrylic records and applied pressure until the casts closed down to the same distance as that measured in the mouth. The pressures exerted on the casts were then read from a gauge in the system. He found that the average pressure exerted on the teeth with the mandible closing in the maximum intercuspation position (in an unspecified number of subjects) was 110 pounds. (See Chapter 11.) When the mandible was shifted just a few millimeters to a lateral position, the maximum pressure exerted dropped to 10 pounds. When the subjects protruded a few millimeters, the pressure measured 55 pounds; when they closed back in the centric relation closure arc toward retruded contact, they could exert only 19 pounds. These data indicate that the proprioceptive receptors of the stomatognathic system are very effective in limiting the contraction of the mandibular elevators so as to protect the structures of the temporomandibular joint in the retruded contact position of the condyle and the teeth when they are occluding on inclines instead of on stable centric stop positions of opposing teeth.

SUMMARY

Many of the complicated and intricate interactions of the structures of the stomatognathic system have been studied and described so that the dentist is now able to measure or closely approximate its normal function in his treatment of the abnormalities of the mouth and jaws. There is, on the other hand, a large part of stomatognathic function that we do not understand. This void in our knowledge daily faces the dentist in his practice and limits his ability to properly diagnose and plan the treatment of his patients.

The movement space of the mandible, telling us where the patient can move his jaws under various conditions, is understood today and we are able to use some of this information in dental treatment procedures. Posselt has demonstrated that most patients have a centric relation closure arc in which the mandible can rotate about an imaginary axis with the condyles positioned superiorly and posteriorly in the glenoid fossae. In some patients this position is established by the seating of the condyle medial poles into facets in the medial wall of the fossae. The tissues in the posterior of the joint are not firm or stable enough to establish the posterior, superior position of the condyle. Most patients can maintain the centric relation closure arc only for the first 2 cm. of jaw-opening, at which point the condyles must translate down and forward out of the fossae. The identification of this deflection point in the posterior border movement of a patient's jaw serves as an excellent landmark for determining centric relation in our patients. Most patients with natural teeth, when closing the jaws in the centric relation closure arc, occlude in a retruded contact position and slide up and forward approximately 1 to 2 mm. into a maximum intercuspation position. Their mandible moves down and slightly backward from maximum intercuspation to its rest position. In the movement from maximum intercuspation to rest position the condyles translate down and forward approximately 1 mm. and rotate a small amount.

The retruded contact position is usually not used in the masticatory cycle, but most patients close back into this position when swallowing and cleansing the mouth. At the top of the masticatory cycle, the teeth first contact in the working bite relationship, slide up into maximum intercuspation, and then move on into a balancing relationship on the bolus side. More pressure is exerted between the teeth when they have reached the balancing relationship than in the earlier occlusal positions when tough foods are being masticated. This finding may explain the observation that few people have balancing contacts of their natural teeth.

Electromyographic studies have shown that the posterior temporalis muscle is usually showing electrical activity at the clinically determined rest position of the mandible. The muscles that have been examined have revealed a resting range of approximately 11 mm. instead of a single rest position of the jaws. The concept that the mandibular muscles are relaxed when the jaw is in its rest position does not seem to be true. Rest position and occlusal vertical dimension both represent a dynamic balance between the opposing forces that close and open the jaws. Many factors such as the addition of a palatal base plate will affect the rest position of the mandible.

When one is considering increasing the occlusal vertical dimension in a patient with temporomandibular joint pain syndrome, one should carefully examine for joint pathology, muscle trismus, interferences or lateral deviation in the slide from retruded contact to maximum intercuspation, balancing side interferences, and uneven centric stops before opening a patient's bite.

There are three general types of occlusal function for the dentist to consider in his diagnosis and treatment planning. These include balanced occlusion, working side occlusion, and cuspid protected occlusion. Any one of these occlusal function patterns may be bilateral or unilateral, and their recognition in a crown and bridge patient is vital to accurate treatment planning.

The proprioceptive mechanism of the stomatognathic system is still poorly understood, but several unique features of the mechanism have been described. There are no muscle spindles in the lateral pterygoids and few or none in the anterior belly of the diagastric. There is, therefore, a deficiency of muscle spindles in the mandibular depressors, but the elevators are richly supplied with spindles. It has been shown, however, that the periodontal membranes of the teeth in animals are well innervated with directionally oriented proprioceptive endings. The attachment of the superior belly of the lateral pterygoid into the joint meniscus and the joint capsule are also richly suplied with Golgi tendon organs. It seems, therefore, that the very organs that must be protected from excessive forces of mandibular elevation are those that house the proprioceptive receptors required to trigger that protection.

SELECTED REFERENCES

1. Posselt, U.: Studies in the mobility of the human mandible, Acta Odont. Scand. **10**:10, 1952.
2. Posselt, U.: Range of movement of the mandible, J.A.D.A. **56**:10, 1958.
3. Beyron, H.: Occlusal relations and mastication in Australian aborigines, Acta Odont. Scand. **22**:597, 1964.
4. Kydd, W. L., and Sander, A.: A study of posterior mandibular movements from intercuspal occlusal position, J. Dent. Res. **40**:419, 1961.
5. Hodge, L. C.: A study of mandibular movement from centric occlusion to maximum intercuspation, Thesis, Emory University School of Dentistry, 1965.
6. Ramfjord, S. P.: Dysfunctional temporomandibular joint and muscle pain, J. Prosth. Dent. **11**:353, 1961.
7. Cobin, H. P.: The temporomandibular syndrome and centric relation, New York Dent. J. **18**:393, 1952.
8. Kyes, F. M.: Temporomandibular joint disorders, J.A.D.A. **59**:1137, 1959.
9. Shohet, H.: The treatment of ear, facial, head and other pains associated with pathologic temporomandibular joint, J. Prosth. Dent. **9**:80, 1959.
10. Hodge, L. C., and Mahan, P. E.: A study of mandibular movement from centric occlusion to maximum intercuspation, J. Prosth. Dent. **18**:19, 1967.

11. Kabcenell, J. L.: Effect of clinical procedures on mandibular position, J. Prosth. Dent. **14:** 266, 1964.
12. Graf, H., and Zander, H. A.: Tooth contact patterns in mastication, J. Prosth. Dent. **13:** 1055, 1963.
13. Moore, E. E.: Movies and slides demonstrating the chewing of various foods with and without deflective occlusal contacts: chewing and centric—clinical lecture, A.D.A. Annual Session, Dallas, Texas, 1966.
14. Ingervall, B.: Retruded contact position of mandible, a comparison between children and adults, Odont. Revy. **15:**130, 1964.
15. Ingervall, B.: Retruded contact position of mandible in the deciduous dentition, Odont. Revy. **15:**414, 1964.
16. Bennett, N. G.: A contribution to the study of the movements of the mandible, Proc. Royal Soc. Med. I:79, 1908.
17. Nevakari, K.: An analysis of the mandibular movement from rest to occlusal position, Acta Odont. Scand. Suppl. 19, 1956.
18. Garnick, J., and Ramfjord, S. P.: Rest position: an electromyographic and clinical investigation, J. Prosth. Dent. **12:**895, 1962.
19. Preiskel, H. W.: Some observations on the postural position of the mandible, J. Prosth. Dent. **15:**625, 1965.
20. Ingervall, B.: Relation between retruded contact, intercuspal, and rest positions of mandible in children with angle class II, division 1 malocclusion, Odont. Revy. **17:**28, 1966.
21. Young, P.: A cephalometric study of the effect of acrylic test palatal piece thickness on the physiologic rest position, J. Philipp. Dent. A. **19:**5, 1966.
22. Vaughn, H. C.: The external pterygoid mechanism, J. Prosth. Dent. **5:**80, 1955.
23. Moulton, G. H.: Centric occlusion and the free-way space, J. Prosth. Dent. **7:**209, 1957.
24. Posselt, U.: Physiology of occlusion and rehabilitation, Philadelphia, 1962, F. A. Davis Co.
25. Zola, A.: Morphologic limiting factors in the temporomandibular joint, J. Prosth. Dent. **13:**732, 1963.
26. McCollum, B. B., and Stuart, C. E.: A research report, South Pasadena, California, 1955, Scientific Press.
27. Moulton, G. H.: The importance of centric occlusion in diagnosis and treatment planning, J. Prosth. Dent. **10:**921, 1960.
28. Beck, H. O.: Clinical evaluation of the Arcon concept of articulation, J. Prosth. Dent. **9:**409, 1959.
29. Schallhourn, R. G.: A study of the arbitrary center of the kinematic center of rotation for face-bow mountings, J. Prosth. Dent. **7:**162, 1957.
30. Fox, S. S.: The significance of errors in hinge axis location, J.A.D.A. **74:**1268, 1967.
31. Weinberg, L. A.: A cinematic study of centric and eccentric occlusions, J. Prosth. Dent. **14:**290, 1964.
32. Conant, J. R.: Sound transmission used for studying masticatory force distribution patterns, J. Periodont. **33:**322, 1962.
33. Schuyler, C. H.: Factors contributing to traumatic occlusion, J. Prosth. Dent. **11:** 708, 1961.
34. Jarabak, J. R.: An electromyographic analysis of muscular and temporomandibular joint disturbances due to imbalances in occlusion, Angle Orthodont. **26:**170, 1956.
35. D'Amico, A.: Canine teeth—normal functional relation of the natural teeth of man, S. Calif. Dent. A.J. **26:**6, 1958.
36. Jerge, C. R.: Organization and function of the trigeminal mesencephalic nucleus, J. Neurophysiol. **26:**379, 1963.
37. Kizior, J. E., and others: Functional and histologic assessment of the sensory innervation of the periodontal ligament of the cat, J. Dent. Res. **47:**59, 1968.
38. Stuart, C. E., and Stallard, H.: Diagnosis and treatment of occlusal relations of the teeth, Texas D. J. **75:**430, 1957.
39. Isaacson, D.: A clinical study of the Bennett movement, J. Prosth. Dent. **8:**641, 1958.
40. Aull, A. E.: Condylar determinants of occlusal patterns, J. Prosth. Dent. **15:**826, 1965.
41. Matthews, P. B. C.: Muscle spindles and their motor control, Physiol. Rev. **44:**219, 1964.
42. Matthews, B. H. C.: Nerve endings in mammalian muscle, J. Physiol. **78:**1, 1933.
43. Corbin, K. B.: Observations on the peripheral distribution of fibers arising in the mesencephalic nucleus of the fifth cranial nerve, J. Comp. Neurol. **73:**153, 1940.
44. Corbin, K. B., and Harrison, F.: Function of mesencephalic root of fifth cranial nerve, J. Neurophysiol. **3:**423, 1940.
45. Friemann, R.: Untersuchungen über Zahl und Anordhung der Muskelspindeln in den Kaumuskeln des Menschen, Anat. Anz. **100:** 258, 1954.
46. Karlsen, K.: The location of motor end plates and the distribution and histological structure of muscle spindles in jaw muscles of the rat, Acta Odont. Scand. **23:**521, 1965.
47. Kawamura, Y., and others: Reciprocal relationships in the brain-stem among afferent

impulses from each jaw muscle on the cat, Jap. J. Physiol. **10**:585, 1960.

48. Thilander, B.: Innervation of the temporomandibular joint capsule in man, Trans. Roy. Schools Stockh. Umed No. 7, 1961.
49. Griffin, C. J.: Inhibition of the linguo-mandibular reflex, part I: Golgi type organs of the pes menisci, Aust. Dent. J. **10**:376, 1965.
50. Leff, A.: Gnathodynamics of four mandibular positions, J. Prosth. Dent. **16**:844, 1966.

GENERAL REFERENCES

Awazawa, Y.: Electron microscope investigation of the dentin with particular regards to the nature of the area surounding the odontoblast process, J. Nipon Univ. School Dentistry **5**: 31, 1962.

Barber, D., and Massler, M.: Permeability of active and arrested carious lesions to dyes and radioactive isotopes, J. Dent. Child. **31**:26-33, 1964.

Beveridge, E. E., and Brown, A. C.: The measurement of human dental intrapulpal pressure and its response to clinical variables, J. Oral Surg. **19**:655, 1965.

Bjorn, H.: Periodontal viewpoints on crown and bridge prosthodontics, Sverige Tandlakarforb Tidn **58**(12):497-504, 1966.

Bulow, F.: Histochemical and electronmicroscopical aspects of human buccal mucosa, Acta. Path. Microbiol. Scand. **66**:409-425, 1966.

Croft, L., and Stanley, H. R.: The effect of a chilled water spray on the human pulp during cavity preparation, Oral Surg. **22**:66-71, 1966.

Diamond, R. D., Stanley, H. R., and Swerdlow, H.: Reparative dentin formation resulting from cavity preparation, J. Prosth. Dent. **16**:1127-1134, 1966.

Eidelman, E., Finn, S. B., and Koulourides, T.: Remineralization of carious dentin treated with calcium hydroxide, J. Dent. Child. **32**:218-225, 1965.

Frank, R. M.: The ultrastructure of the tooth from the point of view of mineralization, demineralization and remineralization, Int. Dent. J. **17**(4):661, 1967.

Held-Wydler, E.: Natural (indirect) pulp capping, J. Dent. Child. **31**:107, 1964.

Henry, P. J., and Mitchel, D. F.: Tissue changes beneath fixed partial dentures, J. Prosth. Dent. **16**:937-947, 1966.

Jacobs, R. M.: Effect of the mechanism of muscle tonus on mandibular rest position, J. Canad. Dent. Assn. **32**(10):594-598, 1966.

Kawamura, Y., and Majima, T.: Temporomandibular joint's sensory mechanisms controlling activities of jaw muscles, J. Dent. Res. **43**:150, 1964.

Koulourides, T., Cueto, H., and Pigman, W.: Rehardening of softened enamel surfaces of teeth by solutions of calcium phosphates, Nature **189**:226-227, 1961.

Koulourides, T., Feagin, F., and Pigman, W.: Remineralization of dental enamel by saliva in vitro, Ann N. Y. Acad. Sci. **131**(2):685-730, 1965.

Krysinski, Z.: Individual variability of mastication efficiency, Czas Stomat **20**(3):299-306, 1967.

Linden, L., and Brannstrom, M.: Fluid movements in dentine and pulp, Odontologisk Revy, Vol. 18, 1967.

Loe, H.: Reactions of marginal periodontal tissues to restorative procedures, Int. Dent. J. **18**(4):759, 1968.

Luostarinen, V., and Scheinin, A.: Dynamics of repair in the pulp, Acta Physiol. Scand. **68**: 126, 1966.

Marcum, J. S.: The tissue response to different crown marginal depths, J. Kentucky Dent. Assn. **20**:21-28, 1968.

Mjor, I. A.: Histologic studies of human coronal dentine following the insertion of various materials in experimentally prepared cavities, Arch. Oral Biol. **12**:441, 1967.

Nyborg, H.: Healing processes in the pulp on capping: a morphologic study, Acta Odont. Scand. **13**:9-130, 1955.

Skinner, C. N.: Physiology of the occlusal coordination of natural teeth, complete dentures, and partial dentures, J. Prosth. Dent. **17**(6): 559-565, 1967.

Stanley, H. R., and Swerdlow, H.: An approach to biologic variation in human pulpal studies, J. Prosth. Dent. **14**:365-371, 1964.

Storey, A. T.: Sensory functions of the temporomandibular joint, J. Canad. Dent. Assn. **34**(6): 294-300, 1968.

Van Huysen, G.: The microstructure of normal and sclerosed dentine, J. Prosth. Dent. **10**:976, 1960.

Weiss, M. B.: Histological effects of silver nitrate on adult pulps, J. Indiana S. Dent. Assoc. **39**: 294-299, 1960.

Wooten, J. W.: Physiology of the temporomandibular joint, Oral Surg. **21**:543-553, 1966.

Chapter 8

The elderly person who requires crown and fixed partial prosthodontics*

The title of this chapter contains two new concepts that may appear strange in a work that dental practitioners use mainly to learn the best procedures in prosthodontic treatment. First, the person is given preference over the prosthodontics, to conform with the lesson that dentistry is gradually adopting from medicine—the person who has a health problem is at least as important as the problem that he has. Second, we are considering the person who "requires" the prosthodontic care as well as the one who "demands" it. If all the people who need oral rehabilitation would request or demand it, we would not have so many young men rejected from military service for being unable to eat army chow. Nor would we, as dentists, be offended by the misfit mouths of many of the prominent people whom we see on the television screen, people who are educated and do not lack the wherewithal to pay for dental service.

A NEW ERA OF OLD PEOPLE

For our immediate purpose, let us proceed to consider the elderly person of today who needs crown and bridge prosthodontics to improve his masticatory function and oral comfort and to acquire a better looking mouth with a more pleasing expression. From a dental point of view, these people are not the same as the oldsters of the early 1900's, a period that is less than one lifetime ago. At the turn of the century there were three million people in the United States who were 65 years of age and older; they constituted 3 percent of the total population, with a proportion of one hundred males to ninety-eight females. By 1965 the number of people who reached and passed the arbitrary compulsory retirement age of 65 years had increased to almost nineteen million; they accounted for 10 percent of the total population, and there were 129 females to one hundred males. Moreover, the number of elderly people is increasing rapidly as the general population "explodes." Statisticians have extrapolated that the elderly will always constitute about 12 percent of the total population. A significant statistic is that only 4 percent of those who are 65 years old and older are ill enough to be confined in domiciliary institutions,[1] which means that 96 percent of them are comparatively well or are not too badly incapacitated. This, in turn, implies that there will always be some older individuals seeking service in most of

*Text by Arthur E. Elfenbaum, D.D.S.; Professor Emeritus, Northwestern University School of Dentistry and University of Illinois School of Dentistry, Chicago, Illinois.

the dental offices of the United States; most of them will be women, who have always had the reputation of being more particular than men about their appearance (Chapter 9).

Less edentulous oldsters

Two generations ago there was a "dental fatalism" that convinced people—dentists, too—that in old age teeth had to be sacrificed, even if a few of them were still good, and complete dentures were accepted as an essential prosthodontic appliance in the later years. There is every indication today that within the coming half-century we will have a large population of elderly individuals who drank fluoridated water during their childhood years when their teeth were developing; in their old age they will have an acceptably good dental economy that they will want to preserve for the rest of their lives. Almost every medium of public communication has, at some time or other, mentioned the importance of oral health, so that the older people of today are much more informed on the subject than their immediate ancestors. Geriatric dentistry has a meaning for them, and it implies much more than the need for more complete dentures for more old people.

Old individuals are individual

The dentist, too, has changed his thinking in recent years. His patient is no longer an articulator with legs. An old man is not a secondhand copy of his son, no more than a child is a vestpocket edition of his parent. Every person is the sum total of his experience in life, and since more people are living to advanced ages than ever before, each oldster has accumulated many more experiences than his parents and grandparents. Inasmuch as no two old people can claim to have gone through the same events in life, however, each one is different from all others, and he has to be treated as an individual.[2] When he enters the dental office, he is not, to put it bluntly, a hole in a tooth that needs to be plugged up, or a vacant space between two teeth that has to be bridged, or an empty mouth that requires dentures. He is a vast totality that the dentist must understand before he looks into the mouth. A patient's mouth is an integral part of his body, and any disease or discomfort in it may be the cause or the effect of a disorder in any other part of the body.

The elderly in the garden of life. For an everyday objective view of the old people who have to or want to visit the dental office, one does not have to be an academic gerontologist to know that the bodies and minds of people undergo aging changes as the years advance. Some oldsters are vigorous and active, and deserve to be called the hardy perennials in the garden of life despite their minor ailments, which many of them regard as a challenge to their ability to adapt themselves to senescense (Fig. 8-1). At the other end of the spectrum of aging changes there are the chronically ill and truly aged persons who cannot adapt themselves to the aging changes that stimulate their hardy counterparts; these people regress into a more

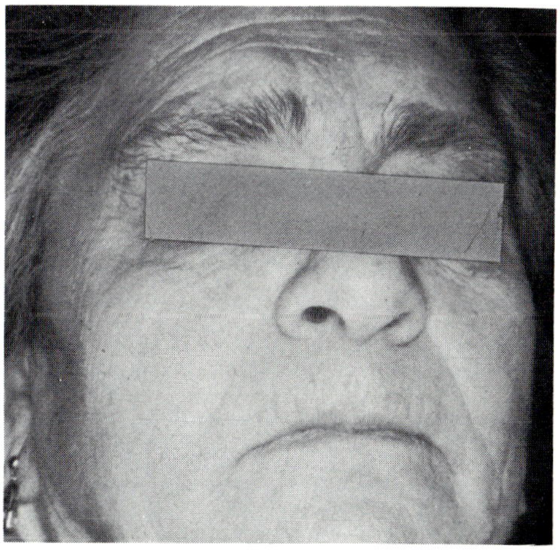

Fig. 8-1. Healthy 70-year-old woman; benign regressive aging changes may be seen.

elementary stage of life by a degenerative process known as involution,[3] the antithesis of evolution, known in the vernacular as "second childhood." They are best described as the broken blossoms in the garden of life (Fig. 8-2).

Between these two extremes in the images of the spectrum of senescence, there are many millions of people who are old, and they have every shade of health and illness; we must not forget that they include those who were formerly hardy, not broken down. Now comes geriatric dentistry to remind us that all old people have oral senescent peculiarities, in addition to the accepted physical and psychologic aging changes that have been amply documented in medical literature.[4] Their aging changes have not been given enough attention by the dental practitioner, but the time has come for every dentist to observe them in every old person, whether his aging process is chronologic, biologic, psychologic, or determined by his level of maturity. The changes can be seen in the occlusion, the teeth, the oral soft tissues, the jawbones, the saliva, the perioral structures, and the entire stomatognathic system, and the dentist must take them into account in geriatric diagnosis, treatment planning, prognosis, case presentation, patient management, and practice administration.

Application in crown and fixed partial prosthodontics

Inasmuch as we are discussing the special considerations to be given to fixed partial prosthodontics in rehabilitating the mouths of the elderly, we shall approach the subject in a scientific and systematic manner, just as it should be practiced at the dental chair. We must assume that the patient has been observed as he entered the reception room, as he appeared in the doorway of the operatory, and as he walked to the dental chair and sat himself in it.[5]

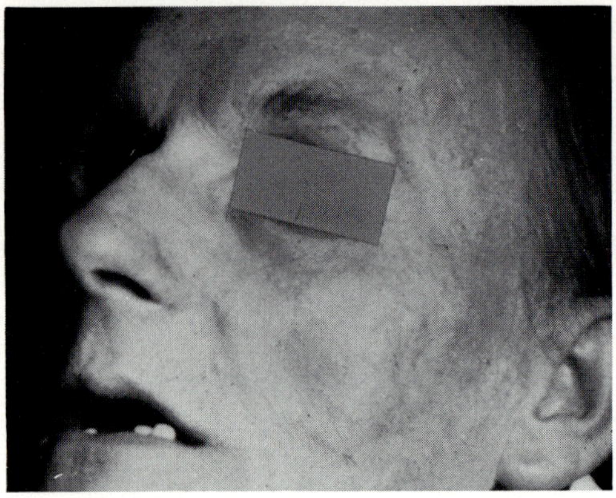

Fig. 8-2. Sixty-year-old man; cyanotic face and ear are indicative of polycythemia, hazard in oral surgery.

To dramatize the importance of understanding a person before examining his mouth, let us imagine that the first patient is a hardy business man, an executive, who keeps his appointments on time and who demands that the dentist, too, be punctual. His whole life is dominated by his mesomorphic personality, one attribute of which is an intense dislike for anything artificial; in his estimation a removable denture is despicable. Without looking into his mouth, it may be inferred that he keeps it clean, but his jaw is set and he no doubt grinds his teeth. The incisal edges are probably chipped, the enamel cracked and stained. Restorations would have to allow for dental abrasion, cusps would have to be "shoed," and it is almost certain that the patient would object to gold showing when the prostheses were placed. It would not take more than a glance at the patient to observe and infer all this—and more.[6, 7]

Another patient, let us say a debilitated old lady who has rheumatoid arthritis, walks with a stoop because of osteoporosis of the spine. She came to consult the dentist soon after she had fallen (as old people often do) and her maxillary central incisor was evulsed. She was more concerned about her appearance than the

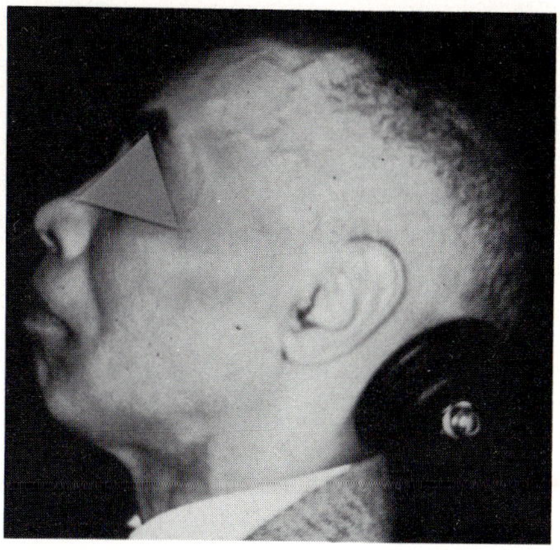

Fig. 8-3. Sixty-year-old man with Paget's disease; head has grown larger by two hat sizes in 5 years; lips show vigorous pull needed to cover enlarged maxillae.

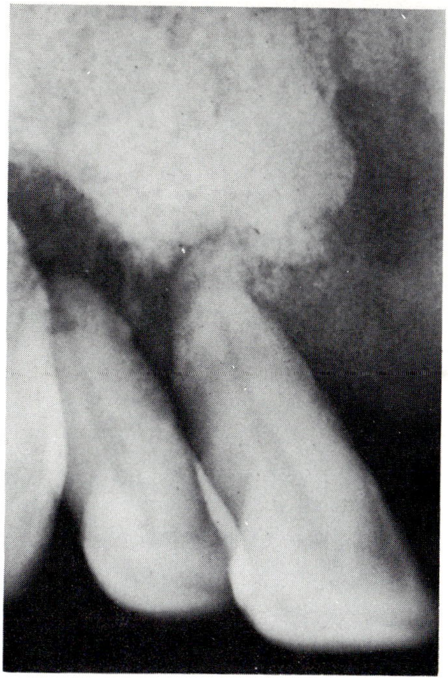

Fig. 8-4. "Cottonwool" bone, characteristic of Paget's disease.

damage to the tissues, but the dentist would have to give some thought to the possible harm done to the adjacent and opposing teeth, the integrity of the gingiva, the character of the bone as it will be revealed in the roentgenograms, the indications and contraindications for a fixed or removable prosthesis, whether multiple retainers would be needed, and several other matters, including, to be realistic, the fee.

The gait in parkinsonism should warn the dentist that the patient's "pill-rolling" fingers are a hazard in oral hygiene. The paralyzed hand of a hemiplegic who has suffered a stroke would make it difficult to manage a removable prosthesis without breaking it. An emaciated old woman who had told the receptionist that she cannot wear her denture because her jawbone hurts, may have a squamous cell carcinoma of the mandible, metastatic from a cancer of the breast that was removed 2 years previously. (All of these are actual clinical cases.) A patient may appear in the doorway of the operatory for only a second or two, but the dentist should make myriad pertinent observations that have intraoral correlations. Thus begins the building of a syndrome, a group of signs and symptoms which, when they occur together, establish a diagnosis.

A person who has a cyanotic complexion and edematous hands and feet and has to sit upright on the edge of the dental chair for a few minutes before he can lean back probably has heart failure. He cannot be put into a supine position for treatment. Orthopnea is the ability to breathe only when upright; difficult breathing is known as dyspnea. Treatment for a patient with cardiac disease should not extend beyond the point of fatigue; lengthier procedures that do not consider the patient may precipitate angina pectoris or other cardiopathy.

When the patient is seated in the chair, he may be observed at closer range. If his head appears to be enlarged and he states that he has to wear a larger hat than before, he probably has Paget's disease (Fig. 8-3). The images of "cottonwool" bone (Fig. 8-4) deposits in the dental and skull roentgenograms will help to confirm

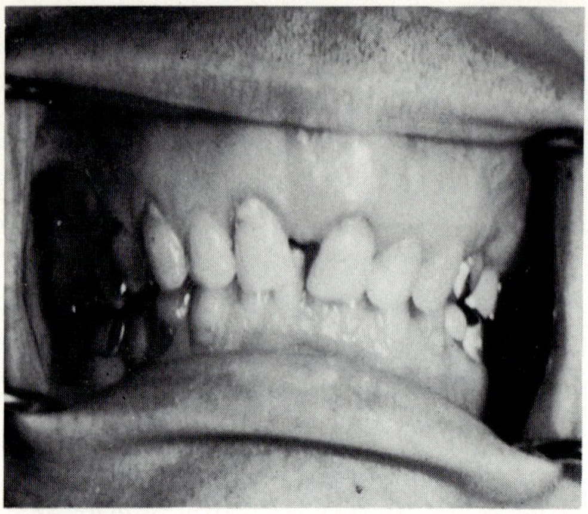

Fig. 8-5. Fifty-one-year-old patient with Paget's disease.

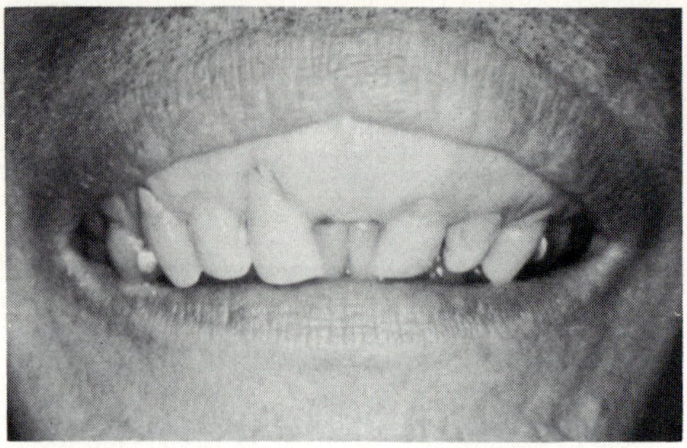

Fig. 8-6. Same patient as in Fig. 8-5, 15 years later; maxillae greatly enlarged.

the impression, but consultation with a physician should be sought before the final diagnosis is made. If it is substantiated medically, there is a possibility that the maxilla will continue to grow, and the roots of the anterior teeth will spread apart (Figs. 8-5 and 8-6). With such a prospect a maxillary anterior fixed bridge is contraindicated.

Bloodshot eyes (Fig. 8-7) are really a plexus of venous capillaries in the cornea, and they may signify a vitamin B complex deficiency that has to be verified later when the patient's diet and nutrition are investigated. Nutritional deficiencies of thiamin chloride, riboflavin, and niacinamide, to name some of the vitamin B complex components, are a hazard to the success of prosthetic rehabilitation. No oral prosthesis can be successful if the environment in which it has to function is not wholesome. The impact of this axiom will become more impressive as we proceed.

As a person ages, the body tissues tend to lose moisture, elasticity, and fat. Dental treatment will be hampered if such a phenomenon is seen in perioral skin and muscles. The skin of the lips wrinkle in vertical lines around the mouth, and the muscles become fibrous and lose their former suppleness (Fig. 8-8). The oral opening is not as extensive as it used to be, mastication is retarded, and the muscles take longer to prepare the bolus of food for deglutition. The extent of the oral opening is important in planning fixed partial prosthodontics. If the "purse-string" mouth restricts the oral opening, it may permit the use of gold crowns on the maxillary first premolars, which otherwise would be objectionable from the esthetic point of view.

Club fingers, in which the bones of the distaphalanges become exostosed, are generally associated with cardiac and pulmonary diseases or with polycythemia. We have referred to the management of the cardiac patient. Treating a patient with a pulmonary disease is an occupational hazard for the dentist who must protect himself from contracting an infection when the patient coughs. Polycythemia, an abnormally high increase in the number of red blood cells, presents a surgical risk. If teeth have to be extracted, or if extensive periodontal surgery is necessary in preparation for the construction of a fixed partial denture, all measures to avoid excessive postsurgical hemorrhage must be taken.

Unusually large feet may be part of the syndrome in acromegaly, an acquired hyperpituitarism in which all the extremities are enlarged. One of the distinguished anomalies of the disease is the massive mandible in which the teeth gradually

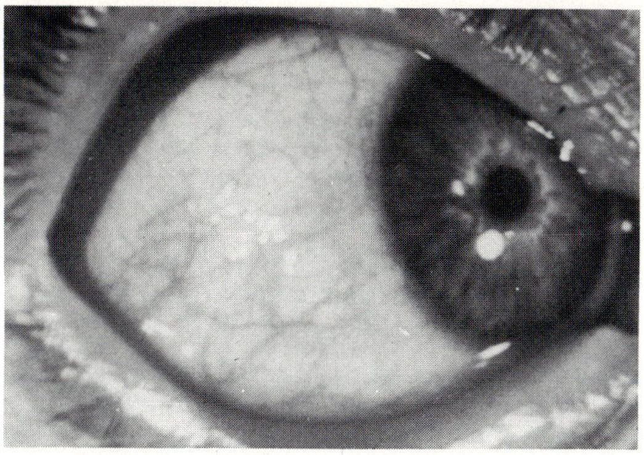

Fig. 8-7. Plexus of venous capillaries in cornea is part of vitamin B complex syndrome. Concomitant oral manifestations may hinder success of prosthesis.

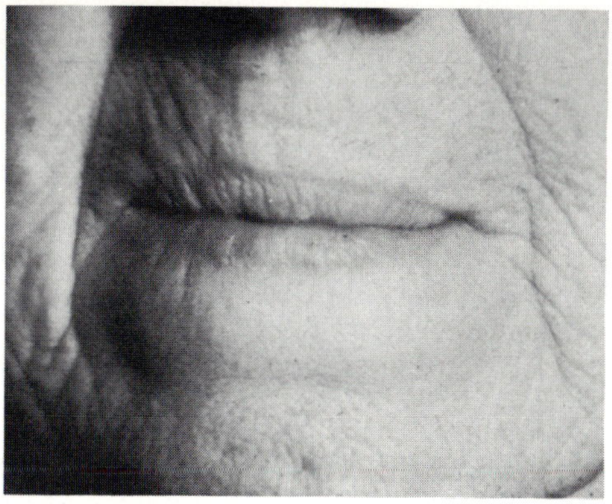

Fig. 8-8. Aging changes evident in "purse-string" perioral skin; mouth cannot be opened as wide as in younger years.

spread apart like the wickets in a fence. If the disease is in an active stage, and a dental bridge is indicated for the lower anterior region, a fixed appliance is not appropriate.

The interview

It is interesting to note here that the dentist has not yet examined the mouth, and although we have omitted many of the details in the observation of the patient up to this point, the actual passage of time is minimal.

With discreet prompting and guiding by the dentist, the history of the patient's previous dental and medical experiences can be elicited. The dentist should also obtain information about the drugs used by the patient and about his diet and nutrition. If there is any oral-systemic correlation in the history, it should not take long for the dentist to learn about it. During the interview he should have been formulating an evaluation of the patient's personality, behavior pattern, temperament, and attitude, not forgetting that the patient is also evaluating him at the same time. If necessary, the dentist should speak slowly to accommodate the conversation to the person's retarded perception and should speak in a low voice, since the elderly do not hear high tones well.[2] During the anamnesis the dentist should sit at the same eye level as the patient and should touch or hold his hand occasionally. The laying on of hands is still good therapy, if used with discretion.

Everything that is worth remembering should be recorded. Further information is to be obtained from additional diagnostic aids such as a preliminary oral survey, pulp vitality testing, transillumination, roentgenography, study casts, photographs, medical laboratory tests, and consultation with the family and the family physician. At a subsequent visit, a critical clinical examination with roentgenographic interpretation is made, and all the findings are recorded on a chart. The dentist should then determine the treatment plan and its prognosis, present the case to the patient and the patient's family, and proceed to make arrangements for appointments and for the payment of fees. There should also be a definite understanding at this time that the patient will respond to a recall notice. Recalls for the elderly should be more frequent than for younger people. Minor adjustments always obviate larger ones. It also gives the dentist an opportunity to observe noxious changes before they become too serious. Furthermore, it is therapeutic for an elderly person to know that the dentist or his assistant will always find a minute's time to say a kind word when it is needed. A preventive program in geriatric dentistry is as important, if not more important, as in pedodontics.

BIOLOGIC CONCEPTS IN TECHNICAL PROCEDURES

The technical details of crown and bridge construction are not of the essence in this chapter, and they could not be presented any better than they are in this textbook. However, there are certain biologic details that should be emphasized because they apply only in geriatric dentistry. From all indications it is not essential for a gerodontist to be a specialist, unless it means that he devotes his entire time to a dental service for old people in a nursing home or in a clinic that caters to the elderly. There is also an increasing demand for dentistry for the homebound, and many maunfacturers have designed portable equipment with which almost every phase of clinical dentistry can be practiced away from the conventional dental office, although it must be admitted that from the technical and financial point of view, geriatric dentistry in an established and fully equipped office is the practitioner's preference. The homebound who cannot possibly come to the dental office or be transported there are not always in the indigent class; some of them live in luxury. It is also worth mentioning that many of the old people in our population have an incurable feeling of insecurity that worsens as they age, especially if they were poor in their childhood days. When the dentist states his fee, he may be greeted with extremely uncomplimentary remarks about highway robbery and the like, but the solution is not to offer a cheaper type of prosthesis or invite the patient to shop around. The dentist will save himself a great deal of aggravation by referring the entire matter to a member of the family who knows the circumstances.

The oral examination

Let us consider the *aging changes* that one must know in order to practice geriatric dentistry as a biologic science rather than only as a mechanical art.

Occlusion. As far as possible, the dentist should give instructions to an elderly patient in a few well-selected simple words. The mouth examination should begin by observation of the occlusion, but the dentist should avoid verbosity in explaining how the patient should move the mandible through protrusive and lateral excursions. By saying, "Close your teeth like this—now move them like this," he will communicate more effectively. The temporomandibular joints are then palpated, and the dentist shows the patient how to open and close the mouth slowly.[8] The purpose of all this is to determine whether there are any frank occlusal interceptions, any clicking in the joints, any muscle spasm, any locking that prevents lateral excursion, or any mandibular deviations in opening the mouth. If the dental economy is fairly good, the old person will have abraded the cusps enough to level off the occlusal

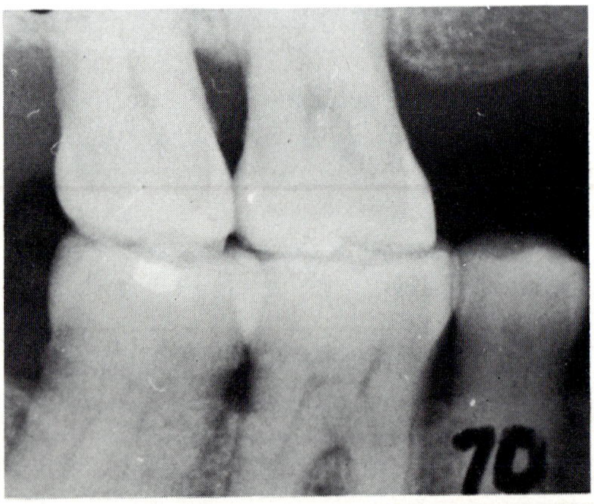

Fig. 8-9. Roentgenogram of patient in Fig. 8-1; no drifting or elevating of teeth, character of bone is excellent, and prognosis for prosthesis is encouraging.

interferences and to permit free lateral excursions. If occlusal interceptions appear after the rehabilitation is completed, they must be attributed to iatrogenic neglect.

Teeth. Missing teeth have significance only if the reason for their absence is known. In the partial anodontia of ectodermal dysplasia, cleidocranial dysostosis, and craniofacial dysostosis, some of the missing teeth may still be embedded in the bone. For some mysterious reason they do not erupt, even when the edentulous area is stimulated by the saddle of a removable partial denture. If given the proper care, erupted teeth may survive into old age, and in response to patient education, there may be a demand for a fixed partial prosthesis.

If the missing teeth were extracted because of dental caries, the prognosis for a fixed restoration is probably favorable, because in such cases the character of the jawbone is frequently good (Fig. 8-9). The patient may need some extra instruction in maintaining oral hygiene and in dietary requirements.[9] More thought must be given to the treatment planning if periodontal disease caused the loss of the missing teeth (Fig. 8-10); whatever caused the disease may still be active. It may be, or may have been, a local or a systemic factor, or the two may have interacted to the detriment of the periodontium. Teeth that have drifted or tipped may have to be treated orthodontically, but only if a study of the bone in the dental roentgenogram indicates that the prognosis warrants it. Telescoping crowns on thimbles have been recommended for a tipped tooth that has to serve as a bridge abutment; while it facilitates the placement of the bridge, however, it does not solve the problem of the masticatory force that is directed in a biologically incorrect direction. Masticatory force stimulates a tooth only when it is directed in line with the long axis of the tooth, an unlikely phenomenon if a tooth is tipped.

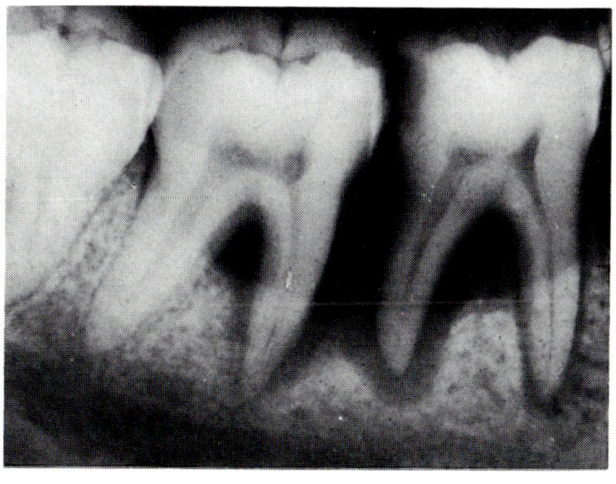

Fig. 8-10. If periodontally involved teeth are to be extracted, prognosis for fixed prosthesis is not good because of patient's history of diabetes.

Attrition and abrasion. Attrition of the cusps of teeth is physiologic in old age (Fig. 8-11). If the teeth show no signs of attrition, the patient no doubt has an overbite and is locked in occlusion, making an unhindered lateral excursion almost impossible. In many such cases the patient (usually a female) is a highly nervous person who clamps her teeth, especially in sleep; since everybody moves or tries to move the mandible while asleep, the clenching of the teeth rocks them out of their sockets. The abnormal direction of the pressure causes a resorption of the alveolar bone and a loosening of the teeth. Most people with such an occlusion and such a clamping habit usually lose all their teeth before they reach 65 years of age, unless they follow the instructions of a periodontist to the letter.

Teeth that are abraded by other than normal masticatory forces are generally "equilibrated" by the abrasion, so that the alveolar bone is not resorbed, but tooth substance is lost. As cusp height is lost by abrasion, the teeth continue to erupt passively en masse, and they are accompanied by the entire periodontium, thus maintaining the vertical dimension of the lower face when the teeth are

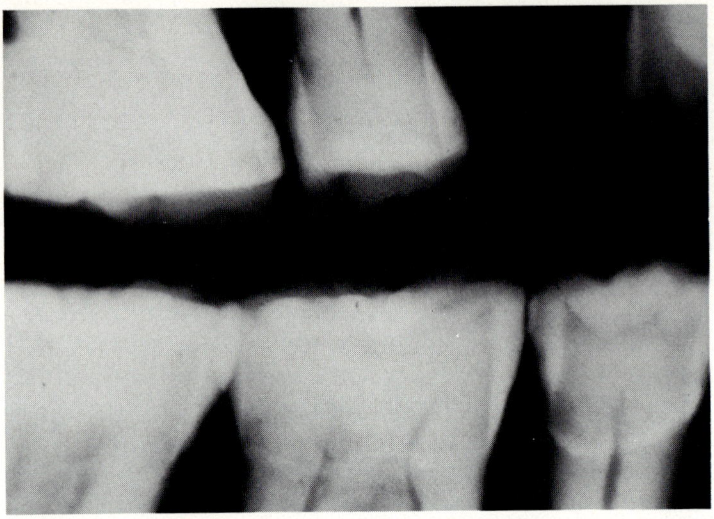

Fig. 8-11. Attrition of teeth in old age is normal; it facilitates lateral excursion of mandible, which elderly people usually favor for mastication.

occluded. But—and this is important—if the perioral skin and muscles, like the rest of the face, have lost their moisture, elasticity, and fat, and if the outside of the mouth has the characteristic dehydrated, "purse-string" appearance and a fibrosis of the tissues, nature cannot restore the vertical dimension completely (Fig. 8-12). The freeway (intermaxillary) space may be increased to some extent, enough to permit food to be introduced into the mouth, and to give more room to let the fibrotic masticatory muscles roll the food slowly into a bolus so that it can be ensalivated and swallowed.

There are instances, however, in which the teeth are severely abraded but there is no compensatory supraeruption of the teeth with their periodontium. The tip of the nose dips and the chin ends in a turned-up ball, resembling the face that characterizes Punch and that artists use to caricature an old person. The constant overclosure often strains the temporomandibular articulations and causes an uncomfortable and painful dysfunction. The same symptom, and for the same reason, is observed in edentulous people who will not or cannot wear dentures, and they "chomp their gooms," as Li'l Abner says.

When abrasion wears down the hard enamel of the cusps, it continues at a much faster rate into the dentin, which is softer than enamel. The dentin is cupped out, and the abraded surface resembles a saucer with a sharp enamel edge that often nips the cheeks, lips, and tongue. The sharp edges should be rounded off liberally so that the occluding width of posterior teeth is narrowed. A broad flat surface of an abraded posterior tooth affords a grinding area that is far in excess of what an elderly person needs. It is not compatible with the reduction in the masticatory force of the muscles that appears to be normal for old people.

If a person has a fairly good complement of teeth that have been abraded, the gradual friction often equilibrates the occlusion, but if there is an amalgam or hard gold restoration in the occlusal surface, its hardness prevents it from being abraded at the same rate as the enamel and dentin (Fig. 8-13). Over a period of many years, the equilibration is upset because the amalgam stands up above the level of the abraded occlusal of the tooth, and results in what has been called a split-level occlusion.[9] Now that more people are living to advanced ages with their own teeth, we are beginning to see more cases of such uneven occlusal abrasion. If no adjustment is made, the prominent amalgam will eventually abrade the interproximals of the opposing teeth and open up the contact areas. The amalgam will then become a piston and pack food between the opposing teeth and will initiate a periodontal pathosis in a mouth that had no sign of it previously. The point to be made here is that it is only because more people are living to advanced ages that such circumstances are on the increase.

The prominent amalgams should be re-

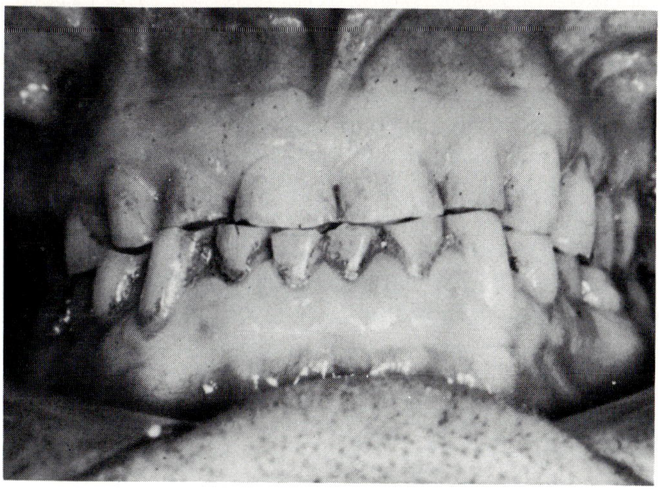

Fig. 8-12. As teeth are abraded, simultaneous loss of vertical dimension is compensated by their passive eruption and their periodontium, but not to same dimension it had in early years. In prosthodontics, slightly increased freeway space may be necessary.

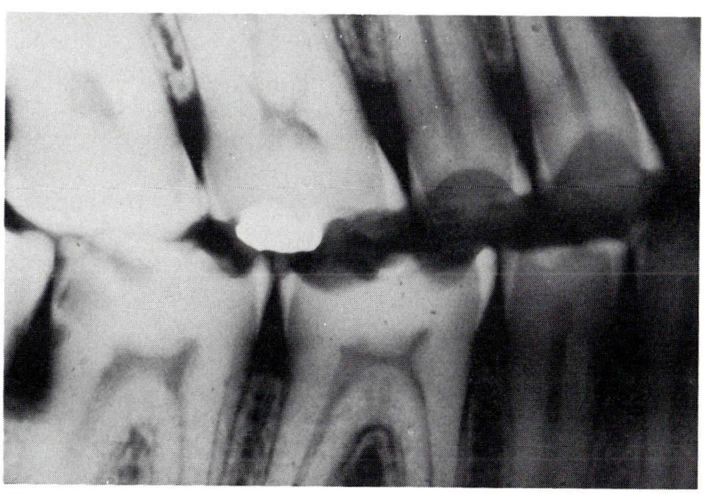

Fig. 8-13. Silver amalgam restorations do not abrade as fast as enamel or dentin. Metal will eventually abrade opposing enamel and probably guide food into interproximal space and initiate periodontal pathosis.

moved. Since, in most cases, secondary or reparative dentin has accumulated on the surfaces of the pulp spaces of the teeth, causing the pulp to recede, new cavities can be cut to a greater depth. The new restorations should be made of gold, which will abrade at about the same rate as the dentin. By the same token, it would seem that the occlusal surfaces of crowns and bridges should not be cast in hard gold unless the entire mouth is being rehabilitated. In any case, the patient should be recalled regularly for adjustment of the occlusion by equilibration.

Pathosis without inflammation. There are instances, however, in which heavy deposits of secondary dentin do not form on the walls of the pulp space and there is little pulpal recession. Occasionally the abrasion exposes the pulp, and when a roentgenogram is taken at a later date, a radiolucency at the apex presents an enigma because the patient cannot recall any pain when the pulp died (Fig. 8-14). In general, the elderly seem to be less sensitive to pain than they were in their younger days.[10] The pathogenicity appears to be another phenomenon that is peculiar in geriatric dentistry and is happening more frequently, not only in endodontics, but also in periodontics. Whenever an irritant exceeds the stimulation state, nature reacts with an inflammation. In the early or active (arterial) hyperemic stage, the inflammation may be regarded as a physiologic process. Leukocytes and other protective agents are summoned to the scene in the pulp space, and the battle begins. If nature is victorious at this stage, the inflammatory process is a healing device, and in the case of pulpal pathosis, the pulpitis is reversible. If it fails, passive (venous) hyperemia and degeneration ensue, and it results in a suppurating acute abscess that can eventually become a granuloma, an atrophic chronic abscess, or a cyst. But in elderly people, the initial inflammatory process is short-lived or it does not occur, and the degeneration proceeds quickly to atrophy, without pain.

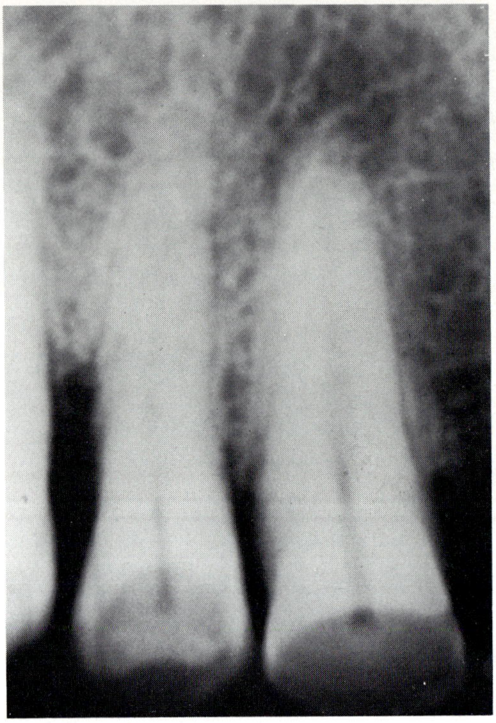

Fig. 8-14. Pulp of canine tooth was exposed by abrasion and lost its vitality, but patient did not experience any pain. Note periapical radiolucency.

This peculiar pathogenic phenomenon has long been known in geriatric medicine. An old person treats himself with cathartics and enemas for a nagging but not extremely painful stomachache, but eventually he has to submit to a medical examination. Roentgenograms are taken, and exploratory surgery is prescribed. The surgeon is not surprised to find that what started as a bothersome appendicitis became gangrenous.

Interproximal abrasion

Before we leave the subject of dental abrasion in the teeth of the elderly, consideration must also be given to the constant, lifelong wearing down of the interproximal surfaces of the teeth at the contact areas. It is assumed to be an inevitable consequence of the physiologic movement of teeth as they are held in their sockets by the hammock-like periodontal ligaments. When a person reaches old age, the total amount of interproximal abrasion is only minimal, but as the surfaces wear down over a period of many years, the teeth are moved mesially toward the midline by what is known as the anterior component of force, and a normal occlusion becomes an edge-to-edge bite. All crown and bridge restorations should then conform to the acquired occlusion, and no attempt should be made to push the mandible back. This acquired edge-to-edge bite should not be confused with the protrusive convenience bite, which many old people like to adopt for various reasons and which has to be critically considered in the construction of complete dentures.

Abrasion and prosthodontics. Complete coverage for abraded teeth is a recommended treatment if the patient can afford the fee, but it presents a number of biologic and technical problems. If the abrasion is the result of bruxism (the excessive diurnal and nocturnal stress exerted by the patient even when not chewing), it is probably an emotional compulsion,[12] for which reason some call it bruxomania. It is sometimes so violent that the messeter muscles become enlarged and the temporomandibular joints are traumatized.

Special care must be exercised not to "raise the bite" beyond a comfortable posture for the type of person who has bruxism. He cannot tolerate even the correction of a bad habit once he has become accustomed to it. A trial acrylic splint or bite plane might help to some extent. If the person is elderly, a prosthesis that restores much of the vertical dimension of the lower face that he had in his youth will improve his appearance, but he may not be able to accustom himself to it, and the prosthesis will be a failure.

It is doubtful whether unprotected porcelain on the occlusal and incisal surfaces of restorations for a person with bruxism could withstand the excessive grinding of the teeth, and a protective gold layer may be objectionable. Someday there may be a porcelain that can take such punishment. Acrylic is totally unsuitable to withstand bruxism. It does not fracture easily, but it flows under stress; it warps at the margins, letting the cement crumble away; and it invites caries to attack the teeth.

If there is a valid objection to the gold crown, a three-quarter crown or mesiocclusodistal (MOD) inlay may be considered, but the cusps must be covered to protect them against fracture. The cusps of old people are especially vulnerable. Like most of the body tissues, they lose moisture. They also become more calcified and extremely fragile with advancing age. The edges of the enamel chip and vertical cracks appear in the labial surfaces, and they are stained yellow. It should be noted that in the construction of pontics and veneers for crowns, the darker shades are more appropriate, even if the little old lady insists that her new teeth must match "the little white pearls that her teeth looked like when she was a girl." Tooth color saturation is attributed to the formation of secondary dentin and to the accumulation of flourides from food, in addition to those found in drinking water. Flourides may contribute to the immunity to dental caries that older individuals are said to have.

RAMPANT DENTAL CARIES IN ADVANCED AGE

A new problem of dental caries in the teeth of old people is beginning to loom large. One of the most destructive phenomena in the mouths of the elderly is xerostomia, which is also known as dry mouth, asialorrhea, hyposalivation, and aptyalism. The epithelial lining of the ducts of the salivary glands undergoes metaplastic changes in old age.[13] It is replaced by fatty cells, which retard the salivary flow. Saliva has serous (thin, watery) and mucous (thick, ropy) components. As age advances, the flow is restricted, but more in the serous secretion than in the mucous flow, with the result that the saliva in old age is much more mucinous than in the younger years. This is the gummy fluid that covers the mucosa in the edentulous mouths of the elderly, and it is the bane in the life of the complete denture prosthodontist. It should be cut by a mucinase before the impression is made.

The lack of saliva is one of the many noxious factors in the postclimacteric syndrome (post-menopausal syndrome in women). Its paucity not only reduces the buffering capacity of the anticaries enzymes in the secretion, but it encourages the formation of plaques that provide the bulk of the evidence for the chemicoparasitic theory of dental caries. Without belaboring the two sides of the theory, the end result is that the teeth of people who are almost octogenarians and have some natural teeth are developing a carious condition that attacks not only the enamel and dentin but also the cementum that is exposed by gingival recession. The decay extends along the surfaces of the tooth and along the dentinoenamel junction, rather than directly into the pulp space, as it does in young teeth. The destruction is almost beyond repair. This is one of the newer problems in gerodontics (Fig. 8-15). It was not of much concern when people sacrificed their remaining teeth in their late middle age, and dentists did not protest too much against such "dental fatalism," but in recent years a practical and reasonable treatment for rampant dental caries of advanced age is being utilized. The carious cavities are carefully excavated without exposing the pulp. Antiseptics are applied to the cavity walls, which are then washed with hydrogen peroxide, alcohol, and water. The cavity is mopped with cotten, and a gentle flow of warm air is used to dry it without dehydration. There is some discussion about the efficacy of these measures, but the clinician can make his own decisions about the matter. A small amount of calcium hydroxide is placed on the floor of the cavity,[14] and a layer of thickened zinc oxide–eugenol paste is placed over it. Some operators are so convinced that the treatment is valid that they fill the rest of the cavity with silver amalgam, and, all other things being equal, they are prepared to crown the

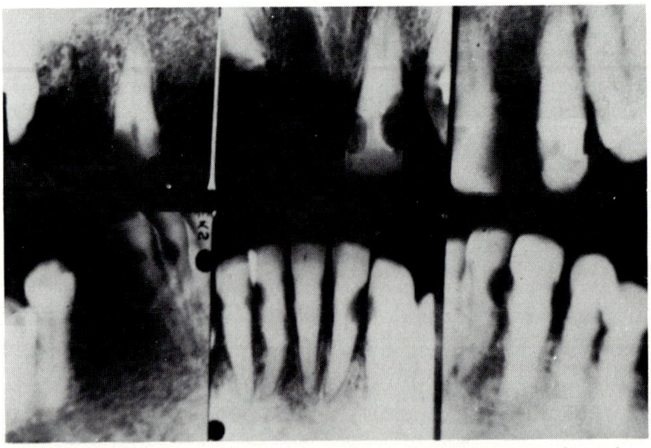

Fig. 8-15. Radiogram of teeth of 75-year-old male. Rampant dental caries probably initiated by loss of buffering action of saliva when its flow was retarded.

tooth, if necessary, or use it as one of the bridge abutments.

To those who are willing to learn by clinical research, it is suggested that cement be used to fill the remainder of the cavity instead of the silver amalgam. After about 2 months, all the contents of the cavity should be removed. It will be found that the alkalinity of the calcium hydroxide has neutralized the acidity of the carious material and that the residual soft dentin has become harder. The calcium hydroxide and the zinc oxide–eugenol stimulate the deposition of reparative dentin, which reinforces the thin part of the cavity dentin where the pulp was almost exposed. A vitality test should be used to determine the integrity of the pulp, and a roentgenogram should be taken to make sure that the root has an acceptably good image of the alveolar lamina dura and that there is no evidence of an abnormal periapical radiolucency. In an elderly person it is possible for a pulp to die painlessly and without inflammation, as mentioned previously.

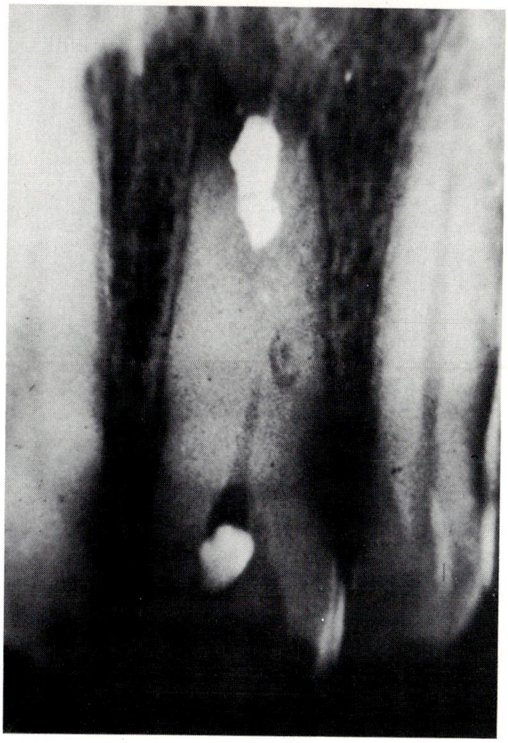

Fig. 8-16. When obliterated canal could not be probed by conventional methods, apical foramen was sealed with zinc-free amalgam. (Courtesy Dr. Franklin B. Weine.)

ENDODONTICS

Endodontic treatment for the elderly is difficult if the pulp canal is occluded by secondary dentin and diffuse fibrillar calcification of the walls of the blood vessels, both commonly seen in the pulp spaces of the teeth of older people. By removing the organic contents of the canals by chelation, it may be possible to obtain access for an acceptable preparation for a dowel (or posts) to be followed by a crown built on a core or amalgam base. If the occluded canal cannot be penetrated, root canal filling by the apical approach may be considered (Fig. 8-16). For multirooted teeth, root amputation has been used with good results.[15] Irrespective of the type of crown to be used for an anterior tooth, the root must be braced with a cast coping (collar or rim) like a hoop that holds the staves of a barrel

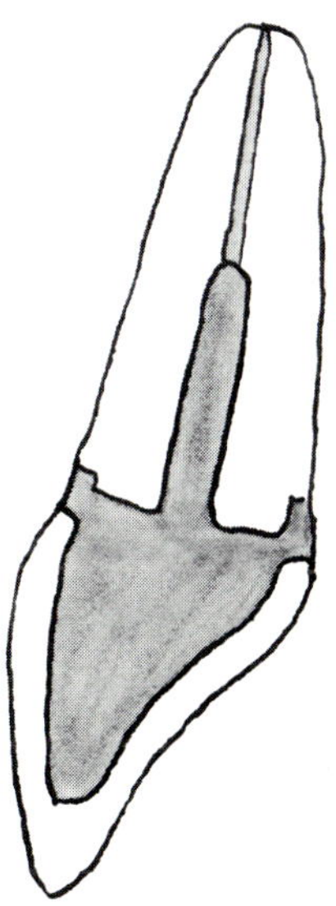

Fig. 8-17. Dowel with cast coping encircling root to prevent it from splitting.

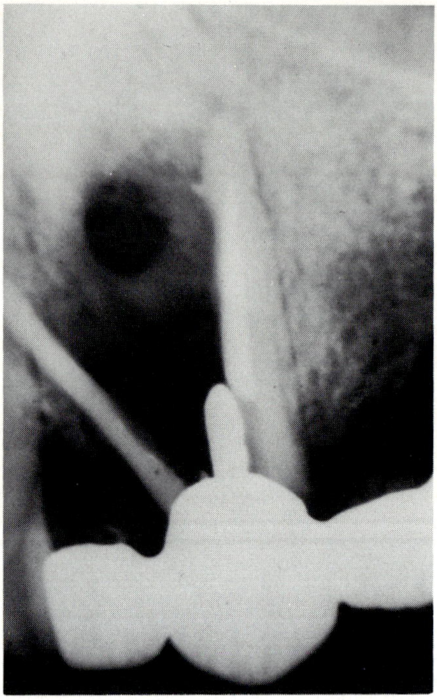

Fig. 8-18. Root split vertically several years after it was prepared for dowel coping minus circular collar reinforcement.

together (Fig. 8-17). It must not be forgotten that endodontic treatment increases the dryness of a tooth that in an older person has already lost some of its moisture and elasticity. A dowel in the canal may split the root vertically a few years after the crown is cemented in place (Fig. 8-18). At the moment we are not prepared to say whether the insertion of pins to anchor an amalgam base to them can cause fracture lines in the dry and less elastic dentin in an older tooth. The gingival marginal collar of a cast gold crown should be effective as a precaution against such an occurrence.

PERIODONTICS AND PERIOPROSTHODONTICS

No crown and bridge prosthodontics should be considered before the surrounding and supporting tissues of the tooth are free from periodontal disease and a favorable prognosis has been established for the prosthesis after a thorough clinical and roentgenographic evaluation has been made. Any foreseeable mishap must be discussed with the patient and the family to avoid any subsequent misunderstandings. If nothing is said at the case presentation, and if at some future time (the passage of time often fools the memory) the prosthesis fails, no explanation, no matter how scientific it is, can be any better than an alibi. An expert architect can view a piece of vacant land and can visualize a building that will take into account the soil, the subsoil, the needs of the owner and his assets and liabilities, the present and future neighborhood environment, and many more intangibles. A dentist should be able to give his patient a service that is just as considerate.

The mobile tooth

If an individual tooth is to be crowned, it must be in a condition that is good enough to accept the prosthesis. The tooth should not be excessively loose or become subject to factors that will loosen it or tend to make it more mobile than it is. If a loose tooth must be crowned, its occlusion may be modified so that when the completed restoration is inserted, the estimated masticatory force will not exceed the limit of the physiologic tolerance of the periodontium. The art of splinting loose teeth involves a biologic understanding of the various forces and stresses that affect them. When a bridge is made to replace one tooth between two that are biologically in good condition, one connector may be of the key and keyway, or so-called broken-stress, type. If there is some looseness in one or both of the abutments, the connectors should be rigid to approach an immobilization status for the teeth, and, if necessary, one or both abutments should be splinted to the adjacent tooth. Immobilization in other parts of the body is used to promote healing, and it can do the same where it is applicable in perioprosthodontics.

One should not be too readily terrified when the roentgenogram shows that a tooth is held by only a small amount of bony socket. If the residual socket has a definite roentgenographic alveolar lamina dura that continues over the crest of the interdental septum of bone and if the bone appears to be well trabeculated with regularly arranged marrow spaces, the prognosis for the preservation of the tooth is still good, if the occlusal circumstances are favorable and if the tooth does not feel too loose. Such a periodontal picture is seen in old people who have what has been called "physiologic senile atrophy."[16] The condition is far from being uncommon. A more serious matter is the crown-to-root ratio. If the leverage on the part of the tooth that is visible clinically is not too great in proportion to the amount of root still in the socket, it should be saved. Additional reinforcement by splinting to another and firmer tooth is optional. The preparation to receive the crown can preserve the esthetics of the prosthesis. Care must be exercised in cementing the crown in place; too much finger pressure may evulse the tooth.

The space to be spanned

If a fixed partial denture is being contemplated for an elderly person, the space to be occupied by the pontics has to be prepared, and the pontics have to be contoured according to the prevailing oral conditions. At the moment we are concerned with the aging tissues with which the pontics have to make contact, and also with the total environment in which the prosthesis has to function.

Pontic-to-tissue contact. Normal gingival mucosa in older people often changes from masticatory type to a less keratinized variety. The stippling tends to smoothen out, and the mucosa becomes more fibrous and less vascular. Like most of the other soft tissues of the body, it responds to low-grade irritations by producing a fibrosis rather than by inflammation and suppuration. If traumatized, it shows rapid signs of degeneration, or it acquires a protective hyperkeratinization. It is imperative that pontics must never press into the mucosa. If their porcelain ridge lap has to be ground, it must be reglazed before final cementation. The ridge lap must not be a shelf that will gather food debris. The fermentation products would be too irritating to the aging, impoverished tissues. The use of acrylic is contraindicated because it absorbs fluids and retains noxious products of fermentation. Porcelain pontics for mandibular posterior bridges should be of the tip type variety rather than the ridge lap type. The extended tips of anterior pontics must not be fitted into the fresh extraction sockets for old people, even if the porcelain is highly glazed. The risk involves probable irritation to which the tissues cannot react well physiologically. The technique produces a beautiful effect in the mouths of young people, but the tissues of the elderly, like the people themselves, must be respected.

Design of preparations

The occlusal and incisal surfaces of bridge retainers and pontics should simulate the wear pattern of the other teeth in the mouth. It may please the eye to see a bridge on a plaster model with well-demarcated cusps, deep grooves, and prominent ridges, but it would be incongruous in a mouth with abraded teeth. Nevertheless, buccal and lingual grooves should be carved into the axio-occlusal edges to act as sluiceways for food. As mentioned previously, the occlusal apex of the pontics should be reduced to conform with the lessened occlusal force of older people. Narrowing the mesiodistal dimensions of the lingual half of the occlusal surface of the pontic will accomplish that. The contact areas and all the embrasures must be designed biologically to facilitate cleansing.

Cantilever pontics

For elderly people we can be more liberal with cantilever pontics if they are needed for mastication or for esthetics, but the dimensions of their occlusal surfaces should be curtailed. To afford more room for an atonic or atrophic tongue, it is not essential to provide masticatory surfaces beyond the first molar. A cantilever pontic may also be used if it opposes a tissue-borne portion of a removable partial denture or if it occludes with a complete artificial denture, because the masticatory force is reduced when it is exerted against a removable prosthesis. Under similar circumstances the span of a fixed bridge for an elderly person may be a little longer than if it had to occlude with natural teeth or with another fixed bridge. In the final analysis, it means that planning crown and fixed prosthodontics for older individuals needs the common sense and the discretion that come with experience rather than the advice of a laboratory man who has nothing but models on an articulator to guide him.

Cementation

The cementation of a prosthesis, especially of a fixed partial denture, for an elderly person also requires special attention. The dentist should know how to mix the cement and how to overcome the trapping of air inside a crown that is being cemented to place. Of greater concern is the strain on a newly crowned abutment tooth when it is called upon to withstand masticatory stress after it has been out of function for some time. The proprioceptive attribute of the periodontal ligament may register a complaint, and if the bridge has to move the tooth even slightly and resorb some of the bone of the socket on the pressure side, it may cause a temporary continuous pain. The fixed restoration should be adjusted before the final cementation, and it should be set with a temporary cement. If the recovery of the tooth is painful, the bridge should be left off occasionally to let the tissues rest while nature readapts them to the new circumstances. Serial roentgenograms may show that the typical narrowing of the periodontal ligament space, the thinning of the alveolar lamina dura, and the disuse radiolucency of the atrophied periapical bone of a tooth that has been out of function for some time gradually return to normal when the functional capacity of the tooth is regained. In fact, it sometimes happens that nature actually reinforces the periapical bone by increased calcification.

The dentist must also remember that many elderly patients cannot exert enough force with their masticatory muscles to force a bridge to place by biting on a cotton roll. Temporary cementation may facilitate the permanent placement.

A special plea is being inserted here against making crown preparations as if the teeth had been put through a pencil sharpener and replaced into their sockets. An anesthetized tooth cannot object to severe cutting, and sometimes the pulpal horns are cut through, even in the older teeth in which it may be assumed that the horns are calcified. The pulps may die, and periapical abscesses or granulomas may form without pain (Fig. 8-19). The conical shape of the abutment preparations helps the bridge go to place without a struggle, but the prosthesis loosens more easily. Dental cement is not glue. Moreover, a crown is a more successful prosthesis if it is held with some frictional resistance to displacement.

A SILENT TONGUE CAN SPEAK

At the risk of being repetitious, we must say again that no prosthetic restoration can be successful if the environment in which it has to function is not wholesome.

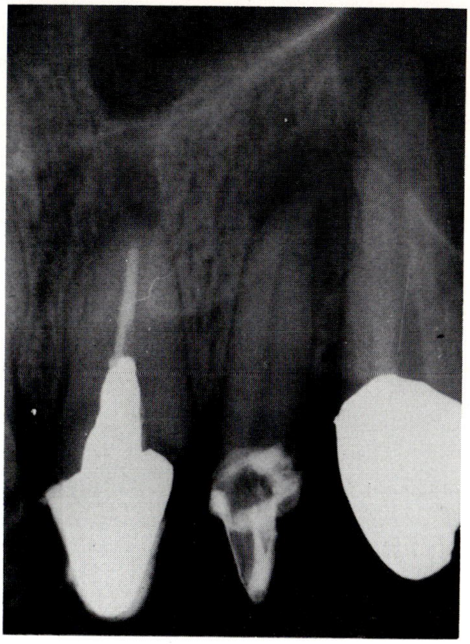

Fig. 8-19. Radiolucency at apex of lateral incisor is result of improper preparation.

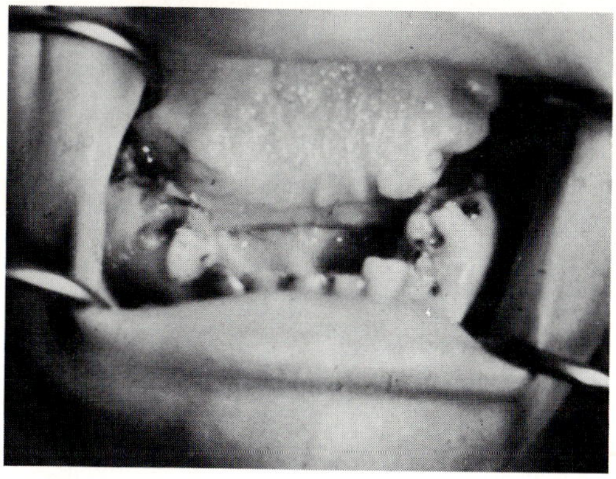

Fig. 8-20. Atonic, crenated tongue of diabetic patient usually lies limp in floor of mouth; prosthesis generally causes discomfort.

It occasionally happens that a few days after an oral rehabilitation is completed and inserted for a post-menopausal patient, she becomes aware that her tongue burns. The symptom probably existed long before dental treatment was instituted, but it was hidden away in her unconscious mind. The new prosthesis in some way pulled a trigger, and the glossodynia (glossopyrosis) was propelled up into the conscious level.[17] The realization may have been caused by the very presence of the prosthesis, by a minor discomfort due to a slight raising of the bite, by one tooth that the patient imagines is out of line, or by some kind neighbor who told her that the fee was excessive. In all probability the sad experience could have been avoided if the dentist had concentrated on the patient who needs the rehabilitation rather than on the prosthesis itself. In taking the history he may have found that the patient was always subject to an imbalance of the sex hormones, that she had had dysmenorrhea since the menarche or a traumatic experience at the onset of the menopause, or that she had to submit to a hysterectomy in her forties. Her oral discomforts may have been associated with an estrogen deficiency.

The patient may have a history of severe anemia, or she may be a person who is easily upset emotionally. A simple question that was asked about the usual breakfast may have disclosed that the protein intake was deficient. The few details we have just mentioned may be enough to determine the true cause of the burning tongue. Of course, if the burning tongue had not been a symptom at the time of the initial interview, it would be dangerous to mention it and cause a phobia, probably of cancer, but the subject could have been discussed with someone in the family or with the physician.

Had the dentist examined the tongue as part of the oral survey, he may have noticed that it was atonic or atrophic. An atonic tongue lies limp in the floor of the mouth, and when it is extended, it literally hangs out of the mouth. It generally becomes enlarged and feels cramped (Fig. 8-20). The suggestions made about reducing the occlusal dimensional areas of pontics as much as possible or omitting second molars afford a little more comfort to the tongue. Similarly, first premolar

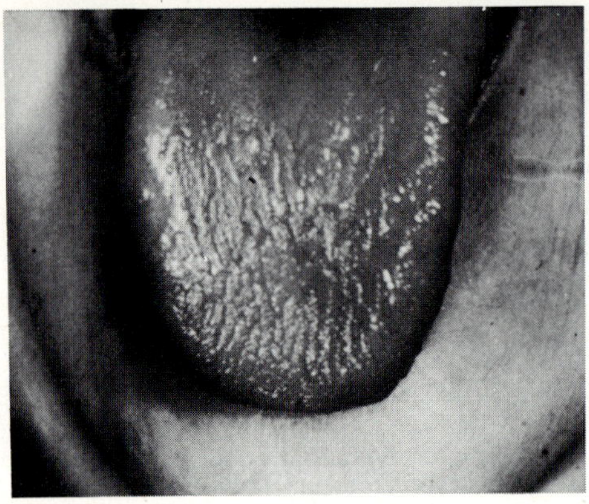

Fig. 8-21. Atrophic, burning tongue; note loss of papillae and red shiny dorsal surface.

crowns and pontics may be constructed with reduced or without lingual cusps, if possible.

An atonic tongue loses its covering of filiform papillae and sometimes also of its fungiform papillae, leaving the taste buds exposed and confused in their ability to report taste sensations to the brain. An atrophic tongue is usually shrunken, its dorsal surface is red, beefy, smooth, and shiny, and it burns (Fig. 8-21). Its hypersensitiveness makes it exaggerate every little contour, and the patient often demands that all the teeth and pontics be ground down. A silent tongue is able to speak, and there is an art in listening to it.

In examining the mouth of an elderly person, the dentist may learn that an oral rehabilitation was completed several years previously, and it may be found that everything is in good order. If the prosthesis had been a failure, it would no doubt have been due, not to a lack of skill, but to a lack of basic biologic knowledge. If it is clinically evident that the health of a patient and of his oral tissues definitely contraindicates the construction of extensive rehabilitation prostheses, the dentist should have the courage not to provide them, although the patient is ready and willing to pay the fee for them. Sometimes the best service a dentist can render is to do no more than to remove all the pathosis from the mouth, and if necessary, leave it edentulous.

Primum non nocere means "Above all else, do no harm." This admonition has been handed down in medicine for centuries; nobody knows its origin, but it is good advice that every gerodontist should accept.

SELECTED REFERENCES

1. American Medical Association: A new concept of aging, Chicago, 1966, The Association.
2. Birren, J. E., and others: Human aging, Public Health Service Publication No. 986, Washington, D. C., 1960, U. S. Department of Health, Education, and Welfare.
3. Bromley, D. B.: The psychology of human ageing, Baltimore, 1966, Penguin Books, Inc.
4. Shock, N. W., editor: Aging, Washington, D. C., 1960, American Association for Advanced Science.
5. Elfenbaum, A. E.: Diagnostic procedures, practical dental monographs, Chicago, 1964, Year Book Medical Publishers, Inc.
6. Hyman, H. T.: Handbook of differential diagnosis, ed. 3, Philadelphia, 1965, J. B. Lippincott Co.
7. Elfenbaum, A. E.: From the doorway to the chair in dentistry for the elderly, J. Amer. Soc. Geriat. Dent. **2**:2, 1967.
8. Shore, N. A.: Occlusal equilibration and temporomandibular joint dysfunction, Philadelphia, 1959, J. B. Lippincott Co.
9. Cheraskin, E., and others: Diet and disease, Emmaus, Pennsylvania, 1968, Rodale Press.
10. Dummet, C. O.: Periodontal consideration in rehabilitation of the aging gnathostomatic system, J. Dent. Med. **20**:1, 1965.
11. Tylman, S. D.: Theory and practice of crown and bridge prosthodontics, ed. 5, St. Louis, 1965, The C. V. Mosby Co.
12. Cheraskin, E., and Langley, L. L.: Dynamics of oral diagnosis, Chicago, 1956, Year Book Medical Publishers, Inc.
13. Burket, L. W.: Oral medicine, Philadelphia, 1965, J. B. Lippincott Co.
14. Weiss, M.: Pulp capping in older patients, New York Dent. J. **32**:326-329, 1966.
15. Weine, F. B.: Endodontic treatment for the geriatric patient, J. Amer. Soc. Geriat. Dent. **2**:1, 1967.
16. Glickman, I.: Clinical periodontology, Philadelphia, 1964, W. B. Saunders Co.

17. Elfenbaum, A. E.: 36 dentures and no relief, Dent. Digest **74**:5, 1968.

GENERAL REFERENCES

Balogh, K.: Significant oral changes in the geriatric patient, Dent. Digest. **72**:352-354, 1966.

Bernick, S.: Effect of aging on the nerve supply to human teeth, J. Dent. Res. **46**(4):694, 1967.

Collins, J. W.: Programs of dental care for the aged and chronically ill, J. Pub. Health Dent. **25**:116-119, 1965.

Elfenbaum, A. E.: Crown and bridge prosthodontics for the elderly, J. Prosth. Dent. **18**(4): 337, 1967.

Elfenbaum, A. E.: Dentistry for the long-term patient, Chart **62**:7-13, 1965.

Haim, G.: Electron microscopic study on the marginal periodontal binding tissue in relation to age, Deutsch. Zahnaerztl. Z. **20**:1021-1027, 1965.

Leathers, L. L.: Modification of prosthetic procedures for the ill and aged, J.A.D.A. **72**:369-372, 1966.

Orens, P. A.: Oral rehabilitation and the geriatric patient, Ann. Dent. **2**:57-60, 1968.

Schabel, R. W.: Practical prosthetic treatment for chronically ill and aged patients, J. Calif. Dent. Assn. **44**(2):135-138, 1968.

Shepherd, R. W.: Prosthetic treatment for the older patient, Aust. Dent. J. **12**(4):339-342, 1967.

Stanley, H. R.: The factors of age and tooth size in human pulpal reactions, Oral Surg. **14**: 498, 1961.

Stanley, H. R.: Traumatic capacity of high speed and ultrasonic dental instrumentation, J.A.D.A. **63**:749-766, 1961.

Thomas, B. O. A.: Gerodontology: the study of changes in oral tissues associated with aging, J.A.D.A. **33**:207-213, 1946.

Waldman, H. B.: Dental care for the homebound aged patient, Geriatrics **21**:139-145, 1966.

Chapter 9

Distribution of abutments, crowns, and fixed partial dentures relative to patient's sex and age

As long as the dental arches are complete, we may expect them to function in a normal way, both mechanically and physiologically. However, when one or more of the natural teeth are lost or missing either through caries, accident, or some other cause, an immediate impairment of their functions takes place in proportion to the number of teeth missing and their relative importance in the arch. Although the loss of a tooth is harmful to the continued welfare of the masticatory mechanism, the dangers of such a condition may be mitigated or prevented to a large degree by replacing the tooth with a prosthetic appliance at the earliest possible time.

Because a patient continues to take food and apparently leads a normal, natural, and healthy existence does not alter the fact that the efficiency of his chewing mechanism has been disturbed and that additional strains have been placed upon the remaining natural teeth. Since unnatural conditions develop from the loss of teeth, it is logical to expect a new environment and the development of new stresses. Nature cannot always accommodate herself to a new arrangement, and, unless rehabilitated by means of prosthetic appliances, the entire arch may be eventually destroyed.

LOSS OF ONE TOOTH

It is, therefore, the duty of every dentist to appraise in the patient not only the mechanical deficiencies which result from the loss of a single tooth, but also the biologic changes which follow such a loss and which extend their destructive local influences to involve the entire upper and lower arches. Such disturbances in the dental structure and the resulting malpositions of teeth may be found in every mouth in which an edentulous area has been permitted to exist for any length of time without being reconstructed.

It has been estimated that the loss of one tooth, particularly the lower first molar, results in a 10 percent decrease in the function of the dental arch. This instant decrease in function may be increased to 30 percent if immediate steps are not taken to replace the lost tooth and thus to maintain normal functions and relationships.

Fig. 9-1 presents a condition that has resulted from the extraction of a lower molar. Because the lost tooth was not immediately replaced, we find a mesial drifting and tilting of the posterior teeth; this results in the loss of most of their chewing efficiency since they contact the opposing arch only in the area of the distal marginal ridges. Such an occlusal relationship

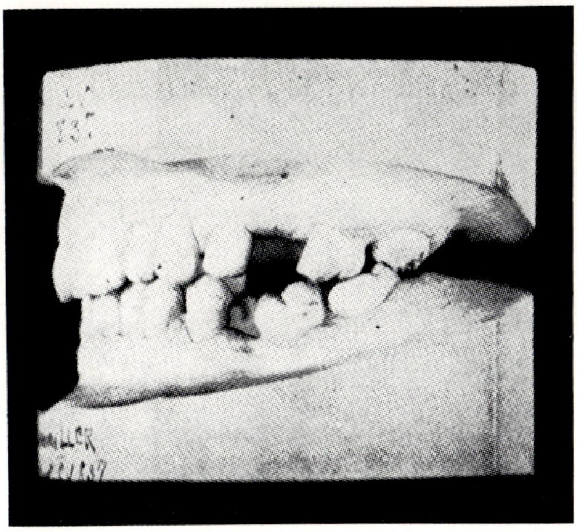

Fig. 9-1. Shifting and tilting of teeth caused by extraction of first molars in upper and lower arches.

is traumatic in its possibilities, creating a predisposition toward periodontal disease and pulp involvement. Because the contact areas on the distal surfaces are also lost, we find a tendency for food impaction and the development of pockets.

With the continued forward inclination of the tooth, the alveolar process on the mesial surface, together with the periodontal membrane in this area, is destroyed, leaving the cementum of the tooth exposed; such a condition makes this area vulnerable to sensitiveness and caries. Eventually a deep pocket develops, necessitating the removal of the tooth.

Because the lower first molar is the most frequently lost tooth in the arch, it is usually found that the second molar moves forward and is subject to the symptoms and changes just described. It is also noticed that the bicuspids sometimes move distally into the edentulous space. There are times when the distal movement of the second bicuspid equals the full width of the tooth. Because a tendency also exists for lower molars to incline lingually, excessive destruction of the periodontal membrane and alveolar process on this surface is frequent. If the lingual inclination of the tooth becomes excessive, it may not only prove a handicap to speech but may also result in an inflammation of the soft tissues of the tongue.

That the deleterious changes are not limited to the individual or adjacent teeth is shown by the fact that teeth in the opposing arch also become directly involved. The removal of a lower tooth causes the loss of occlusal function with an opposing upper tooth; hence the upper tooth gravitates beyond its normal occlusal plane. In so doing, it changes or loses its contact with its proximating teeth, and the resultant unusual egression promotes pathologic possibilities, since it produces an unusually rapid and extensive epithelial detachment and cementum exposure. Moreover, such egressed teeth later prove serious obstacles when the restoration of the edentulous condition is undertaken.

Because patients are less prone to chew their food on a partially edentulous side, the disuse of these teeth will assist in the development of an unhygienic condition. Such a habit frequently is a predisposing cause of caries and excessive calculus formation with its accompanying gingivitis. As previously indicated, teeth not used habitually or used only to a minor degree induce definite tissue changes. Not only is the structural form of the alveolar process changed or modified, but also the lack of functional stimulation results in an area of lowered resistance, making the periodontal membrane and the gingival tissues easy prey for infective organisms.

LOSS OF SEVERAL TEETH

Noticeable changes in the facial contour of patients frequently may be traced to the loss of several teeth and to the edentulous space which was permitted to remain for a long time. Such unnatural oral conditions are very often reflected unfavorably in temporomandibular joint disturbances. Several investigators[1-5] have indicated an apparent relationship between the two conditions.

The majority of reports dealing with the loss of permanent teeth invariably indicate that the first molar is the tooth most frequently lost; this is especially true of the lower first molar. This view is also substantiated by data which have been compiled from clinical records of several thousand crown and bridge clinic patients extending for a period of over 40 years.

The following discussion concerns itself with, first, those teeth restored with crowns, and, second, those missing teeth which were restored with bridges during the first 17 years of the research. A recent recapitulation shows no appreciable deviation in the sex and age distribution of patients or in the teeth or types of restorations involved. Our clinical data and observations cover 12,000 crowns and 6,000 fixed structures made by students. An analysis of the first 17 years of clinical data presents the following findings.

CROWNS AND FIXED PARTIAL DENTURES

There were 1,075 crowns for teeth having vital pulps. These were placed for 378 men and 574 women patients.

Tables 9-1 and 9-2 indicate the distribution and location of the teeth restored. It is significant that for upper teeth with vital pulps the greatest number of crown restorations are placed on the central and lateral incisors. This is due largely to the use of complete porcelain veneer crowns subsequent to operative restorations. In the lower arch the first and second bicuspids, also the first molar, are the teeth most frequently crowned. This is due largely to the fact that biscuspids with vital pulps are very freqeuntly retained and crowned in order that they may be used as direct retainers for removable partial dentures. In studying this group of patients, it is found that all except 126 patients had normal occlusion; 60 percent were in good health; 39 percent, in fair health; and 1 percent, in poor health. These patients were divided almost equally between those who were and those who were not susceptible to caries.

Table 9-3 shows the sex and age distribution of patients requiring crowns on teeth with vital pulps.

It is interesting to note that, while the

Table 9-1. Crowns for teeth with vital pulps—distribution of restored teeth

	Upper																
Times restored	3	17	26	32	21	31	51	62	81	59	22	19	23	28	21	9	
Tooth	8	7	6	5	4	3	2	1	1	2	3	4	5	6	7	8	
R	*Lower*																L
Tooth	8	7	6	5	4	3	2	1	1	2	3	4	5	6	7	8	
Times restored	3	26	45	45	56	22	4	5	6	3	27	65	54	40	23	8	

Table 9-2. Crowns for teeth with vital pulps—location of restored teeth

Upper teeth		*Total*	*Order*	*Lower teeth*		*Total*	*Order*
Central	(1)	143	1	Central	(1)	11	5
Lateral	(2)	110	2	Lateral	(2)	7	6
Cuspid	(3)	53	5	Cuspid	(3)	49	4
First bicuspid	(4)	40	6	First bicuspid	(4)	121	1
Second bicuspid	(5)	55	3	Second bicuspid	(5)	99	2
First molar	(6)	54	4	First molar	(6)	85	3
Second molar	(7)	38	7	Second molar	(7)	49	4
Third molar	(8)	12	8	Third molar	(8)	11	5

quantity of the work was done for patients between the ages of 20 and 40 years, the maximum for women occurred in the 30- to 39-year period, while for men it was in the 20- to 29-year group.

There were placed 1,350 crowns on teeth without pulps, 707 for women and 506 for men patients.

In studying Tables 9-4 and 9-5 it will be noted that the majority of crowned pulpless teeth are also in the upper arch. Again, the two upper incisors predominate in the frequency of their restoration, while in the lower arch the first molar is the tooth most frequently restored; the cuspid and the two bicuspids follow next in order. The occlusion of these patients is normal in all but 220 patients. Approximately 70 percent of the patients were susceptible to caries, while 75 percent were in good health, 24 percent in fair health, and 1 percent in poor health. It is significant that here again the largest percentage of restorations was placed for patients between 20 and 40 years of age.

It is observed in Table 9-6 that the

Table 9-3. Crowns for teeth with vital pulps—sex and age distribution of patients

	Age of patient				
	17-19 years	*20-29 years*	*30-39 years*	*40-49 years*	*50 years and over*
Male	51	89	76	41	33
Female	78	92	157	93	41

Table 9-4. Crowns for pulpless teeth—distribution of restored teeth

	Upper																
Times restored		40	55	42	54	56	88	100	104	120	55	65	50	47	37		
Tooth	8	7	6	5	4	3	2	1	1	2	3	4	5	6	7	8	
R	*Lower*																L
Tooth	8	7	6	5	4	3	2	1	1	2	3	4	5	6	7	8	
Times restored	4	30	58	38	43	42	15	3	3	10	42	38	40	65	33	2	

Table 9-5. Crowns for pulpless teeth—location of restored teeth

Upper teeth		*Total*	*Order*	*Lower teeth*		*Total*	*Order*
Central	(1)	204	2	Central	(1)	6	7
Lateral	(2)	208	1	Lateral	(2)	25	6
Cuspid	(3)	111	4	Cuspid	(3)	84	2
First bicuspid	(4)	119	3	First bicuspid	(4)	81	3
Second bicuspid	(5)	92	6	Second bicuspid	(5)	78	4
First molar	(6)	102	5	First molar	(6)	123	1
Second molar	(7)	79	7	Second molar	(7)	63	5
Third molar	(8)			Third molar	(8)	6	7

Table 9-6. Crowns for pulpless teeth—sex and age distribution of patients

	Age of patient				
	17-19 years	*20-29 years*	*30-39 years*	*40-49 years*	*50 years and over*
Male	114	154	122	61	55
Female	170	202	193	107	37

highest percentage of restorations for men is between 20 and 29 years of age, while for women the requirements are almost equally divided between the 20- and 30-year groups.

Tables 9-7 and 9-8 are concerned with 853 fixed partial dentures constructed for 462 female and 391 male patients. Here again we observe the distribution of women requiring dental service; it is evident that the upper teeth are more frequently restored than the lower teeth. Since the upper cuspid is common to the anterior, median, and posterior bridge components, it is the tooth most frequently employed as an abutment. Because of the frequent loss of the first molars, we find that the second bicuspids and the second molars are next in the frequency of their use as abutments. As expected, the lateral incisors and third molars are the teeth least used as abutments.

A study of the lower arch presents a slightly different situation, for the second molars and the second bicuspids are the teeth most frequently used as abutments; the first bicuspid is next in order. That the third molar is used as often as it is may at first seem incredible. Yet, it is recalled that the lower first molar is the tooth most frequently lost and that the second molar has a high mortality because of mesial tilting; as a result there frequently is no alternative left except to use the lower third molar for the bridge abutment. The significant fact is that the lower first molar is used the least number of times as a bridge abutment.

Of the total number of abutments used for fixed bridges, 1,439 were teeth with vital pulps, while 300 were pulpless. While the ratio of vital to pulpless teeth is nearly 5:1, periodic examinations, both clinical and roentgenographic, have shown that the pulpless tooth may be used satisfactorily as a bridge abutment, provided: first, that the prognosis for treatment is favorable; second, that the treatment and filling of the root canal are carried out under aseptic and controlled conditions; and third, that the treated tooth is kept under periodic surveillance.

The 1,739 abutment teeth supported 1,559 pontics. This gives a ratio of 1.7:1.5

Table 9-7. Fixed partial dentures—distribution of restored teeth

	Upper																
Times restored	7	88	65	64	60	190	42	59	49	37	162	66	91	58	98	13	
Tooth	8	7	6	5	4	3	2	1	1	2	3	4	5	6	7	8	
R	*Lower*																L
Tooth	8	7	6	5	4	3	2	1	1	2	3	4	5	6	7	8	
Times restored	43	113	18	109	60	30	8	3	49	37	30	44	80	14	91	37	

Table 9-8. Fixed partial dentures—location of restored teeth

Upper teeth		*Total*	*Order*	*Lower teeth*		*Total*	*Order*
Central	(1)	108	6	Central	(1)	52	6
Lateral	(2)	79	7	Lateral	(2)	45	7
Cuspid	(3)	352	1	Cuspid	(3)	60	5
First bicuspid	(4)	126	4	First bicuspid	(4)	104	3
Second bicuspid	(5)	155	3	Second bicuspid	(5)	189	2
First molar	(6)	123	5	First molar	(6)	32	8
Second molar	(7)	186	2	Second molar	(7)	204	1
Third molar	(8)	20	8	Third molar	(8)	80	4

of abutment tooth to pontic. A further analysis discloses 706 four-tooth bridges and 147 three-tooth restorations. Although the ideal bridge has two abutment teeth for every restored tooth, clinical evidence indicates that the four-tooth restoration is a biologically acceptable restoration.

The occlusion was normal in 35 percent of the patients; 80 percent kept their mouths habitually clean, while slightly more than 50 percent were susceptible to caries. Moreover, 75 percent of these were in good health, 24 percent, in fair health, and 1 percent, in poor health.

Table 9-9 again emphasizes that crown and bridge prosthesis is primarily a service for the 20- to 40-year age group. It will again be noted that the maximum requirement for men is in the 20- to 29-year period; for women it lies within the 30- to 39-year span.

In the semifixed bridges, employing a flexible or nonrigid connector at one terminal, we find that of 683 restorations of this type 355 were constructed for women, while 287 were made for men.

A study of the data in Tables 9-10 and 9-11 indicates that this type of bridge is used most frequently to restore an upper first bicuspid and upper lateral incisor, for we find that the second bicuspids, cuspids, and central incisors are used most frequently as abutments. We also find evidence here of the frequent restoration of the upper first molar, since the second molar is used eighty-four times as an abut-

Table 9-9. Fixed partial dentures—sex and age distribution of patients

	Age of patient				
	17-19 years	*20-29 years*	*30-39 years*	*40-49 years*	*50 years and over*
Male	24	153	104	54	33
Female	35	120	153	81	22

Table 9-10. Semifixed partial dentures—distribution of restored teeth

	Upper																
Times restored		44	21	75	32	68	12	38	35	15	68	26	74	23	40	3	
Tooth	8	7	6	5	4	3	2	1	1	2	3	4	5	6	7	8	
R	*Lower*																L
Tooth	8	7	6	5	4	3	2	1	1	2	3	4	5	6	7	8	
Times restored	9	105	22	98	29	7	1	—	2	—	4	22	96	15	100	10	

Table 9-11. Semifixed partial dentures—location of restored teeth

Upper teeth		*Total*	*Order*	*Lower teeth*		*Total*	*Order*
Central	(1)	73	4	Central	(1)	2	7
Lateral	(2)	28	7	Lateral	(2)	1	8
Cuspid	(3)	136	2	Cuspid	(3)	11	6
First bicuspid	(4)	58	5	First bicuspid	(4)	51	3
Second bicuspid	(5)	149	1	Second bicuspid	(5)	194	2
First molar	(6)	44	6	First molar	(6)	37	4
Second molar	(7)	84	3	Second molar	(7)	205	1
Third molar	(8)	3	8	Third molar	(8)	19	5

Table 9-12. Semifixed partial dentures—sex and age distribution of patients

	Age of patient				
	17-19 years	*20-29 years*	*30-39 years*	*40-49 years*	*50 years and over*
Male	34	128	57	26	8
Female	30	100	125	48	10

ment. The tabulation likewise emphasizes the infrequent use of the upper lateral incisors and third molars as bridge abutments.

In the lower teeth we find that the first molar is most frequently restored by means of a bridge. The second molars and second bicuspids are most frequently used, while the central and lateral incisors are employed the least number of times as abutments.

Of the abutments used, 1,070 had vital pulps, while 221 were pulpless. These teeth supported 944 pontics, with a ratio of 2 abutment teeth to 1.5 of pontics. In this instance it is found that of the total number of bridges constructed 66 percent are the three-unit type, i.e., two teeth supporting one pontic. Of these patients 80 percent had normal occlusion and 75 percent of them kept their mouths habitually clean. The records disclose that fully half of the patients were susceptible to caries, while 75 percent were in good health, 15 percent, in fair health, and 10 percent, in poor health.

Table 9-12 again emphasizes the 20- to 40-year bracket for this type of service; likewise, the fact that the male requirement has its optimum in the 20- to 29-year group, while the women find their greatest need in the 30- to 39-year period.

The foregoing data are factual; what, if any, biologic significance is attached to these findings remains for future investigators to determine.

Since the ratio of teeth with vital pulps to pulpless teeth is approximately 5:1, it is frequently necessary to decide whether a pulpless tooth should be retained or extracted, and, if retained, what the possibilities are of its giving satisfactory service. Although it is unquestionably true that a tooth with a vital pulp is better than one without it, the decision should be made by ascertaining what the response has been and what service the patient has obtained from his or her previously treated teeth. If radiographic evidence indicates an unfavorable biologic reaction to treated teeth, then it is unwise to employ such teeth for additional bridge abutments.

SELECTED REFERENCES

1. Hildebrand, G. Y.: Studies in mandibular kinematics, D. Cosmos **68**:449, 1936.
2. Hildebrand, G. Y.: Studies in the masticatory movements of the human lower jaw, Berlin, 1931, Walter De Gruyter & Co.
3. Hildebrand, G. Y.: Studies in dental prosthetics, Stockholm, 1937, A. B. Fahlcrantz' Boktryckeri.
4. Brodie, A. G.: The temporo-mandibular joint, Illinois D. J. **8**:2, 1939.
5. Maves, T. W.: Radiology of the temporo-mandibular articulation with correct registration of vertical dimension for reconstruction, J.A.D.A. **25**:585, 1938.

GENERAL REFERENCES

Anderson, D. J.: Measurement of stress in mastication, J. Dent. Res. **35**:664, 1956.

Brekhus, J. J.: Dental disease and its relation to the loss of human teeth, J.A.D.A. **16**:2237, 1929.

Cheyne, V. D., and Drain, C. L.: Dental caries and permanent tooth extraction: a study of age, sex and location of the incidence of first permanent molar extraction in 8,677 school children, J. Dent. Res. **19**:570-584, 1960.

Finn, S. B.: Prevalence of dental caries, Publ. 225 National Academy of Sciences, Washington, D. C., 1952, National Research Council.

Grewe, J. M., and Meskin, L. H.: Loss of teeth, Northwest. Dent. **46**(3):156-158, 1967.

Knutson, J. W., and Klein, H.: Studies on dental caries, IV: tooth mortality in elementary school children, U. S. Public Health Reports **53**:1021, 1938.

Lundquist, C.: Tooth mortality in Sweden: a statistical survey of tooth loss in the Swedish population, Acta Odont. Scand. **25**:289-322, 1967.

McCollum, B. B.: Is it necessary to replace missing teeth? J.A.D.A. **24**:442, 1937.

Salzmann, J. A.: A study of orthodontic and facial changes, and effects on dentition attending the loss of first molars in five hundred adolescents, J.A.D.A. **25**:892, 1938.

Silness, J.: Distribution of crowns and bridges, Bergen, Norway, 1968, University of Bergen.

Weinberg, L. A.: Force distribution in mastication, clenching and bruxism, D. Digest **63**:58, 72, 1957.

Westin, G., and Wold, H.: 1942 ars tandmonstring av innskrivningsskyldiga, Odont. T. **51**: 487-616, 1943.

Chapter 10

Movements of abutment teeth related to the fixed partial denture

Chapters 11 and 13 consider the principles involved in the preparation of teeth for intracoronal retainers and crowns and their relationship to the forces of mastication. When a retainer is part of a fixed partial denture and is united to another more or less distantly located retainer by means of an intervening rigid piece of metal, it is subjected to a new series of forces. Each tooth is capable of individual and combined movements in several directions: buccolingually, distomesially, and vertically. When two teeth are rigidly united, the forces of mastication are transmuted into new reactions, and, unless recognized and provided for, they may result in the loosening and failure of the most skillfully constructed fixed partial denture.

When two abutment teeth are rigidly connected with a fixed bridge and force is applied linguobuccally to the structure, there is little danger that either of the bridge retainers will be dislodged, provided both teeth move an equal distance in the buccal direction. If, however, one of the teeth is loose, it will rotate buccally to a greater degree than the other and a severe strain is set up in the latter tooth because of its more restricted mobility.*

BUCCOLINGUAL MOVEMENT

Since the buccolingual movement of a tooth describes an arc with its center of rotation located near the apical region of the root as shown in Fig. 10-7, a torsional strain is set up in the retainer of the more rigid tooth; this tends to rotate shallow castings out of the cavity (Fig. 10-1, *A*). The preparation of parallel buccal and lingual proximal walls of sufficient depth counteracts this rotary, dislodging force (Fig. 13-11, walls *A* and *B*, and Fig. 10-1, *B*).

Where one of the abutment teeth is loose, there is still another displacing force present. If a bicuspid is the abutment having an exceptional amount of movement, any force applied to it will swing the bridge out buccally on a radius whose rotation center is the buccal margin of the

*The author wishes to acknowledge and give credit to the pioneer work done along these lines by H. W. C. Bödecker, *The Metallic Inlay,* Berlin, 1911, Hermann Muesser.

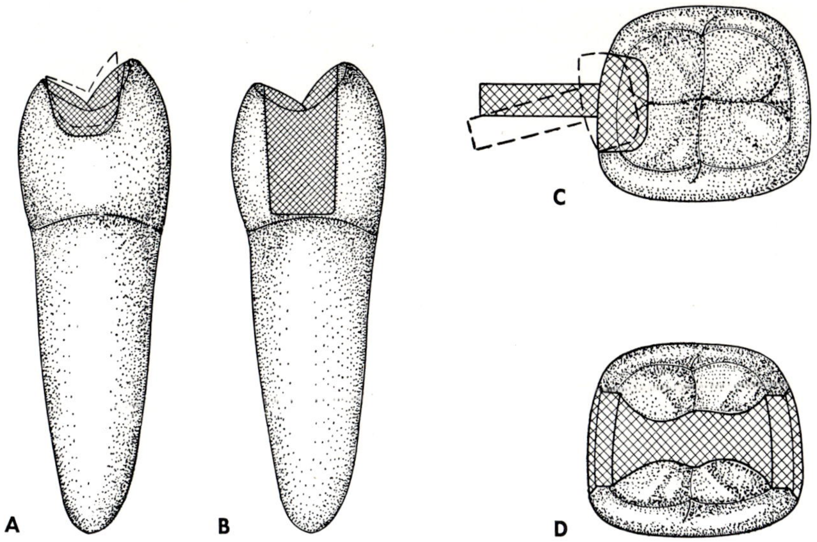

Fig. 10-1. Incorrect and correct preparations of cavity to resist displacement.

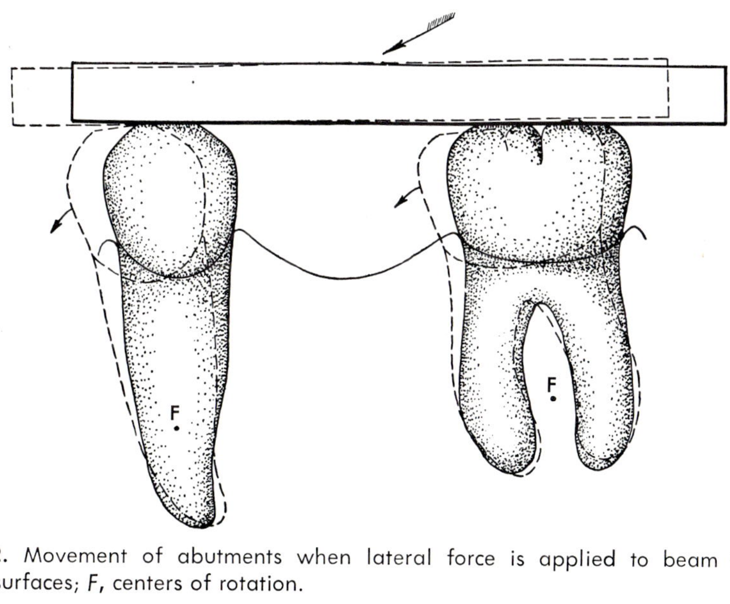

Fig. 10-2. Movement of abutments when lateral force is applied to beam resting on occlusal surfaces; *F*, centers of rotation.

retainer in the molar tooth (Fig. 10-1, *C*). If, however, the retainer holds, the tendency exists to rotate the firm molar tooth. To resist displacement at the proximal portion of the retainer, it is essential that the cavity be extended sufficiently buccolingually and that all buccal and lingual walls, gingivoclusally and mesiodistally, parallel each other within 2 to 5°. Additional resistance to displacement is obtained by extending the preparation across the occlusal surface and involving the opposite proximal surface of the tooth; the mechanical grip of a staple or a wrench with parallel jaws is thus obtained (Fig. 10-1, *D*). The three-quarter partial veneer retainer and the complete veneer crown afford the best resistance to torsional and lateral strains.

The forces exerted upon such a retainer lodged in a firm abutment are very destructive, during both the horizontal and the lateral displacements of the bicuspid. The danger inherent in such a situation is more evident when it is recalled that during lateral movements power is usually applied at the most destructive position mechanically, i.e., at the cusp points.

DISTOMESIAL ROTATION

Abutment teeth may also move distomesially (see Figs. 10-2 to 10-4). This latter direction is more common due to the

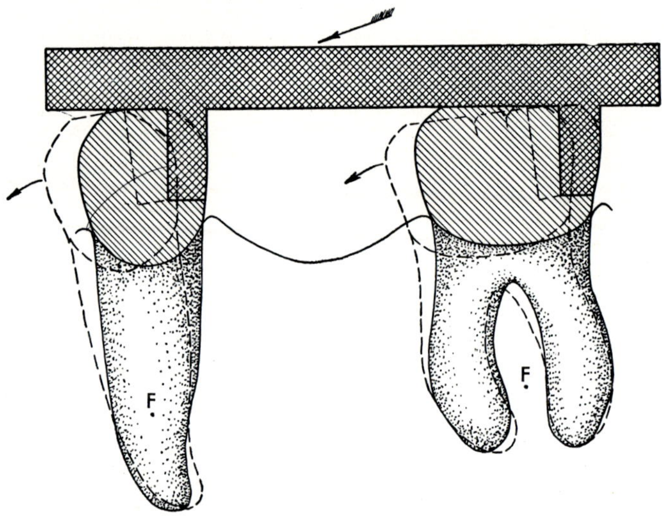

Fig. 10-3. Displacement of two-surface castings when attached rigidly to bar and subjected to lateral force.

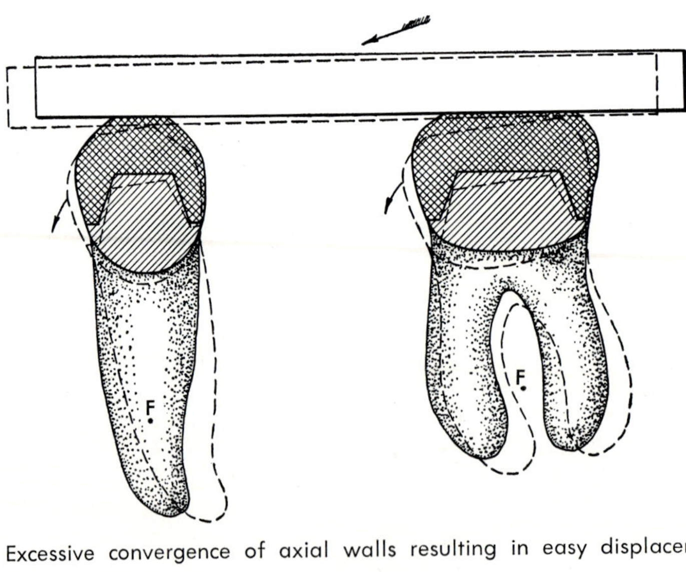

Fig. 10-4. Excessive convergence of axial walls resulting in easy displacement of cast retainers.

anterior component of force which drives the buccal teeth anteriorly. The effect of only the horizontal component of force is discussed, without consideration of the frictional coefficient between the teeth. In Fig. 10-2 a lower second molar and a second bicuspid support a solid bar which extends across the occlusal surfaces. When diagonal force is applied to the bar so as to move it mesially, both teeth tilt mesially, rotating on their centers of rotation *F*, and the bar rests on the distal portions of both teeth on their distal marginal ridges. If shallow proximal cavities are prepared (Fig. 10-3) and inlay bar extensions carried into these, the rotation of the teeth will also displace these shallow inlays.

Even where the cavity is extended gingivally to a greater depth, if the mesial

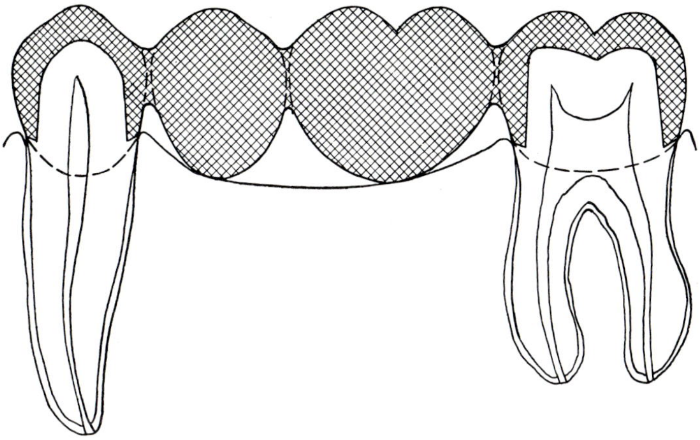

Fig. 10-5. Axial walls within 2 to 5° of parallelism give maximum retention.

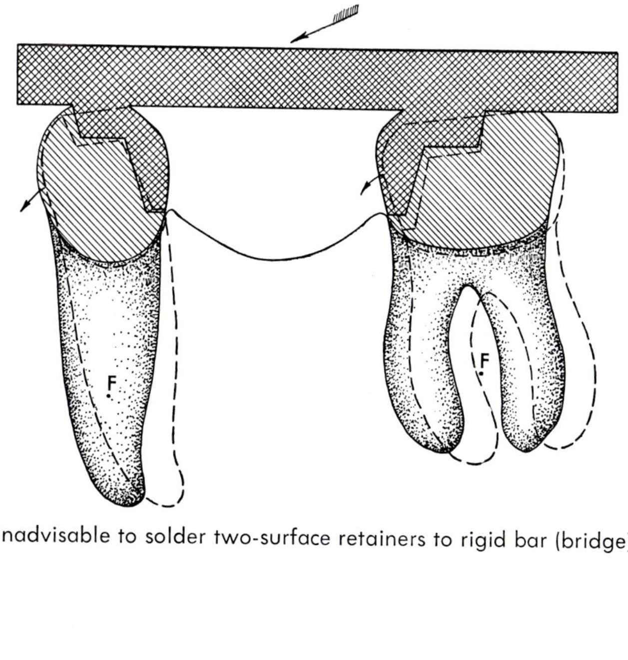

Fig. 10-6. It is inadvisable to solder two-surface retainers to rigid bar (bridge).

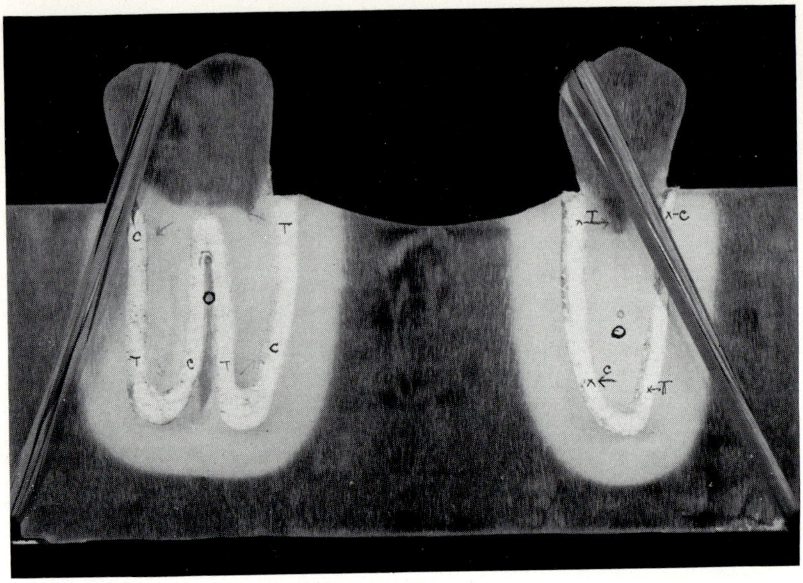

Fig. 10-7. T, area of tension; **C,** compression; **O,** centers of rotation in separate abutments.

and distal axial walls of the preparations converge excessively (Fig. 10-4), a bridge with such retainers will be rotated out of its abutments. It is only when the axial walls are prepared, as shown in Fig. 10-5, i.e., with a convergence not exceeding 2 to 5°, that the bridge will prevent the tipping of the teeth mesially.

Fig. 10-6 illustrates why it is inadvisable to construct a fixed bridge which employs only a distoclusal inlay retainer in the anterior abutment and a mesioclusal type in the posterior tooth; the rotation of the teeth mesially may dislodge the bridge.

This also helps to explain why it is impractical to employ a fixed bridge having a three-quarter retainer in the bicuspid with a mesioclusal inlay in the molar and, similarly, why the broken-stress type of connector is not employed between the pontic and the posterior retainer.

If the forces of mastication were always distributed equitably and only in a direction parallel to the long axes of the roots, there would be very little difficulty experienced with fixed bridges, even in those cases having extensive spans. This ideal situation, however, rarely exists (Fig. 10-8).

MOVEMENT OF THE BRIDGE AS A WHOLE

For many bridges there is some area (usually in the edentulous ridge between abutment teeth) through which pass the resultants of the three sets of forces acting on the bridges. These three sets are (a) the occlusal load on the bridge and (b and c) the reactive forces induced in the embedded portion of each abutment. When resultants do so intersect at a point, the bridge, as a unit, may not rotate with respect to this point, since none of the forces has any leverage with respect to it. In order to better understand the difference in the movement of two individual abutments when forces are applied and when they are united by means of a fixed beam or bridge in a unit structure, it must be kept in mind that the roots are confined in the alveoli of the jawbone with a periodontal membrane interposed between the alveolus and the cementum of the root.

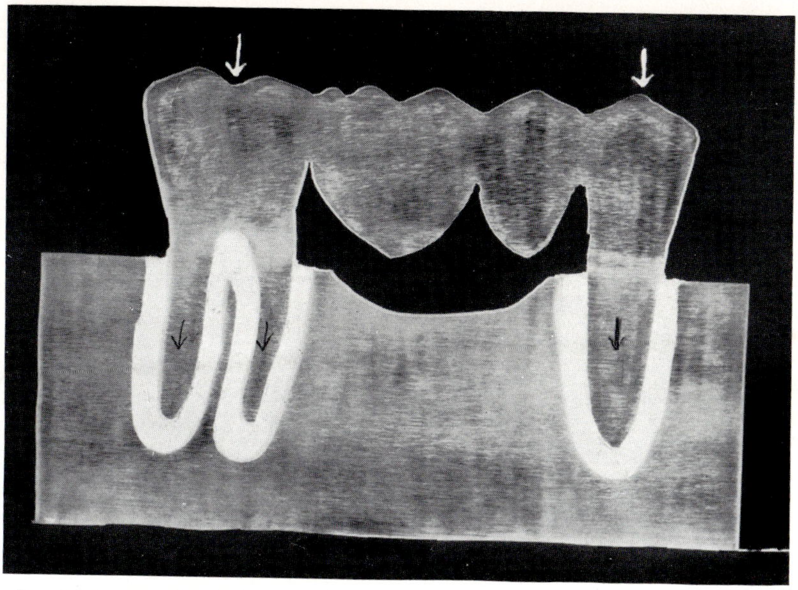

Fig. 10-8. Ideal but infrequent force application of occlusal forces to bridge.

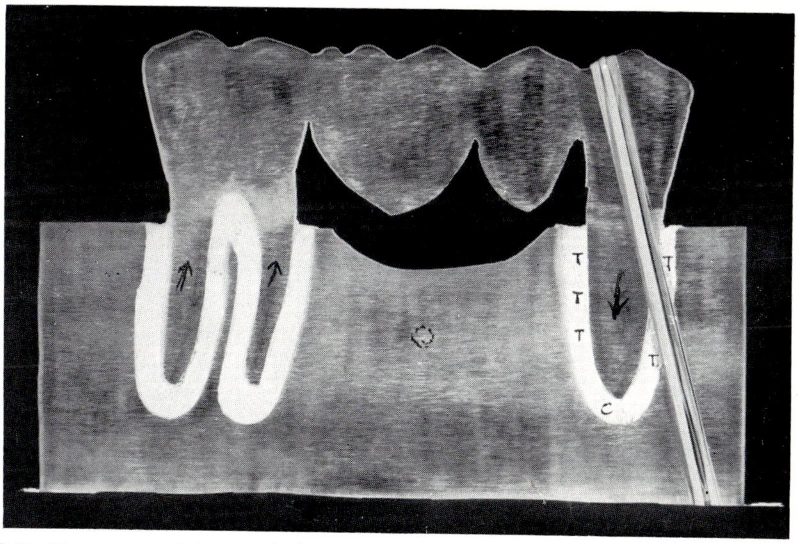

Fig. 10-9. Movement of bicuspid changes when it is rigidly united to bridge; center of rotation for bridge lies in bone of edentulous area between two abutments.

Any movement of one of the abutment teeth must now affect all other abutment teeth, also through the elastic deformation of the intervening connecting beam or bridge.

If, however, the bridge still attached to the abutments were a free structure in space detached from its sockets, and then if forces were applied to one of the abutments, the center of rotation of the bridge, as a whole, would shift to the center of gravity of all forces applied to the bridge. Such a center might be that shown in Figs. 10-9 and 10-10. If it be assumed that the

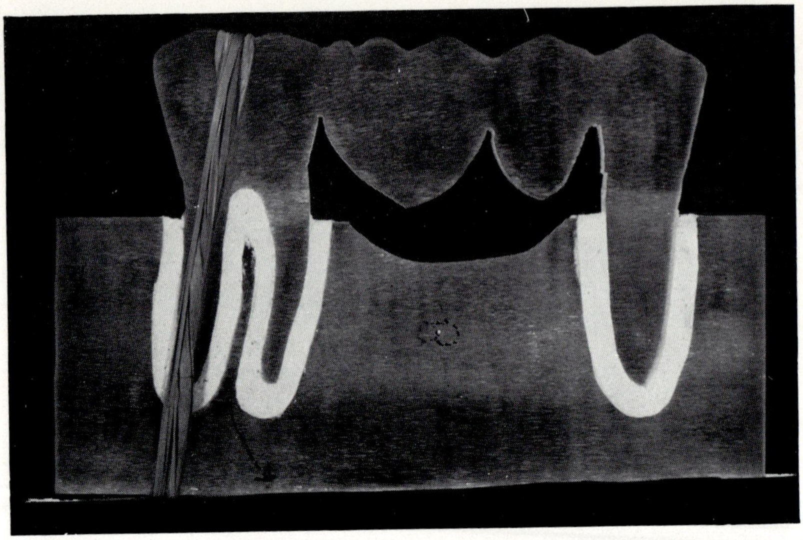

Fig. 10-10. Change in movement of molar when rigidly united to bridge; center of rotation of bridge lies in bone of edentulous area between two abutments.

abutment teeth are replaced in their sockets and the influences of the periodontal membrane are removed in the abutments, then the effects of the membranes on the abutment teeth must be added to the external forces on the bridge, which will cause some change in the point of rotation of the bridge previously indicated but which cannot be definitely established without taking into account the elastic deformation of the beam or bridge.

Fig. 11-1 shows the movements of an individual bicuspid buccolingually and mesiodistally when forces are applied to its coronal portion. It is observed that on one side there is an area of tension in the periodontal membrane and on the opposite side of the tooth an area of compression. The conditions prevail in the gingival and in the apical third regions. It is also noted that the center of rotation is not at the apex but somewhere between the apical and middle thirds of the tooth (Fig. 10-7). In the molar the point of rotation lies in the inter-radicular alveolar bone between the crest and the base of the bone. When occlusal pressure is applied distally, the distal root is depressed and the mesial root is raised in its socket; the periodontal membrane is tensed alongside the distal root and relaxed on the mesial root (Fig. 10-7).

If a vertical force is applied equally and simultaneously on the bicuspid and the molar teeth rigidly united by means of a bridge or beam, there would be an apical thrust of the teeth resulting in a tensing of all of the periodontal fibers, except those at the apices, which would be under compression (Fig. 10-8). Such equal and uniform distribution of forces does not usually occur. On the contrary, during function, abutment teeth are subjected to both vertical and horizontal forces.

Under these conditions we find that the bicuspid functioning as an abutment of a bridge reacts differently from a bicuspid which is unattached. Now the center of rotation changes from the individual teeth to a point between the two abutments and at a plane level with the middle third of the root lengths. As a result, the bicuspid is depressed apically and the molar rises occlusally (Fig. 10-9). Since the bicuspid is the load-bearing abutment, nature is prepared biologically to meet the new

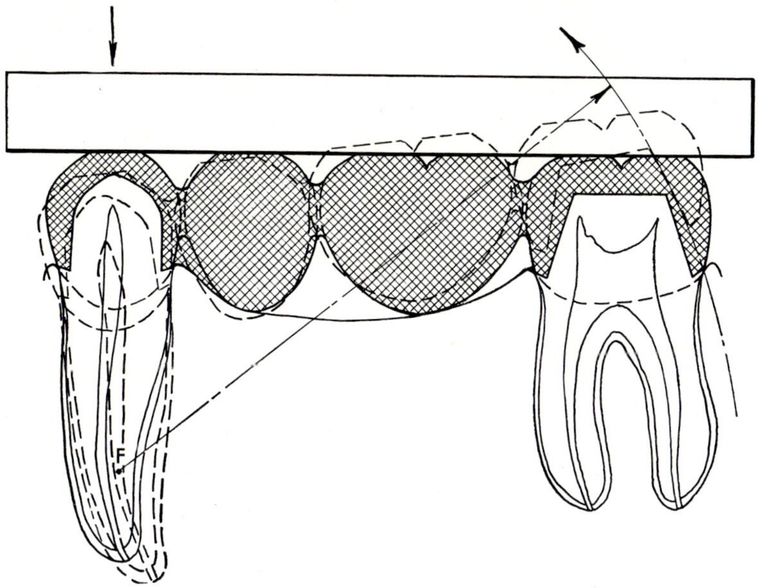

Fig. 10-11. Possibility of displacing bridge is increased if one of abutment teeth is lacking in normal, firm retention.

situation, for now instead of having two favorable areas of tension and two unfavorable areas of compression (Fig. 11-1), the fixation of the bicuspid abutment with the fixed bridge has placed the periodontal fibers into tension. Only the small periapical area is compressed. Since bone responds favorably to tensile forces, the lamina dura is stimulated to meet its new environment by depositing new bone if necessary. The adjacent trabeculated bone also responds to this increased favorable tension by reshaping its architectural form.

If the force is directed primarily upon the molar abutment (Fig. 10-10), depressing it within its socket, only a small amount of movement in the apical direction takes place before the root starts to exert a compressive force on the periodontal membrane of the mesial surfaces of the roots. If the roots of the lower molars were curved mesially, depressing the molar would enable it to move favorably, but since the roots curve distally, the amount of tolerable depression is very slight.

Fig. 10-11 represents a four-tooth bridge in which the biscuspid is extremely loose but the molar is firm. An occlusal force directed anteriorly and applied to the bicuspid has a tendency to raise the distal portion of the bridge out of the molar. If a bridge is employed under such conditions, the posterior abutment should be prepared with wide proximal surfaces parallel to each other gingivoclusally, as shown in Fig. 10-5; buccal and lingual surface boxing should also be employed.

There are times when it is necessary to use, as an abutment, a lower molar which is mesially inclined considerably beyond its normal vertical position (Fig. 10-12, *A* and *B*). A bridge placed upon such a tooth will have a tendency to tip the tooth mesially and rotate it from under its retainer. Whenever such a tooth is used, a retainer should be employed which furnishes at least two flat mesial and distal surfaces of sufficient width and length to hold the tooth firmly and to prevent its tipping mesially.

Usually, it is advisable to extend a half-

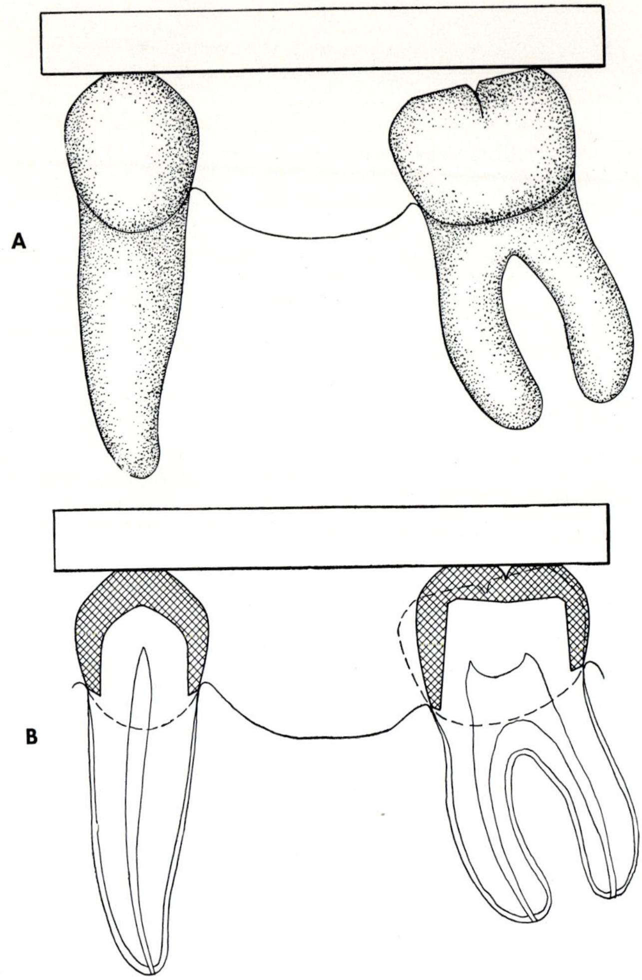

Fig. 10-12. Mesially inclined lower molar requires specially designed preparation to ensure retention and to prevent further mesial tipping.

crown veneer buccally and lingually including the grooves and carry each extension gingivally on these surfaces, to or slightly below the gingival crest. The mesial one-half crown is ideal for such conditions (Fig. 10-13). Where there is no danger of pulp exposure, the proximal dovetail keyway may be incorporated. Fig. 10-14 shows the use of such a preparation in the lower arch; Fig. 10-15 as it is used in the upper arch.

If, instead of using retainers with nearly parallel walls, a preparation is made with greatly converging axial walls, as in the molar (Fig. 10-16), a small force moving the bicuspid mesially will dislodge the MOD retainer from the rotating molar.

A force exterted distally or mesially will not dislodge the bicuspid retainer, due to the near parallelism of its axial walls (Fig. 10-17). Fig. 10-18 shows a bridge with a nonrigid connector (broken-stress) within an anterior retainer. It is obvious when such a connector should not be used: (1) if one of the abutments is excessively mobile, and (2) if a preparation cannot be made on it with nearly parallel walls.

If the molar is loose and mobile and

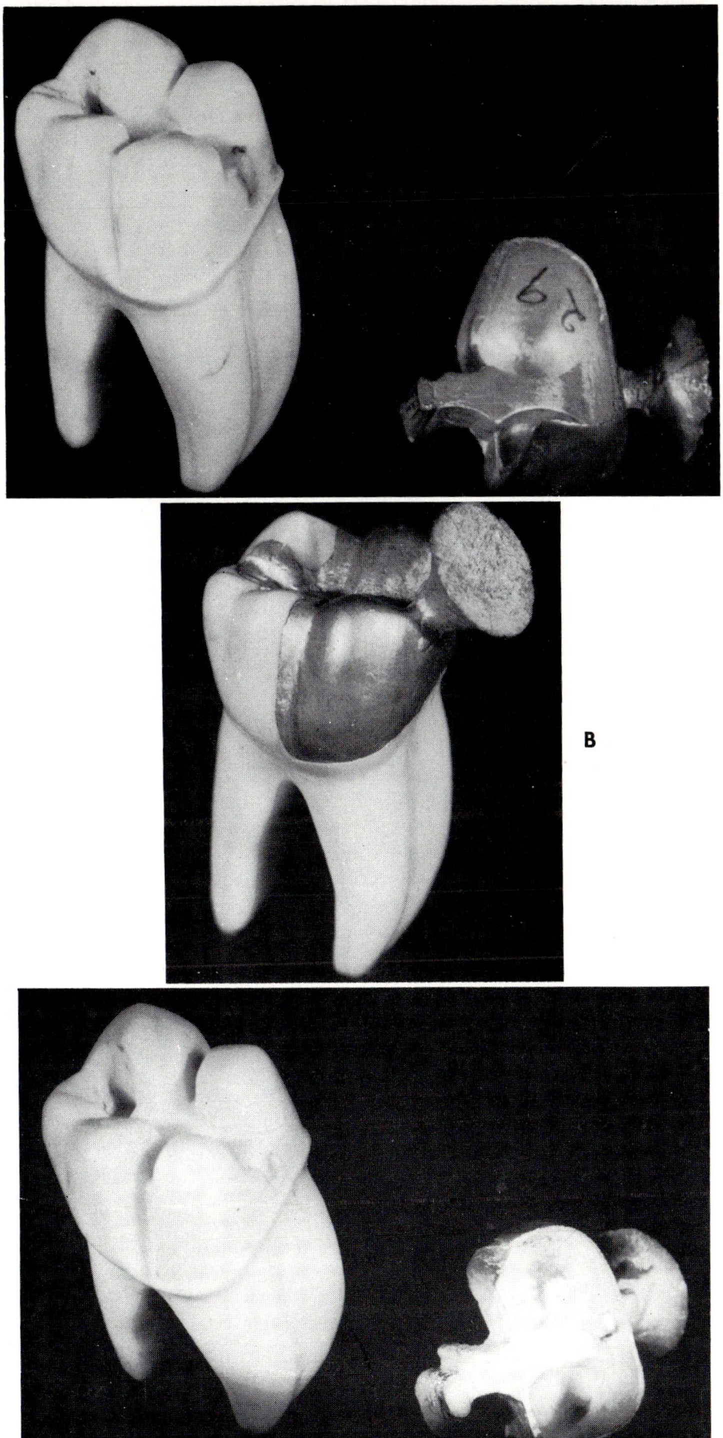

A

B

C

Fig. 10-13. Mesial one-half veneer crown useful on tilted lower molars.

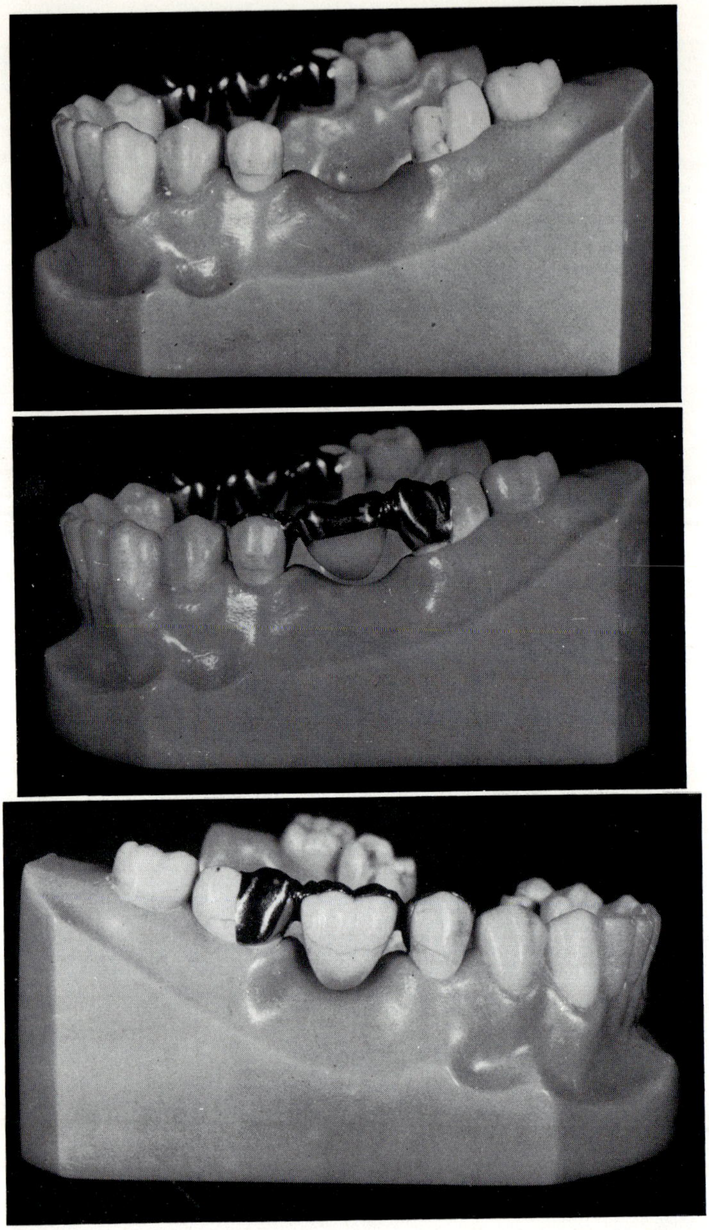

A

B

C

Fig. 10-14. Bridges using mesial one-half veneer crown as retainer.

still a strong retainer can be made, then the movement of the molar will cause the key to move in and out of the keyway in the bicuspid inlay. Also, it will subject the bicuspid to a mesial or distal thrust with its resultant two areas of compression and tension. If the molar is loose and quite mobile and the axial walls converge excessively (Fig. 10-18), the slightest force exerted in a distal direction on the tooth will rotate the molar abutment out of the MOD retainer.

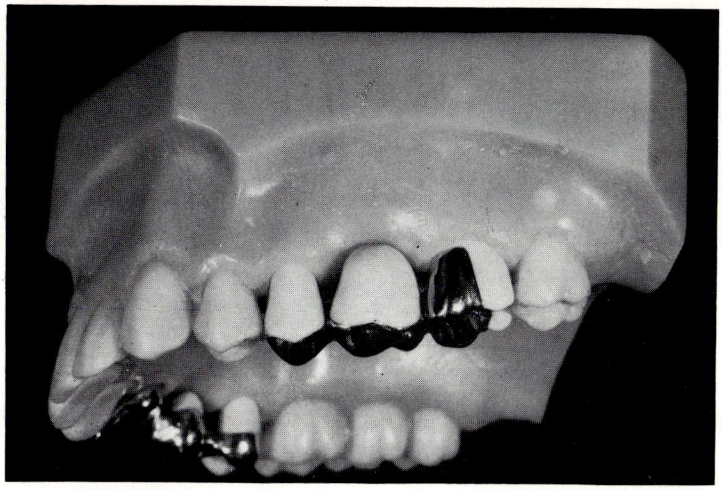

Fig. 10-15. Mesial one-half veneer crown used as bridge retainer on upper molar.

Attention was called by the author in 1940 to the relationship which exists between engineering principles and dentistry. Since then, Brumfield,[1] Gabel,[2] and Smyd[3, 4] have discussed the structural laws of engineering from an engineer's viewpoint and have indicated how these also apply to dentistry. Their writings are recommended to those wishing an explanation of the principles involved in structural problems from the engineer's viewpoint.

Definitions and engineering principles. The following definitions are by Brumfield[1]:

Beam: A beam is any bar whose curvature changes under load.

Reaction: The reaction of a beam is the external force induced due to load, at a point of support. The reaction prevents lateral movements of the beam.

Support: The support of a beam prevents movement when loads are applied to it. Three types of support should be mentioned:

1. *Fixed support*—Permits no rotation of the beam due to load at its support point, nor any lateral translation.
2. *Free support*—A free support permits perfect freedom of rotation at the support point but no lateral movement.
3. *Restrained support*—The first two support types mentioned are mathematically idealized. A restrained support permits some freedom of rotation at the support point but not perfect freedom. It permits no lateral movement.

Cantilever beam: A beam with one fixed support only, at one of its ends.

Simple beam: A beam with two free supports only, one at each of its ends.

Continuous beam: A beam with more than two free supports or with one free support and one or more fixed supports.

Concentrated load: A load applied over such a small area that for practical purposes it may be considered as applied at a point.

Distributed load: A load applied over a sufficiently large area that it may not be considered as applied at a point. If its pressure over this area is equally distributed it is said to be a uniformly distributed load; otherwise, it is a varying or non-uniformly distributed load.

Shear: The shear at any section of a beam is equal to the net sum of all the normal forces (reactions included) which act on the beam to one (either) side of the section.

Bending moment: The bending moment at a section of a beam is equal to the net sum of the moments of all forces acting on the beam (reactions included) to one (either) side of the section, these moments being taken about the section.*

To illustrate the importance of having a sufficient thickness of gold in a bridge in its occlusogingival depth, let us consider Fig. 10-16. It will be observed that in this model the depth of the gold through the soldered joint between the

*From Brumfield, R. C., C.E.: Dental gold structures, New York, 1949, J. F. Jelenko & Co.

A

B

C

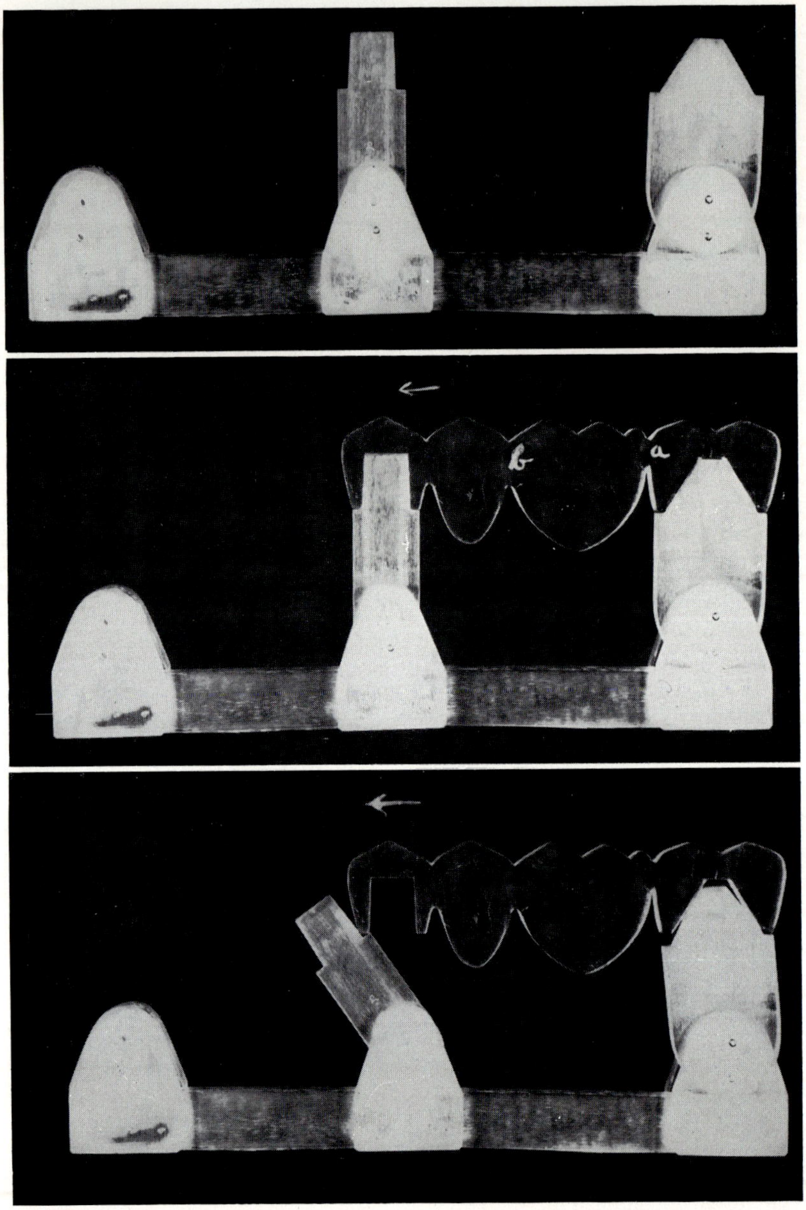

Fig. 10-16. Ease with which molar retainer is displaced from preparation with excessively tapered axial walls.

first molar pontic and the second molar retainer, *a,* is half of that between the second bicuspid and first molar, *b.*

The following demonstrating models show in simple form how certain known laws of physics and engineering are applicable and important in dental practice.

It is known that when a load is applied to a beam (and a dental bridge is a beam of nonuniform section) the beam bends; it is deformed temporarily or permanently, depending upon the load and many other

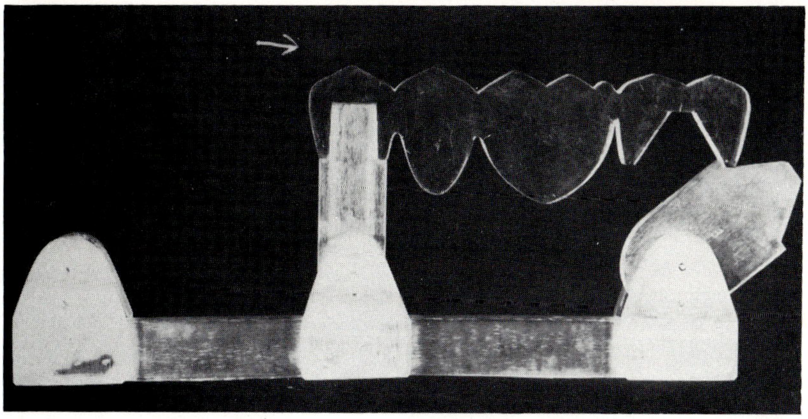

Fig. 10-17. Bicuspid preparation having nearly parallel axial walls prevents displacement of bridge retainer.

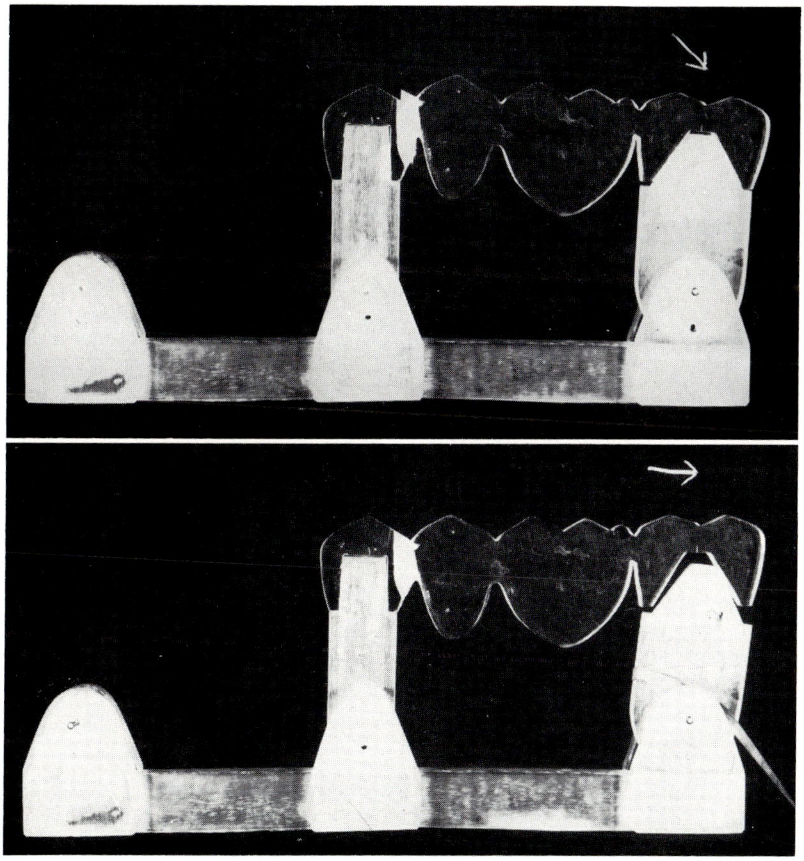

Fig. 10-18. Inadvisability of using nonrigid connector (broken-stress) when one of abutments is very mobile in its socket.

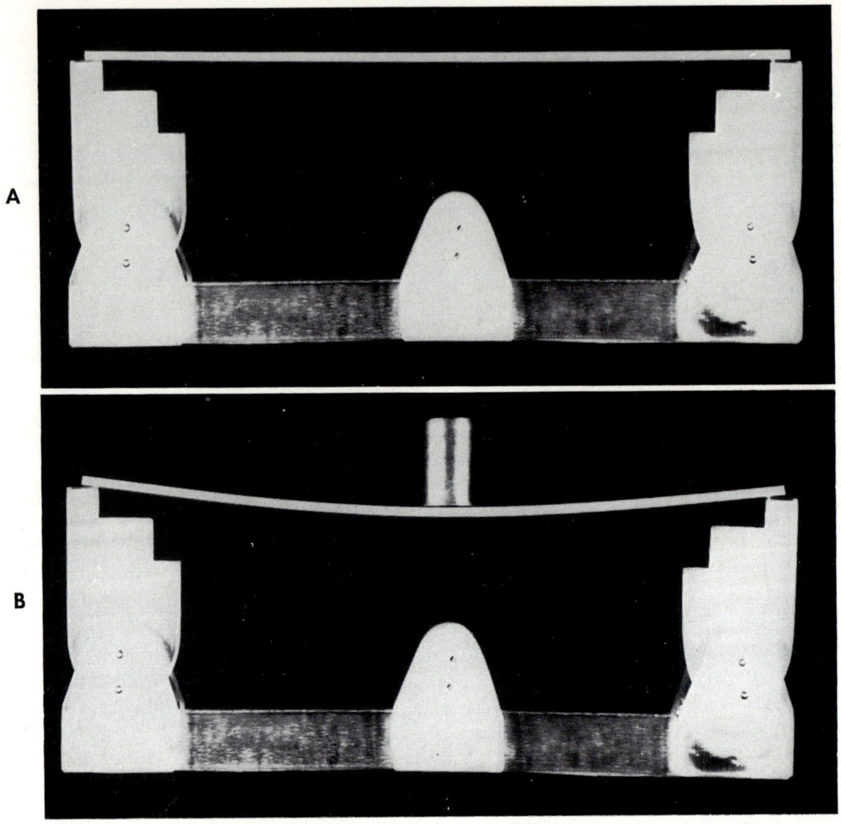

Fig. 10-19. Beam of given thickness, material, and distance between its terminal supports bends certain amount under given load.

factors. The amount of bending or deflection of the beam varies according to its thickness. In Fig. 10-19, we see a beam of a given thickness; the beam bends or is deflected to a certain amount. Let us assume that the thickness of this beam is comparable to the thickness of the connector or joint *(b)* between the second bicuspid and the first molar (Fig. 10-16, *B*). Therefore, under a given load the bridge would bend a certain amount at this point.

In Fig. 10-20, the beam is of identical material and is supported by two abutments the same distance apart as Fig. 10-19. The only difference is in the thickness of the beam; it is half of that in Fig. 10-19. In Fig. 10-20, the same load is applied as in Fig. 10-19. This thickness of the beam is comparable to the thickness of the soldered joint between the first and second molars (Fig. 10-16, *B, a*). The question arises: How much more will a beam bend which is half the thickness of the other? Engineers tell us it will bend eight times more because deflection or bending varies inversely as the cube of the depth, provided the same amount of load is placed on each beam and the stresses of either beam are not beyond the elastic limit of the material.

A bridge, therefore, having its soldered connectors the thickness of that between the molars, would bend eight times more than one having connectors the thickness of that between the molar and the bicuspid.

In Fig. 10-21, the same material and

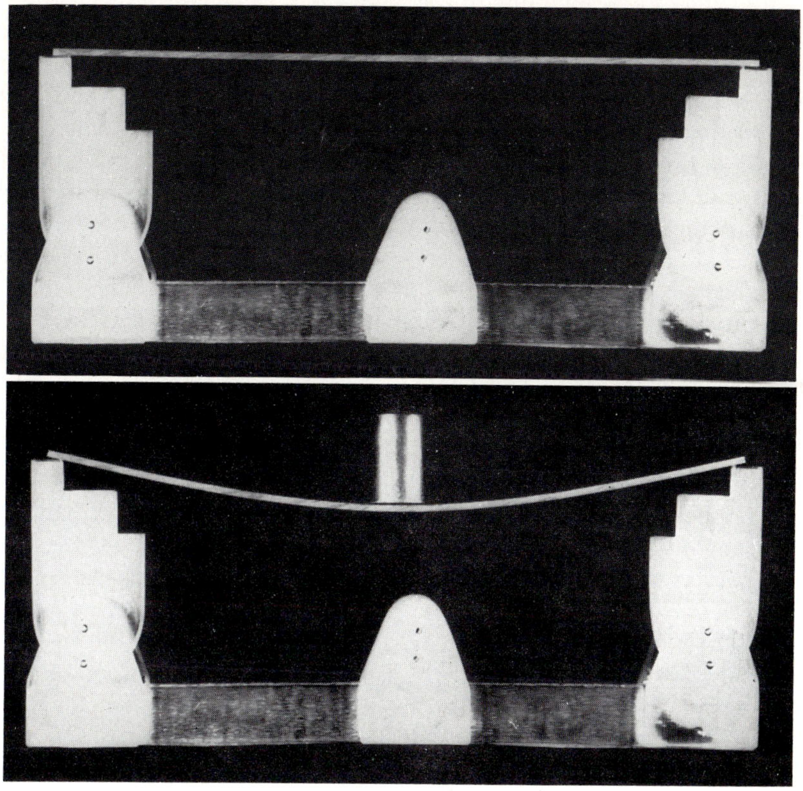

Fig. 10-20. Varying only one factor, that of reducing thickness of beam by half, will increase amount of bending eight times.

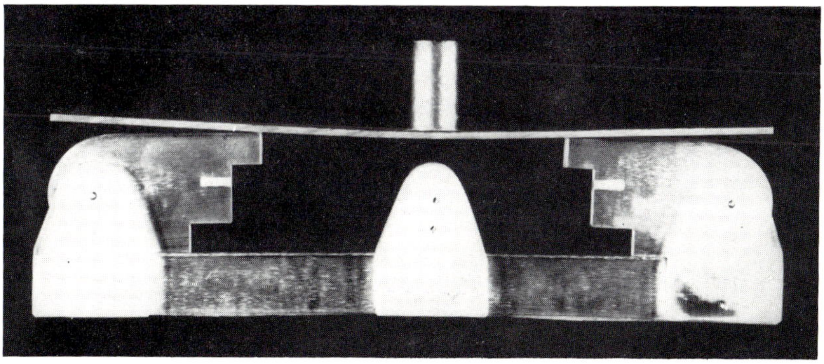

Fig. 10-21. Reducing distance by half between abutment supports reduces amount of bending by eight times.

thickness of beam is used as that in Fig. 10-20. The same load is used; the only difference is that the distance between the two supports has been shortened from twelve inches to six. The question arises: How much more does the beam deflect at the twelve-inch spacing than at the six? The answer again is eight times, for engineers have determined that the potential angle of rotation of the beam at the abutment varies directly as the cube of the length. In their clinical application, these engineering facts caution us that a four-tooth bridge, such as seen in Fig. 10-18, will bend eight times more under the same load than will a three-tooth bridge from cuspid to second bicuspid, which is approximately half the length. It is immediately evident that a thicker metal beam (bridge) is indicated.

Angular rotations of bridge sections at abutments.* Fig. 10-22, *(a)*, represents a dental bridge of span length *L* (center to center of free supports). An occlusal load *P* is applied at the center of the bridge. When the bridge bends under the influence of the applied load, its ends rotate through some angle θ, as shown. If, instead of a free support at the ends, the retainer were a cemented crown on the abutment, which is soldered to the bridge, this rotation would be partially prevented by the abutment and this restraint, in turn, would tend to rupture the cement by which the crown is held to the abutment. Comparisons will be made as to the amount of this angular rotation for: (a) the depth of the beam halved; and (b) the length of the beam halved and the depth allowed to remain constant. The load is always at the center.

For any span, loaded as shown, the angle θ at the support is equal to the area of the M/EI diagram lying between the center and one of the supports. (See cross-hatched area.)

$$\theta = \frac{PL}{4}\ \frac{L}{2}\ \frac{1}{2}\ \frac{1}{EI} = \frac{PL^2}{16\,EI} = \frac{PL^2}{16\,E\,C\,bd^3} \quad \text{(a)}$$

Where *C* is the Modulus Constant for the bridge section.

*This section written by R. C. Brumfield, C.E.

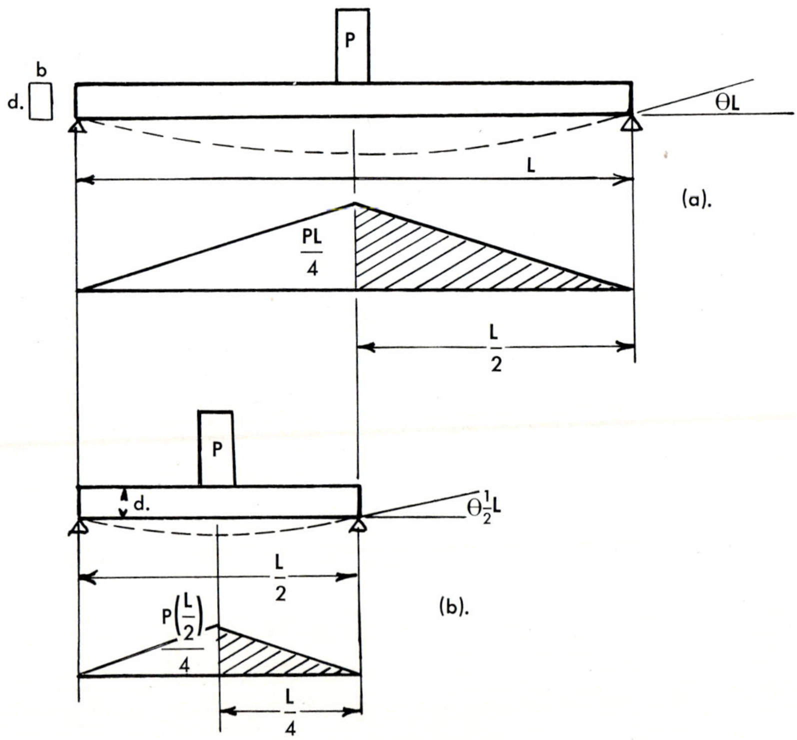

Fig. 10-22. Influences of beam depth and span length on rotations and bending moments. (Courtesy R. C. Brumfield, C.E.)

Bridge depth halved. If the depth of the bridge is halved and no other dimension or load changed, then the only dimension changed in Equation (a) is d, which becomes d/2. Making this substitution in Equation (a):

$$\theta_{\frac{1}{2}d} = \frac{P\ L^2}{16E\ C\ b(\frac{d}{2})^3} = \frac{P\ L^2}{2\ E\ C\ bd^3}$$

or

$$\theta_{\frac{1}{2}d} = 8\ \theta_d \qquad (b)$$

Thus it is seen that if the depth of the bridge be halved and no other dimension or load be changed, the potential angular rotation at the abutment is eight times what it would otherwise be.

Span length halved. If the span length be halved and no other dimension or load be altered [see Fig. 10-22, *(b)*], then from Equation (a):

$$\theta_{\frac{1}{2}L} = \frac{P(\frac{L}{2})^2}{16\ E\ C\ bd^3} = \frac{P\ L^2}{65\ E\ C\ bd^3}$$

or

$$\theta_{\frac{1}{2}L} = \frac{\theta_L}{4} \qquad (c)$$

Thus, halving the length of the span reduces the potential rotation of the bridge at the abutment by 75 percent.

Bending moments at soldered abutment connections. In the final analysis the influence which tends to break the cement bond between the MOD or crown and the abutment is the bending moment induced, due to the restraint which the abutment offers to rotation of the beam end. If it may be assumed that the abutment offers perfect restraint, then these moments (potential maximums) may be computed. The computed bending moment at the support for perfect restraint is:

$$M = -\frac{P\ L}{8} \qquad (d)$$

This maximum potential influence tending to break the cement bond at the abutment would be lessened by rotation of the abutment in its alveolar fundus, toward the edentulous area. (See Fig. 10-25.)

Halving the span length. If the span length be halved, the bending moment of Equation (d) becomes PL/16, or half what it is in Equation (d); and:

$$M_{\frac{1}{2}L} = \frac{M_L}{2} \qquad (e)$$

Bending moment, bridge depth halved. If the bridge depth be halved the bending moment at the abutment is in no way affected, for depth does not enter into the expression for bending moment. This statement assumes that when depth is halved, stresses in the bridge remain within the proportional limit of the material.

In Fig. 10-23, the beam has distal and mesioaxial extensions resting on the gingival walls of the two abutments.

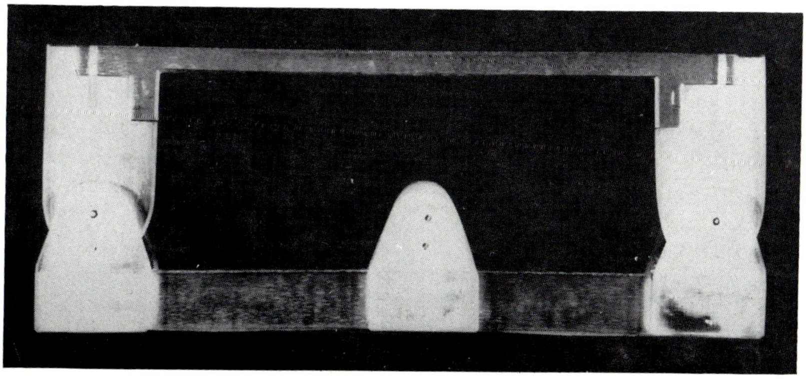

Fig. 10-23. Beam representing bridge with two-surface retainers as terminal supports.

In Fig. 10-24, a load is applied to the beam, causing it to bend. The end of the beam on the right side has risen vertically so that its distal portion has risen out of the cavity and forced the tooth to rotate distally. On the left side that portion of the beam representing the retainer has been secured with a dowel extending through the beam and into the abutment. This has prevented the distal portion of the beam from rising. The same retention may be secured by extending ribs of gold in a cast retainer which fit into grooves or keyways prepared on the buccal or lingual surfaces (Fig. 10-13).

Fig. 10-25 demonstrates the importance of extending the dowel or axial retention grooves in the retainer well below the level of the pulpal wall. On the left, the extension gingivally is adequate; hence there is no dislodgment of the retainer. On the right, the dowel extension is too short and the dowel hole is too wide; hence there is no resistance to displacement of the retainer.

LOOSE ABUTMENTS

The placement of a fixed bridge is sometimes recommended as a therapeutic measure in those instances in which one of

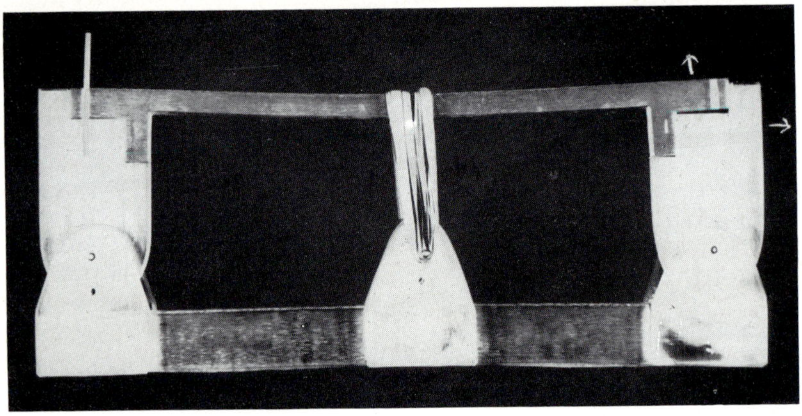

Fig. 10-24. Bending of beam by applied load displaces right retainer; left one is locked into abutment, which moves in its socket.

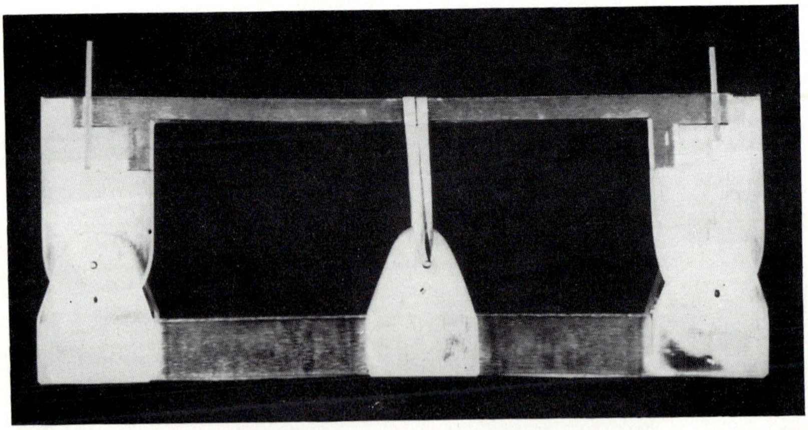

Fig. 10-25. When left terminal retainer is securely locked into abutment, bending of beam causes abutment to rotate without dislodging terminal retainer; right retainer is dislodged from abutment due to inadequate retention.

the abutment teeth is extremely loose in its socket. Consider again the simple experiment of placing a bar across the occlusal surfaces of a lower second molar and a second bicuspid, which, in this case, is the loose tooth. When pressure is applied vertically in the bicuspid region, the bicuspid is depressed in its socket, causing the distal end of the bar to rise with the mesial margin of the molar acting as the fulcrum. If a three-quarter or complete crown retainer is now fixed to the bicuspid or mesial end of the bar and the bar is extended distally over the molar as an MOD inlay retainer, which becomes a part of the distal end of this bar, it will be dislodged on the distal end, unless the dislodging force is counteracted by a broad resisting surface on the mesial surface of the firm molar and the two fingerlike extensions on the buccal and lingual surfaces. It is evident, however, that the strain upon the firm tooth will be so great that within a short time it also will loosen, due to the destruction of the gingival investing tissues with pocket formation on the mesial surface and the crushing of the apical periodontal membrane on the distal surfaces of the root. It is inadvisable, therefore, to employ any tooth as a bridge abutment that lacks a degree of firmness comparable to its healthy neighbor. There are times, however, when the usefulness of a relatively loose tooth may be extended for many years if it is stabilized. This is usually accomplished by preparing multiple abutments and soldering the retainers of the bridge. This type of fixation by means of multiple terminal supports acts as a splint for the loose teeth, which frequently show remarkable recovery both from the standpoint of stability and function.

USE OF PIER (INTERMEDIATE ABUTMENT)

The vertical displacement of abutment teeth merits special attention in those restorations in which more than two supporting teeth are used as abutments or piers. Fig. 10-26 illustrates a five-tooth bridge having two abutments and one pier as the supporting members of the structure. All three

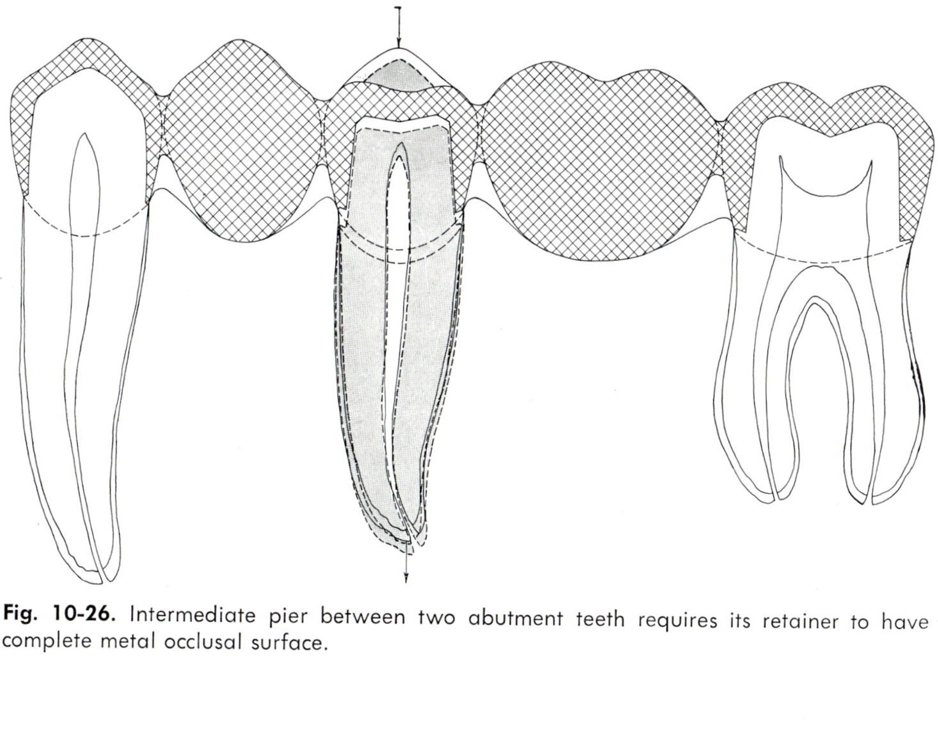

Fig. 10-26. Intermediate pier between two abutment teeth requires its retainer to have complete metal occlusal surface.

teeth are normal and are so prepared that the three retainers resist displacement equally in every direction except in the vertical.

If each of the three cast retainers is of a type having the entire occlusal surface of the tooth restored in metal, there is less danger of dislodgment, even in the vertical direction. If, however, the bicuspid carries an intracoronal type of retainer, such as an MOD, whose buccal and lingual cusps are not covered by the gold casting, a vertical pressure exerted upon one of the uncovered natural cusps could possibly depress the tooth into the socket and out of its retainer. The likelihood of such an occurrence increases in proportion to the looseness of the tooth. Therefore, in all instances in which an intermediate pier is employed in a fixed bridge, its entire occlusal surface should be covered by the casting.

SELECTED REFERENCES

1. Brumfield, R. C.: Dental gold structures, New York, 1949, J. F. Jelenko & Co.
2. Gabel, A. B.: The American textbook of operative dentistry, Philadelphia, 1947, Lea & Febiger.
3. Smyd, E. S.: The mechanics of dental structure, J.A.D.A. **44**:187-193, 1952.
4. Smyd, E. S.: Mechanics of dental structures; guide to teaching dental engineering at graduate level, J. Prosth. Dent. **2**:668-692, 1952.

GENERAL REFERENCES

Bodecker, H. W. C.: The metallic inlay, Berlin, 1911, Hermann Meusser.

Jepsen, A.: Root surface measurement and a method for x-ray determination of root surface area, Acta Odont. Scand. **21**:35-46, 1963.

Johnson, E. W.: A three dimensional photoelastic investigation of stress concentrations in operably deformed human teeth, Thesis, University of Alberta, Edmonton, 1965.

Stuteville, O. H.: The movements of teeth subjected to pressure, Chicago Dent. Soc. Bull. **14**:20-23, 1933.

Chapter 11

Biologic interpretation of physical and mechanical principles

The vital, biologic processes must be correlated with the basic laws of physics and engineering. The occlusion of the carnivora is characterized by shearing action associated primarily with the vertical opening and closure of the mandible; that of the herbivora is characterized by a definitely horizontal movement of the jaw, producing its accompanying milling action; that of the human being is characterized by the omnivorous type of mastication, which combines both the shearing and milling actions of the teeth. The shearing is accomplished by points, moving along the convex surfaces, which touch each other at various points of occlusal contact, and by the contact of the marginal ridges. The crushing and the milling of food are accomplished by the cusps of the teeth when they reach their positions in their respective fossae. In such a complex mechanism we may expect to find forces present which with their associated resultants will produce various biologic reactions not only in the individual teeth but also in the natural dentition, contiguous tissues, muscles, and temporomandibular articulations.

TYPES OF FORCES

While the tooth is sometimes regarded as a one-armed lever, the more generally accepted theory is that it functions as a two-armed lever. When a single-rooted tooth is subjected to a vertical force, it is found that the tooth is depressed toward the fundus of the alveolar socket in a direction parallel to its long axis. When this occurs, most of the periodontal fibers are subjected to tensile stress. Since alveolar bone responds most favorably to tension, it may be safely stated that a force parallel to the long axis of the tooth is the most favorable direction in which a tooth may be moved. Since the law of Nature is "response to demand" and since it is found that the bulk of the periodontal fibers is of the oblique group, which primarily resists a vertical force, it is evident that Nature has responded to the physical demands through the biologic design of its periodontal membrane.

The other type of force, the diagonal, is directed sidewise against a part of the peripheral surface of the tooth and is directed obliquely against the long axis of the tooth. Whenever horizontal components of force are present, the tooth is tipped in its alveolar socket. In such cases the center of rotation is not located at the root end, but it is situated at a point somewhere between the apex and the middle of the clinical root. Fig. 11-1 discloses that when a tooth is subjected to diagonal force, the periodontal membrane area consists of two general regions, one part lying apically to the center of rotation, the other occlusally to it.

The center of rotation of a tooth about an axis perpendicular to its longitudinal axis is that point on the longitudinal axis

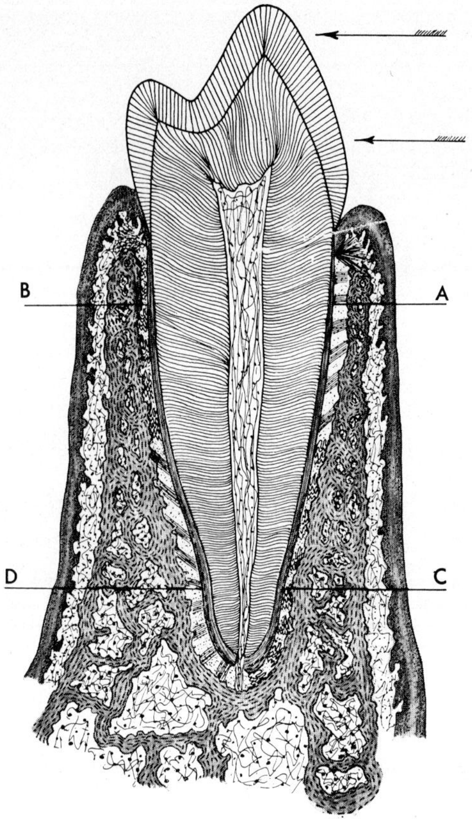

Fig. 11-1. Areas of tension, **A** and **D,** and those of compression, **B** and **C,** in periodontal membrane; center of rotation lies between apical one-third and occlusal two-thirds of root.

which has no lateral movement when the tooth rotates. That portion of the tooth above this point moves in one direction during rotation and the portion below in the opposite direction. This center of rotation is often referred to as a "fulcrum."

The *longitudinal axis of a tooth* is arbitrarily defined as the line connecting the center of rotation of the tooth and the center of gravity of the sectional area of the tooth, cut off by a plane, parallel to the occlusal plane and tangent to the cervical line at its higher proximal crest.

When the force is applied from the buccal surface, it is observed that the buccal region of the marginal area, *A*, is in tension, while on the lingual surface, *B*, opposite to the buccal area, the periodontal fibers are under compression. Similarly, it will be observed that from the center of rotation apically the fibers on the buccal surface are compressed, *C*, while those on the lingual surface are tensed, *D*.

Centers of rotation in teeth

Examination of a histologic section of the periodontal membrane in these areas shows that it is narrower in the rotation region, from whence it widens out apically and gingivally. This is in harmony with other observations that the periodontal membrane is wider in a functioning tooth or area than in one out of function or having a diminished function.

It is well to remember that, while the center of rotation of a tooth is in the apical region of the root, it is usually nearer the middle part than the apex of the root.

In two-rooted teeth, when a diagonal force is applied mesiodistally, the center of rotation does not lie in either root, but is situated in the inter-radical alveolar bone at a point midway between the crest and the base of the bone (Fig. 11-2). If occlusal force is applied in such a way that a tooth is forced distally, the distal root is depressed and the mesial root is raised in its socket. Likewise, the distal surfaces of both the distal and mesial roots have the periodontium compressed in the occlusal regions and stretched in the apical area. On the mesial surfaces the periodontal fibers are stretched on both the distal and mesial roots. When the oblique or diagonal forces are applied simultaneously in a mesiodistal direction on both the mesial inclined planes of such a tooth, it is found that the tooth does not act as a tilting body, but that the entire tooth moves bodily in a distal and downward direction. In such a case it will be noted that the periodontal membrane on the distal surfaces of both mesial and distal roots is compressed, while on the mesial surfaces it is relaxed or stretched.

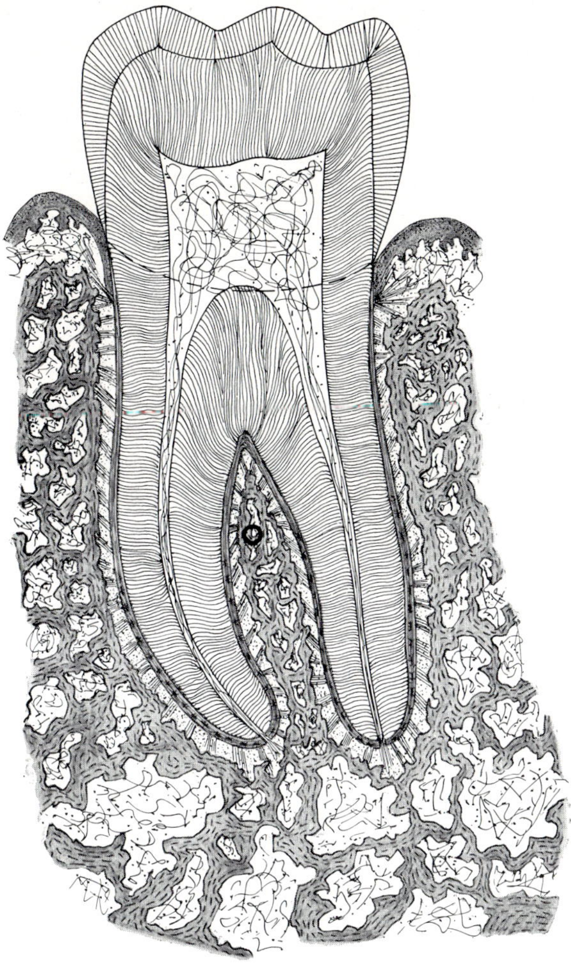

Fig. 11-2. Center of rotation lies in inter-radicular alveolar bone midway between crest and base.

These facts and experiments were well demonstrated by Schwarz.[1]

While it is true that bone responds more favorably to tension than it does to compression, it is likewise true that bone has the capacity of resisting and sustaining compressive force. The reaction of bone to force is dependent upon the amount of its application. If it is slight and intermittent, no resorption of bone occurs. If it is more intense and sustained, it is quite likely that a certain amount of resorption will occur; whereas, if the amount of force is excessive and sustained, it may result in an acute resorption or may even terminate in areas of necrosis and loss of function.

It has been suggested that the hydraulic systems of blood and lymph act as a protective measure to counteract the forces of mastication. Too great a pressure may produce an interference with the capillary system, resulting in a lowered resistance of the traumatized area with the possibility of infection setting in. It is evident that a close relationship exists between physical laws and biologic reactions.

The prognosis of a physiologic or a pathologic reaction lies not so much in the nature of the force as (1) in the scope of this reaction, be it mechanical, bacterial, or chemical and (2) in the ability of the tissues to respond favorably to a new environment. If a force is normal, it acts as a stimulant to the tissues; if it is abnormal, it may be temporary or continuous, resulting in either an acute or a chronic irritation.

Under normal conditions the application of proper force is not to be avoided; in fact, it is essential to the well-being of the tissues. Nature has so arranged the supporting tissues that, with each closure of the mouth, each act of deglutition, and during the process of mastication, the teeth are constantly subjected to intermittent pressure, which is stimulating in its effect. It induces an increased circulation and prevents a tendency toward stasis.

While it is generally true that the disturbance of a normal arch may result in abnormal forces, the abnormal conditions may react quite differently in two individuals. In the one having the vital capacity for adjustment, there will be no breakdown of tissues; while in the other not possessing such power of compensation and adaptability, there may be a serious breakdown of tissues.

The loss of one or more of the natural teeth generally creates an abnormal oral condition with accompanying abnormal functions and forces. An increased load is placed on some teeth, while others suffer through a loss or diminution of function. The deleterious change from normality, while slow, is continuous and may become progressively worse with the lapse of time. The chewing habits of the patients are frequently modified, and, in turn, exert forces which may develop to a degree where the entire dental mechanism is thrown out of equilibrium and effective use.

Forces of mastication

Hildebrand[2] and Tholuck[4] classified forces of mastication first into the absolute or theoretical, by which is implied the combined forces exerted by all of the masticating muscles; and second, the actual or masticating force, namely, that which can be exerted by any given individual to a maximum degree. Hildebrand pointed out that the actual force depends upon "the extent of the opening of the mouth, that is, the distance between the relative teeth; the point of application of the force; the extent of the force area, and the sensitiveness of the periodontium."[2]

While the problem of measuring the physical forces used in mastication has been approached from many angles, the device most frequently employed involves the use of the gnathodynamometer.

Klaffenbach in a study of gnathodynamics listed eight factors as possible variables which enter into the problem in any effort to obtain the measurements of forces of mastication: "(1) the kind of gnathodynamometer used and the technic employed; (2) sensitivity and condition of the periodontal membrane; (3) individual habits of mastication; (4) fulcrum (anterior or posterior); (5) osseous structure; (6) close approximation of opposing teeth; (7) pathological conditions; (8) cooperation of patient."[3]

Effects on biting force

The published reports of Hildebrand,[2] Tholuck,[4] Klaffenbach,[3] Jepsen,[8] and the author[5] dealing with the biting force of patients are significant in that their findings point to similar conclusions: (1) the loss of one or more of the natural teeth reduces the recorded biting pressure on the partially edentulous side; (2) the poundage exerted continues to drop progressively with the lapse of time; (3) an unfavorable reaction takes place in the investing and supporting tissues adjacent to the edentulous area; (4) normal, proximal, and occlusal relationships are disturbed; (5) the replacement of a lost tooth with a fixed prosthesis restores to a large degree the biting pressure normal to that area; (6) in time the biting forces gradually increase up to a certain amount; (7) the original biting pressure is never quite fully regained; (8) the biting force indicated on the gnathodynamometer is a measure of the tolerance of the periodontal membrane, rather than an indication of the combined efforts of all of the muscles of mastication; (9) of the different types of prostheses, the fixed partial denture is capable of exerting the highest biting pressure; (10) abnormal force and not overload is the most frequent cause of failures in fixed partial dentures; (11) patients of greater physical power usually exert greater pressure; (12) women achieve less pressure than men; (13) the optimum age period for maximum pressure is 20 to 40 years; and (14) habitual vigorous use of teeth increases pressure capacity.

What frequently has been attributed to overload rightfully should have been ascribed to the ill effects of leverage. Even excessive vertical forces accidentally exerted on a tooth may not cause permanent injury; rather, it is the unnatural buccolingual or torsional movements that cause the harm. It is true that the muscles of mastication are capable of exerting a maximum pressure of 200 to 300 pounds, yet it is the exception, rather than the rule, for a patient to bite regularly on any one tooth in excess of 100 pounds. This is so not because the muscles of mastication are incapable of maximum effort, but because the periodontal membrane becomes painful beyond a certain degree of force. Teeth will endure, with difficulty, pressure greater than that for which they are suited, the membrane acting as the safety gauge. It has been shown, however, that the periodontal membrane has the capacity to sustain additional moderate pressure and that this tolerance gradually increases with the continued presence of the new load, provided it is within physiologic limits.

Biting force in partially edentulous mouths

It is stated authoritatively that the average normal biting force of a patient is 175 pounds; our survey of unselected, consecutive cases, covering a period of many years, has given a slightly different result in partially edentulous mouths. In reviewing the poundage data of clinic bridge patients, some interesting facts are disclosed. An analysis reveals that in women the average bite on the restored side of a partially edentulous mouth is 48 pounds, while on the corresponding natural teeth on the opposite side it is 52 pounds. These figures for women are based on bridges of both types, namely, rigidly fixed at both abutments and the semifixed type. It is interesting to find that the average bite pressure recorded is greater in the fixed than in the semifixed partial dentures.

For men we find the averages are slightly higher; on restored teeth the average registration of biting force was 55 pounds, while on the natural teeth the average was 64 pounds. Here again, the fixed bridges average a higher bite pressure than the semifixed. Again the averages are based upon both types of bridges, fixed and semifixed. Such a marked variance between the 175 pounds which G. V. Black[6] gave as the average for the normal mouth and the 58 pounds which is the general average for mouths having partial restorations is indeed significant. These figures suggest that, just as Nature gradually increases her powers of endurance when additional loads are added, so also does she decrease these powers in proportion to the disuse of the teeth. Since it is Nature's law that disuse results in atrophy, edentulous areas should not be permitted to remain for any length of time without being restored with prostheses. It has been found, almost without exception, that, during periodic recordings of the bite poundage on the gnathodynamometer, the increase in tolerance takes place in teeth with vital pulps as well as in those that have had their pulps removed. With such assurance of favorable reaction on the part of Nature, every effort should be made by the prosthetist to have the design and placement of the appliance restore and maintain tolerable forces which will result in favorable biologic tissue reactions.

Table 11-1 shows the bite poundage sustained by 642 semifixed partial dentures.

Table 11-2 shows the bite poundage sustained by 853 fixed partial dentures.

The upper row of figures in each horizontal column indicates the average poundage recorded by each of the different abutment teeth. It will be observed that with few exceptions the upper row of figures shows a smaller force than the lower row, which represents the average poundage recorded by the corresponding natural teeth on the opposite side of the mouth. It should be noted that these figures represent the tolerance of the periodontal membrane to pressure.

Klaffenbach has calculated that, if a total bite pressure of 50 pounds is recorded on the gnathodynamometer and if the total area of contact on a mesioclusodistal inlay in an upper second bicuspid is 0.0379 square inch, the intensity of force equals 1,319 pounds per square inch. The

Table 11-1. Bite poundage averages for semifixed partial dentures

								Female (355)								
								Upper								
	8	7	6	5	4	3	2	1	1	2	3	4	5	6	7	8
Abutment teeth Natural teeth	—	53- 65	55- 54	50- 60	55- 57	35- 40	44- 46	28- 37	38- 34	21- 22	44- 52	41- 41	46- 53	54- 61	63- 65	— —
								Lower								
Abutment teeth Natural teeth	56- 52	50- 53	60- 61	47- 52	48- 60	—	—	—	—	—	15- 15	46- 53	51- 54	52- 60	55- 60	—
								Male (287)								
								Upper								
	8	7	6	5	4	3	2	1	1	2	3	4	5	6	7	8
Abutment teeth Natural teeth	—	75- 65	60- 82	62- 64	54- 65	46- 51	30- 28	43- 47	30- 34	23- 26	48- 52	73- 70	67- 68	66- 70	70- 82	20- 38
								Lower								
Abutment teeth Natural teeth	45- 130	68- 67	65- 76	69- 59	60- 76	51- 47	31- 48	— —	40- 40	— —	57- 81	65- 75	63- 68	82- 89	70- 73	49- 62

Table 11-2. Bite poundage averages for fixed partial dentures

								Female (462)								
								Upper								
	8	7	6	5	4	3	2	1	1	2	3	4	5	6	7	8
Abutment teeth Natural teeth	—	49- 95	125- 126	50- 48	51- 63	119- 136	29- 28	29- 43	34- 39	29- 34	40- 47	45- 48	51- 53	54- 54	56- 62	58- 55
								Lower								
Abutment teeth Natural teeth	42- 50	46- 54	53- 57	45- 51	44- 47	25- 26	30- 34	30- 30	30- 30	80- 85	39- 49	44- 52	51- 54	50- 40	43- 47	44- 44
								Male (391)								
								Upper								
	8	7	6	5	4	3	2	1	1	2	3	4	5	6	7	8
Abutment teeth Natural teeth	39- 38	70- 72	59- 96	55- 62	61- 73	48- 46	34- 44	38- 41	33- 47	55- 45	47- 53	60- 70	57- 65	64- 72	84- 91	70- 80
								Lower								
Abutment teeth Natural teeth	65- 94	70- 85	90- 90	57- 63	51- 65	60- 65	— —	— —	— —	32- 52	41- 37	67- 69	52- 59	32- 45	63- 68	61- 66

averages listed in Tables 11-1 and 11-2 afford a basis for further comparative studies.

It is recommended that the reader review Chapter 39 at this time to facilitate integration of the pertinent mechanical principles with the following and subsequent discussions as they relate to clinical dentistry.

The following is an approximate analysis by Brumfield of the effects of an incisal force on an upper central incisor (Fig. 11-3). The force is assumed to be

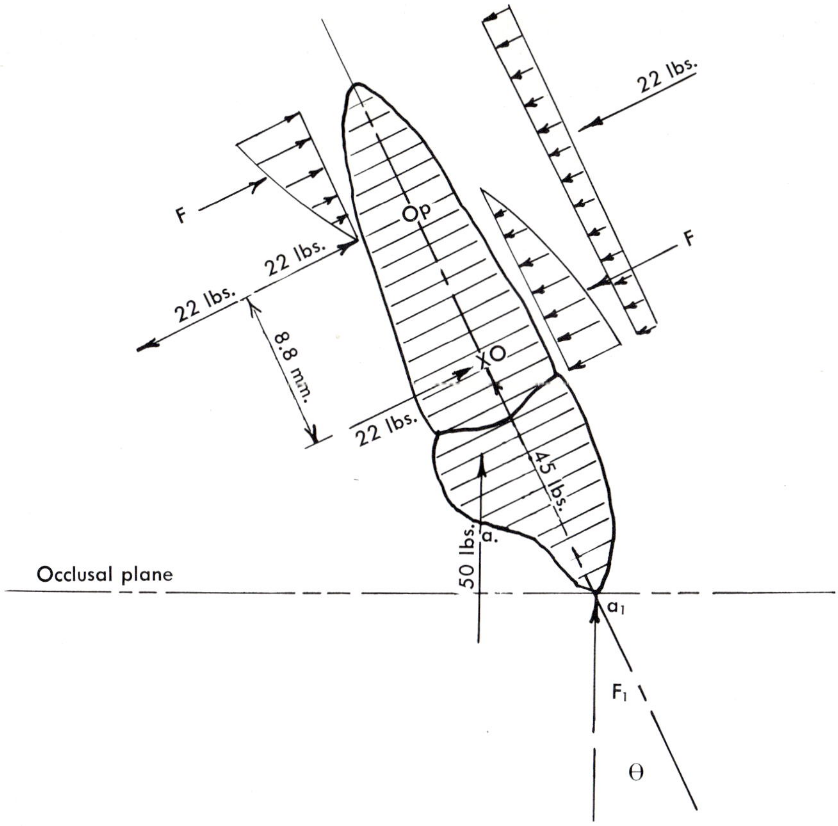

Fig. 11-3. Analysis of effects of incisal force on upper central incisor. (Courtesy R. C. Brumfield, C.E.)

applied by the abutting lower incisor, and to have a direction perpendicular to the occlusal plane. The direction of this force, with respect to the longitudinal axis of the central incisor is shown by the angle θ. This force is first applied to the central incisor at a_1, near the incisal edge of the tooth. It is of unknown but probably relatively small intensity at this point. As the lower central incisor slides down the incisal angle of the upper incisor, intensity increases until it reaches an assumed maximum value of 50 pounds at *a* when the bite is closed.

Produce the line of action (Fig. 11-3) of the 50-pound force at *a* until it intersects the longitudinal axis of the central incisor at *o*. Here resolve the force into components, as shown, of 45 pounds along the axis of the tooth and 22 pounds perpendicular to this axis. The 45-pound load produces no bending or lateral force in the tooth, because it acts along the axis. Its effect is to induce reactions (not shown) in the periodontal membrane and the fundus, which are approximately parallel to the axis, and equal in total to the 45-pound component.

The 22-pound transverse component acting at *o* produces bending in the central incisor in the same manner as the load on a cantilever beam produces reactions in its clamp. The center of rotation of the tooth, in its socket, is assumed to be at point *p*, 8 mm. from the upper apex of the tooth. This represents best present dental opinion of its approximate location for this type of root structure. Through the point *p* apply two equal and opposite forces of 22 pounds each, parallel to the 22-pound force at *o*. These forces can have no effect on the tooth, since each is the equilibrant of the other. Acting opposite to the direction of the 22-pound force at *o* and 8.8 mm. from it, one of these forces, when taken in conjunction with the force at *o*, constitutes a couple, which tends to rotate the tooth in a counterclockwise direction. The moment of this couple is 22 × 8.8 mm. pounds. The other force at *p* acts in the same direction as the 22-pound force at *o*, and passes through the center of rotation at *p*. It can therefore have no turning moment on the tooth, having no lever arm.

The couple, whose turning moment is 22 × 8.8 mm. pounds, induces bending in the tooth. This bending causes reactive forces in the bony structure of the fundus, increasing from zero at the point *p*, by an unknown law, to a maximum at the lower apex, and another maximum at the cervical plane, as shown. These forces are not unit stresses, but total stresses, resisting turning. The center of gravity of the resisting forces on each side of the center of rotation is indicated, and a force is shown, marked *F*, to represent the sum of all the resisting forces on that side. The exact location of either force *F* cannot be known, for the law of variation of individual stresses is unknown. These two resultant forces, however, constitute a couple whose lever arm is about 12.2 mm., as scaled from the drawing.

Now from the laws of equilibrium, the resisting couple must equal the applied couple. Therefore:

$$\begin{aligned} 12.2\ \mathrm{F} &= 22 \times 8.8 \\ \mathrm{F} &= 15.9 \text{ pounds} \end{aligned}$$

Thus the total resistance to turning, between the center of rotation and the lower apex, and that between the center of rotation and the cervical plane, are both the same—about 16 pounds. The manner of distribution is unknown. If some reasonable assumption be made such as parabolic or approximately triangular, some idea as to unit pressures may be obtained by taking into account variations in areas of root structure of the tooth.

Whether or not all this resisting force is exerted as compression between the root structure and the walls of the fundus, or whether part of it is exerted as tension in the periodontal membrane on the opposite surface, is not surely known. An intelligent guess would seem to place most of the force on the compressive side. It will be remembered that stress is the result of movement or distortion in material. The small movement possible for the tooth in its socket would not seem to indicate great total tension in the periodontal membrane. For the purposes of the discussion, it is immaterial whether or not part of the total force is developed as tension on sides opposite to the compression indicated.

The independent effect of the 22-pound force at *p*, which causes no turning, is indicated separately on the labial side of the tooth. These are total forces, and again their exact manner of distribution cannot be known. It is surely known, however, that the center of gravity of this set of forces lies at *p*, since there is no turning effect.

The normal denture maintains its equilibrium and state of health only so long as it remains in a state of dynamic balance. The presence of all of the natural teeth or their properly constructed substitutes is one of the important factors in maintaining this balance; these must have their opposing, occlusal, inclined surfaces properly interrelated. It will be found that where this condition is lacking or disturbed, the function and health of the dental tissues are also proportionately impaired.

CAUSES OF ABNORMAL FORCES

However, a well-balanced and properly related denture will also be thrown out of equilibrium if abnormal forces and relationships develop. Such disturbances are usually started when a lower first molar is extracted. Unless immediately restored with a prosthesis, the opposing upper first molar drops below its normal occlusal plane and the lower second molar tips anteriorly into the space formerly occupied by the first molar.

When only a part of the tooth is lost by caries, such as the mesial surface of a lower first molar, if the cavity is permitted to remain, the tendency is for the first molar to move anteriorly through a tipping action of the tooth. The second molar also then tips forward, its long axis inclined mesially. If the amount of tooth destroyed by caries is extensive, the relationships of the upper first and second molars are likewise disturbed.

During the adolescent period, while permanent teeth are replacing the deciduous teeth, the premature loss of a deciduous tooth will sometimes result in the anterior movement of those permanent teeth which lie posterior to the extracted tooth.

Similarly, it has been observed that in adult patients, those beyond middle age, the contacts between the proximal surfaces of the posterior teeth are no longer rounded and do not touch with a convex contact; these, during the course of years, have been worn flat so that their proximal surfaces touch with flat surfaces. This change of a convex surface to a flat one naturally reduces the mesiodistal diameter of the tooth. Since the cumulative amount of wear on all the teeth from the second molar to the median line is considerable and since in a normal mouth teeth are in proximal contact with each other, it is evident that some functional force is present, driving the posterior teeth forward in order to maintain this contact between the teeth.

There is one other condition which merits our attention. Fig. 2-5, *A*, shows the occlusal surfaces of two upper bicuspids in which inlays have been placed with improper contact position and contour. Under such circumstances it has been observed that the second bicuspid, because of the lingual placement of the contact area, has a tendency to rotate lingually; while the first bicuspid, because of the position of the contact on its distal surface, has a tendency to rotate bucally.

Fig. 2-5, *B*, shows another condition frequently encountered due to the improper contour and placement of a proximal contact. In this instance the vertical relationship of the contact to the marginal ridge is such that there is a tendency to depress the lower second bicuspid and to elevate the first bicuspid.

Fig. 11-4 shows a similar unfavorable and unnatural reaction; here the lower cuspid, a natural tooth, because of its improper mesial contact relationship with the lateral incisor has been forced labially and anteriorly.

It is apparent from these examples that an inherent driving force that has a tendency to move teeth forward is present in the natural dentition. Fig. 2-12 shows that

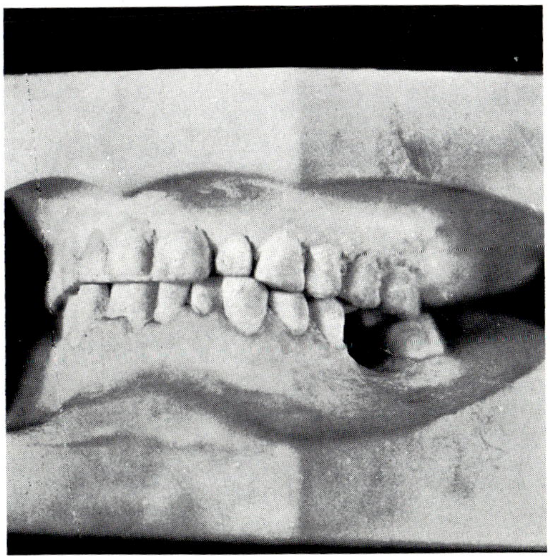

Fig. 11-4. Lower left cuspid has moved anteriorly, having slipped its mesial contact with lateral incisor.

the long axes of the upper and lower posterior teeth are not in the same plane; neither are the axes of the teeth at right angles to their occlusal surfaces; rather, the axes incline distally. The gingivoclusal height of the crown is not the same in its distal and mesial halves. Moreover, the roots of the buccal teeth incline distally.

ANTERIOR COMPONENT OF FORCE

In referring to Fig. 11-5 it is observed that the long axis, *X*, of the upper first molar meets the long axis, *Y*, of the lower first molar to form a vector line, *Z*, which is directed anteriorly. The anterior component of force is the functional force which drives the buccal teeth anteriorly; it becomes effective immediately upon the eruption and occlusion of the two permanent upper and lower molars.

That this force is not negligible clinically is evident through its daily manifestations. This force is not self-limiting. To resist this ever-present anterior force, Nature has set up an efficient and well-balanced muscular counterforce. This restraining force of the muscles is exerted backward against the incisors and canines, as well as posteriorly against the bicuspids and molars, in such a way that a state of equilibrium is maintained between the two forces.

This equalization presupposes that the forward and backward forces neutralize each other by passing through properly

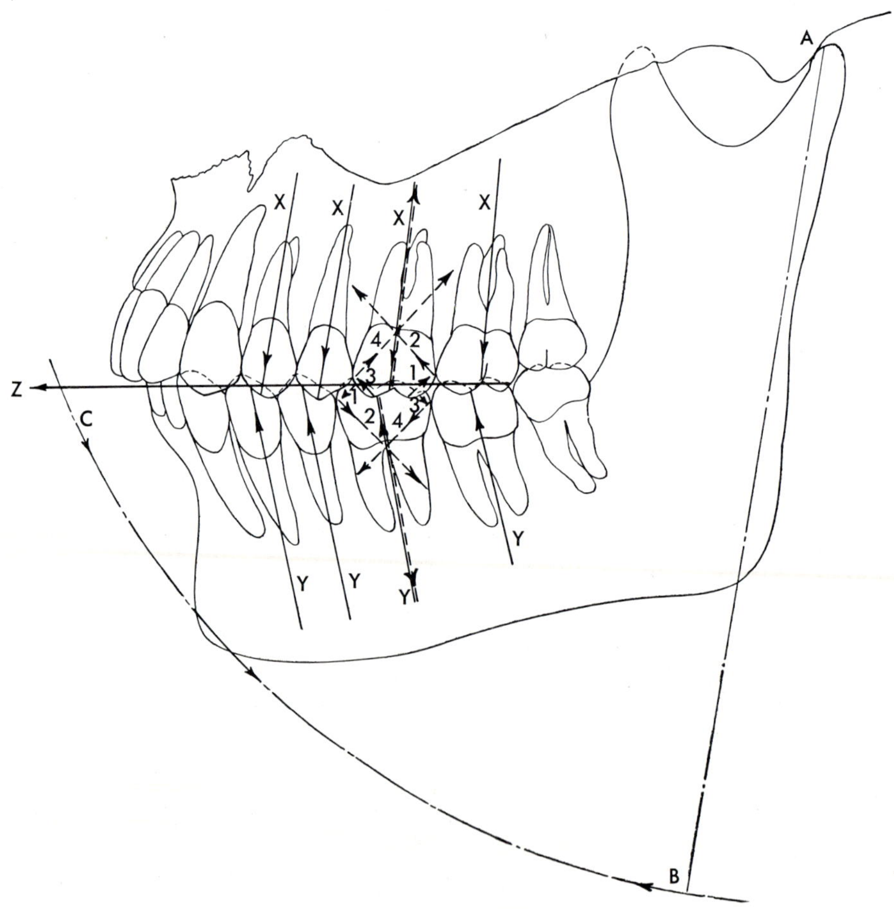

Fig. 11-5. Anterior component of force. (After R. A. Jentzsch.)

contoured and related proximal contact areas of the teeth. Fig. 2-4 shows (1) a diagram of the forces which pass through the contact areas in a line forming an arch where the two forces are neutralized and (2) an arch wherein the continuity of the line is broken and the equalization of the two forces is lost.

The anterior movement of teeth is definitely disclosed upon examining microscopic sections of teeth with their investing and supporting tissues. It is known that bone responds to pressure by resorption and that new bone is laid down in response to tension. Since the anterior movement of teeth exerts pressure on the anterior surfaces of the roots, and a pulling force on the distal surfaces, the presence of osteoclasts and areas of resorption may be expected on the mesial surface; whereas, the distal areas should disclose layers of newly formed bone. These changes usually take place.

Stein and Weinmann[7] attribute the distal curvature of the root apices to this anterior "wandering" of the teeth. It is their opinion that the anterior movement begins before the formation of the root is completed. They believe that, while the crown of the tooth is moving anteriorly, the formative organ of the root remains at its original position and thus the root, while forming, maintains an inclination toward the distal side. Normally, this anterior movement of teeth takes place bodily if there is an equitable distribution of all the forces of occlusion.

Intra-alveolar movement of teeth

Along with this anterior movement of teeth, clinical observation discloses that the functional movement of the individual tooth which is best tolerated by the supporting tissues is the intra-alveolar; this is produced by pressure parallel to the long axis of the tooth. That the major stress of a tooth is directed into its alveolar socket is confirmed by the fact that Nature responds to this directional force by developing a periodontal membrane having four-fifths of its fibers of the oblique type, which is built primarily to accept this kind of force. Fig. 11-5 explains the equalization of the various occlusal forces which drive the tooth into its alveolar socket, resulting in a tensing of the periodontal fibers.

As the jaw moves forward along the line, *BC*, the initial force is exerted by the sliding of the cusps. The resultant forces are numbered *1*. The reactive pressure to this force occurs at the contact area and is numbered *2*. At the initial contact of the cusp, the apex of the upper molar has a tendency to move anteriorly and the lower to move distally.

As the jaws are closed completely, opposite forces are developed and are indicated by *3*. These, likewise, meet reactive pressure at the contact areas and produce resultants, *4*. This force tends to move the apex of the upper molar distally and that of the lower molar anteriorly. Thus, the actions of *2* and *4* result in a reciprocating action on the tooth. By taking the vector of *2* and *4*, we get lines *X* and *Y*, which are parallel with the long axes of the teeth. The final vector of *X* upper and *Y* lower is the anterior component of force line *Z*.

Shape of roots

In addition to the continuous arch form with its properly placed contacts and the muscular resistance of the facial muscles, Nature has taken other precautionary steps to offset the forces imposed upon the teeth. Because the crowns of all teeth are not the same shape and because they do not receive their forces in the same direction or of the same magnitude, it is found that the root system of each tooth with its periodontal attachment has been developed to meet the individual requirements of each tooth. Since the force on an upper central incisor is directed from

Table 11-3. Average poundage exerted by natural and restored teeth (columns 1 to 5); root surface areas available for periodontal membrane attachment (columns 5 to 9)

1	2	3	4	5	6	7	8	9
Average bite poundage for men								
Relative order	*Restored*	*Natural*	*Relative order*	*Tooth*	*Peridontal membrane*	*Relative sizes*	*Total ratings*	*Average*
				Upper				
7	38	42	7	Central	139	7	21	7
8	35	35	8	Lateral	112	8	24	8
5	47	50	6	Cuspid	204	3	14	4
2	62	69	3	First bicuspid	149	5	10	3
4	60	64	4	Second bicuspid	140	6	14	5
2	62	80	1	First molar	335	1	4	1
1	74	77	2	Second molar	272	2	5	2
6	43	52	5	Third molar	197	4	15	6
				Lower				
7	40	40	8	Central	103	8	23	8
8	31	50	7	Lateral	124	7	22	7
6	52	57	6	Cuspid	159	4	16	6
3	61	71	4	First bicuspid	130	6	13	4
4	60	62	5	Second bicuspid	135	5	14	5
2	67	75	2	First molar	352	1	5	1
1	68	73	3	Second molar	282	2	6	2
5	55	88	1	Third molar	190	3	9	3

the lingual direction and the distal direction, it is found that the root is pyramidal in shape, affording a maximum periodontal attachment on the mesial, distal, and lingual surfaces. The same is true of the lateral surface, only to a less degree due to the smaller size of the tooth. In the lower incisors, due to the fact that the teeth are part of a closed arch and the forces are directed primarily in a lateral direction, we find that the roots are flattened on the mesial and distal surfaces, an arrangement affording the greatest amount of resistance to such forces. The same morphologic response to forces is manifest in the cuspids, both upper and lower; the cuspid must largely resist forces from the mesial and the distal directions, and consequently its greatest root surface areas are the mesial and distal.

An examination of the upper molar will disclose a similar adaptation of the roots to the existing forces. It is readily seen that the two buccal roots by their flattened mesial and distal surfaces afford large areas of periodontal membrane attachment against mesial and distal forces. The lingual root, on the other hand, in order to meet the buccolingual forces, has the larger areas for periodontal attachment on the buccal and lingual aspects of its root.

The same general adaptation of root shapes to applied forces is found in the lower teeth.

As a basis for comparison only, in Table 11-3 the root surface areas of periodontal membrane attachments of the average normal teeth have been computed in an effort to determine what, if any, relationship exists between this factor and the average poundage which was exerted by 678 partially edentulous male patients requiring fixed partial dentures.

The vertical columns 1 and 2 in Table 11-3 indicate the relative order and magnitude of the average bite pressure exerted

Table 11-4. Results of measurement of root surface areas*

Type of tooth	*1 Average (area sq. mm.)*	2 *Standard deviation*	3 *Coefficient of variation*	4 *Number of measure-ments*	5 *Relative sizes*	6 *Tylman and Tylman (1960)*	7 *Boyd (1958)*
Superior							
I^1	204	31.4	15.4	19	6	139	204.5
I^2	179	24.9	13.9	25	7	112	177.3
C	273	43.9	16.1	26	3	204	266.5
P^1	234	33.7	14.4	20	4	149	219.7
P^2	220	39.0	17.7	19	5	140	216.7
M^1	433	40.9	9.4	15	1	335	454.8
M^2	431	62.5	14.5	10	2	272	416.9
Inferior							
I_1	154	26.5	17.2	10	7	103	162.2
I_2	168	21.5	12.8	10	6	124	174.8
C	268	42.2	15.7	18	3	159	272.2
P_1	180	27.2	15.1	24	5	130	196.9
P_2	207	26.6	12.9	17	4	135	204.3
M_1	431	59.5	13.8	15	1	352	450.3
M_2	426	69.7	16.4	10	2	282	399.7

*From Jepsen, A.: Acta Odont. Scand. **21**:35, 1963.

by the upper teeth indicated in column 5; columns 3 and 4 indicate similar values for the corresponding unrestored natural teeth. Columns 6 and 7 indicate the average total surface area in square millimeters of the root systems of the various teeth, also their relative sizes.

By averaging the order of magnitudes in columns 1, 4, and 7, we observe in column 9 that a certain relationship exists between the area of periodontal membrane attachment and the actual or masticating forces exerted by patients. With but few modifications, these results correlate quite closely with clinical findings. However, great caution and reserve are essential whenever an attempt is made to interpret biologic phenomena entirely by mathematical measurements and computations. These may vary slightly, depending largely on the type of technique and measuring instruments used.

More recently Jepsen[8] published the results of his excellent research and they are summarized in Table 11-4.

The thought must prevail in constructing crowns and fixed partial dentures that, unless the restoration is biologically compatible with the rest of the natural dentition, it may seriously hinder the normal functioning of the mouth. On the other hand, many mouths are so badly damaged that even the best mechanical restoration can restore a normal function to a partial degree only.

Nature possesses such powers of compensation and adaptability that in the course of a few years new forces are gradually balanced, increasing the functional value of the restoration. Such an adjustment can take place, however, only if the new forces are not traumatic, excessive, or beyond the physiologic limits of tissue adjustment.

SELECTED REFERENCES

1. Schwarz, A. M.: The movement of teeth subjected to pressure, Ztschr. Stomatol. **1**: 40, 1928.
2. Hildebrand, G. Y.: Studies in dental prosthetics, Stockholm, 1937, Fahlcrantz.

3. Klaffenbach, A. O.: Gnathodynamics, J.A.D.A. **23**:371, 1936.
4. Tholuck, H. J.: The force of mastication, Deutsche Zahnarztl. Wchnschr. **51**:24, 1923.
5. Tylman, S. D.: Clinical and radiographic observations on fixed and semi-fixed bridgework, J.A.D.A. **14**:1379, 1927.
6. Black, G. V.: Operative dentistry, Chicago, 1917, Medico-Dental Publishing Co.
7. Stein, G., and Weinmann, J.: The physiological wandering of teeth, Ztschr. Stomatol., p. 733, 1925.
8. Jepsen, A.: Acta Odont. Scand. **21**:35, 1963.
9. Schwarz, A. M., and Gratzinger, M.: Removable orthodontic appliances, ed. 1, Philadelphia, 1966, W. B. Saunders Co.
10. Brumfield, R. C.: Personal communication, 1968.

GENERAL REFERENCES

Adlet, P.: Sensibility of teeth by loads applied in different directions, J. Dent. Res. **26**:279, 1947.

Anderson, D. J.: Measurement of stresses in mastication, I and II, J. Dent. Res. **35**:664-670, 1956.

Anderson, D. J., and Picton, D. C. A.: Masticatory stresses in normal and codified occlusions, J. Dent. Res. **37**:312-317, 1958.

Ardran, G. M., and Kemp, F. W.: Biting and mastication; a cineradiographic study, Brit. Soc. Study Orthodont. Tr., pp. 17-28 (disc. pp. 28-30), 1960.

Baker, C. R., Brekhas, D. J., and Dowell, R. L.: Brinell hardness method as applied to the registration of vertical intermaxillary force, J. Dent. Res. **19**:314, 1940.

Beke, A. L.: Margins of safety for forces on the human dentition, J. Prosth. Dent. **18**:261, 1967.

Boos, R. H.: Intermaxillary relation established by biting power, J.A.D.A. **27**:1192-1199, 1940.

Brawley, R. E., and Sedwick, H. J.: Gnathodynamometer, Amer. J. Orthodont. **24**:256-258, 1938.

Finnegan, F. J.: Determination of maxillomandibular force generated during deglutition, J. Prosth. Dent. **17**:134-143, 1967.

Granger, E. R.: Practical procedures in oral rehabilitation, Philadelphia, 1962, J. B. Lippincott Co.

Howell, A. H., and Brudevold, F.: Vertical forces used during chewing of food, J. Dent. Res. **29**:133-142, 1950.

Howell, A. H., and Manley, R. S.: An electronic strain gauge for measuring oral forces, J. Dent. Res. **27**:705-712, 1948.

Johnson, A. L., and Hatfield, H. K.: A study of the relations of dental conditions, biting force and the hand-grip, D. Cosmos **59**:599-609, 1917.

Jorgensen, K. D.: Relationship between retention and convergence angle in cemented veneer crowns, Acta Odont. Scand. **13**:35, 1966.

Klaffenbach, A. O.: Gnathodynamics, J.A.D.A. **23**:371-382, 1936.

Lucia, V. O.: Modern gnathological concepts, ed. 1, St. Louis, 1961, The C. V. Mosby Co.

Muhlemann, H. R.: Ten years of tooth-mobility measurements, J. Periodont. **31**:110, 1960.

Neumann, H. H., and DiSalvo, N. A.: Compression of teeth under the load of chewing, J. Dent. Res. **36**:286, 1957.

Osborn, J. W.: Investigation into the interdental forces occurring between the teeth of the same arch during clenching the jaws, Arch. Oral Biol. **5**:202, 1961.

Parfitt, G. J.: Dynamics of a tooth in function, J. Periodont. **32**:102, 1961.

Picton, D. C. A.: Tilting movements of teeth during biting, Arch. Oral Biol. **7**:151, 1962.

Picton, D. C. A.: Vertical movement of check teeth during biting, Arch. Oral Biol. **8**:109-118, 1963.

Schwarz, M. A.: A further contribution to the question of movement of burdened teeth, Ztschr. Stomatol. **27**:499, 1929.

Smyd, E. S.: Role of mechanical stress in dentistry, New York J. Dent. **28**:227, 1958.

Smyd, E. S.: Dental engineering applied to inlay and fixed fabrication, J. Tennessee D. A. **31**:123, 1951.

Smyd, E. S.: Mechanics of dental structures, J.A.D.A. **44**:187, 1952.

Smyd, E. S.: Role of torque, torsion, and bending in prosthodontic failures, J. Prosth. Dent. **11**:95, 1961.

Tylman, S. D.: Relationship of the structural design of dental bridges to their supporting tissues, Internat. D. J. **13**:303, 1963.

Watt, D. M., and others: Preliminary investigation of the support of partial dentures and its relationship to vertical loads, Dent. Pract. **9**:2-15, 1958.

Worner, H. K.: Gnathodynamics: the measurement of biting forces with a new design of gnathodynamometer, Australian J. Dent. **43**:381-393, 1939.

Yurkstas, A. A.: Occlusal forces used during food consumption, J. Dent. Res. **31**:489, 1952.

Chapter 12

Stomatognathic pathologic physiology related to crown and fixed partial prosthodontic therapy*

It has been found that the menisci from chronically painful temporomandibular joints are vascularized in the central portion, which is avascular in the normal joint.[1] In his study, Davidson found all sixteen of the painful joint menisci to be vascularized. It is possible that compression of this vascularized meniscus results in a wave of pressure being communicated directly along the blood vessels to the richly innervated region of the posterior meniscus giving rise to pain. Two types of perforations of menisci from temporomandibular joints in cadavers have been reported.[2] The first type occurs in the thin, central portion of the meniscus and has a raised, vascularized border. The second type occurs just above the lateral pole of the condyle and has a thin, knife-edged border. This type is not vascularized and resembles a defect that has been produced by sanding the mensicus until it is perforated.

Clicking of the temporomandibular joint may or may not be associated with pain dysfunction syndrome. The mechanism of the clicking is poorly understood today but there is good evidence that a disturbed relationship between the meniscus and the condyle is involved in many cases. When the normally tight attachments of the meniscus to the lateral and medial poles of the condyle have been torn or stretched, it becomes possible for the condyle to quickly slip over the thick border of the meniscus.[3] With arthritic changes of the joints the menisci become frayed and roughened and may break up into separate tags and pieces. These meniscal changes are also probable causes of crepitation in the joint. Painful clicking of the temporomandibular joint has been reported[4] as a major complaint in a patient who had a large bony projection medially. This exostosis would not have been discovered without radiographic examination of the joint. Temporomandibular joint radiographic examination is indicated for accurate diagnosis of a clicking joint problem.

Calcification of the stylohyoid ligament is a rare condition but often causes limited opening of the jaws with pain that may resemble temporomandibular joint pain dysfunction syndrome.[5, 6] Approximately 40 percent of the patients with temporomandibular joint pain syndrome have limited opening of the jaws.[7] It has been found that patients with a maximal incisal opening of 35 mm. or less should be examined to rule out abnormal function

*Text by Parker E. Mahan, D.D.S., Ph.D., F.A.C.D.; Associate Professor of Dentistry, Emory University School of Dentistry, Atlanta, Georgia.

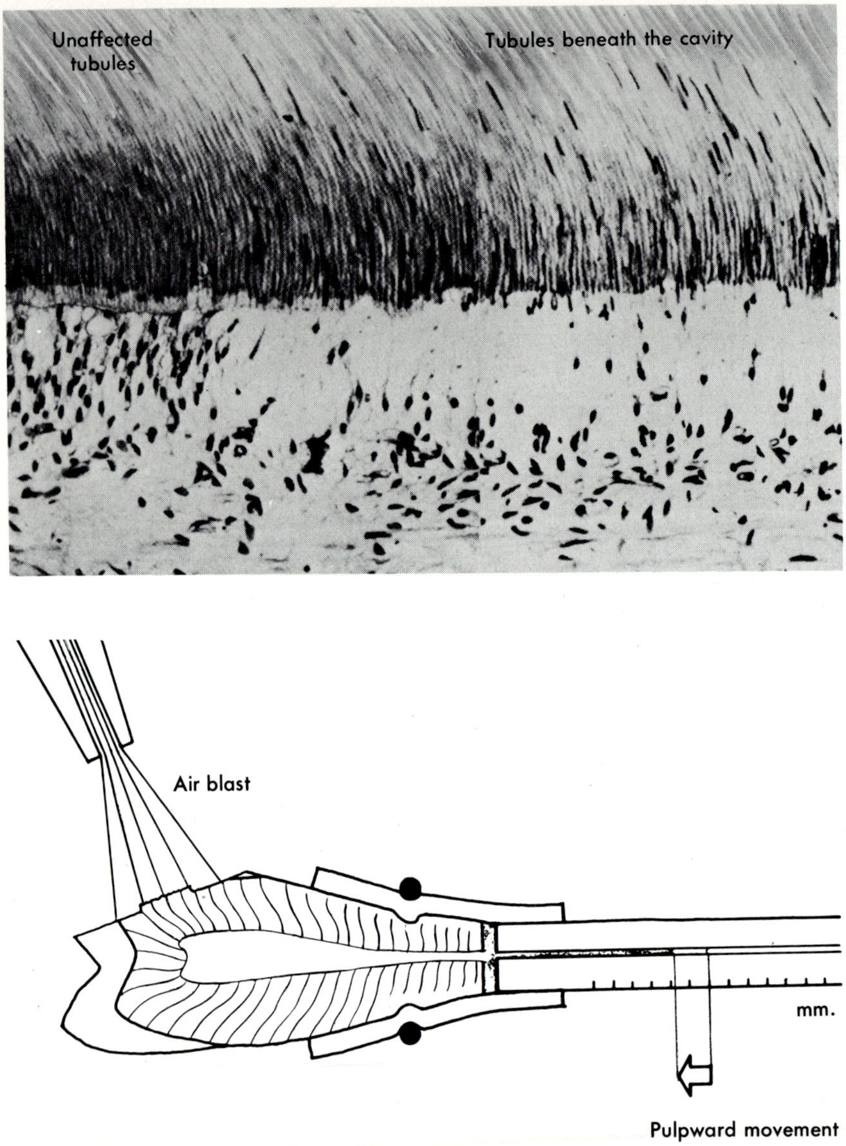

Fig. 12-1. A and **B,** Pulp and dentin adjacent to cavity exposed to airstream for 30 seconds. Odontoblast nuclei in dentinal tubules. Tooth was extracted after 5 minutes. (From Brännstrom, M.: Acta Odont. Scand. **18**:17, 1960.)

or pathology. The average maximal incisal opening for adults with no history of temporomandibular joint pathology is 45 to 50 mm.; that for young children, surprisingly, equals the average in adults. The average maximal opening in a study of 124 patients with temporomandibular joint pain was only 26 mm.[7]

Histologic examination of the temporomandibular joint from an elderly osteoarthritic man has demonstrated the effects of trauma to the jaws in such patients.[8] This 71-year-old man was bronchoscoped with some difficulty; when he died 24 hours later, examination of his meniscus revealed laceration of the vessels in the

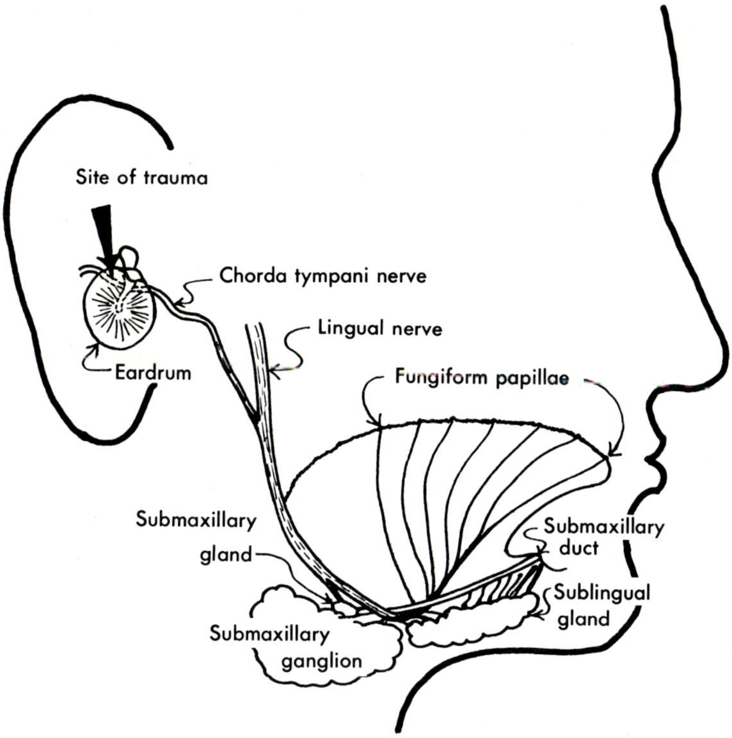

Fig. 12-2. Fibers from chorda tympani nerve join lingual nerve as shown. Some of these fibers enter submaxillary ganglion and continue to discrete Langley's ganglia in submaxillary gland, which they innervate. Fibers that synapse in ganglion rejoin lingual nerve and then innervate sublingual gland. Other fibers from chorda tympani continue in lingual nerve to innervate taste buds associated mainly with fungiform papillae on anterior two-thirds of tongue. When surgical approach for stapedectomy is through eardrum, chorda tympani may be cut or stretched at location indicated, thus causing altered taste and saliva flow.

bilaminar zone with fresh hemorrhage into the area. Blackwood[8] has pointed out that when rheumatoid arthritis affects the temporomandibular joint, it first affects the condyle and may progress either to partial or to complete fibrous ankylosis of the joint. Osteoarthritis, on the other hand, causes erosion and perforation of the meniscus with eburnation and osteophyte formation of the condyle; it rarely results in ankylosis.

Travell[9] has pointed out that pain from severe muscle spasm is almost always referred a distance from the affected muscle. She injected hypertonic saline into potential trigger areas of the head and neck muscles and mapped out the pain reference patterns. She found that injection of the deep belly of the masseter, the middle temporalis, and the lateral and medial pterygoids referred pain to the temporomandibular joint.

An unusual case of muscle function has been reported in a 56-year-old denture patient.[10] When the patient was 9 years old he had meningitis and afterward had to support his chin against his chest in order to masticate food. When he was not able to chew with his second dentition his dentist discovered that his mandibular elevators were paralyzed. Later the patient was able to masticate food using the muscles of facial expression to elevate the mandible, after the vertical dimension of the denture was greatly increased.

It has been found that drying the exposed dentin of a tooth with an air blast will aspirate odontoblast nuclei into the dentinal tubules[11-14] (Fig. 12-1). It follows, therefore, that the odontoblasts may usually be damaged by routine crown and bridge therapy. It has been found that coating prepared teeth with petroleum jelly or some similar compound before inserting tooth-colored, quick-cure acrylic over the teeth in the construction of a temporary crown or bridge will help prevent adverse pulpal changes.[15] Coating the prepared teeth with a cavity varnish will also protect the pulp from the acid in crown and bridge cement.

Epitheloid or glomus cell arteriovenous anastomoses have been identified in the human temporomandibular joint meniscus and periodontal membrane. Tumors of these structures are known to give rise to local or referred pain of variable intensity. The pain is often intermittent and is accompanied by a blanching of the part. Glomus tumors have been reported in the temporomandibular meniscus[16] and in the periodontal membrane.[17]

The surgical approach for operations in the middle ear is commonly through the tympanic membrane. In these operations, such as the stapedectomy, it is often necessary to cut or traumatize the chorda tympani nerve to gain adequate access to the operative field. Eighty percent of 126 poststapedectomy patients in one study[18] experienced symptoms of altered taste and dryness of the mouth. These patients commonly complained of a metallic taste in the mouth. The chorda tympani contains the taste nerves to one side of the anterior two-thirds of the tongue and the secretomotor nerves to the ipsilateral submaxillary and sublingual glands as shown in Fig. 12-2. In the stapedectomy patients the fungiform papillae on the operated side atrophied to the midline of the tongue. There was no reinnervation from the chorda tympani of the opposite side. Many of these patients did not associate altered taste sensation with their ear operations and went to their dentists, thinking they had carious teeth or gingivitis.

SELECTED REFERENCES

1. Davidson, A. S.: Hemodynamic theory of pain production in temporomandibular joint syndrome, J. Oral Surg. **22**:39, 1964.
2. Gregg, R. V.: Anatomy and histopathology of temporomandibular joints with perforated discs, I.A.D.R. Program and Abstracts of Papers, Washington, D. C., 1967.
3. Dixon, A. D.: Structure and functional significance of the intra-articular disc of the human temporomandibular joint, Oral Surg. **15**:48, 1962.
4. Grossman, E.: An unusual case of clicking jaw, Brit. J. Oral Surg. **3**:158, 1966.
5. Bruni, A.: Calcification of the stylohyoid ligament, J. Oral Surg. **21**:67, 1963.
6. Balasubramanian, S.: Ossification of the stylohyoid ligament and its relation to facial pain, Brit. Dent. J. **116**:108, 1964.
7. Sheppard, I. M., and Sheppard, S. M.: Maximal incisal opening—a diagnostic index, J. Dent. Med. **20**:13, 1965.
8. Blackwood, H. J. J.: Arthritis of the mandibular joint, Brit. Dent. J. **115**:317, 1963.
9. Travell, J.: Temporomandibular joint pain referred from muscles of the head and neck, J. Prosth. Dent. **10**:745, 1960.
10. Payne, A. G. L.: Mandibular elevation by the facial muscles: a case report, Dent. Pract. **14**:333, 1964.
11. Marsland, E. A., and Shovelton, D. S.: The effect of cavity preparation on the human dental pulp, Brit. Dent. J. **102**:213, 1957.
12. Brännstrom, M.: Sensitivity of dentine, Oral Surg. **21**:517, 1966.
13. Brännstrom, M.: Dentinal and pulpal response, II: application of an air stream to exposed dentine; short observation periods, Acta Odont. Scand. **18**:17, 1960.
14. Brännstrom, M.: The effect of dentin desiccation and aspirated odontoblasts on the pulp, J. Prosth. Dent. **20**:165, 1968.
15. Berk, H., and Stanley, H.: Human pulp response to full crown procedures, I.A.D.R.

Program and Abstracts of Papers, Washington, D. C., 1967.

16. Griffin, C. J.: Glomus tumor in the bilaminar zone of the human temporomandibular meniscus, Aust. Dent. J. **7**:377, 1962.
17. Harris, R., and Griffin, C. J.: Glomus tumor of the periodontal tissues, Aust. Dent. J. **10**: 33, 1965.
18. Bull, T. R.: Taste and the chorda tmypani, J. Laryng. **79**:479, 1965.

GENERAL REFERENCES

Ackerman, J. B.: A new approach to the treatment of bruxism and bruxomania, New York Dent. J. **32**:259-261, 1966.

Barber, D., and Massler, M.: Permeability of active and arrested carious lesions to dyes and radioactive isotopes, J. Dent. Child. **31**:26, 1964.

Binns, W. H., Jr.: Resorption of bone, its mechanism and control: a review, Bull. Phila. Dent. Soc. **31**:5-10, 1966.

Brännstrom, M.: Physio-pathological aspects of dentinal and pulpal response to irritants. In Symons, N. B. B., editor: Dentine and pulp, London, 1968, E. & S. Livingstone Ltd.

Brännstrom, M.: The effect of dentin desiccation and aspirated odontoblasts on the pulp, J. Prosth. Dent. **20**(2): 165, 1968.

Brudevold, F., Amdur, B. H., and Messer, A.: Factors involved in remineralization of carious lesions, Arch. Oral Biol. **6**:304, 1961.

Clarke, J., and Hampson, E. L.: Effect of cavity preparation and filling materials on the human dentine, Brit. Dent. J. **124**:456-461, 1968.

Corbett, M. E.: The incidence of secondary dentine in carious teeth, Brit. Dent. J. **114**:142, 1963.

Craig, R. G., and others: Compressive properties of enamel, dental cements, and gold, J. Dent. Res. **40**:936, 1961.

Fisher, F. J.: The viability of micro-organisms in carious dentine beneath amalgam restorations, Brit. Dent. J. **121**:413, 1966.

Franks, A. S.: Masticatory muscle hyperactivity and temporomandibular joint dysfunction, J. Prosth. Dent. **15**:1122-1131, 1965.

Fröhlich, E.: Pathologic-anatomical aspects of the relationship between gingival margin and artificial crowns, Deutsch. Zahnaerztl. Z. **22**(10): 1252-1258, 1967.

Glickman, I., and Smulow, J. B.: Effect of excessive occlusal forces upon the pathway of gingival inflammation in humans, J. Periodont. **36**:141, 1965.

Hassan, E. H., Van Huysen, G., and Gilmore, H. W.: Deep cavity preparation and the tooth pulp, J. Prosth. Dent. **16**(4): 1966.

King, J. B., Crawford, J. J., and Lindahl, R. L.: Indirect capping: a bacteriologic study of deep carious dentine in human teeth, Oral Surg. **20**: 663, 1965.

Langeland, K.: Dentin and pulp reactions to cavity and crown preparation: survey of literature, Amer. Inst. Oral Biol. Ann. Meet. **23**:73-88, 1966.

Malone, W. B., Bell, C., and Massler, M.: Physicochemical characteristics of active and arrested carious lesions of dentin, J. Dent. Res. **45**:16, 1966.

Mongini, F., Preti, G., and De Fabianis, E.: Functional disturbances of the temporomandibular articulation (etiology, pathogenesis, and symptomatology), Minerva Stomat. **17**(1):23-28, 1968.

Mylen, W. K., and Quigley, M. B.: Internal resorption of the dentine with extensive osseous metaplasia of the pulp, Oral Surg. **21**:75-82, 1966.

Nyborg, H., and Brännstrom, M.: Pulp reaction to heat, J. Prosth. Dent. **19**(6):605, 1968.

Ostrom, C. A.: The trauma of cooling in operative dentistry, Dent. Progress **3**:138-144, 1963.

Robinson, M. J.: The influence of head position on temporomandibular joint dysfunction, J. Prosth. Dent. **16**:169-172, 1966.

Slaughter, D. P.: Symposium on minor surgery: superficial tumors of the head and neck area, Surg. Clin. N. Amer. **28**:69-81, 1948.

Wei, S. H. Y., Kaqueler, J. C., and Massler, M.: Remineralization of carious dentin, J. Dent. Res. **47**(3):381, 1968.

Zach, L., and Cohen, G.: The biology of high speed rotary operative dental procedures, I.: correlation of tooth volume removed and pulpal pathology, J. Dent. Res. **37**:67-68, 1958.

Chapter 13

Mechanical principles in preparing teeth for intracoronal, extracoronal, and complete crown retainers

For a bridge retainer to be acceptable biologically and satisfactory mechanically, the tooth upon which it rests must be so prepared that the retainer will receive sufficient support and adequate retention against displacing forces. Any cavity design which removes more tooth structure than is absolutely necessary for purposes of retention and prevention of caries or which jeopardizes the health of the tooth and its supporting tissues, either during its preparation or subsequently, should not be used.

IDEAL ABUTMENT

The ideal abutment tooth contains a vital pulp. It must not be inferred from this that a treated tooth with a properly filled root canal is not suitable as a bridge abutment; clinical evidence indicates that in properly selected cases such treated teeth have rendered years of valuable service to the patient without any harmful effects. Nevertheless, the first requisite in preparing vital teeth for the reception of bridge retainers is pulp conservation. Every effort should be made during the cutting operations to avoid overheating or irritating the pulp so as to prevent its future degeneration or death. Those preparations are contraindicated which bring the metal too close to the pulp, thus exposing it to continuous thermal shocks; if existing conditions indicate the probability of such an occurrence, every precaution should be taken to reduce the danger to a minimum.

To be suitable for use as an abutment, a tooth must have sufficient bulk to withstand the forces to which it will be subjected after the bridge is attached to it. This physical requirement is sometimes compromised in the effort to conserve the pulp of an extensively decayed tooth.

As previously indicated, abutment teeth sustain forces of a type and magnitude which an individual tooth is not required to bear; hence, the type and amount of periodontal membrane attachment are items of importance and should be determined separately for each abutment tooth. Although the ideal abutment is one which has a normal amount of periodontal attachment, many teeth lacking one-third or slightly less of the normal amount, when judiciously selected, have rendered satisfactory service. Where the detachment greatly exceeds this amount, it is questionable whether such a tooth should be used as an abutment. The amount of alveolar bone is determined by the extent of periodontal attachment, and the type of bone present reflects its degree of function.

In operative dentistry cavities are prepared primarily to receive fillings which restore that part of the tooth lost by caries or accident. In fixed partial denture prosthesis a large proportion of the teeth receiving bridge retainers are sound and noncarious; occasionally a monocarious tooth is used. Polycarious teeth, those with more than one carious lesion, are often restored with a complete crown instead of with the intracoronal or extracoronal type of retainers. The location of a cavity in an abutment tooth is also a determining factor.

Questionable abutments

While most abutments can be restored with complete crowns, the employment of intracoronal or extracoronal type of retainers has definite limitations. Before approving a tooth to serve as an abutment, its degree of calcification should be established; enamel that has not been properly calcified, but that is soft and chalky, will not furnish a suitable wall against which the margin of the casting may be finished. Some teeth have opalescent dentin; these are questionable for use as abutments to carry retainers other than complete crowns. In polycarious teeth the suitability of an abutment is determined to a large degree by the amount and distribution of healthy tooth structure that is left after the carious parts have been removed.

The construction of a bridge retainer, other than a complete crown, frequently offers serious mechanical and biologic problems on a severely abraded tooth. Due to the reduced coronal height of such a tooth, little opportunity is found to develop sufficient mechanical retention and still not endanger the pulp. It is much better, when such teeth are encountered, to employ the complete veneer type of retainer with certain modifications.

At times teeth egress beyond their normal occlusal plane to a point where, to use them as bridge abutments, it is necessary to grind down a considerable portion of the occlusal third of the tooth. Such teeth are not usually in occlusal contact with the opposing arch. The amount of such vertical displacement varies from 1 mm. to a point where the teeth touch the mucosa of the opposite arch. Where the egression of such a tooth has exceeded one-third the normal height of its crown, its use as an abutment usually requires that the pulp be removed. Where the necessary amount of reduction can be made without encroaching upon the pulp, the same physical and biologic handicaps prevail as in the case of an abraded tooth. An egressed tooth is further handicapped since it does not have a periodontal membrane of normal, functional width; neither does it possess a supporting bone of normal structure. Such teeth are of questionable value when used as abutments.

A malposed or malrelated tooth is not necessarily contraindicated as an abutment. The deciding factors are whether a suitable retainer can be prepared for it and whether the forces which will be transmitted to the tooth after the bridge is placed will be of a magnitude and direction which can be tolerated by the tooth and its investing tissues. The malpositions may be varied, such as a tilting of the tooth mesiodistally or buccolingually; a rotation of the tooth about its own axis; and a migration bodily of teeth into new positions and malrelations in the arch.

There is no objection to the use of anomalies as abutments, provided they have a sound biologic relationship with the investing and supporting tissues and that their coronal contour is such as to afford sufficient mechanical retention. Such teeth, however, are rarely employed for intra coronal or partial veneer types of retainers; the complete crown is preferred.

Where an abutment is loose, the etiology for the existing condition should be determined. If it is due to periodontal infection, excessive bone destruction, or other similar causes, its use as a bridge abutment should not be considered until the existing conditions have been corrected and their causes removed. The mechanical disadvantages inherent in the use of a loose tooth for a bridge abutment are discussed in Chapter 10.

Occasionally there is the possibility of using a tooth with a resected or a fractured root as an abutment. While such a condition curtails the probable life of a bridge, there are times when such a procedure is justified. The prognosis is more favorable in those cases in which the root is used to carry only an individual crown. Fig. 2-17 shows the use of a fractured root for a bridge abutment; the conditions under which fractured roots may be used are described in previous parts of the text.

Root length of abutment

In the ideal abutment a proportionate relationship exists between the lengths of the crown and the root. Where the root is excessively short, either congenitally or due to a resorption, it cannot furnish the necessary support to the crown or resistance to the forces of mastication developed during the various movements of the mandible. The additional forces inherent in a bridge will cause such teeth to fail as abutments.

The acceptable abutment, therefore, must be a healthy tooth, both individually and in relationship to its environment; it must be capable of supporting the additional forces to which it will be subjected as part of the fixed partial denture; its preparation must be such that its retentive power will be sufficient to resist the displacing forces to which it will be exposed; it must maintain and safeguard the normality of the pulp and ensure the continued integrity of the tooth structure against fracture or caries.

While the prime mechanical function of a retainer is to unite the body of the bridge with the abutment, it must also restore the form, function, and the esthetics of the latter, at the same time forestalling any future harm to both the tooth and its adjacent tissues. While most retainers furnish retention as well as support to a bridge, some are primarily a support even though they assist indirectly in its retention. An example of this type of a retainer is the two-surface intracoronal retainer, which contains a recessed keyway into which is fitted a cast, tapered key, or rest (see Chapter 38).

CLASSIFICATION OF RETAINERS

Retainers are classified in two classes and six types.

Class I contains four types.

- Type 1—Anterior intracoronal retainer (Chapter 15)
- Type 2—Posterior intracoronal retainer (Chapter 16)
- Type 3—Anterior extracoronal retainer (Chapter 17)
- Type 4—Posterior extracoronal retainer (Chapter 18)

Two or more surfaces may be involved in all types; they also may use intermediate retention (Chapter 19)

Class II contains two types.

- Type 1—Complete crown; gold, porcelain, or a combination; without dowel; usually used on a vital tooth (Chapter 23)
- Type 2—Complete crown with metal dowel; used on endodontically treated tooth with filled root canal (Chapter 27)

Both types may be fabricated of metal, porcelain, or a combination of both.

Class I, Types 1 and 2. As the name indicates, the prepared cavity and its cast retainer lie largely within the body of the coronal portion of the tooth and within the contour of the crown. The retention or resistance to displacement is developed between the casting and the internal walls of the prepared cavity; the distoclusal, mesiolingual, and similar retainers are examples.

Class I, Types 3 and 4. As the name indicates, the preparation of the tooth and its cast retainer lie largely externally to the body of the coronal portion of the prepared tooth and complement the contour of the crown. The retention or resistance to displacement is developed between the inner surfaces of the casting and the external walls of the prepared tooth. The three-quarter partial veneer and the proximal one-half veneer are examples of this type of retainer.

Class II, Type 1 (crown without dowel). The retention or resistance to displacement is developed between the inner walls of the casting and the external walls of the prepared tooth. The complete cast gold crown and the complete porcelain veneer crowns are examples of this type of retainer.

Class II, Type 2 (complete crown with dowel). The dowel type of retention is usually confined to the root portion. The retention or resistance to displacement and shear is developed by extending an attached metal dowel into the root canal of the tooth. Examples are the complete gold crown, the coping types of crowns, and the complete porcelain veneer crown with a cast core.

The ideal retainer

The ideal retainer can be constructed and retained in the mouth without injury to the pulp or the investing tissues; it should protect the pulp against thermal and galvanic shocks; this also implies safety during the lifetime of the restoration. Retainers which involve the least amount of tooth cutting and change of tooth contour and the least number of surfaces are more desirable and ideal than are those which are more extensive in these respects. The ideal retainer is also capable of resisting distortion and displacement by the forces of mastication and at the same time protect the tooth against fracture.

The ideal retainer is so designed that it has sufficient strength with a minimum of bulk and that its margins are capable of being finished in areas which will prevent the irritation of soft tissues and the recurrence of caries. The ideal retainer is self-cleansing or readily cleansable; it does not corrode or tarnish; neither does it discolor the abutment; it is esthetic; finally, it can be prepared by the average operator.

Selection of type

The type of retainer selected for a specific case depends upon many factors. The mouth hygiene habits or the diet of the patient may preclude the use of the intracoronal types of retainers which have long marginal lines; the complete veneer crown is preferable under such conditions. Distinction should also be made between those patients who are immune to caries and those actively susceptible to it.

Abnormalities in the alignment, contour, or articulation of the abutments are frequently the deciding factors in determining not only the outline form but even the type of the retainer employed.

It was shown in Chapter 9 that the amount of force which patients are capable of exerting on fixed partial dentures varies with the age and sex of the patient. It is important, therefore, to select the type of retention best suited to the particular individual.

The importance of the esthetic factors of a retainer depends largely on the occupation of the patient and the functional position of the lip line. People constantly before the public are in greater need of the esthetic values than those who are not.

While the periodontal membrane of the abutment teeth determines the limit of force which a bridge can endure, the length of the bridge span and the type of bridge used also determine the type of retainer selected. A two-surface intracoronal retainer is capable of supporting an occlusal tapered key in a three-tooth bridge; yet this type of retainer would be inadequate to serve as the terminal support of a bridge extending from the upper first molar to the upper cuspid.

A retainer not only is part of a mechanical structure replacing lost teeth, but it also is intimately related to the vital tissues; it is the medium through which mechanical and physical forces are transmuted into physiological functions and biological reactions in living tissues.

An understanding of the materials used in constructing a retainer, together with a knowledge of their correct manipulation, is also an important factor in the success or failure of a retainer. More will be said regarding this phase of bridge prosthesis in those chapters describing the construction of fixed partial dentures.

PRINCIPLES OF INTRACORONAL PREPARATIONS

Class I, types 1 and 2

The principles of cavity preparation were classified by G. V. Black[1] over half a century ago and, while they were formulated primarily for gold foil restorations, with but few modifications, they are basically applicable in the construction of cast retainers. It was not until 1907, however, when W. H. Taggart[2] made his epoch-making contribution to the dental profession, that present-day bridge prosthesis received the impetus and the means enabling it to attain its present status. It is hoped that sometime in the future the dental profession will recognize in a suitable manner the great contribution made by him to the advancement of better dentistry. Following Taggart's introduction of the casting process, men in various parts of this country and the world at large carried on further studies; these they reported to the profession in an effort to correlate the new casting technic with the accepted principles of cavity preparation extant at that time. The contributions of Price,[3] Ward,[4] and Bodecker[5] are prominent in the advances made in this early period. Price[1] made a noteworthy contribution in 1908 relative to the materials, procedures, and phenomena involved in the casting process.

Three systems. Brown[6] has called our attention to the fact that three basic systems of cavity preparation have been developed for the cast gold inlay. The *first system,* devised by Taggart, was based almost entirely upon the principles of cavity preparation as outlined by Black; it stipulated a cavity prepared with parallel axial walls, which were at right angles, or nearly so, to the pulpal and gingival walls. To obtain the necessary strength, the inlays were bulky, since the material invariably used was 24-karat gold. To allow for the withdrawal of the wax pattern from the cavity, a flare of 2 to 5° from parallelism was incorporated in the vertical walls.

Because of the inherent contraction of metal castings, there was some difficulty in fitting the larger and more complicated types of inlays. To overcome this difficulty, Ward suggested a modified cavity preparation. He devised a preparation wherein the flare of the wall was increased to 8 to 20 percent per inch. This modification helped to seat the castings more easily within the cavities.

An American dentist, H. W. C. Bodecker,[5] practicing at the time in Europe, suggested in 1911 a "slice" type of cavity preparation in which the convexity of a tooth was removed from the proximal surface and the margin extended gingivally so that it finished below the crest of the gum tissue. In 1911 he reported the use of the "channel" type of retention, which consisted of a groove anchorage extending into the cavity walls.

The *second system,* a further development and application of the groove principle of retention, becomes evident in the various forms of one-half and three-fourth partial veneer retainers which have been gradually developed and improved, culminating in the modern type of partial veneer retainers. This latter type is primarily extracoronal in character. A portion of the outer surface of the tooth is removed; nearly parallel axial grooves are placed on opposite surfaces of the tooth; the anchorage is obtained by uniting the ribs of cast metal which fit into these grooves by means of a metal veneer, which covers the outer surfaces of the tooth.

The *third system* and final development was the use of the casting process to construct complete veneer metal crowns and their many modifications.

The outline of the cavity form has changed considerably since 1907; therefore, it is well to see if the principles underlying cavity preparation have correspondingly changed. For this reason the principles as outlined by Black are here briefly reviewed.

Black's principles of cavity preparation

In considering the principles of cavity preparation, the seventh edition of Black's *Operative Dentistry* gives the following definitions: "The term 'cavity preparation' is applied to that mechanical treatment of dental caries and other diseases and injuries of the hard tissues of the teeth as will best fit the remaining part of the tooth to receive a restoration to its original form, give it strength, and prevent recurrence of decay in the same surface."[1]

The first point of difference between operative and prosthetic procedures is noted. The operations in operative dentistry relate only to diseased teeth; in prosthodontics normal and sound teeth, in addition to carious teeth, are prepared to receive crowns and bridges.

A certain order of procedure has been listed by Black in the preparation of cavities, frequently referred to as "steps in cavity preparation": (1) Obtain the required outline form; (2) obtain the required retention and resistance; (3) obtain the required convenience form; (4) remove any remaining carious dentin; (5) finish the enamel wall; (6) make the toilet of the cavity."[1]

Outline form. In the "outline form" is included all of the tooth surface area, encompassed within the enamel margins of the finished preparation. The extent to which the outline is carried depends upon several factors. In the occlusal area, Black stated, the outline form is controlled: "(1) by the extent to which the enamel has been involved by direct penetration of acids; (2) by the lateral spread of decay along the dento-enamel junction; (3) by extensions that must be made along fissures to secure smooth margins; (4) by inclusion within the outline, such portions of the surface as are especially liable to decay in the future; (5) a dovetail for good anchorage which may require extensions along grooves which are not fissured."[1]

On the proximal surfaces the outline is controlled: "(1) in the gingival direction, by the position of the crest of the healthy gingiva, which should cover the entire length of the gingival margin of the restoration. Consideration should be given to the probability of future recession, depending upon the age of the patient. (2) In the buccal or labial, and lingual directions, by the dentist's estimate of the extent of the area and liabilities to surface extension of decay near the line of the margin of the gingivae."[4]

Let us consider briefly whether these rules laid down by Black for operative procedures also hold true for determining the outline form of bridge retainers. Obviously, the requirements are the same for both, with the addition that in the case of persons who are 20 years of age or younger it is unwise, at times, to place the gingival margin of a retainer entirely beneath the crest of the healthy gingiva. It has been shown in patients of this age group that the enamel epithelium or epithelial attachment in a large majority of cases is still attached to the enamel, and the gingival crevice is practically of zero depth. In older patients, those for whom incidentally the largest percentage of bridge restorations is placed, it is found that the epithelial attachment lies below the cementoenamel junction, and the average depth of the gingival crevice is 0.8 mm. Under these conditions the rule formulated by Black for operative work applies with equal force to prosthetic restorations.

It should be stated that, in addition to the buccal or labial and lingual extensions of the outline form for purposes of caries prevention, it is frequently found necessary in bridge prosthesis to extend these margins even farther, especially those surfaces proximating the pontic of a bridge. In either operative or prosthetic restorations, where the enamel is undermined by lateral decay and must be removed, it is often necessary to extend the margins beyond the normal outlines.

It is apparent from this that the factors governing outline form are applicable not only to the intracoronal type of retainers, such as the distoclusal inlay, but also to the extracoronal, partial veneer crowns.

Retention and resistance form. In discussing "retention form and resistance form," Black made the following stipulation: "The cavity should have such retention form that (1) the restorations will be firmly held in place; (2) the cavity should also have such resistance form that the restoration will withstand the stress without being dislodged."[1]

The basic need for such requirements is self-evident, and a consideration of the means available for developing these qualities appears later in the chapter.

Convenience form. While "convenience form" in operative dentistry relates particularly to those modifications in cavity preparation which make the placing of a gold foil filling easier and more accessible, this term is not without its significance in prosthetic dentistry. Some walls of a cavity and occasionally the entire preparation are

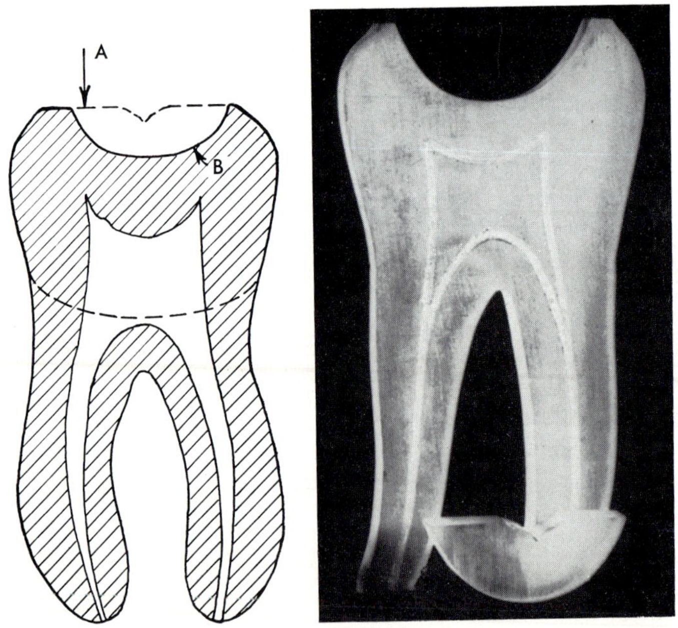

Fig. 13-1. Cavities with rounded pulpal and axial walls. (From McMath, J. F.: D. Cosmos **67:**1162, 1925.)

modified either to facilitate the removal of a wax pattern from the tooth or to help parallel the line of insertion of bridge retainers.

Removal of carious dentin. The fourth step, the "removal of remaining carious dentin," is not always present in crown and bridge prosthodontics, for very often the teeth used as abutments are sound, noncarious teeth. Where this procedure is required, however, it should be one of the first to be performed. If there is any question of possible pulp exposure, the rubber dam should be applied first and then the carious tooth structure carefully removed. In this step of cavity preparation, the use of a bur at either high or low speed to remove carious dentin is contraindicated. The spoon-shaped, hand cutting excavators are indicated. If the pulp should be exposed, the tooth is then ready for immediate endodontic treatment.

A treated tooth which is to be used as a bridge abutment should always be given a period of rest subsequent to the filling of its root canal. Following a period of clinical and roentgenographic observation for a reasonable length of time, a decision can be made as to its fitness for use as a bridge abutment.

Finish of the enamel wall. The fifth step, "the finish of the enamel wall," is of equal importance in both operative and prosthetic procedures. This step also includes the beveling of the gingival cavosurface angle. Operative procedures demand that this operation be carried out with the rubber dam in position, particularly when a gold-foil or an amalgam restoration is to be placed immediately thereafter. The necessity for a dry field is obvious. The rubber dam should be used, too, to enable the operator to make a final inspection and examination of the cavity, determining whether all carious tooth structure has been removed, whether any undercuts exist, and whether all enamel walls are supported by sound dentin. These observations can be made more readily when the tooth is dry than when

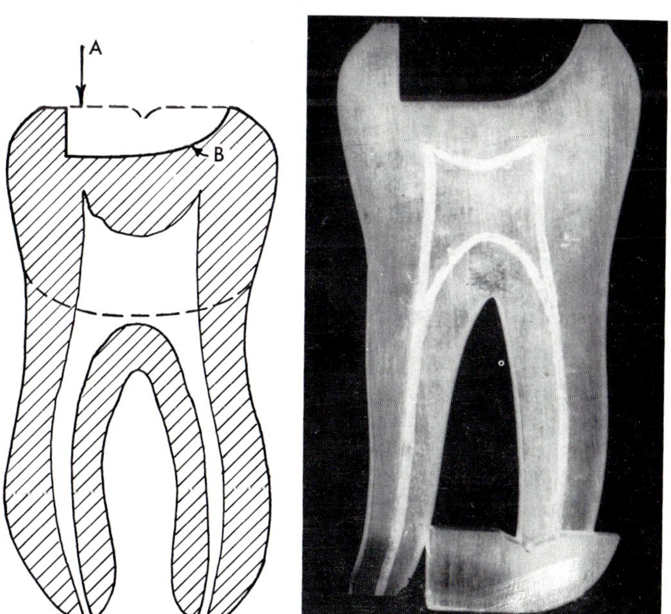

Fig. 13-2. When vertical force is applied at **A**, curved wall **B** offers no resistance to displacement. (From McMath, J. F.: D. Cosmos **67**:1162, 1925.)

it is flooded in saliva. While it is not necessary to use the rubber dam for this step on sound, noncarious teeth, its use is strongly urged in polycarious teeth.

The following rule relative to the enamel wall and the cavosurface angle of the cavity was expressed by Black with reference to operative procedures:

"The cavosurface angle of the cavity in every part of its outline should receive attention. The plane of this enamel wall should be as nearly as practicable in the line of the length of the enamel rods, or such as will certainly cut more from the outer than the inner ends of the rods, and should be perfectly smooth. When this has been satisfactorily accomplished, the cavosurface angle of the enamel should, if necessary, be cut to a sufficient bevel outward. The depth of this bevel should generally not include more than ¼ of the thickness of the enamel wall, although in some cases, as occlusal fillings, the entire wall may be cut at such an angle in relation to the direction of the rods to fully meet the requirements. The angle of the bevel should be from 6 to 10° C. from the plane of the enamel wall for gold foil restorations, but should be less for all others. The object is, first, to cut away any loose ends of enamel rods that might afterwards fall away and render the margin imperfect and, second, to strengthen the cavosurface angle of the enamel as a safeguard against possible checking in the condensation of gold."*

A careful study of this statement discloses that the principles enunciated therein apply with equal force to most intracoronal retainers, as well as to those surfaces of the extracoronal retainers where it is necesary to cut through the enamel wall into the dentin (Figs. 13-20 to 13-27, 13-29, and 13-30).

Toilet of cavity. The sixth and final step, "making the toilet of the cavity," is a procedure involving the removal of all debris and loose particles, leaving the cavity absolutely clean. Under microscopic examination, walls of dentin and enamel prepared

*From Black, G. V.: Operative dentistry, ed. 7, Chicago, 1936, Medico-Dental Publishing Co., vol. 2, pp. 137-147, 155-158.

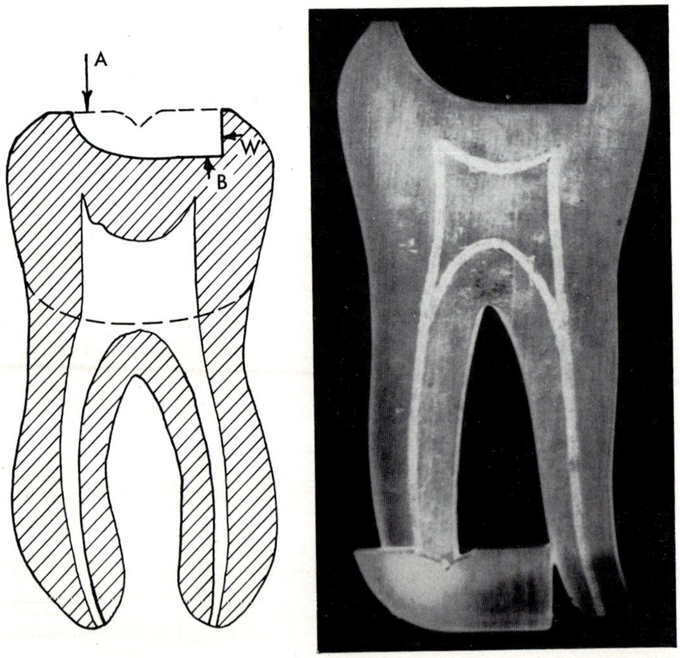

Fig. 13-3. Flat walls, **B** and **W**, resist displacing force, **A.** (From McMath, J. F.: D. Cosmos **67:**1162, 1925.)

with diamond stones or burs, especially the cross cut type, leave serrations of varying depths. It is well to finish surfaces, especially those against which wax patterns are to be made, with fine mounted points of Arkansas-stone or the multi-bladed Tinker type of polishing burs. Orange wood points with wet alumina polishing powder are also effective.

Modifications of retention and resistance form

While the principles discussed here are generally true, it is equally true that the order and method of their application may be modified to meet different conditions and requirements. Because the cast inlay has been put to new uses, the one step that has undergone most modifications relates to the retention and resistance to displacement forms.

Since the retention of an inlay and its resistance to displacement are primarily mechanical problems, some of the factors involved may be properly considered at this time. A grasp of the principles of retention in bridge retainers is based on an understanding of the forces of mastication and an analysis of the stresses which develop in the abutments and concentrate in the restorations.

Let us first consider force applied at right angles to the flat surface of a filling not cemented in the cavity. A typical cavity (Fig. 13-4) presents such a surface to vertical forces. If one of the walls, the pulpal, is rounded as in Fig. 13-1, a force at *A* has a tendency to dislodge the filling by rolling it out of the cavity, as indicated in the direction *B*. In a series of experiments, McMath[9] indicates the different degrees of retention obtained, depending upon the relationship of the pulpal and axial walls. While the resistance to displacement is increased by the junction of the vertical wall near *A* with the floor of the cavity (Fig. 13-2), it offers less resistance to the same displacing force, *A*, than the preparation shown in Figs. 13-3 and 13-4.

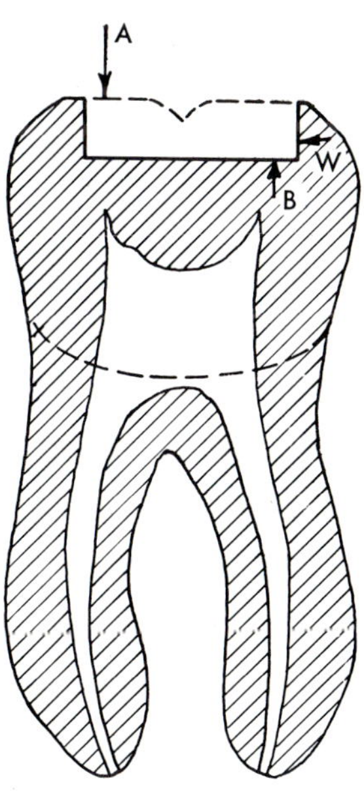

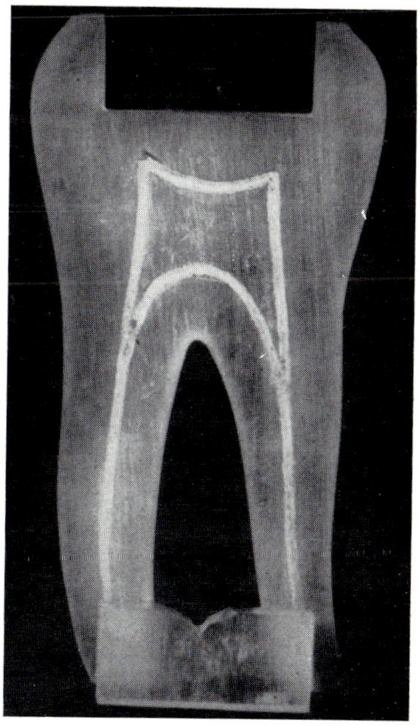

Fig. 13-4. Vertical force, **A**, meets maximum resistance to displacement due to vertical axial walls. (From McMath, J. F.: D. Cosmos **67:**1162, 1925.)

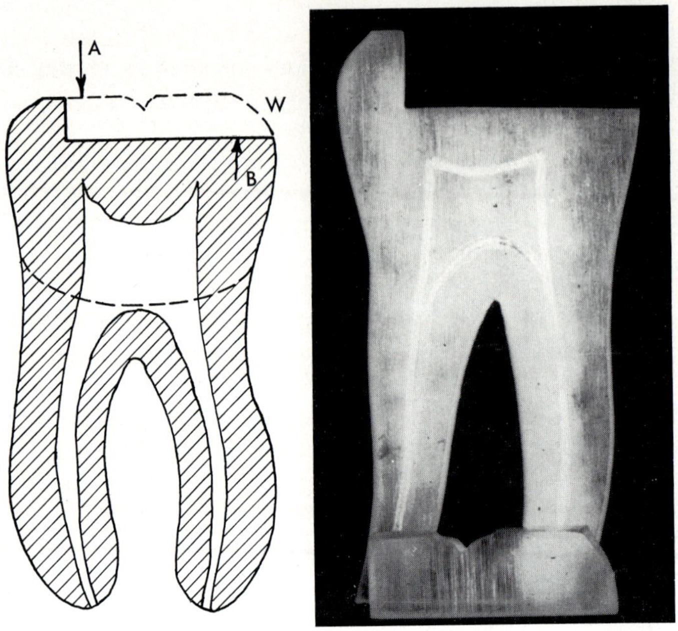

Fig. 13-5. Vertical force at **A** will cause displacement at **B**. (From McMath, J. F.: D. Cosmos **67**:1162, 1925.)

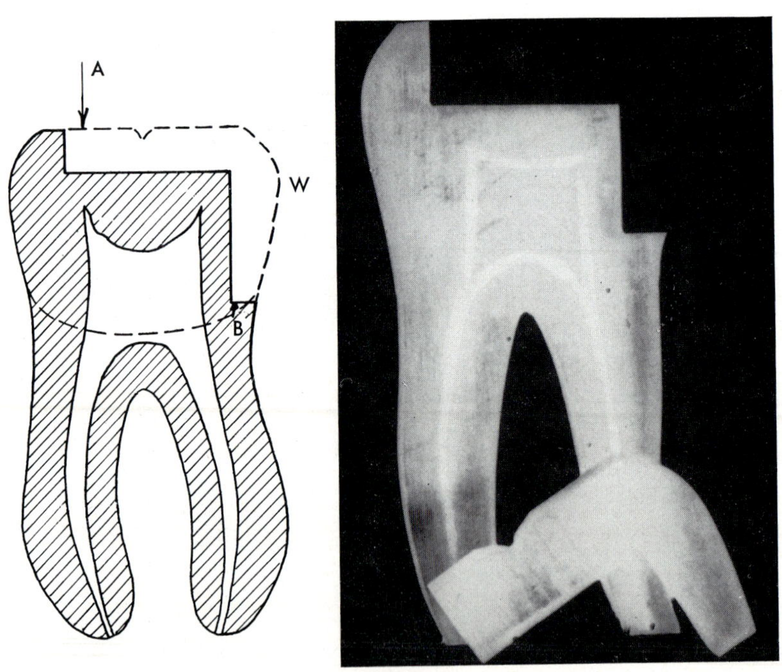

Fig. 13-6. Force **A** tends to dislodge filling at **B**. (From McMath, J. F.: D. Cosmos **67**:1162, 1925.)

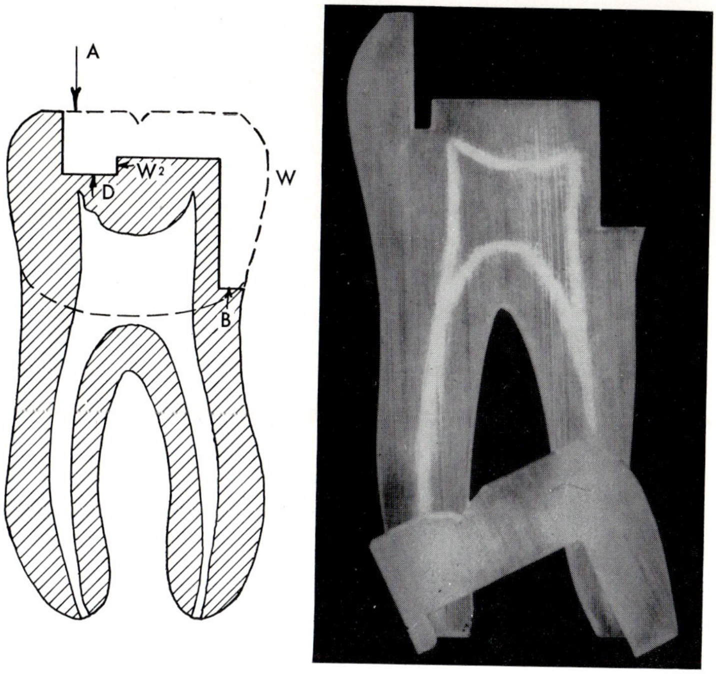

Fig. 13-7. Addition of channel, **D**, produces slight resistance to displacement at **W**. (From McMath, J. F.: D. Cosmos **67:**1162, 1925.)

While these illustrations refer to a simple box type of occlusal cavity, the same principles apply when a vertical concentrated force is applied to the occlusal surface of a proximoclusal inlay.

As seen in Fig. 13-5, elimination of one of the vertical parallel walls considerably reduces the resistance to displacement.

Even though a gingival extension is made in this cavity preparation, nothing will be added to the retentive qualities of the cavity (Fig. 13-6).

Fig. 13-7 shows a modification of the cavity appearing in Fig. 13-6, made to the extent that the pulpal wall has been dropped in area *D*, thus replacing to a small degree the resistance to displacement at W^2, which was lost when the vertical wall *W* was cut away, as shown in Figs. 13-3 and 13-4. As McMath[9] pointed out, the wall W^2 does not retain that portion of the inlay at *W* directly, but only because and as a result of its being attached to and a part of that portion of the inlay near *A*, which is the occlusal portion. This same statement holds true of the dovetail anchorage at *T* shown in Fig. 13-8.

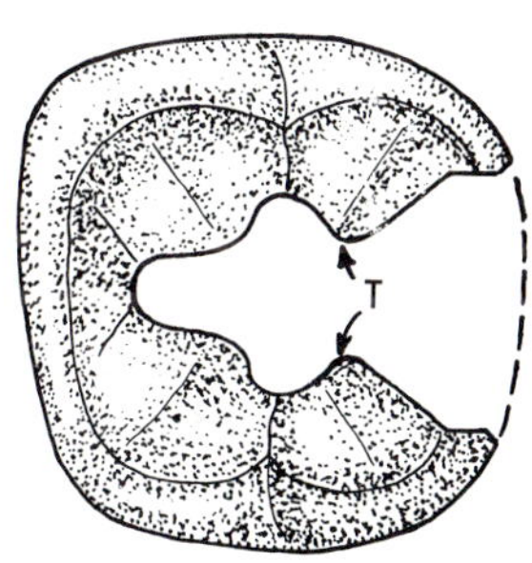

Fig. 13-8. Effect of dovetail in resisting lateral displacing forces. (From McMath, J. F.: D. Cosmos **67:**1162, 1925.)

Fig. 13-9 is similar to Fig. 13-6, with the exception of a groove *G* placed in the gingival wall. Here the wall W_1 in a lesser degree resists the same displacement force that the wall *W* did in Fig. 13-3.

Instead of having a vertical force applied to Fig. 13-6, the force is directed

A

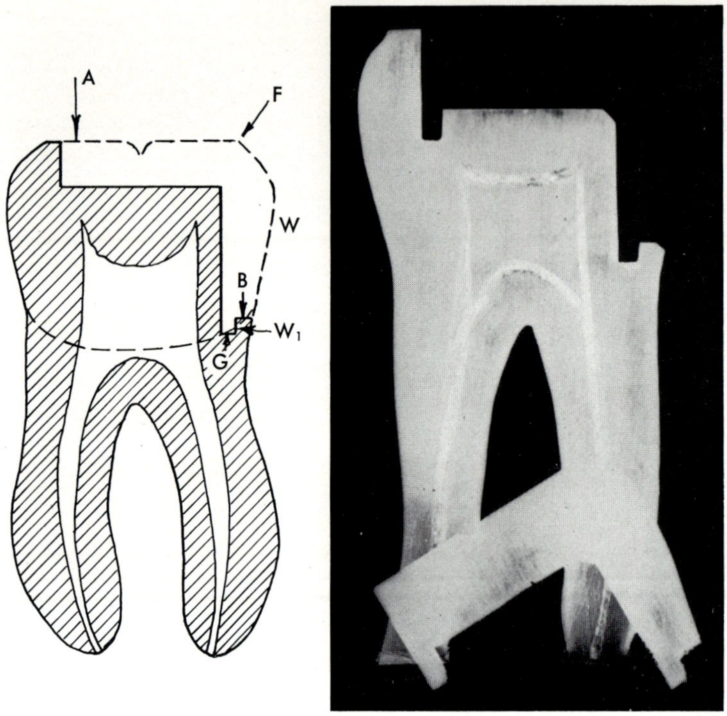

B

Fig. 13-9. A, Channel placed in dentin of gingival wall, $\mathbf{W_1}$, gives added retention to filling. (From McMath, J. F.: D. Cosmos **67:**1162, 1925.) **B**, Preparation in which occlusal and gingival channels are employed.

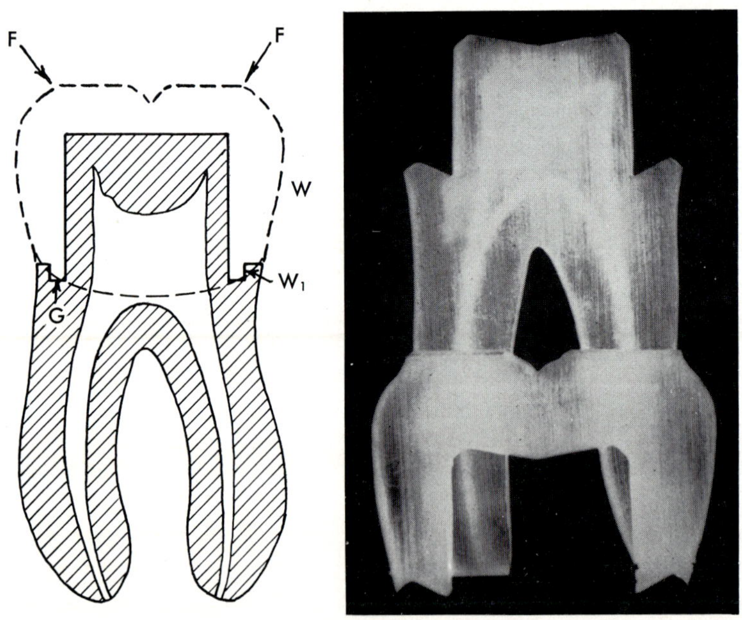

Fig. 13-10. Use of grooves or inclined planes in gingival walls to obtain added retention. (From McMath, J. F.: D. Cosmos **67:**1162, 1925.)

horizontally on the angle of the filling as indicated by *F* (Fig. 13-9). Note the reaction to this force. In Fig. 13-7, because of the added retention which is obtained by the lowered wall *D*, the casting would respond to this diagonal force with a tendency for the L shaped metal casting to straighten out; this would cause the metal at the wall *B* to move out laterally at the gingiva. To resist this lateral spreading at the gingival wall, provision is made (Fig. 13-9) for the depression of the wall *G* and the creation of the wall W^1. Fig. 13-10 illustrates the application of the foregoing principles in a three-surface retainer.

Gingival groove. It is apparent that in cavities involving two or more surfaces the gingival groove simulates to a certain extent the retentive form of a simple occlusal cavity. McMath suggests that the gingival groove be not wider than half the width of its gingival wall and that the depth of the groove be equal to its width.

Axioproximal walls. The compressive forces resulting from vertical pressure have an important bearing on the retention of the inlay; this bears on the relationship of the vertical axial walls, both the buccal and lingual (Fig. 13-11, *A* and *B*), and the mesial and distal proximal walls in dentin. The question arises whether they should flare axioproximallly or parallel each other, at least those parts of the wall lying within the dentin. Peyton[6] reported the following physical properties for dentin:

A. Modulus of elasticity, 1.67 × 10^6 psi.
B. Proportional limit, 24,000 psi.
C. Compressive strength, 36,000 psi.

See general references also for recent investigations conducted at the National Bureau of Standards.

Fig. 13-11 illustrates a horizontal cross section of a tooth slightly above the gingival wall. It will be observed that walls *A* and *B* are parallel, while walls *C* and *D* diverge outwardly. It must be kept in mind that these cavities also flare gingivoclusally and, therefore, may be considered as sections of a tapering keyway into which will fit a cast tapering key.

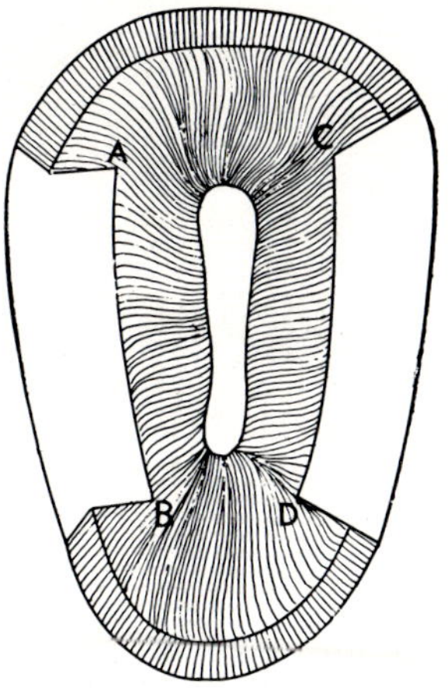

Fig. 13-11. Left, proximal preparation of tooth for bridge retainer, **A-B. Right,** Cross section of cavity usually used for single operative inlay type of restoration, **C-D.** Opposing walls in dentin at **A** and **B** utilize retentive stress on cast retainer due to elasticity of dentin when compressed by cast inlay.

Fig. 13-12, *A*, represents a buccal-lingual cross section view of dentin in the proximal cavity, *A-B*, in Fig. 13-11. There are three possible relationships of wall *A* to wall *B* in the gingivoclusal direction. In model *1*, the walls are parallel to each other; in *2*, they are widely divergent; in *3* the gingivoclusal divergence does not exceed 5° from a vertical plane.

Let us consider briefly the degree of resistance to displacement offered by each type of preparation and how it is attained. In Fig. 13-12, *B1*, *F* repreesnts the rotation center when a rotational force is applied by means of the bar in a counterclockwise direction to the casting. In the mouth this might be a buccolingual or a linguobuccal rotation. It is seen that the tendency for point *X* to rise occlusally on arc *XY* is resisted by the dentin lying within the area *XYZ*.

The same rotational force applied to Fig. 13-12, *B2*, finds no resistance to point *X* rotating right out of the cavity. The di-

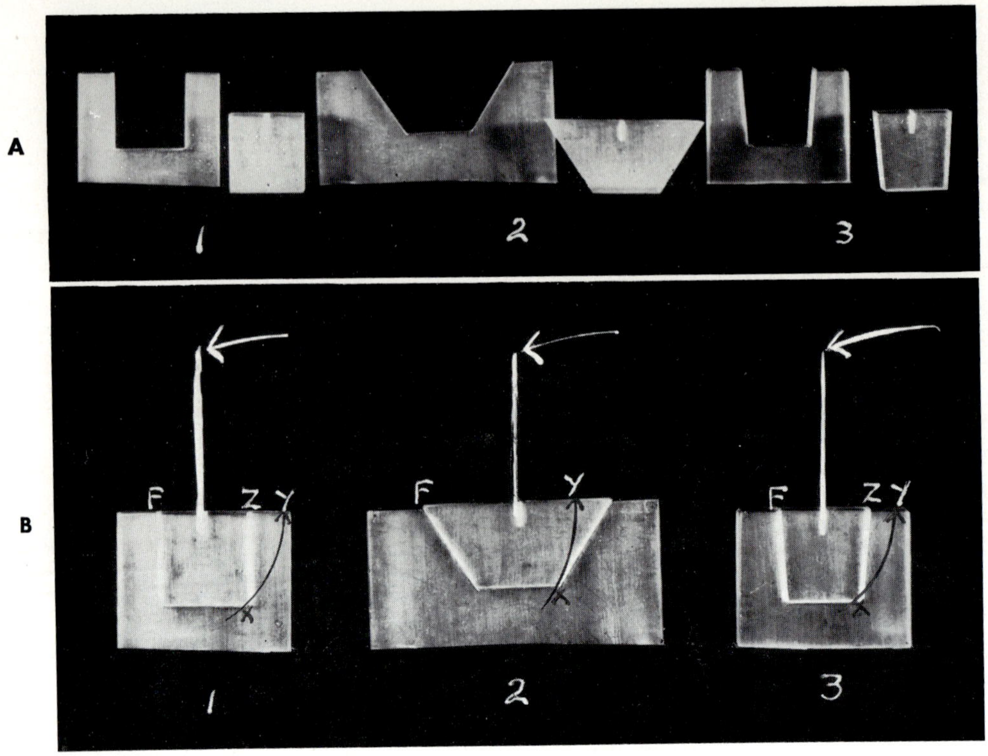

Fig. 13-12. Amount of retentive force exerted by dentin on casting depends on amount of divergence from parallelism of axial walls (see text).

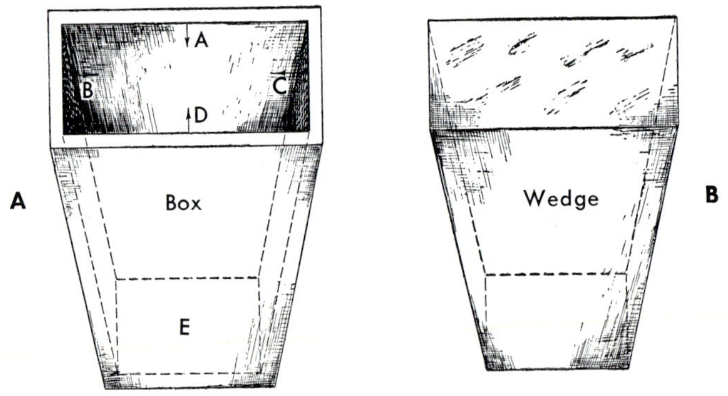

Fig. 13-13. Metal wedge, or key, and keyway principle in dentin walls of intracoronal cavity and casting. **A,** Mesial; **B,** buccal; **C,** lingual; **D,** distal; **E,** gingivoproximal or occlusopulpal wall.

vergence of the buccal and lingual walls is too great to prevent the displacement buccally or lingually.

In Fig. 13-12, *B3*, the force is applied as before but the filling does not roll out of the cavity. Again the rotation center is at *F*, but when point *X* in the filling tries to dislodge along the arc *XY*, it meets resistance in the bulk of dentin contained within the area *XYZ*.

Therefore, while parallelism of the walls offers the maximum rotational resistance

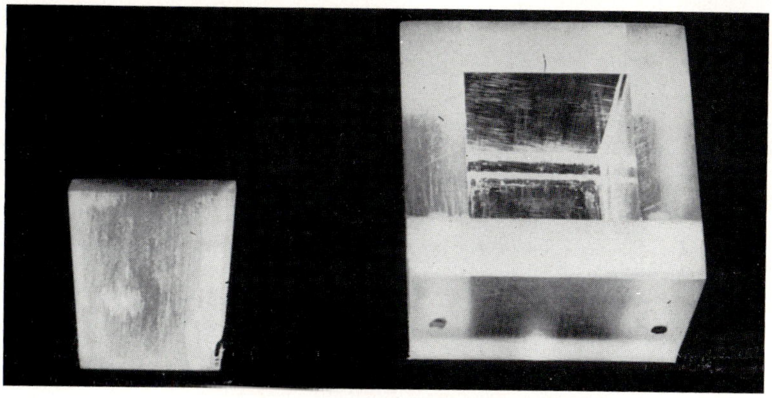

Fig. 13-14. Acrylic resin key and keyway.

from a clinical standpoint, it is difficult to attain and not necessary, since a slight divergence of 2 to 5° from parallelism will furnish the necessary resistance to buccolingual torque displacement.

These same principles also apply to the buccal and the lingual walls of the occlusal dovetail of inlays in Fig. 13-8.

Fig. 13-13, *A*, shows a rectangular box or cavity in dentin that tapers to a smaller size at its bottom. Fig. 13-13, *B*, shows a key or wedge metal casting that fits the keyway accurately. After the cast inlay has been seated in the keyway, its four sides are in contact with the axial surfaces or walls of the boxed keyway. In addition to this, the bottom of the key rests upon the bottom of the tapered keyway or cavity. When force is applied vertically or occlusally to the top of the key placed within the tapered cavity, there is a tendency to force it through the bottom, *E* (Fig. 13-13, *A*). However, since the walls converge gingivally, the wedging effect of the metal tends to distend the lateral walls of the keyway outwardly. If the bottom and the side walls of the keyway consist of elastic material (Fig. 13-14), the lateral pressure of the wedgelike key presses against all lateral keyway walls, creating opposing stresses that grip the sides of the key, thus making its dislodgment upward or occlusally difficult.

THE INLAY AND ITS CAVITY (FORCES, STRESSES, AND RETENTION)

The stresses of retention developed in the proximo-occlusal dentin walls of a properly prepared cavity resist any tensile forces of displacement by tacky foods or dental floss. Depending entirely upon cement for retention is a gamble; cement serves other useful purposes. Because inlay metal is relatively hard and tooth tissue relatively elastic, let us briefly discuss the engineering principles illustrated in Fig. 13-15.*

Fig. 13-15 shows a proximal view of an MOD inlay not quite seated in its cavity. The width of the inlay is *w*, at about its vertical center. Contact is assumed to have been made between the inlay and the walls of the cavity. After contact, the inlay is further forced downward an amount *dh*, as shown at left. The walls of the cavity make an angle with the vertical.

Let it first be assumed: that the tooth structure, which surrounds the inlay, is artificially prevented from deformation so all shortening of *w*, due to *dh*, is forced to take place in the gold of the inlay. Under this condition, the total shortening per unit of width becomes:

$$E_g = \frac{dh \tan \theta}{w} \qquad (a)$$

*Text by R. C. Brumfield.

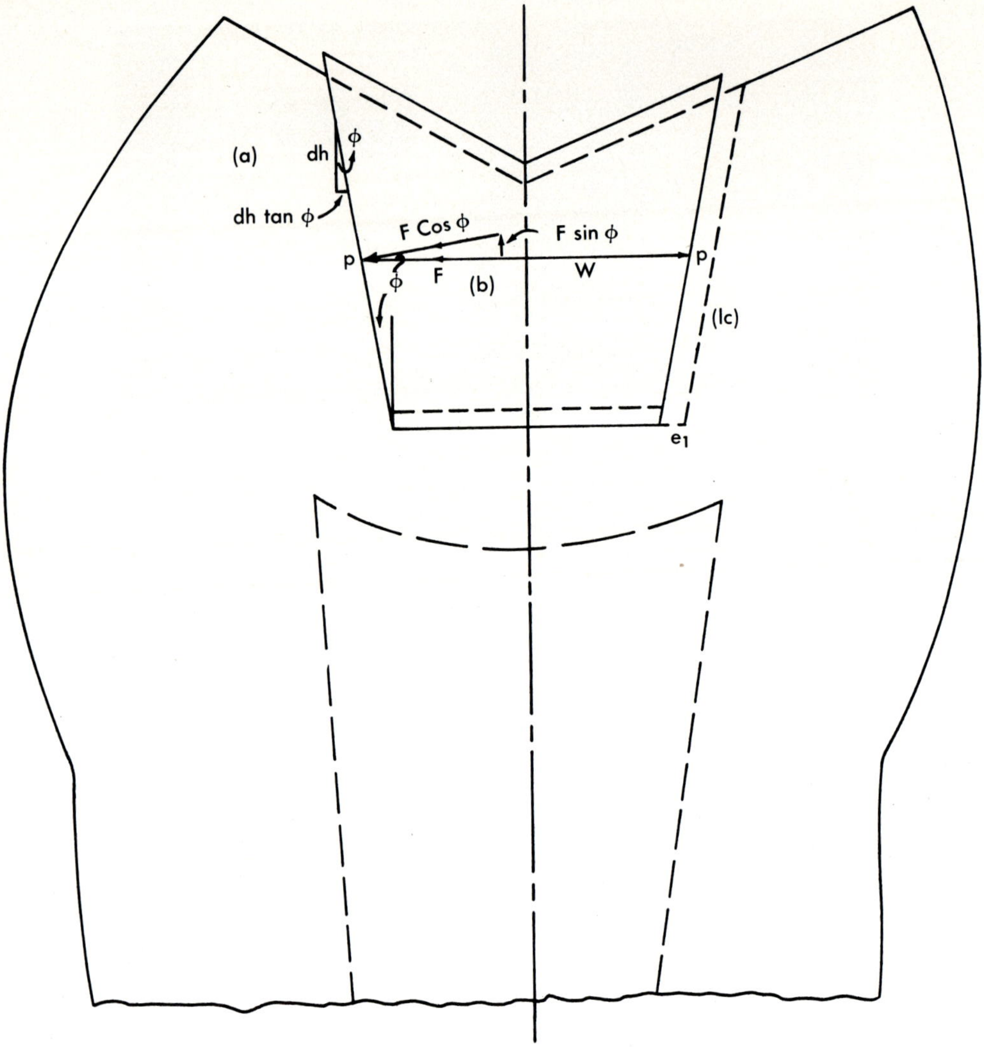

B

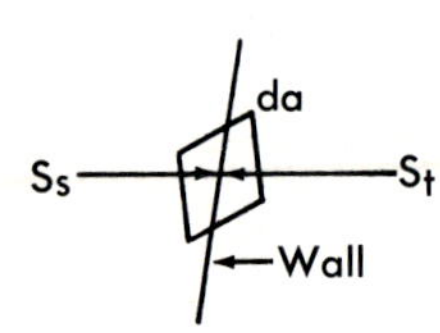

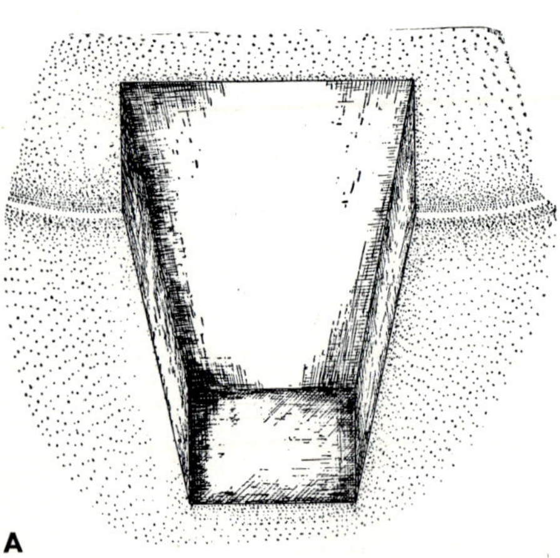

A

Fig. 13-15. A, Proximal segment removed from box-type cavity; **B,** proximal view of inlay to be seated in cavity.

The unit stress in the gold of the inlay then becomes:

$$S_g = E_g \Sigma_g = E_g \frac{dh \tan \theta}{w} \qquad (1)$$

The unit stress, whose value is given in Eq. (1), is not perpendicular to the cavity wall but is parallel to *w*, the direction of the shortening. The unit stress or the total stress may now be resolved into components, one of which, *F* cos *θ*, is perpendicular to the cavity wall and the other, *F* sin *θ*, is parallel to the wall (see Fig. 13-15, *B*).

If it be assumed that the coefficient of friction, between the gold of the inlay and the tooth structure, is *μ*, then *μ*F cos *θ* is the frictional force between the gold and the tooth structure, which tends to prevent movement of the two with respect to each other.

It will be noticed that the component of F, F sin *θ*, is parallel to the cavity wall and tends to push the inlay back out of the cavity. Then, under any value of *θ*, the total force of frictional retention tending to hold the inlay in its cavity is:

$$R_F = \mu F \cos \theta - F \sin \theta \qquad (2)$$

Eq. (2) shows that, as the angle *θ* is varied, it has a value at which these two opposing forces will become equal; that is, the force tending to stop the inlay being pushed farther into the cavity will exactly equal the force of friction tending to hold it there. For greater values of *θ* the inlay will bounce out of the cavity when it is driven. This angle is known as the "critical angle," θ_c. If the wall-angle is made slightly larger than θ_c, the inlay would simply be pressed into place and retention would be wholly that furnished by the cement.

The value of θ_c, in degrees, may be determined as follows. Since the critical angle is reached when the right side of Eq. (1) becomes zero, its value may be established by equating the positive to the negative values of the right-hand side of the equation. Thus:

$$\mu F \cos \theta = F \sin \theta, \text{ or } \mu = \frac{\sin \theta}{\cos \theta} = \tan \theta_c \quad (3)$$

Eq. (3) shows that the critical angle occurs when the coefficient of friction is equal to the tangent of the critical angle θ_c. If *μ* is known, by experimentation, the value of the critical angle may be obtained at once from any set of trigonometric tables. If the value of θ_c is known instead, the value of the coefficient of friction may be found with equal facility.

Turning to the original assumption that the tooth structure, in which the cavity was formed, was artificially held from movement under the force *F*, it will be interesting to determine what stress is induced in the gold of the inlay under this artificial condition.

Let the angle *θ* be 2°, as is frequently used in dental practice; the value of dh be 0.01 in.; the value of E_g be 12,000,000 psi; and the value of w be 0.15 in. Using these values and substituting in Eq. (1):

$$S_g = 12{,}000{,}000 \times \frac{0.01 \times 0.349}{0.15} = 27{,}800 \text{ psi}$$

This unit stress would be high, even for hard inlay golds. Of course, it would be quite excessive for the material of the tooth. It must be remembered that the deformation was assumed to be forced wholly within the gold, and that the tooth structure was not allowed to deform. The demonstration has little practical value, except to show the great power of the wedging action at these small angles for cavity wall sides.

Since we have been dealing with a hypothetical artificial condition, it will be profitable to consider what happens when artificial restraints are removed and the tooth structure is allowed to return to its natural state of participating in the deformations resulting from wedging action.

Two positions are shown for the wall in Fig. 13-15, *B;* the first, solid line at the left is artificially held and was considered in the foregoing. The second is shown to the right of this, by the dashed line. The space e_1 between them represents the compression of the tooth structure together with other secondary effects and also the outward expansion of the gold of the inlay due to removal of restraints. As restraint is removed, the gold of the inlay expands, maintaining contact with the tooth structure. While expansion proceeds, the tooth structure compresses, inducing stresses within it, while the gold expands an equal amount, relieving stresses within itself. This proceeds until a point has been reached where the induced unit compressive stress in the tooth structure is exactly equal to the residual compressive unit stress in the gold of the inlay. At this point movement stops. Equilibrium has been attained. The unit stresses in the tooth structure and the gold are exactly equal.

Here a differential unit area of the inclined wall of the inlay cavity, in its final position at the dashed line, has been removed and is shown as a free body. The residual unit stress in the gold is shown acting rightward and the induced unit compressive stress in the tooth structure acting leftward, opposing the force from the gold. If these two unit stresses are not equal, movement of the differential area would continue, which violates the original assumption that the dashed line represents the final position of the cavity wall, after equilibrium is attained. (Of course this conclusion ignores such secondary effects as bending of the tooth structure, tension in the cavity bottom, and others, even though these may be present to some extent.)

It may be shown, by making certain assumptions, that the law expressed in the following equation is valid:

$$e_1 = \frac{dh \tan \theta}{1 - \frac{E_t}{E_g}\frac{w}{w_t}} \qquad (4)$$

In this equation, the numerator of the fraction has the same significance as in Eq. (a). In the denominator, E_t and E_g are the respective moduli of elasticity of the tooth structure and the gold. Both are substantially constants; w has the same meaning, and w_t is in no sense a width or thickness of tooth structure as it exists in the mouth. It is rather a hypothetical attribute of the tooth, in the following sense: w_t is the thickness of tooth structure required to give the compressive shortening e_1, when the common residual unit stress has been reached and equilibrium has been established.

In Eq. (4) the only variables are e_1 and w_t. Other factors are constants. It should be remembered the e_1 is the movement causing relief of the maximum stress in the gold, under restraint, to the point where equilibrium is attained.

If the surrounding tooth structure was infinitely massive, it would offer infinite resistance to the finite force induced in the gold by wedging. Therefore e_1 would be zero, there would be no movement, and w_t would also be zero because there is no relief to the gold. When the surrounding tooth structure is only relatively massive, some relief would be obtained, but less than if the tooth structure was light in bulk. Therefore, the less bulky teeth would be accompanied by a relatively large w_t and the more bulky teeth by a smaller w_t. It can be seen from Eq. (4) that, when w_t is large, the denominator of the equation becomes smaller, and that when it is zero, e_1 becomes zero.

One more aspect of the situation requires mention. Living bone acts more or less like a plastic, under force and stress. It gives permanently before these influences. It is probable that this yielding also holds for tooth structure. It is certain that any such gradual yielding would relieve some of the initial stresses in both the gold and the tooth structure.

If one of the walls, *D*, in Fig. 13-13 is

now removed from the keyway (Fig. 13-15, *A*), the key reinserted (Fig. 13-16), and the vertical or occlusal force again applied, opposite retentive stresses are again developed as in the previous instance, except that now the wedge is effective in only two of its surfaces, *B* and *C;* whereas the gripping power has been lost in the direction *AD* because of the removal of the wall *D*. Not only has the

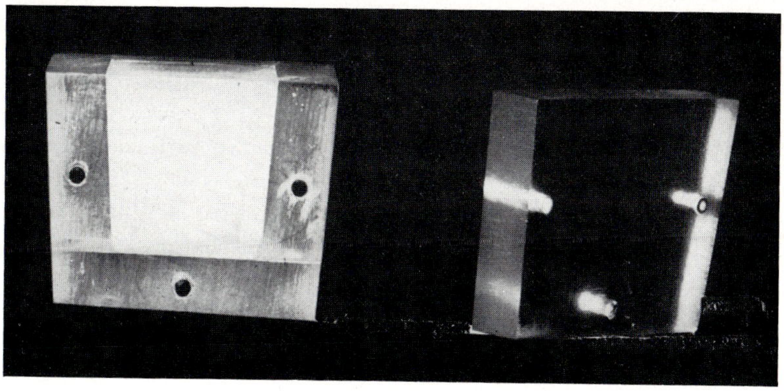

Fig. 13-16. Retention due to elasticity of dentin is still effective when proximal wall of cavity is missing.

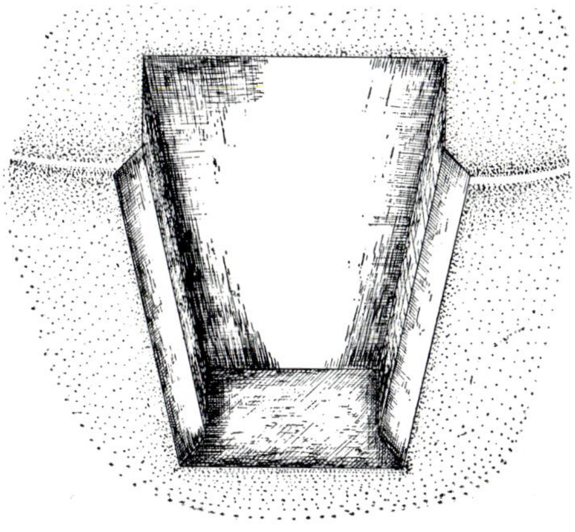

A

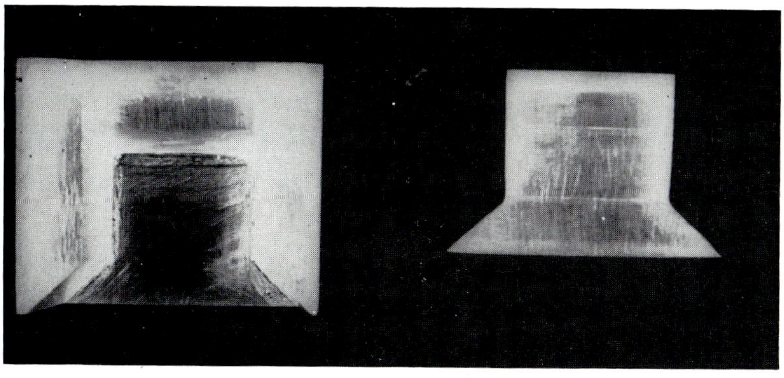

B

Fig. 13-17. Flaring enamel of proximal walls has little effect on retention of casting.

gripping action been lost in the direction *AD* (Fig. 13-15, *A*), but there is now present a force tending to push the tapering key out through the opening made by the removal of wall *D*, as seen in Figs. 13-15, *A*, and 13-16. This displacing force is counteracted by the retaining stresses present in walls *BC* and can be supplemented clinically by placing a gingival groove in the gingival wall. By adding an occlusal dovetail lock (Fig. 13-8), the lateral displacement of the key is then resisted by the additional tensile stresses developed in the occlusal lock.

Fig. 13-17, *A* and *B*, shows a simple cavity with the wall *D* removed, but the buccal and lingual axial walls, instead of flaring from the axial line angles to the cavosurface margin in a continuous plane, are now changed into two narrower and two smaller diverging planes. It is evident from this that, even with such a modification of the buccal and lingual proximal walls, it is possible to retain the retentive stresses of a preparation since the supplementary diverging planes are mostly in the enamel leaving the balance of the walls (Fig. 13-13, *A* to *C*) in the elastic dentin.

Fig. 13-17 is similar to Fig. 13-16, with the two walls diverging in a continuous plane from the axial line angles to the cavosurface bevels. If walls *A*, *B*, and *C* in Fig. 13-13, *A*, diverge excessively occlusally from the gingival wall, *E*, the reacting stresses in the dentin will tend to dislodge the key or inlay outward, since all the forces now react as displacing stresses. The best means of retaining the key or filling in a cavity of this design is by placing a gingival groove in the gingival wall and by adding an occlusal dovetail lock to the occlusal wall. By referring to Fig. 13-18, it is apparent that every effort should be made to approach parallelism not exceeding 2 to 5° gingivocclusally.

Referring to Fig. 13-19, *A*, it is seen that by converging two axial walls toward each other a mortise type of preparation results, giving the maximum retention. This principle should be modified into a groove or a channel (Fig. 13-19, *B*). When this is done, care must be taken that a sufficient amount of dentin is present to support the two converging walls in order to prevent their being fractured by the wedging action of the tapering key.

Having considered some of the results of vertical force when applied at right angles to the surface of a filling, what are the reactions when forces are applied to the surface of a filling at an angle other than a right angle?

When this occurs, the force is resolved into two forces, one of which reacts in its effectiveness at right angles to the surface; this force is not opposite in direction nor is it equal in magnitude to the original force. The tendency in a tooth is for the cusp of the opposing tooth to slide down the inclined plane and for an inlay to be pushed out of the cavity in a horizontal plane.

Resistance to horizontal displacing forces. A study of Fig. 13-20 discloses that the application of a vertical force to the inclined plane will dislodge a filling hori-

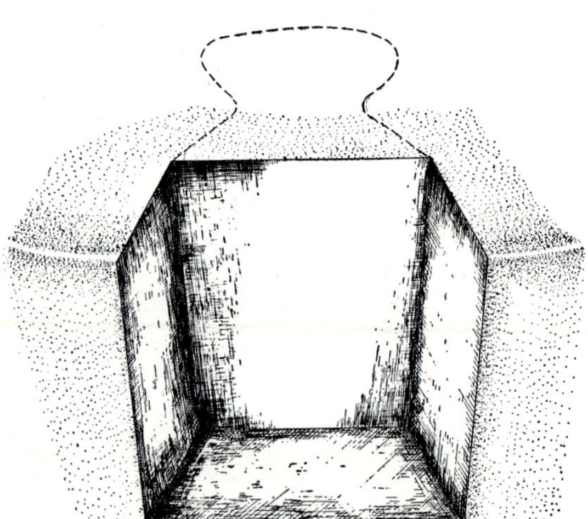

Fig. 13-18. Proximal retention is minimal when walls diverge gingivocclusally and buccolingually; it is therefore necessary to use occlusal dovetail.

zontally even in a cavity prepared with flat pulpal and gingival walls.

Fig. 13-21 illustrates the reaction of a filling to vertical force when applied to a proximal extension. The filling is rotated occlusoproximally out of its cavity, the rotation point being the gingival marginal wall.

These forces are always effective unless counteracted by an opposing moment. The latter is obtained in four ways: first, by means of a properly prepared occlusal lock; second, by the proper preparation of the gingival wall; third, by the proper preparation of the pulpal wall; fourth, by a properly contoured and placed contact area.

Occlusal dovetail. The tensile stress de-

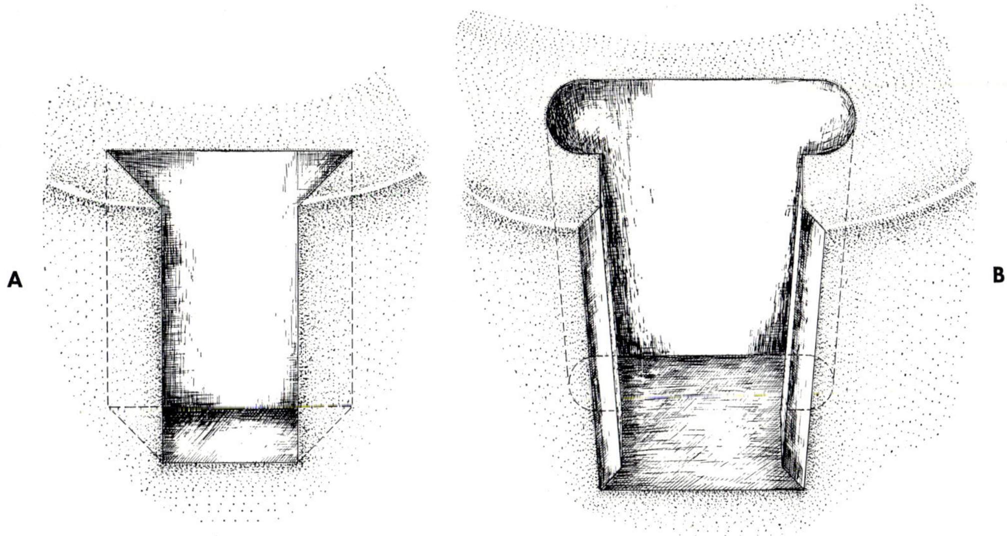

Fig. 13-19. A, Incorrect design of mortise principle. **B,** Correct use of mortise principle with grooves.

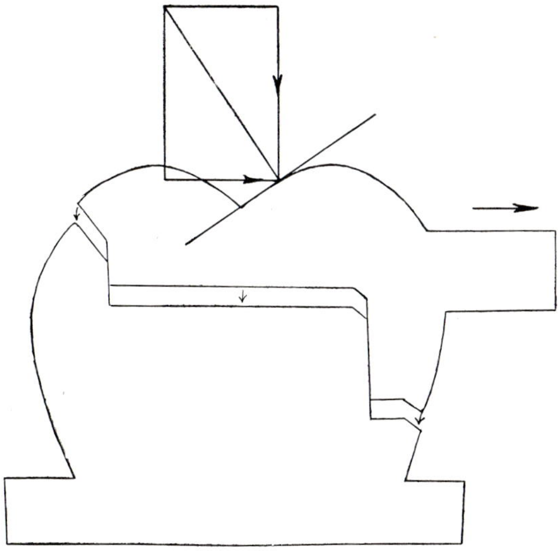

Fig. 13-20. Direction of displacement due to vertical force on inclined plane.

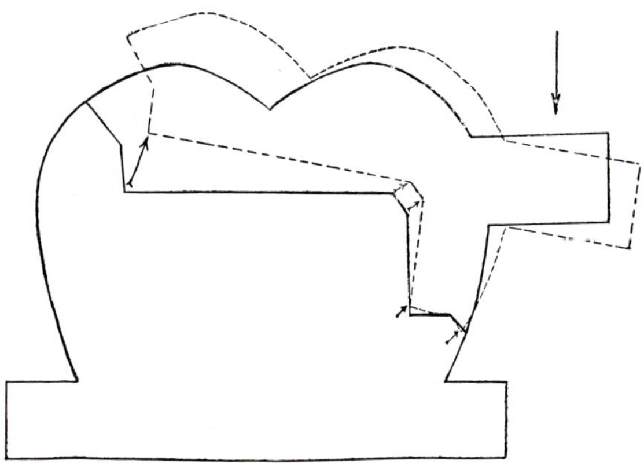

Fig. 13-21. Rotating displacement of filling when vertical force is applied to attached beam.

veloped by the occlusal lock or dovetail is one of the strongest means of resisting the displacement of an inlay. Clinical precaution demands that the two cusps, the buccal and the lingual, which extend into the isthmus of the occlusal lock, *T* (Fig. 13-8), be sound cusps with a sufficient amount of supporting dentin; if these are lacking, there is likelihood of fracture of one or both of the cusps whenever the inlay is subjected to horizontal forces. Likewise, the axial dentin walls of the occlusal dovetail should approximate 2 to 5° parallelism.

Gingival wall. The second method of resisting horizontal displacement is the proper preparation of the gingival wall. In Figs. 13-9 and 13-10 it was shown how a properly placed gingival groove assists in preventing the lateral displacement of an inlay, wall W_1 acting in a direction opposite to the displacing force. Because of the inherent weakness of the gingival groove, the possible fracture of the thin wall of tooth structure between the groove and the cavosurface angle, many operators prefer the inward beveling of the gingival wall, forming an acute angle between the axial and gingival walls.

Figs. 13-22 and 13-23 show a gingival wall with two planes, cavosurface and axial. It is evident that when the horizontal displacing force is applied to the occlusal inclined plane as in Fig. 13-20, lateral displacement of the filling will be resisted by the triangular wedge portion of the inlay, which extends into the acute angle formed by the axiogingival walls. The resistance to displacement is positive until the inlay is raised vertically sufficiently to clear ridge *B* of the gingival wall (Fig. 13-22).

It is not enough, however, to prepare a gingival wall with an inward and downward slope; this must be placed at a certain angle to resist the dislodging forces which are applied at point *1* (Fig. 13-23). Here the fulcrum point is the cavosurface bevel of the gingival wall, *F*.

In Plate 4 the axial wall Gf is prepared so that it has an angle of –2° from the line *AB*. Line *F*AB represents: (1) AB, the typical gingival wall; (2) the bevel of the cavosurface plane represented by A*F*. The wall AB lies in a horizontal plane, 90° from vertical. Using point *F* as the rotation point, the line *F*B represents the radius of rotation of a filling with a gingival wall shaped *F*AB. When a horizontal displacing force *M* is applied to the ocolusal surface of the inlay, that part of the casting lying

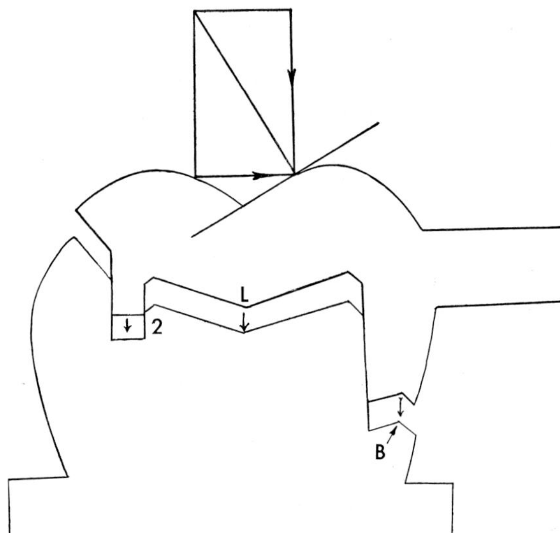

Fig. 13-22. Horizontal displacement of filling prevented by channel, **2**, and inward beveled gingival plane, **B**.

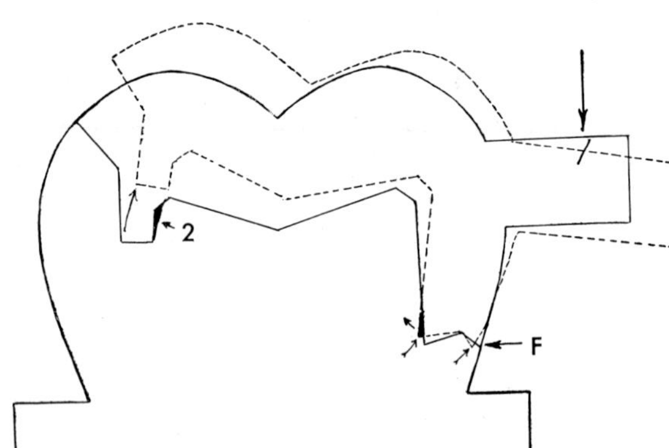

Fig. 13-23. Shaded areas of dentin resist rotatory displacement of inlay.

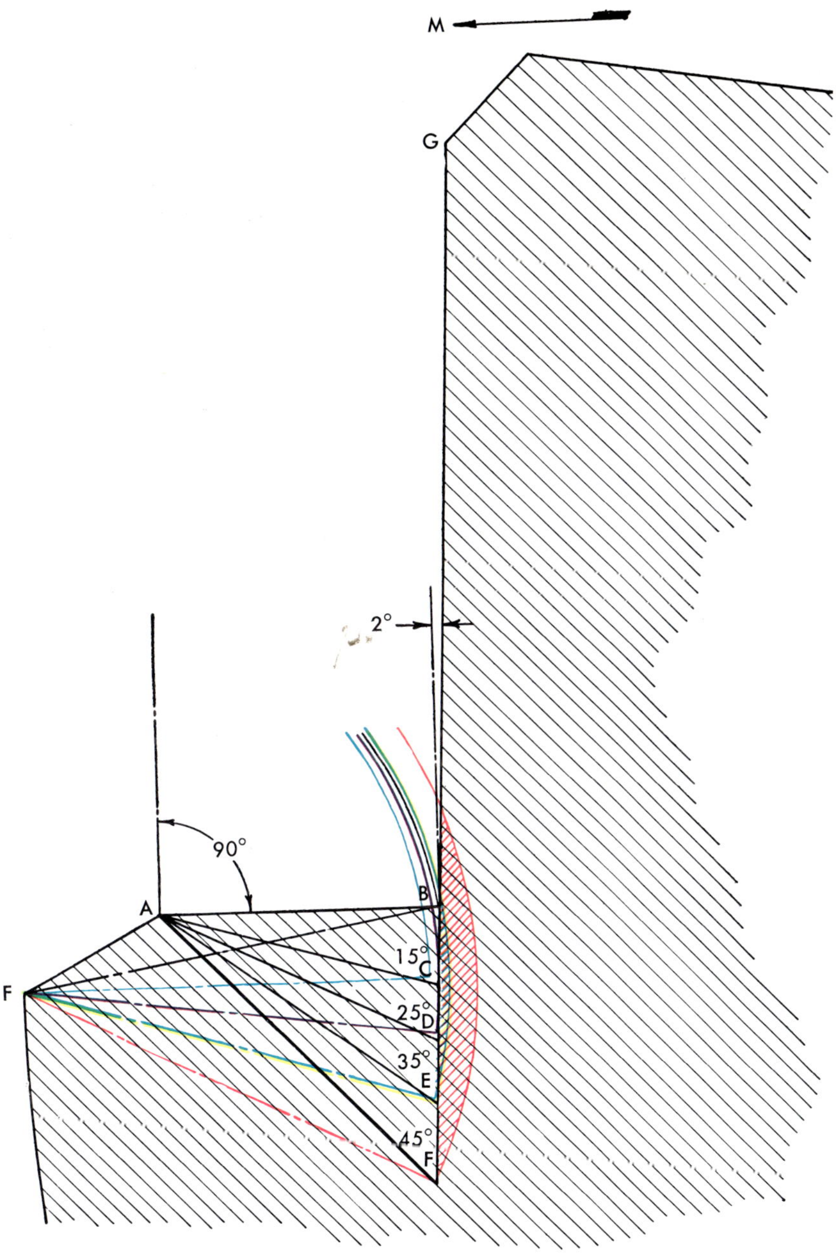

Plate 4. External gingival bevel and internal inclined plane. (Drawn by E. Bannister.)

at point B rotates outwardly without meeting any resistance from the axial wall BG.

What benefits, if any, are derived from including the gingival wall apically 15° from the horizontal plane, as represented by line *F*AC? It is observed here, as in the previous preparation, that the filling may also be rotated out of the cavity because no resistance to displacement is offered by the axial wall CG, since the point C is on the same horizontal plane as the rotation center; consequently, the radius *F*C, to be effective, must be lengthened and dropped below the plane of the rotation point.

By lowering the bevel of the gingival wall to 25°, the gingival wall assumes the shape *F*AD. With *F* as the rotation center, the radius *F*D will meet resistance in the path of its arc in that portion of the dentin represented by the smaller purple area in the chart.

Increasing the angulation to 35 and 45°, the resistance to displacement is shown by those portions of the dentin enclosed within the arcs formed by the radii *F*E (green) and *F*F (red). It is seen from this that the ideal depth of bevel should be approximately 45° from the horizontal plane.

Pulpal wall. The third method of obtaining opposing moments to horizontal displacing forces is by establishing planes of resistance in the pulpal wall. While the pulpal wall shown in Fig. 13-20 offers no resistance to horizontal displacement other than that of friction, Fig. 13-22 shows a similar cavity with the pulpal wall prepared with two planes. The inclined planes of the pulpal wall will prevent the lateral dislodgment of the inlay until point *L* rises above the axiopulpal planes of the cavity preparation.

Another modification of the pulpal wall consists of lowering grooves or pinholes whose walls are parallel within 2°. Wall 2 (Fig. 13-22) in such a preparation resists horizontal displacement of an inlay, since first it must be raised out of its cavity before any lateral movement can take place. Wall 2 also resists rotary displacement (Fig. 13-23) because of the frictional resistance of the dentin in this part of the cavity.

Fig. 13-24 shows an extension of this principle to the typical mesioclusodistal type of bridge retainers.

Vertical resisting walls may also be employed in the form of groove extensions on the buccal and lingual surfaces.

In addition to the increased mechanical retention resulting from slight modifications of cavity preparations, it is essential that suitable gold alloys be used and that castings made of such alloys be properly heat-treated in order that their maximum physical properties are made available. It is conceivable that, even with a correctly

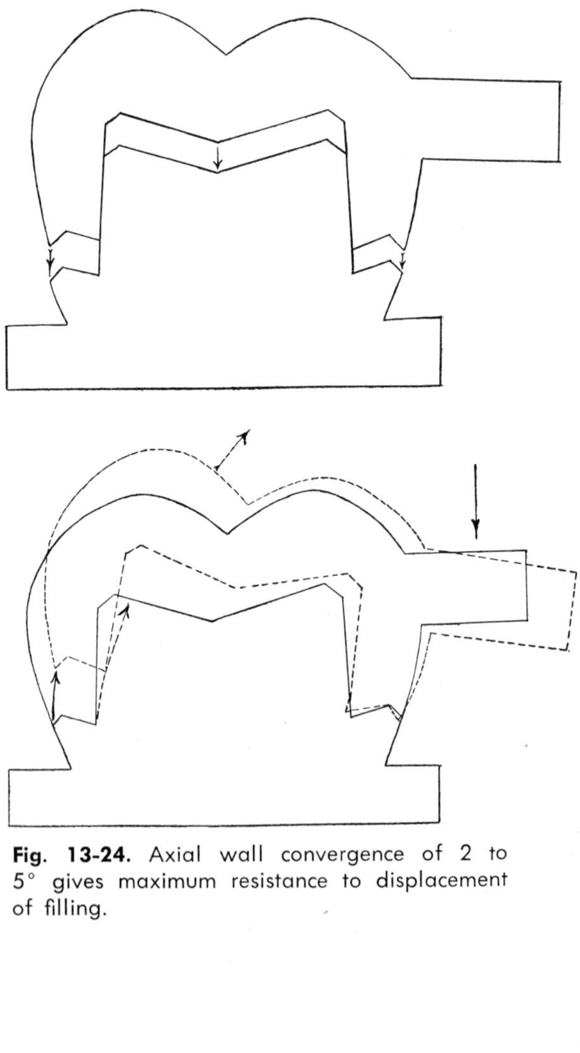

Fig. 13-24. Axial wall convergence of 2 to 5° gives maximum resistance to displacement of filling.

prepared cavity and an accurately fitting casting, failure may result if the retainer does not possess the necessary tensile strength, hardness, and other physical qualities necessary for it to withstand the forces of daily use.

PRINCIPLES OF EXTRACORONAL PREPARATIONS

Anterior partial veneer retainers; class I, type 3

In the upper central incisors and cuspids, the three-quarter partial veneer retainer, as its name indicates, is an extracoronal type of preparation. Since vertical occlusal forces usually have horizontal resultants, the displacing forces tip or rotate a filling out of its cavity.

Usually the tipping is in a lingual direction and the rotation occurs mesiolingually or distolingually. The retention form of the partial veneer retainer is more readily understood, if the method used to resist both the lingual tipping and the torsional displacement or rotation is analyzed.

In Fig. 13-25, *A*, observe the proximal groove, *ab;* if a force *P*, directed lingually, is applied at the incisal edge, it will have a tendency to tip the casting out of the cavity, turning on the center of rotation often designated as the fulcrum point. The resistance to this displacement is furnished by the rib of gold which lies in the axial groove *ab;* also by that part of the axial wall lying lingually to the axial groove and encompassed between arcs *c* and *f*.

It will be observed that the lingual wall of the incisal groove does not furnish any resistance to lingual displacement since the plane of this wall lies in the tipping path of arc *c*. For this reason, the incisal portion of the preparation is usually prepared with one plane instead of a two-plane groove (see Fig. 17-20).

Fig. 13-25, *B*, discloses an incisal view of the same three-quarter partial veneer preparation and a bevel at the cervical margin. When force *P* is applied mesiolingually to the marginal ridge of the upper central, the tendency is to rotate the filling out of the cavity mesiolabial wall, point *F*, acting as the center of rotation. It is observed that the resistance to this rotational displacement is furnished by the distal proximal groove and that portion of the proximal surface lying within the arcs R^1 and R^2.

Analogous resisting forces are present when the forces are in a distolingual direction; then the distolabial wall acts as the point of rotation and the mesial proximal groove and wall furnish the resistance.

The incisal groove is indicated when its lingual wall is needed to resist lingual displacement under torsional forces and when the tooth is relatively thick labiolingually.

In Fig. 13-25, *C*, we find a horizontal force *P* applied mesially to the incisal area; this has a tendency to tip the casting mesially, rotating on point *F*. This displacing force is resisted by the proximodistal groove and that portion of the proximodistal surface lying between the arcs R^1 and R^2.

Posterior partial veneer retainer; class I, type 4

By referring to Fig. 13-26, it will be observed that the same general displacing forces are manifest, but the ability of this retainer to resist displacement is more favorable than in the anterior teeth. In *A* the occlusal force may be occlusal, horizontal, or any one of the other component forces as indicated by letter *P*. No problem exists when the force is vertical, for the reaction is equal and opposite. When the force tends to displace the casting lingually, it does so along the paths R^1, R^2, and R^3, with its rotation center at point *F*. Resistance to this displacing force is furnished by the ribs of gold lying within the axial groove *ab* and by that portion of the proximal surface extending lingually from the proximal groove and lying within the arcs R^1, R^2, and R^3. In addition to this, the occlusal surface lying in the plane R^2-R^3 offers resistance.

Fig. 13-26, *B*, shows horizontal and occlusal views of the same preparation. When force *P* is applied in a mesiolingual direction, the tendency is to rotate the casting meisodistally, the rotation center being point *F*, the mesiobuccal wall. The resistance to this displacing force is developed by the rib of gold lying in the distal proximal groove and by the portion of the casting coming in contact with the proximodistal surface lying between the arcs R^1 and R^2. Additional resistance to displacement is offered by the occlusal inclined planes, R^3, R^4, and R^5.

Fig. 13-26, *C*, illustrates occlusal force *P* being directed in the distal direction. The tendency is to rotate the casting occlusally, dislodging it out along the arcs R^1 and R^2, *F* serving as the point of rotation. The resistance to this displacing force is furnished by the rib of gold lying in the mesioproximal groove, also by the

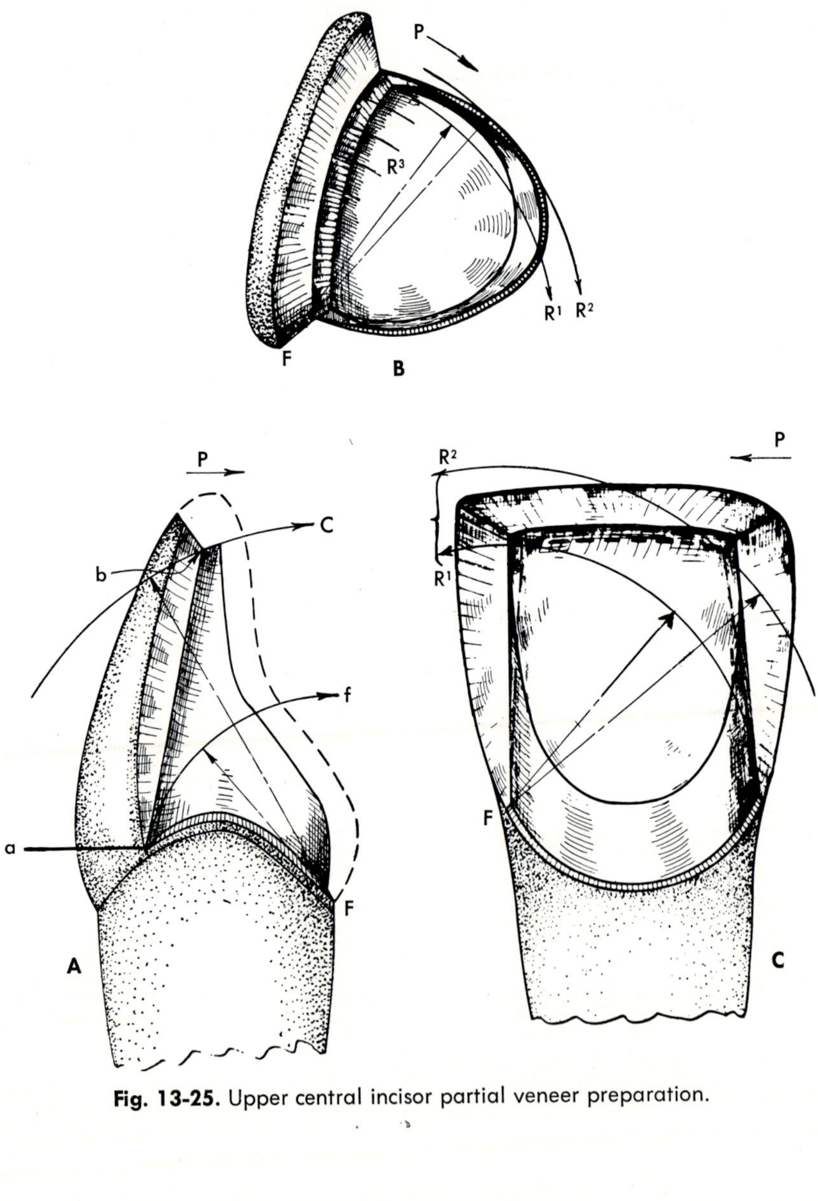

Fig. 13-25. Upper central incisor partial veneer preparation.

buccal and the mesioproximal walls lying within the areas R^1 and R^2.

The displacement of a bridge retainer in a direction opposite to its line of insertion is resisted by (1) the cement holding the retainer in position, (2) an accurate fit of the casting, and (3) axial walls prepared as nearly parallel as possible to 2 to 5° convergence.

There are likewise available the right-angle pin locks, which are described in Chapter 19.

In making intracoronal and extracoronal preparations for the reception of retainers, the contour of two or more, but not all, of the surfaces of a tooth are involved, while preparations for complete veneer or solid crowns involve the contour of the entire coronal portion of the tooth.

The mechanical retention in partial and complete veneer crowns is obtained mainly by the internal stresses developed between the external axial walls in the dentin of the preparation and the internal sur-

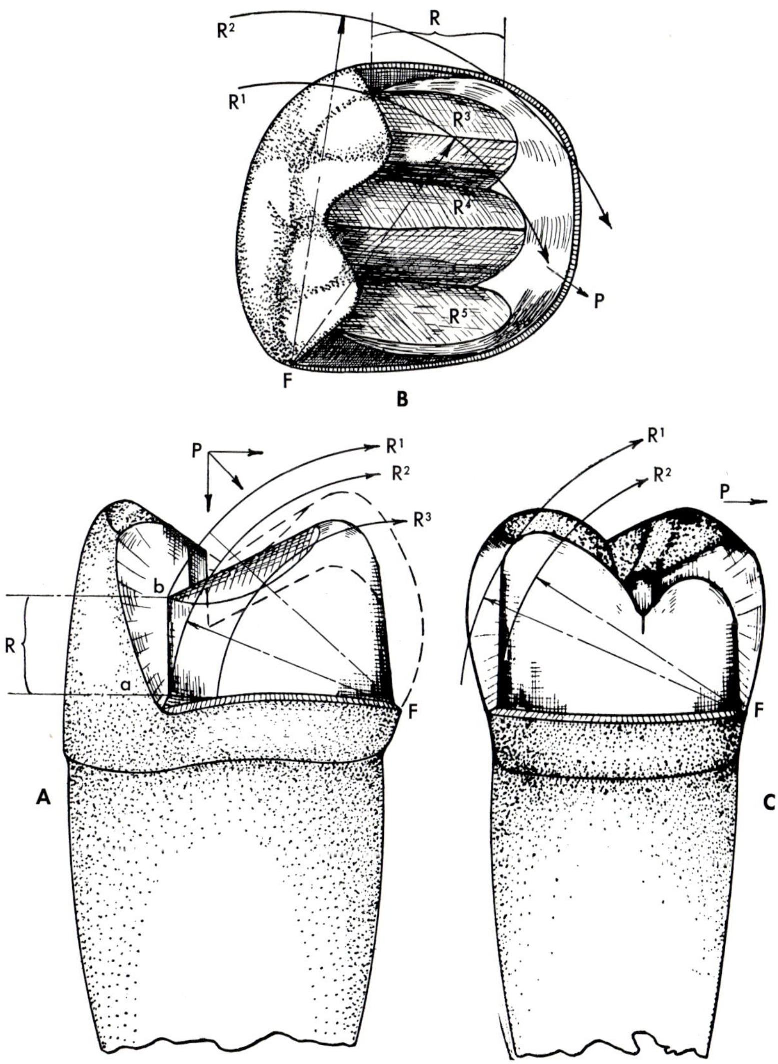

Fig. 13-26. Upper molar partial veneer preparation.

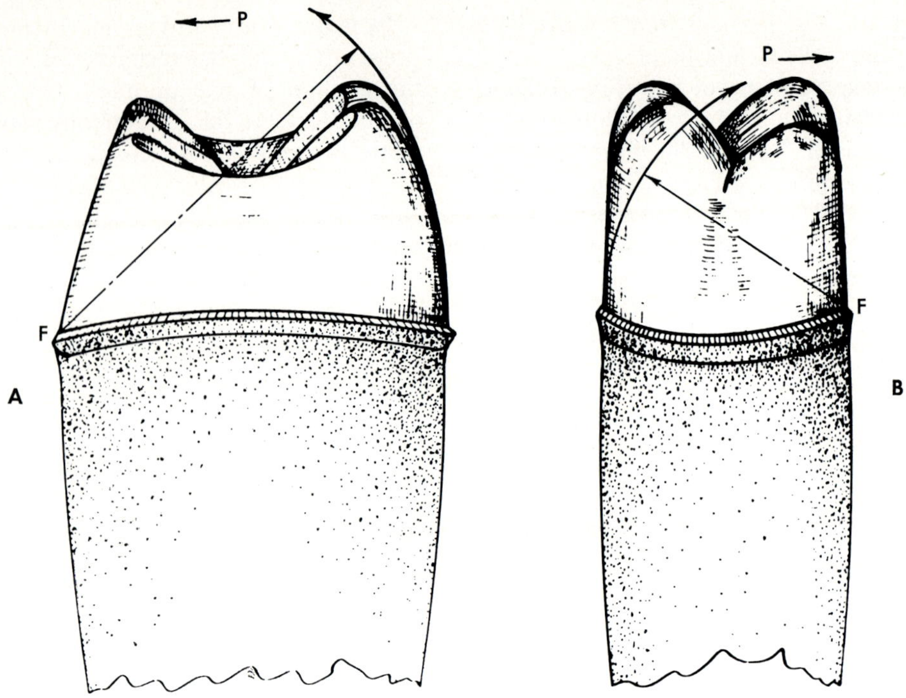

Fig. 13-27. Complete veneer preparation with gingival chamfer on vital tooth for cast gold crown.

faces of the metal retainer when the restoration is cemented and maintained under steady pressure. In those instances in which the coronal portion of a tooth has been destroyed or is missing and in which no axial wall resistance is available, the use of a dowel placed in the root canal will afford the major means of retention and resistance to displacement. The effectiveness of a dowel is frequently augmented by the use of a root coping, which furnishes a limited axial retention. A dowel counteracts shearing as well as tipping forces. The horizontal dowel retention may likewise be employed (see Figs. 19-3 and 19-4).

Complete cast gold retainers; class II, type 1

Figs. 13-27 and 13-28 show types of complete veneer preparations. It is observed in Fig. 13-27 that the mesial and distoproximal walls are most favorable for developing near parallelism essential to stress retention. The buccal and lingual surfaces, due to their natural contour, do not afford the same opportunity. Where possible, the occlusal planes are reproduced at a lower level; these planes help considerably to resist buccal or lingual displacement. Where it is impossible to reproduce the normal occlusal anatomy, usually in a pulpless tooth, a buccal and a lingual occlusal plane are prepared, as shown in Fig. 13-28; these offer resistance to lingual or buccal forces. When necessary and where indicated, additional resistance form may be obtained by preparing a gingival plane or shoulder at right angles to the axial surfaces of the preparation.

In Fig. 13-28, *A*, it is seen that, if an occlusal force P^1 is directed buccally, the lingual portion of the crown tends to be dislodged occlusally and bucally with the

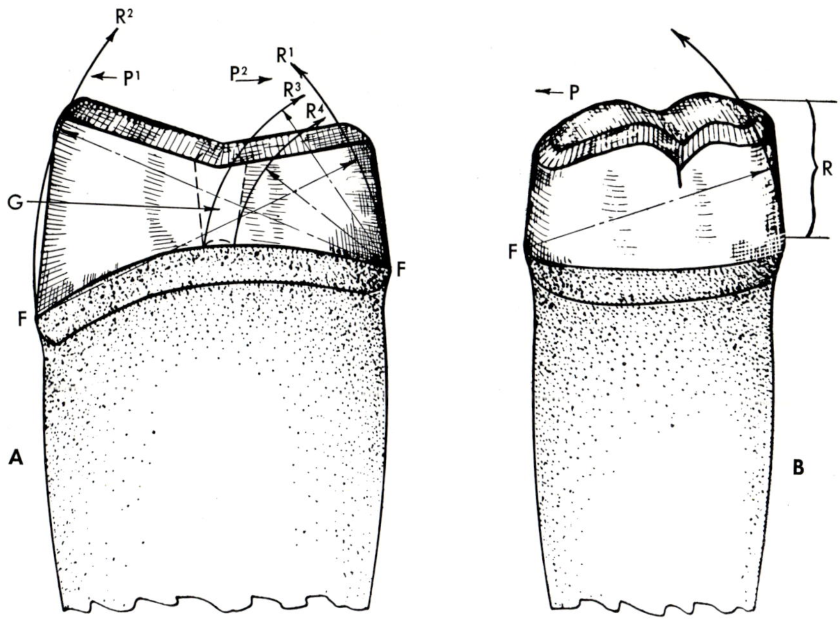

Fig. 13-28. Complete veneer shoulderless preparation on pulpless tooth for gold crown.

point of rotation situated at *F;* this displacement is resisted by the lingual surface lying outside the arc R^1.

On the other hand, an occlusal force P^2 directed lingually is liable to dislodge the crown lingually, since the buccal wall of the preparation lies within the tipping path of the arc R^2. When such a condition prevails either in the buccal or lingual wall, resistance to displacement can be developed by placing two proximal shallow keyways or grooves at *G* in the mesial and distal surfaces.

In Fig. 13-28, *B,* it is evident that an occlusal force *P* directed mesially will not dislodge the crown, since the distal wall of the preparation lies outside the tipping path of arc *R*.

ROLE OF ENAMEL IN PREPARATION OF RETAINERS

Cutting the enamel wall

One other factor merits thoughtful consideration in preparing teeth for all types of retainers, namely, the enamel wall. This problem may be considered from two angles: first, the relationship of the histologic structure of enamel to the cutting operations; and second, the requisites for a sound enamel wall capable of resisting fracture and deterioration of its exposed surfaces.

Methods of cutting enamel. The cutting of enamel may be accomplished in three ways: first, by cleavage; second, by the process of planing; and third, by the process of abrasion or disintegration.

When a substance possesses the property of cleavage, it discloses the tendency to split readily in a definite plane or direction with the result that a more or less smooth surface results nearly always parallel to actual or possible crystal faces. This is due primarily to the fact that the structural cohesion is lowest in the direction of the cleavage plane itself. As is well known, enamel will usually cleave in the direction of the enamel rods and within the interprismatic cementing substance, since the latter has the minimum value of cohesion. Such cleavage will occur only so long as the enamel rods are relatively straight and parallel; when gnarled enamel is encountered, the cleavage, if any, will be irregular and difficult.

Cleavage is usually accomplished by the use of a wedge-shaped cutting instrument, such as a chisel or enamel hatchet, and by exerting force in the direction of the enamel rods. Enamel that is unsupported by sound dentin cleaves very readily. As a rule, enamel rods emerge upon the outer surfaces of the tooth at right angles to that surface. Knowledge of the cleavage lines of enamel on its various surfaces is of considerable assistance in the preparation of cavities for bridge retainers. Such information is usually acquired by the study of ground sections of teeth and by clinical observations while cutting teeth.

Cleavage. In the preparation of teeth, cleavage of enamel is employed mostly in carious teeth or in those sound teeth being prepared for intracoronal retainers. Where the surface of a tooth is sound, enamel cleavage is usually preceded by an undermining of the enamel with a bur at the dentinoenamel junction.

Planing. Cleaved surfaces are not always smooth, nor are they always parallel to the plane of cleavage; hence it is necessary to pare off the inequalities of the surface by planing with sharp chisels or enamel hatchets. This planing, which reduces all elevations and eliminates depressions, may be done in any direction, since the prime purpose of this operation is to establish smooth plane surfaces.

Abrasion. The third method of cutting enamel is by abrasion. By abrasion is meant the removal, wearing down, or disintegration of a substance or its surface, such as enamel, by small amounts through the frictional use of an abrasive, such as carborundum, diamond, or pumice, which scores the surface of the material with a series of scratches, causing it to separate into integrant parts.

Instruments and methods of cutting enamel. The instruments used for this abrasion are cutting stones of various sizes, shapes, and materials. This method of removing tooth substance is employed largely in preparing teeth for partial and complete veneer crowns, or in cutting through the walls of a sound and noncarious enamel. While the cutting by cleavage or planing is done with straight-edge steel instruments and a reciprocating stroke, that done by abrasion is usually accomplished with a rotary motion of round abrasive stones held against the tooth with light pressure and high speeds under a stream of water.

Dental burs. The dental steel or carbide bur, in reality, is a planing instrument, since it consists of a series of cutting blades that remove tooth structure in the form of chips or shavings. It is said that the spear-shaped drill or bur was introduced by Cornelius von Solingen in 1686, and the ball-shaped bur by Fauchard in 1728. Originally designed for hand operation, both were gradually modified and adapted for use with the electric motor of the present day having 12,000 to 300,000 revolutions per minute. The latter high speed is used with the diamond stone.

While the use of stones for smoothing and polishing objects of art dates to ancient times, their use for dental purposes received an impetus when in 1870 a bonding material was developed which made it possible to manufacture synthetic stones by bonding the abrasive granules or crystals into a solid mass which could then be shaped to any desirable size and form.

The use of steel burs on enamel surfaces is ineffective at the low speeds because the revolving cutting edge of the bur blade cannot be effectively applied to the cleavage planes of the enamel rods. Since a revolving bur removes tooth structure in the form of chips or shavings, it is apparent, first, that sufficient pressure is necessary on the cutting edge of the blade to allow it to penetrate sufficiently into the tooth to enable it to remove chips of a sufficient size; and second, that sufficient time must be allowed for the blade to penetrate into the material which it is cutting. For these reasons, the hardness and the structural form of the material being ground determine the relative cutting efficiency of a bur. Where the speed of a revolving bur and the hardness of the material are such that the blades are unable to penetrate appreciably into the structure, considerable heat is developed with little cutting efficiency. Steel burs were primarily intended to cut dentin at a lower rate of speed with moderate pressure.

In proportion, as the size of a bur was increased, it was necessary to lower the speed of the motor and increase the amount of pressure. In spite of the great advances made in the design of dental cutting burs, many operators still prefer the bibeveled drill in preference to the multibladed bur. The noise sometimes created by the vibration of the straight-bladed fissure bur may be reduced or eliminated if burs are used with spiral blades.

Because enamel is much harder than dentin, and since at times it is necessary to remove only the outer length of the enamel rods in preparing teeth for retainers, it is rather difficult to accomplish this by the process of cleavage. Such partial removal of the enamel is best accomplished by the use of abrasive stones, followed by plain finishing burs and fine sandpaper disks.

Dental cutting stones. The cutting efficiency of stones is dependent upon several factors: (1) the type of abrasive crystal used; (2) its shape; (3) the nature of the bonding material in which the crystals are imbedded and held; (4) the arrangement of the crystals in the imbedding material; (5) the speed of the revolving stones; and (6) the amount of pressure exerted by the stone against the tooth. (See Chapter 14.)

Of the many abrasives used for this purpose, carborundum, silicon-carbide, and the diamond are the ones most generally used today. Of these, the diamond is the most desirable, because it is hardest, highly resistant to wear, and it maintains its crystalline structure; it also retains its abrasive edges, even though divided into the smallest sizes of crystals. The main objection to its more general use is its relatively higher cost. Carborundum and other synthetic abrasives are not nearly as efficient although less expensive. (See Chapter 14 for different types and sizes of stones.)

The degree of pressure required in cutting with burs is not necessary with stones, since the sharp edges and points of the crystals score and scratch the surface of the enamel with the slightest amount of pressure. The disintegration occurs rapidly and increases as the speed of rotation is accelerated. Because there is a minimum of surface contact between the long, sharp points of the crystals and the surface of the enamel, very little heat of friction is generated. It is clear that those stones having the hardest crystals with sharp points and applied with a minimum of pressure will do a maximum of cutting. Hence, the final cutting with stones should be accomplished with stones having crystals of a small size and with smaller abrasive points and edges. The use of stones having softer and smaller crystals for the final polishing of surfaces is also recommended; the final finish may be obtained by the use of a fine alumina powder applied by means of a revolving, soft wood prophylactic polishing point, or by very fine sandpaper disks. Mounted Arkansas stones are excellent for this purpose from the engineer's viewpoint.

Good grinding technic also demands that the handpieces and mandrels used to hold the abrasive stones be true and in excellent mechanical condition. A stone that is eccentric in its periphery or a mandrel whose axis is bent will strike a jarring blow with each revolution and may result in serious damage to the tooth and to its contiguous structures. When using abrasives, it is necessary to protect the mechanism of the handpiece.

If the crystals imbedded in the bonding material of a stone are placed too closely together, so that there is no opportunity for the particles of enamel to clear the surface of the stone during the cutting operation, it gradually becomes clogged to a degree that a flat surface contacts the enamel, producing excessive heat but little cutting.

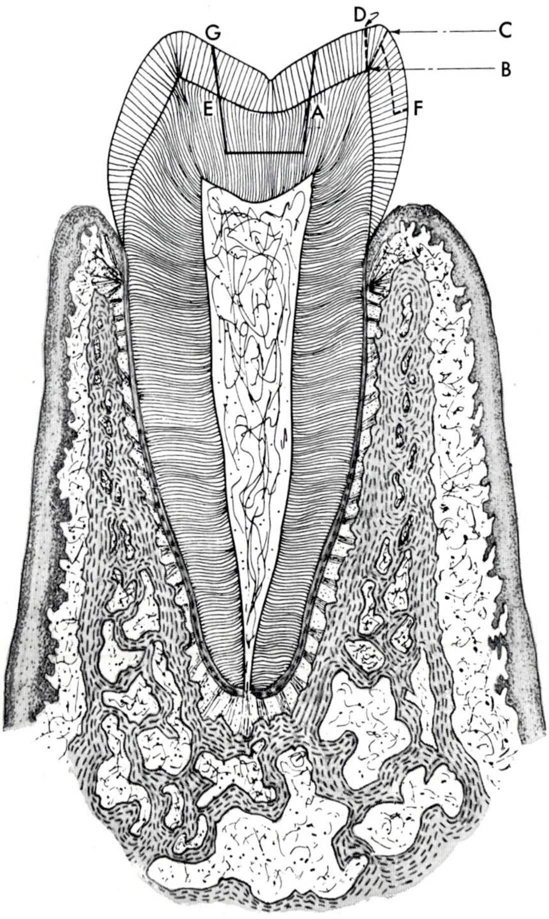

Fig. 13-29. Lower molar showing position and direction of enamel rods in relation to dentin in occlusal and cusp areas.

Wet grinding. The question of the relative efficiency of wet or dry grinding is important. The use of cocoa butter in conjunction with a stream of warm water (110° F.) has been advocated as a means of increasing cutting efficiency and as a protection against possible injury to the pulp from overheating the tooth during the cutting operations. Kruel,[7] in an exhaustive study, has shown that the maximum amount of material is not removed when the cutting is done in a dry field, but when a stream of water is used. During grinding operations, water should be used in a quantity sufficient to carry away the particles of tooth structure loosened during each revolution of the stone. Water serves the additional function of dissipating frictional heat.

The use of cocoa butter on stones serves a similar function, acting as a vehicle for the debris and a cooling agent at the same time.

The final step in preparing the outer surface of an enamel wall reduced with abrasive stones consists in smoothing the surface by means of fine alumina powder, prophylactic polishing points, and finishing burs, such as the Tinker, Krause, and Maves types and fine Arkansas stones.

Structural requirements for enamel walls

Many years ago, Noyes[8] pointed out that there were certain structural requirements for strong enamel walls: that the enamel must rest on and be supported by sound dentin; that those rods facing the cavosurface angle rest upon sound dentin; and in certain operative procedures that the cavosurface angle be trimmed or beveled.

It has been clinically demonstrated that enamel, unsupported by sound dentin, when subjected to pressure will fracture along cleavage planes. For this reason the outline form of a cavity should always extend beyond areas of unsupported enamel.

At this time, it is well to repeat that

portion of Black's statement which relates to the cavosurface angle of enamel: "The depth of the bevel should generally not include more than one-fourth of the thickness of the enamel wall, although in some cases, as occlusal cavities, the entire wall may be cut at such an angle in relation to the direction of the rod, as to fully meet the requirements. The angle of the bevel should be from 6 to 10° C. from the plane of the enamel wall for gold foil restorations, but should be less for all other. The object is first to cut away any loose ends of enamel rods that might afterwards fall away and render the margin imperfect, and second, to strengthen the cavo-surface angle of the enamel as a safeguard against possible checking in the condensation of gold."[1]

A third point may be added, the safeguarding of the enamel margins during the fitting and finishing of the retainer margins after the restoration has been cemented to place. While the cavosurface bevel is primarily indicated for gold foil operations, if used in bridge preparations, it is also necessary that all rods facing the cavosurface angle be supported by sound dentin. Due to the direction of the enamel rods, particularly in the region of pits and fissures, the cavosurface bevel is not ordinarily employed on the occlusal cusps, since the slope of the enamel walls is usually such that there are no unsupported enamel rods.

Fig. 13-29 shows the relative direction of the enamel rods on the various surfaces of the lower molar. The convergence of the enamel rods is characteristic of the fissure regions. By cutting the buccal enamel wall in the direction shown, *EG*, it is seen why there are no unsupported enamel rods.

The danger of extending cavity margins into areas of weakness should be avoided. Noyes has pointed out that the dentin cusps and marginal ridges do not lie at points directly below corresponding areas on the surface of the enamel, but are situated closer to the long axis of the tooth. When, therefore, the margin of a filling lies between the area *D-C* (Fig. 13-29), it should be carried or extended beyond the point *C* onto the lingual surface. Very frequently in the case of bridge retainers, such marginal extension is not obtained by the removal of the entire enamel wall, but by cutting away only a part of the outer surface of the enamel and terminating the margin at point *F*. The casting then covers this area as a veneer beyond point *D* to point *F*.

In studying the inclination of the enamel rods in relation to the inclined occlusal

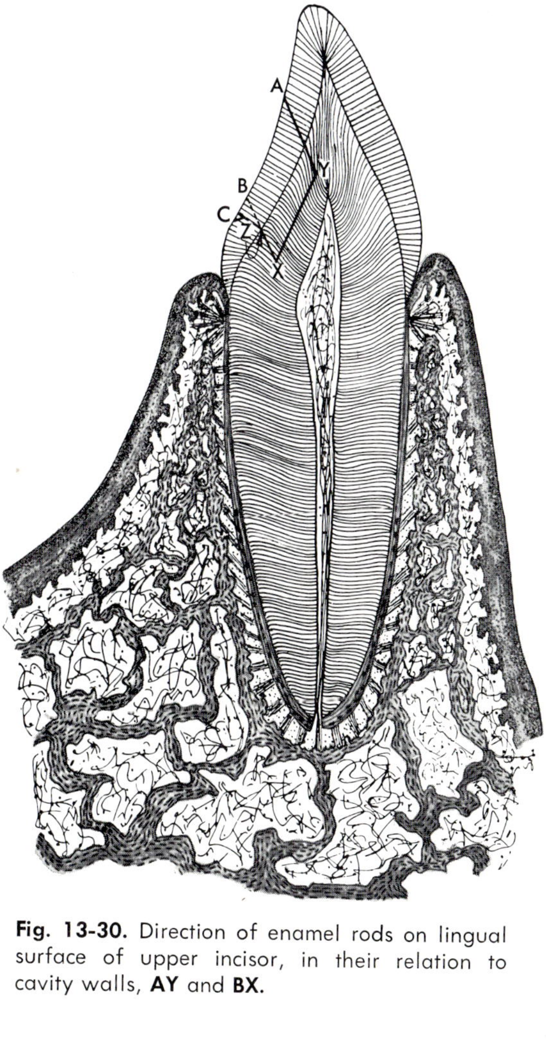

Fig. 13-30. Direction of enamel rods on lingual surface of upper incisor, in their relation to cavity walls, **AY** and **BX**.

surfaces of teeth, it is interesting to note that the axes of the enamel rods usually parallel the reacting resultants of the occluding forces in these areas.

In Fig. 13-30 enamel walls are shown extended in two different planes. The lingual incisal wall is cut diagonally through the enamel rods in such a way that no unsupported enamel is found in the plane *YA*. On the other hand, if the lingual gingival wall is carried in the same direction from *X* to *B*, it is seen that those enamel rods lying in the area *CBZ* are entirely unsupported by dentin; hence it is necessary to place the plane of this enamel wall in the direction *ZC*.

SELECTED REFERENCES

1. Black, G. V.: Operative dentistry, ed. 7, Chicago, 1956, Medico-Dental Publishing Co., Vol. 2.
2. Taggart, W. H.: A new and accurate method of making cast gold inlays, D. Cosmos **49:** 1117, 1907.
3. Price, W. A.: Laws determining casting or fusing results, their control and a new rational technic, D. Items Int. **30:**363, 1908.
4. Ward, M. L.: American textbook of operative dentistry, ed. 6, Philadelphia, 1926, Lea & Febiger.
5. Bodecker, H. W. C.: The metallic inlay, Berlin, 1911, Hermann Mensser.
6. Peyton, F. A., Mahler, D. B., and Hershenov, B.: Physical properties of dentin, J. Dent. Res. **31:**366-370, 1952.
7. Kruel, P.: Grundlegende Erkenntnisse über das Schleifen von Harstoffen, Braunschweig, 1935, Friedrich Vieweg and Gohn.
8. Noyes, F. B.: Dental histology and embryology, ed. 2, Philadelphia, 1915, Lea & Febiger.
9. McMath, J. F.: The gingival groove in gold inlay preparations, D. Cosmos **67:**1162, 1925.
10. Brown, R. K.: A system of cavity preparation and wax manipulation for a cast gold inlay, J.A.D.A. **25:**1974, 1938.

GENERAL REFERENCES

Bowman, D. C., and Nakfoor, P. M.: Evaluation of the human subject's ability to differentiate intensity of forces applied to the maxillary central incisors, J. Dent. Res. **47**(2):252-259, 1968.

Burnell, S. C.: Obtaining harmony between retainers and abutment teeth in bridgework, J.A.D.A. **66:**668, 1963.

Charbeneau, G. T.: Planning for the restoration of nonvital teeth, J. Michigan D. A. **42:**75, 1960.

Craig, R. G., and Peyton, F. A.: Elastic and mechanical properties of human dentin, J. Dent. Res. **37:**710, 1958.

Dietz, W. H.: Means of saving mutilated teeth, J. Prosth. Dent. **11:**967, 1961.

Dietz, W. H.: Modified abutments for removable and fixed prosthodontics, J. Prosth. Dent. **11:** 1112, 1961.

Davidson, G. B.: A method for three dimensional photoelastic stress analysis of the remaining tooth structure associated with various cavity preparations, abstracted, J. Dent. Res. **43:**912, 1964.

Eisenbrand, G. F.: Method for constructing a fixed bridge with an extremely tipped abutment, D. Digest **68:**514, 1962.

Fujii, T.: Experimental study concerning the roughness of cut surface of human teeth, J. Nihon Univ. School Dent. **2:**184, 1960.

Gabel, A. B.: Present-day concepts of cavity preparation, Dent. Clin. N. Amer. p. 3, March, 1957.

Granath, L. E.: Further photoelastic studies on the relation between the cavity and the occlusal portion of class II restorations, Odont. Rev. **15:**290-298, 1964.

Granath, L. E.: Photoelastic model experiments on class II cavity restorations of dental amalgam, Odont. Rev. **16:**7-38, 1965.

Gray, H. S.: Retentiveness of bridge retainers, J. Dent. Res. **47:**1030, 1968.

Guard, W. F., Haack, D. C, and Ireland, R. L.: Photoelastic stress analysis of buccolingual sections of class II cavity restorations, J.A.D.A. **57:**631-635, 1958.

Haskin, R. C., Haack, M. S., and Ireland, R. L.: A study of stress pattern variations in class II cavity restorations as a result of different cavity design, J. Dent. Res. **33:**757-766, 1954.

Klaffenbach, A. O.: An analytic study of modern abutments, J.A.D.A. **23:**2275, 1936.

Klaffenbach, A. O.: Retention factors in fixed bridge prosthesis, Iowa D. Bull. **34:**224, 1948.

Leander, C. T.: Preparation of abutments for fixed partial dentures, Dent. Clin. N. Amer., pp. 59-72, March, 1959.

Linkow, L. I.: Abutments for full mouth splinting, J. Prosth. Dent. **11:**920, 1961.

Linkow, L. I.: Mesially tipped mandibular molars, J. Prosth. Dent. **12:**554, 1962.

Maxwell, E. L., and Wasser, V. E.: Debate: full vs. partial coverage as the abutment of choice in fixed bridgework, J. Dist. Columbia D. Soc. **36:**9, 1961.

Morrison, R. L.: Laws of physics and engineering applied to dentistry, D. Survey **22**:678, 1946.

Pruden, W. H., II: Today's approach to fixed partial denture prosthesis, J. New Jersey D. Soc. **32**:11, 1960.

Smyd, E. S.: Dental engineering applied to inlay and fixed bridge fabrication, J. Prosth. Dent. **2**:536, 1952.

Stanford, S. W., and others: Compressive properties of hard tooth tissues and some restorative materials, J.A.D.A. **60**:746, 1960.

Stanford, S. W., and others: Determination of some compressive properties of human enamel and dentin, J.A.D.A. **57**:487, 1958.

Stevenson, S. B., Jr.: Variables of crown and cavity preparations and their effect on the human pulp, Pennsylvania D. J. **64**:48, 1960.

Chapter 14

Methods of cutting teeth and preferential use of instruments

Newer materials, equipment, and biologic knowledge have enabled today's dentist to mold his professional services to conform with better understanding of present-day mechanical, engineering, and biologic principles. These principles have always existed, but we are progressively recognizing and applying them piecemeal and sometimes are prone to designate them as "modern" concepts.

The problem may arise of deciding which type of cutting instrument to use in preparing an abutment tooth for a retainer. It depends primarily on the tooth substance to be cut; it may be hard, brittle, and highly calcified enamel, or it may be the relatively softer and less calcified dentin. Consideration must also be given to the neurovascular relationships of each tissue being cut and to the characteristics of their physical structure.

The blade of a wood-plane readily shaves wood but does not do so well on plate glass, due to differences in their composition and physical structure. However, a diamond crystal easily disintegrates glass by scratching its surface lightly. Cutting wood requires a definite amount of pressure on the edge of the blade to remove the softer material in the form of wood chips or shavings. Diamond crystal points penetrate and disintegrate the hard glass surface into powder under very light pressure and high cutting speed.

A carbide steel bur revolving even at accelerated speeds and applied with increased pressure to a smooth glass surface will have little, if any, cutting effect on glass. It will chatter, vibrate, heat, and sometimes fracture the glass and chip the edge of the steel cutting blade. However, the same bur applied to dentin, under reduced cutting speeds and pressure, removes chips without chatter, vibration, heat generation, or injury to the pulp.

Formerly, the conventional cutting speeds ranged from 4,000 to 6,000 rpm. Dentin was removed with steel burs rotating at the lower speeds, and a pressure of 2½ to 4 pounds was applied to the cutting instrument. Enamel was usually undermined at its dentinoenamel junction and then removed in small sections by means of enamel hatchets and chisels. Cutting into a sound external surface of enamel was done by using abrasive wheels containing either carborundum or diamond crystals. Thus steel cutting instruments were designed and intended primarily for cutting dentin, while carborundum or diamond stones were used for the removal of enamel. In the 1930's the greater efficiency of the diamond cutting instrument was more fully utilized by the dental profession. This took place when cutting speeds were increased to 100,000 rpm and over.

Early investigators in Germany and the United States realized that the successful use of the diamond instrument depended upon high speed and light pressure. It was recognized that the bur removed dentin in small chips, whereas the diamond stone disintegrated the enamel by scoring and pulverizing the rods of the enamel. It was recognized that, coincident with the higher speeds and lighter pressure, there was less heat produced. To safeguard the health of the tooth tissues, particularly the pulp, the use of a stream of water applied during the cutting process is necessary and recommended.

Certain advantages accrued with the use of increased speeds: (1) smaller stones could be used at the increased speeds; (2) less fatigue resulted both for the patient and the operator; (3) the control of the instruments by the operator was better; (4) due to the high speed, very light pressure was required; (5) less vibration was felt by the patient; (6) the dentist required less chair time for a given preparation; (7) there was a reduction in trauma to the pulp; (8) the efficiency and life of the cutting tool were increased; (9) there was greater ease of control of the instrument because smaller tools were used; (10) the removal of old amalgam and gold restorations was simplified.

Accompanying these advantages are certain disadvantages. The increased speed creates increased temperatures in the tooth; therefore, some method of cooling the tooth more efficiently is required not to injure the pulp. This necessitates additional equipment. When a dentist changes from the conventional lower speeds, which utilize a pressure in pounds, to high speeds which need only a pressure in ounces, he must develop a new technic and retrain himself to a new tactile sense. To operate at the higher speeds, good visibility of the cutting instrument is necessary due to the danger of overcutting and overextension of the cavity. Dut to the ease with which tooth tissue is removed, caution must be taken not to injure the proximal enamel of the adjacent healthy tooth. High speeds create higher temperatures, which might damage the pulp. With some of the newer high-speed handpieces an unpleasant noise level may be developed. High speeds result in greater wear on the working parts of the handpiece, necessitating more frequent repairs and replacements, in addition to a more exacting and a more frequent care. Finally, unless properly used, high speeds have a tendency to create striations on a tooth surface.

Notwithstanding the disadvantages of high speeds, the method has so many compensating advantages that it is at present the accepted procedure by the profession. However, it must be stated that its sole objective is not speed per se, but that the biologic objectives and principles of procedure in preparing the tooth still remain the same; namely (1) that the operator removes the least amount of tooth tissue consistent with necessary mechanical retention; (2) that he does this with the least harm to the periodontal tissues and the pulp; (3) that it be done with the least discomfort to the patient; and, finally, (4) that no pathologic reactions be initiated in the pulp.

There is some question as to the dividing line between low, intermediate, and high speeds. Generally, it is accepted that speeds up to 10,000 rpm are regarded as low speeds; those 25,000 to 45,000 rpm as intermediate; and those 50,000 to 100,000 rpm as high speeds. Since many handpieces attain speeds of 100,000 to 400,000 rpm they are designated as the super- or ultra-high speeds.

Kilpatrick[1, 2] has classified the ultrahigh-speed handpieces into three classes: type I, the gear-driven contra-angle handpiece, up to 125,000 rpm; type II, the belt-driven contra-angle handpiece, up to 200,000 rpm; and type III, turbine-driven air contra-angle handpiece, up to 300,000 rpm and higher.

Another step in the successful application of high speeds was the introduction of

A complete size range to fill virtually every dental need

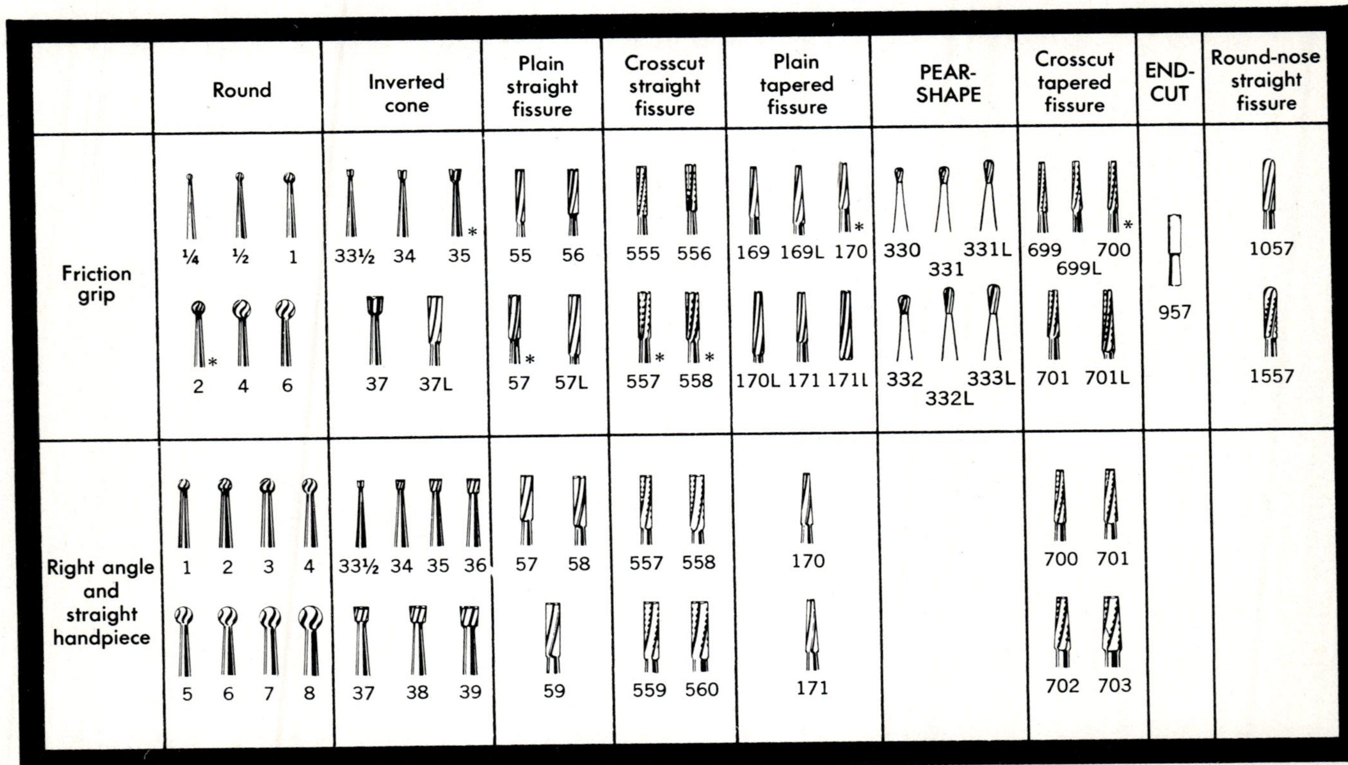

*Available in short shank

Fig. 14-1. Kerr carbide steel burs.

the carbide tipped bur, about 1947. While the greater cutting efficiency of this type of bur over the steel bur was immediately recognized, its optimum values were not realized until greater rotational speeds were developed along with handpieces that were designed to tolerate such speeds. Recognizing this need in dental equipment, manufacturers set about developing handpieces capable of higher speeds. Research revealed that the improved stones and burs (Figs. 14-1 to 14-4) removed tooth tissue three times as fast at 60,000 rpm as at 3,000 rpm and also at $\frac{1}{30}$ of the required pressure.[3] As the speeds were increased it became evident that handpieces with friction-sleeve bearings were inadequate due to the heat which developed, also because of the necessity of frequent celaning and lubrication. Similarly, the higher speeds resulted in greater wear, which produced more vibration.

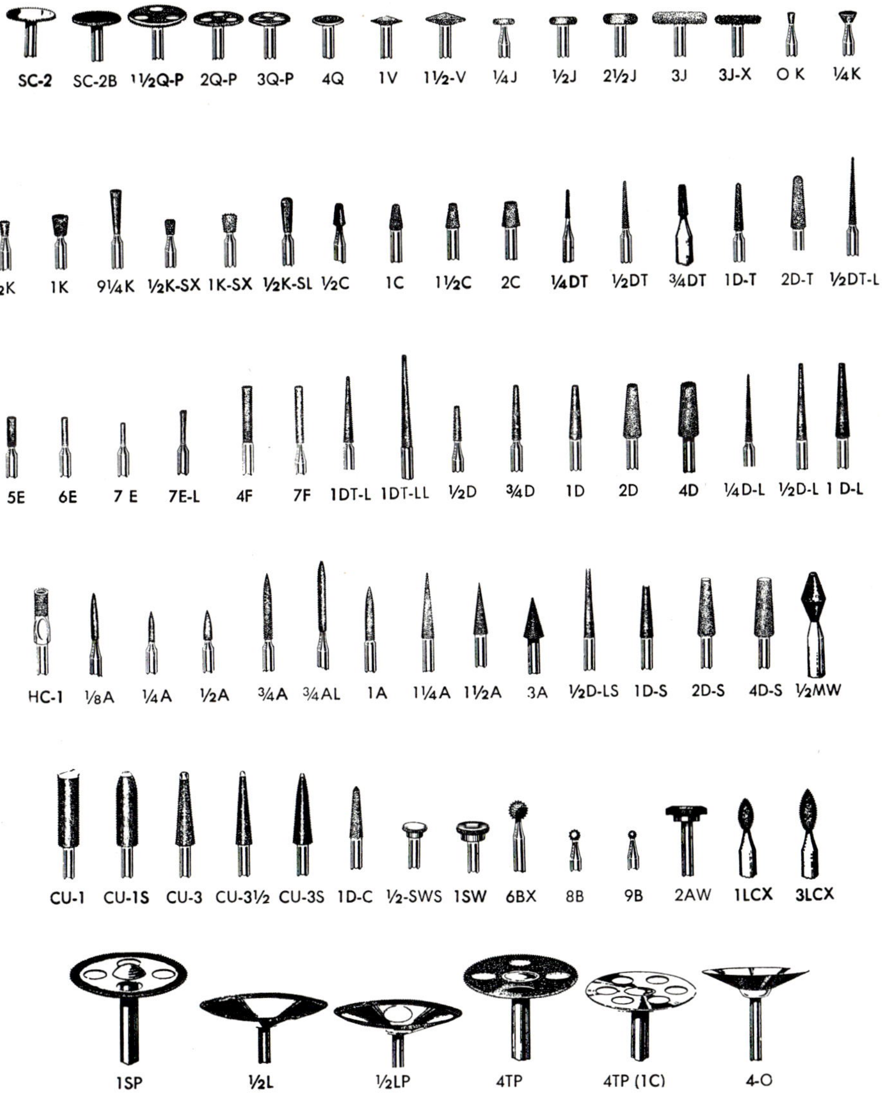

Fig. 14-2. Densco diamond stones.

Improvements were made in handpieces whereby speeds 25,000 to 30,000 rpm were usable for short intermittent periods of time. These contained polished-glass or steel ball bearings.

It was recognized that the solution to higher speeds would come with further development of the contra-angle handpiece, because the greater number of operations performed in the mouth utilize the contra-angle. Such contra-angles are now available.

Concurrently, a new approach was made to solve the problem of high speed handpieces. The first of these was the water turbine type developed by Nelsen,[4, 5] which attains a speed of approximately 50,000 rpm. Subsequent to this, air turbine types were developed capable of generating speeds of 300,000 to 400,000 rpm. Although

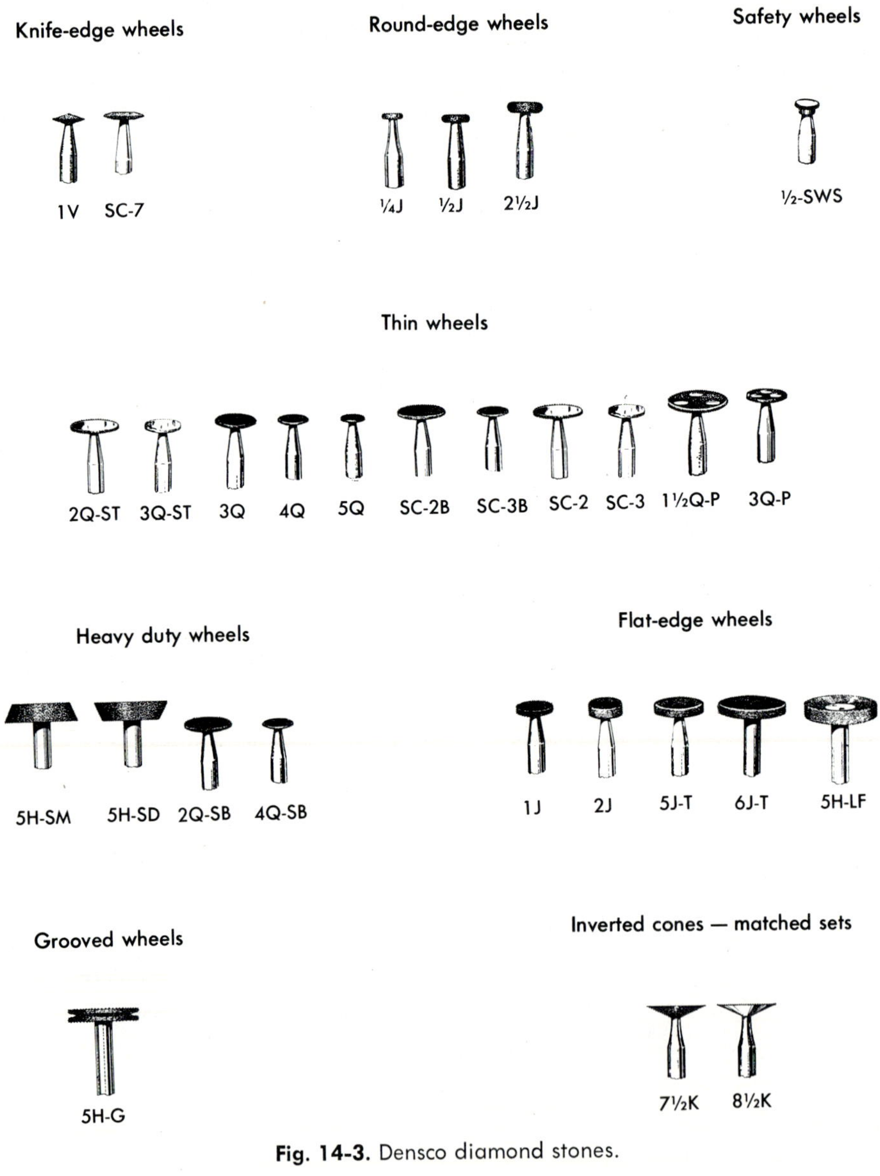

Fig. 14-3. Densco diamond stones.

the latter type of handpiece is capable of delivering high speeds, it possesses a lower torque. This is said to be an advantage because it prevents the application of excessive pressure on the cutting instrument during the preparation of the tooth. At the present time there is a difference of opinion as to the relative values of the high-speed gear-driven, belt-driven, and turbine types of contra-angle handpieces regarding the situations in which each of these may be best used.

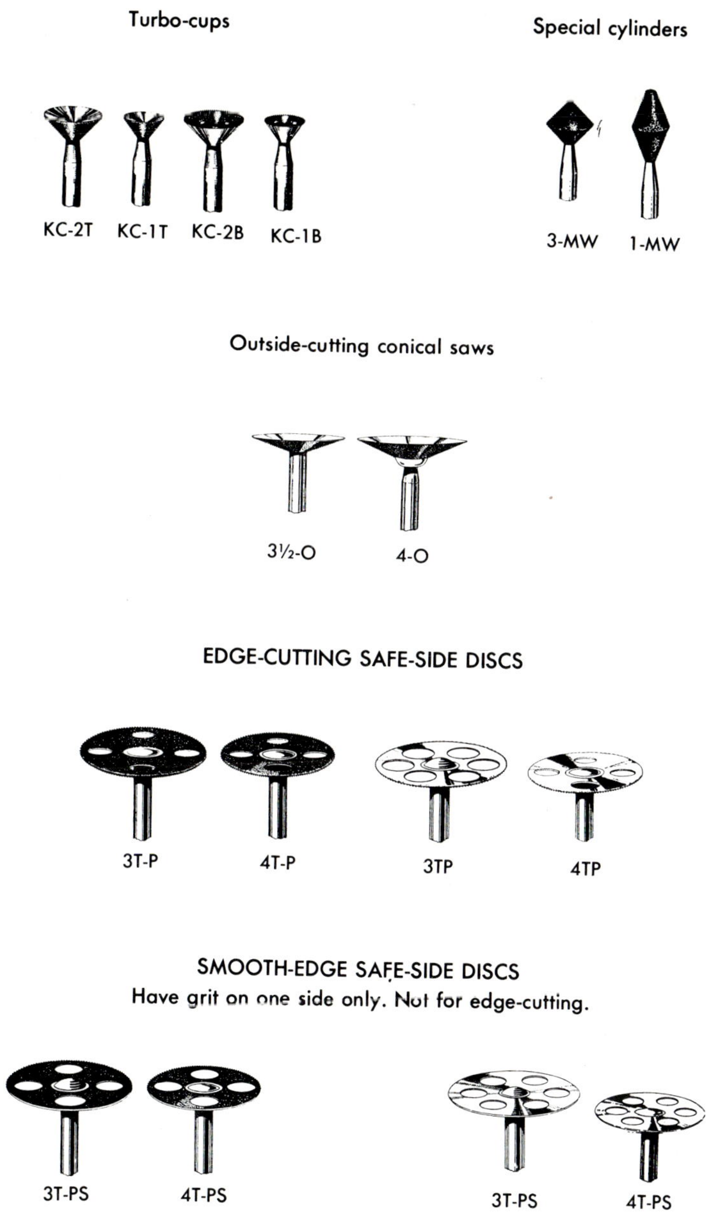

Fig. 14-4. Densco diamond stones.

HEAT GENERATION

Hudson and associates[6, 7] have shown that in cutting human dentin with dental burs the rise in temperature ranged from 150 to 275° F. This increase in temperature actually represents the release of the energy that bonds the molecules of the tooth structure. This is accomplished by the cutting action of the bur blades or the diamond crystals of the stone.

There are many factors that influence the rise in temperature which takes place in cutting operations—first, the speed of rotation of the cutting tool: the faster the tool revolves, the higher the resultant temperature. It has been found that a temperature rise is developed within 10 to 12 seconds after the cutting operation is started. Second, the size of the cutting instrument has an important bearing on heat generation, since its diameter affects the cutting speed at its periphery. A third factor in heat generation is the pressure applied by the dentist during cutting operations. It is known that as the pressure is increased in the cutting tool, the temperature rises in the substance cut. It is almost axiomatic that as the speed is increased, the pressure should be decreased. The size of the bur and the size of the stone are also relevant factors since the product of the pressure and the linear distance traveled by the rim of the cutting instrument represents the work done (Fig. 14-5).

In the selection of diamond stones, it is necessary to observe certain details of their manufacture, such as the type of crystals, their distribution, their size, and their sharpness. It is on these factors that the excessive generation of heat may depend. Similarly in the selection of burs, the same observations should be made as to the type of blade, its angulation, and the quality of its material.

An important consideration is the speed with which the generated heat is dispelled before it can affect the pulp adversely; this depends somewhat on the nature of the tooth tissue being cut, whether it is dentin or enamel that is being removed. The temperature differences result from a difference in their individual thermal conductivity and in their relative hardness. A cutting instrument primarily designed for cutting by lateral pressure should not be used for vertical cutting. It is important to estimate the proximity of the cutting operation to the pulp, for cutting the pulpal wall causes the increased temperature to reach the pulp sooner and in greater

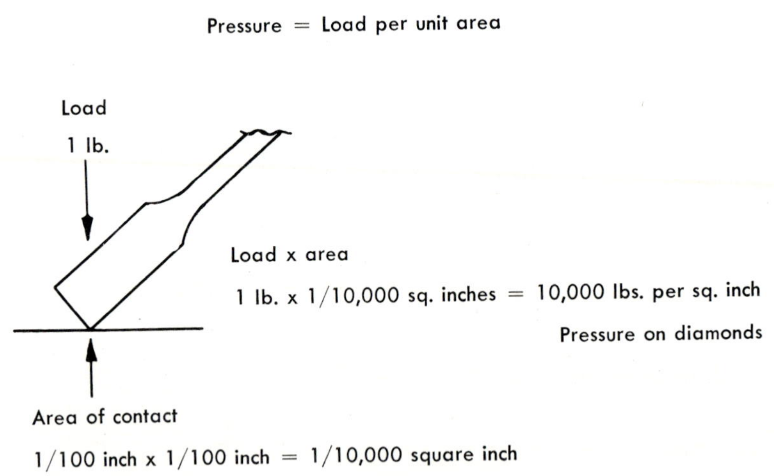

Fig. 14-5. Size of cutting instrument, speed, and pressure are relevant to work done. (Courtesy Dr. R. J. Nelsen.)

intensity than when the same temperature rise develops on the external surface of the enamel.

Coolants

Every means should be employed to keep the temperature down as much as possible during cutting operations. Coolants must be employed which, to be effective, should be applied at the *point of contact* between the cutting instrument and the tooth tissue. There are three types of coolants usually employed in dental practice: (1) water, (2) a spray of air and water, and (3) air alone. Peyton[8, 9] has shown that at speeds ranging from 30,000 rpm to 170,000 rpm and with an application of four ounces of pressure, a temperature rise within the tooth of less than 15° F. occurred when water or air-water sprays were employed. He also found that even with a water coolant, excessive temperatures developed when large diameter instruments or excessive forces were applied with increased operating speeds. This indicates that the mere use of a coolant, per se, does not eliminate the danger of excessive temperature rise.

A reduction in concentration of the amount of water used during the cutting procedure shows the significant temperature rise. The minimum volume of water to be applied was estimated at 1.5 ml. per minute. Increasing the applied load to the cutting instrument definitely affected the temperature rise.

The question whether water in spray form should be used at mouth or room temperature seemed to have no significance insofar as temperature rise in the tooth was concerned. Our experience has been that if the water reservoir is kept at 100° F., it is most comfortable to the patient, less liable to be harmful to the pulp, and still reduces the heat of friction during cutting.

Other problems have arisen with the use of the high-speed cutting tools. Most handpieces are so designed that a spray or stream of water is directed from the head of the handpiece directly onto the cutting operation. Where the water strikes the tooth and the stone directly, full benefit is obtained from the coolant. Where, however, the abrasive on the wheel is on the surface away from the stream of water, water does not flood the tooth surface being cut, resulting in excessive temperature rise. To overcome this difficutly, perforated disks have been developed which permit the water to go through the openings and lubricate the disk and tooth on the cutting side. The use of a perforated disk results in less temperature rise. Consequently where disks are nonperforated and when the stream of water cannot be directed to the cutting contact area, they should be used at speeds not exceeding 10,000 rpm.[10, 11]

Another advantage of a water coolant lies in the fact that the tooth debris from cutting is removed rapidly, preventing the clogging of the diamond stone. This results in greater cutting efficiency of the stone; also it prolongs the life and effectiveness of the instrument. It is essential that the water be in intimate contact with the revolving instrument and the tooth tissue. To do this more effectively, Nelsen[5] recommended the addition of a wetting agent to the water spray.

Because the high-speed technic requires a larger quantity of water as a coolant, there is the problem of removing this water from the mouth. To have the dentist stop frequently to allow the patient to spit out the excess water is time consuming; the customary saliva ejector has insufficient removal capacity.

The washed field technic as presented by Thompson[12] solves this problem. Evacuators possess definite advantages over the generally used saliva ejector. First, a most important advantage is that they permit the use of larger volumes of water to reduce temperature rise during the

Table 14-1. Physical properties of Vacudent versus aspirator*

	Vacudent	*Aspirator*
Mercury pull	3-4 inches	29.92 inches
Airflow: cu. ft. per min.	10.9	.33
Air velocity	120 mph	Slight
Pick up of water from air	75%-95%	None
Water "bridge"	12 mm.	3 mm.
Water removal (1 pint)	2 sec.	11-13 sec.
Pick up of solids	100%	Negligible
Effect on tissue	Gentle	Harsh
Tendency to clog	No clogging	Clogs easily

*From Better Dentistry, Denver, Colo., Densco, Inc.

cutting operation. Second, a steady stream of water may be applied so that it floods both the cutting instrument and the cut tooth surface; at the same time, the water is drawn across the operating field, keeping it clear and clean. Water is not permitted to accumulate in the floor of the mouth because it is immediately evacuated. While the normal saliva ejector may become clogged with small solid particles of debris, the high-velocity, negative airstream draws these away immediately. The airstream pulls 8 to 10 cubic feet per minute at a rate of about 125 miles per hour; however, it has a low mercury pull and for this reason does not suck in the soft tissues. (Table 14-1). Another advantage is that bacteria-laden cuttings and sprays are not blown into the atmosphere to be inhaled by the dentist or patient. There are several models of this equipment: the mobile-table type, the permanently attached wall type, and the small type that may be attached to the unit.

VIBRATION

Cutting a tooth may be very annoying and unpleasant to the patient but still not be painful. In pain, there is usually an involvement of the nerve endings, either by trauma or extreme irritation, resulting in an acute, painful reaction. Most patients, however, associate the sensations of vibration, noise, pressure, and the slight increase in cutting temperature with the sensation of pain.[5] Consequently, if the factors of vibration, heat, and pressure are reduced to a minimum, the patient usually concludes that the factor of pain has also been reduced or eliminated. Next in importance to reducing or eliminating heat in cutting comes that of reducing or eliminating vibration and excessive noise.

One of the mechanical factors that influences vibration is the dental handpiece, whether it is friction-bearing, ball-bearing, high-speed belt-driven, or the turbine ultra-speed type. When the friction-bearing, conventional type of handpiece is used at a speed of 4,500 rpm to 6,000 rpm it is connected by the conventional belt-and-pulley system of the dental motor. We may expect a high order of vibration depending upon the condition of the various mechanical parts, their adjustment, and speeds of their operation. Idler pulleys on the engine-arm that are worn, likewise a worn belt, or an improperly adjusted belt will cause vibrations that are transmitted down to the cutting tool. Similarly, handpieces which do not hold the cutting tool properly, which have worn bearings, or are out of adjustment will also cause vibration.

The investigations of Walsh and Symmons[13] showed that vibration, when applied to teeth, produced the most unfavorable responses when the frequency was between 100 cycles per second (cps) and 200 cps. When the frequencies were above 1,000 cps they were generally beyond the upper threshold of perception of the average patient. It is the lower frequencies, in the range of 100 to 200 cps, that are usually developed at the lower speeds, especially if the equipment is worn and maladjusted.

The importance of having concentricity in the cutting tool was reported by Hudson and associates.[6, 7] They found that eccentric burs when rotated at 6,000 to 10,000 rpm produced a lower frequency in the range of 100 to 200 cps, whereas a true running bur at 10,000 rpm produced vibrations in a frequency range above the unpleasant plateau. Tanner[14] pointed out that only a part of an eccentric bur or stone is used as it rotates, thus causing unfavorable impacts and vibrations which fall into the most annoying frequency range. Disks and stones that are unmounted and are screwed onto a mandrel very frequently are eccentric and therefore should not be used in high-speed cutting operations; the permanently mounted instruments are indicated in preference to the unmounted type.

Poorly built burs with blades not evenly cut or chipped will likewise cause vibration. In using new carbide burs, it is very important to see that none have chipped blades.

Correct adjustment of the belt is very important in the reduction and elimination of vibration. A belt that is too loose increases the vibration pattern transmitted directly to the tooth.

In the ultrahigh-speed handpieces the metal chuck holding the cutting instrument often is replaced by a rubber or plastic chuck. This lessens the vibration transmitted to the cutting instrument and facilitates the more rapid cutting action.

Cutting with a water turbine handpiece at 45,000 rpm the intensity of vibrations was well tolerated by the patient; he gave this an annoyance factor of four.

When the speed of cutting was increased to 80,000-120,000 rpm Hartley found that while the removal of tooth tissue was most effective, the frequency of vibrations was annoying to the patient. He assigned an annoyance factor of five to these speeds.[15]

Morrison and Grinnell[16] made the following informative observations:

> The deleterious effects of vibration are twofold in origin: (1) amplitude, and (2) undesirable modulating frequencies. If we can minimize or eliminate these factors, we can then reduce the undesirable effects of vibration.
>
> *Amplitude.* The wave of vibration consists of frequency and amplitude [Fig. 14-6]. At conventional speeds, amplitude is greater but frequency is less. At higher speeds the reverse is true. The greatest harm is caused by the amplitude of vibration which is the factor most destructive of instruments and which causes the most apprehension in the patient and the greatest fatigue in the dentist. By increasing operating speeds, the amplitude and its effects are reduced, and a more satisfactory result is attained.
>
> Vibration waves are measured in cycles per second. It has been shown that rotation of approximately 6,000 r.p.m. sets up a vibrational wave of approximately 100 cycles per second. This has been demonstrated to be the range most annoying to the patient and dentist. As the revolutions per minute are increased, the cycles per second of the fundamental vibration wave are increased until, at ranges of 100,000 r.p.m., we have a vibration wave of 1,600 cycles per second. In experiments conducted in vivo, it has been demonstrated that at wave of vibration of over 1,300 cycles per second, vibration is practically imperceptible to the patient [Fig. 14-7]. The reason for this is not fully understood, but

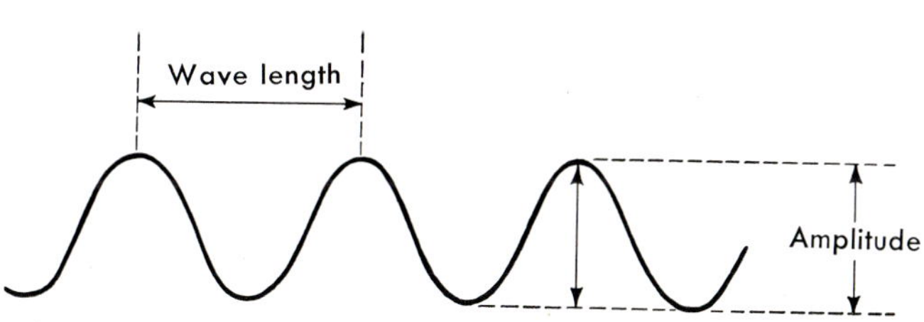

Fig. 14-6. Two factors causing undesirable effects of vibration. (From Morrison, A. H., and Grinnell, H. W.: J. Prosth. Dent. **8**:297, 1958.)

there are two theories for this phenomenon: (1) the Wedensky inhibition phenomenon holds that where stimulation occurs during the refractory period of recovery of the perceptor mechanism, no further reaction will be evident, and (2) due to light pressure and high speed, the chronaxie (the amount of stimulation multiplied by the frequency of stimulation necessary for a reaction) needed for vibratory perception, has not been attained [Fig. 14-8].

Thus it can be concluded that, the more the r.p.m., the less the amplitude, and the greater the frequency, vibratory perception will be lost in the ultra speed range of 100,000 r.p.m or more.*

*From Morrison, A. H., and Grinnell, H. W.: Theoretical and functional evaluation of higher speed rotary instrumentation, J. Prosth. Dent. **8:** 297, 1958.

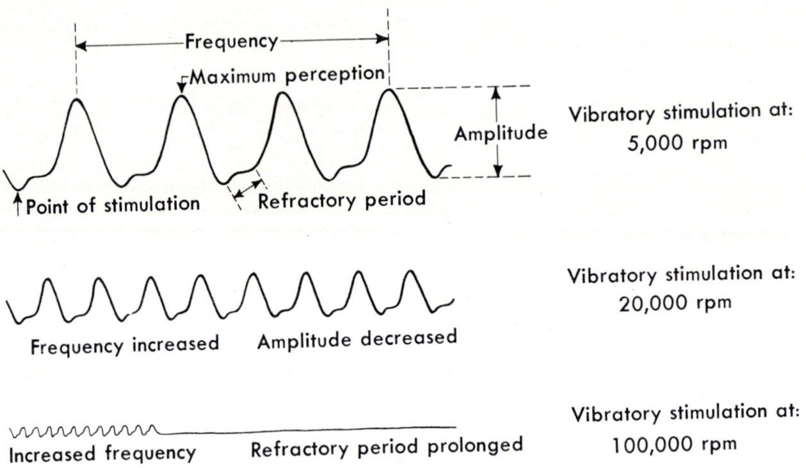

Fig. 14-7. Vibration waves increased in cycles per second. (From Morrison, A. H., and Grinnell, H. W.: J. Prosth. Dent. **8:**297, 1958.)

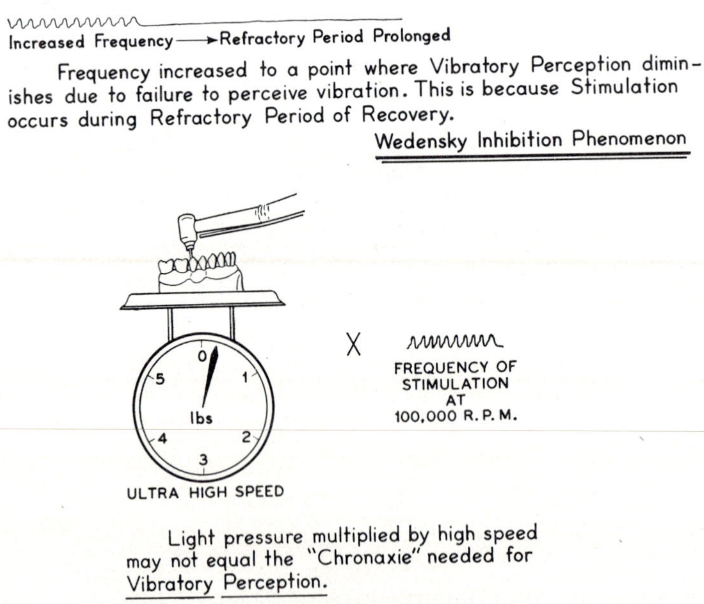

Fig. 14-8. (From Morrison, A. H., and Grinnell, H. W.: J. Prosth. Dent. **8:**297, 1958.)

SIZE OF CUTTING INSTRUMENT AND CUTTING SPEEDS

It has been pointed out by Peyton,[8, 9] Nelsen,[4, 5] and others that "*the important factor of increased operating speeds is the instrument surface speed in feet per minute rather than the revolution per minute of the instrument.*" The larger the diameter of the cutting instrument, the slower the speed required at the spindle. For example, in order to have surface speed of 5,000 feet per minute, it will require 300,000 rpm when using a 1/16 inch bur or stone. However, the same surface speed can be attained with a 3/4 inch disk at 30,000 rpm. Therefore, the specific phase in the preparation of a cavity or an abutment should determine the size of the cutting tool and the rpm that should be used. Employing super speeds for all operations, under all conditions, places unnecessary strain and danger upon the patient and equipment. If the same effect can be accomplished by using a larger instrument at a lower speed but still remaining above the threshold of perception, this should be done. *However, oversized cutting tools should not be used at super speeds due to the difficulty of instrument control and accuracy of cutting.*

It has been pointed out by Nelsen[4, 5] that each tool has its individual maximum cutting capacity, largely determined by the design of the tool and the manner in which the operator uses it.

In cutting at high and super speeds, the tools usually are carbide burs and diamond stones. McEwen[17] reported that the six-bladed carbide burs are very efficient at cutting speeds of 100,000 rpm and over. He believed that the most effective results are obtained when the carbide burs are used with a planing action rather than a milling action, and that burs utilized for extracoronal preparations need not be larger than No. 557.

For the diamond stones he recommended that the tapered cylinder stones should not exceed 2 mm. in diameter, the wheel stones not over 5 mm. in diameter, and the diamond disk when used should not exceed 1/2 inch in diameter.

Nelsen[5] recommended the use of an assortment of ten diamond stones and a cross-cut fissure bur No. 701. He added that where the small internal refinements in anterior and posterior cavities are necessary, very small steel burs may be used for this purpose at very slow speeds. Likewise, where decalcified tooth tissue is to be removed, round burs should be used.

Recognizing the many advantages which accrue with the present high-speed equipment and the accompanying diamond stones and carbide burs, "updating" instrumentation does not justify eliminating the use of the lower cutting speeds or the use of hand cutting instruments when indicated.

The rising percentage of need for endodontic treatment of teeth during the past 40 years may bear some relationship to the possible biologic pejorative reactions of the pulp to the misuse of super-high speeds with burs and stones.

THE BIOLOGIC RESPONSES OF THE PULP TO HIGH-SPEED CUTTING

The use of high speeds has focused greater attention upon the reactions of the tooth tissues to the accelerated cutting processes, particularly that of the pulp.[18, 19, 23] When cutting speeds did not exceed 6,000 to 10,000 rpm and concentric cutting tools were employed with a water spray, there was less worry about the reactions of the pulp. At these lower speeds and using the water spray, there might have been an initial discomfort of a temporary nature due to a slight pulpal reaction. This was usually a reversible reaction and within a few days the tenderness and slight inflammation of the pulp, if any developed, soon subsided with no serious, unfavorable reactions. As a matter of record, a clinical and roentgenographic study and recorded data over a period of 42 years, the number of pulps that died under such extensive restorations as complete, gold, porcelain, and porcelain fused to gold crowns has been less than 1 percent in the hands of dental students.

When high and super-high speeds are used improperly, danger to the pulp tissue arises. To employ high speeds safely, the specifications of the burs and stones used must meet very accurate standards: first, that of concentricity; second, that of size and shape of the crystals or the blades of a bur; third, whether the bur is made of good quality steel or tungsten carbide. Another factor endangering the pulp is the pressure applied to the cutting tool and the length of time that the cutting is done continuously.[5] An excess of either will influence the degree and rapidity of temperature rise both in the hard tissues and in the pulp. Finally, the proper type, temperature, and amount of coolant must be used to dissipate any temperature rise created during cutting.

Although the depth of the pulpal floor and its proximity to the pulp is always a vital concern, it is even greater with high speeds because of the rapidity with which tooth tissue is removed and the added danger of inadvertently cutting away more dentin than is desired. There still remains an unknown factor, namely, the individual resistance of the pulp to the cutting operation.

Limit of heat tolerance of the pulp

Although the upper limit of heat trauma which a pulp can withstand has not been definitely established, experiments[10] have shown that irreversible heat changes in the pulp may begin at 110° F. On the other hand, they also have demonstrated that a tooth may be heated up to 600° F. for a period of 10 seconds and still have the pulp recover as evidenced by a subsequent formation of secondary dentin. To avoid any injury to the pulp due to heat, some form of effective *coolant must be used.*

Not only does a coolant dissipate the heat generated but it also enables bringing the floor of the cavity closer to the pulp when necessary. The research of Swerdlow and Stanley[11] shows that when a preparation was brought to within 0.3 mm. of the pulp with the use of a coolant, there was no abscess formation. On the other hand, when the distance of the pulpal floor was placed twice as far from the pulp, namely, 0.6 mm., but no coolant was used, there was evidence of abscess formation, in addition to acute and prolonged unfavorable pulpal responses.

The pulp responds to any stimulus, and the nature and type of its response to a stimulus depends upon the intensity and length of time that the stimulus is applied. If it is a sustained and intense irritation, then an irreversible type of pulp injury may result.

ASPIRATED OR MISPLACED ODONTOBLASTS

A phenomenon associated with pulpal injury is the so-called "aspirated" odontoblast, where the nucleus is carried into the dentinal tubule, usually in three degrees: first, part of the nucleus moves into the tubule; second, the entire nucleus moves into the predentin tubule; finally, there is a third stage wherein the nucleus may travel any distance into the tubule.[18] One explanation given for this phenomenon is that in a severe irritation of the pulp, there is a crowding of the pulpal tissues within the confines of the pulp chamber causing a pressure against the odontoblastic layer; this is caused by hyperemia, edema, and inflammatory exudation. For this reason Swerdlow and Stanley prefer to use the word "displaced" rather than "aspirated," to designate those odontoblasts whose nuclei have been found in the dentinal tubules.[11, 18]

In 1957, Marsland and Shovelton prepared cavities in thirty-four teeth with tungsten-carbide burs at speeds ranging from 1,000 to 15,000 rpm.[19] They extracted the teeth at time periods of up to 28 days and compared their pulpal histology with that of control teeth. They found odontoblastic nuclei aspirated into the dentinal tubules under the cavities. Extensive vacuolization of the odontoblast layer was also demonstrated.

Brännstrom cut cylindrical cavities on the buccal aspects of teeth scheduled for extraction and connected a vacuum pump to the cavities.[20-22] Reduced pressure was applied for 2 to 3 minutes and the teeth were immediately extracted. Many odontoblast nuclei were found in the tubules beneath the cavities. He found that the application of an airstream for up to 2 minutes also caused aspiration of odontoblast nuclei. When he applied steam for 45 seconds to cavities he rarely found aspiration, while application of dry heat at 100° C. routinely caused aspiration. Brännstrom concluded from these findings that evaporation of moisture from the tubules resulted in a capillary force, which displaced the contents of the tubules outward. The evaporation of water created opened tubules at the cavity floor, making the development of capillary force possible.

Brännstrom found that a 30-second blast of air will aspirate nuclei approximately 100 microns into the tubules. In a later study he found that the cells aspirated at the time of dentin desiccation disappear from the tubules after 6 to 24 hours. He postulated that the cell nuclei present in the tubules after 24 hours may not be the same as those aspirated at the time the cavities were first cut. He believed that secondary aspiration results from leaky restorations until reparative dentin caused the formation of dead tracts in the dentin. He found reparative dentin forming under the cavities after 1 to 3 months.

It is generally assumed that pulp temperatures rise during cutting operations of the tooth, even more when done without a water spray. These conclusions are based largely on experiments performed on extracted teeth. Bhaskar and Lilly undertook an investigation to determine if preparations in vivo with the high speeds would produce significant temperature changes within the pulp itself.[23]

Under conventional methods of cavity preparation they found a drop in the intrapulpal temperature. They concluded that there were factors other than heat which might be causing changes in pulp tissues. These might be the drop in temperature, desiccation, or the cutting of the odontoblastic processes. They noticed that, the deeper the cavity was cut toward the pulp, the lower was the temperature attained in the pulp. They concluded that pulpal changes are not necessarily due to heat production in cavity preparation. The possible other causes of pulpal injury they list as dehydration under an air blast and the severance of the odontoblastic extensions in the dentin.

Nelsen[4] observed, with due respect to histologic investigations reported in the literature, that "the evaluation of cutting procedures histologically by describing a pulp 'reaction' without carefully stating the energy applied, in terms of total dose and dose rate, is as meaningless as the evaluation of a sun lamp singularly in terms of skin reaction without stating total exposure, rate of exposure, wave lengths of the light used, and the type of skin irradiated. Not until 'histopathological evaluations' are qualified by adequate descriptions of the total cutting procedure, in terms of quality and quantity of energy applied, will they have any greater values than the conclusions of the clinicians about the relative merits of one cutting procedure and another."[5]

Carefully kept clinical records for over 40 years testify to the unusual recuperative powers of the pulp following the cutting of a tooth. When the usual precautions, correct instruments, and a careful technic are employed, the pulp need not be injured permanently.

As with all newer materials, instruments, and methods, the high-speed technics will prove their value only if they are understood and properly used.

SELECTED REFERENCES

1. Kilpatrick, H. C.: Problems and solutions in high speed dentistry, J. Connecticut D. A. **31**:20, 1951.
2. Kilpatrick, H. C.: High speed and ultra speed in dentistry, Philadelphia, 1959, W. B. Saunders Co.
3. Walsh, J. P., and Symmons, H. F.: Comparison of heat production and mechanical efficiency of diamond instruments, stones and burs at 3,000 and 60,000 r.p.m., New Zealand D. J. **45**:28, 1949.
4. Nelsen, R. J.: Turbine hydraulic handpiece; its use in operative dentistry, New York J. Dent. **26**:308, 1956.
5. Nelsen, R. J., and Nelsen, A. E.: The patient, the tooth and the dentist: a modern perspective of tooth preparation, J.A.D.A. **58**:1, 1959.
6. Hudson, D. C., and Sweeney, W. T.: Temperatures developed in rotating dental instruments, J.A.D.A. **48**:127, 1945.
7. Hudson, D. C., Sweeney, W. T., and Dickson, G.: Methods for evaluation of rotating diamond-abrasive dental instruments, J.A.D.A. **54**:637, 1957.
8. Peyton, F. A.: Effectiveness of water coolants with rotary cutting instruments, J.A.D.A. **56**: 664, 1958.
9. Peyton, F. A.: Response to shaping cavities in teeth, Bull. Chicago Dent. Soc. **38**:11, 1957.
10. Kennedy, J. J., Buckman, N., and Proffit, W. R.: Biological response to high speed instruments, J.A.D.A. **58**:35, 1959.
11. Swerdlow, H., and Stanley, H. R., Jr.: Human pulpal reactions following 20,000 r.p.m. preparations with and without coolants, Int. Dent. **31**:10, 1957.
12. Thompson, E. O.: Clinical application of the washed field technic in dentistry, J.A.D.A. **51**:703, 1955.
13. Walsh, J. R., and Symmons, H. F.: Vibration perception and frequencies, New Zealand D. J. **45**:28, 1949.
14. Tanner, H. M.: Greater efficiency through modern instruments and higher speeds, Ann. Dent. **15**:34, 1956.
15. Hartley, J. L., and others: Comparative evaluation of newer devices and technics for the removal of tooth structure, J. Prosth. Dent. **8**:170, 1958.
16. Morrison, A. H., and Grinnell, H. W.: Theoretical and functional evaluation of higher speed rotary instrumentation, J. Prosth. Dent. **8**:297, 1958.
17. McEwen, R. A.: High speed preparations, Dent. Clin. N. Amer., March, 1957.
18. Stanley, H. R., Jr., and Swerdlow, H.: Aspiration of cells into dentinal tubules, Oral Surg. **11**:1007, 1958.
19. Marsland, E. A., and Shovelton, D. S.: Displacement of odontoblasts associated with cavity preparation, J.A.D.A. **59**:1257, 1959.
20. Brännstrom, M.: Dentinal and pulpal response, I, application of reduced pressure to exposed dentin; an experimental study, Acta Odont. Scand. **18**:1, 1960.
21. Brännstrom, M.: Dentinal and pulpal response, II, application of an air stream to exposed dentin; short observation period, Acta Odont. Scand. **18**:17, 1960.
22. Bränstrom, M.: Dentinal pulpal response, III, application of an air stream to exposed dentin; long observation periods; an experimental study, Acta Odont. Scand. **18**:234, 1960.
23. Bhaskar, S. N., and Lilly, G. H.: Intrapulpal temperature during cavity preparation, J. Dent. Res. **44**(4):644, 1965.

GENERAL REFERENCES

Agnew, R. G.: Rationale for the pain problem in dental practice, Dent. Clin. N. Amer. pp. 565-581, July 1959.

Alonso, H. M. D., Van Huysen, G., and Johnston, J. F.: Changes in pulp and periodontal tissues of teeth subjected to crown prosthesis, J. Prosth. Dent. **10**:350, 1960.

Anderson, D. J., and Naylor, M. N.: Sensation in human dentin, J. Dent. Res. **40**:1275, 1961.

Aplin, A. W.: A modified cutting procedure using the air-turbine handpiece, J. Kentucky Dent. Assn. **19**:13-17, 1967.

Arnim, S. S.: Conservation of the dental pulp—cavity preparation, J. Prosth. Dent. **9**:1017, 1959.

Arnim, S. S., and Hagerman, D. A.: effect of periodontal treatment on the connective tissue fibers of the marginal gingiva: II, J.A.D.A. **58**:60, 1959.

Arnold, M. L.: Tips on how to maintain a dry field, D. Survey **38**:42, 1962.

Awazawa, Y.: Electron microscopy of carious dental enamel, 2: with reference to incipient caries, J. Nihon Univ. School Dent. **4**:25, 1961.

Ball, J. S., and Davidson, C. W.: Estimation of air turbine rotational speed under clinical conditions, Brit. D. J. **112**:208, 1962.

Belting, C. M., Haberfelde, G. C., and Juhl, L. K.: Spread of organisms from dental air rotor, J.A.D.A. **68**:648-651, 1964.

Benfield, J.: Work simplification in dental practice. In Kilpatrick, H.: Applied time and motion studies, Philadelphia, 1963, W. B. Saunders Co.

Berk, H.: Preservation of the dental pulp in deep seated cavities, J.A.D.A. **54**:226, 1957.

Berke, J. D.: Further studies on the nature of the organic matrix of human enamel, New York D. J. **27**:59, 1961.

Bernier, J. L., and Knapp, M. J.: Methods used in evaluation of high-speed dental instruments and some results, Oral Surg. **12**:234, 1959.

Bernier, J. L., and Knapp, M. J.: A new pulpal response to high-speed dental instruments, Oral Surg. **11**:167-183, 1958.

Bissell, S. L.: Study of air turbine versus conventional handpiece on odontectomies, J.A.D.A. **72**:645-647, 1966.

Bouschor, C. F., and others: A four-year clinical study of teeth restored after preparation with an air turbine handpiece with an air coolant, J. Prosth. Dent. **16**:306-309, 1966.

Brown, R. V.: Bacterial aerosols generated by ultra high-speed cutting instruments, J. Dent. Child. **32**:112-117, 1965.

Brunel, A. L., and Griffie, R. A.: Spectrometric evaluation of emissions from air-driven handpieces, D. Progress **2**:85, 1962.

Brunel, A. L., and Griffie, R. A.: Chief benefits of high speed reaped by operative work, crown and bridge, D. Survey **38**:50, 1962.

Burhani, H.: Protection of dentist's health against air turbine dangers, Rev. Dent. Syrie **3**(1): 5-14, 1967.

Cantwell, K. R., Tunturi, A. R., and Manny, V. R.: Noise from high speed dental handpieces, J.A.D.A. **61**:571-577, 1960.

Cantwell, K. R., Tunturi, A. R., and Sorenson, F. M.: Noise levels of a newly designed handpiece, J. Prosth. Dent. **15**:356-359, 1965.

Charbeneau, G. T.: Use of ultrasonic techniques for cleaning instruments and appliances, J. Prosth. Dent. **11**:573, 1961.

Charbeneau, G. T., and Berry, G. C.: Simple and effective autoclave method of handpiece and instrument sterilization without corrosion, J.A.D.A. **59**:732, 1959.

Charbeneau, G. T., and others: Profile characteristics of cut tooth surfaces developed by rotating instruments, J. Dent. Res. **36**:957, 1957.

Christensen, G. J., and others: The use of ultrahigh speed handpieces in restorative dentistry, J. Kentucky Dent. Ass. **18**:18-24, 1966.

Cleveland, L. L.: Sensitivity and desensitization of tooth structure, J. A. D. Hyg. A. **32**:20, 1958.

Collins, E. M.: Desensitization of hypersensitive teeth, D. Digest **68**:360, 1962.

Cooperman, H. N., and others: Radiated noise from high speed dental handpieces, D. Digest **71**:404-407, 1966.

Craig, R. G., and Peyton, F. A.: Elastic and mechanical properties of human dentin, J. Dent. Res. **37**:710, 1958.

Craig, R. G., and Peyton, F. A.: Microhardness of enamel and dentin, J. Dent. Res. **37**:661, 1958.

Custer, F., and Andersen, R.: New method of sterilizing handpieces, New York J. Dent. **38**: 8-17, 1968.

Dachi, S. F., and Stigers, R. W.: Pulpal effects of water and air coolants used in high-speed cavity preparations, J.A.D.A. **76**:95-98, 1968.

Degering, C. I.: Physiologic evaluation of dental-pulp testing methods, J. Dent. Res. **41**:695, 1962.

Eichner, K.: Investigation on cutting and grinding procedures on the hard tooth structure and ivory, Australian D. J. **10**:214-216, 1965.

Eichner, K.: Practical results of scientific investigations of high speed cutting, Internat. D. J. **11**:293, 1961.

Fraser, E. D.: High speed and the dentist's responsibilities, Roy. Canad. D. Corps Quart. **1**: 13, 1961.

French, G. H. T.: Class I and II preparations with air turbine, Texas D. J. **77**:3, 1959.

Gardner, A. F., and Hecht, A.: High speed—what does it do to the dental pulp?, J. Dent. Child. **29**:72-84, 1962.

Grundy, R. J.: Enamel aerosols created during use of the air turbine handpiece, J. Dent. Res. **46**:409-415, 1967.

Grundy, J. R.: Symptoms attributed to the air turbine, Dent. Pract. **17**:17-20, 1966.

Hamilton, A. I., and Kramer, I. R. H.: Cavity preparation with and without water spray, Brit. Dent. J. **123**:281-285, 1967.

Hartley, J. L., and Hudson, D. C.: Modern rotating instruments: burs and diamond points, Dent. Clin. N. Amer. pp. 737-745, Nov., 1958.

Hartnett, J. E., and Smith, W. F.: Production of heat in the dental pulp by use of the air turbine, J.A.D.A. **63**:210, 1961.

Hauler, W. J., Jr., and Madden, R. M.: Microbiologic comparison of dental handpieces, 2: aerosol decay and dispersion, J. Dent. Res. **45**:52-58, 1966.

Hesselgren, S. G., and Forstell, G.: Chemical disinfection of handpieces and contra-angles, Svensk Tandlak. T. **55**:211, 1962.

Holden, G. G. P.: Some observations on the vibratory phenomena associated with high speed air turbines and their transmission to living tissue, Brit. D. J. **113**:265, 1962.

Hunter, H. A., and Madlener, E. M.: Disinfection of dental instruments, Internat. D. J. **11**:312, 1961.

Ingraham, R.: Evaluation of turbine, belt and gear driven type handpieces for producing ultra high speeds, J. South. California D. A. **27**: 86, 1959.

James, V. E., and others: Biology of the pulp and its defense, J.A.D.A. **59**:903, 1959.

Johnston, C. M.: Sterilization of dental handpieces, Brit. D. J. **110**:205, 1961.

Kaminszcik, I., Jarer, E., and Salvatori, J. M.: Trauma acustico provocado por las turbinas de alta velocidad en los odontologos, Rev. de la Associacion Medica Argentina **80**:625-634, 1966.

Kaminszcik, I., Salvatori, J. M., Pettinari, M., and Sanz, S.: Trauma acustico por ultrasonidos, Fonoaudiologica **10**:228-230, 1964.

Kasloff, Z.: Continuing study of cracks in teeth associated with various rotary cutting instruments, J. Canad. D. A. **28**:244, 1962.

Kasloff, Z., Swartz, M. L., and Phillips, R. W.: An in vitro method for demonstrating the effects of various cutting instruments on tooth structure, J. Prosth. Dent. **12**:1166, 1962.

Kazantzis, G.: Air contamination from high speed dental drills, Proc. Roy. Soc. Med. **54**:242-244, 1961.

Kennedy, F. F., Hansen, L. S., Scofield, H. H., Neilsen, A. G., and Buckman, N.: Pulpal response to various high-speed cutting instruments, Dent. Progress **3**:6-12, 1962.

Kilpatrick, H. C.: Ultra-speed and auxiliary equipment in fixed partial denture construction, J. Prosth. Dent. **10**:574, 1960.

Kohari, S., and Bona, K.: Study of enamel and dentin in persons of different ages, D. Abst. **6**:468, 1961.

Kondo, S., and Hori, Y.: Study on transaction of changes in pulp observed after cavity preparation, especially that of clinical findings, Bull. Tokyo D. Col. **2**:1, 1961.

Kramer, I. R. H.: Changes following cavity preparation usuing turbine handpieces, J. Dent. Res. **39**:1100, 1960.

Kramer, I. R. H.: Changes in dentin during cavity preparation using turbine handpieces, Proc. Roy. Soc. Sec. Odont. **54**:244-248, 1961.

Kramer, I. R. H.: The effects of cavity preparation on the dental pulp, Aust. Dent. J. **12**(6): 565-569, 1967.

von Krammer, K. R.: High speed equipment and dentist's health, J. Prosth. Dent. **19**(1):46, 1968.

Langeland, K.: Tissue changes incident to cavity preparation; an evaluation of some dental engines, Acta Odont. Scand. **19**:397, 1961.

Langeland, K., and Langeland, L. K.: Cutting procedures with minimized trauma, J.A.D.A. **76**:991-1005, 1968.

Larato, D. C.: Sterilization of the high-speed dental handpiece, D. Digest **72**:107-109, 1966.

Larato, D. C., Ruskin, P. F., and Martin, A.: Effect of dental air turbine drill on the bacterial counts in air, J. Prosth. Dent. **16**:758, 1966.

Madden, R. M., Hausler, W. J., Jr., and Leaverton, P. E.: Study of some factors contributing to aerosol production by the air-turbine handpiece, J. Dent. Res. **48**(3):341, 1969.

Massler, M., and Servaty, M.: Effects of different cutting procedures on dentin apposition in rat incisors, J. Dent. Res. **39**:619, 1960.

Morrant, G. A.: Noise of air turbine handpiece related to acoustic trauma, J. Dent. Res. **39**: 1109, 1960.

Morrant, G. A., and Kramer, I. R. H.: The response of human pulp to cavity preparations using turbine handpieces, Brit. D. J. **115**:99-110, 1963.

Morrant, G. A., and Stephens, R. R.: Development and application of modern methods in cavity preparation, Brit. D. J. **109**:42, 73, 114, 155, 1960.

Muntz, M. L., Gilmore, R. W., and Pigman, W.: Microhardness studies of intact surface enamel, J. Dent. Res. **36**:732, 1957.

National Naval Medical Center: Noise levels of higher speed dental equipment, Navy M. News Letter **38**:30, 1961.

Nixon, G. S., and Tilston, D. R.: Inhalation of oil particles from air turbine handpieces, Brit. D. J. **119**:114-117, 1965.

Peyton, F. A., and Morrant, G. A.: High speed and other instruments for cavity preparation, Internat. D. J. **9**:309, 1959.

Pistocco, L. R., and Bowers, G. M.: Demonstration of an aerosol produced by the air water spray and air turbine handpiece, Navy M. News Letter **40**:24, 1962.

Plischka, G., and Dimeg, K.: Studies of optimal particle size of diamond instruments in dentistry, Zahnaerztl Rundsch **77**(1):9-12, 1968.

Prevedello, P., Luksich, G., and Faggian, I.: Osservazioni sul trauma acustico determinato dall' uso di trapani a turbina nella pratica odontoiatrica, Ann. Stomat. **13**:543-557, 1964.

Riley, R. L., and O'Grady, F.: Air-borne infections: transmission and control, New York, 1961, The Macmillan Company.

Schubert, E. D., and Glorig, A.: Noise exposure from dental drills, J.A.D.A. **66**:751-757, 1963.

Schuchard, A. S.: Evaluation of high and ultrahigh speed cutting equipment, J. California D. A. **37**:99, 1961.

Schuchard, A.: Action of water coolants with ultra-high rotating speeds, J. Prosth. Dent. **12**: 559, 1962.

Schuchard, A., and others: Comparative efficiency of rotary cutting instruments, J. Prosth. Dent. **15**:908-923, 1965.

Schuchard, A., and Watkins, E. C.: Cutting effectiveness of tungsten carbide burs and diamond points at ultra-high rotational speeds, J. Prosth. Dent. **18**(1):58-65, 1967.

Schuchard, A. S., and Watkins, E. C.: Temperature response to increased rotational speeds, J. Prosth. Dent. **11**:313, 1961.

Schuchard, A., and Watkins, E. C.: Thermal and histologic response to high speed and ultra high-speed cutting in tooth structure, J.A.D.A. **71**:1451-1458, 1966.

Semmelman, J. O., Kulp, P. R., and Kurlansik, L.: Cutting studies at air-turbine speeds, J. Dent. Res. **40**:404, 1961.

Shima, Y., and others: Study on cavity preparation, I: appearance of cut tooth surfaces developed by the use of a chisel 15 and instruments at varying rotating speeds of operation, D. Bull. Osaka Univ. **1**:35, 1960.

Stanley, H. R.: Traumatic capacity of high speed and ultrasonic dental instrumentation, J.A.D.A. **63**:750, 1961.

Stephens, R. R.: Symposium on the use of high speeds in cavity preparation, Proc. Roy. Soc. Med. Sec. Odont. **54**:239, 1961.

Stevens, R. E., Jr.: Preliminary study—air contamination with microorganisms during use of air turbine handpieces, J.A.D.A. **66**:237-239, 1963.

Stevenson, S. B., Jr.: Variables of cavity and crown preparations and their effect on the human pulp, Pennsylvania D. J. **64**:48, 1960.

Swerdlow, H., and Stanley, H. R., Jr.: Reaction on the human dental pulp to cavity preparation, part II: at 150,000 r.p.m., with an air-water spray, J. Prosth. Dent. **9**:121, 1959.

Taylor, W., Pearson, J., and Mair, A.: The hearing threshold levels of dental practitioners exposed to air turbine drill noise, Brit. D. J. **118**: 296-310, 1965.

Travaglini, E. A., and Larato, D. C.: A disposable dental face mask with a plastic eye shield for operating with the air turbine drill, J. Prosth. Dent. **15**:525-527, 1965.

Travaglini, E. A., Larato, D. C., and Martin, A.: Dissemination of organism-bearing droplets by high-speed dental drills, J. Prosth. Dent. **16**: 132-139, 1966.

Troxell, R. R.: High speed technics in crown and bridge prosthodontics, New York J. Dent. **28**: 222, 1958.

Zach, L., and Cohen, G.: Thermogenesis in operative techniques: comparison of four methods, J. Prosth. Dent. **12**:977, 1962.

Chapter 15

Tooth preparations and instrumentation: class I, type 1—anterior intracoronal retainers

Prior to constructing a fixed partial denture, the dentist must make a comprehensive examination of the existing oral condition as well as the general condition of the patient. Complete clinical and roentgenographic records and a set of correctly mounted diagnostic casts are prime requirements for a meaningful diagnosis and for determining sound biologic and mechanical plans of treatment before, during, and after oral rehabilitation. The preoperative steps were discussed in Chapters 2 and 3 and, as indicated, may involve many procedures. Not only is the preparation of the teeth for crowns or bridge retainers important, but likewise evaluation of the type of the existing occlusion, of disorders of the temporomandibular articulation, of surgical removal of teeth or other tissues, and of the treatment of pathologic conditions of the supporting and contiguous soft tissues is needed. Frequently this may also entail the splinting of functionally impaired teeth.

Diagnostic study casts mounted in centric relation in an adjustable articulator and utilizing a hinge axis facebow are very often helpful in determining the design and method of preparing a tooth for a crown or bridge retainer.

Having appraised the biologic tolerance of the abutment teeth, the periodontal membrane, and bone support clinically and radiographically, the physical and mechanical engineering aspects of the prosthesis require equal consideration.

First among the latter is the total structure itself: (1) the number, size, position, and anatomic integrity of each abutment tooth (see Chapter 2); (2) the length, dimensions, and curvature of the bridge span and the forces that may be placed upon the structure; (3) the materials, and their manipulation, of which the appliance is to be made; (4) the design of the supporting retainers to tolerate the anticipated displacing forces of occlusion; (5) instrumentation and steps of procedure; (6) construction of pontics; (7) methods of connecting the component units of the bridge (connectors); and, finally, (8) the methods of fixation and postoperative procedures.

Bridge retainers are classified into two general groups, the intracoronal and the extracoronal. The intracoronal retainers may be placed in the anterior and the posterior teeth and involve two or more surfaces: the DL, ML, MO, DO, and MOD, as well as the MODL and similar types are examples of this class (Chapter 13).

Intracoronal retainers

An intracoronal retainer is one that is largely or entirely confined within the contour of the crown and whose retentive forces are effective within the body of the tooth; its exposed surface area is generally less than that lying within the cavity.

INDICATIONS

The indications for intracoronal retainers are determined to some extent by the age of the patient. Although fixed partial denture prosthesis is primarily a service for patients between 20 and 55 years of age, there are numerous instances in which younger patients also require it.[1] When planning restorations for the latter group, extreme caution must be exercised not to use a retainer whose preparation requires the removal of relatively large amounts of tooth structure, since such a requisite brings the pulp into close proximity to the restoration. Unless the position and size of the pulp chamber are such as to preclude the possibility of subsequent pulp irritations from thermal shock, the intracoronal types of retainers should not be used; instead, some form of extracoronal retention should be employed.

A clinical condition that frequently confronts the dentist is the loss of a lower first molar in a patient 12 to 14 years of age whose second molar is erupted. In the desire to maintain normal alignment and space between the second molar and the second bicuspid, dentists sometimes construct space maintainers with intracoronal retainers, when, for example, an MOD is placed in a recently erupted second molar. Unless extreme care is taken, the pulp or its pulpal horns may be exposed during the preparation of the cavity for the MOD inlay. In such cases it is much safer to use a removable appliance, which does not require the cutting of the molar and bicuspid; if a fixed space maintainer is unavoidable, some form of extracoronal retention should be employed.

Similar dangers exist when one of the anterior teeth in young patients is accidentally lost. If teeth adjacent to an edentulous space are cut into for intracoronal retainers, there is great danger of pulp exposure or at least of severe pulp irritation; hence it is better to construct some type of removable partial denture, which the patient may use until such time as it will be safe to cut into the teeth.

Intracoronal retainers, both anterior and posterior, are primarily indicated in short span prostheses. Where two or more teeth are replaced, it is very doubtful whether the standard intracoronal retainer can be successfully used without some modification of its retentive form. It is questionable whether the intracoronal retainer should be used when three missing teeth are replaced anteriorly.

The two- and three-surface intracoronal retainers are indicated in a three-tooth bridge that restores one lost tooth. In such a restoration one of the retainers, which may be a two-surface inlay, is grooved to receive a tapered key used in conjunction with the broken stress principle.

Where used, the intracoronal types of retainers require abutments that are physically suitable for their reception; namely, teeth that are sufficiently long gingivoincisally or gingivoclusally and teeth that are sound and not weakened by excessive decay. Where the teeth are abraded or short or where the cusps are not supported by healthy dentin, the intracoronal type of retainer is contraindicated.

INTRACORONAL RETAINERS IN PULPLESS TEETH

Clinically, it has been observed that those teeth from which the pulp has been removed are not capable of withstanding torque and other stresses developed in a bridge as well as teeth with vital pulps.

Consequently, the extracoronal type of retainers is indicated for pulpless teeth. Where intracoronal retainers are used in *pulpless teeth,* particularly in the posterior region, the buccal and lingual cusps should *always* be protected on the occlusal surface by covering and including them within the casting.

Where conditions are favorable for the reception of an intracoronal retainer, the esthetic values are usually more easily attainer than with the extracoronal types.

Two- and three-surface intracoronal retainers may be used in the upper anterior teeth, including the incisors and cuspids. The two-surface intracoronal retainer is employed only to support a tapered nonrigid connector; rarely is this type of retainer soldered to a pontic. When a central incisor or cuspid is sufficiently long gingivoincisally and is of normal labiolingual thickness, a three-surface intracoronal retainer, such as the MLD, may also be successfully used. Moreover, under very favorable conditions a pin modified three-surface retainer may be soldered to the pontic.

In preparing an anterior tooth for a two-surface retainer, for example a DL inlay, the access to the distal surface is simplified since there is an edentulous space next to the tooth. Where, however, the proximating tooth is still present, as in the immediate replacement type of bridge prosthesis, it is necessary that separation be first secured between the distal surface of the abutment and its neighbor.

REMOVAL OF CARIES

When caries is present, it should be removed first, in preference to other steps, in order to determine its extent; likewise, the presence of any undermined enamel is ascertained. With rare exceptions, all such enamel should be removed. Where the possibility of pulp exposure exists, it is advisable to apply the rubber dam before removing all of the carious tooth structure.

In removing tooth decay, the dentist is confronted with the decision of what constitutes carious tooth structure and to what extent the dentin should be removed when it is stained or discolored.

Without question, all carious dentin that is soft and leathery should be excavated; this is usually done with spoon-type hand instruments or very cautiously with a larger round bur at very low speed, the former being preferred. When dentin is encountered which is hard and offers the same resistance to the cutting edge of an instrument that other normal dentin does,

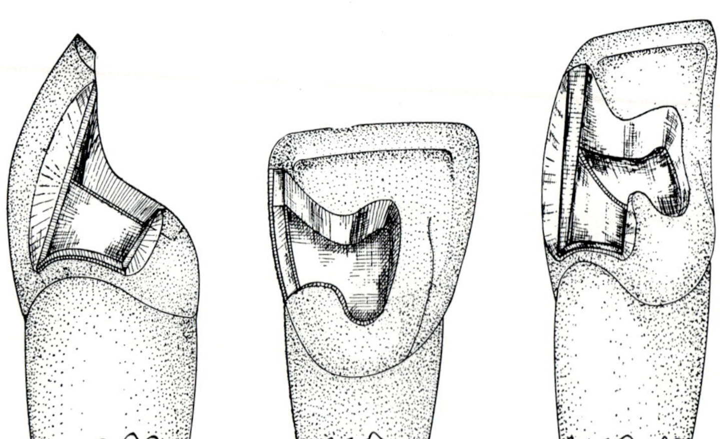

Fig. 15-1. Intracoronal retainer preparation used primarily with broken-stress principle.

it is safe to assume that sound tooth structure has been reached, even though it may show some discoloration. While the investigations of Beust[2] and others indicate that the dentinal tubules extending from such areas to the pulp are modified structurally, and the pulp responds by laying down secondary dentin opposite the terminations of these tubules, it is reasonable to assume that this is a protective mechanism established by Nature to ward off and forestall the deleterious effects of caries. Discolored but sound dentin may be retained provided: first, that it does not lie so close to the pulp that the pulp is already involved; second, that it is thoroughly cleaned and sealed; third, that a protection against termal shock be supplied by covering it with a suitable nonirritating base. Many of the suggestions offered in Chapter 4 are also applicable here.

Clinical evidence indicates that discolored but sound dentin exerts no apparently harmful effect on the pulp. Under no circumstances, however, is there justification for leaving decayed dentin beneath a permanent restoration.

STEPS IN THE PREPARATION OF AN ANTERIOR CLASS I, TYPE 1, INTRACORONAL RETAINER

Outline form

While the outline form of a DL or an ML inlay in an anterior tooth is more limited than that of an extracoronal retainer, special care should be taken to extend the margin sufficiently in a labial direction so that it can be readily cleaned or be made self-cleansable after the installation of the bridge (Fig. 15-1). So frequently in overemphasizing the esthetic factors, sufficient labial extension is not obtained, with the result that recurrence of caries ultimately occurs in this area.

Lingually (Fig. 15-2), the outline form is less extensive in this type of retainer because of the wide embrasure which is usually present between the proximal surfaces of the abutment and the adjoining pontic; the gingival margin, however, should be dropped so that it extends slightly below the crest of the gingiva into the gingival crevice. This extension, however, is contingent upon the age of the patient and the amount of epithelial attachment still present; in a situation in which the depth of the gingival crevice is zero, the level of the gingival margin of the inlay terminates above the level of the gingival crest.

Resistance and retention forms

As explained in Chapter 13, the resistance and retention forms of a two-surface

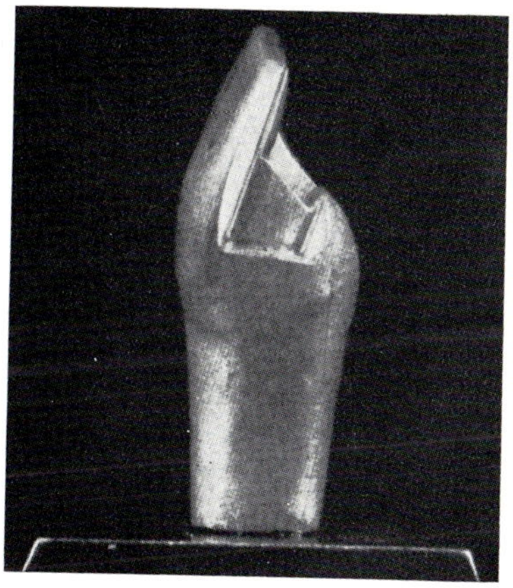

Fig. 15-2. Proximal view showing limited extension of lingual wall.

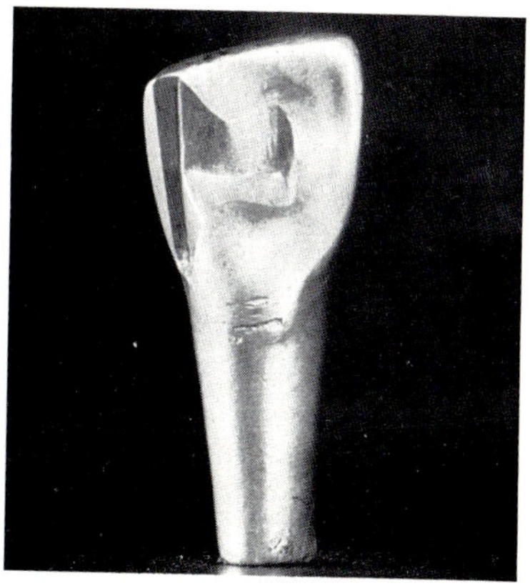

Fig. 15-3. Correct lingual dovetail outline.

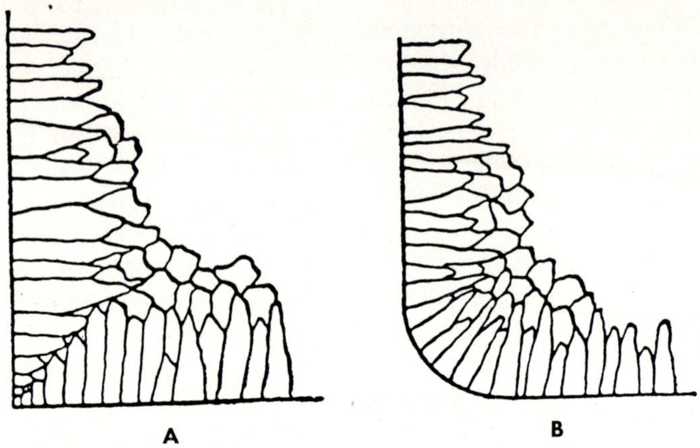

Fig. 15-4. Diagrammatic drawing showing plan of crystal formation in **A,** sharp-angle casting, and **B,** cove-angle casting. Plane of line of porosity from casting corner shown in **A** is lessened when cove is formed at angle in **B.** (From Doan, G. E.: Physical metallurgy, New York, 1935, McGraw-Hill Book Company.)

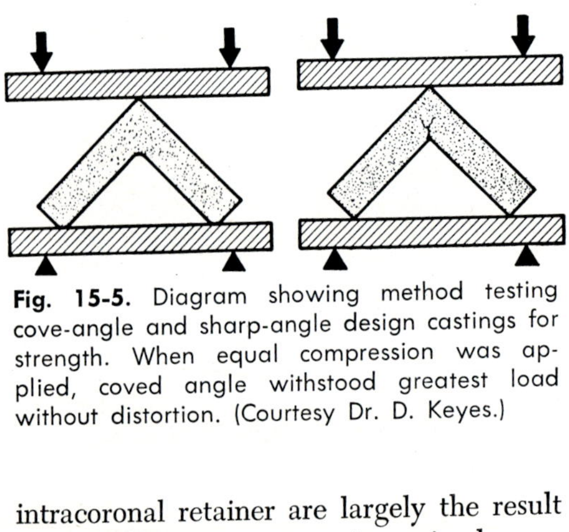

Fig. 15-5. Diagram showing method testing cove-angle and sharp-angle design castings for strength. When equal compression was applied, coved angle withstood greatest load without distortion. (Courtesy Dr. D. Keyes.)

intracoronal retainer are largely the result of developing a correct axioproximal preparation, which has labial and lingual walls in the dentin nearly parallel to each other and with a cervicoincisal convergence of these walls not exceeding 2 to 5° axially. In addition, the gingival wall is prepared so that it slopes axioapically approximately 45° from the horizontal plane (Plate 4).

The retention form is developed further to resist displacement by preparing a lingual dovetail (Figs. 15-1 to 15-3). In younger patients and in those whose teeth are thin labiolingually, the dovetail is made broader and not as deep as in older patients. The line angle formed by the pulpal and axial walls is beveled because (1) it eliminates an inner line angle in the wax pattern which, if retained, tends to trap air bubbles in the investment, resulting in nodules in the cast gold; (2) the sharp corner of investment is liable to fracture during the casting process, resulting in a misfit; and (3) as shown by Keyes[3, 4] the casting will be structurally stronger if the sharp line angle is replaced by a bevel or cove (Figs. 15-4 and 15-5). A sufficient gingivoincisal width is required on the lingual aspect where the isthmus of the dovetail joins the proximal portion of the retainer in order to withstand the lateral tensile stresses which will later develop in the retainer. The inner line angle formed by the pulpal and the lingual walls is slightly acute as opposed to the slightly obtuse line angle formed between the pulpal and labial inner walls. The pulpal wall of the dovetail is slightly dropped as it extends mesially from the axiopulpal bevel. For additional retention in the adult patient a pin or well 1 mm. in depth may be placed at the inner angle of the pulpal and mesial walls.

CLASS I, TYPE I RETAINERS: STEPS IN PREPARATION

With the advent of the high-speed cutting technics which are discussed in Chapter 14 there is the tendency to cut tooth tissue with carbide burs irrespective of whether it is enamel or dentin. To a large extent this is also true of the use to which diamond stones are put. It is our belief that certain tissues are cut better with stones, others with burs. New high-speed instrumentation technics must also be used with caution and discretion. Hence, the proved methods are here given so that the student is trained in a *step procedure of logical sequence.* With increased experience, skill, and judgment he can later avail himself of advantages of the high-speed cutting methods and modified instrumentation. Fundamentally, principles do not change, only their better understanding and better application enable the dentist to apply the knowledge gained from biologic and physical research for the betterment of his services to the patient.

Step 1 (Fig. 15-6) is the removal of the proximal enamel. A small, mounted, diamond stone, cylinder-shaped (Densco 5E)* coated with cocoa butter, is applied to the proximal surface of the tooth and slightly lingually to its contact point; the long axis of the stone is held parallel to the incisal half of the labial surface of the crown. With slight lateral pressure, the revolving stone is raised and lowered axially, making a cut which extends from the gingivae, incisally, past the contact point. The cutting is deepened until the dentinoenamel junction is exposed; this leaves a concave, trough-like depression in the axial surface. If the outline form demands a greater extension of the margins labially or lingually, the stone is carried in these directions during the cutting process, resulting in a wider labiolingual dimension. With due respect to the highly perfected carbide steel burs, it must be emphasized that *steel burs are not indicated mechanically or biologically to cut into smooth, sound, external surfaces of enamel.* Special mutibladed burs may be used to smooth surfaces of enamel previously reduced with diamond stones.

Step 2 (Fig. 15-7) consists in the cutting of the proximal portion of the preparation. By placing a cross-cut, tapered fissure bur (No. 700) at the exposed dentinoenamel

*For numbers, shapes, and sizes of diamond stones and burs, see Chapter 14.

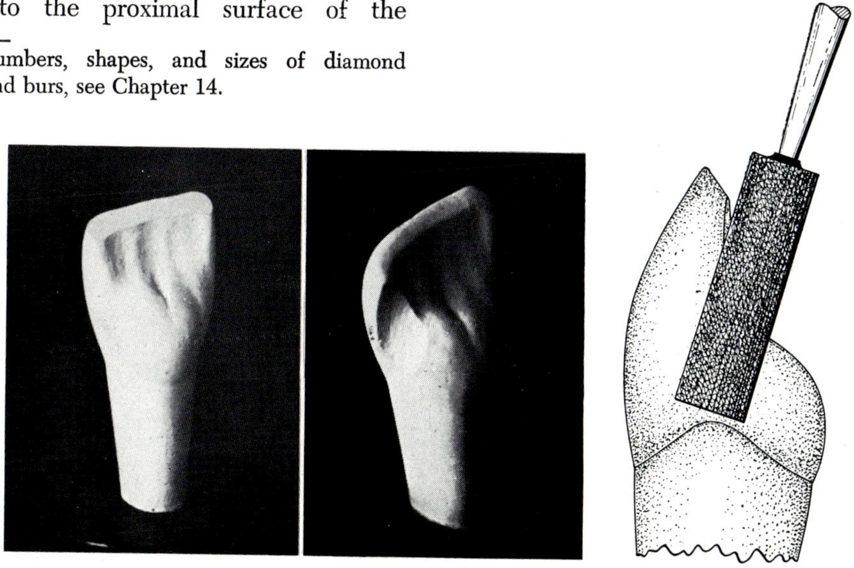

Fig. 15-6. Step 1 in preparing a DL cavity.

junction on the proximal surface, and carrying the bur labially and lingually through the plane of the dentinoenamel junction, the remaining proximal enamel is undermined. In making this cut, every effort should be made not to cut the axial dentin wall flat labiolingually; instead, it should be convex, making its surface equidistant from and parallel to the inner wall of the pulp chamber.

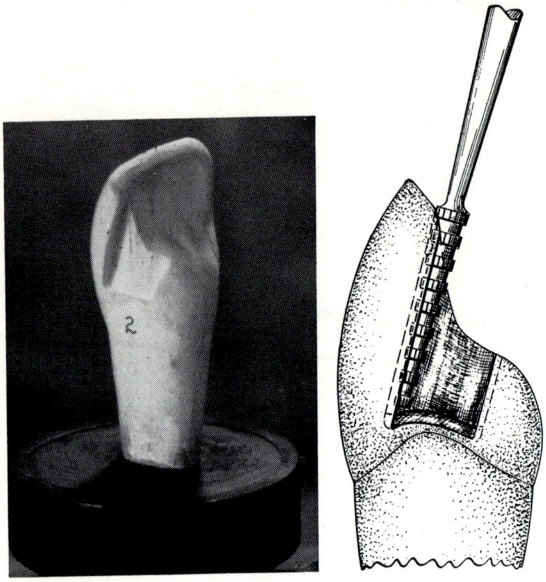

Fig. 15-7. Step 2, extending walls labially and lingually.

In Step 3 parallel proximal walls are next developed labially and lingually in the dentin by the use of straight and binangle chisels (Fig. 15-8). If the dentin walls are flared divergently toward the proximal, the wedge principle of retention of the inlay as considered in Fig. 13-26, *B*, will be lost. The use of a diamond stone at this step may destroy this needed retention.

In Step 4 the remaining undercut enamel is planed on the labial and the lingual sides with straight chisels and enamel hatchets, extending the outline form to the desired area (Fig. 15-9). It may then be smoothed with a multibladed finishing bur of the Tinker type. A fine textured disk is frequently used but care must be taken to avoid creating undercuts.

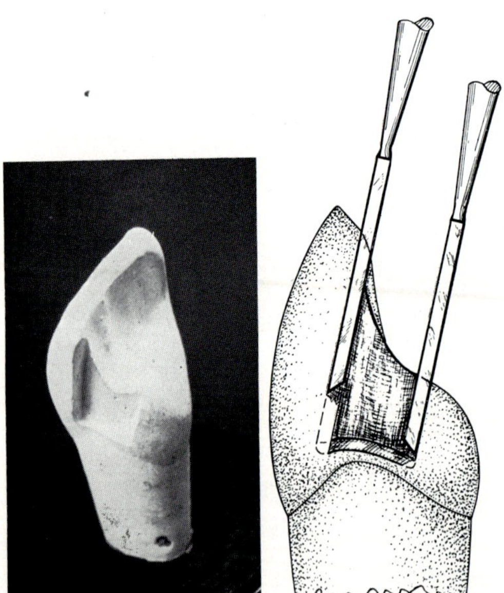

Fig. 15-8. Step 3, paralleling labial and lingual walls in dentin.

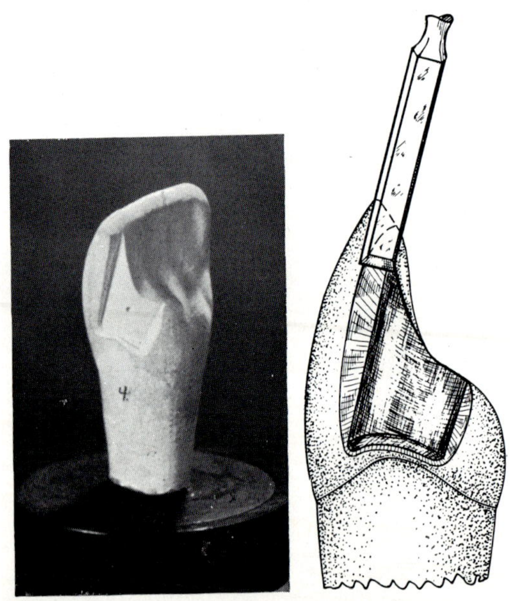

Fig. 15-9. Step 4, extending labial and lingual enamel walls into areas of immunity and cleansability.

Step 5 develops the lingual dovetail. For this purpose the inverted cone bur, chisels, and fine polishing Arkansas stones are used. With the periphery of the base of an inverted cone bur (No. 33 or 34) placed at the dentinoenamel junction on the lingual surface approximately in the center of the proximal cut (Fig. 15-10, *A* and *B*), an inverted cone cut is carried distally, along the labial and lingual walls of the cut. It is well to do this in a series of short cuts, rather than in one uninterrupted cutting operation. As the groove is carried distally (Fig. 15-10, *C*), the bur is occasionally withdrawn, in this way removing some of the enamel. The remaining enamel and dentin (Fig. 15-10, *D* and *E*) are then cut away with binangle chisels (Nos. 10 and 15) or other suitable cutting instruments. The inverted cone bur and a Densco 2C tapered cylinder diamond stone are used to outline roughly the shape of the dovetail (Fig. 15-10, *F*).

In Step 6 the final outline form is developed with tapering fissure burs and suitable planing and polishing instruments (Fig. 15-11, *A*). The pulpal wall of the dovetail parallels the lingual slope of the tooth, while the labial and lingual walls of the dovetail parallel approximately the incisal two-thirds of the labial surface with a 2 to 5° divergence (Fig. 15-11, *B*).

Although a divergence of 2 to 5° from parallelism is established between these two walls, Fig. 15-11, *C*, indicates (1) that an obtuse angle exists between the labiopulpal walls, while (2) an acute angle is developed between the linguopulpal walls.

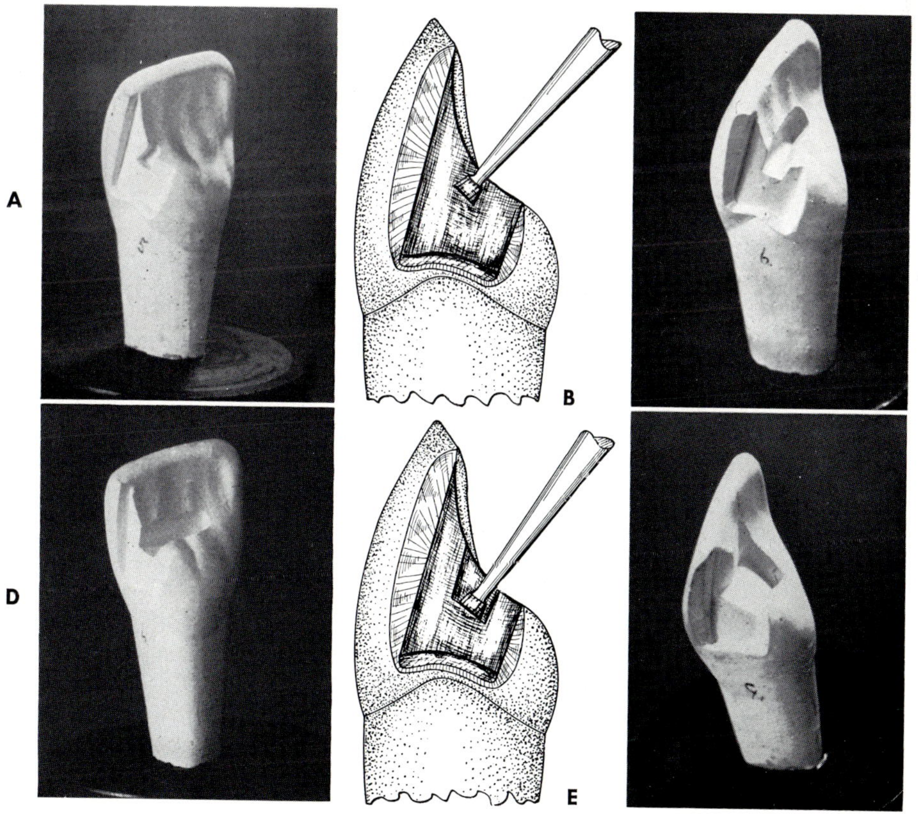

Fig. 15-10. Step 5, developing lingual dovetail.

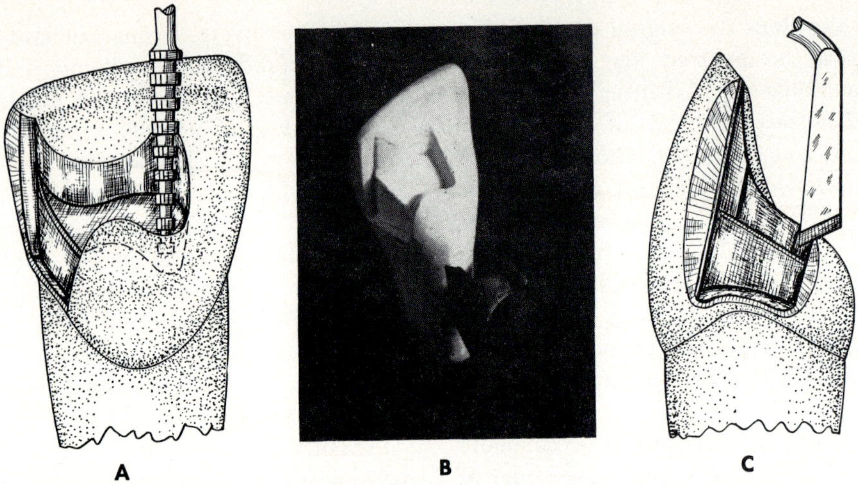

Fig. 15-11. Step 6, final outline and finish of cavity walls.

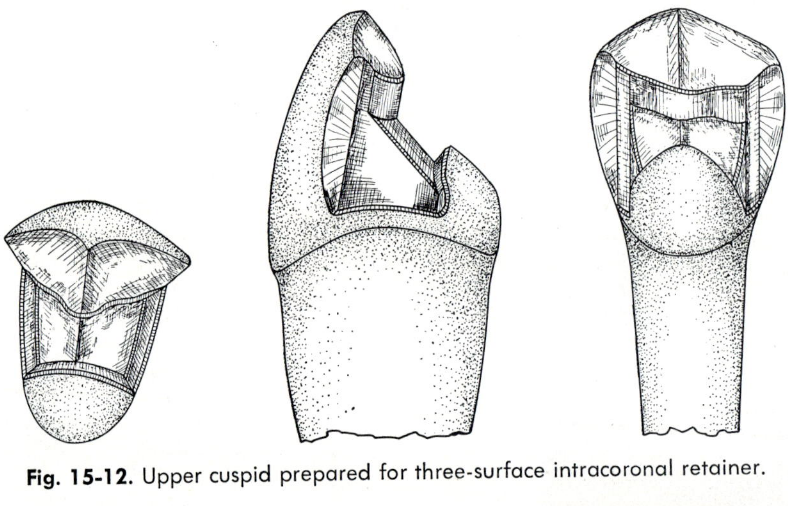

Fig. 15-12. Upper cuspid prepared for three-surface intracoronal retainer.

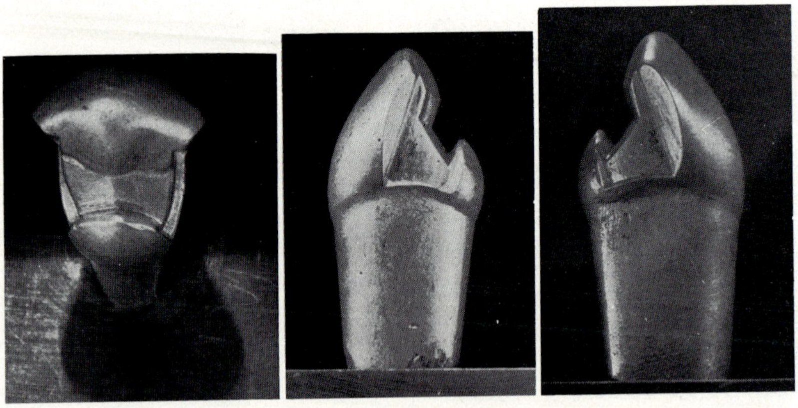

Fig. 15-13. Model of three-surface anterior intracoronal retainer on upper cuspid.

Much of the retentive value of such a preparation is lost if the lingual wall is flared excessively to a point where an obtuse angle is formed. The depth to which the distal part of the pulpal wall is lowered pulpally varies according to the type of tooth and the age of the patient. As previously stated, in older patients and in thick teeth the slope may be carried lower than in young patients. This wall should be in dentin.

Where the lingual proximal wall, cavosurface line angle joins the dovetail on the lingual surface, a lingual (Fig. 15-10, *C*) gingival bevel is developed largely in the enamel wall to afford strength and a greater bulk of metal to the retainer.

The gingival wall is lowered to the desired level with a No. 700 or 701 crosscut taper fissure bur, or a Densco 10 tapered cylinder diamond stone, followed by enamel hatchet (No. 10 and No. 15, R and L).

The gingival cavosurface enamel is beveled with gingival marginal trimmers, and the plane of the gingival wall is sloped axioapically at an angle of 45° from the horizontal (Plate 4). The lingual cavosurface margin of the dovetail is also beveled as shown in Fig. 13-30, line C-Z; this is accomplished with a hoe (No. 8-4-12) or an enamel hatchet (No. 10 or 15). The incisal and the distal cavosurface enamel of the dovetail are not beveled on the lingual surface.

In this type of three-surface retainer (Figs. 15-12 and 15-13), the other proximal surface is usually in contact with the adjacent natural tooth; precautions must be taken not to injure the contacting area of the other tooth while preparing the cavity.

A thin steel strip may be slipped between the two contacting teeth prior to making a cut through the abutment that is being prepared. A space may also be created with a mechanical separator. Thirdly, the lateral lingual cut made in Step 3 (Fig. 15-10) may be extended farther until the marginal enamel ridge is undermined, but the bur does not perforate through the enamel wall.

A crosscut tapered fissure bur (No. 700) is placed on the exposed dentinoenamel junction and slowly lowered gingivally between the mesioproximal plate of enamel and the dentin. While the bur is cutting gingivally, it is also tilted laterally in a labiolingual direction, care being taken to leave the axial dentin wall convex labiolingually, rather than a flat surface.

After the mesial plate of enamel has been undermined on the proximal side, a No. 12-5-6 hatchet or a No. 10 enamel hatchet is inserted in the opening between the undermined enamel and the dentin; then with a prying motion the enamel is readily fractured and the cavity is extended to the gingival floor.

The alternative method is to insert a Densco ½D tapered diamond stone between the enamel and dentin surfaces and cut through both labially and lingually, into immune or self-cleansing areas. The remaining proximal wall of enamel will readily fracture at the gingival level. Use of this method will leave the enamel of the proximating tooth intact.

Where necessary, a further gingival extension may be made until the desired depth of cavity has been established. The labial and lingual planes of enamel are prepared as before and the walls of dentin are planed and squared, using the same instruments and technic as described in the preparation of the distal wall; the form of the gingival wall is similar to that prepared in the distal surface.

In younger patients, the pulpal floor of dentin is usually prepared in two planes, meeting at a higher level in the center of the preparation and sloping down to their respective pulpal axial line angles (Figs. 15-12 and 15-13). This will leave a thicker floor of dentin covering the pulp, in addition to giving added resistance to displacement of the casting from the cavity.

Under microscopic examination, walls of dentin and enamel prepared with diamond stones or burs, especially the crosscut type, leave serrations of varying depths. It is advisable to finish cavity surfaces against which the wax pattern will be made, with mounted fine point Arkansas stones or with the multibladed Tinker type of polishing burs. Tapered orangewood points using a slurry of alumina powder is also effective in obtaining smooth walls.

Many modifications have been suggested to increase the retentive factors in this intracoronal retainer; these usually take the form of supplementary pins and grooves placed in the axial, pulpal, or gingival walls. Such retentive aids, however, should be used with great caution, because of the danger to the pulp in preparing the pinholes for the pins (see Chapter 19).

The types of retainers discussed are indicated primarily for anterior teeth in the upper arch, since here the functional forces are directed in a labial and gingival direction; in other words, the forces applied in function usually tend to seat the retainer more firmly in the tooth.

On the other hand, when the same type of retainers is employed in the lower arch, the masticating forces usually resolve themselves into displacing forces, since they are directed lingually from the labial aspect. Hence, in the lower anterior teeth the two-surface intracoronal retainer is usually contraindicated.

SELECTED REFERENCES

1. Osborne, J., Brill, N., and Hedegard, B.: The nature of prosthetic dentistry, Int. Dent. J. **16**:(4):509, 1966.
2. Beust, T. B.: Reactions of the dentinal fibrils to external irritation, J.A.D.A. **18**:1060, 1931.
3. Keyes, D. A.: Effect of cavity and pattern design on structure, stress, strain and density of castings, J.A.D.A. **30**:1432, 1943.
4. Keyes, D. A.: A study in casting density, J.A.D.A. **32**:25, 1945.

GENERAL REFERENCES

Bodecker, C. F.: Cavity preparation based on histologic and biologic principles, J.A.D.A. **28**: 540, 1941.

Greenberg, Alvin: Cavity outline form with a minimum of contact and a maximum of control, J.A.D.A. **64**:603, 1962.

McCollum, B. B.: Tooth preparation in its relation to oral physiology, J.A.D.A. **27**:701, 1940.

Meyer, F. S.: Inlays, crowns and full cast bridges, Am. D. Surgeon **53**:33, 73, 1932.

Segat, L.: Protection of prepared abutments between appointments in crown and bridge prosthodontics, J. Michigan D. A. **44**:32, 1962.

Smith, D. E.: Abutment preparations, J.A.D.A. **18**:2063, 2075, 1931.

Smith, D. E.: Twenty-five years of fixed bridgework, J. South. California D. A. **3**:794, 1936.

Thom, L. W.: Principles of cavity preparation in crown and bridge prosthesis, J.A.D.A. **41**:284, 443, 541, 1950.

Vedder, F. B.: Grief in fixed bridge work, J. Michigan D. Soc. **16**:532, 1934.

Waerhaug, J.: Histologic considerations which govern where the margins of restorations should be located in relation to the gingiva, Dent. Clin. N. Amer., March, 1960, pp. 161-176.

Zander, H. A.: Bacteria in the dentin after cavity preparation, Illinois D. J. **9**:207, 1940.

Chapter 16

Tooth preparations and instrumentation: class I, type 2—posterior intracoronal retainers

The anterior intracoronal preparation discussed in Chapter 15 was originally intended and designed as a single operative restoration. When gold alloys with better physical properties and casting technics were developed, the cavity design was modified to allow limited use as a retainer. If three surfaces are included in the preparation, it is still used cautiously even when resistance to displacement increases from the use of pins, screws, and grooves. If retentive sufficiency is questionable, the extracoronal retainer is preferred. However, intracoronal preparations have been designed and used successfully for retainers on posterior teeth supporting fixed partial prostheses.

The posterior teeth best suited for the reception of intracoronal retainers are the first and second molars and the first and second bicuspids. Occasionally the third molar is used, but in most instances this tooth requires either a partial or a complete cast crown. While the intracoronal retainers may be employed both in carious and noncarious teeth, they are placed and usually indicated in those abutments having some decay; they may also be used either in pulpless teeth or in those having vital pulps.

Retainers of the MO, DO, or even MOD types are more generally used as supports for tapered keys with the broken-stress principle; rarely is a two-surface retainer soldered directly to the pontic.

A three-surface retainer, such as the MOD, is sometimes used to furnish the retention for a bridge; this design is acceptable provided more than one missing tooth is not replaced in the restoration. Where two or more teeth are missing, the partial or the complete cast crowns are preferred.

INDICATIONS

Because the intracoronal retainer lies within the body of the tooth, it approaches the pulp more closely than an extracoronal type. Although it is usually contraindicated in young patients, it may be used with reasonable safety in older patients whose pulps are fully formed, and where there is likely to be secondary dentin in the pulp chambers.

Because of the limited area of the internal cavity walls affording resistance to displacement, teeth should be selected for this type of retention whose crowns are sufficiently long gingivoclusally and sufficiently thick buccolingually. Teeth that are short, severely abraded, or whose structural form is such that sufficient mechanical retention cannot be obtained should not be used. Where a tooth is in normal alignment, its occlusion is normal, and the strength of the bite is average, intracoronal retainers in posterior teeth will fulfill their requirements satisfactorily.

One of the frequent causes of failure of three-surface intracoronal retainers may be attributed to their use in abutments which are extensively decayed or whose buccal and lingual cusps are unsupported. With the mistaken idea of preserving such cusps and in the effort to establish maximum esthetic values, the enamel of cusps and other surfaces unsupported by sound dentin is frequently retained after having been reinforced with cement. While this practice is sometimes permissible in those areas not exposed to compressive forces or torque, this procedure is fatal when used in regions exposed to the direct forces of mastication. It is much better to recognize a condition of existing weakness and take the necessary steps to develop the required protection and retention by using some other type of retainer.

Where occlusal decay has penetrated deeply without exposing the pulp, but where the buccal and lingual cusps are separated by a deep cavity, such a tooth, when used for an MOD retainer, should have its occlusal outline extended so that the casting will include and cover both cusps. Clinical experience confirms the view that a three-surface intracoronal retainer, when used in a pulpless tooth, should *always* have its entire occluding surfaces restored in metal; if this precaution is not taken, one or both of the natural cusps very likely will be fractured at a later time.

When a tooth is prepared to receive a two-surface intracoronal retainer, there is usually an edentulous area approximating it; hence, there is access for the preparation of the proximal surface. However, when there is an adjacent tooth in contact with the abutment, separation of the teeth may be necessary first; this is accomplished by the methods discussed in Chapter 2.

STEPS IN THE PREPARATION OF A POSTERIOR INTRACORONAL RETAINER

The initial step in the preparation of a carious tooth for the reception of an intracoronal retainer is the removal of the decay and the determination of the extent to which the caries has destroyed the remaining tooth structure. Where there is reasonable doubt of a possible pulp exposure, the rubber dam should be applied before the complete removal of the decay. This precaution is extremely important in the event that the pulp is exposed.

Where the depth of decay approaches the pulp closely, it is safer and less painful to use hand-cutting instruments instead of rapidly revolving engine burs to remove the decay. In all abutments having extensive decay, but no involvement of the pulp, it is well to place an intermediate base of calcium hydroxide; cement then should be sealed over the base. Where possible, the cement filling should be allowed to remain in the tooth for a week or more to determine the possibility of any unfavorable pulp reaction; if none occurs, it is safe to assume that the pulp is biologically safe.

Outline form

The outline form of an intracoronal retainer in a biscuspid or a molar is developed in two phases—the proximal and the occlusal. Exclusive of its limited retention, one of the most frequent criticisms of this type of retainer is the susceptibility of its proximal margins to recurrent caries. In operative procedures involving the restoration of an individual inlay, this recurrence of decay is less frequent because an adjacent natural tooth usually furnishes normal contact and normal surface contours, making it simpler to locate the correct buccal and lingual outlines of the restoration. When an edentulous space exists next to the abutment, no such natural landmarks are present; consequently, there is more likelihood of underextending the buccal and lingual margins of the preparation. Later, when the pontic is in position, there is danger of marginal recurrence of decay, due to the insufficient extension bucally or lingually of the margins into a cleansable or immune area. In the posterior teeth, particularly those distal to the first bicuspid, it is a cardinal rule to extend the buccal margins of intracoronal retainers boldly into the buccal surfaces. This does not mean the unnecessary cutting away of buccal tooth structure, but an extension of the margins into cleansable areas. The only possible objection to such a procedure is the sacrifice of some esthetics; however, this loss does not actually play an important role because the position of these margins lies beyond the range of normal visibility.

On the lingual side it is not necessary to extend the margin to the same extent, since in a bridge restoration there usually exists a wide lingual embrasure between the pontic and the abutment. Marginal extension in the lingual direction is mainly determined by the amount of cutting necessary to obtain the required mechanical retention. One of the best guides to the correct placement of the buccal and lingual margins in the proximal portion of a cavity is the position of the axial surface angles of the tooth. By placing the buccal and lingual margins of the cavity near these angles, a sufficient extension is usually obtained. Later, if the soldered joint between the retainer and the pontic is properly placed and contoured, and if their approximating surfaces curve properly toward the buccal and the lingual walls, the excursion of food and brushing will keep the margins of the filling clean.

In extending the preparation gingivally, the same general procedures prevail as in other types of bridge retainers. In those teeth which have a normal depth of the gingival crevice, the margin of the casting is brought slightly beneath the crest of the gum tissue. Where a clinical examination discloses that the depth of the gingival crevice is zero, a condition usually prevailing in younger patients, the alternative exists, either of detaching the epithelial attachment and dropping the margin gingivally to the desired depth, or of leaving the epithelial attachment intact and terminating the margin of the casting slightly above the gum tissue. While no set rule can be given for predetermining the exact level at which the gingival margin should lie, nothing should be done to impair the biologic integrity of the investing tissues; yet, where a fixed bridge must be placed, it is necessary that the preparation be extended into such areas and to a depth sufficient to obtain the necessary mechanical retention. As a rule, for patients of the adolescent age and those in the early twenties, it is wise to avoid any epithelial detachment; however, in older patients there may be a justification for the extension of margins gingivally, even though it results in a slight detachment of the epithelium. Existing conditions will indicate the best procedure for each specific case.

The second phase in the development of the outline form includes the preparation of the occlusal dovetail. In a distoclusal inlay, for example, the margin of the occlusal outline begins at the buccal and lingual proximal walls. From there it continues mesially, narrowing into an isthmus as it rounds the buccal and lingual triangular ridges; then, as it approach distally, it again widens and includes the distal pit and groove. Care must be exercised, in extending the distal wall of the dovetail, that the distal marginal ridge is not undercut.

One of the frequent mistakes in planning the outline form is the tendency to cut a straight-walled occlusal groove from mesial to distal through the triangular ridges, thus sacrificing, unnecessarily, valuable tooth structure. This procedure also endangers the pulp because of the proximity of the casting to it.

In older patients the pulpal wall of the preparation may be dropped deeper than in younger individuals; in the latter the pulpal wall is usually made more shallow.

The pulpal wall slopes pulpally as it continues toward the distal wall. In older patients additional retention may frequently be obtained by countersinking a slight oval depression in the pulpal wall in the distal part of the dovetail. Similarly, pins of varying diameters and lengths may be countersunk in the same region to furnish a supplementary retention.

Resistance and retention forms

Resistance and retention forms are developed largely by a properly prepared proximal boxing which has its buccal and lingual dentin walls nearly parallel to each other axioproximally and a cervicoclusal flare that does not exceed 2° axially. The resistance to displacement is further augmented by a properly beveled gingival wall, as previously explained (Plate 3). The retention form is completed by a properly outlined and prepared occlusal dovetail lock, whose width at the isthmus of the lock does not ordinarily exceed one-third the buccolingual width of the occlusal surface. Since the weakest part of this type of retainer is found where the occlusal dovetail unites with the proximal portion, the buccal and lingual occlusal walls in this limited area are flared widely in the enamel, extending well onto the crest of the buccal and lingual cusps. This results in an additional bulk of metal, thereby precluding distortion at this point caused by tensile forces. Proceeding distally, however, the buccal and lingual walls again assume their near-parallel relationship.

The flaring of a part of the buccal and lingual occlusal walls is indicated in the pontic side of an MOD inlay which lies next to the bridge. This furnishes the strength necessary to resist the torque forces of a bridge.

Retention at the gingival margin is gained by sloping the gingival wall axially from the cavosurface bevel, an angle of 45° horizontally. Some obtain this additional retention by cutting a groove or by placing short dowels, pits, and pins in the gingival wall.

Instrumentation. In those instances in which a two- or three-surface intracoronal bridge retainer is used, the proximal surface is usually next to an edentulous space; hence, there is good access to the abutment. The first step, therefore, is the removal of the proximal surface; this technic is similar for the bicuspid (Fig. 16-1, *A*) or the molar (Fig. 16-1, *B*). A small, mounted, cylinder-shaped Densco 2F stone is applied to the proximal surface of the tooth approximately in the region of the contact area. The long axis of the stone is parallel to the long axis of the crown. Lateral pressure is applied, and, while the stone is revolving, it is slowly raised and lowered occlusogingivally, making a buccolingual, furrow-shaped cut which extends from the occlusal surface to the crest of the gingiva. The cutting and increased pressure are continued until the stone has cut through the proximal enamel and exposed the underlying dentinoenamel junction (Fig. 16-1, *C*). The buccal and lingual marginal extensions are determined at this time, and, if necessary, the concave cut is extended buccally and lingually with the same stone to the desired distance. In making this cut, the axial wall is maintained convex buccolingually and lies mostly in dentin; next, a flat gingival wall is established level with the crest of the gum tissue.

The next procedure in the completion of the proximal preparation consists in removing the balance of the proximal enamel. This is done with a suitable bur, usually a No. 700 or 701. While rotating,

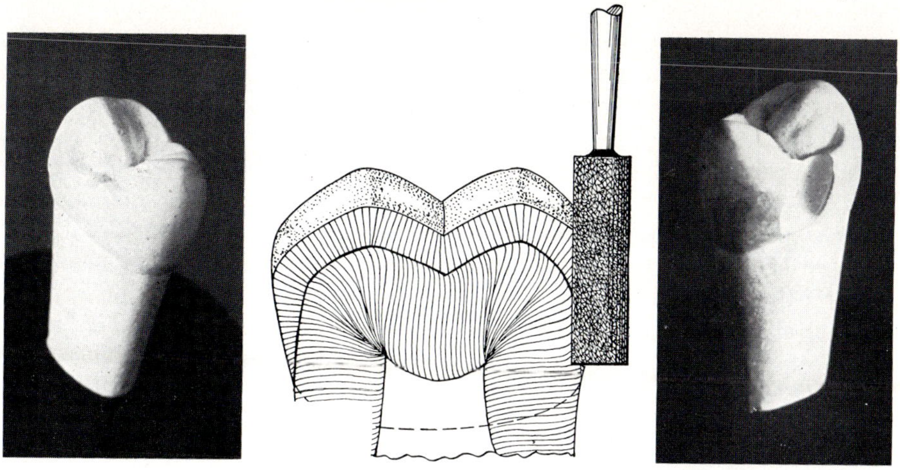

A **B** **C**

Fig. 16-1. Step 1 in preparation of posterior tooth for intracoronal retainer.

the bur is pressed gently into the dentin at the dentinoenamel junction, just behind the enamel; then it is carried laterally in a buccolingual direction, the cutting being done in the dentin (Fig. 16-2). In making this cut, the dentinal axial wall should be left convex buccolingually. After the enamel is undermined, enamel hatchets of suitable size are used to cut away the unsupported buccal and lingual segments of the enamel wall. During the same operation, it is frequently possible to carry the end of the bur gingivally, undermining the gingival enamel wall. This is then removed with enamel hatchets and other suitable hand-cutting instruments to the level of the gum tissues.

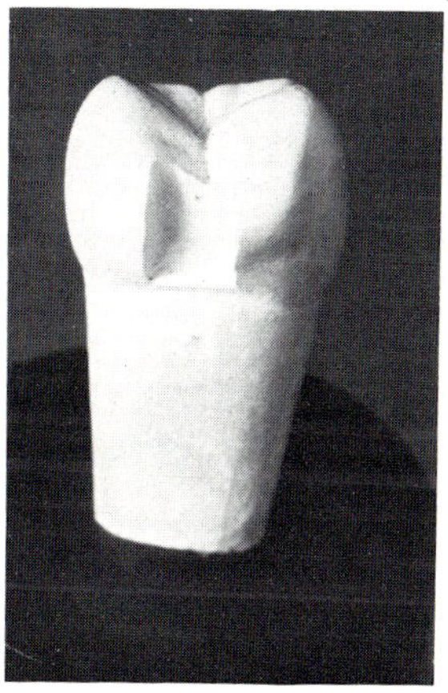

Fig. 16-2. Step 2 in preparation of posterior tooth for intracoronal retainer.

Following the removal of the undermined enamel, the widths of the buccal and lingual walls are planed either with enamel hatchets or chisels of suitable size (Fig. 16-3, *B*). The tendency is to use a mounted tapering diamond stone to accomplish this. If done, flat planes and sharp angles are usually not obtained. Those parts of the buccal and the lingual walls lying within the dentin are planed and squared with chisels and enamel hatchets, so that two near-parallel planes, axioproximally, are established having a cervicoclusal flare not exceeding 2° axially. This procedure is similar to that shown in Fig. 15-8.

In planing the enamel walls buccally and lingually, it is necessary that their cavosurface margins be extended sufficiently into cleansable or self-cleansable areas in order to prevent the recurrence of caries.

The gingival wall is lowered axioapically 45° horizontally (Plate 3); the final preparation of the gingival wall consists in beveling the cavosurface angle approximately 2 to 6° from the horizontal plane; this is done to preclude the possibility of leaving any unsupported enamel rods. Black's marginal trimmers No. 15-80-8-12 or 15-95-8-12 or a special set of Gillet's chisels may be used.

The next step in the preparation of a two-surface intracoronal retainer is the development of the occlusal portion. Two methods are available in making the initial cut or groove through the occlusal surface.

A small, Densco 1-V stone may be employed to start the occlusal cut. The edge of the stone is placed on the occlusal surface at the margin of the proximal surface, and, while revolving under a stream of water, it gradually cuts through the enamel to the dentinoenamel junction (Fig. 16-3, *A*). The cut is extended distally to within 1 mm. of the distal marginal ridge (Fig. 16-3, *B*). If a bicuspid is being prepared, care should be taken not to cut away too much of the buccal or lingual triangular ridges; if a molar, the cuts follow the general direction of the occlusal developmental grooves. Here, also, every precaution must be taken to preserve as much of the triangular or transverse occlusal ridges as possible.

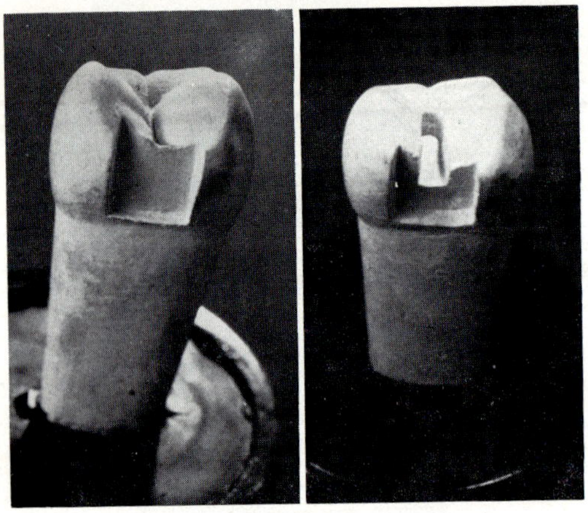

A **B**

Fig. 16-3. A and B, Step 3 in preparation of posterior tooth for intracoronal retainer.

The groove cut by the stone is enlarged with a carbide fissure bur No. 700 or 701. At this time the general outline form of the occlusal portion of the cavity is prepared by extending the cuts into the desired pit and fissure areas.

Another method sometimes used to develop the occlusal portion starts with the use of an inverted cone bur No. 34 (Fig. 16-4). The periphery of the base of the bur is placed at the exposed dentinoenamel junction on the proximal surface; while revolving, the bur is gently pressed into the

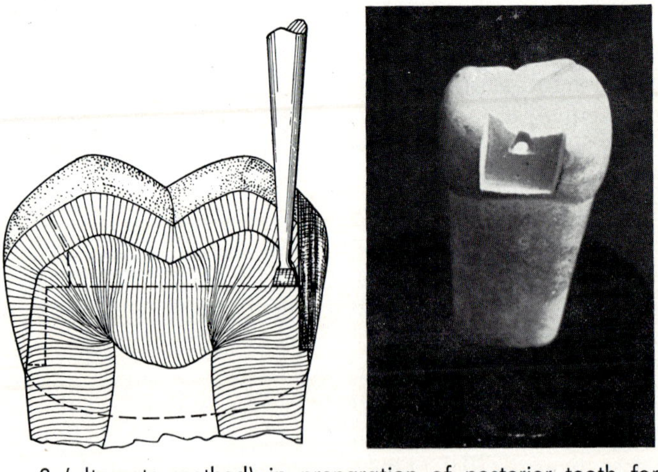

Fig. 16-4. Step 3 (alternate method) in preparation of posterior tooth for intracoronal retainer; dotted line, extension of initial cut for three-surface intracoronal preparation.

dentin, in close contact with the undercut enamel. When the bur has penetrated its full diameter into the tooth structure, it is then drawn occlusally, cutting through the overlying enamel. In doing so, the blades of the bur are shaving away the enamel rods lengthwise along their interprismatic substance. The bur is reinserted and again another cut is made laterally and drawn occlusally. This operation is repeated, the cuts following the general direction of the occlusal grooves.

Following this initial undermining of the enamel, lateral cuts are made with a larger inverted cone bur (No. 35 or 37) along the dentinoenamel junction—first along the buccal, then the lingual walls, thus undercutting the enamel (Fig. 16-5, *A*). The undercut enamel is next cut away with chisels and enamel hatchets of suitable sizes and angles (Fig. 16-5, *B*). While endeavoring to retain as much of the tooth structure as possible, the occlusal outline of the preparation is extended so that the margins of the filling will include those areas which will permit the proper finishing of the gold in smooth surfaces and not in deep pits or fissures (Fig. 16-5, *C*).

In those instances in which separation has not been previously made, the preparation of the occlusal surface may be started with a bibeveled drill or a No. ½ round bur or a 700 cross-cut tapered fissure bur placed in the mesial pit or fissure (Fig. 16-6, *A*). While rotating slowly, the instrument is lowered pulpally to the dentinoenamel junction (Fig. 16-6, *B*).

A No. 33½ or 34 inverted cone bur is now lowered to the bottom of the opening, and by cutting laterally toward the proximal surface, the enamel is undercut (Fig. 16-7, *A*). In doing so, the bur is also raised occlusally, cutting away the overhanging enamel (Fig. 16-7, *B*). This process is continued until the inner surface of the proximal enamel wall is reached (Fig. 16-7, *C*). A No. 700 cross-cut fissure bur is substituted, and, by cutting laterally, buccolingually, and gingivally, the proximal plate of enamel is undercut and removed by the same technic and with the same instruments as previously described (Fig. 16-8, *A*).

The pulpal wall should not be cut deeper than is necessary when making the cuts through the occlusal surface into the dentin; 1 mm. should be considered the maxi-

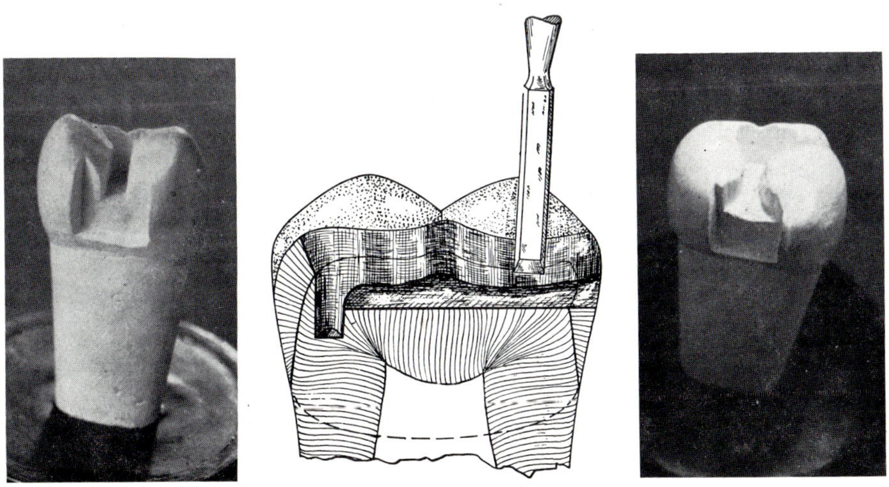

A B C

Fig. 16-5. Step 4 in preparation of posterior tooth for intracoronal retainer.

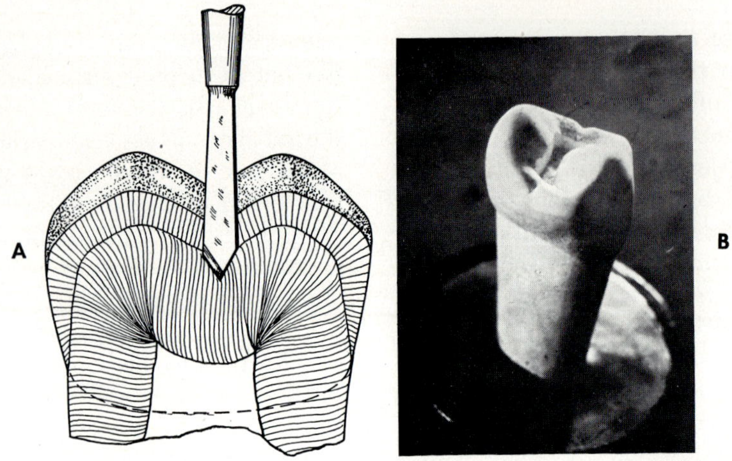

Fig. 16-6. Where proximal separation has not been obtained, Step 1 starts in occlusal surface.

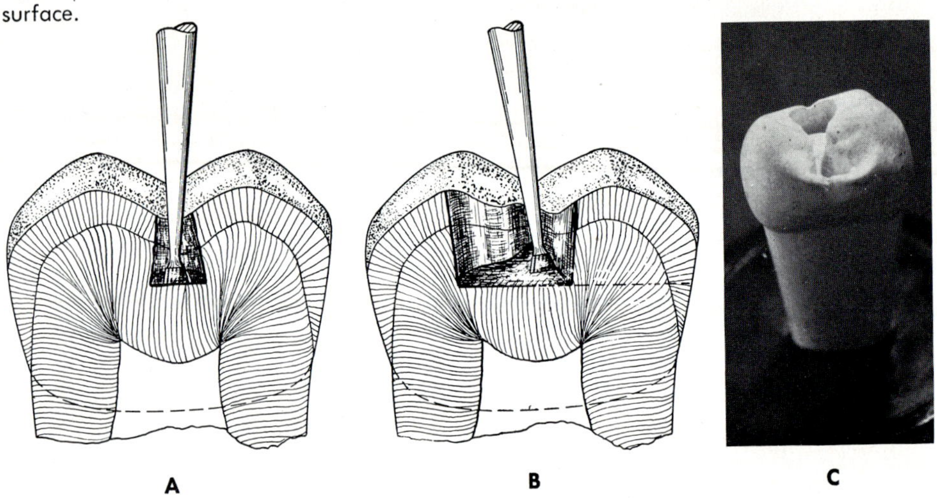

Fig. 16-7. Step 2, where initial opening is made through occlusal surface and extended proximally.

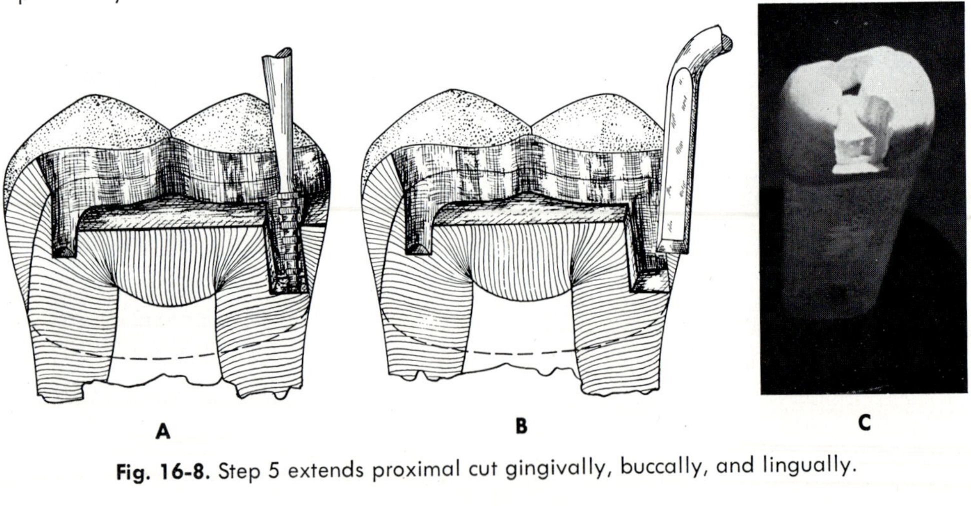

Fig. 16-8. Step 5 extends proximal cut gingivally, buccally, and lingually.

mum depth, because, if the cuts are made deeper, there is the possibility of pulp involvement.

Following the removal of the undercut gingival and occlusal dentin and enamel (Fig. 16-8, *B* and *C*), the next step consists in finishing the preparation of the proximal, buccal, and lingual walls. These are customarily extended in one plane from the pulpoaxial line angles to the axial cavosurface margins in operative dentistry (Fig. 16-9, *A*). In fixed prosthodontics two planes are prepared; one extends in dentin from the pulpoaxial line angle to the dentinoenamel junction, the other flares outwardly from this line to the cavosurface margins; the degree of flare depends upon the direction of the enamel rods in those areas (Fig. 16-11).

It is seen in Fig. 13-29 that the direction of the enamel rods varies in different locations of the occlusal surface; hence, it is essential to understand the histologic arrangement and structure of the enamel peculiar to each area. As a rule, the occlusobuccal and lingual walls diverge gingivocclusally 2 to 5° from parallelism.

The arrangement of occlusal enamel rods in the region of pits and fissures usually makes it unnecessary to bevel the occlusal cavosurface margins.

In extending the pulpal wall from one proximal surface toward the other in a two-surface preparation, additional retention may be obtained by lowering the dovetail portion of the pulpal wall. In older patients additional retention is sometimes obtained by countersinking an oval depression in the distant portion of the pulpal wall (Fig. 16-10, *B*). In doing so, however, extreme caution must be exercised not to jeopardize the pulp.

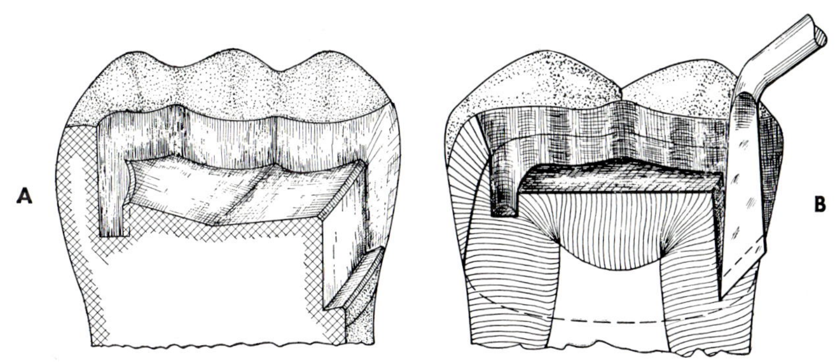

Fig. 16-9. Step 6, beveling of internal line angles and cutting pulpally inclined plane of gingival wall.

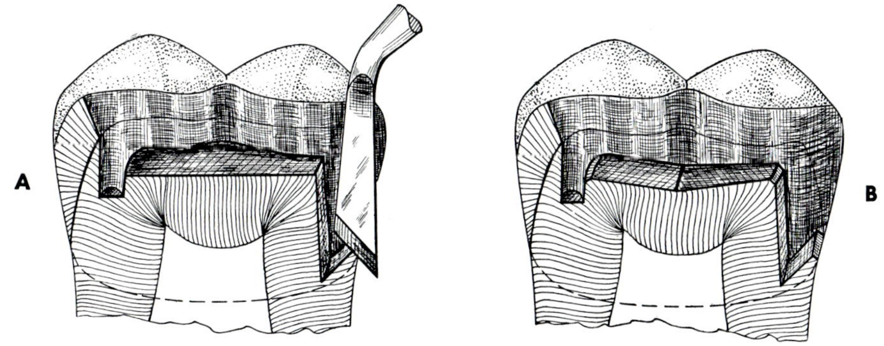

Fig. 16-10. Step 7, beveling of cavosurface angle of gingival enamel wall.

When the pulpal wall in a molar tooth extends mesiodistally, it frequently is prepared in two or more planes which alternately drop and rise. Such a modification affords additional resistance against a horizontal displacement.

The next cutting operation in preparing an intracoronal retainer involves the pulpoaxial line angles. It consists of creating a bevel between the pulpal and the proximoaxial wall (Fig. 16-9, *A*). The enamel hatchets or the gingival marginal trimmers of suitable size, used with a lateral cutting motion, are used in making the bevel at an approximate angle of 45°. The final step is the preparation of the gingival wall (Figs. 16-9, *B*, and 16-10, *B*) and the bevel of the gingival cavosurface angle (Fig. 16-10, *A*). This is fully discussed in Chapter 13. Others are shown in Fig. 16-11; the finished preparations in a molar are also shown in Fig. 16-11, upper left.

Where a mesial two-surface, intracoronal

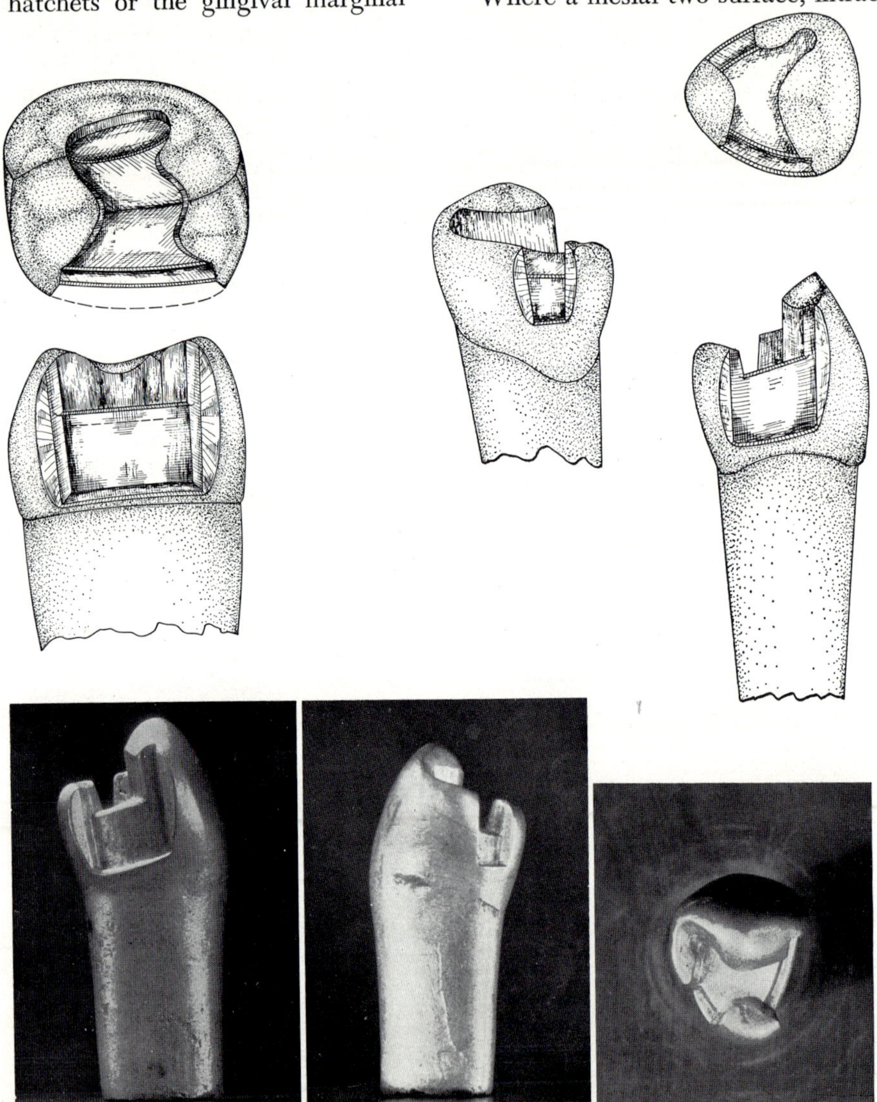

Fig. 16-11. Other types of intracoronal tooth preparations for bridge retainers.

retainer extends into the opposite or disto-proximal surface, the operative steps are as follows: instead of terminating the occlusal cut just short of the distal marginal ridge, as in Fig. 16-10, it is carried distally until the distoproximal dentinoenamel junction is exposed (see Fig. 16-4, *A*). A No. 33 inverted cone bur, a No. ½ round, or a No. 700 cross-cut tapered fissure bur is now gently lowered into the dentin at the distal dentinoenamel junction and, while revolving slowly, is carried gingivally, at the same time being held lightly against the inner surface of the proximal enamel wall. While it is moved back and forth buccolingually, the bur is slowly raised and lowered, cutting a convex well between the distoproximal enamel wall and its axial dentinal wall. Here again care must be taken to shape the dentin wall, convex buccolingually.

After the distal plate of enamel has been undercut, a suitable instrument of the hatchet or chisel type is inserted into the opening to pry off the enamel quite readily. By an alternative method a tapering

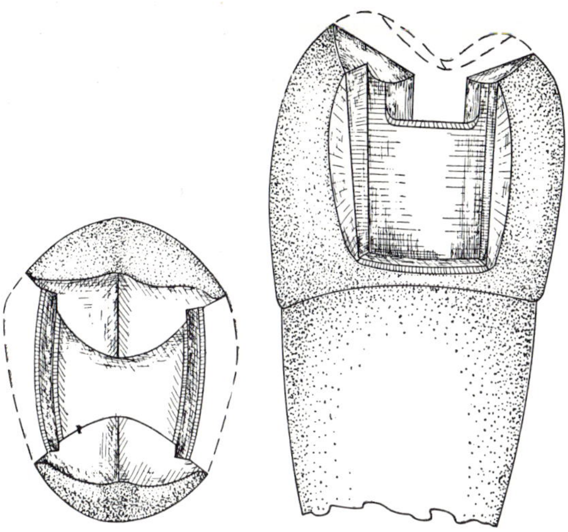

Fig. 16-12. MOD intracoronal preparation in upper devitalized bicuspid, with both cusps restored in casting.

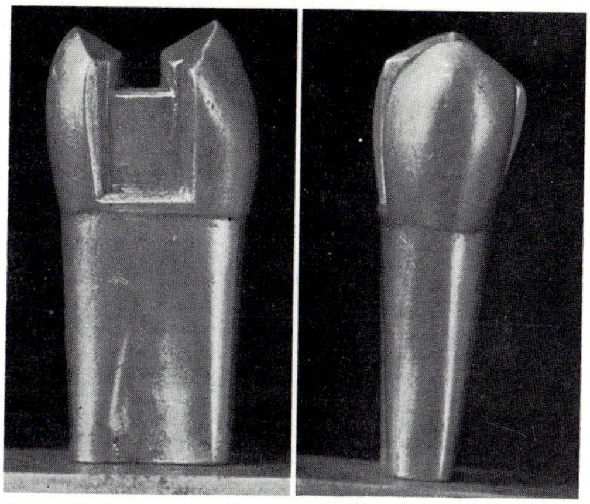

Fig. 16-13. Proximal and lingual views of MOD intracoronal preparation; both cusps to be restored in retainer.

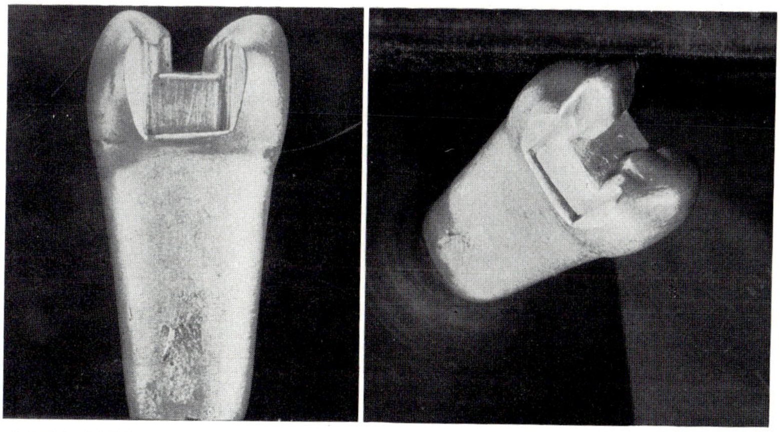

Fig. 16-14. MOD preparation with cusps left intact, proximal and occlusal views.

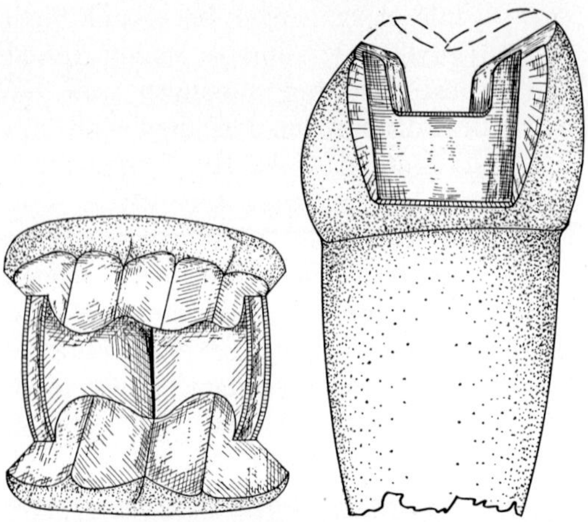

Fig. 16-15. MOD preparation with cusps involved.

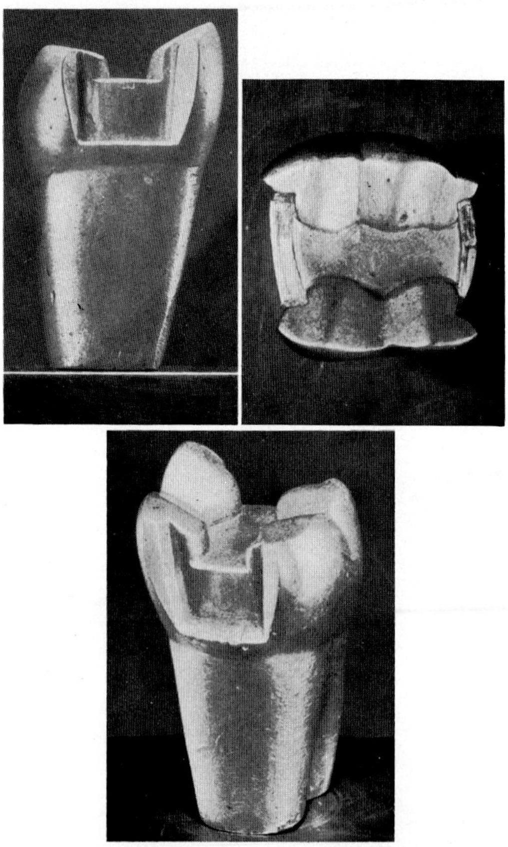

Fig. 16-16. Lower molar, intracoronal preparation for complete occlusal coverage.

Densco 1D diamond stone may be lowered into the opening and carried out buccally and lingually as previously done in the anterior DL preparation. The buccal and lingual walls are next planed with chisels and enamel hatchets, care being taken (1) to establish a near parallelism in two walls of dentin and (2) to obtain a sufficient extension of the cavosurface enamel margins to prevent recurrence of caries. The distal gingival wall is finished in the same manner as the mesial wall. Figs. 16-12 through 16-16 show views of bicuspid and molar MOD preparations.

Where, for example, a molar abutment contacts two approximating teeth, the approach to the preparation of the proximal surface differs somewhat. The proximal wall of enamel may be removed by using thin, steel ½ inch diamond separting disks after sufficient proximal separation has been previously obtained. After the proximal enamel has been reduced with disks to a depth where the dentinoenamel junction is exposed, the instruments used and the steps of the procedure are similar to those previously described.

MODIFICATIONS

There are many modifications of the typical three-surface MOD intracoronal retainer just described. In some cases, additional resistance against displacement is obtained by extending the cavity outline and casting into the buccal and lingual grooves. When used, these fingerlike extensions need not be wide, but they should have their opposing axial walls as close to parallelism as it is possible to make them within 2 to 5°; likewise, they must be sufficiently strong to resist any torsional forces to which they may be subjected. They must be extended gingivally below the level of the pulpal wall by several millimeters.

A very satifactory modification of the MOD is shown on an upper bicuspid and a lower molar preparation in Figs. 16-17 and 16-18. Castings on prepared abutment teeth are seen in Fig. 16-17. Fig. 16-19 shows the lingual aspect of the second bicuspid where the gold casting covers the lingual cusp and half of the lingual surface. The lingual margin ends in a chamfer placed at the greatest convexity of this surface. Fig. 16-20 shows a bridge on the opposite side, where the second bicuspid's cervical margin is below the gingiva.

The slice preparation

The so-called slice preparation is a modification of the typical intracoronal retainer. When properly prepared and used where indicated, the slice type has rendered satisfactory service. It differs from the standard type preparation mainly in its proximal design (Fig. 16-21). As the name indicates, this preparation removes a slice of the proximal convexity and as much of the tooth as is necessary to carry the buccal and lingual margins into immun or cleansable areas; it also establishes a cervical finishing facet or bevel. The slice is made by the use of small diamond disks such as the Densco 3½ D stone (Fig. 16-22). Among the advantages claimed for it are: first, the quickness and

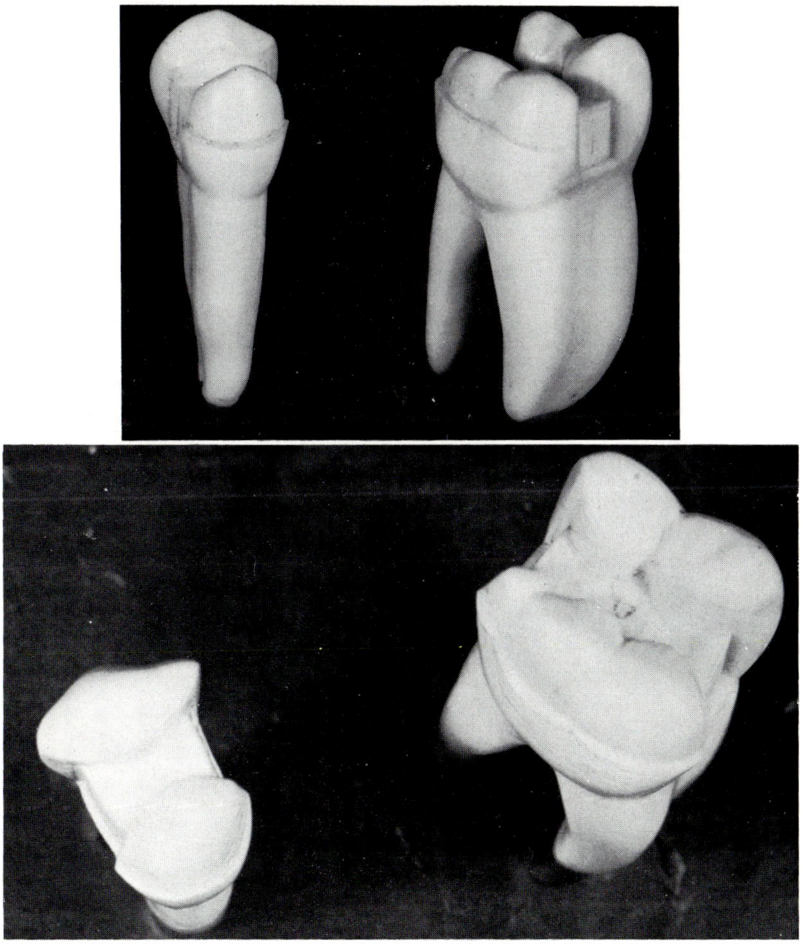

Fig. 16-17. Modified intracoronal preparations extended to include part of lingual surface on upper bicuspid and part of buccal surface on lower molar.

ease with which the proximal outline form may be prepared; second, the conservation of tooth structure; and, third, the assurance that the marginal enamel rods are supported and properly protected.

There are two types of the slice modification: the "lock" slice and the "channel" slice. The former was systematized by Knapp,[1] while the latter was developed into a system by Gillett and Irving.[2] It is interesting to find, however, that the principle of the slice preparation was advo-

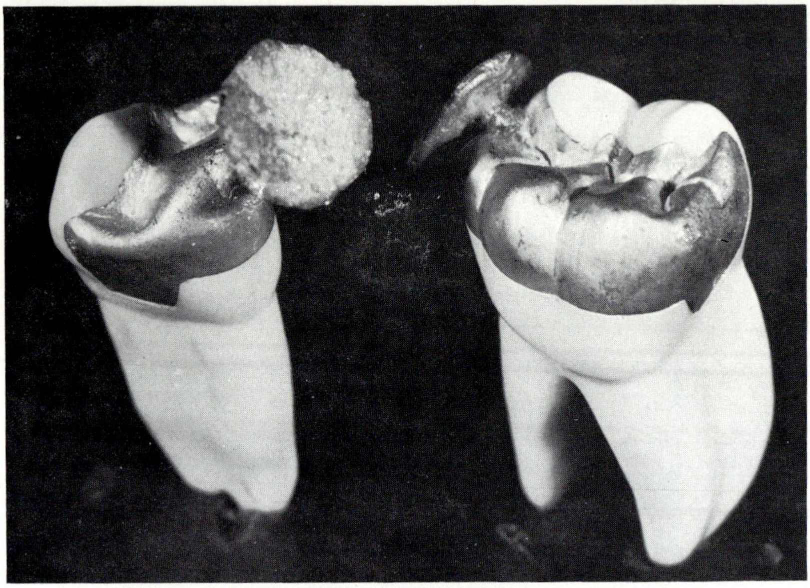

Fig. 16-18. Castings for prepared teeth seen in Fig. 16-17.

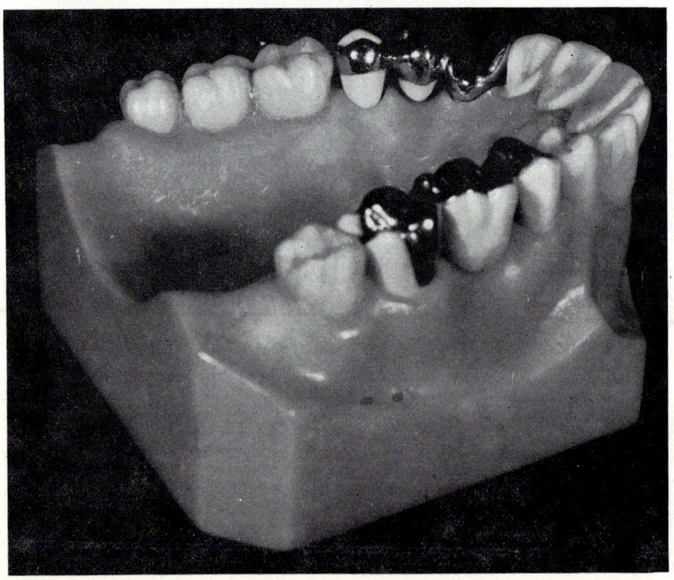

Fig. 16-19. Upper bridge with modified lingual extension on second bicuspid intracoronal retainer terminating its lingual cervical margin above gingiva.

cated as far back as 1911. At that time Bödecker[3] showed a picture of a lower bicuspid containing a mesioclusal cavity of the "slice" type with the following accompanying description: "The mesial surface of the tooth has been flattened with a diamond disk. The margin of the enamel in this case should not be beveled. Retention is obtained by means of a strong fissure anchorage, or if preferred, by cutting a dovetail in the distal part of the occlusal surface."[3] That the slice preparation has not been more extensively used since first suggested many years ago may be attributed to the fact that a systematized technic and present-day instrumentation were not available until recently.

The occlusal dovetail retention is common to both the "lock" and the "channel" slice preparations (Figs. 16-22 to 16-26).

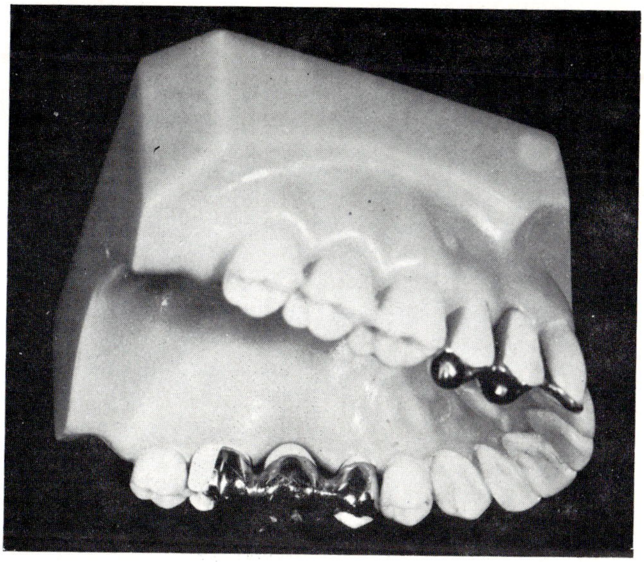

Fig. 16-20. Upper bridge with typical extracoronal partial veneer retainer on second bicuspid having its cervical margin below gingiva.

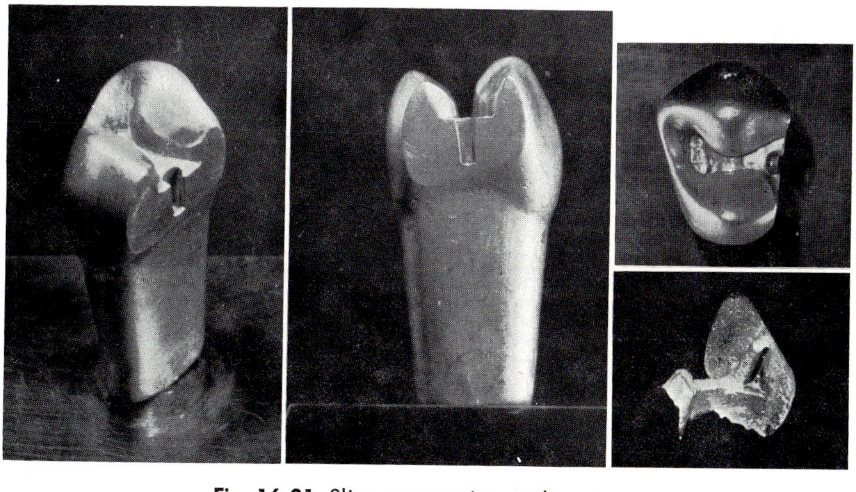

Fig. 16-21. Slice preparation and casting.

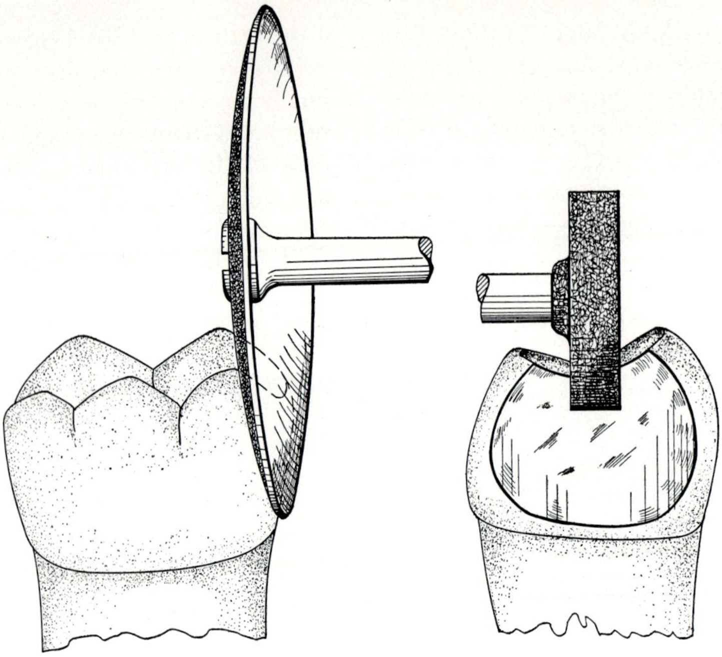

Fig. 16-22. Initial steps of slice preparation.

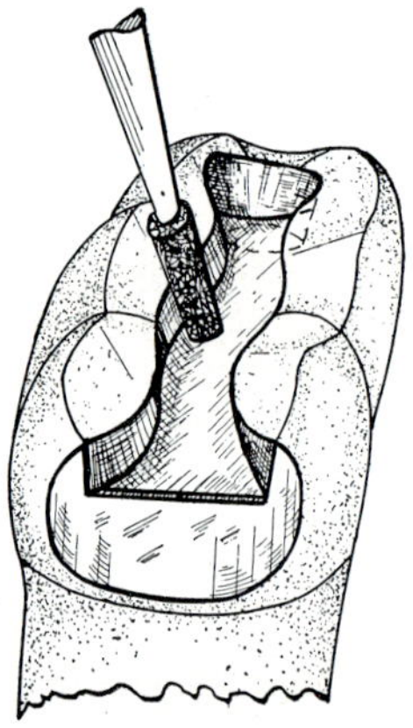

Fig. 16-23. Cutting occlusal dovetail to outline form.

Proximal retention in the lock type is obtained by cutting a tapered keyway in the proximal surface and extending it occlusally from the gingival to the pulpal wall (Fig. 16-24). This keyway is cut into the tooth so that more than half of its circumference lies within the dentin tooth structure. This keyway may be either round or oval-shaped. It is prepared by placing a No. 701 cross-cut tapered fissure bur against the proximal surface after the slice has been made, and gradually pressing it into the tooth structure, the axis of the bur being held parallel with the line of withdrawal of the occlusal dovetail walls. In making the initial cut, the bur is placed midway between buccal and lingual margins and is imbedded to its full diameter within the tooth (Fig. 16-24).

Next, a No. 700 cross-cut tapered fissure bur, which is smaller in size than the No. 701, is placed into the cut made by the No. 701 bur; with the No. 700 bur revolving slowly, it is inclined laterally first buccally, then lingually, so that the tapered keyway assumes an oval shape.

After the retainer is cast, the tapered key which fits this keyway and which is a part of the casting interlocks so that a mechanical lock results. No effort is made in the slice preparation to establish a definite gingival wall similar to that found in the typical intracoronal retainer.

In addition to its customary use as a restoration for the individual tooth, the

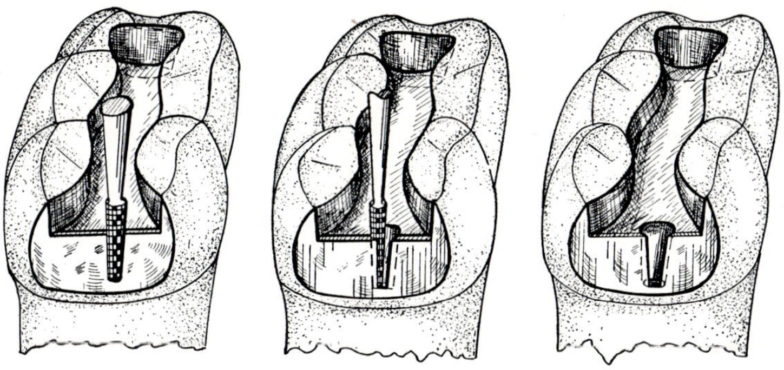

Fig. 16-24. Steps in preparation of proximal keyway (lock type) slice retainer.

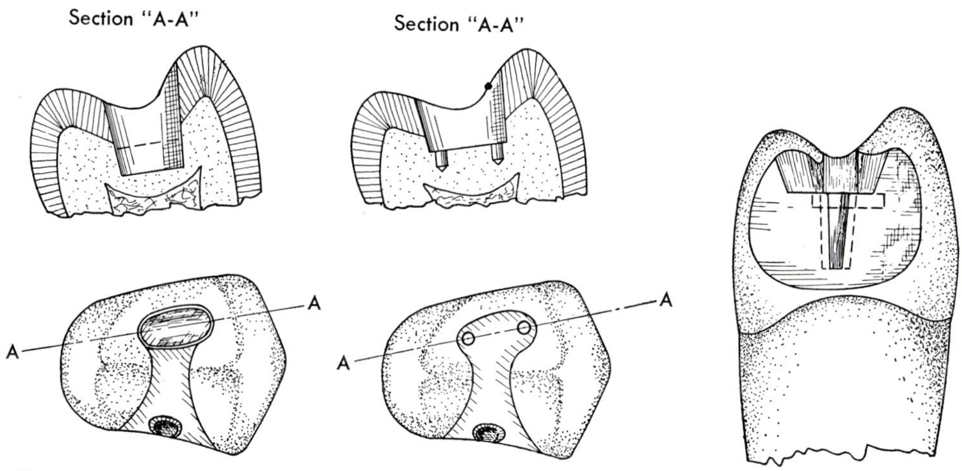

Fig. 16-25. Cross sections of slice preparation (lock type), showing use of depression or pins in pulpal wall and keyway on proximal surface.

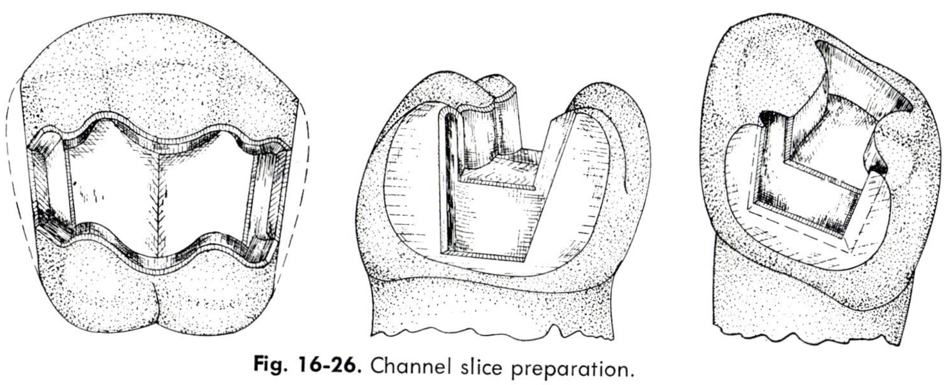

Fig. 16-26. Channel slice preparation.

slice preparation has also been recommended as a bridge retainer.

Fig. 16-25 shows a typical slice preparation having its pulpal wall modified by a countersunk pulpal depression or by pins for the purpose of securing additional retention.

The channel slice preparation. The channel slice differs primarily from the lock slice in that it has two keyed grooves or channels; one is placed in the dentin of the buccal wall and the other is placed in the lingual wall (Fig. 16-26). This modification differs from the typical intracoronal retainer in that its proximal contour has also been removed, leaving a flat or a slightly concave surface. Whereas the regular intracoronal preparation has two walls parallel axioproximally, the channel preparation contains two tapering keyways or grooves (Fig. 16-27).

The degree of divergence of these grooves cervicoclusally varies proportionately with the height of the proximal portion of the preparation; where it is shallow, the divergence is so slight that it is nearly parallel; where, however, the height of the proximal surface is considerable, a greater degree of flare or gingivoclusal divergence is permissible.

Although the channel wall is usually rounded, the same mechanical effect may be obtained by preparing two flat walls which converge axioproximally. Since the latter is more difficult to prepare and since nothing additional is gained mechanically by doing so, channels are usually prepared with cross-cut, tapered fissure burs, No. 700 or 701, and finished with fine polishing stones or burs.

In cutting the channel keyway, precaution must be taken that a sufficient bulk of tooth structure forming the dentin wedges remains between the inside surface of the channel and the sliced surface opposite to it; if the amount is insufficient, there is great danger of fracture occurring through these rib-like dentin locks.

In order to strengthen the casting where the proximal and occlusal portions meet and to eliminate the sharp angles in the occlusal cavosurface margins, that portion of the wedge-shaped tooth structure lying on the occlusal portion between the channel and the slice is rounded and flared back, establishing one continuous curved cavosurface margin between the channel and the proximal cavosurface angle.

A basic rule of the slice preparations is that the amount of gingivoclusal flare or divergence of slice and channel walls is in proportion to the depth of the cavity and the length of the coronal portion of the tooth; the shorter the distance or height, the closer should these walls approximate parallelism.

When starting a proximal slice, it is well to remember that the diamond disks used for this purpose are dangerous instruments unless kept absolutely under the operator's control. These disks should always be used in conjunction with cocoa butter, and a copious stream of water at body temperature should be directed upon the

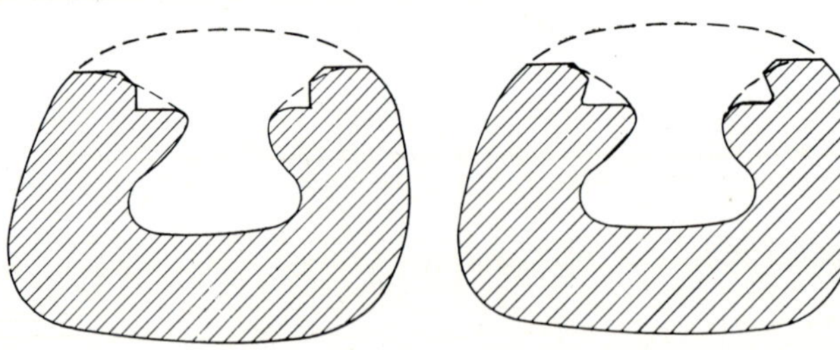

Fig. 16-27. Cross section of regular two-surface inlay, with parallel axioproximal walls on left; dovetail locks or grooves in slice type preparation. (After Gillet and Irving.)

tooth during the cutting operation. A disk revolving at high speed, but applied with light pressure, is more efficient and less painful than the same disk applied at a lower rate of speed, but with greater pressure. Cutting of a tooth with a disk should not be done as one continuous, uninterrupted procedure; rather, it should be accomplished by intermittent applications and withdrawals of the disk, thus reducing to a minimum the tendency of the disk to cumulate frictional heat.

If separation of teeth has been previously provided, a thin, diamond disk can be applied easily to the proximal surface of a tooth. The contour of the tooth, the type of embrasures present, the axial inclination, and the type of slice preparation that is being prepared (i.e., the lock or the channel type) all determine to a large extent whether a flat or a concave disk is to be used.

Where no preliminary separation of teeth has been provided, the initial cut is made by locating the disk over the occlusal surface in the region of the marginal ridge to be included in the casting; the disk is placed approximately 0.5 to 1 mm. from the proximal surface and tilted toward the central fossa; the slice is so directed that, when it emerges cervically, its gingival margin will terminate at or slightly beneath the crest of the gingival tissue, without leaving a shoulder. In making these proximal cuts, every precaution must be taken not to injure the proximal surfaces of sound adjacent teeth. After the proximal surface has been sliced, the slice cut usually exposes the dentinoenamel plane.

From here the usual technic is employed in developing the proximal boxlike preparation, with the added preparation of the buccal and lingual channels. The occlusal

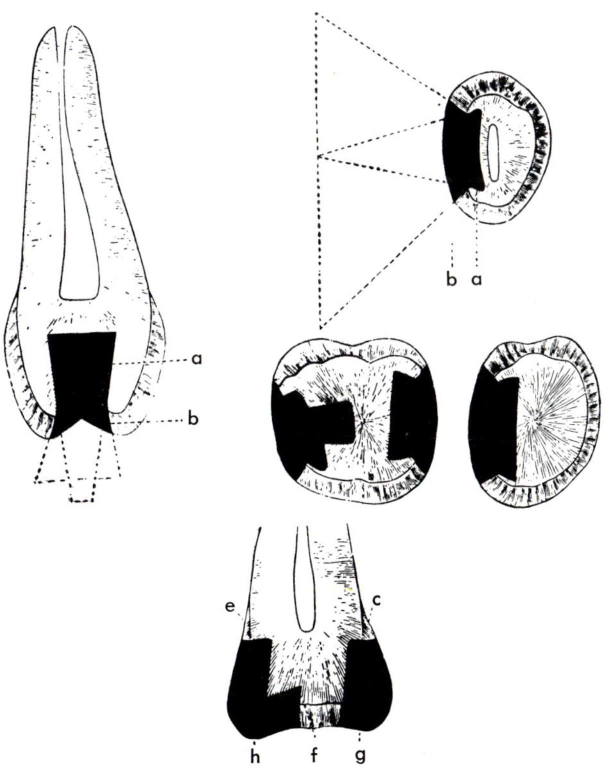

Fig. 16-28. Principles of slice and channel retentions, illustrated in 1894 by Weeks.

dovetail is prepared similarly to that of the typical intracoronal retainer.

The mechanical merits of the channel and the slice preparations were recognized many years ago. Fig. 16-28 is reproduced from a page taken from a manual published in 1894 by Thomas E. Weeks,[4] showing that these mechanical, engineering, and biologic principles were recognized before the casting process, high-speed cutting, and porcelain fused to metal restorations came into general use. Sometimes these principles are designated as "modern."

SELECTED REFERENCES

1. Knapp, K. W.: Modern fixed bridge abutments for vital teeth, Illinois D. Soc. Tr., p. 16, 1925.
2. Gillett, H. W., and Irving, A. J.: Gold inlays by the indirect system, Brooklyn, 1932, Dental Items of Interest Publishing Co.
3. Bödecker, H. W. C.: The metallic inlay, Berlin, 1911, Hermann Meusser, p. 80.
4. Weeks, T. E.: Manual of operative technics, Chicago, 1894, H. D. Justi and Son.

GENERAL REFERENCES

Blackwell, R. E.: Cavity preparation for inlays to be used as bridge abutments in fixed bridgework, J.A.D.A. **17**:1446, 1930.

Hollenback, G. M.: A plea for a more conservative approach in certain dental procedures, J. Alabama D. A. **46**:16, 1962.

Klaffenbach, A. O.: An analytic study of modern abutments, J.A.D.A. **23**:2275, 1936.

Meyer, F. S.: Inlays, crown and full cast bridges, Am. D. Surgeon **52**:33, 73, 1932.

Nuttall, E. B.: Abutment preparations using high speed instruments, J. Kentucky D. A. **13**:161, 1961.

Smith, D. E.: Fixed bridge restorations with the tilted mandibular second or third molar as an abutment, J. South. California D. A. **6**:131, 1939.

Tinker, E. T.: A fixed bridge, Minneapolis Dist. D. J. **23**:18, 1939.

Chapter 17

Tooth preparations and instrumentation: class I, type 3—anterior extracoronal partial veneer retainers

GENERAL CONSIDERATIONS

The cast partial veneer retainer is almost universal in its application; it may be used on most of the anterior or posterior teeth of the upper and lower arches. Its virtue lies in the fact that maximum retention may be obtained with the least danger to the normality of the pulp and minimum sacrifice of tooth structure. Its esthetic values permit its use in the anterior as well as the posterior regions, while, from a mechanical or retentive standpoint, it very closely approximates the values of a complete veneer crown.

INDICATIONS

Although it is primarily indicated on sound normal teeth, it may be employed on those teeth whose pulps have been removed and on teeth having small carious lesions on the proximal or lingual surfaces.

The general acceptance of this type of retainer is largely due to the facts that (1) the preparation conserves most of the enamel of the tooth; and (2) the clamplike locking effect of the three-quarter design minimizes the possibility of a tooth fracturing from the forces of mastication, which is frequently the situation with the intracoronal type of retainers.

As the name "partial veneer" indicates, the retainer covers several but not all of the external surfaces of the crown portion of the tooth. In upper anterior teeth it ordinarily involves all surfaces except the labial, and in the upper posterior teeth all surfaces but the buccal are included. In the lower molar teeth the buccal surfaces are included instead of the lingual.

Although most lower molars can accept a three-quarter veneer casting individually, when used as bridge retainers their actual relationship to the anterior abutment tooth make the path of insertion of a fixed bridge difficult or impossible. In such situations, a mesial one-half veneer retainer (Fig. 18-32) or a complete crown is preferable.

Three-quarter partial veneer retainers can be used as units of a bridge if the long axis of the preparation can be aligned axially with the other abutment, or it can be used as an individual restoration. To use this type of restoration successfully, it is essential that a sufficient amount of dentin and enamel be available to prepare grooves and planes to resist displacing forces.

It has been found that the square type of anterior teeth, relatively thick labiolingually, are more suitable for this type of retainer than the ovoid, which are not as thick in their incisal third. This type of retainer is contraindicated in those carious anterior teeth in which considerable caries extends from the proximal surfaces onto the labial surface. Due to its relatively long cavosurface margin it is usually contraindicated in patients with high caries susceptibility.

As previously stated, the partial veneer retainer is used primarily in bridge prosthesis when one, two, or more missing teeth are restored. This retainer requires, in addition to the correct placement of the proximal grooves and walls, that the gold alloy used be of the proper type and that it be properly heat treated before the bridge is permanently cemented in place. Failure of this type of retainer may be attributed in most instances to the improper preparation of the tooth, to the use of improper alloys, or to the improper or lack of heat treatment of the finished casting.

SEPARATION

Where an abutment requires a partial veneer retainer, one surface of the tooth usually approximates the edentulous area, while the other is in contact with a natural tooth. To make a satisfactory preparation and yet not injure the adjacent tooth, it is advisable to develop separation by one of the several methods previously discussed, after which it is safe to proceed with the cutting operations. Even where separation has been established, it is frequently advisable to protect the adjacent tooth by means of a thin steel strip to avoid injuring it.

REMOVAL OF DECAY

In abutments having some proximal caries, it is advisable to remove any decay to determine whether enough of the natural tooth remains to allow the preparation of typical proximal grooves, or whether the preparation must be changed to a complete crown. Where the lingual half of the proximal surfaces is destroyed by caries and where the labial surface has extensive caries gingivally or across the labioproximal line angle, a typical three-quarter partial veneer retainer is not recommended.

OUTLINE FORM

Before any cutting is undertaken on an anterior tooth, the outline form, especially that of the labial and proximal surfaces, should be accurately determined. This is extended into an immune area, but at the same time there should be no unnecessary display of metal after the bridge has been placed. To avoid this undesirable display of gold, the exact locations of the labioproximal and the incisal margins should be determined from the labial aspect. The incisal margin should not be carried onto the labial surface so that it is visible; it should terminate at the line where the labial and incisal surfaces meet.

While it is essential that the proximal margins be carried labially into cleansable or immune areas, this can be done without an excessive display of gold if they terminate in the area where the proximal surface breaks lingually at the proximolabial line angle.

Locating the position and outline of the gingival margin is governed by the same rules and conditions that govern the placement of the gingival margin of an intracoronal retainer; the margin is placed slightly beneath the crest of the gum tissue in those instances in which a gingival crevice exists; the curve of the gingival margin generally parallels the curvature of the crest of the gum tissue.

In those instances in which the gum tissue has receded, exposing the cementoenamel junction, no attempt is made to carry the margin below this line; instead it terminates in a cleansable area and is placed at a uniform distance from the cementoenamel junction.

Before undertaking any cutting operation, it is well to have determined the direction in which the finished bridge will be inserted so that the grooves and axial surfaces may be prepared parallel to it. The dentist should also determine the type of occlusion present and the location and amount of tooth structure to be removed from the incisal, lingual, or occluding surfaces to allow sufficient gold alloy in these areas in the finished casting.

GUM RETRACTION AND REMOVAL

It is necessary in some instances to retract the gingival tissues before the gingival outline and position of the preparation can be determined. This may be done by the use of temporary crowns of copper-band material having gingival, marginal rolls of low fusing metal with beveled, flaring wall; however, this is a slow method. A more acceptable method is the use of cotton cord as described by Thompson[1] (Figs. 21-15 to 21-17). Other methods include the crimped copper-band and washer method of Pagenkopf[2] (Figs. 21-18 and 21-19), the rubber dam and clamp technic recommended by Selberg[3] (Fig. 17-17), and the electrosurgery method of Malone.[4] The metal retractor serves a dual purpose; first, it presses back the soft gingival tissues; and second, it may be used as a temporary covering to protect the tooth after the tooth has been prepared and during the time that the bridge is being constructed. When gum retractors are employed, they usually accomplish their purpose within 24 hours; if they are left longer on the tooth, there is danger of inducing permanent recession of the gum tissues. Either the Selberg method or the Thompson method is usually used.

Before describing the technic of preparing an anterior tooth for a three-quarter retainer, let us consider what bearing tooth morphology or anatomy has on the type of preparation that is to be made. The following review summarizes the 1951 study and report of LeHuche.[5]

In his study of the anatomy of over 2,000 natural teeth, he found great variance in three of their dimensions, all of them having a definite influence on their preparation for a three-quarter retainer. The shapes vary from the extreme tapering to the square types, with an intermediate type. Each type enables the dentist to determine the length and depth of the axial grooves, whether the incisal groove can or should be used, and also what modifications are indicated in selected circumstances.

The *first* dimension to be considered is the *mesiodistal.* By comparing the widest mesiodistal width in the contact regions with that in the cervical area it is possible to classify the tooth into its type: square, tapering, or average.

The *second* dimension is considered in its *labiolingual* direction. Whether a tooth is thin or thick in its incisal third will make a difference in the preparation, also the amount of abrasion that exists in the incisal third. The measurement is taken at a labiolingual plane 4 mm. from the incisal edge of a normal, nonabraded tooth. Here it is found that the thickness varies from 2.6 to 4 mm.

The depth of the lingual concavity at this level is also taken into consideration with reference to the height of the mesial and distal marginal ridges.

In this respect the presence of incisal abrasion is important, since its presence determines the type and amount of incisal retention that may be developed. Abrasion of the lingual surface lying above the cingulum and extending incisally makes the ideal preparation even more difficult because of the proximity of the pulp.

The *third* dimension to consider is the

axial. A nonabraded tooth with a high gingival attachment is not as favorable a tooth as one in an older patient having slight abrasion and gum recession.

One other consideration is the *gingivo-incisal curvature* of the crown of the tooth. The length of the axial groove is reduced in proportion to the increased curvature of the crown.

This work of LeHuche will be referred to later.

RESISTANCE AND RETENTION FORMS

The resistance and outline forms of the anterior partial veneer type of retainer are discussed and described in Chapter 13. This resistance to displacing forces is largely related to properly prepared and placed proximal and incisal grooves and axial surfaces (Fig. 17-1). The following technic applies to the average type of tooth bordering on the square type. Variations available in the other types will also be discussed.

Incisal groove

The anterior partial veneer retainer is frequently prepared with an incisal groove (Fig. 17-2). It has been found that this may be dispensed with in many instances. The groove is especially contraindicated in those teeth which are thin labiolingually, at which time the incisal plane or bevel is used. One of the disadvantages of the incisal groove, often encountered but not necessarily, is the blue-gray color effect that sometimes accompanies this type of incisal preparation; there is also the possibility of a weakened enamel margin at the incisal edge that is likely to be fractured during the interval between the preparation of the abutment and the final setting of the bridge. An incisal bevel or plane of 45° provides the necessary incisal protection without the liabilities just mentioned (Fig. 17-3). Such an angle is usually at right angles to the applied forces of mastication (Fig. 17-8). The lingual margin of the plane should have a minimum clearance of 1 mm. from the opposing occluding teeth; this will allow for enough metal in the incisal portion of the casting to give it rigidity and permanence.

Proximal grooves

The direction of insertion and position of the proximal grooves can be determined on the diagnostic study casts by means of the dental surveyor. These can then be verified and, if satisfactory, penciled on the natural tooth prior to cutting the grooves.

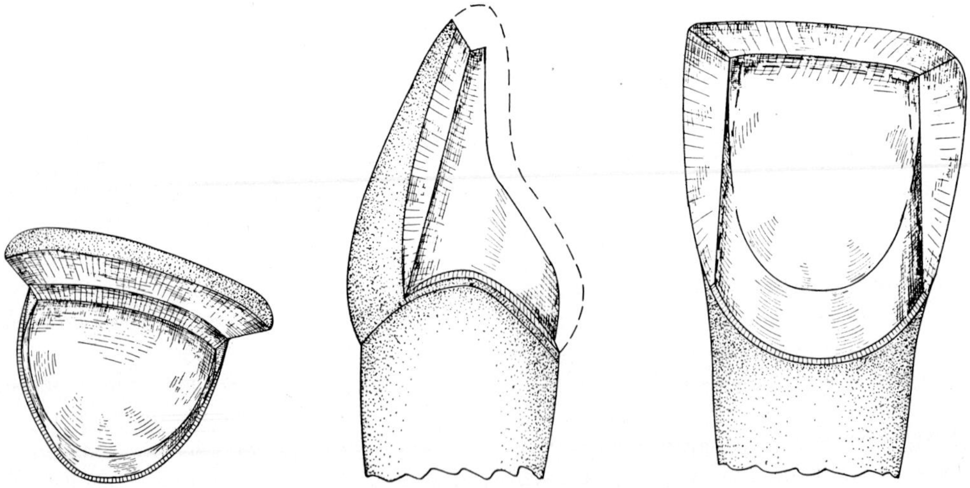

Fig. 17-1. Upper central incisor prepared for partial veneer extracoronal retainer.

In order that the proximal grooves in anterior teeth exert their maximum resistance to displacement, it is necessary for them to be so placed that: first, they parallel the incisal two-thirds of the labial surface (Fig. 17-1); second, these grooves, in their gingivoincisal relationship to each other, are nearly parallel (Fig. 17-1); and third, their convergence cervicoincisally does not exceed 2° from parallelism. By observing these principles, a clamp-like grip furnishes resistance to lingual displacement immediately when the proximal ribs or keys of the cast retainer enter the proximal grooves or keyways of the prepared tooth. Placing the proximal grooves parallel to the incisal two-thirds of the labial surface results, first, in a retainer that automatically enables its labial margins to be extended into a cleansable area; second, it gives a retainer that encompasses three-fourths of the circumference of the tooth; and third, it furnishes proximal grooves that are comparatively longer, and hence stronger, than grooves placed parallel to the long axis of the crown (Fig. 17-15).

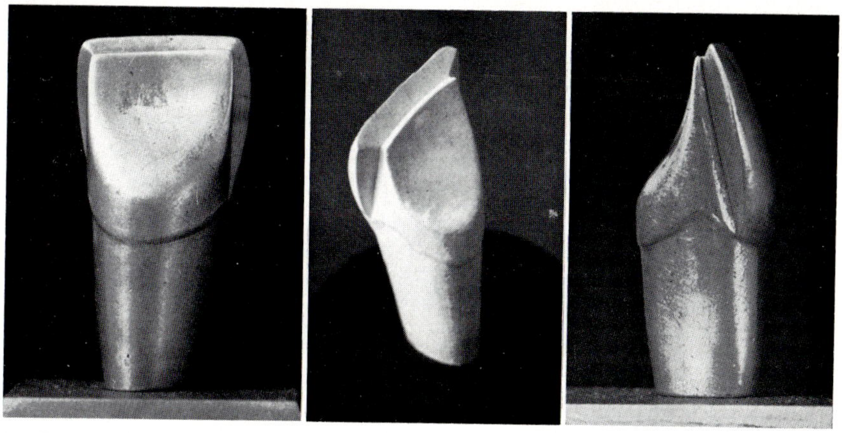

Fig. 17-2. Lingual and proximal views of partial veneer extracoronal preparations on upper incisors having incisal grooves.

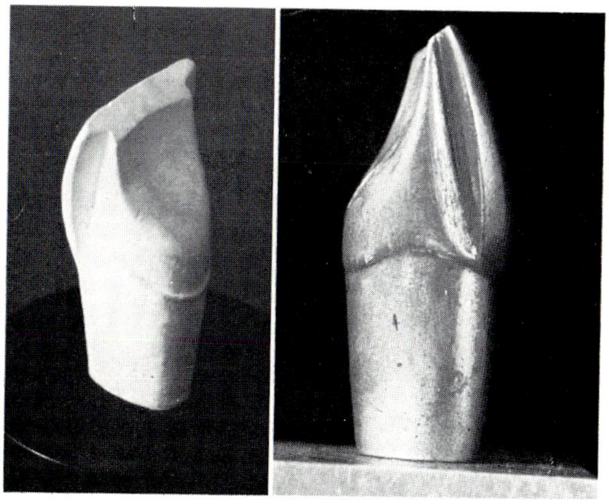

Fig. 17-3. Lingual and proximal views of partial veneer extracoronal preparation on upper incisors having incisal planes.

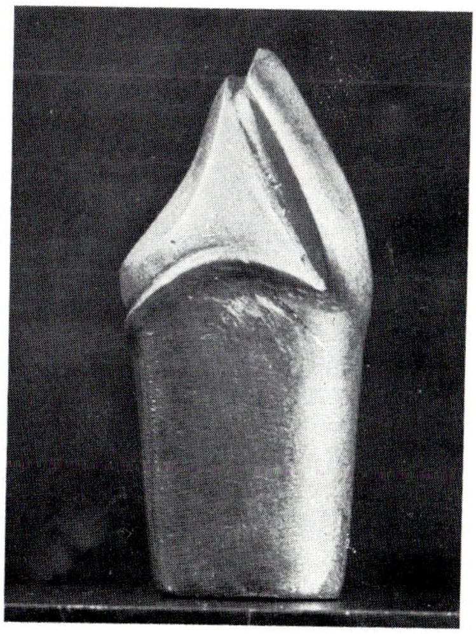

Fig. 17-4. Proximal view of partial veneer extracoronal preparation on upper cuspid with incisal groove.

Axial walls

Every effort should be made to prepare the opposing proximal walls as close to parallelism as possible; at any rate, the convergence should not exceed 2°. Such near parallelism will add greatly to the retention qualities of the preparation.

One of the frequent errors observed in the preparation of this type of retainer is the excessive reduction of the lingual axial wall in the region of the cingulum (Fig. 17-10). Only enough of this convexity should be removed to permit the withdrawal of the pattern. If a near parallelism is established between this wall, the proximal grooves, and the axis of the preparation, a considerably increased retention will result (Figs. 17-4, 17-12, and 17-14).

In this type, as in other types of bridge retainers, care should be observed not to overheat the tooth while cutting and not to cut away more tooth structure than is absolutely essential to obtain the required mechanical retention. Cocoa butter applied to stones and a stream of water played on the tooth during cutting operations are recommended as precautionary measures.

STEPS AND INSTRUMENTATION OF PREPARATION

The technic of making a three-quarter partial veneer retainer for an anterior tooth consists of six steps.

Preparation of proximal surfaces

The first step, the preparation of the proximal surfaces, while comparatively simple, unless properly made may be the ultimate reason for a lack of retentive and esthetic qualities in the finished retainer. The cuts that remove the proximal contours of the tooth are usually made with a ½-inch, safe-sided, thin, diamond disk, Densco 4T-PS (Fig. 17-5).

In order to use the thin diamond disk on the surface that approximates the adjacent tooth without injuring it, a temporary mechanical separation of the teeth may be made while the initial slice is being cut. As a precaution, a piece of thin steel-matrix material is interposed for protection. Another method of gaining access safely through the interproximal contact is to apply cocoa butter to the contacting areas and to carefully insert a thin diamond-coated steel strip between the teeth. This is gradually worked through the contact area with a sawing motion under light pressure, keeping the cutting surface toward the abutment tooth and the smooth side of the disk against the adjacent contacting tooth. In using cutting speeds of less than 6,000 rpm in making the proximal cuts, every effort must be made to retain as much of the tooth structure as possible, especially the mesiodistal width of the labial surface (Fig. 17-6); the two cuts, while inclined slightly toward the lingual surface, should have their planes cervicoincisally near-parallel to the long axis of the preparation. When these cuts are being made, they are brought from the lingual toward the labial surface, through the contact area, care being taken not to cut away too much of the cingulum (Fig. 17-7). The labial margins of the

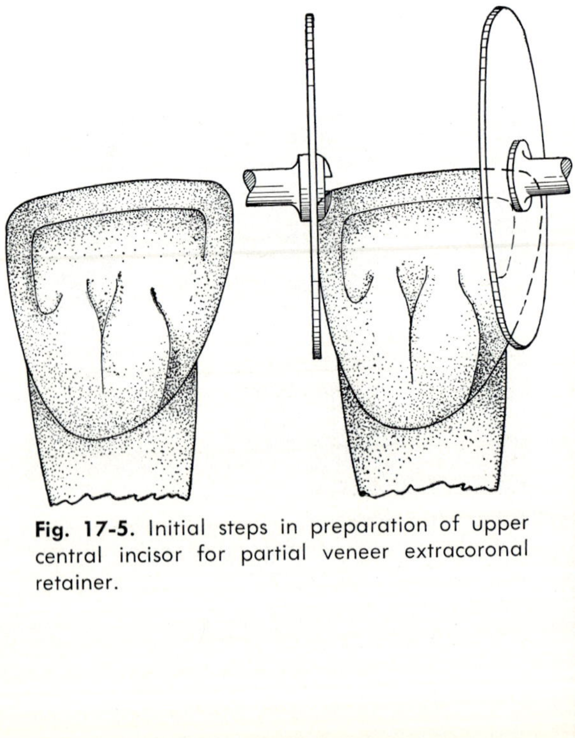

Fig. 17-5. Initial steps in preparation of upper central incisor for partial veneer extracoronal retainer.

cuts should terminate near the self-cleansing or cleansable areas, just short of the incisal plane (Figs. 17-7 and 17-8). The amount of curvature of the gingivae and the type of tooth, whether square or tapering, will determine to a large degree the extent of the first proximal cuts gingivally.

If the disk cuts are incorrectly made (Fig. 17-6), i.e., parallel linguolabially, an unnecessary amount of the labial surface will be removed, resulting in an unnecessary display of gold. Care must also be exercised to avoid undercutting the tooth at the gingival margin.

Incisal cut

The second step involves the preparation of the incisal surface. A flat plane is cut labiolingually and extends mesiodistally between the two proximal surfaces. The purpose of the inclined plane is to give the incisal portion of the tooth a sufficient minimum bulk of gold alloy, approximately 1 mm., to protect it against fracturing when incising food (Fig. 17-8, *C*). The labial margin of this plane is so positioned that gold will not be visible from the labial aspect (Fig. 17-8, *A*). The angle of the plane labiolingually is ap-

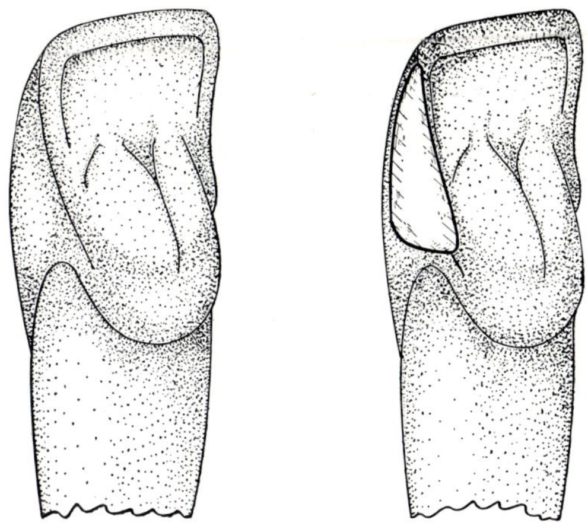

Fig. 17-7. Amount of enamel removed in initial cut.

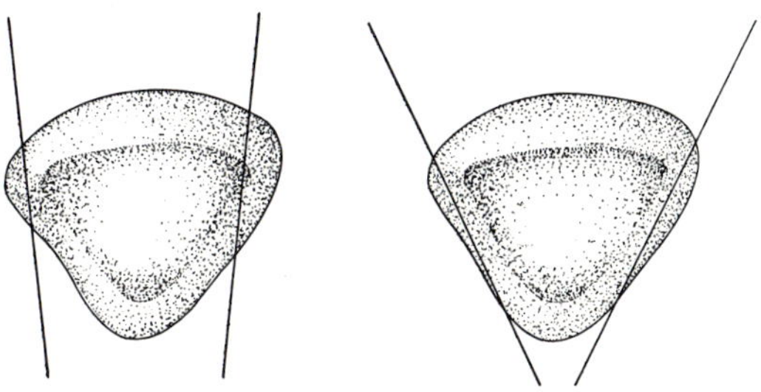

Incorrect Correct

Fig. 17-6. Incorrect and correct initial proximal cut angulation.

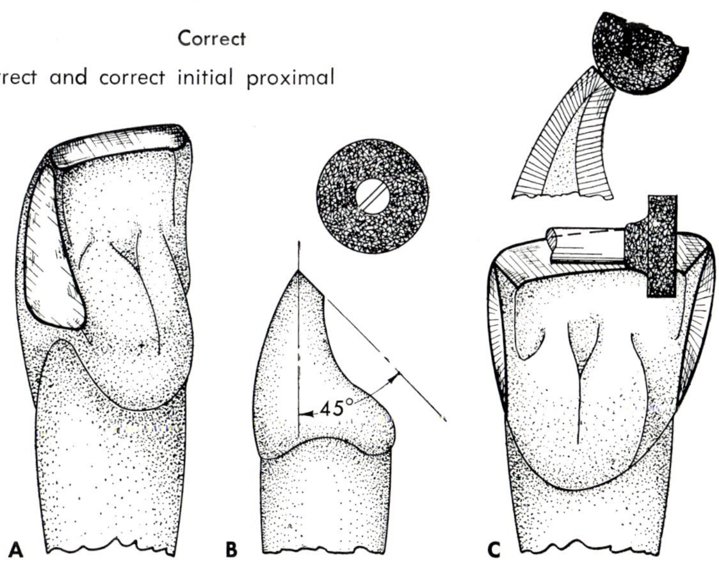

Fig. 17-8. Second step is preparation of incisal plane.

proximately 45° to the long axis of the tooth (Fig. 17-8, *B*). A small mounted diamond stone, Densco 5J-T, may be used for this purpose with a cutting speed of 10,000 rpm. (Fig. 17-8).

Lingual cuts

The third step consists in the reduction of the lingual surface; this is usually accomplished in two phases (Fig. 17-9). The first involves the removal of the enamel on the lingual surface to a minimum depth of 0.5 mm. extending from the crest of the cingulum to the lingual margin of the incisal plane. The general contour of the lingual surface is followed (Fig. 17-9, *A*). The precaution must be taken to create sufficient space to allow 1 mm. thickness of gold in those areas on the lingual surface and the incisal plane that the diagnostic casts disclosed came in functioning contact with the opposing teeth in all positions of the mandible. It is neither necessary nor desirable to remove the entire thickness of enamel on the lingual surface (Fig. 17-10); only enough is removed to create room for 0.5 mm. of gold in the finished casting in this area.

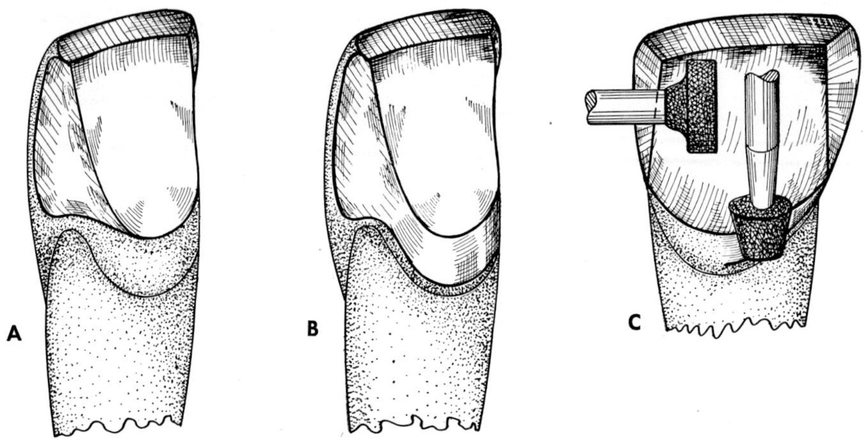

Fig. 17-9. Third step involves preparation of lingual surface.

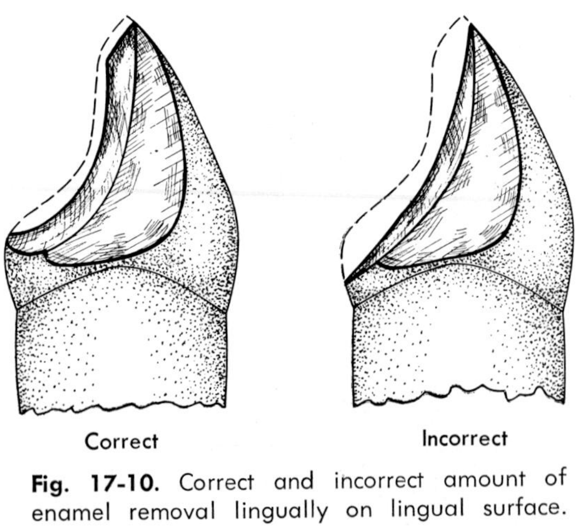

Fig. 17-10. Correct and incorrect amount of enamel removal lingually on lingual surface.

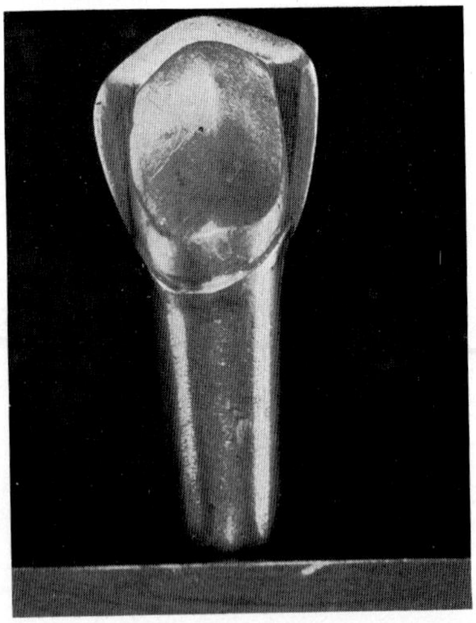

Fig. 17-11. Lingual aspect of upper cuspid prepared for partial veneer extracoronal retainer.

Deeper cutting than this is unnecessary and may jeopardize the health of the pulp. During the lingual reduction, if the general contour of the tooth is followed, it will be found that in an upper central incisor the surface is concave incisogingivally and mesiodistally (Fig. 17-2); whereas in a cuspid the lingual surface will consist of two planes that rise and meet in a central lingual ridge (Figs. 17-11 and 17-12).

The preparation of the lingual surface (Fig. 17-9) may be accomplished by the use of barrel-shaped, mounted stones (Densco 1MW) or the wheel-shaped, round-edge stone (Densco 2½J at 60,000 rpm).

The second phase of the lingual preparation consists of reducing the lingual enamel lying between the crest of the cingulum and the crest of the gingiva; it extends from one proximal cut to the

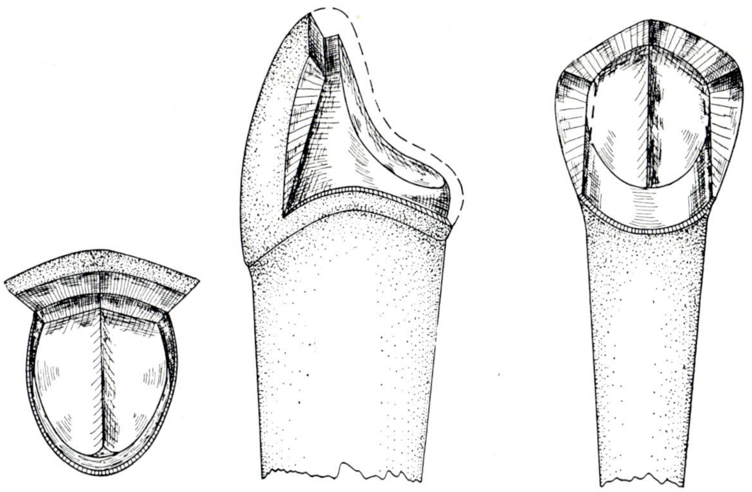

Fig. 17-12. In upper cuspid partial veneer extracoronal retainer two planes are prepared on incisal and lingual surfaces; one plane slopes mesially, the other distally.

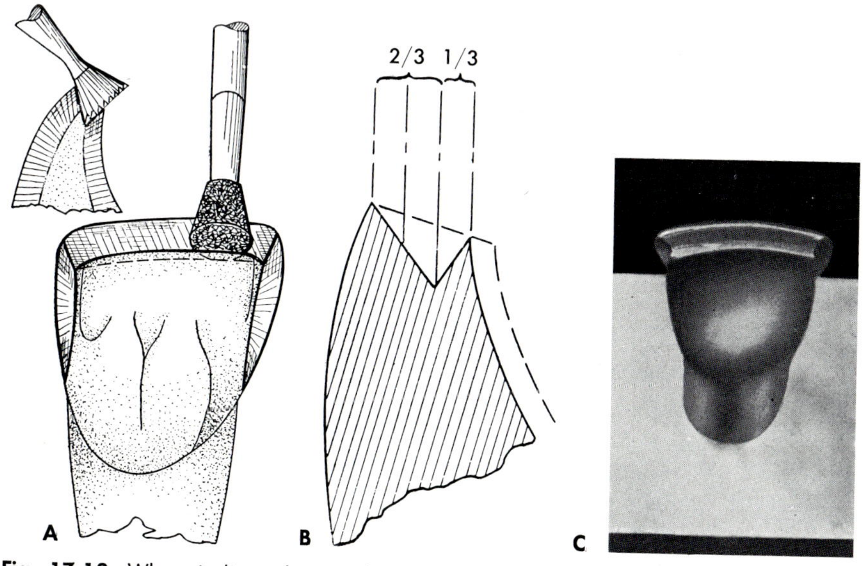

Fig. 17-13. When indicated, incisal plane is modified by forming incisal groove.

other (Fig. 17-9, *B* and *C*). Care must be exercised in reducing this part of the lingual wall so that it is made near-parallel to the long axis of the preparation and yet does not converge excessively toward the incisal edge. If desired, this second phase of the preparation may be postponed until after the proximal grooves have been prepared. When properly prepared, the wall will later be parallel to the proximal grooves, which, in turn, are parallel to the incisal third of the labial surface of the tooth; this arrangement results in retentive qualities of considerable measure.

The instruments used are the smallest mounted, tapered stone (Densco 1C) or the pointed stone (Densco safe-end tapered 1D-S).

Incisal groove

Where an incisal groove is indicated instead of the incisal plane, its preparation constitutes the fourth step (Fig. 17-13). The incisal groove is not an indefinite crevice made in the flat incisal surface; it is formed by two very definite planes, a labial and a lingual, which meet at a right or at a slightly acute angle. This angle at the bottom of the groove lies in dentin just lingual to the labial plate of enamel. The labial plane of the step extends from the bottom of the groove to the labioincisal edge and is approximately twice the height of the lingual plane. The incisal groove is not in a straight line mesiodistally; instead, it parallels the general contour of the labial incisal edge. In the central and lateral incisors the labial and lingual planes of the incisal groove extend in a continuous curve mesiodistally; in the cuspid these rise from the mesial and distal slopes and merge at the cusp (Fig. 17-14).

In starting the incisal groove, a small, inverted cone diamond stone (Densco 1K-5X) is placed in the center of the incisal plane in such a position that the base of the cone faces lingually and the sides of the cone face toward the labial plate of enamel (Fig. 17-13, *A*). Held in this position, the revolving stone is moved from the mesial to the distal proximal cuts, gradually cutting a V-shaped groove between the labial and lingual plates of enamel. The labial wall being approximately twice as high as the lingual, care must be exercised to have a supporting dentin wall back of the projecting enamel plate. The height of the lingual wall should have a minimum clearance of 1 mm. with the opposing teeth. This will give the casting a sufficient bulk and rigidity and will

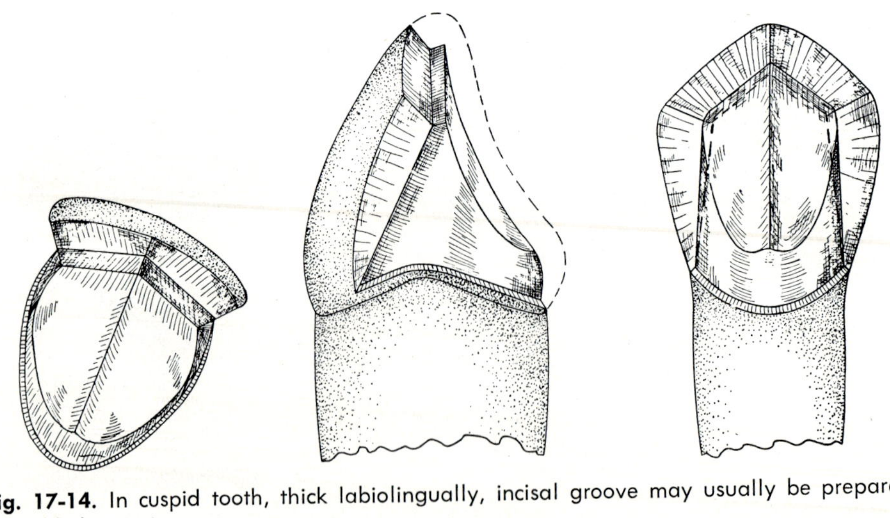

Fig. 17-14. In cuspid tooth, thick labiolingually, incisal groove may usually be prepared for added retention.

allow for any necessary slight occlusal adjustment.

After the cut has been carried to the desired depth with the diamond stone, the labial and lingual planes may be finished with an inverted cone bur No. 35 or No. 34 and fine sandpaper or garnet disks. No jagged edges or sharp angles should be left along the incisal or axial margins of the enamel (Fig. 17-13, *C*).

Axial proximal grooves

The fifth step consists in the preparation of axial grooves in the proximal surfaces. Since the proximal grooves furnish the major retention of a partial veneer retainer, it is essential that they be prepared properly and be placed correctly in relation to the axis of the preparation (Fig. 13-25).

In the original Carmichael preparation, which is the prototype of the present partial veneer retainer, the proximal grooves were placed midway labiolingually and parallel to the long axis of the tooth (Fig. 17-15, *B* and *C*). Such a direction resulted in relatively short proximal grooves cervicoincisally; it also had the disadvantage of encompassing only half or less of the circumference of the tooth. Because of the lingual position of the grooves, it was extremely difficult to carry the labial margins of the finished preparation into the cleansable or immune areas of the labial surface.

When Tinker[6, 7] and others developed the Carmichael retainer and refined it to its present state of efficiency, they repositioned the proximal grooves (Fig. 17-15, line *B-B*) so that many mechanical and biologic advantages resulted.

The present-day partial veneer retainer, largely because of esthetic requirements, is so prepared that it sheds from the gingival area in an incisal direction. Such a direction eliminates the necessity of including little, if any, of the labial surface of the enamel, thus avoiding the unpleasant display of gold. Best results are obtained when the proximal groove extends incisally from the gingival, line *B-B*, parallel to the incisal third or half of the labial surface, line *A-A*.

Assistance may be had in determining the correct labial marginal outline of the preparation if the dentist has previously selected the proper facing and has ground it to the desired contour and position on

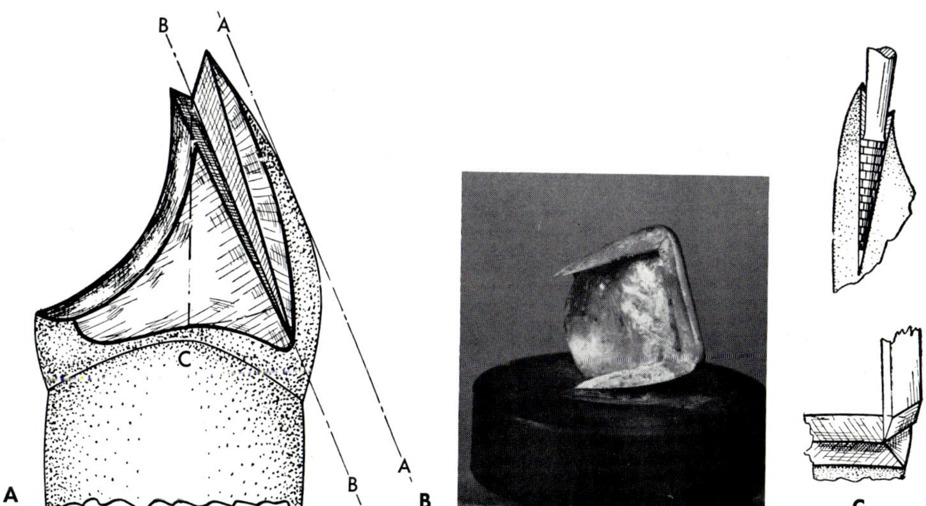

Fig. 17-15. Correct shape, direction, and relative parallelism of axial grooves are important in obtaining maximum retention in retainer.

the edentulous area on the diagnostic study casts. The facing is attached to a temporary shellac or resin baseplate and is tried in the mouth; this furnishes the operator with guidelines for the labial marginal outline and positions.

The depth of the groove must lie in dentin and in the region of the contact areas, which usually encompasses the widest portion of the tooth mesiodistally (Fig. 17-15). Proximal grooves so located enable the completed retainer to encircle three-fourths of the circumference of the tooth.

The groove has two walls—the labial, which is a flat plane, and the lingual, which is a convex surface. Labially, the flat plane is prepared incisogingivally to extend from the depth of the groove to the labial cavosurface margin. The inner portion of this plane lies in dentin, while the outer lies largely in the enamel structure.

In paralleling the direction of the two proximal grooves with the incisal two-thirds or half of the labial surface, every effort should be made to parallel the grooves with each other within a 2 to 5° convergence cervicoincisally. The proximal groove is started at the bottom of the incisal groove (Fig. 17-15) and is directed incisogingivally so that it terminates at or slightly below the crest of the gum tissue (Fig. 17-15, *B*).

A pilot groove is started with a Densco ½DT tapered diamond stone, which is placed midway along its length in contact with the bottom of the incisal groove at low speed. It is brought into the tooth structure to a depth of its full diameter. All cutting with diamond stones is done under a stream of water and light pressure. The groove is extended gradually from the incisal, in the gingival direction, becoming shallower as it nears the gingival area but without forming any definite shoulder cervically at this time (Fig. 17-15, *B*). The stone is then replaced with a No. 699 or 700 cross-cut fissure bur and the depth of the groove is increased, depending upon the size of the abutment tooth worked on.

When the two proximal grooves have been verified as to parallelism to the direction of the labial surface and to the correct degree of mutual convergence, the labial walls are made smooth either by the use of straight chisels No. 15 and 20 (Fig. 17-15, *C*) or with very fine tapering polishing stones (Densco ½DTL).

Krause files are frequently used to accentuate the triangular shape of the axial grooves.[8] In planing the labial wall of enamel, care must be exercised not to overextend the labial cavosurface margins and yet ensure that the margins are in areas of cleansability.

Some operators prefer to end the groove in a definite shoulder or step at the gingival margin, thereby getting a stronger rib of gold in the finished cast retainer. This mechanical advantage is offset, however, by the resulting closeness of the gold casting to the pulp and the necessity of cutting away a greater amount of tooth structure.

The lingual wall of the proximal groove has been left curved labiolingually by the cutting surface of the No. 700 bur. To expedite the making of a wax pattern, any sharp lingual margin of this wall is either rounded off with a No. 170 or 171 finishing bur or it is beveled slightly with a chisel, No. 10, 15, or 20. The flat Krause file may also be used for this purpose. If paper disks are used to smooth and round off the angle, care must be taken not to develop undercut facets.

CERVICAL MARGIN PREPARATION

The sixth and final step is accomplished in two phases; the first consists of reducing the small triangular area of enamel that is lingual to the gingival termination of the axial groove and cervical to the gingival margin of the initial proximal cuts

(Fig. 17-16). This may be accomplished at speeds of 25,000 to 50,000 rpm with a small tapering diamond stone ½DL or with a Tinker finishing bur.

The second phase establishes the cervical margin, which normally is placed slightly below the crest of the gum tissue and extends around the lingual surface from one axial groove to the other. This is done after the soft tissues have been retracted by one of several methods. A technic suggested by Selberg[3] for both three-quarter and complete veneer crown preparations utilizes the rubber dam and a suitable rubber dam clamp.

A piece of rubber dam of the proper size is selected and the holes are punched so that at least one tooth on either side of the abutment is included. For the posterior teeth, the bicuspids and molars, a No. 208, 200, or 205 S. S. White clamp is selected. For the anterior teeth a clamp, similar to No. 211 S. S. White, is used. This type of clamp has two wings adjacent to the jaws of the clamp. These extensions serve a very useful purpose.

The bow of the clamp is slipped through the hole in the dam designated for the abutment tooth and the clamp and dam are placed over the abutment with the clamp forceps. The clamp is lowered on the tooth until the curved jaws on the buccal and lingual surfaces rest in the gingival crevice (Fig. 17-17). The rubber dam is now slipped over the two wings of the clamp. In doing so the rubber dam depresses the free gingival tissue, thus exposing that part of the cervical enamel that normally lies in the gingival crevice in contact with the gingiva. The dam is now applied over the remaining teeth.

By this method, it is now possible to prepare the chamfer below the plane that the crest of the gum tissue normally occupies.

After the chamfer is prepared and the clamp and dam are removed, the gum tissue springs back to its normal position, leaving the cervical margin of the preparation lying 0.5 mm. below the gingival crest.

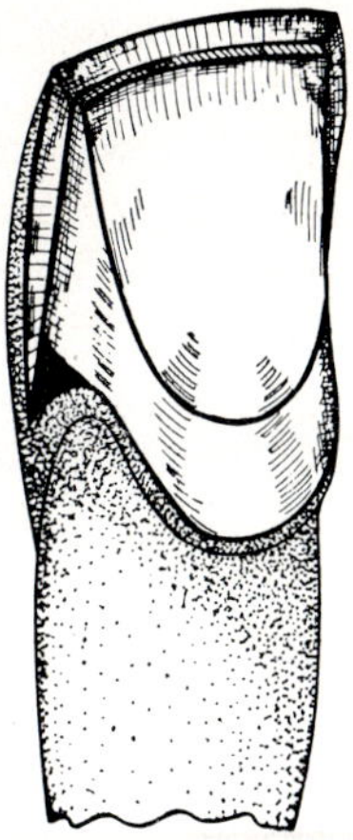

Fig. 17-16. Triangular area of enamel is removed with tapering stone or bur.

In cutting the chamfer, the stones and burs are prevented by the metal wings of the clamp from accidentally injuring the soft tissues. The same technic may be used when cutting a shoulder for a shoulder crown.

The gingival margin of a partial veneer retainer does not end in a definite shoulder as does a porcelain veneer crown (Fig. 24-30); neither does it fade away indefinitely as does the shoulderless crown (Fig. 13-28, *B*). In the partial veneer retainer an effort is made to establish a chamfer or bevel, which is cut in the enamel by means of a tapered stone (Densco 1D-T), and finished with a Tinker type, finishing bur, No. 650-L or 651-L, at 100,000 rpm (Fig. 17-18, *A*). The shape of the bur is such that, when it is held axially against the proximal and lingual surfaces, the cone-shaped end-cutting portion of the bur creates a chamfer or bevel whose gingival margin extends slightly beneath the crest of the gum tissue (Fig. 17-18, *A* to *D*). The gingival bevel or chamfer starts at the gingival termination of one proximal groove and is extended to the lingual surface and thence to the other axial groove. A study of the cavosurface angle of a typical intracoronal retainer shows that the bevel is approximately 6 to 12° from the horizontal plane, whereas the angle of the chamfer made with the Tinker finishing bur averages between 22 and 45° from the horizontal

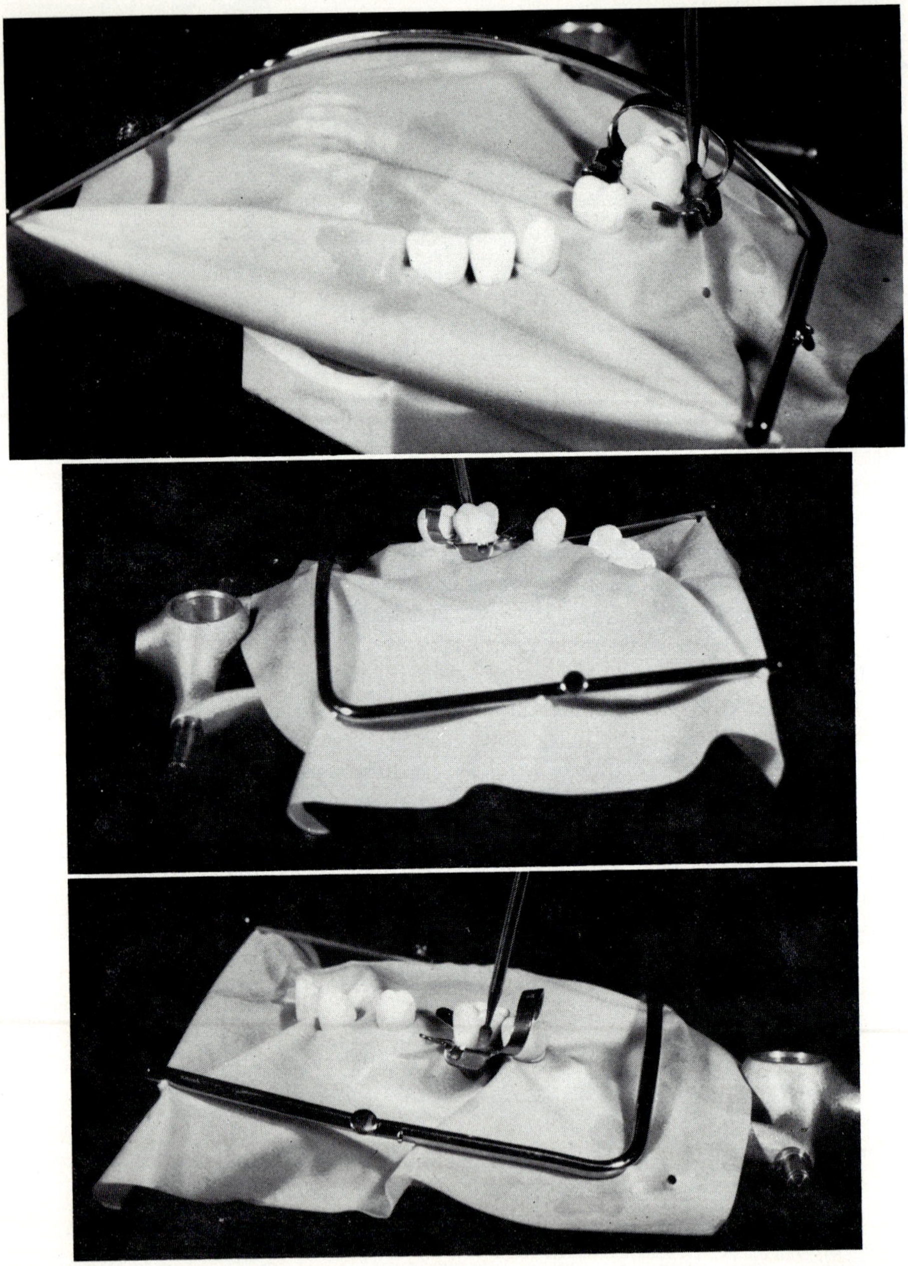

Fig. 17-17. Rubber dam and clamp are used to depress gum tissue to allow extending cervical margin of preparation below gingival crest.

plane (Fig. 17-19). Attention is called to the fact that *in the intracoronal retainer the gingival bevel usually involves the entire length of the enamel rods; whereas the gingival bevel of the partial veneer extracoronal retainer involves only the outer ends of the enamel rods.*

The advantage of using even a narrow chamfer lies in the fact that it affords a definite finishing margin for the wax pattern and the casting, yet at the same time eliminates cutting away considerable portions of tooth structure.

After the instrumentation has been completed, it is well to go over the tooth carefully with finishing stones, burs, and disks to make certain that all undercuts are eliminated and that all surfaces and margins are properly finished (Fig. 17-20). For modifications of the anterior extracoronal partial veneer retainers, see Chapter 19.

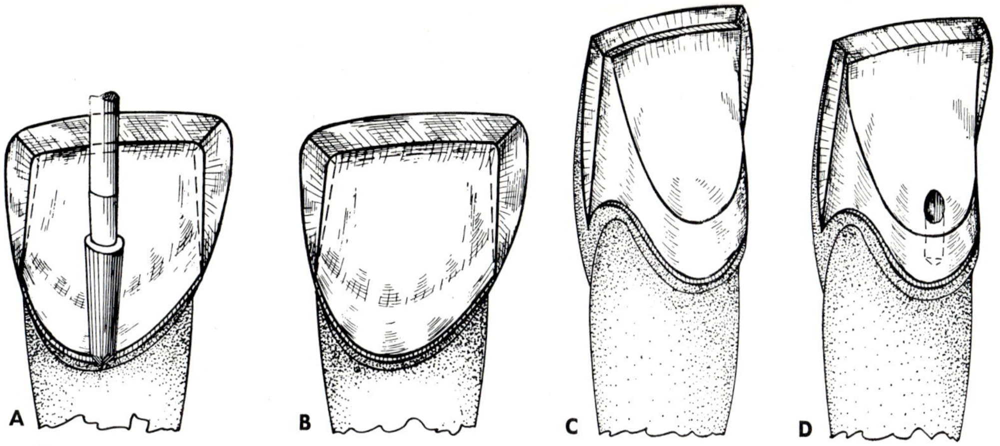

Fig. 17-18. Preparation and finished chamfer at cervical plane of upper central incisor.

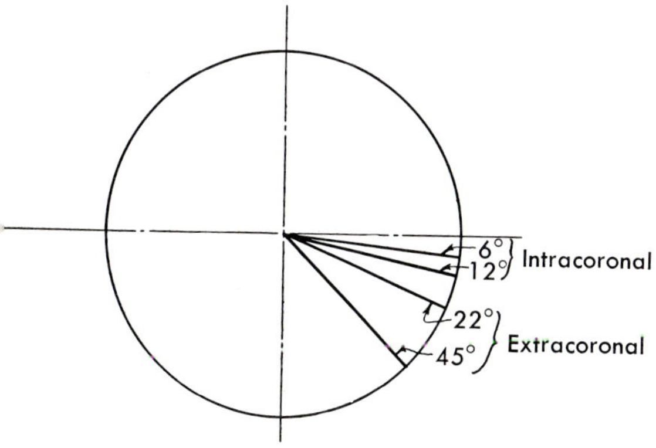

Fig. 17-19. Different angles of gingival bevels of intracoronal and extracoronal retainers.

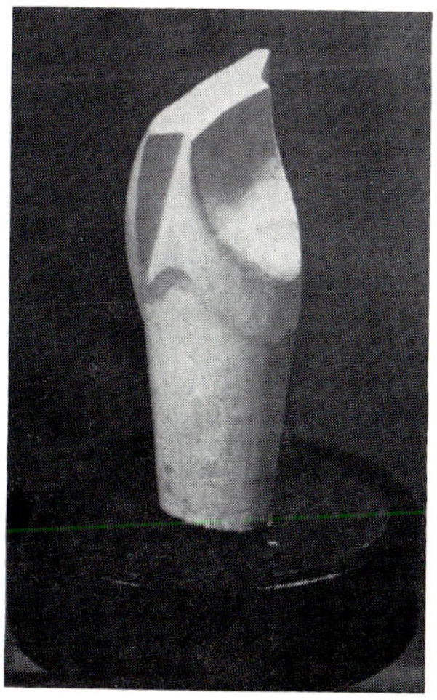

Fig. 17-20. Finished preparation of upper incisor for partial veneer extracoronal retainer with incisal plane.

SELECTED REFERENCES

1. Thompson, M. J.: Exposing the cavity margin for hydrocolloid impression, J. South. California Dent. Ass. **19**:17, 1951.
2. Pagenkopf, A. A.: Hydrocolloid method: if not, why not? Northwest Dent. **34**:93, 1955.
3. Selberg, A.: Cast gold crowns, J. Tennessee D. A. **29**:21, 1949.
4. Malone, W.: Interceptive periodontics through electrosurgery, J. Prosth. Dent. **22**:135, 1969.
5. LeHuche, R.: Inlays and onlays, bridges on living teeth, Paris, 1951, Julien Prélat.
6. Tinker, E. T.: Some of the fundamentals in the construction and application of crown and bridge restorations, J.A.D.A. **12**:1347, 1935.
7. Tinker, H. A.: Three-quarter crown in fixed bridgework, J. Canadian D. A. **16**:125, 1950.
8. Krause, O. G.: Cast attachments for bridgework, with special reference to vital teeth, J.A.D.A. **21**:4, 1934.

GENERAL REFERENCES

Alpert, C. C.: Anterior pin-ledge abutment, J. Dist. Columbia D. Soc. **34**:11, 1959.

Baker, C. R.: Replacement of lost mandibular incisor or incisors: 1. fixed; 2. removable appliances, Int. Dent. J. **5**:287, 1955.

Baum, L.: New cast gold restorations for anterior teeth, J.A.D.A. **61**:1, 1960.

Brigadier, L. R.: The anterior one-half pin-lay, D. Digest **45**:448, 1939.

Burgess, J. K.: The pinledge attachment, D. Items Int. Quart. Rev. **4**:33, 1920.

Carlson, N. C.: Selection of proper abutments for anterior bridges, J. Kansas City Dist. D. Soc. **30**:12, 1954.

Carpenter, E. E.: Pinledge attachments for anterior bridgework, D. Items Int. **72**:132, 1950: Indiana D. Rev. **20**:67, 1951.

Chechik, M. M.: Retention simplified: employing prefabricated tapered gold pins, D. Digest **61**:386, 441, 1955.

Cowger, G. T.: Retention, resistance and esthetics of the anterior three-quarter crown, J.A.D.A. **62**:167, 1961.

Falkner, P. L.: Anterior bridges—full or partial coverage? Roy. Canad. D. Corps Quart. **2**: 7, 1961.

Fisch, G. M.: The three-quarter crown as a filling for anterior teeth, J.A.D.A. **18**:2393, 1931.

Gade, E.: Function and aesthetics of anterior bridges, Int. Dent. J. **12**:18, 1962.

Hoelzel, S. H.: Dowel pin locators for hydrocolloid impressions, North-West Dent. **41**:100, 1962.

Kaloyiannides, T.: A method for the attainment of parallel grooves on three-quarter crown construction, Acta Stomat. Hellen. **2**(1):3-13, 1967.

LaForgia, A.: Tissue retraction for fixed prosthesis, J. Prosth. Dent. **11**:480, 1961.

Linkow, L. I.: Reconstruction of anterior teeth with an extreme vertical and horizontal overlap, J. Prosth. Dent. **12**:947, 1962.

McAdam, D. B.: Maxillary cuspid three-quarter crown preparation of increased retentive form, J. Canadian D. A. **28**:291, 1962; D. Digest **68**:522, 1962.

Nally, J. N.: Fixed bridge for anterior teeth, Int. Dent. J. **12**:1, 1962; Chir. Dent. Fr. **22**: 57, 1962 (Fr.).

Peterka, C. A.: A modern three-quarter veneer crown, J.A.D.A. **27**:1175, 1940.

Pruden, K. C.: A hydrocolloid technique for pinledge bridge abutments, J. Prosth. Dent. **6**:65, 1956.

Rudin, B. M.: Conservative abutment restoration for anterior fixed partial dentures, J. Prosth. Dent. **11**:272, 1961.

Shapiro, F. M., and Rosen, B. S.: Fixed splint for lower anterior teeth, J. New Jersey D. Soc. **33**:95, 1961.

Shooshan, E. D.: Pin-ledge casting technique—its application in periodontal splinting, Dent. Clin. N. Amer. pp. 189-206, March, 1960.

Chapter 18

Tooth preparations and instrumentation: class I, type 4—posterior extracoronal partial veneer retainers

The posterior partial veneer retainer does not differ fundamentally from the anterior, since the principles of its retention and preparation are similar to those of the anterior teeth. While in the anterior retainers the proximal grooves are placed parallel to the incisal two-thirds of the labial surfaces, in the posterior teeth the axial grooves are made parallel with the long axes of the crowns (Fig. 18-1). In posterior retainers, the two proximal, the occlusal, and the lingual surfaces are involved on all teeth with the exception of the lower molars. The reason for this difference in the lower molars, according to Tinker,[1] is the natural inclination that is found in these teeth and that would necessitate a great deal of tooth cutting if the lingual surfaces were to be included.

In preparing a posterior tooth to receive a partial veneer retainer, an effort should be made to place the proximal grooves so that three-fourths of the circumference of the tooth will be encompassed within the casting; therefore, the grooves are placed in the buccal third of the tooth (Fig. 18-2). Such positioning of the grooves will sufficiently extend the proximal outline of the preparation to the buccal vestibule that the margins will lie in a cleansable area.

Because of their location in the arch and because of poor visibility, greater

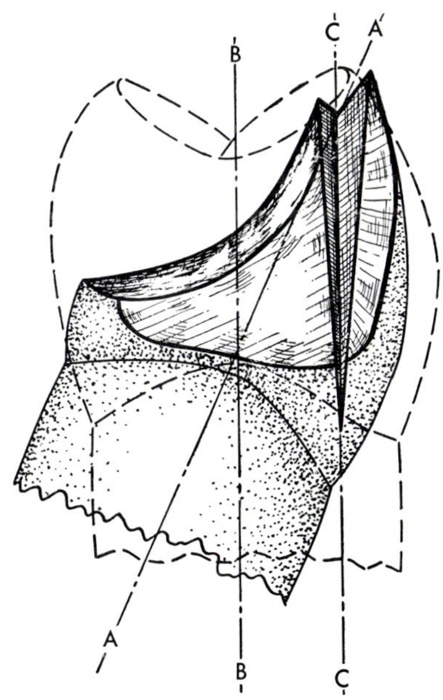

Fig. 18-1. Directions of axial grooves in anterior and posterior teeth prepared for partial veneer retainers. **A-A,** Long axis of cuspid. **B-B,** Long axis of molar. **C-C,** Direction of axial groove with reference to labial or buccal surfaces of cuspid or of molar.

latitude is permitted in the buccal extension of the margins of the posterior retainers than in that of anterior retainers.

As in the anterior teeth, the proximal grooves in the posterior teeth in their relationship to each other should not converge gingivocclusally from parallelism more than 2 to 5° if maximum retention is to be obtained. They usually terminate beneath the crest of the gum tissue. Where the epithelium is still attached to the enamel, it should not be severed if it is at all possible to avoid doing so.

There is a difference between the gingival termination of the grooves placed in posterior and anterior teeth. It is recalled that in anterior teeth the gingival end of the proximal groove usually fades away into the labiogingival area without any definite shoulder or step formation; in the bicuspids and molars the proximal groove terminates gingivally in a flat, V-shaped gingival wall (Fig. 18-3, *A*). There are occasions when this triangular, proximal groove in the bicuspids and molars is modified into a box-like form (Fig. 18-4).

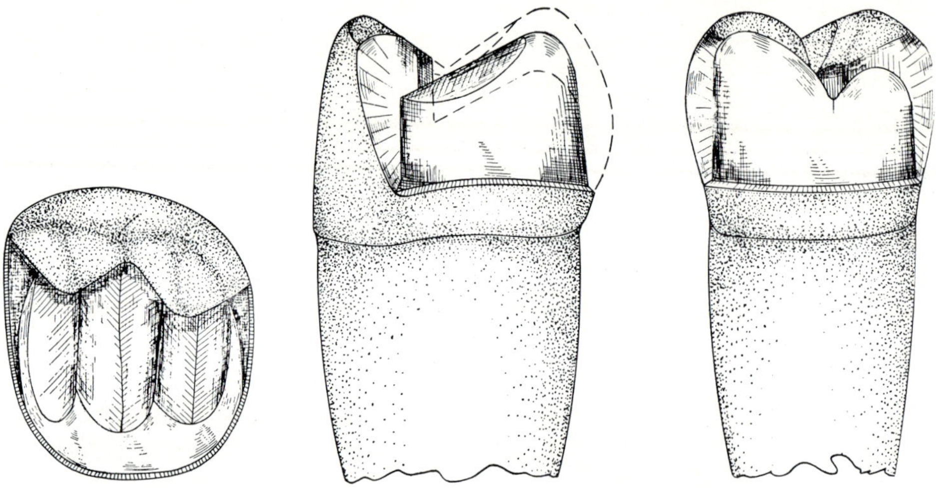

Fig. 18-2. Typical partial veneer preparation for upper molar.

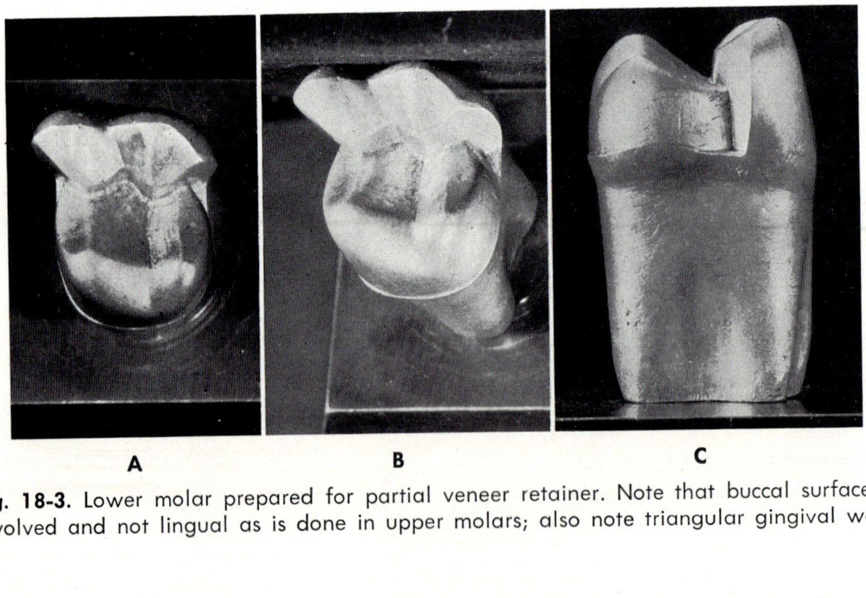

A **B** **C**

Fig. 18-3. Lower molar prepared for partial veneer retainer. Note that buccal surface is involved and not lingual as is done in upper molars; also note triangular gingival wall.

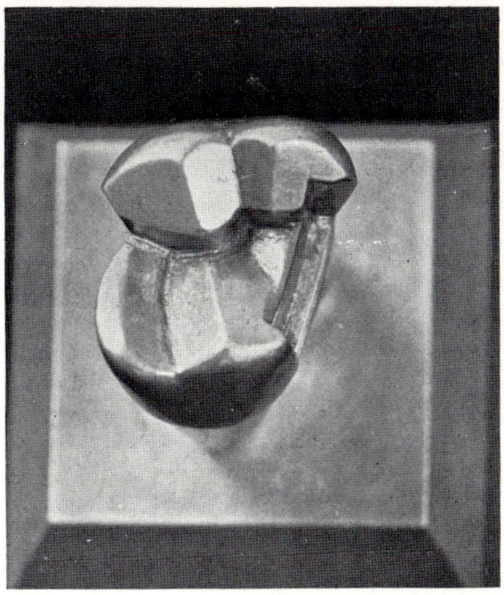

Fig. 18-4. Upper molar partial veneer preparation with box-like mesial modification.

This is usually done if caries is present in the proximal surfaces of the abutment tooth. If the retainer is to receive an interlocking key used with the semifixed principle, the proximal surface facing the edentulous space is also modified with the box-like form (Fig. 18-5).

It is generally accepted that the V-shaped groove is used only in those teeth that are more or less round in cross section; whereas the box-like proximal modifications are used in those teeth that are of parallelogram shape.

INDICATIONS

While the partial veneer retainers may be used on most posterior teeth having a

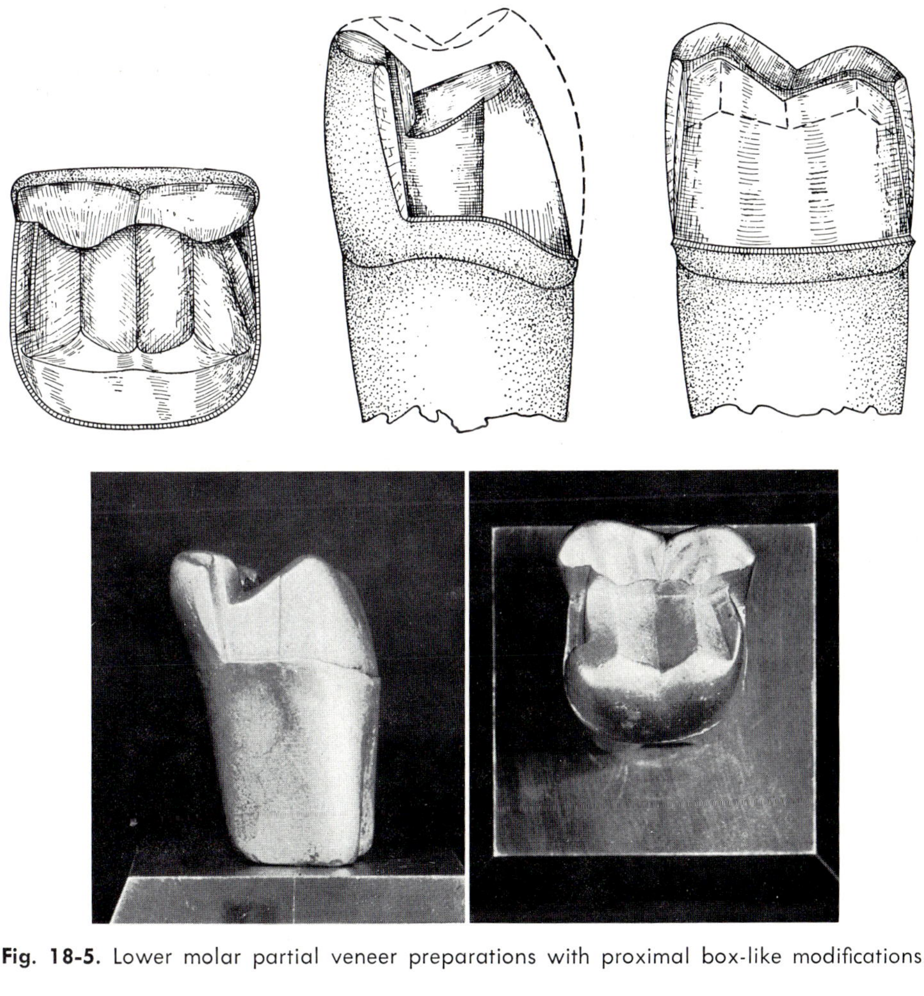

Fig. 18-5. Lower molar partial veneer preparations with proximal box-like modifications.

sufficient amount of tooth structure, their use is indicated primarily on teeth having vital pulps.

Because this type of preparation is shallow, because it is confined mostly to the outer portion of enamel, because the retentive grooves are remotely removed from the pulp, and because with all these advantages it still possesses sufficient mechanical retention, this type of retainer during the past 50 years has been universally employed.

Dressel[2] has indicated that in those teeth of average length and in those that are likely to be subjected to average forces, the typical, triangular proximal grooves will suffice; however, in those teeth of medium or short length the box type of proximal modifications is recommended.

Where a posterior tooth is to serve as a bridge abutment, the same procedures are carried through in obtaining separation of teeth and gum retraction as described previously for the anterior teeth. Because a greater amount of tooth structure is removed than in an anterior tooth and because of more difficult access to posterior teeth, greater precautions are required and more time is consumed in making the posterior types of veneer retainers.

Where caries is present, it is advisable to first remove the decay in order to determine its extent and to enable the den-

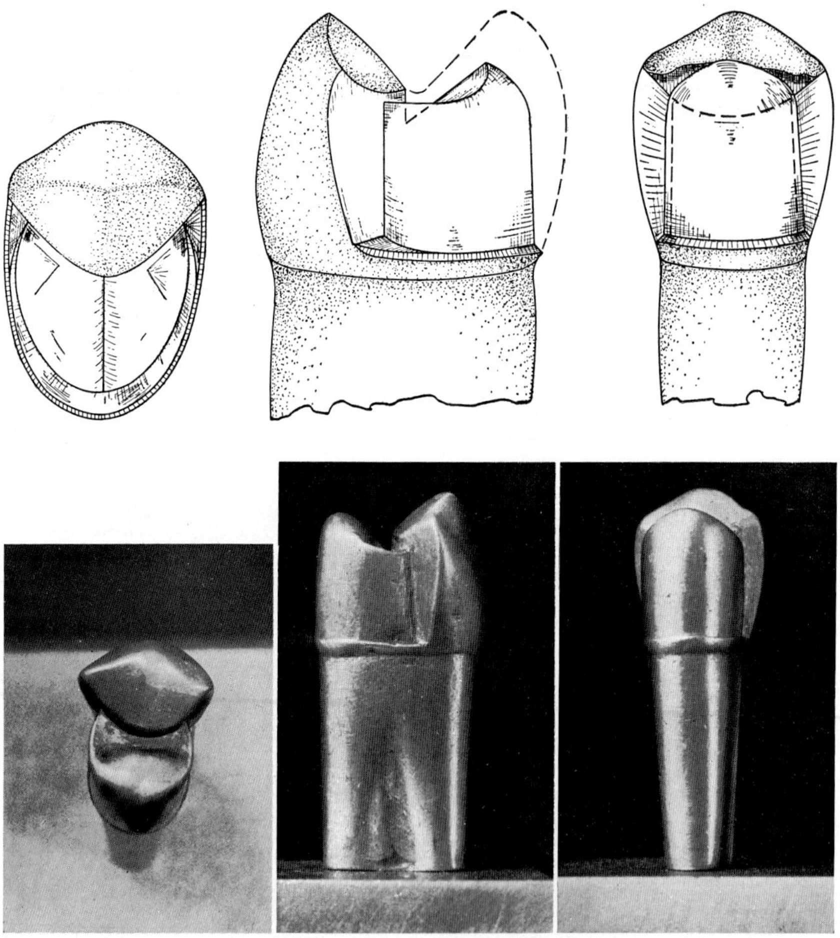

Fig. 18-6. Typical partial veneer preparations for upper bicuspids.

tist to decide what deviation from the normal type of preparation must be made, if any.

OUTLINE FORM

Since all surfaces of the crown but one are usually involved in the preparation, the normal outline form for upper posterior teeth brings the buccal margins well out on the buccal surface; also, the gingival margin is normally carried slightly below the crest of the gum tissue into the gingival crevice. The location of the occlusal margin varies with the type of preparation

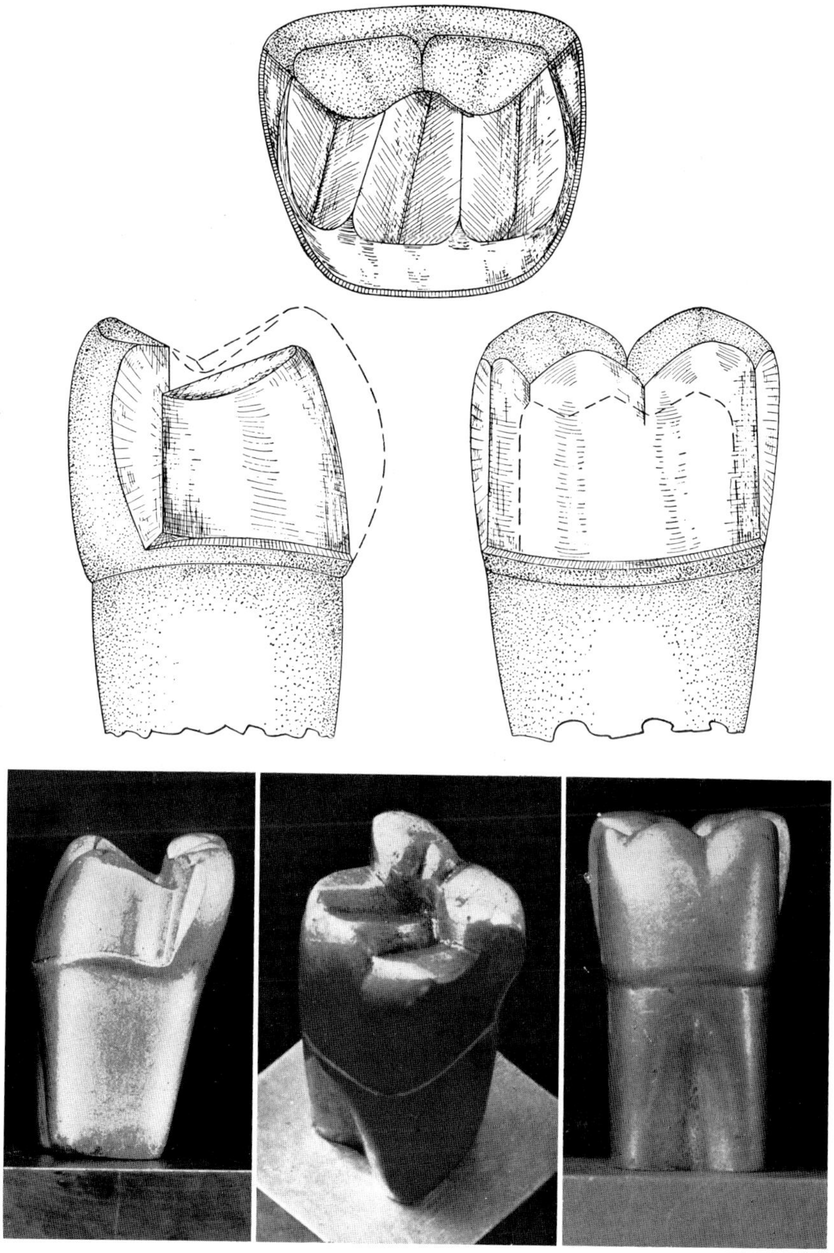

Fig. 18-7. Typical partial veneer preparations for lower molars.

made; in an upper bicuspid (Fig. 18-6) or molar that is noncarious and that contains a vital pulp, the buccal cusps are not usually included and the occlusal buccal margin extends from one proximal groove to the other in a curved line that leaves intact as much of the buccal cusps as possible. Where a tooth is pulpless, however, clinical experience has shown the necessity of also covering the buccal cusps in the casting. A large percentage of fractures occurs in those teeth whose pulps

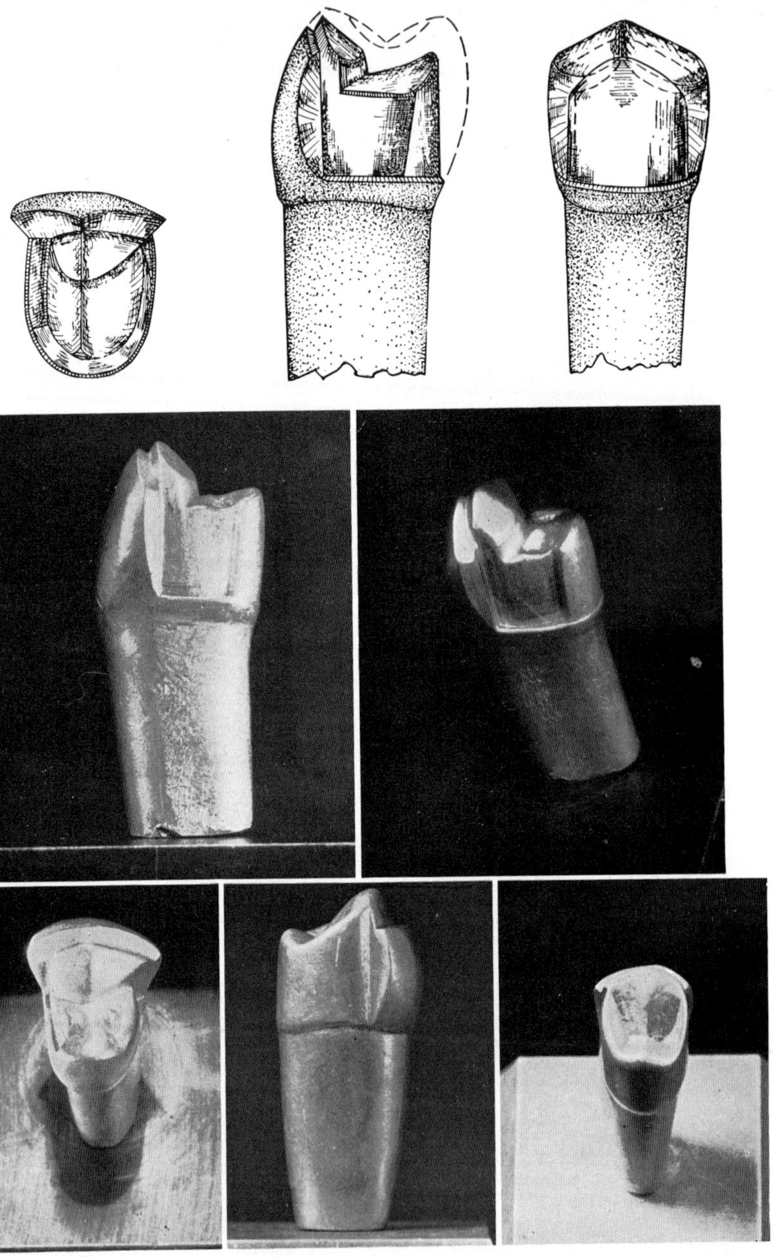

Fig. 18-8. Partial veneer preparations on lower bicuspids that include part of buccal surface as well as all of lingual surface.

have been removed and whose cusps have been left unprotected with metal.

RESISTANCE AND RETENTION FORMS

The resistance and retention forms of this type of retainer are discussed in Chapter 13. It is recalled that the major resistance to displacement is developed by the two opposing proximal grooves, by the opposing axial walls that are nearly parallel, and by correctly formed occlusal planes.

In the lower molars the buccal surface is the fourth surface involved instead of the lingual (Fig. 18-7). The lower bicuspids, because of their contour, frequently necessitate extending the retainer into a fifth surface, the buccal. Fig. 18-8 shows a slight buccal extension of the lower bicuspid. Where the tooth is small, the buccal margin is frequently extended cervically to two-thirds of its buccal distance (Fig. 18-9).

The same modifications of cusps and surfaces are frequently employed with lower molars (Fig. 18-10).

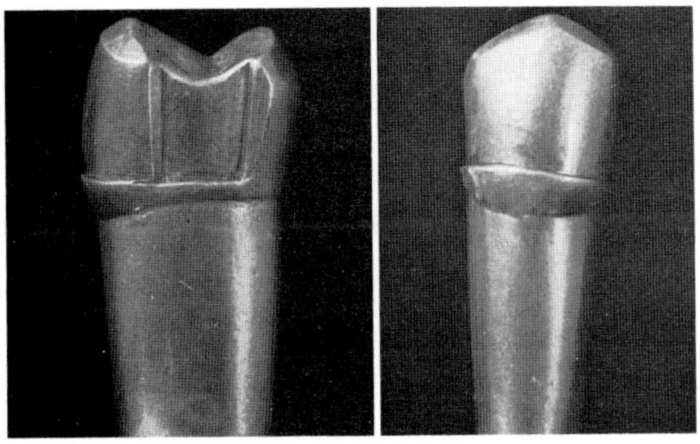

Fig. 18-9. Occasional type of preparation that covers all of buccal and part of lingual surfaces.

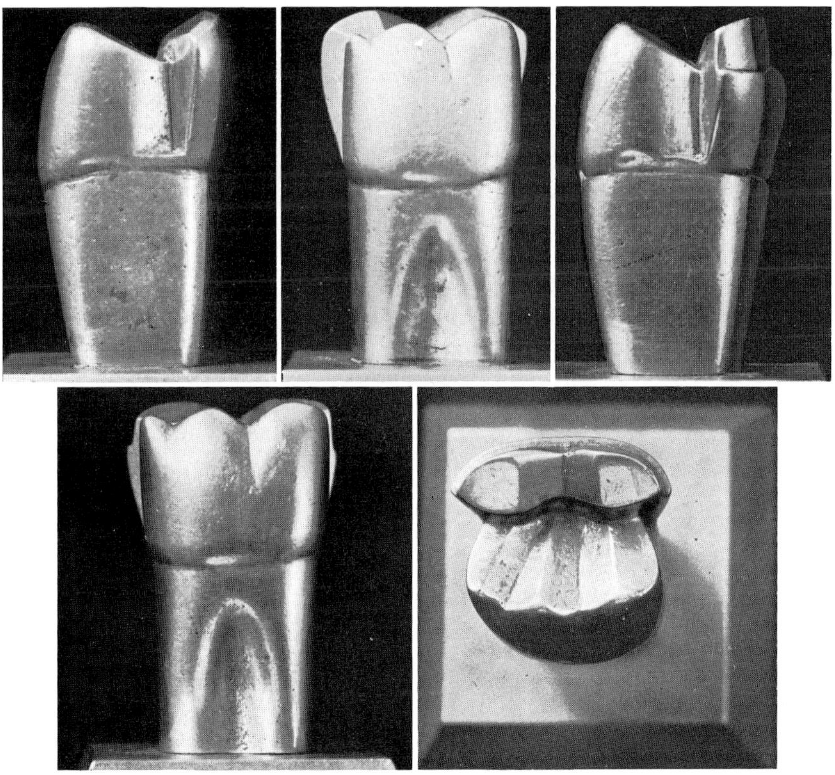

Fig. 18-10. Lower molar partial veneer preparations in which part of lingual surface is also included.

It is not always desirable or necessary to lower the lingual cervical margin on the upper molars or the buccal cervical margin on the lower molars below the crest of the gingiva; these margins are often placed in a self-cleansing area away from the gingival tissues there. The proximal margins, as a rule, are brought below the gingival crest, except in those instances in which recession of the gums has progressed beyond the cementoenamel junction.

While the procedures and instrumentation in the preparation of a posterior partial veneer retainer have been somewhat modified since they were first presented by Tinker,[1] they are fundamentally still the same. In most instances it makes little difference which technic is employed, provided the steps are carried through in sequence and with suitable instruments so that the finished preparation is fundamentally correct.

UPPER ABUTMENTS

Steps of preparation

Proximal cuts. The first step of the technic in preparing an upper bicuspid for a partial veneer retainer involves making the proximal cuts (Figs. 18-11 and 18-12). The mesial and distal contours of the tooth are first removed with a ½ inch, safe-sided, perforated diamond disk, 4T-PS, under a steady stream of water. The cut is carried from the lingual surface toward the buccal, maintaining a slight convergence toward the *lingual;* the cut is made occlusogingivally so that a flat plane is produced parallel to the long axis of the crown; sometimes it converges very slightly gingivocclusally (Fig. 18-13). The gingival termination of this cut ends at or slightly beneath the crest of the gum tissue without, however, forming a shoulder at this point. It is well at this time to ascertain that the buccal outlines of the cuts are carried sufficiently buccally into self-cleansing or cleansable areas. This operation is performed first on the mesial and then on the distal surfaces, or visa versa.

When making these cuts on the upper molars, care should be exercised to remove as little of the tooth as possible at the mesiolingual and distolingual angles, because the widest mesiodistal width of the preparation is found through this dimension (Fig. 18-14).

When making proximal cuts on the lower molar, the planes are cut buccolingually, so that they have a slight convergence *buccally* instead of lingually, as is done in the upper teeth.

Occlusal surface. The second step consists of the preparation of the occlusal surface. Some operators, however, prefer to reduce the lingual surface as the second

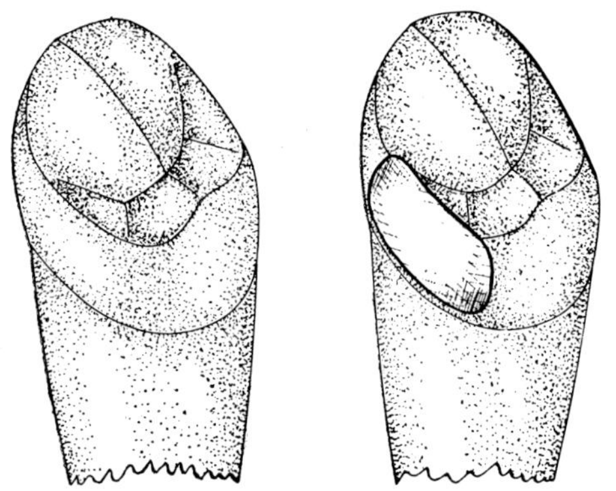

Fig. 18-11. Initial steps in preparation of upper bicuspid or upper molar for partial veneer retainer.

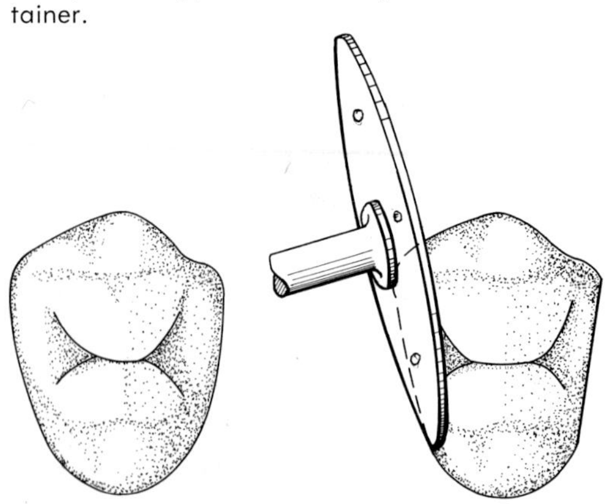

Fig. 18-12. Position of disk in making initial proximal cuts.

step. In the preparation of the occlusal surface, the condition of the tooth largely determines whether the entire occlusal area will be reduced or whether any cusps are left uncut. Clinical practice has shown that the entire occlusal surface of all pulpless posterior abutments should be restored in metal in order to prevent fracture of the buccal cusps in the upper teeth and the lingual cusps in the lower teeth. Where a posterior abutment contains a vital pulp and where the length of the bridge span is short and the occlusion is normal, the retainer does not require inclusion of the additional cusp within the casting.

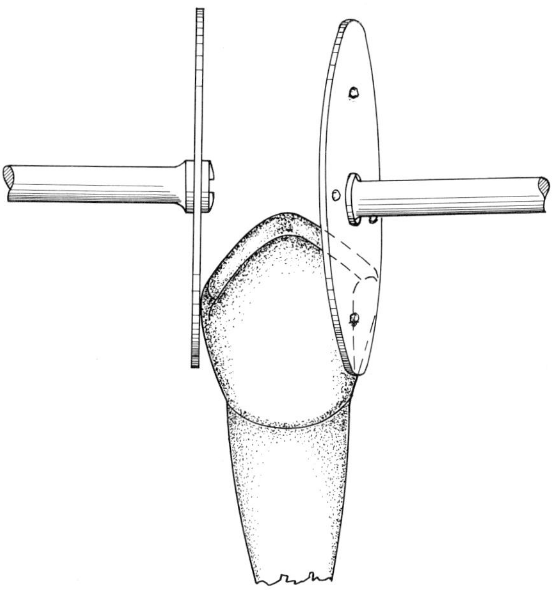

Fig. 18-13. Position of disks in making initial proximal cuts.

Where the entire occlusal surface is involved in the preparation, it is uniformly reduced to a depth of 1 to 1.5 mm. In doing so the inclined occlusal slopes and the grooves are retained in their general contour and position, and there is little danger of exposing pulpal horns.

Where the bicuspid buccal cusp is not involved, the buccal margin of the occlusal surface of the partial veneer retainer is similar to that of a typical mesiodistoclusal preparation.

Reduction of the entire occlusal surface and maintenance of its general anatomic form is best done with small, mounted stones of the following shapes and numbers: inverted cone (Densco 1K); wheel (Densco 5Q and 2½J); cylinder (Densco 3MW); tapering stones (Densco 1D-S and 4D-S) (Fig. 18-15).

In preparing the occlusal inclined slope, a small, knife-edged stone (Densco 5Q) is so placed that its edge is in contact with the marginal ridge of the tooth; the stone is then carried to the opposite proximal surface, at the same time cutting a groove through the occlusal surface into the den-

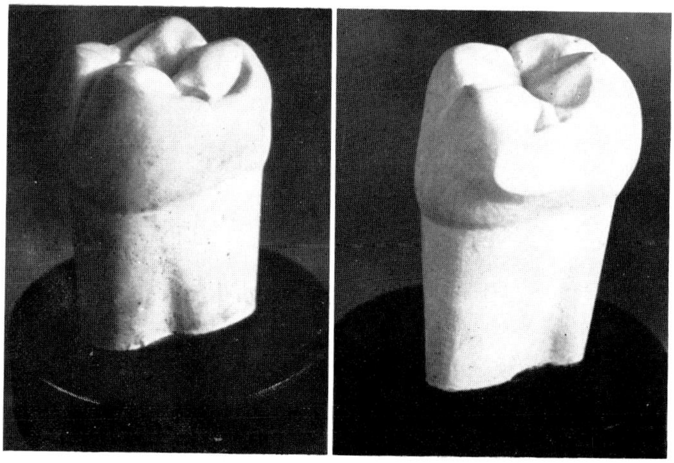

Fig. 18-14. Initial proximal cut made on upper molar.

tin; the cut extends in a curved line through the marginal ridges. The occlusal planes of the lingual cusp are then prepared with an inverted cone stone (Densco 1K). The buccal wall of the occlusal step is finished with the cross-cut tapering fissure bur, No. 701; and the finishing burs, Nos. 169 and 169 L.

The inclined slope is one of the factors that help to resist the lingual displacement of the retainer (see Fig. 13-26, *A*).

Proximal grooves. The next step consists of placing the proximal retention grooves parallel to the long axis of the crown (Fig. 18-16). The proximal grooves, one on the mesial and one on the distal surface, are placed buccally at the junction of the buccal and middle thirds of the tooth. Every effort should be made to keep the grooves as nearly parallel to each other as possible. The proximal grooves in the bicuspids and molars have a definite gingival wall; whereas in the anterior teeth the gingival termination of the grooves usually fades into the labiogingival area without forming a definite gingival wall.

In placing the grooves toward the buccal third as indicated, the greatest amount of tooth structure is encompassed lingually within the grip of the retainer, thus resisting from the upper teeth any tendency toward lingual displacement. In the lower molar teeth the proximal grooves are placed at the junction of the lingual third and the buccal two-thirds of the tooth, since in the lower molars the buccal surface is included in the preparation instead of the lingual.

To prepare the groove, a No. 700 cross-

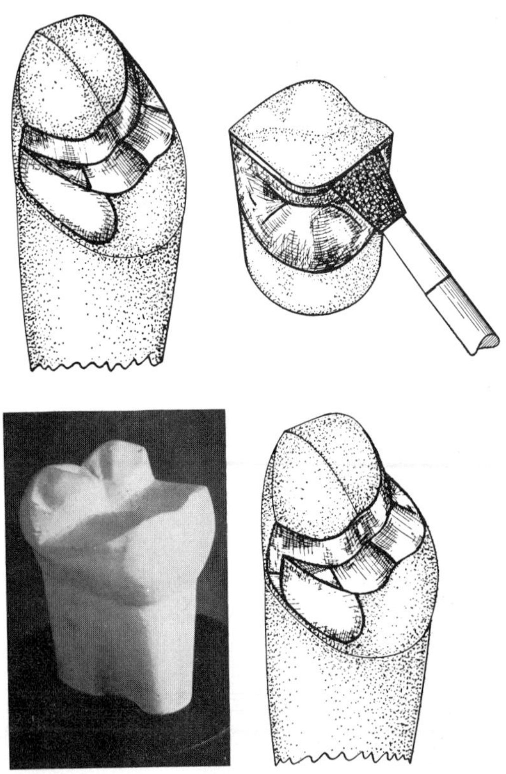

Fig. 18-15. Occlusal surface prepared in upper bicuspid and in upper molar.

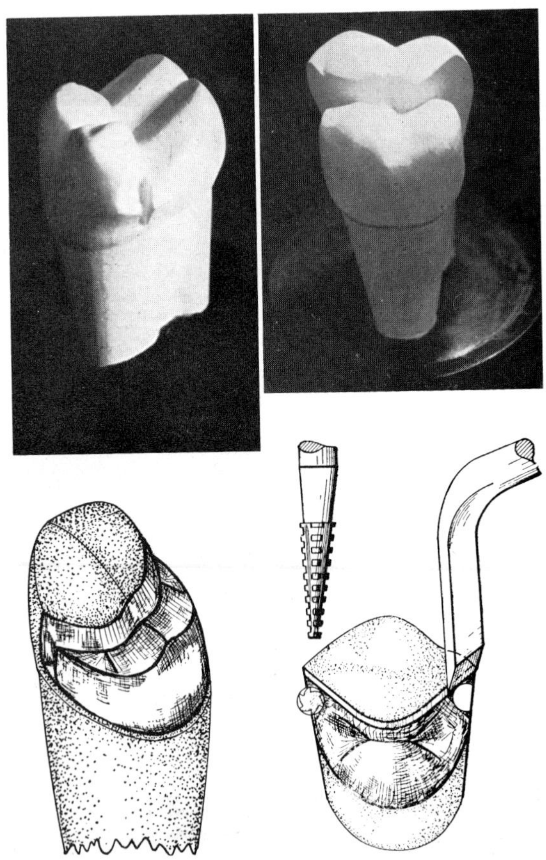

Fig. 18-16. Initial step in preparing proximal grooves.

cut tapering fissure bur or a Densco ID tapered cylinder stone is placed parallel to the long axis of the tooth between the buccal and the middle thirds of the tooth and is carried gingivally so that it terminates in a flat gingival plane slightly beneath the crest of the gum tissue. The groove at the occlusal end inclines into the dentin to a depth of approximately 1 mm. (Fig. 18-16).

Following the initial cut with the bur or stone, the buccal surface of the groove is planed from the inner angle of the groove buccally so that the buccal margins are extended into cleansable or self-cleansing areas (Fig. 18-16). This is done with Nos. 15 and 20 chisels, with an enamel hatchet, No. 15 or 20, or with the Densco ID-S tapered cylinder diamond stone. If the access is good, some operators finish these walls with fine sandpaper disks; when these are used, care must be taken not to undercut the walls.

The lingual surface of the groove is now rounded proximolingually, removing the sharp angle; the preparation takes on the shape of a horseshoe, opening buccally in the upper teeth (Fig. 18-17). This is best accomplished by using the safe-end tapered cylinder stone (Densco 1DS) and finishing by the use of Tinker finishing burs, Nos. 650-L and 651-L (Fig. 18-17, right).

Where a definite, triangular-shaped proximal groove is desired, it may be readily obtained by using the Krause[3] files, which are designed for this specific purpose (Fig. 18-17, left).

The typical proximal groove is used in most of the posterior teeth, particularly those that are rounded in their horizontal plane (Fig. 18-18, *A*). Where a molar has proximal caries or where the shape of the molar in its horizontal plane is generally that of a parallelogram, it is recommended that the typical triangular, or V-shaped groove be substituted with a box-like form (Fig. 18-18, *B*). Such a modified proximal retention takes care of the proximal decay; moreover, the bulk of metal and the additional frictional walls increase the retentive qualities of the preparation considerably.

Whether the V-shaped groove is used or the box-like modification, it is usually desirable to bevel the cavosurface margin of the gingival wall of enamel approximately 6° from the horizontal plane, just as it is done in the typical intracoronal preparation. This bevel removes any unsupported enamel rods at the gingival wall margin and is continuous with, and blends into, the

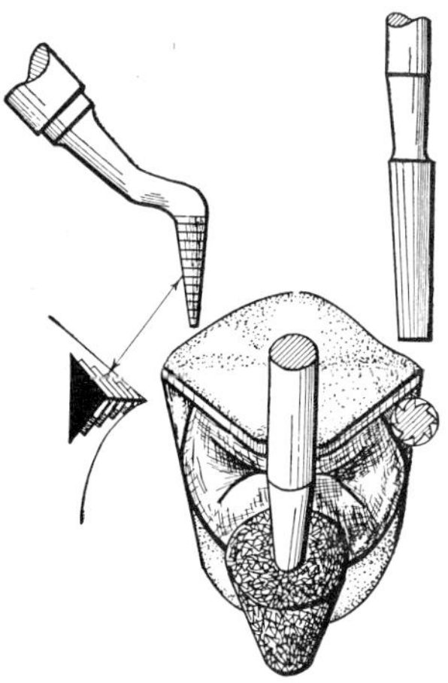

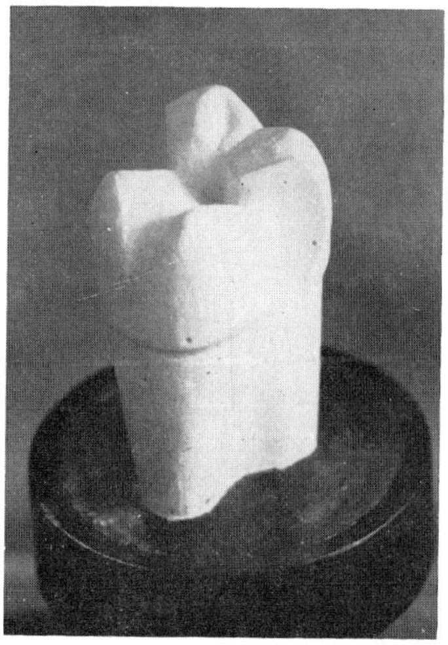

Fig. 18-17. Finishing axial grooves with files and finishing burs.

A 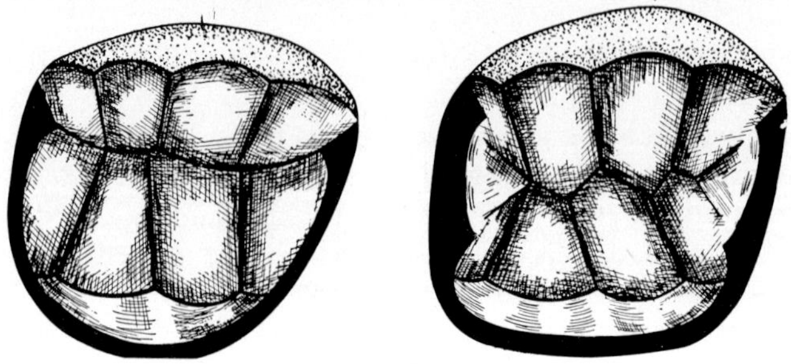 B

Fig. 18-18. Substituting box-like proximal modifications for typical grooves.

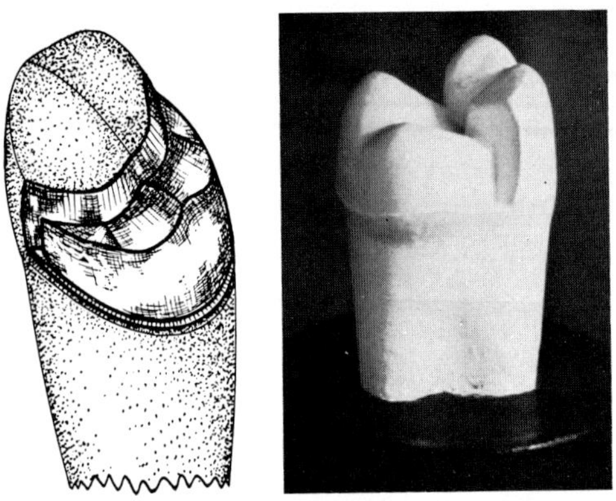

Fig. 18-19. Undercut areas on lingual and proximal surfaces eliminated.

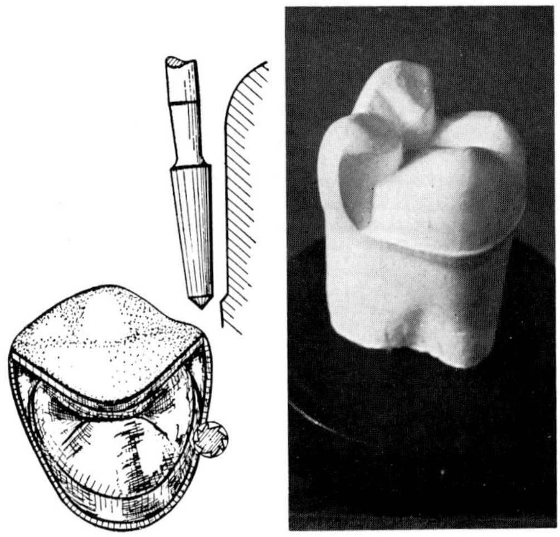

Fig. 18-20. Establishing cervical chamfer using Tinker bur.

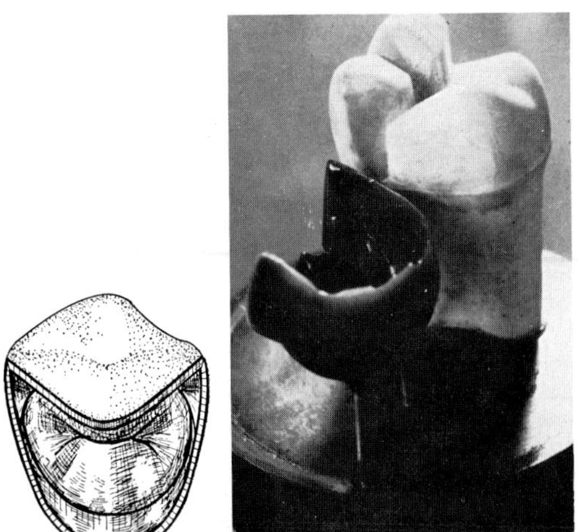

Fig. 18-21. Finished partial veneer preparations on upper bicuspid and upper molar.

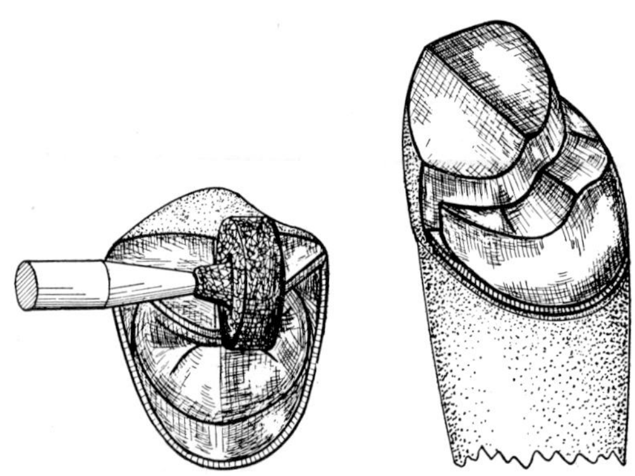

Fig. 18-22. In pulpless teeth both cusps are included in preparation and covered by cast retainer.

gingival chamfer or bevel, which is subsequently established around the lingual wall (Fig. 18-20).

Lingual cuts. On an upper posterior tooth, the next step involves the removal of the lingual convexity. In carrying out this procedure, no effort is made to remove all the enamel; in fact, every effort is made to retain as much of it as possible. Only enough of the enamel is removed to make the preparation slightly convergent gingivocclusally. No effort is made at this time to lower the axial preparation beyond the crest of the gum tissue; this is done as the final step. If the access is unusually difficult, the lingual surface may best be reduced by using a small Densco 2DS tapering diamond stone (Fig. 18-19).

Gingival chamfer. It is well at this point in the preparation of the tooth to examine all the axial surfaces to see if any undercuts exist and to determine the amount of occlusal convergence needed in these walls in order to permit the withdrawal of the wax pattern. Having established the correct degree of convergence, the final step is undertaken, that of establishing the finishing chamfer or bevel in the gingival area. The rubber dam and clamp are placed on the tooth in order to depress the free gingiva and expose the enamel lying in the gingival crevice (Fig. 17-17). The chamfer is now prepared. The diamond stone is used first to cut into the enamel surface, followed by the Tinker finishing bur, No. 650-L or 651-L. They are held parallel to the axial surface and are brought from the proximal groove on the mesial around the lingual to the proximal groove on the distal (Fig. 18-20). Because this bur has an end-cutting cone, it not only cuts laterally into the axial walls, but also establishes a gingival chamfer. This cut usually terminates in the gingival crevice slightly below the crest of the gum tissue; the gingival margin of the retainer is finished flush against it. This chamfer is continuous with and merges into the bevel of the gingival enamel wall at the proximal grooves.

Toilet of preparation. The final step in the preparation consists of finishing all the axial and occlusal walls to remove any sharp angles or undercuts (Fig. 18-21). If disks are used care must be taken to avoid creating undercut areas. To remove superficial striae and scratches created by the diamond stones or burs, a slurry of fine alumina powder with an orangewood prophylactic point will produce a smoother inner surface in the wax pattern. Also, there is less danger of injuring the enamel margins of the preparation. The rubber dam and clamp are now removed.

In pulpless teeth, the buccal cusp is reduced 1 to 1.5 mm. with a mounted stone (Densco 2J flat-edge wheel stone) (Fig. 18-22). The cast veneer then restores the entire occlusal surface. Where additional retention is desired, the buccal margin of the preparation may be lowered gingivally as a veneer with a chamfer margin: this terminates in a caries-immune area.

LOWER ABUTMENTS

As previously stated, in the lower molar the buccal surface is included in the preparation instead of the lingual. This is due to the anatomy as well as the position of the tooth in the arch. The lower first bicuspid, because of its size and position, very often requires an additional gingival extension of its buccal surface extending one-third to two-thirds its length. When the crown is exceedingly short, this buccal extension may even be carried to the gingival crest; then it practically becomes a complete veneer cast crown (Fig. 18-9).

ONE-HALF VENEER CROWN

A frequently used modification of the extracoronal partial veneer retainer is the proximal, one-half partial veneer crown, sometimes called the "Kennedy modified

Carmichael." This preparation is especially valuable on those abutment teeth that are sound and have a good contact area on both proximal surfaces. This modified crown is particularly indicated in the mesial aspect of the upper first and second molars and in the lower molars. It is exceedingly valuable in those lower molars tilted mesially to such an extent that all occlusal contacts have been lost with the exception of the distal cusps and the marginal ridge. Its use not only affords an attachment for the pontic, but also is a convenient means of restoring the mesial one-half or two-thirds of the occlusal surface to proper occlusal relationship with the opposing teeth.

In this preparation the partial veneer retainer is rotated one-quarter turn so that the entire mesial surface and the mesial halves of the buccal and lingual surfaces are included also. On the mesioclusal surface a typical intracoronal cavity is prepared so that it extends into and includes all pits and fissures (Fig. 18-32).

Steps of construction

The first step in this preparation involves the reduction of the mesial proximal surface by using a diamond (Densco 4T-PS) perforated disk on the lower molar (Fig. 18-23) and on the upper molar (Figs. 18-23 to 18-25). The cervicocclusal inclination of the cut usually has a slight distal tilt. The cut is brought sufficiently buccolingually that the margins are in cleansable or self-cleansing areas. Gingivally it terminates at or slightly below the gingival crest (Figs. 18-23 and 18-26).

The occlusal step is started by placing an inverted cone bur, No. 34, against the dentin of the proximal surface slightly be-

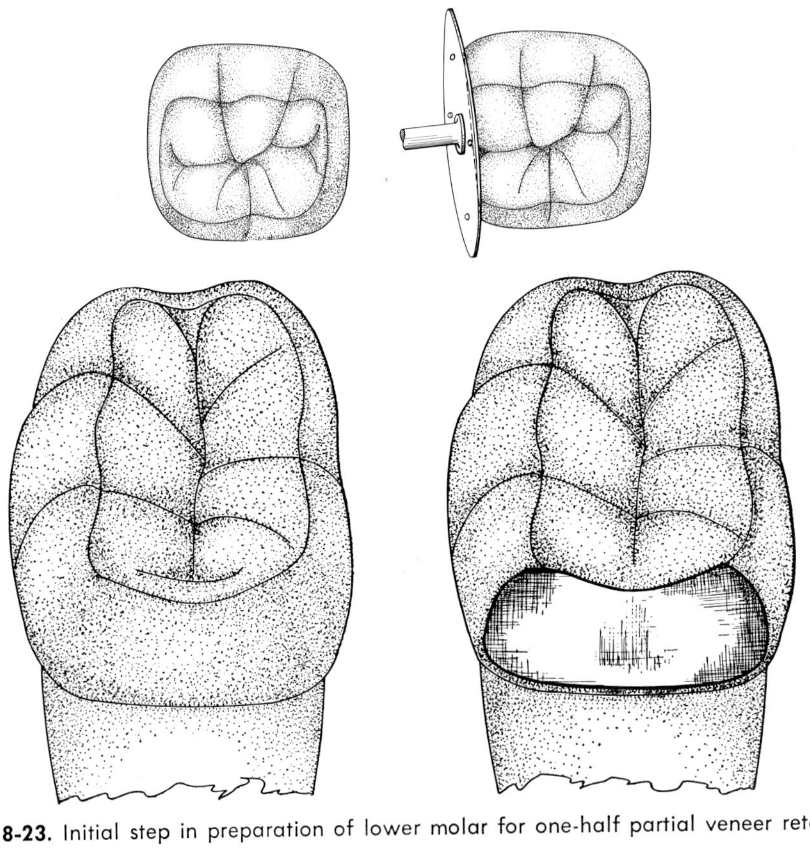

Fig. 18-23. Initial step in preparation of lower molar for one-half partial veneer retainer.

low the occlusal dentinoenamel interface (Fig. 18-26, left); while the bur is revolving it is carried across the occlusal surface following the general direction of the fissures and grooves (Fig. 18-26). Because the occlusal enamel has been undermined while cutting through the dentin, the enamel has been mostly disintegrated and also removed. If any remains it may be easily removed with chisels, hatchets, or a fine tapered diamond stone, Densco 4D (Figs. 18-26 and 18-27).

The next step is cutting occlusal grooves buccally and lingually through the buccal and lingual fissures (Fig. 18-28). The groove-cut starts at the level of the pulpal dentin wall and opens into the buccal surface. A knife-edge wheel stone (Densco 1½V) is utilized first; it is then followed by a tapered cylinder-type stone, Densco 2D (Fig. 18-28).

From the level of the pulpal wall, the groove is continued bucally and lowered gingivally through the enamel wall 1 mm. into the dentin; the groove parallels the general slope of the surface of the tooth. It should drop cervically 3 to 4 mm. below the level of the pulpal wall and be a minimum of 2 mm. in width.

The line angles in dentin between the pulpal wall and the buccal and the lingual grooves should be beveled.

With a small wheel (Densco 2J), the enamel on the occlusal surface of the mesiobuccal and mesiolingual cusps is next reduced to an approximate depth of 0.5

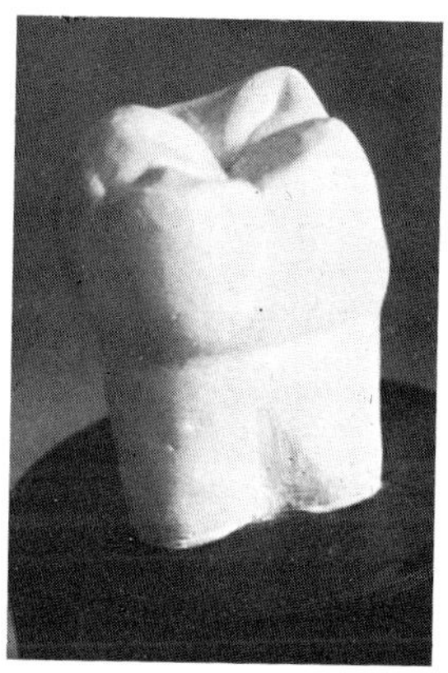

Fig. 18-24. Initial step prepared in upper molar.

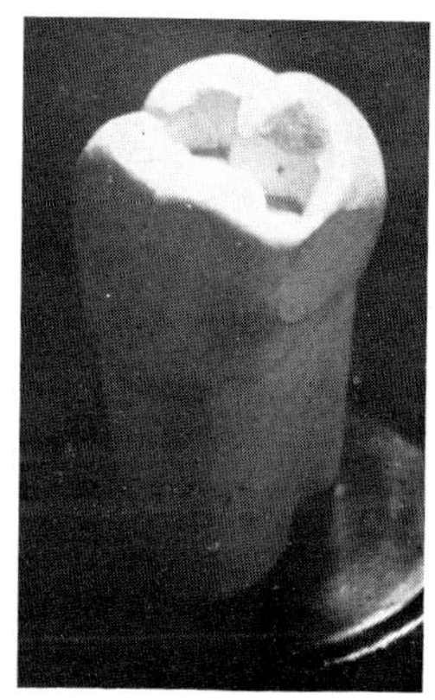

Fig. 18-25. In addition to proximal cut, occlusal outline has also been prepared.

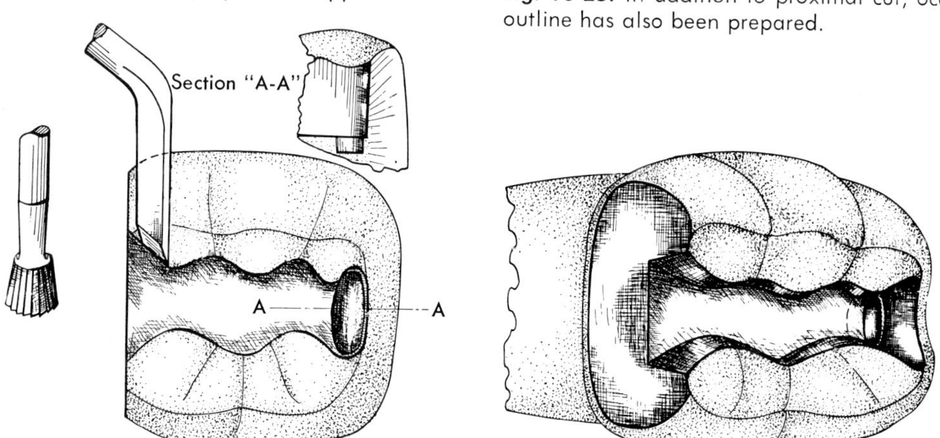

Fig. 18-26. Uniting occlusal portion of preparation with proximal cut in lower molar.

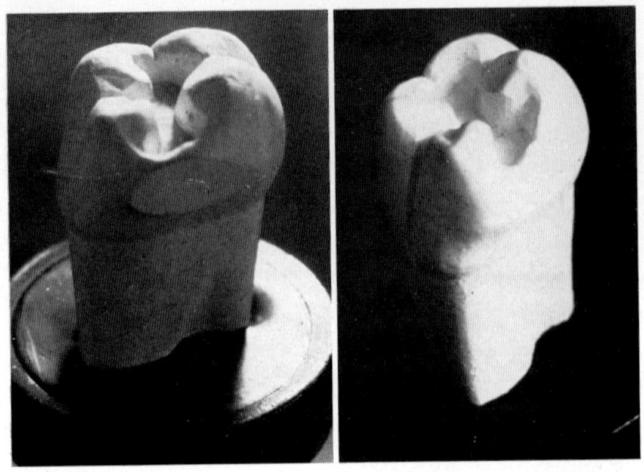

Fig. 18-27. Same procedure as in Fig. 18-26, on upper molar.

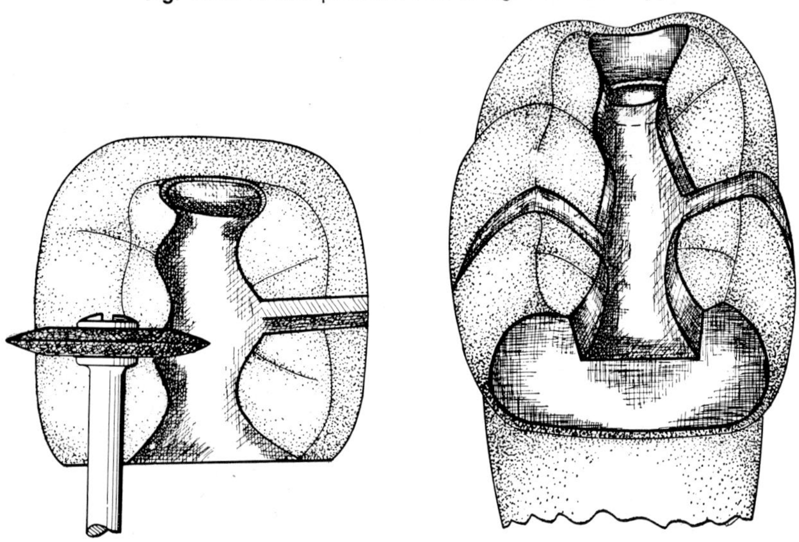

Fig. 18-28. Grooves cut buccally and lingually through occlusal fissures of lower molar.

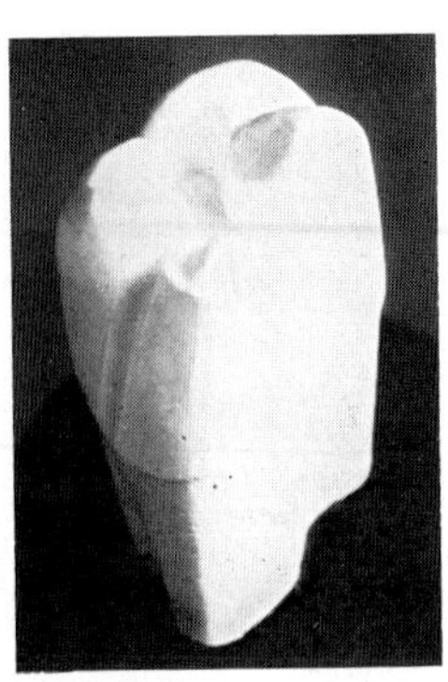

Fig. 18-29. Same step as in Fig. 18-28, accomplished in upper molar.

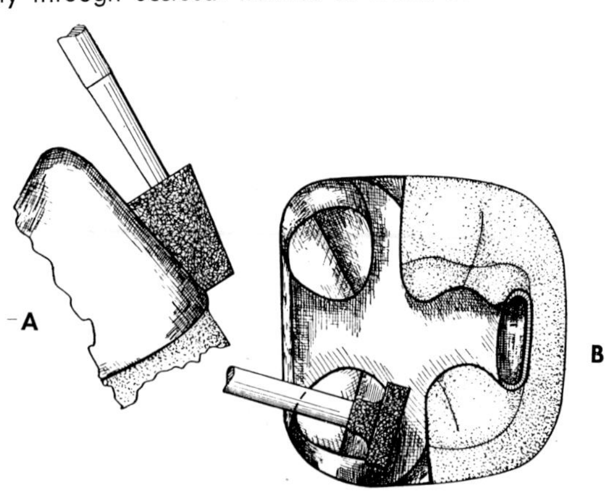

Fig. 18-30. Where necessary, mesial cusps are reduced 0.5 to 1.0 mm. and axial enamel in lower molar mesial cusps is reduced 0.5 to 1.0 mm.

to 1.0 mm. (Fig. 18-30, *B*). With a tapering stone (Densco 5D-S), the enamel is reduced 0.5 mm. from the buccal and lingual surfaces of the buccal and lingual cusps down to the crest of the gingiva; the cutting extends from the initial proximal slice to the buccal and the lingual grooves (Fig. 18-30, *A*).

For additional retention, a proximal keyway or lock may be prepared in the mesial surface; the same instruments and technic are used as for the tapered dovetail groove made for a typical slice preparation (Fig. 18-32). Usually, a depression or well is also sunk in the distal portion of the pulpal wall (Figs. 18-31 and 18-32).

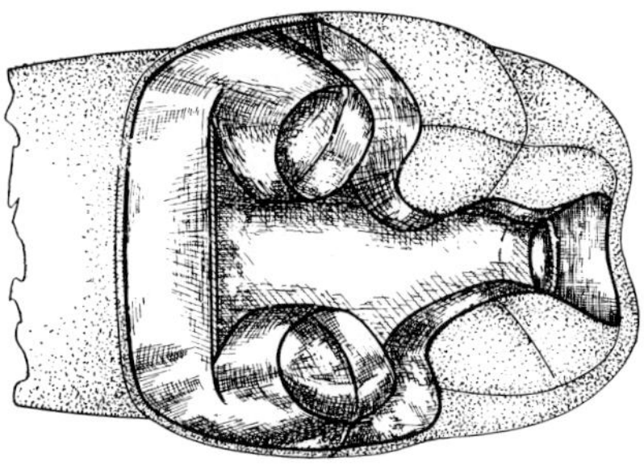

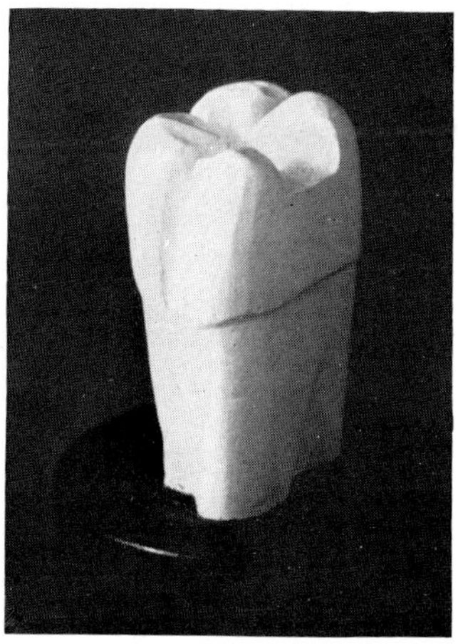

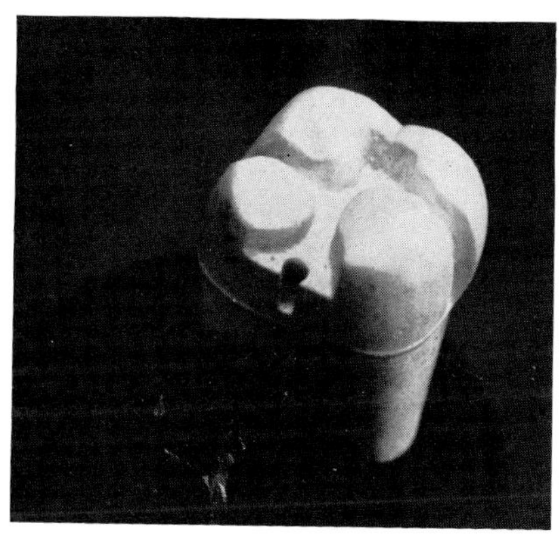

Fig. 18-31. Finished one-half veneer preparations on lower molar and upper molar.

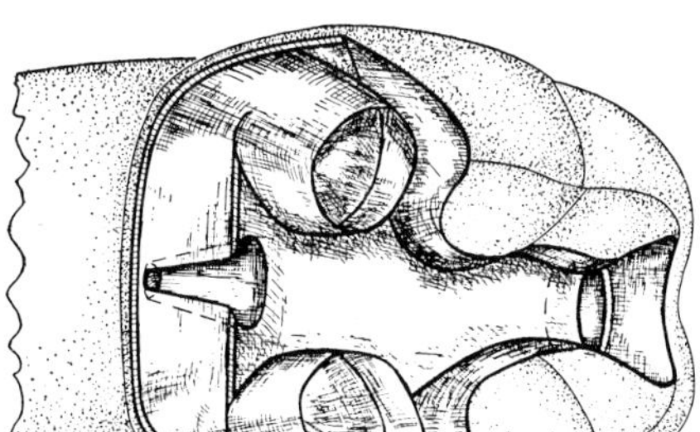

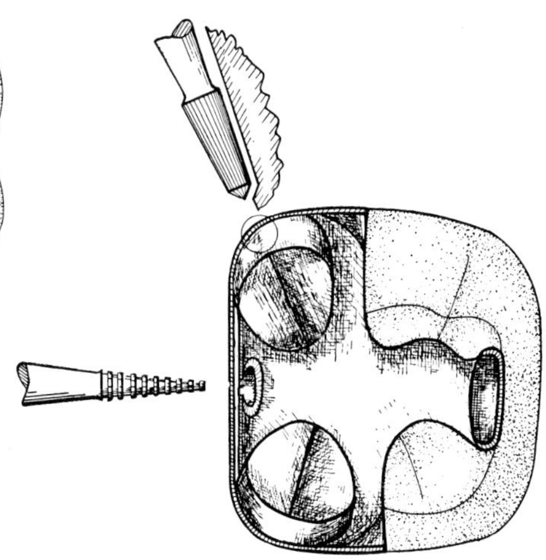

Fig. 18-32. Addition of proximal keyway and occlusal well gives added retention to retainer.

The final step of the preparation consists in establishing a gingival chamfer on the buccal and lingual surfaces, which unites with a similar bevel made on the proximal surface. The preparation of the chamfer in the cervical enamel is not easily accomplished unless a definite technic has been developed and followed. The following is suggested and recommended for the final step in the tooth preparation.

Up to this point, the enamel on the buccal, lingual, and mesial surfaces has been reduced with diamond 1½V and safe-end tapered cylinder-type stones (Densco 5D-S), but only to the crest of the gingival tissues. Generally, the

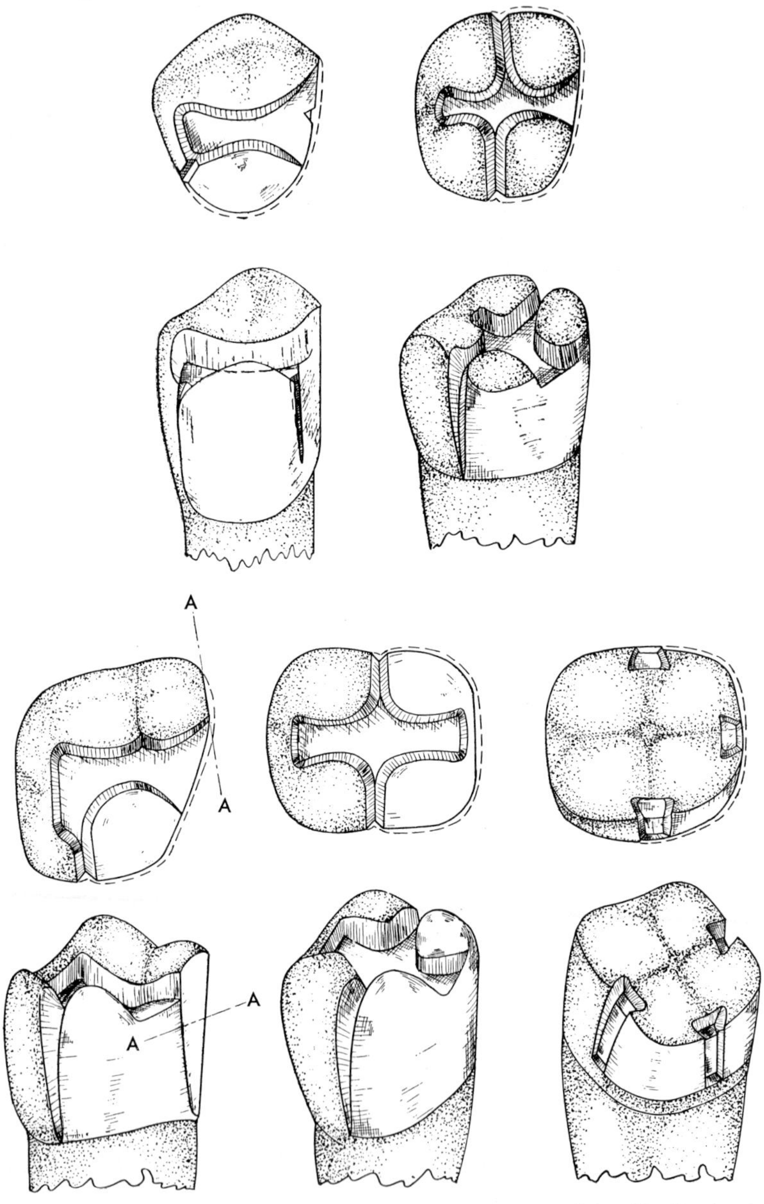

Fig. 18-33. Modifications of partial veneer principle suggested by MacBoyle. In **B, left,** note acute angle between plane **A-A** and mesioaxial surface.

chamfer is lowered slightly below the gingival crest if it can be done without injury to the soft tissues. To do so, the gingiva may first be retracted with cord to expose the cervical enamel; better still, the method recommended by Selberg[4] may be employed, in which the rubber dam and clamp are utilized. The rubber dam method not only depresses the gingiva but it also protects it from mechanical injury. With the rubber dam in place it is a matter of minutes to prepare the chamfer with a Densco 1D-T tapering and beveled diamond stone, which is followed by the Tinker finishing bur (Fig. 18-32, top left). A dovetail keyway cut in the mesial proximal dentin surface gives additional retention to the retainer (Fig. 18-32, lower right).

MacBOYLE TYPE

Another type of modification of the posterior partial veneer retainer is the MacBoyle[5] preparation. Reference is made in Chapter 19 to its principle of construction and retention. Fig. 18-33 shows five views of typical MacBoyle posterior retainers. It is evident, upon studying these preparations, that fundamentally they are similar to the one-half proximal veneer crown previously described. The third preparation shows an extreme adaptation of this retainer, wherein the proximal and parts of the buccal and lingual surfaces are involved, yet without including any of the occlusal surface. This type of preparation is recommended for the extreme, close-bite geriatric patients. It is conceivable that this preparation might be extended to the distal proximal surface so that the entire tooth circumference would be encompassed, the four axial locks and grooves furnishing the main means of resisting displacement.

SELECTED REFERENCES

1. Tinker, E. T.: Fixed bridgework, J.A.D.A. **7:**579, 1920.
2. Dressel, R. P.: Principles of fixed bridge construction, D. Cosmos **72:**565, 730, 853, 941, 1173, 1272, 1930: **73:**130, 253, 342, 1931.
3. Krause, O. G.: Cast attachments for bridgework with special reference to vital teeth, J.A.D.A. **21:**2104, 1934.
4. Selberg, A.: Cast gold crowns, J. Tennessee D. A. **29:**21, 1949.
5. MacBoyle, R. E.: Crown and fixed bridgework, from the point of view of our present knowledge, J. Nat. D. A. **8:**635, 1921.

GENERAL REFERENCES

Abramowsky, Z. L.: Fixed partial dentures by one-piece casting, J. Prosth. Dent. **10:**938, 1960.

Boitel, R. H.: Parallelometer, a precision instrument for the prosthetic laboratory, J. Prosth. Dent. **12:**732, 1962.

Dietz, W. H.: Means of saving mutilated teeth, J. Prosth. Dent. **11:**967, 1961.

Dietz, W. H.: Modified abutments for removable and fixed prosthodontics, J. Prosth. Dent. **11:**1112, 1961.

Guyer, S. E.: Partial veneer crowns: preparation alignment, Washington Univ. D. J. **26:**72, 1960.

Hollenback, G. M.: Fixed bridgework which meets functional physiologic and esthetic requirements, J.A.D.A. **29:**1179, 1942.

Klaffenbach, A. O.: Basic considerations in fixed partial denture prosthesis, J. D. Soc. New York **8:**31, 1942.

Knapp, K. W.: A modern conception of proper bridge attachments for vital teeth, J.A.D.A. **14:**1027, 1927.

Leander, C. T.: Preparation of abutments for fixed partial dentures, Dent. Clin. N. Amer., pp. 59-72, March, 1959.

Schnepper, H. E., and Baum, L.: Miniature parallel pins for retention of cast restorations, J. Prosth. Dent. **11:**772, 1961.

Smith, D. E.: Fixed bridge restorations with the tilted mandibular second or third molar as an abutment, J. South. California D. A. **6:**131, 1939.

Smith, D. E.: Fixed bridgework in the various phases of dental practice, J. South. California D. A. **9:**13, 1942.

Smyd, E. S.: Advanced thought in indirect inlay and fixed bridge fabrication, J.A.D.A. **31:**759, 913, 1052, 1944.

Sturdevant, R. E.: Choice of bridge retainers, J. South. California D. A. **14:**16, 1947.

Tylman, S. D.: Fixed partial denture prosthodontics, Int. Dent. J. **10:**58, 1960.

Vedder, F. B.: The place of the fixed bridge in restorative dentistry, J.A.D.A. **29:**1973, 1942.

Chapter 19

Intermediate retention of retainers

Up to the present, the resistance of a retainer to displacement is shown to be dependent largely upon the retention form developed by the tooth itself. In other words, a properly made inlay, when placed in its prepared tooth, even without the intervention of cement, would be able to resist displacement in almost every direction except that opposite to its insertion (Fig. 13-12, *B*). Tension or pull under ordinary circumstances will lift a casting out of its cavity. The only resistance to such displacement is developed by utilizing some intermediary substance placed between the casting and the cavity walls; this is usually done with cement.

CEMENT

When two dry, flat surfaces are brought together under pressure, such as two pieces of glass, it is difficult to separate them by applying forces in opposite directions at right angles to their surfaces (Fig. 19-1, *A*). The resistance to separation arises from imbalanced air pressure between outer surfaces and the contacting surfaces. The adhesion between the two surfaces is even greater if some intermediary substance such as a film of water is placed between them. Two such planes of glass can be separated only by sliding one surface horizontally over the other in opposite directions. The addition of water or oil helps to exclude the air between the two surfaces more perfectly, thus the unbalanced pressure between the plates could be increased to a possible maximum of some 14.2 pounds per square inch, the normal air pressure (Fig. 19-1, *B*). If cement is used many of the interposed crystals of cement attach themselves to both surfaces of glass and thus augment their powers of retention by their resistance to tensile, compressive, and shearing forces.

The fact that low tensile strength may be the real cause of failure of soldered joints would provide a reason for making the cementing layer as thin as possible, i.e., as thin as is consistent with making usable joints, particularly at the interfaces (Fig. 19-1, *B*). This is because the small movement necessary as an accompaniment to failure cannot take place as readily in a thin layer as in a thick one without also involving some of the stronger material in the parts being cemented, and thus bringing into play their superior properties as an aid to the perhaps weaker adhesion at the interface.

Where a restoration is exposed to a tensile displacing force only, as in a labial porcelain or gold inlay, then the contiguous surfaces of the inlay and of the cavity wall may be modified as in Fig. 19-1, *C* and *D*.

If an inlay is loosened in its cavity, rupture ordinarily occurs in the cement layer that lies between the cavity and the metal walls. Since the cement layer is the location of weakness in the assembly and rupture occurs here, if the inlay is to be loosened in its cavity, it seems appropriate that some discussion be given to how the load on the occlusal surface is transmitted to the layers of weakness and of its effect on the cementing material, the purpose of which is to hold the metal of the inlay securely to the tooth. Rupture cannot occur in these layers unless the ultimate strength of the cementing material is exceeded.

Any material has three types of strength —compressive, tensile, and shearing. The usual primary load applied to the occlusal surface induces either compressive stress or shearing stress in the material at the surface. Compressive stress is induced when the movement of the mandible is normal to the occlusal plane, and shearing stress when its is parallel to that plane. Tensile stress at this point is occasionally induced when chewing sticky food such as a caramel.

However, since rupture ordinarily occurs at the cementing layer between the cavity walls and the metal of the inlay, consideration must also be given to the *stresses induced in cementing material at the cavity floor* by bending action or by the occlusal loads in the vertical cavity walls (Fig. 13-15, *B*).

Dental cement is rated as a brittle material. Brittle materials as a rule are critically low in tensile strength when compared to their compressive and shearing strengths. Therefore, our interest lies specifically in the points of induced tensile strength in the cementing material. But since each of the three sorts of stress induces each of the others, it interests us to know not only where the greatest tensile stress occurs in the cement but also where other types of stress exist that might induce damaging tensile stress. We need also to know the relationship that exists between compressive stress and shearing stress and between shearing stress and tensile stress.

Fig. 19-2, *C*, shows a sketch of the metal (upper), an abutment inlay, and the dentin lying between the metal and the pulp chamber (lower). These are shown as solid lines. The dotted lines show the deformation of this combination beam (spanning the pulp chamber) bent into a parabola under the influence of occlusal load. The thin layer of cement that attaches the metal to the dentin layer, covering the top of the pulp chamber, is shown as a double line.

The sketch is in no way meant to provide a basis for the exact analysis of the stresses in the combination beam shown (inlay cemented to the dentin that covers the pulp chamber). The purpose is rather to stimulate the imagination of the reader to an understanding that at all points of the cement lined cavity interior exists a variety of stresses, all of which are in turn

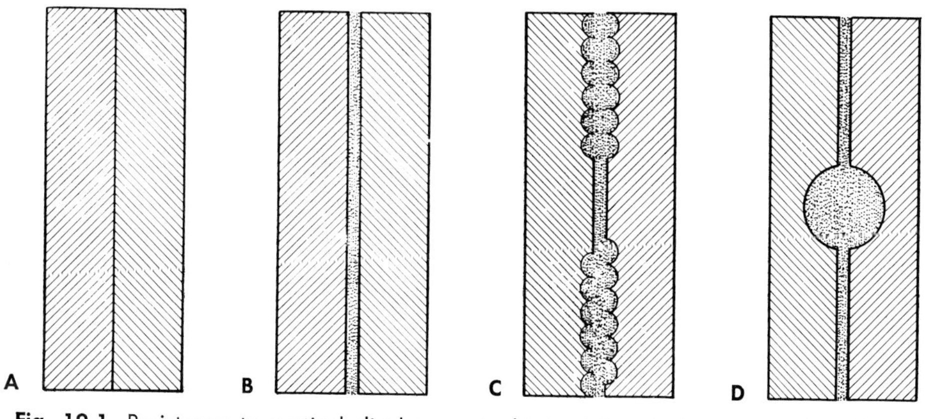

Fig. 19-1. Resistance to vertical displacement obtained by placing cement keys between dentin and metal walls having mechanical locks.

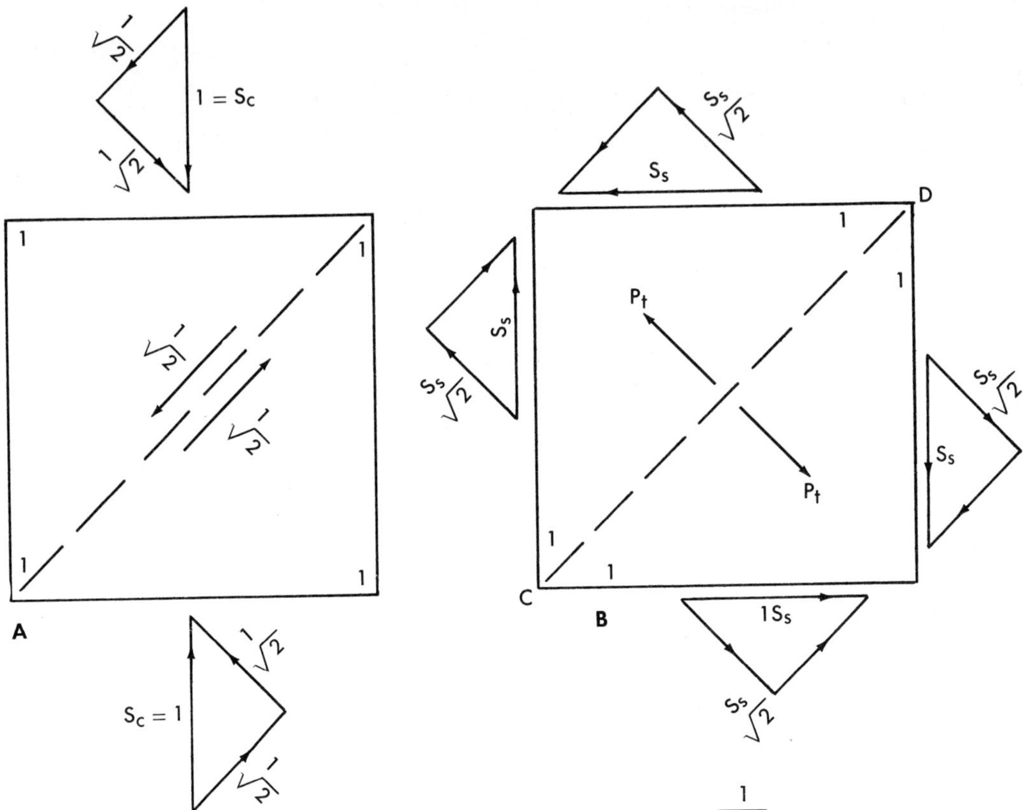

Fig. 19-2. A, Compressive stress and induced shear. $S_s = \frac{\frac{1}{\sqrt{2}}}{\sqrt{2}} = \frac{1}{2}$ in general. $S_s = \frac{S_c}{2}$. **B,** Shearing stress and tensile stress. $P_t = \frac{2\ S_s}{\sqrt{2}}$ (Area CD $= \sqrt{2}$); (Induced) $S_t = \frac{2\ S_s}{\sqrt{2}} \times \frac{1}{\sqrt{2}} = S_s$. **C,** Combination beam action of inlay and dentin covering pulp chamber.

capable of inducing tensile stresses in the cementing material. Resistance of cementing material to tension is apt to be low and therefore tension in the cement layer is a matter of importance to the practitioner.

Let it first be assumed that the dentin is not attached to the metal by cement. In this case the two beams (lower), and metal of the abutment inlay (upper) will act separately. Each will have tension in its lower fibers and compression in its upper fibers, as indicated at the left end of these beams. The lower fibers will lengthen due to the tension in them. The amount of this lengthening is indicated by the symbol e_t at the left end of the metal beam. The upper fibers of the dentin beam will, by a similar token, shorten an amount e_c (shown at the left end of the beam). These movements are deterred only by such friction as may exist at the plane where the lower fibers of the metal beam make contact with the upper fibers of the dentin beam.

In practice, however, a layer of cement exists at this plane of contact. This layer welds the two surfaces together, forcing

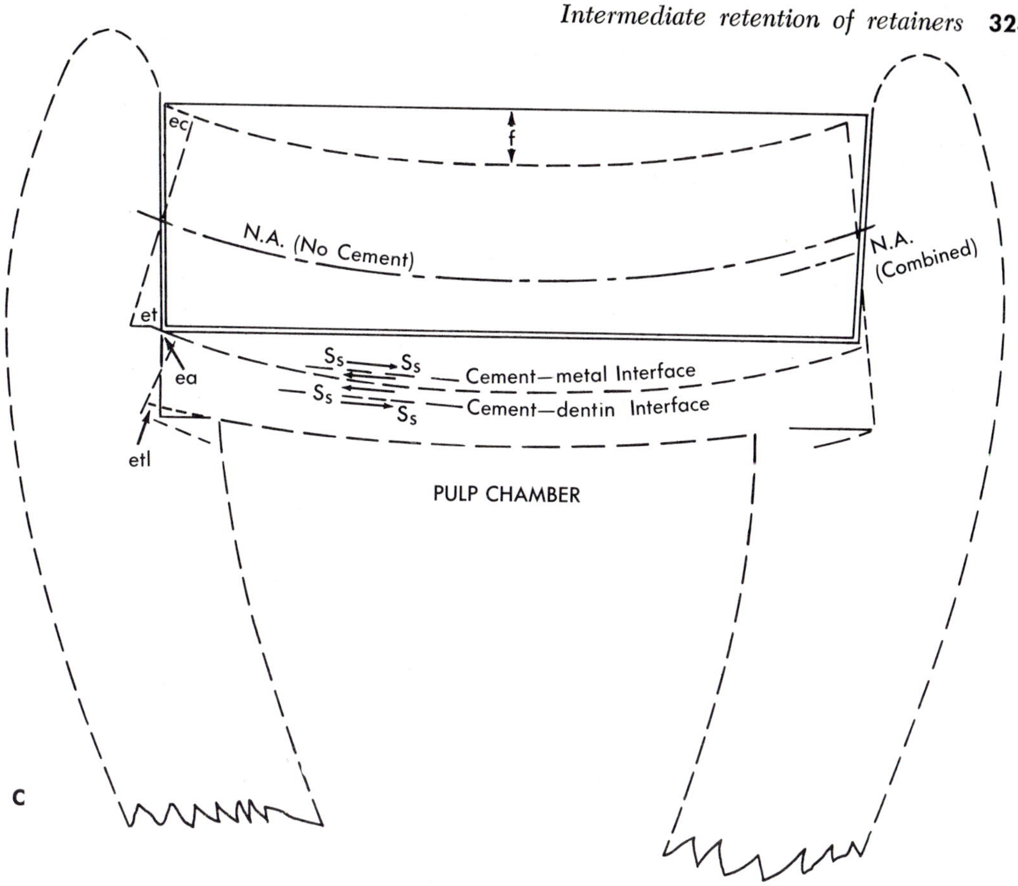

Fig. 19-2, cont'd. For legend see opposite page

the upper fibers of the dentin beam and the lower fibers of the metal beam to remain at the same length, under combination beam action. This condition is shown at the right ends. In order to make this possible, the upper fibers of the dentin beam must have lengthened and the lower fibers of the metal beam must have shortened till they have attained a common length (left end of the beam shown by dotted lines). This coercion of the two beams to maintain a common length at their plane of contact could have only been produced by inducing shearing stresses in the cement layer at this plane, as shown above and below the cement layer. They are labeled "cement-metal" and "cement-dentin" interfaces. These shearing stresses are of course variable in unit values from the point of zero shear of the beam to the supports. It should be also noted that simultaneous compressive stresses exist between these layers, induced by the occlusal loads that come upon the inlay. These shearing stresses, as well as compressive stresses, exist in the cement at the contact layer.

Fig. 19-2, *A*, shows a compressive unit stress axially applied to a cube, each of whose faces is unity in area. This unit force may be assumed to be of differential value and the sides of the cube as of differential length. The applied unit stress (force) may be resolved into components, each of which is at 45° to the applied unit stress. Two of these components (one from the upper force and the other from the lower-equalizing force) are equal in intensity but opposite in direction. The intensity of each of these components is

$\frac{1}{\sqrt{2}}$. These are parallel to the diagonal 45° plane of the cube as shown. They obviously produce a total shearing stress on this plane of $\frac{1}{\sqrt{2}}$. But the area of this plane is $1 \times \sqrt{2}$. Therefore, dividing this area into the total shearing force on the plane, we obtain that the unit shearing stress, induced on the diagonal plane by the unit compressive stress applied to the face of the cube, is equal to $\frac{1}{2}$, or $S_s = \frac{S_c}{2}$. It will be readily seen that the two unused components of the compressive unit stress also induce equal shearing unit stresses on that diagonal plane of the cube, which is perpendicular to the one shown.

We may then write laws as follows:

1. Unit compressive stress in any material induces within the material unit shearing stresses at 45° to the direction of the compressive stress and equal in intensity to half the intensity of the unit-inducing–compressive stress.

And by analogy:

2. Unit tensile stress in any material induces within the material unit shearing stresses at 45° to the direction of the inducing-tensile stress, which are equal in intensity to half the value of unit-inducing–tensile stress.

Consider the cube shown in Fig. 19-2, *B*. We will apply to this cube, on its upper face from right to left, a unit shearing stress, S_s. The cube is not in equilibrium under this single unit stress. The sum of its external horizontal forces is not zero (see second law of equilibrium). A second equal and opposite force must be applied to the lower face to restore horizontal equilibrium. But the forces on the upper and lower faces of the cube constitute a unit couple, whose tendency to rotate the cube is counterclockwise. The cube now satisfies the first two laws of equilibrium. However, the third law of equilibrium is not satisfied, which requires also that there be no tendency to rotate. This deficiency may be supplied by adding an equal and opposite couple to the two vertical faces of the cube as shown. From this discussion comes this law:

3. Pure shear may only exist at a point in a body when shearing stresses of equal intensities exist at right-angled directions.

The cube now satisfies all three laws of equilibrium. Each unit, with external force (stress) on the four cube faces, is now resolved into components, at 45° to the applied original shearing stresses on the cube faces. The components are either perpendicular or parallel to the diagonal plane *CD* of the cube. It will be seen that the pair of components on either side of *CD*, which are perpendicular to it, produce a tension on this plane, whose total value is P_t. By the same reasoning the four components, which are parallel to *CD*, would produce compression on the other diagonal of the cube (not shown), which is at right angles to *CD*.

The total value of P_t is seen to be:

$$P_t = \frac{2\ S_s}{\sqrt{2}} = S_s\sqrt{2} \qquad \text{(a)}$$

But the area of plane CD is $1 \times \sqrt{2}$.

Now if P_t is divided by the area of plane *CD*, we obtain the tensile-unit stress within the material of the cube, which is induced by the unit stresses (external forces) applied to its faces:

$$\frac{P_t}{\sqrt{2}} = \frac{S_s\sqrt{2}}{\sqrt{2}} = S_s \qquad \text{(b)}$$

From Eq. (b) we may write a general law as follows:

4. Any material subject to shearing stress has induced within it a tensile unit stress at 45° to its direction which is equal in intensity to the unit shearing stress that induced it. It also has induced within its material at 45° to the inducing unit shearing stress (and perpendicular of the induced unit tensile stress) a compressive unit stress equal in intensity to the inducing-unit–shearing stress.

It is now established that shearing stresses exist in the cement layer under all conditions of occlusal load. It also has been stated that these stresses are greater near the supports of the beam bridging the pulp cavity than in the middle, and that compressive stresses exist in the cement along the floor of the cavity preparation that result from applied occlusal loads. These compressive stresses also induce shearing stresses in the cement layer. Such compressive stresses should be greater near support areas (vertical walls of the pulp chamber), since the reactions of the beam are there transferred into the dentin. It also seems obvious that direct shearing stresses are induced in the predominantly vertical walls of the cavity preparation as a result of occlusal loads being transferred into the dentin of the vertical cavity walls. All of these eventually lead to tensile stresses at most points of the cement layer. This, coupled with the fact that it is probable the weakest strength characteristic of dental cement is its tensile strength, should suggest that data be established on the specific tensile properties of dental cement.

Thin cement layers are apt to be stronger than thicker ones because in a thin layer failure due to tension is more apt to involve the greater strength of abutting layers than in the case of thicker ones.

METAL PINS

Reverting to Fig. 19-1, it is evident that, if a piece of round wire is substituted for a round cylinder of cement, the inlay would be so locked mechanically that it would resist all effort to dislodge. It is possible to obtain retention of this type by cutting, at right angles to the surface, a round hole or depression 1 mm. wide and 2 to 3 mm. deep on an axial surface between the margins of the casting and the enamel wall (Fig. 19-3, *A*, *B*, and *C*). This

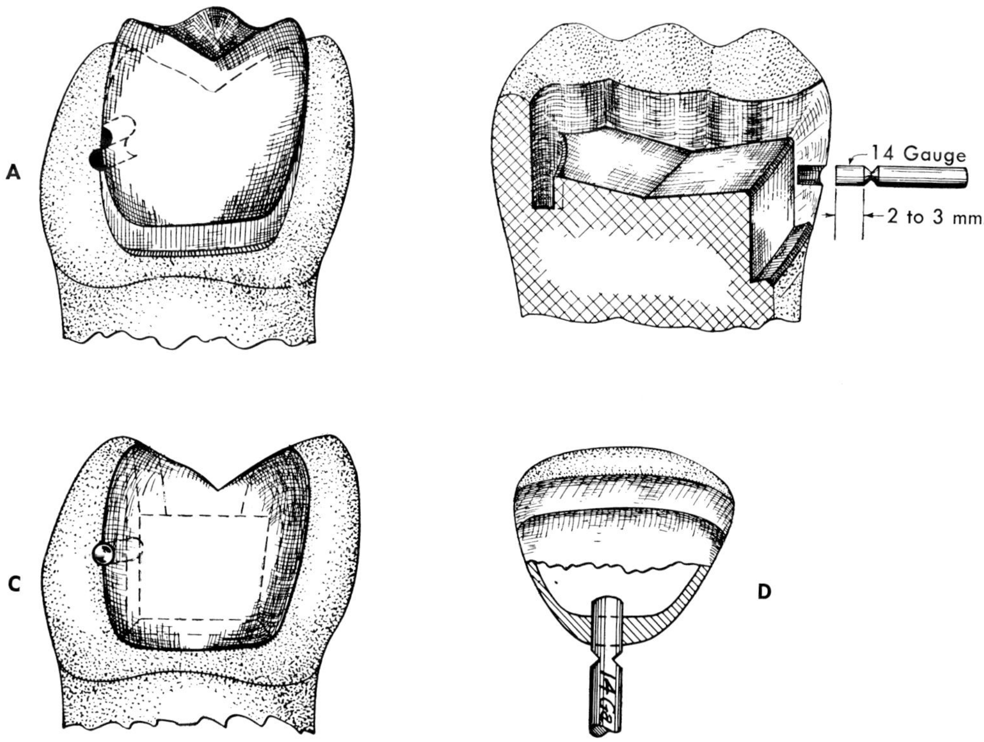

Fig. 19-3. Pin locks placed at right angles to directions of displacing forces.

round groove is enlarged sufficiently to receive a 16- or 14-gauge clasp metal wire, which completely fills the opening. Since half of the circular opening lies within the casting in the form of a semicircular groove and the other half lies as a semicircular groove in the tooth structure, the dislodgment of the inlay occlusally is resisted by the rod of the inserted clasp metal wire. This technic has been described and has been in use many years.[1, 2] It recently was claimed as a new method of retention.

Where a three-quarter partial veneer retainer is used or a complete gold crown, a round opening of suitable diameter is made through the outer surface of the casting; a round depression of the same diameter is then sunk into the tooth structure to a depth varying from 1 to 2 mm. (Fig. 19-3, *D*). A clasp metal wire of the same diameter is inserted and cemented in position at the time that the restoration is permanently cemented. Any excess wire is finished smooth in the final polish. This method of right angle resistance to displacement has also been in use for many years.

Threaded key

To simplify the use of the right angle wire lock just described, several accurately machined types have been manufactured under various names.

The right angle lock or key shown in Fig. 19-4 is typical. The technic for its use is as follows: The device consists of a gold tube, threaded on the inside, a threaded key, and two guide nuts. The purpose of this device is to lock mechanically a fixed retainer in a tooth by means of a wire key placed at an angle to resist the force of displacement. The tube, A^1, consists of a hard, high-fusing gold alloy; it is of thin gauge and is threaded on the inside and knurled on the outside.

The threaded wire key, A^2, or wire has a head at one end designed to receive a wrench or screwdriver (*D* and *E*). The threaded wire key is also made of hard gold to prevent stripping of the threads or bending under stress.

The two small nuts, *A*, are used as guides to register the depth to which the wire key is carried into the recess cut in the tooth; they assist in carrying the threaded wire key into the tooth to a previously predetermined depth.

When attached to a bridge retainer, the threaded tube is placed at an obtuse angle to the prepared lingual surface of the abutment, with its inner end directed toward the incisal or occlusal surface of the tooth, while the outer surface end slopes slightly gingivally.

The tube may be soldered to the attachment after it has been cast, or it may be placed in a wax pattern and cast directly as a part of the retainer. In order that the wire key may exert its maximum gripping power, it is advisable that another juxtaposed surface, groove, pin, or bevel be placed to offer resistance to the locking force of the metal key.

It is necessary that a sufficient amount of tooth structure be removed from the area of the tooth lying opposite the opening of the tube, so that a thickness of metal is present in the casting sufficient to hold the tube firmly in position; at least half the length of the tube should be embedded in the body of the casting (Fig. 19-4, *B*).

If the tube is to be soldered in the retainer, a small hole is first drilled through the wax pattern at the point where the tube is later to be soldered. When the casting is made, the hole is enlarged sufficiently to accommodate the tube and the tube is placed in position, waxed, invested, and soldered.

When the tube is to be attached directly to the retainer in casting, a small opening is made in the wax pattern just as previously; then with a fissure bur the opening is enlarged sufficiently to accommodate the tube snugly. The tube is inserted in the opening and attached with sticky wax and the wax pattern is removed from the abutment. A carbon point is now painted with investment material and inserted into and through the threaded portion of the tube. This will hold the tube in its proper relation when the molten casting gold enters the mold. The wax pattern is invested, burned out, and cast, following which the carbon point is carefully removed from the inner part of the tube. Any investment or carbon that remains and that cannot be readily dislodged can be removed by using a small tap (Fig. 19-4, *C*) which can be worked in and out gently until the

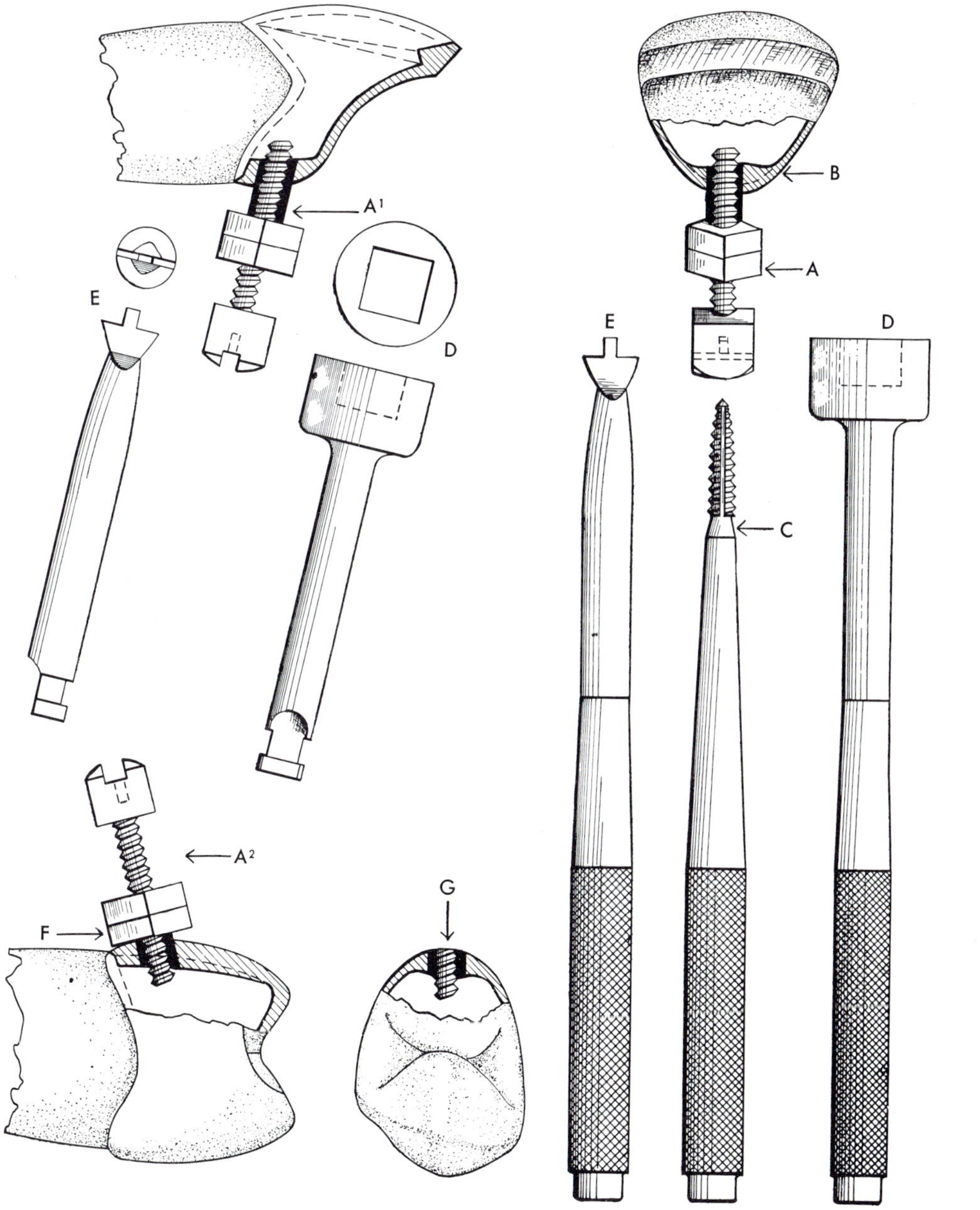

Fig. 19-4. Threaded pin lock key.

obstruction is removed. It is well to use a little oil in performing this operation. The threaded wire key should not be used for this purpose, since there is danger of stripping the threads.

There are several methods of establishing the exact location of the depression in the tooth that is to receive the wire key. In those cases in which the tube is to be soldered into the cast retainer, the retainer is first seated in position on the tooth. With a bur of the proper size, a small hole or depression is cut into the tooth through the opening made in the retainer. The retainer is now removed and the opening in the tooth is enlarged and deepened to the desired size and depth, making sure that, when later the wire key is screwed into position, it will not press against the gingival wall of the pit, causing it to unseat the retainer. After the tube has been soldered to the retainer, the correct relationship of the threaded wire key to the depression in the tooth may be verified and, if necessary, adjusted.

If, on the other hand, the retainer has been completed and the tube is in place, yet no pit or depression has been prepared in the tooth, this may be done by taking a small bit drill that will pass through the tube and slightly beyond its inner end. If the end of the drill previously has been rubbed on articulating paper a mark will be left on the tooth when they are brought in contact. The retainer is now removed and a depression is made in the tooth at the point marked by the end of the drill. The position and size of the opening in the tooth are verified by inserting the threaded wire key through the tube after the retainer has been replaced on the tooth.

It is also possible to locate the exact point opposite the opening of the tube by carbonizing the point of the threaded wire key; by screwing it lightly against the inner surface of the tooth, it will leave a mark similar to the one left by the drill. The retainer is then removed and a depression is cut in the tooth as previously described.

After the pit has been cut in the tooth and its position and size have been verified by carrying the threaded wire key into it, the next step is very important, for it establishes the distance that the wire key extends into the pit. If it fails to extend far enough into the opening, only a small part of its maximum retentive force is utilized; if, however, the threaded wire key is forced too far into the pit, there is danger of lifting the retainer from the prepared tooth. When adjusting the wire key, it should be turned slowly and with little force. Just as soon as the wire key is in place, i.e., in contact with the bottom of the pit, resistance is noted. It is only necessary that the point of the wire key enter the pit and touch the tooth structure at its bottom. Force is likely to spring the attachment from the tooth at the gingiva. The wrenches and screwdrivers (Fig. 19-4, *D* and *E*) supplied are merely a convenience to assist in the manipulation of the nut.

The first step is to screw the two nuts completely against the slotted head of the pin lock key. The assembly is then inserted into the opening of the threaded tube extending from the outer surface of the casting, and then slowly screwed into the tube.

When the point of the wire key has been carried to the bottom of the pit, the first nut is brought in contact with the outside end of the tube (Fig. 19-4, *F*); a small amount of quick-setting cement is placed lightly on the wire key against the nut, whereupon the second nut is brought through the cement against the first nut, thereby cementing both to the wire key. A small amount of cement is also carried between the second nut and the head of the wire key. After the cement has hardened, the wire key and the two nuts cemented to it are unscrewed from the threaded tube sufficiently to allow the retainer to be withdrawn. The nuts are left cemented on the wire key until after the final cementation of the retainer, since they are the guides to the depth that the wire key is screwed through the tube into the pit in the tooth. If in the final cementation the guide nuts do not contact the external opening of the tube, it is evident that the retainer or the wire key has not been fully seated. After final cementation, the excess lengths of wire key, tube, and two guide nuts are cut off and the surface is finished and polished smooth (Fig. 19-4, *G*).

This and other similar types of intermediary retention are indicated on extremely short teeth or on those abutments where very little of the natural tooth structure remains.

The same principle of retention is also utilized in removable fixed bridges, in which the pontic element structure of the restoration is rigidly attached to the retainers by means of threaded metal dowels or pins. This can subsequently be removed by the dentist at any time later for repair or hygienic purposes.

MODIFICATIONS

One of the most frequent modifications of the typical three-quarter partial veneer retainer in an anterior tooth is the substitution of the tapering proximal grooves with a boxlike preparation (Figs. 19-5 and 19-6, *A* to *C*). This is done usually when proximal decay is present or when it is necessary to have a proximal bulk of metal in which a tapered keyway is cut to support an interlocking key used with the broken-stress principle. When such a change is made, the technic shown in Figs. 15-7 and 15-8 is employed to prepare the proximal, box-like modification.

Occasionally, it is deemed necessary to increase the retentive qualities of a retainer which has an incisal plane instead of the incisal step or groove. This may be done by placing a slight pit in the cingulum extending 1 to 2 mm. into the tooth and sufficiently large to accommodate a 20-gauge iridioplatinum pin (Fig. 19-7). The direction of this pit must parallel that of the proximal grooves. The 20-gauge pin may be cast, a plastic pin may be embedded in the wax pattern before casting, or the pin may be soldered after the casting has been made.

At other times, it is more convenient to prepare on each proximal surface a grooved keyway placed lingually to the usual proximal groove (Figs. 19-8 to 19-10). These keyways are made parallel with the axis of the axial grooves or boxing.

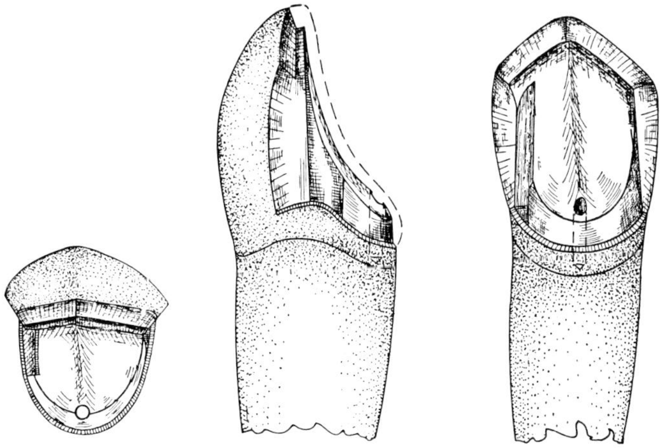

Fig. 19-5. Box-like modification of one of axial grooves.

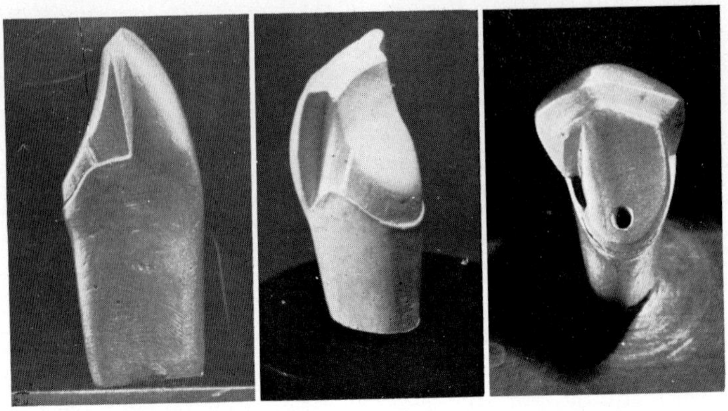

A B C

Fig. 19-6. A to **C,** Box-like modification of one of axial grooves.

To further increase the retention of the retainer, these supplementary lingual keyways may be united with a groove extending across the lingual surface above the cingulum. This creates a supplementary staple-like lock (Fig. 19-9).

In rare instances the esthetic requirements of a restoration are such that no gold may be placed along the incisal edge. In this event the lingual and the two proximal surfaces retain the outline form of a typical partial veneer retainer with the exception that the incisal margin of the retainer terminates on the lingual surface 2 or 3 mm. below the incisal edge of the tooth (Fig. 19-11). Such a preparation, while possessing high esthetic values, lacks the mechanical strength needed for the majority of fixed partial dentures. This type of preparation may also be used in thin teeth where an axial groove is contraindicated. In these circumstances, the Type IV hard casting golds are used.

Lower abutments

Sometimes lower incisors are prepared for partial veneer retainers. Usually no incisal groove is employed; where the teeth are extremely thin, even the proximal grooves may be omitted. In such situations the proximal cuts are carried around onto the labial surface sufficiently to establish a group and bring the margins into a cleansable area. Usually the pinlay or pinledge types are indicated.

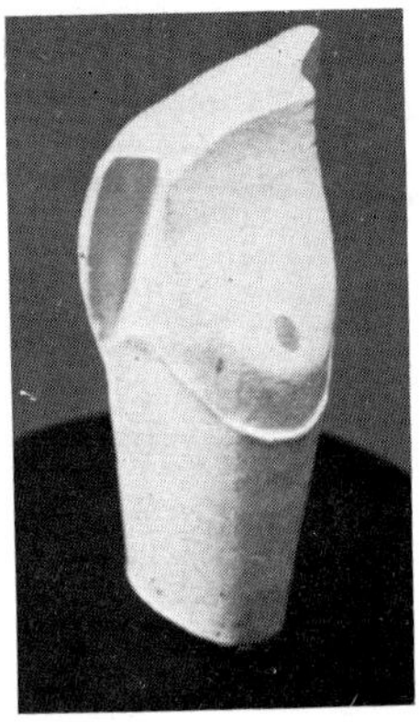

Fig. 19-7. Employing wire pins for supplementary retention.

Kabnick type

Kabnick[1] suggested a "pit-veneer" preparation for anterior teeth wherein one proximal surace and most of the lingual and incisal surfaces are involved (Fig. 19-12). The retention is obtained by placing two pins in the lingual surface, one in the region of the incisal plane and the other in the cingulum. Additional retention is developed by placing a lock groove in the proximal surface, which parallels the direction of the two lingual pins.

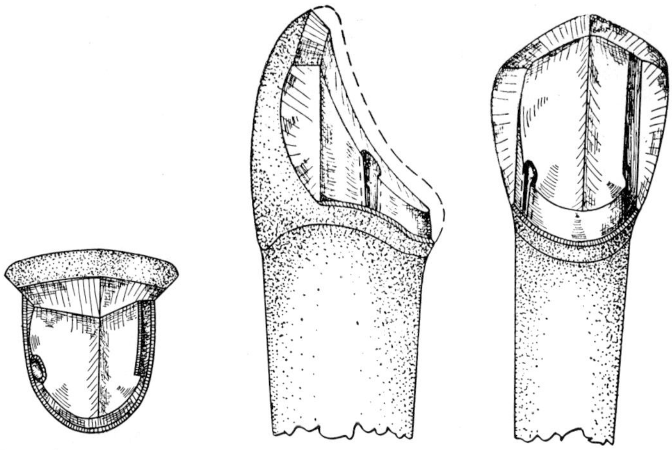

Fig. 19-8. Utilizing supplementary grooves and keyways for additional retention.

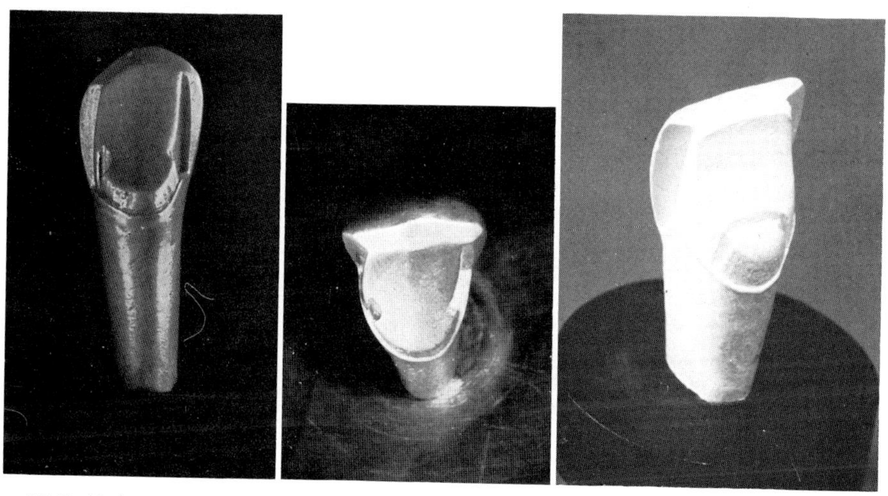

Fig. 19-9. Utilizing supplementary grooves, keyways, and staple for additional retention.

MacBoyle type

MacBoyle[2] in 1921 suggested still another modification of the veneer type of bridge retainer (Fig. 19-13). His description of an ideal fixed bridge retainer for the six anterior teeth in either the upper or lower arches is as follows:

> It is a metal construction covering the lingual, mesial, and distal surfaces of the tooth, perfectly adapted and extending to the gum line, at the mesial and distal, avoiding the gum line at the lingual. This should be anchored by means of two pins located near the incisal area well toward the mesial and distal and extending into small canals drilled into the tooth well removed from the pulp area. These canals are slightly less than one-sixteenth of an inch in depth in the larger teeth, and gauge 20 in size. In the lower incisors, two pins one millimeter in length and gauge 22 are used. If the pins are placed at the incisal area this abutment piece [retainer] is made adaptable to the lower incisors as well as to the larger anterior teeth. This is the logical place for the pins because in both uppers and lowers the pins should be at the place of most stress. It is possible to place a third pin in the area of the cingulum of the tooth, if necessary.
>
> The tooth is but slightly mutilated; there are no grooves cut, and no shoulder at the gingival. The incisal edge is beveled about 45°, and the

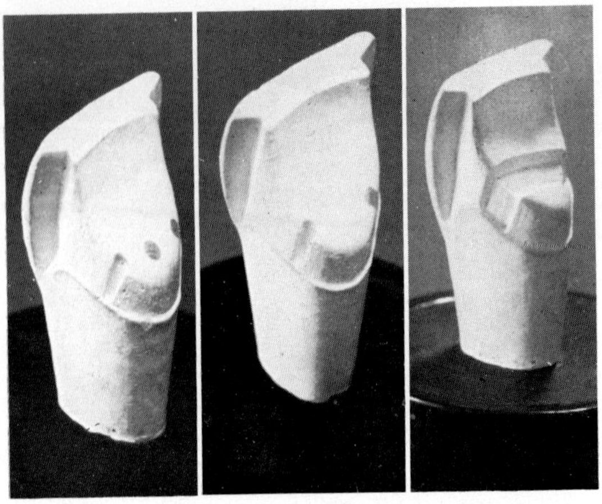

Fig. 19-10. Utilizing supplementary grooves and keyways for additional retention.

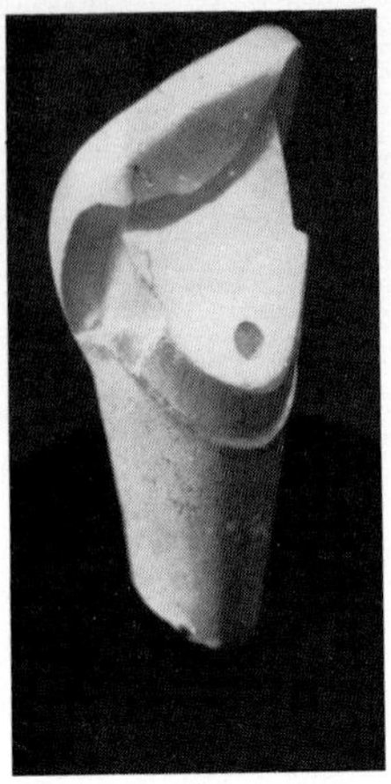

Fig. 19-11. Continuation of intracoronal and pin principles of retention with those of partial veneer retainer utilizing proximal boxings.

metal extends just slightly to the labial of the contact point on the mesial and distal surfaces. The labial contour of the tooth is not impaired but in the preparation any bell shape is removed from the surface covered, so that the adaptation is perfect at all margins. This anterior abutment piece [retainer] is made preferably by the swaging and burnishing method. An impression is taken of the prepared tooth in modeling compound, then a cement model is made from this impression over which pure gold No. 34 gauge is swaged and over this a second piece is put aside until the first piece has been fitted to the tooth in the mouth and the pins soldered to it. After the pins are soldered to the first pure gold backing, it should be placed on the tooth in the mouth and trimmed and burnished perfectly. It should be removed carefully, filled with crown and bridge investment, and the second piece adapted for reinforcement. In the second backing, large holes should be cut to fit over the projecting pins, and a slit in the center of the second backing; in soldering the two plates together, the pieces of solder should be placed in the slit and around the pins. Further reinforcement can be done if desired by sweating solder upon any portion of the structure.

The anterior abutment piece [retainer] may be made by the casting method if desired, in the same way as described for the posterior pieces. The pins should be threaded or roughened and in place in the tooth when the wax impression is taken so that they will be in the proper relation in the model. The fused inlay wax is then placed around the projecting ends of the pins and upon the model to the desired form and contour, the sprue attached, and the case invested, and cast.*

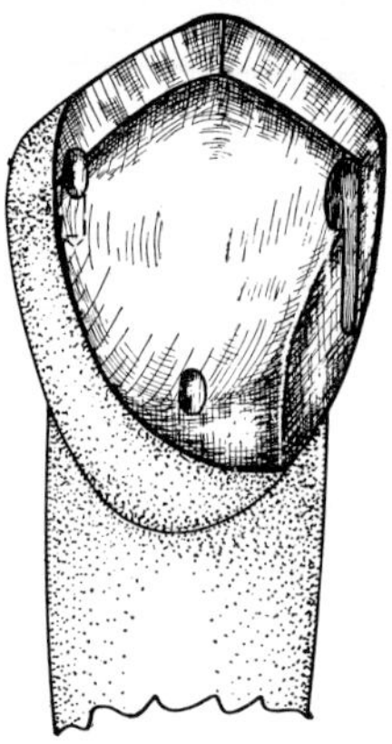

Fig. 19-12. Pin, groove, and partial veneer employed in principles of retention. (After Kabnick.)

PINLAY AND PIN LEDGE RETAINERS

There are other modified forms of the veneer type of retainer for anterior teeth; among those most frequently referred to are the pinlay or pin ledge retainers.

As the name indicates, this type of retainer is the partial veneer type resorting to pins for means of retention (Fig. 19-14).

*From MacBoyle, R. E.: Crown and fixed bridgework, from the point of view of our present knowledge, J. Nat. D. A. 8:635, 1921.

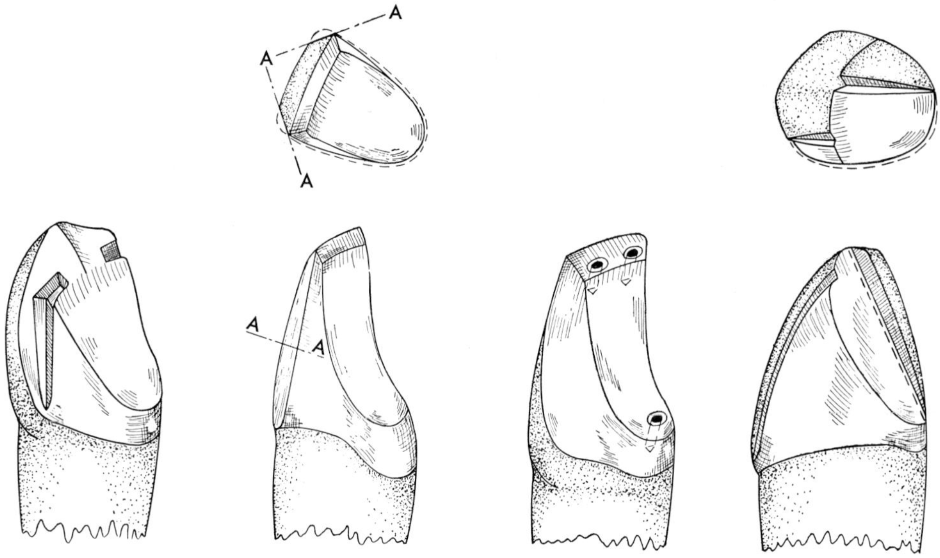

Fig. 19-13. Designs of extracoronal preparations designed by MacBoyle. **A-A** indicates linguolabial convergence of planes.

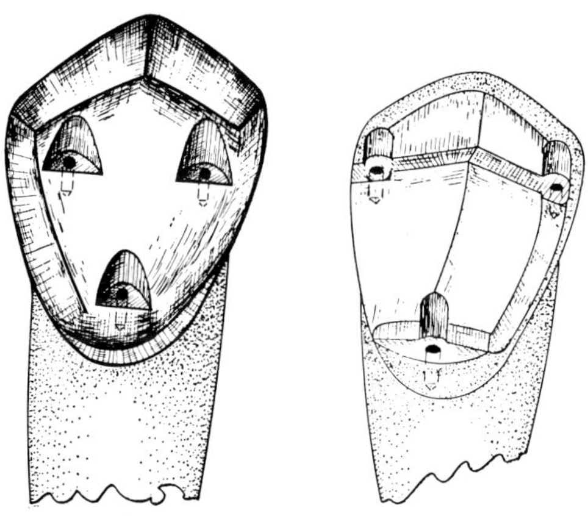

Fig. 19-14. Frequently used pinledge retainer.

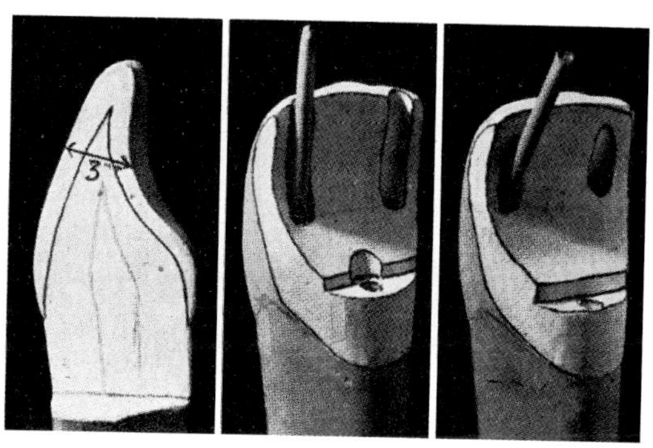

Fig. 19-15. Thin incisor. Comparison of models shows that there is an advantage to drilling pits parallel to labial surface and not parallel to axis of tooth. (Courtesy Dr. R. LeHuche.)

The credit for the development and systematization of this retainer is usually given to Burgess,[3] who presented it to the dental profession over 50 years ago. Since that time many modifications and improvements have been made, notably by Gillett and Irving,[4] Doxtater.[5] A careful study of the preparation discloses that it has certain advantages not possessed by the typical partial veneer retainer, particularly when used in the anterior teeth, especially the mandibular.

By referring again to the relationship existing between tooth morphology and cavity prepaartion, LeHuche pointed out the following facts: In a thin tooth (Figs. 19-15 and 19-16, LeHuche[6]), placing the pins parallel to the incisal half of the labial surface gives better and safer retention than if they were placed parallel to the axis of the tooth.

In a tooth of average thickness (Fig. 19-17), it is also preferable to place the pins parallel with the incisal half of the

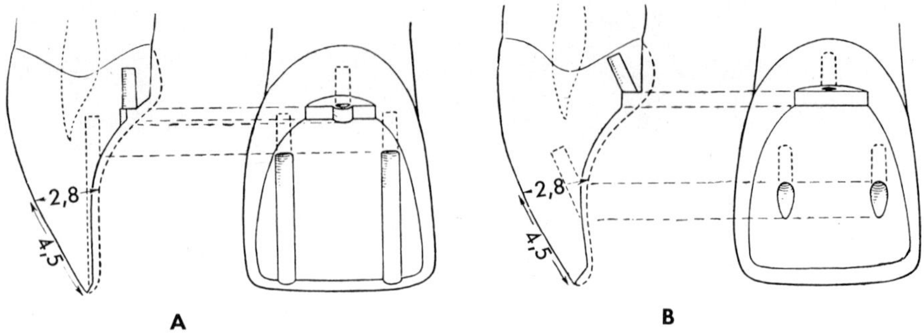

Fig. 19-16. Sketch to scale showing disposition of pits in two suggested directions in Fig. 19-15. **A,** Pits parallel to axis. Triangle formed by orifices of three pits is very small; retention of inlay is very weak. **B,** Pits parallel to labial surface. Retention is better. (Courtesy Dr. R. LeHuche.)

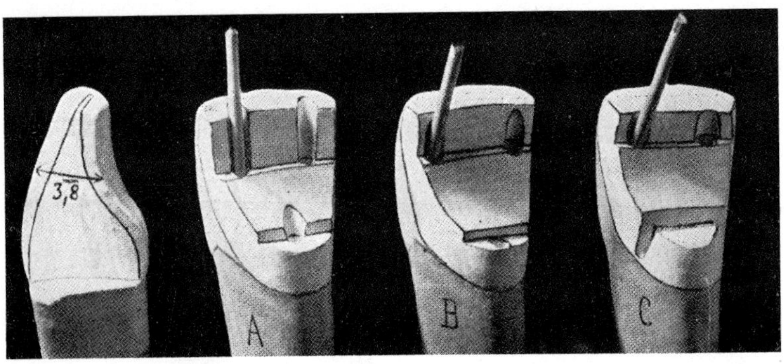

Fig. 19-17. Onlay with pins for tooth of average thickness. There is an advantage to making pits parallel to labial surface. (Courtesy Dr. R. LeHuche.)

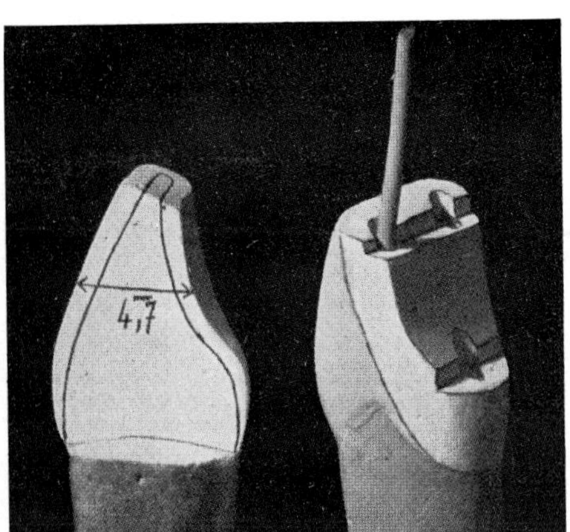

Fig. 19-18. Onlay with pins for very thick tooth. Direction of pits is immaterial. (Courtesy Dr. R. LeHuche.)

labial surface. The best retention is obtained in a tooth thick labiolingually, as shown in Fig. 19-18. The spacing of the pins also gives a triangle with widely separated points, giving greater mechanical retention.

Indications. It is claimed by Iwanson[7] that the teeth best adapted for this type of retention are the cuspids and the incisors of the upper arch; the lateral incisor also may be used if it is a well-developed tooth. Generally those teeth having small crowns should not be used since there is great danger of pulp involvement and a small crown does not provide sufficient room for a sufficiently strong pin retention. It is further claimed[1] that anterior teeth having very thin incisal edges are contraindicated because of cement showing through the enamel opposite the ledges. Because of the characteristic type of its proximal preparation, this type of retention should not be used in those mouths that are susceptible to caries or that are habitually neglected.

It is claimed that this retainer is preferable to the standard partial veneer type, because (1) less tooth structure is sacrificed, (2) less gold is displayed labially, and (3) the danger of pulp involvement is remote. Pruden[8] believed that this type of preparation is well adapted to the indirect technic employing the hydrocolloid impression material.

PIN AND PIN LEDGE RETENTION OF CAST RESTORATIONS

Preparing pinholes—direct method

Many methods have been developed to enable the dentist to prepare pinholes parallel to each other in individual teeth and with those in other teeth in the same arch. This may be possible to do by visual guidance alone in a single tooth. If, however, a series of pinholes must be paralleled with those in a distant abutment tooth, the accomplishment of paralleling becomes more difficult unless some form of mechanical aid facilitates the procedure.

Several methods and paralleling devices have been developed, some using appliances, fixed on teeth in the mouth during the cutting operations; these are usually restrictive and cumbersome.

To gain freedom of movement and better access and vision, a handpiece position finder was designed[9] which contained the parallelizing aid as an integrated part of the handpiece (Fig. 19-19, *A* and *B*). It shall be considered for making parallel pinholes and/or paralleling grooves at various distances and levels by varying the position of the paralleling guide. This may be designated as the direct method of determining and preparing the pinholes. First, the decision must have been made for the desired angle to be given the pinholes in the teeth and the pins in the retainers. The positioner is attached firmly to the handpiece and adjusted so that the red V completely surrounds the air bubble. The operator can

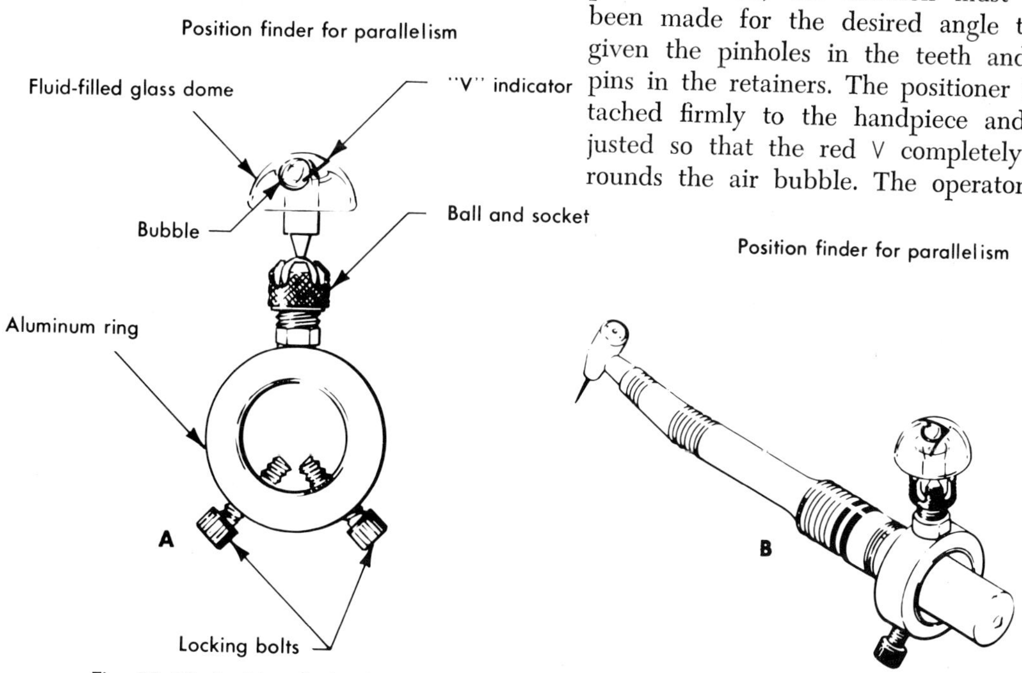

Fig. 19-19. Position finder for parallelism, **A;** attached to handpiece, **B.** (Courtesy E. Klein.)

cut parallel grooves or pinholes on single or multiple preparations. Each additional cutting is done by holding the handpiece so that the bubble is centered between the V and the cross bars.

PINS

Because metal pins are fitted in the holes, certain physical factors of the pins should be considered: composition, shape, length, diameter, surface texture, and number. Reports of investigators who have studied these factors may be summarized as follows:

1. Composition: if pins are to be of the manufactured type they should be of clasp metal type of wrought wire; if the pins are cast, then type IV inlay cast gold or partial denture gold should be used.
2. Shape: threaded pins are more retentive than smooth-sided surfaces.
3. Length: the retention is greater against tensile displacement in the longer pins than in the shorter.
4. Diameter: the larger the diameter of the pin the greater was its resistance to shearing and tensile forces. The 0.75 mm. diameter pin had greatest retention with all lengths on numbers used.
5. Surface texture: the threaded wrought wire pins afford greater resistance to tensile loads then the smooth crest pins.
6. Significant differences in retentive values occur as number of pins used is increased from one to five.

FRIDGE PARALLELING GUIDE*

Consideration shall be given next to the equipment and method developed and described by Dr. David S. Fridge[10] and used by many dentists (Fig. 19-20).

*Paralleling instrument designed by Dr. David S. Fridge. (Figs. 19-20 to 19-34 courtesy Densco Mfg. Co.)

In all fine precision work it is preferable to first lay out and mark work. After preparing the lingual, distal, and mesial surfaces of the abutment teeth, dry tooth surfaces and select and mark sites where pins are to be placed.

On centrals, laterals, and cuspids, ledges are ground (usually with end-cutting carbide burs or diamond points) at selected sites before drilling pinholes. For esthetic purposes, use only the lingual surfaces of the anterior teeth, as pin ledge attachments do not require cutting the mesial or distal surfaces.

The drilling of the primary pilot (first) pinhole is done freehand with the guide removed from the handpiece (Fig. 19-21). This pilot pinhole must be the distal of the most posterior abutment tooth and should be drilled to a depth of 2 to 2.5 mm. as parallel as possible to the long axis of the tooth. (In the lower incisors the pinholes should be no more than 1 mm. deep so as not to endanger the pulp.) Fig. 19-21 also shows the initial drilling.

All pilot or guide holes should be cleansed of any drilling residue before

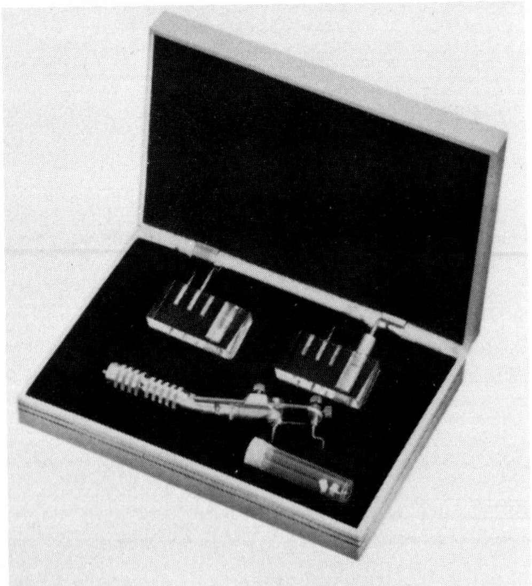

Fig. 19-20. Complete pinledge guide kit.

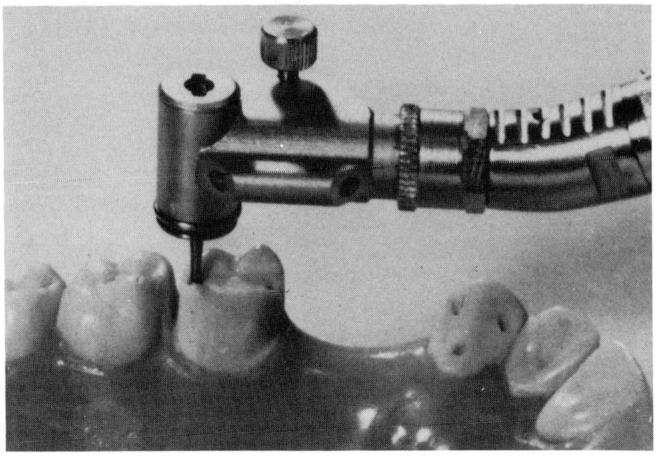

Fig. 19-21. Paralleling guide is removed from handpiece before drilling pilot pinhole or groove. This pinhole or groove is usually drilled freehand as nearly parallel to long axis of tooth as possible on disto-occlusal surface of most posterior abutment tooth.

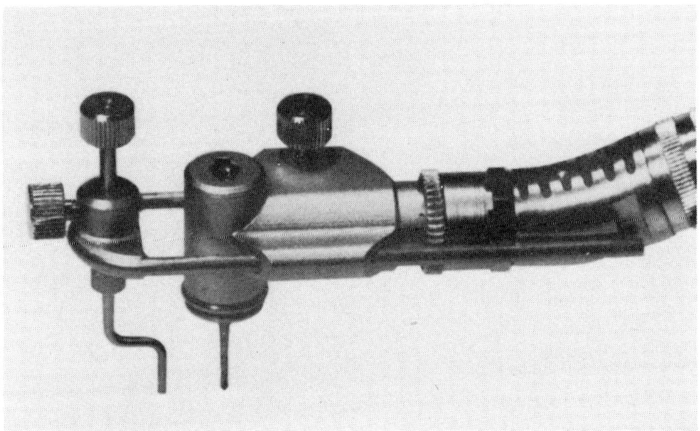

Fig. 19-22. Handpiece with paralleling guide and cutting bur in level position; pinholes on level positions of teeth can be filled with this setting.

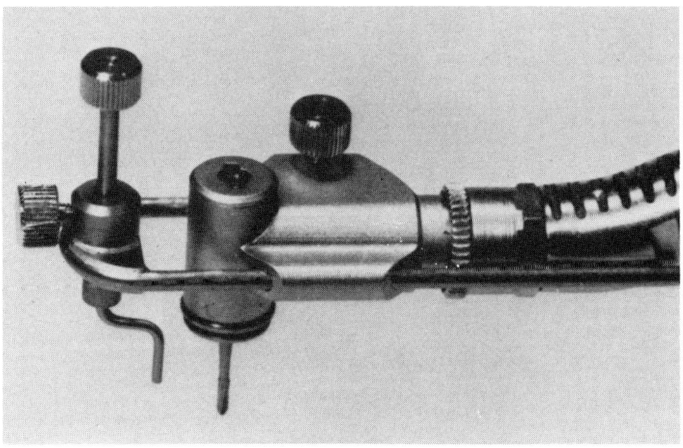

Fig. 19-23. Guide in raised position is placed in predrilled pinhole in incisal or middle third of tooth to drill pinhole in cingulum or gingival surface.

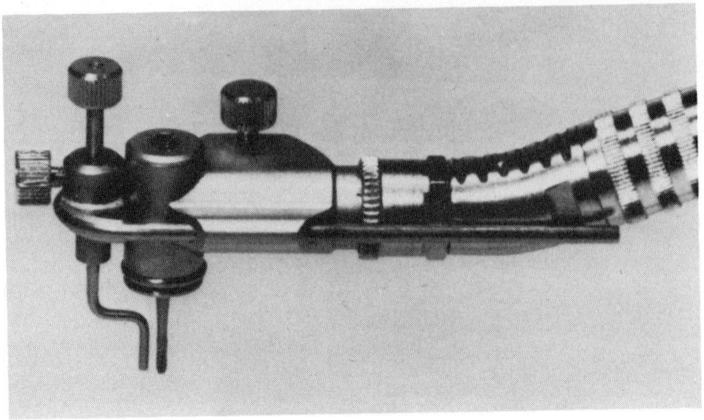

Fig. 19-24. Handpiece with guide in closed position. Short guidepin may be used for easier access in small mouths.

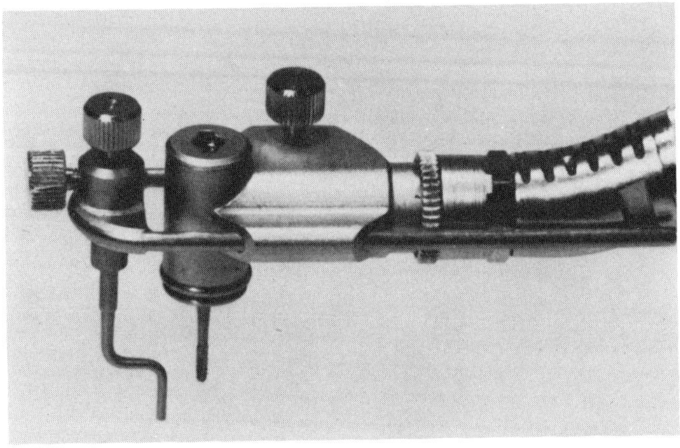

Fig. 19-25. Guidepin in lowered position can be placed in pilot pinhole or groove of molar or bicuspid to drill pinholes in incisal or middle third of anterior teeth.

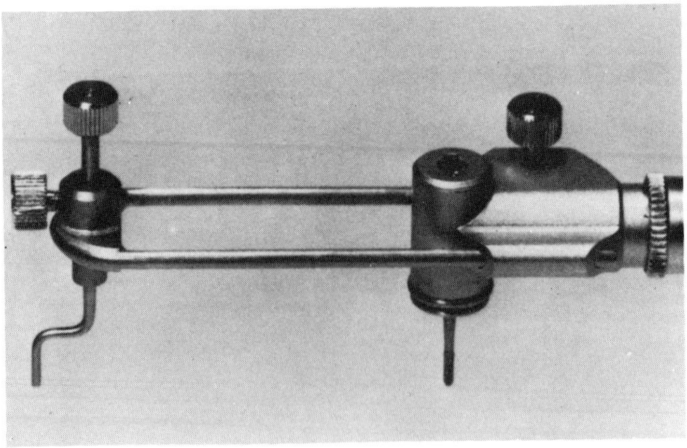

Fig. 19-26. Guide in extended position; used when parallel pinholes or grooves are made from one tooth to another.

placing the guide in them. To prevent binding of bur or guide, teeth should be kept wet at all times during operation, and the bur should be kept turning when withdrawing from the pinhole or groove being formed.

Replace the paralleling guide on the handpiece (Figs. 19-22 to 19-26) with the bur at the predetermined site of the next pinhole to be drilled, and set the guide at proper distance and level. Be sure knurled screws are tight before starting to drill. Place the tip of the guide at the lip of the pilot pinhole. Do not force the guide but let it slip into the pinhole as the bur is revolving (Fig. 19-27). Only gentle pressure should be used.

Use the same method in drilling the initial pinhole in an abutment tooth (Fig. 19-28). Since this pinhole will be parallel with the pilot pinhole, it may be used as a secondary pilot to form other pinholes in the same tooth or in other abutment teeth. Follow the same procedure, always setting the paralleling guide to the proper distance and level, until all pinholes are

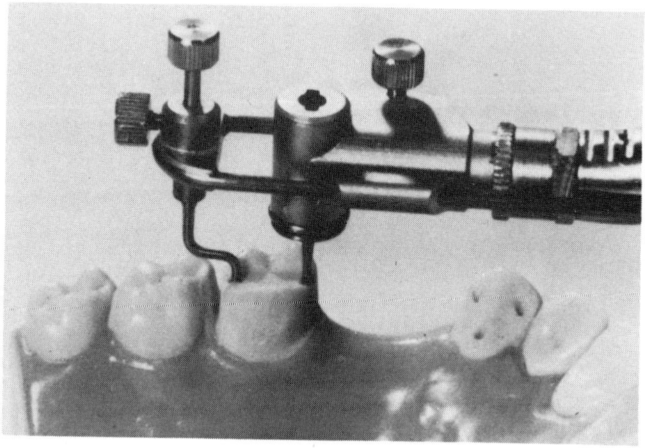

Fig. 19-27. Guide set at proper level and distance for second pinhole, at lip of pilot pinhole. Gentle pressure to revolving drill forms second pinhole to proper depth; guide should not be pushed forcibly into pilot pinhole.

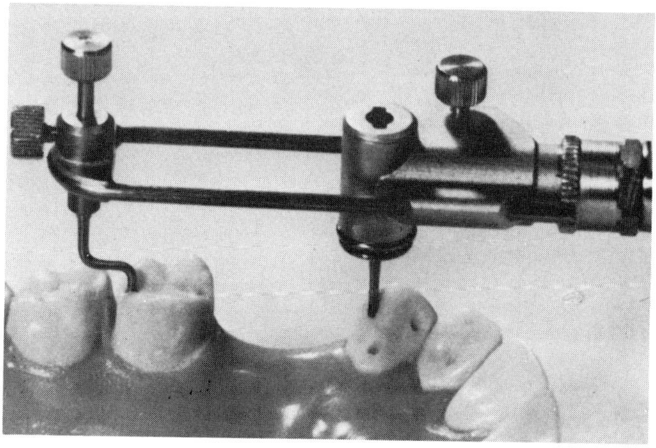

Fig. 19-28. Guide extended to proper distance and lowered into pilot pinhole to form pinhole in incisal third of cuspid tooth.

drilled to a proper depth (Figs. 19-29 to 19-31).

In pinledge work, ledges and pinholes can be made at different levels of teeth, such as from the incisal or middle third of a tooth to the gingival third, or vice versa. The paralleling guide of the handpiece is set as in Figs. 19-23 and 19-24, according to which is needed for a given operation. Pinholes may also be made at different levels from one abutment to another (Fig. 19-32).

Parallel grooves

Grooves for three-quarter crowns are formed in the same manner as parallel pinholes. In fact, if the operator prefers to use a pinhole rather than a groove as a pilot, he may follow the instructions for parallel pinholes with the intent of converting a properly placed pinhole to the desired groove after it is no longer needed as a pilot, or he may proceed as follows: the primary pilot (or first) groove is made freehand with the guide removed (Fig.

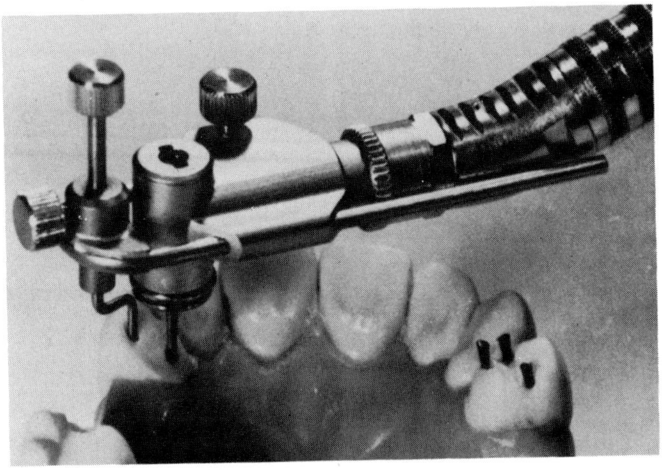

Fig. 19-29. Guide in raised position in pilot pinhole with bur forming pinhole in cingulum area of cuspid.

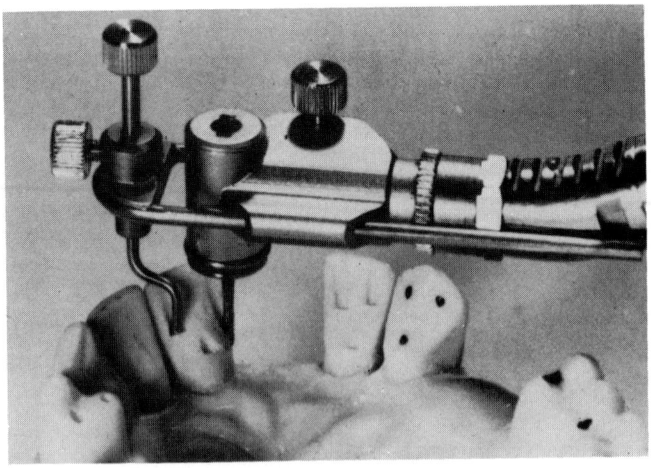

Fig. 19-30. Guide in raised position in pilot pinhole; bur forming groove in mesial surface of same tooth.

19-21) and should be made in the distal surface of the most posterior abutment tooth as near parallel with the long axis of the tooth as possible, and also to the depth of the dentinoenamel junction. Replace the guide and, with bur at predetermined site of next groove (on mesial surface of the same tooth), set guide at the proper distance. Place guide at occlusal edge of distal groove and gently press revolving bur to cut second groove in parallel. Using the mesial groove for the guide, as in Fig. 19-33, follow the same procedure in cutting parallel grooves in abutment teeth. After another parallel distal groove is made, it in turn can be used as a secondary pilot for forming other parallel grooves (Figs. 19-27 to 19-33).

The device can also be used for forming parallel pinholes for splinting teeth (Fig. 19-34).

THE NEY PARALLEL PIN TECHNIC

Another method extensively used was developed by Dr. Frank H. Nealon[11]; the

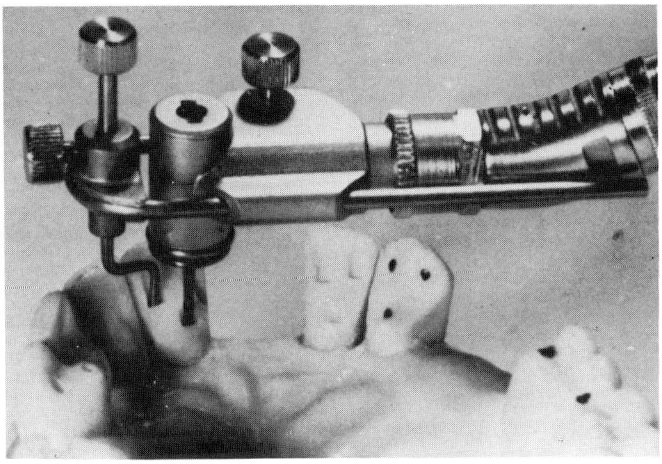

Fig. 19-31. Guide in raised position in predrilled pinhole in middle third of tooth in order to drill pinhole in cingulum or gingival third of tooth.

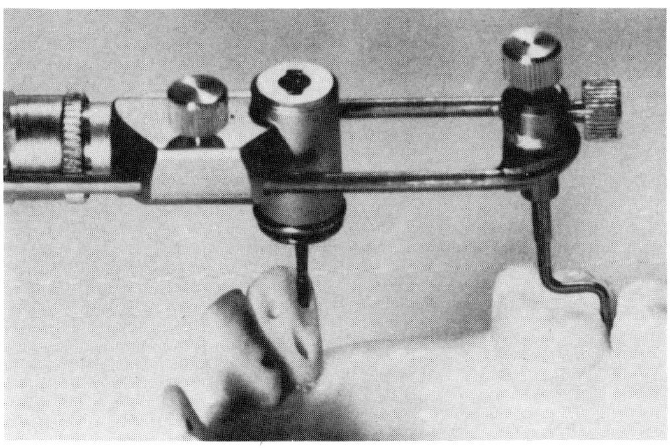

Fig. 19-32. Guide in lowered position in pilot pinhole or groove of molar or bicuspid to drill pinholes in incisal or middle third of anterior teeth at higher level.

equipment comes in the Ney Parallel Pin Kit. It has certain advantages in the precision drilling of parallel pinholes.

Operative procedure*

The abutment tooth or teeth are prepared. The design of the preparation should be such that a minimum of tooth structure is removed. Modification of the conventional three-quarter crown or the overlay-onlay type of preparation is generally used. After the preparation has been completed, a round carbide bur No. ¼ is used to indicate the starting point where the pinhole is to be drilled. A starting point is prepared for each pinhole that is planned. The pinholes are not drilled at this time.

At this point the operator will use his usual procedure for obtaining impressions for crown and bridgework. Any one of the elastic impression materials such as hydrocolloid, rubber base, or silicone may be used. Because the actual pinholes have not been drilled, the very difficult job of pinhole impressions is eliminated in the parallel pin technic.

*Courtesy Dr. F. H. Nealon and J. M. Ney Co., Hartford, Connecticut.

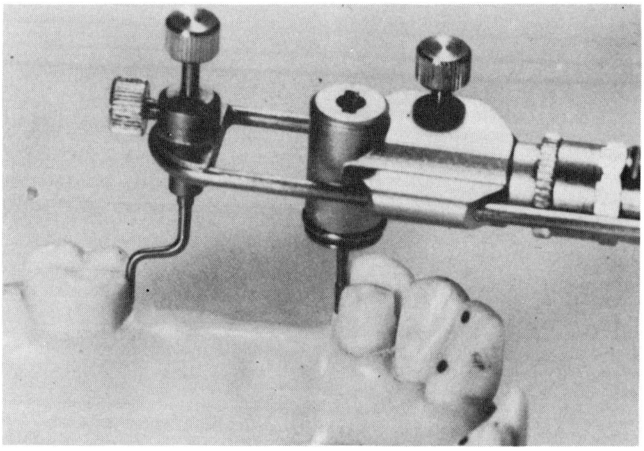

Fig. 19-33. Guide in level position in mesial groove of molar; bur forming distal groove in bicuspid.

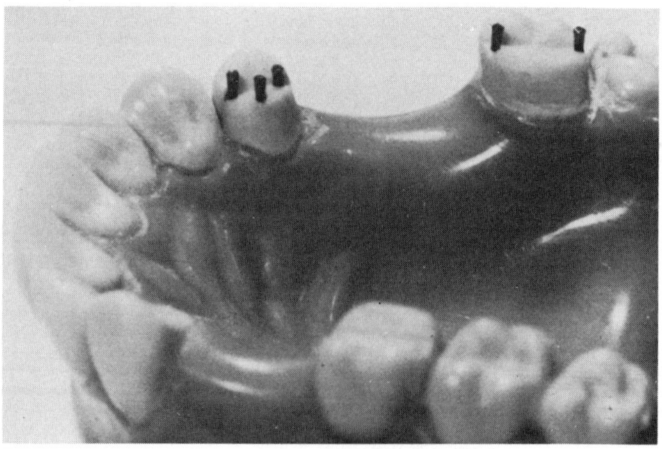

Fig. 19-34. Plastic pins placed in parallel pinholes to be cast in splint prosthesis.

A

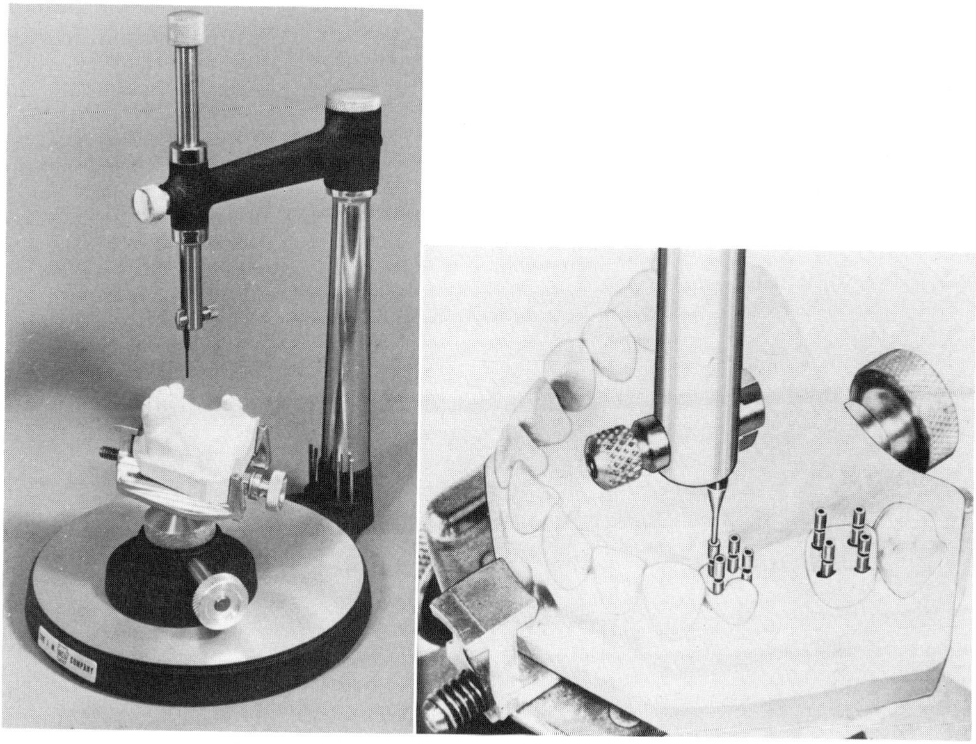

B

Fig. 19-35. A, Ney surveyor. **B,** Paralleling brushings and luting them to cast.

Bite registrations and opposing casts are prepared in the usual manner.

Accurate study casts should be mounted on the survey table of the Ney Surveyor (Fig. 19-35, *A*), and pin direction or path of insertion should be established. X-rays should be used to observe pulpal position so that pinhole positions will avoid involvement of the pulp (Fig. 19-35, *B*).

The factors that indicate the depth of pinholes are the number of pinholes used, proximity of pulp, the direction and position on the tooth, and the functional stress expected.

If short pins are indicated, then the number of pins used should be increased in order to assure good retention of the restoration. Pins should always be placed in dentin. If fillings are present, pins should be selected that will be long enough to pass the filling and reach sound dentin.

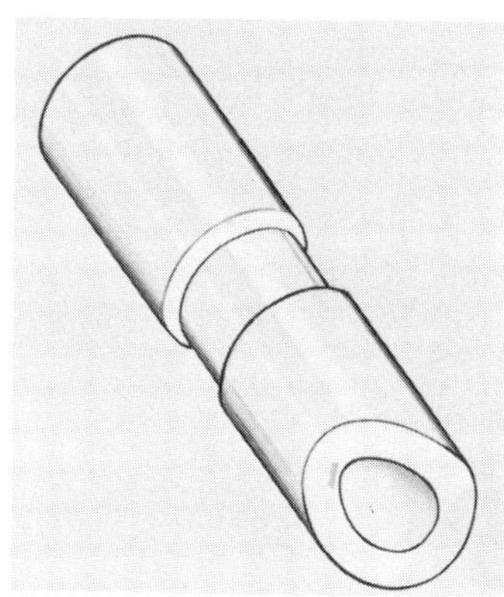

Fig. 19-36. Anterior brushing cut at angle before luting to cast.

When drilling holes in gold, use an oil lubricant.

Laboratory procedure

Make a duplicate model of the master working cast: lock this duplicate cast onto the survey table of the Ney Surveyor (Fig.

19-35, *A*). The need for a precise parallel relationship of the pins negates the use of a "swivel arm" surveyor. The surveyor must maintain a fixed and positive relationship between the paralleling mandrel and the cast.

The duplicate model is lubricated to prevent the self-curing plastic from adhering to the stone. A bushing of the proper length is placed on the mandrel and positioned over the starting point indicated on the die and then luted in

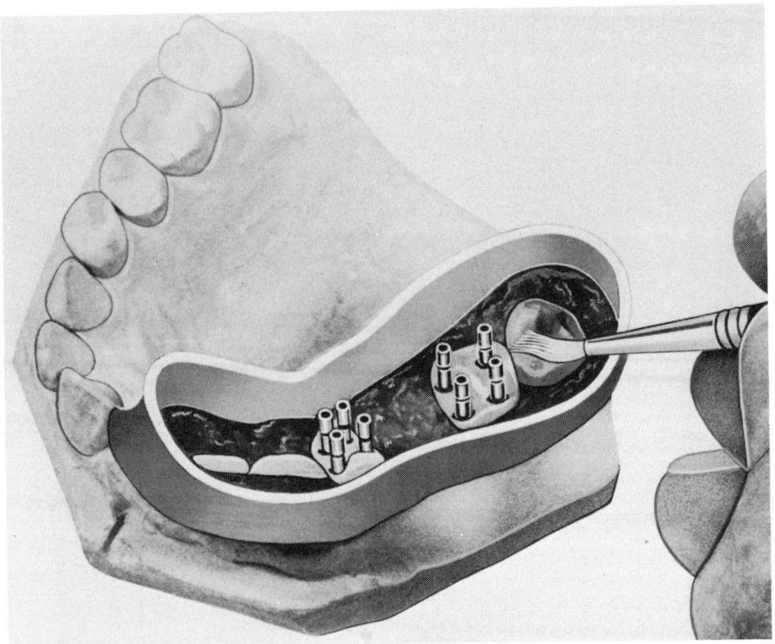

Fig. 19-37. Joining brushing by brush-on method to form acrylic resin matrix.

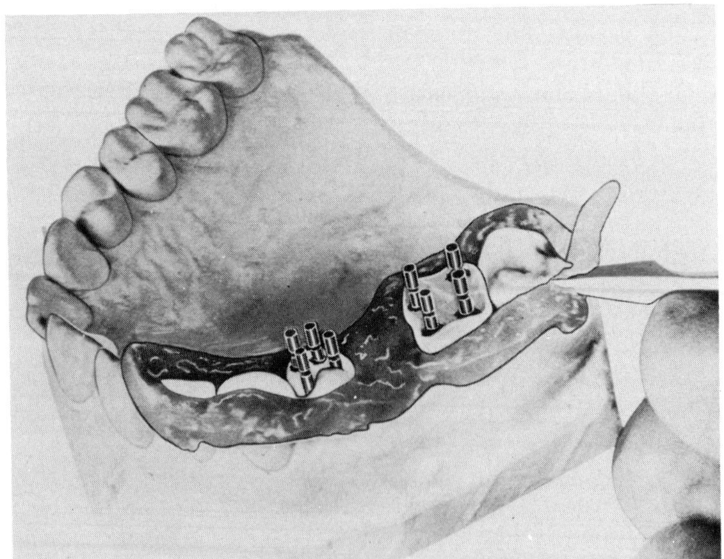

Fig. 19-38. Eliminating undercut areas prior to building up matrix base in resin.

place with a small amount of sticky wax (Fig. 19-35, *B*). Each bushing is then checked for parallel relationship. On anterior teeth, an angle cut should be made at the base of the bushing so that it can be positioned against the lingual surface. Do not alter the length of the bushing (Fig. 19-36).

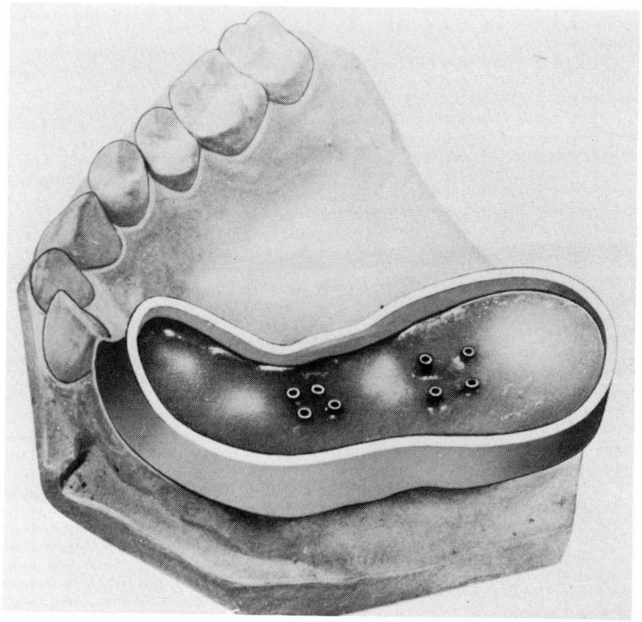

Fig. 19-39. Additional buildup of resin confined in matrix strip.

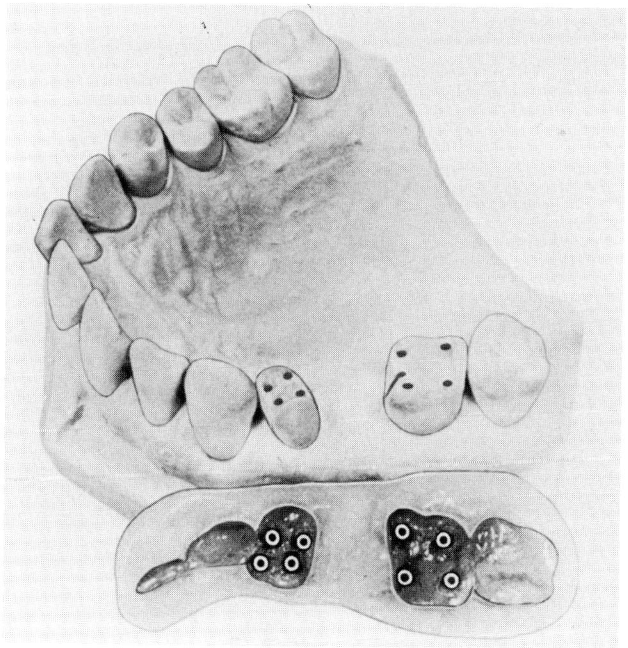

Fig. 19-40. Cured matrix with brushings locked in position removed from cast.

All bushings are joined together by constructing an index or matrix of self-curing acrylic. The brush-on method is recommended (Figs. 19-37 to 19-39). The matrix is extended to include one or more of the approximating teeth as well as at least three-fourths of the prepared surfaces of the teeth that are to contain pinholes. Be certain no undercuts are engaged (Fig. 19-38). When the acrylic matrix has cured (Fig. 19-39) it is removed from the duplicate cast (Fig. 19-40), trimmed of any excess, and placed on the master cast. Check for accuracy of fit (Fig. 19-41).

The P-T drill (Fig. 19-42) is inserted into one of the bushings, and the pinhole is drilled in the stone die by twisting the drill head by hand* (Fig. 19-43). Clean stone dust from drill periodically to prevent a buildup that could chip the die. Additional pinholes are drilled in the same manner.

After all pinholes have been drilled, the index and bushings are removed and the dies are again lubricated and P-T *pins* of the proper length are selected and

*Use handpiece for metal dies at slow speed.

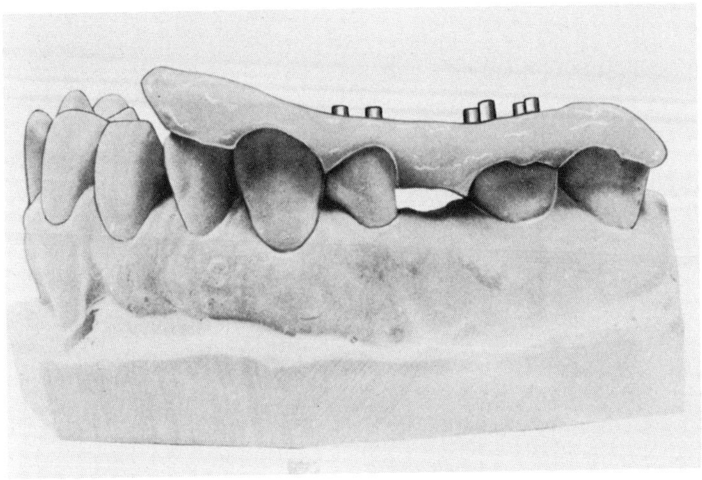

Fig. 19-41. Trimmed matrix with brushings, trimmed and tried on cast for fit.

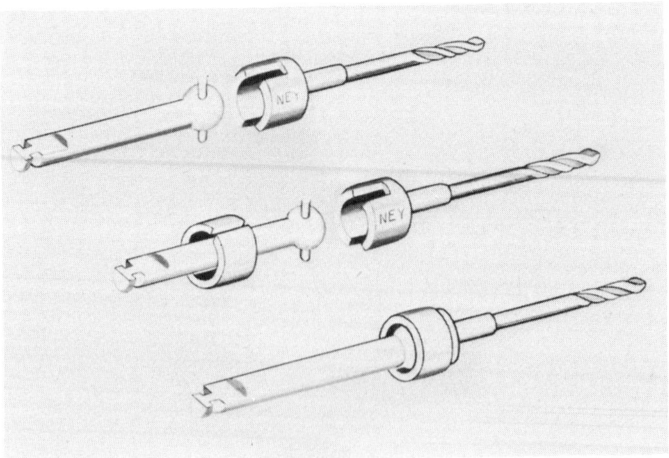

Fig. 19-42. Ney twist drills with drive assembly.

placed in the pinholes. The pins will extend a little above the pinholes. Self-curing acrylic is brushed on in a thin layer engaging the extended ends of the P-T pins. Care should be used in keeping the layer of acrylic away from the margins of the preparation. Before the acrylic completely hardens, the pattern should be lifted slightly from the die and reseated in position to make sure that all pins draw off easily. The margins and coronal form of the pattern may then be completed with a good inlay wax.

Patterns are carefully removed from the dies, sprued, invested, and cast, using the same technic as for conventional inlay and bridgework.

After the parallel pin castings have been made, they are carefully placed back on the dies. Castings should never be forced on the dies. There is a great advantage in using duplicate dies to check castings. When the castings have been placed on their respective dies and are found to fit satisfactorily, the bridgework is then completed, using the type of pontic prescribed.

Placement of the finished restoration

On completion of the bridgework and previous to trying it in, the bushing index is positioned on the teeth (Fig. 19-44). The Ney Parallel Pin Drive Assembly is used with a contra-angle handpiece to drill the pinholes in the prepared teeth. Drilling should always be done at ultra-low speed—300 to 500 rpm.

The drill bushing index will guide the P-T Twist Drill in its flexible drive assembly so that pinholes may be drilled in precise parallel relationship to the proper depth.

When all pinholes have been properly drilled, remove the index and countersink the hole using a No. 4 round bur; then the finished bridgework can be placed in position.

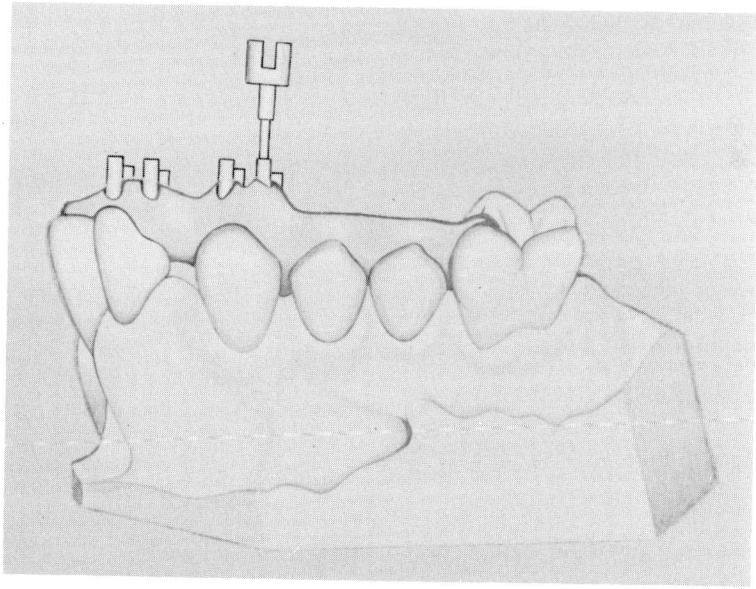

Fig. 19-43. Acrylic matrix with brushings on cast and pinhole drilled by hand in stone die in cast.

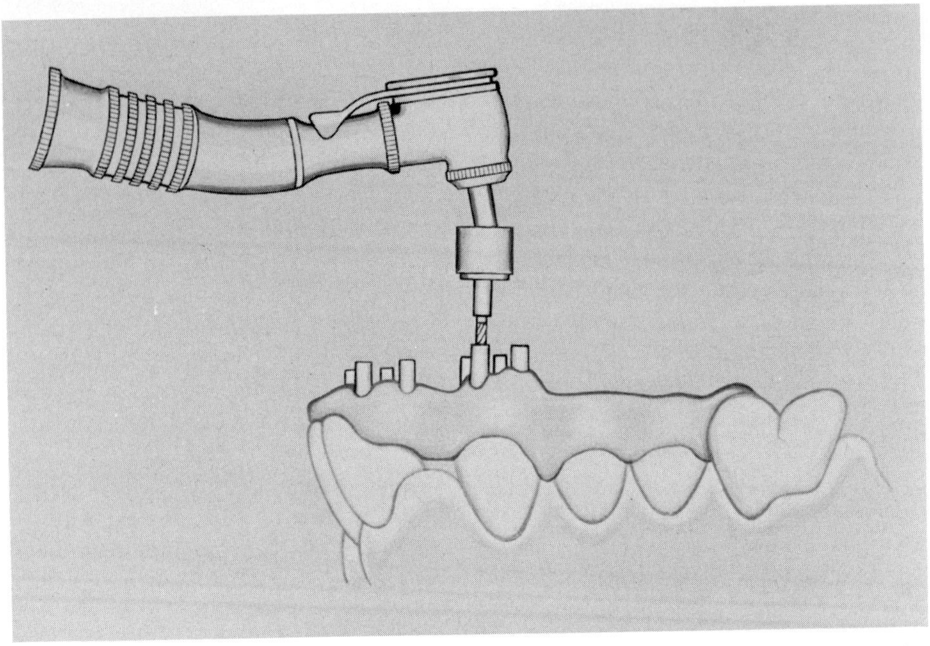

Fig. 19-44. Ney Pin Drive Assembly used with contra-angle handpiece to drill pinholes in prepared tooth.

SELECTED REFERENCES

1. Kabnick, H. H.: The "pinledge" as a cast bridge attachment, D. Items Interest **53**:376, 1931.
2. MacBoyle, R. E.: Crown and fixed bridgework, from the point of view of our present knowledge, J. Nat. D. A. **8**:635, 1921.
3. Burgess, J. K.: The preparation of abutments and construction of pinlay and pinledge attachments for bridge work, Pacific D. Gaz. **24**:559, 1916.
4. Gillett, H. W., and Irving, A. J.: Gold inlays by the indirect system, New York, 1932, Dental Items of Interest Publishing Co.
5. Doxtater, L. W.: Procedures in modern crown and bridgework, New York, 1931, Dental Items of Interest Publishing Co.
6. LeHuche, R.: Inlays and onlays, bridges on living teeth, Paris, 1951, Julien Prélat.
7. Iwanson, R.: The pinledge attachment and its use for fixed bridges, D. Items Int. **46**: 207, 1934.
8. Pruden, K. C.: A hydrocolloid technic for pinledge bridge abutments, J. Prosth. Dent. **6**:65, 1956.
9. Gamer, S., and Zusman, S.: Position finder for parallelism, J. Prosth. Dent. **65**:717, 1965.
10. Fridge, D. S.: Forming pin-ledge holes and paralleling grooves, Denver, 1966, Densco Mfg. Co.
11. Nealon, F. H.: A new approach to parallel pin restorations, Ney Technical Bulletin, 1964.

GENERAL REFERENCES

Alpert, C. C.: Anterior pin-ledge abutment, J. Dist. Columbia D. Soc. **34**:11, 1959.

Arbo, M. A.: A simple technic for castings with pin retention, Dent. Clin. N. Amer., pp. 19-29, 1970.

Baum, L., and Contino, R. M.: Ten years of experience with cast pin restorations, Dent. Clin. N. Amer., pp. 18-41, 1970.

Beck, P. B.: Parallel pins in fixed prosthodontics, J. S. California Dent. Hyg. Ass. **34**:237-240, 1966.

Burns, B. B.: Pin retention of cast gold restorations, J. Prosth. Dent. **15**:1101-1108, 1965.

Courtade, G. L.: The use of pins in restorative dentistry, part II: paralleling instruments, J. Prosth. Dent. **15**:691, 1965.

Courtade, G. L.: Pin pointers, III: self-threading pins, J. Prosth. Dent. **20**:335, 1968.

Courtade, G. L.: Methods for pin splinting the lower anterior teeth, Dent. Clin. N. Amer., pp. 3-17, 1970.

Courtade, G. L., Sanell, C., and Mann, A. W.: The use of pins in restorative dentistry, part I: parallel pin retention obtained without using paralleling devices; part II: paralleling instruments, J. Prosth. Dent. **15**:502-516, 691-703, 1965.

El-Brashi, M. K., Craig, R. G., and Peyton, F. A.: Experimental stress analysis of dental restorations, part V, the concept of occlusal reduction and pins, J. Prosth. Dent. **22**:565-577, 1969.

Fusayama, T., and others: A one-piece cast permanent splint, J. Prosth. Dent. **16**:572-582, 1966.

Gamer, S., and others: Position finder: an improved design for paralleling preparations, J. S. California Dent. Ass. **33**:566-567, 1965.

Karlstrom, G.: Parallel pins and fixed partial dentures, J. Prosth. Dent. **19**:615, 1968.

Lamb, R. T.: Varied applications of direct pin inlays, J. Canadian D. A. **22**:282, 1956.

Lehuche, R.: Molded key inlay lock for bridges, Rev. Stomatol. **41**:533, 1939.

Lorey, R. E., Embrell, K. A., and Myers, G. E.: Retentive factors in pin-retained castings, J. Prosth. Dent. **17**(3):271, 1967.

Manes, R. J.: Pinledges as bridge anchorages, pins and inlays combined, D. Abst. **2**:81, 1957.

Mann, A. W., Courtade, G. L., and Sanell, C.: The use of pins in restorative dentistry, part 1: parallel pin retention obtained without using paralleling devices, J. Prosth. Dent. **15**:502-516, 1965.

Mittleman, G.: Use of pins in difficult cases, J.A.D.A. **49**:163, 1954.

Moffa, J. P., and Phillips, R. W.: Retentive properties of parallel pin restorations, J. Prosth. Dent. **17**:387-400, 1967.

Moffa, J. P., Razzano, M. R., and Doyle, M. G.: Pins—a comparison of their retentive properties, J.A.D.A. **78**:529-535, 1969.

Mollersten, L.: An impression technique for teeth prepared for parallel pins, J. Prosth. Dent. **18**:579, 1967.

Mosteller, J. H.: Parallel pin gold castings, P. D. M. Nove., 1963.

Mosteller, J. H.: Pin castings by a paralleling device and hydrocolloid technique, Dent. Clin. N. Amer., pp. 53-61, 1970.

Nealon, F. H., and Sheakley, H. G.: An extraoral pin technique, J. Prosth. Dent. **22**:638-646, 1969,

Overby, G. E.: Esthetic splinting of mobile periodontally involved teeth by vertical pinning, J. Prosth. Dent. **11**:112-118, 1961.

Parmlid, A.: A new intraoral parallelometer, J. Prosth. Dent. **18**:469-475, 1967.

Rosen, H.: The incisal insertion pin inlay, J. Prosth. Dent. **19**:263, 1968.

Sanell, C.: Vertical parallel pins in occlusal rehabilitation, Dent. Clin. N. Amer. pp. 755-778, 1963.

Sanell, C., Mann, A. W., and Courtade, G. L.: The use of pins in restorative dentistry, part III: the use of paralleling instruments, J. Prosth. Dent. **16**:286-296, 1966.

Shooshan, E. D.: A pinledge casting technique—its application in periodontal splinting, Dent. Clin. N. Amer., pp. 189-206, March, 1960.

Smith, C. L.: Prefabricated parallel pin castings, Dent. Clin. N. Amer., pp. 31-41, 1970.

Sobel, S. L.: A technique for using parallel pins, J. Prosth. Dent. **20**:526, 1968.

Steen, P. M.: Positive pin retention for bridge work and inlays, D. Survey **30**:757, 1954.

Timmermans, J. J., and Courtade, G. L.: Nonparallel threaded pin retention of fixed prosthesis, J. Prosth. Dent. **19**(4):381-392, 1968.

Wagner, A. W.: Pin retention for extensive posterior gold onlays, J. Prosth. Dent. **15**:719-721, 1965.

Willmott, J. T.: Pin retention for indirect inlays utilizing rubber-base impression material, Brit. D. J. **102**:359, 1957.

Chapter 20

Construction of retainers: direct method—materials, equipment, and procedures

HISTORY OF DENTAL CASTING

At the Quinquennial Dental Congress held in London in 1952, Hollenback[1] gave the following brief history of the cast dental restorations:

It is probably true that cast dental restorations were made prior to 1907 by a number of individuals. It is also true that none of these early users of the art of casting had any conception of its great value and the profound effects it would have on all phases of dental restorative procedures.

The first detailed description of a technic for making cast inlays was given by Taggart (1907), who fully appreciated the value of the procedure. He also displayed great wisdom in that he did not divulge his process until he had developed the technic to the point that it was quite easily possible to make cast restorations which compared favourably with the standard of dental practice of that time. Dr. Taggart knew that the metal used in a cast restoration had a certain definite shrinkage after solidification in the mould and the subsequent cooling to room temperature. However, he erroneously assumed that by maintaining the pressure for a minute or two after the mould was filled, that the shrinkage would be prevented.

Those who used the Taggart technic were soon aware of the fact that all restorations cast by this method were appreciably smaller than the wax pattern. Lane (1908), becoming convinced of this fact, attempted to overcome its effect by casting into a red-hot mould, using an expanding investment material. He assumed correctly that in this super-heated state, the mould would be appreciably enlarged and the casting, therefore, being more nearly dimensionally correct than if cast in a mould, would be the exact size of the wax pattern. Van Horn (1910), having arrived at a conclusion similar to that of Lane, and by careful testing having ascertained that none of the investment materials available at that time had a thermal coefficient sufficiently high to compensate for the shrinkage of the metal, developed a technic in which the wax pattern was heated several degrees above mouth temperature, and kept in this heated, and therefore expanded, condition during the entire procedure of investing and until the investment had become thoroughly set. He then heated the investment to a cherry red heat, which no doubt gave the maximum expansion of which it was capable. The thermal expansion of the wax, when added to the expansion of the investment, permitted the making of castings which were quite accurate.

These early investigators were not entirely scientific in their procedures in that, firstly, they had not evaluated the casting shrinkage of the metal used, and secondly, had not evaluated the physical properties of the materials used in forming the mould; that is, the pattern wax and the investment materials. Price (1911) made the first attempt to evaluate the shrinkage of gold. His results, however, do not coincide closely with those of recent investigators, probably owing to the complicated apparatus used and to a somewhat incorrect understanding of the problem. Shell (1923) attempted to evaluate the casting shrinkage of gold by making wax patterns in a metallic die of known dimension. He did not contend that his results were more than relatively correct since too many uncontrolled variables entered into the procedure. Shell's work tended to indicate that linear shrinkage of gold is considerably in excess of 1.25 per cent.

Coleman (1928) carried out an extensive research on the problem of the dimensional changes occurring during the casting of gold and gold alloys. This was the first time that the problem was undertaken in a scientific manner. The linear casting shrinkage of the metal was first determined. The physical properties of pattern wax and investment were ascertained. Particular attention was paid to the thermal coefficient of expansion of these materials. Coleman then used the method of Van Horn, first forming a mould around the heated and expanded wax pattern, then heating the mould to produce its maximum expansion. For instance, assuming the figure of 1.25 per cent was the linear casting shrinkage of the metal used and the thermal coefficient of the investment used was 0.8 per cent, it was then only necessary to expand the wax pattern 0.45 per cent to produce a completely compensated mould.

Later, Coleman concluded that the thermal expansion of the pattern was not a safe procedure in that it was liable to be distorted in this process. He then replaced the silica content of the investment with cristobalite, the thermal coefficient of expansion of cristobalite alone being sufficient to produce adequate compensation.

Maves (1932) carried out an investigation which clearly showed that raising the temperature of a wax pattern only a few degrees above that of the mouth invariably caused distortion.

Wax expansion as a means of compensation was used extensively in the latter twenties, but did not prove satisfactory and has now been almost completely discarded.

Scheu (1932) developed an entirely new method of compensation in which the hygroscopic expansion of the investment was used for enlarging the mould. A small amount of thermal expansion occurred with Scheu's technic. This however was only incidental as hygroscopic expansion alone can be sufficient in amount to produce a compensated mould. Scheu also carried out an investigation in which he determined that there is considerable difference in the casting shrinkage of different alloys of gold. He determined the linear shrinkage of pure gold to be 1.6 per cent.

Hollenback and Skinner (1946) carried out a very extensive investigation on the linear shrinkage of gold and its alloys. This work was done under very carefully controlled conditions, the temperature, and therefore, the dimension of the mould being under complete control during the entire casting procedure. The specimens used were 1 inch in length, measurements being made to an accuracy of 0.0001 inch or 0.01 per cent. In this investigation, the linear casting shrinkage of pure gold was determined as 1.65 per cent; 22 K 'dark' plate 1.50 per cent; Type A soft inlay 1.56 per cent; Type B medium inlay 1.37 per cent; Type C hard inlay 1.42 per cent. This investigation shows there is a wide difference between the linear casting shrinkage of gold and its alloys, the composition of gold alloys undoubtedly having a very marked effect on their linear shrinkage.* [See General References.]

Two methods may be employed in the construction of cast retainers: (1) the direct and (2) the indirect.

The objective of both methods is to obtain a wax pattern of the retainer that (1) is accurately adapted to the prepared abutment; (2) reproduces the correct tooth contour; (3) establishes the correct relationships between the adjacent teeth and the opposing arch; and (4) reproduces the wax pattern in a suitable cast metal alloy so that it is an exact dimensional reproduction.

FABRICATION OF DIRECT RETAINERS—THE DIRECT METHOD

To obtain a wax pattern by the direct method, the wax is adapted directly to the prepared tooth. There is less possibility of mishaps and misfits if several intermediary steps and procedures are eliminated. In those instances in which the preparation involves three or more surfaces; in which it is complicated, in which several teeth are to be prepared and restored in one quadrant of the mouth, in which the access to the tooth is difficult, or in which fixed or removable partial dentures are to be made, the indirect method is employed.

Need for matrix

To bring wax into contact with all the walls and angles of a preparation, it must be confined and surrounded by axial walls.

*From Hollenback, G. M.: The cast gold inlay, Int. Dent. J. 1:67, 1951.

If one or more of these walls is missing in the tooth, they are replaced temporarily with a metal matrix. This matrix helps to confine and conform the wax to the cavity walls.

The metal matrix. Usually, 36- or 40-gauge steel or copper matrix material is used. Because of its workability and ease of adaptation, copper is sometimes used; however, steel is stronger and may be used in thinner gauges.

A matrix formed to the shape of a band may be made for each individual tooth from a strip of metal matrix material, or manufactured bands of various sizes and gauges may be had for this purpose.

If a manufactured band is used, a wire measurement is first taken of the abutment around its greatest circumference. The band must be long enough so that it will extend from the gingival limits of the preparation to a point 3 or 4 mm. beyond the highest part of the occlusal surface. Before adapting the metal band to the tooth, it is well to decide upon the direction to be followed when seating the metal matrix to place; this usually parallels the axis of the preparation.

Fig. 20-1 shows the approximate outline forms of the various teeth at the cervical planes in the upper and lower arches. Having the general outline of the tooth in mind, the metal matrix is shaped approximately to this contour.

In conforming the metal band to the prepared tooth gingivally, care must be taken not to fit it too closely around the tooth cervix. There should be 0.2 to 0.3 mm. clearance around the gingival circumference of the band.

Next, the gingival periphery of the band is trimmed so that it parallels the curvature of the gingival crest next to the preparation. Great care must be exercised during this procedure not to lacerate the gingival tissues nor to cause detachment of the epithelial attachment. If a properly fitted gum retractor has previously been used, or if the rubber dam and clamp are still in place, the gum tissue is pushed back sufficiently to enable the operator to fit the metal band accurately, quickly, and with no injury to the soft tissues.

If the rubber dam is not used, then in the initial trial of the band on the tooth, no effort should be made to depress the band margin below the crest of the gum tissue; instead, it should be brought only to the plane where it touches the highest curvature of the gingiva, which usually occurs in the interproximal regions (Fig. 24-19). A measurement is then made of

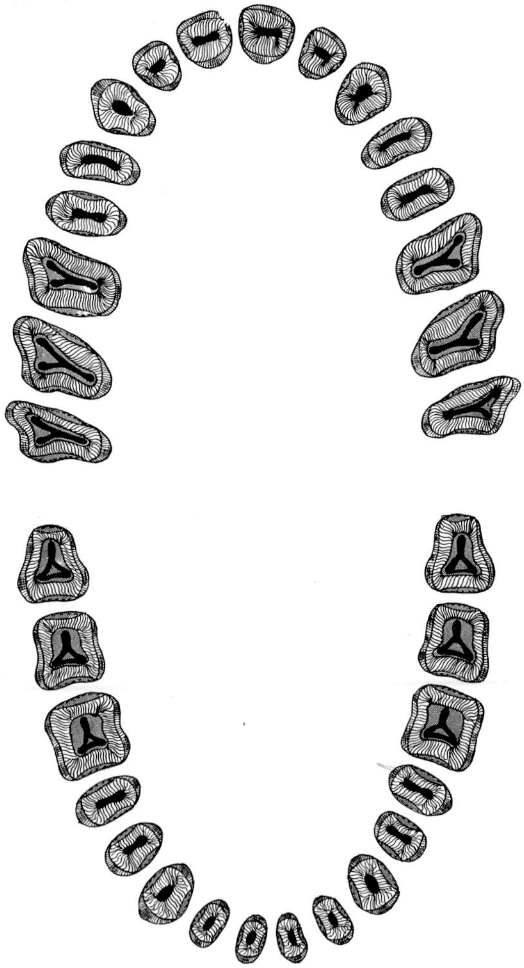

Fig. 20-1. Approximate outline of various teeth at their cervical planes.

the distance between the gingival margin of the band and the highest point of the tissue curvature on the labial and lingual surfaces. A curved line on the proximal sides of the band is then marked this same distance from the margin of the band, the line being parallel to the labiolingual curvature of the interproximal gum tissue. The band is removed and that portion lying within the curved line is cut out with curved shears and the edge is polished with a disk.

When replaced on the tooth, the gingival outline of the band should parallel the contour of the gingival tissues, encompassing the preparation on all sides.

If the matrix just described is to be used for an upper molar three-quarter partial veneer retainer, a rectangular piece at the gingival is cut way from the buccal part of the band, since it is not necessary to confine wax in this area (Fig. 20-2). When this segment of the matrix is removed, provision is made so that the proximal edges of the band next to the buccal opening extend buccally beyond the buccal margins of the proximal grooves. Unless this precaution is taken, the wax may not be carried against the buccal margins of the preparation.

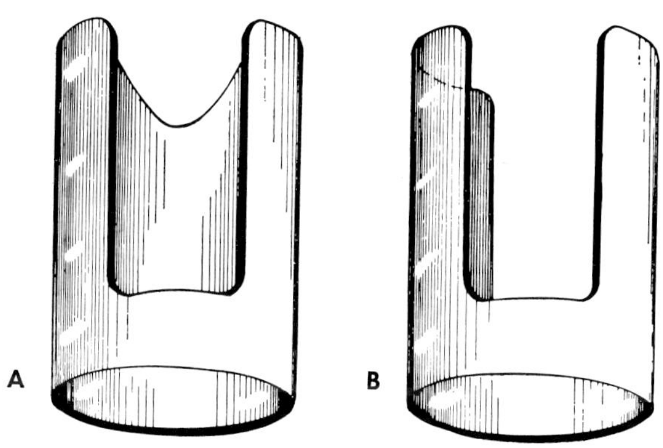

Fig. 20-2. Copper bands cut out for partial veneer and intracoronal tooth preparations.

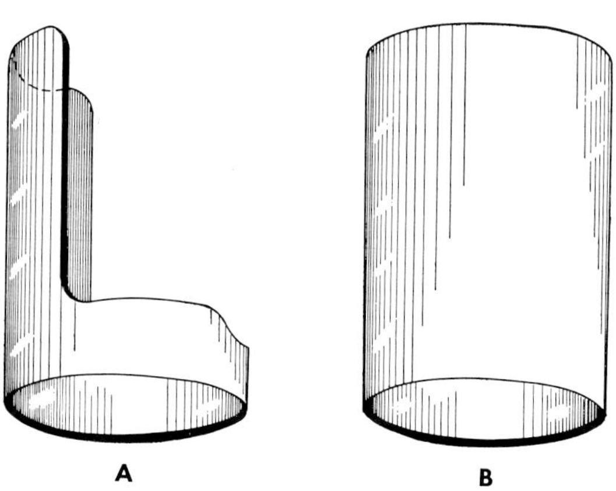

Fig. 20-3. A, Copper band for two-surface preparation. **B,** Seamless copper band used for complete crown preparations.

Where the matrix is to be used for a three-surface intracoronal retainer, another piece is removed from the lingual in addition to that cut from the buccal. In this type of preparation the matrix is required to confine the wax only to the two proximal and the occlusal surfaces (Fig. 20-2, *B*); if a two-surface retainer is involved, the band is cut as shown in Fig. 20-3, *A*.

The band is replaced on the tooth and its occlusal edge is trimmed to a height that will permit the opposing teeth to come into occlusion without striking the band. When this has been accomplished, the copper band matrix is ready to receive the softened inlay wax for making the wax pattern directly in the mouth.

In addition to the manufactured, seamless copper bands (Fig. 20-3, *B*), matrices may also be custom made for each tooth. These handmade metal bands are usually constructed of 36-gauge copper or stainless steel plate and may be either soldered or riveted to form a band.

To construct the soldered type, a wire measurement is taken as previously described and the height of the band is determined. A piece of copper matrix material is cut to the proper length and width and shaped to form a cylinder, and the two ends are soldered by means of low-fusing silver solder. From this point, the procedure is identical with that for the seamless manufactured copper band previously described.

The riveted metal band, as described by Smith and Potter,[2] is simple and inexpensive to construct; it has certain advantages which neither the seamless nor the soldered band possesses (Fig. 20-4).

The first step in constructing a riveted band matrix is to obtain the wire measurement. In determining the circumference of the metal strip for the band, a surplus of 3 to 4 mm. is allowed so that one end of the band will overlap the other by this amount. The pointed end of a No. 141 S. S. White riveting plier is now placed on the inside of the band at the overlap so that, when pressure is applied to the plier, the point pierces the two thicknesses of matrix material. This raises three or four little flanges or lips on the buccal surface of the band. By reversing the pliers and placing the point into the opening through the buccal surface of the band, the little flanges of matrix material on the buccal surface are swaged tightly against the band, uniting rigidly the two thicknesses of band material. If necessary, two such rivets may be made, one toward the occlusal, the other toward the gingival margin of the band.

From this point on, the band is adapted to the tooth and fitted to the tissues as previously described.

The advantage of the riveted type of matrix over the seamless or the soldered type lies in the fact that, after the wax within the matrix has been forced into the cavity and the occlusal relationships have been established, the riveted matrix may be readily removed merely by placing a small, flat instrument between the laps of the band; this readily forces the flanges of the rivet open and loosens the matrix for removal. To remove the seamless or the soldered types of band after the wax has been adapted to the tooth it is first necessary to cut through that portion of the matrix which lies on the buccal surface or else to make a preliminary cut extending part way through the buccal portion of the band before the matrix and wax are carried to the prepared tooth.

A third type of matrix that can be used is the adjustable type (Fig. 20-5) (Siqueland). The band material, either copper or steel, comes in strips of various widths. These are inserted into an adjustable matrix

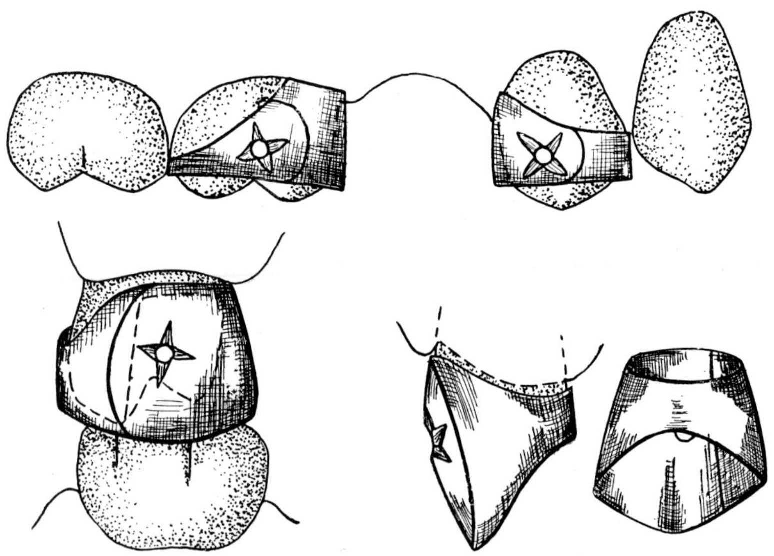

Fig. 20-4. Various types of riveted copper or steel bands made for individual teeth. (After Smith and Potter.)

holder, which permits enlarging or reducing the circumference of the matrix by a simple screw device. The matrix is first fitted snugly to the preparation, then loosened slightly before removal from the tooth, to be filled with the softened inlay wax. The advantage of this type of matrix, which is the one generally used, is that (1) it is quick and simple to fit, and (2) after the wax pattern has been adapted, the matrix is easily loosened and removed without danger of distorting the wax pattern.

It is presumed that sufficient separation of the teeth exists to allow the free passage of the metal matrix around the entire circumference of the tooth. Separation is usually made for those teeth that are to receive a three-surface intracoronal retainer or a partial veneer type that involves the two proximal surfaces. Where the proximal

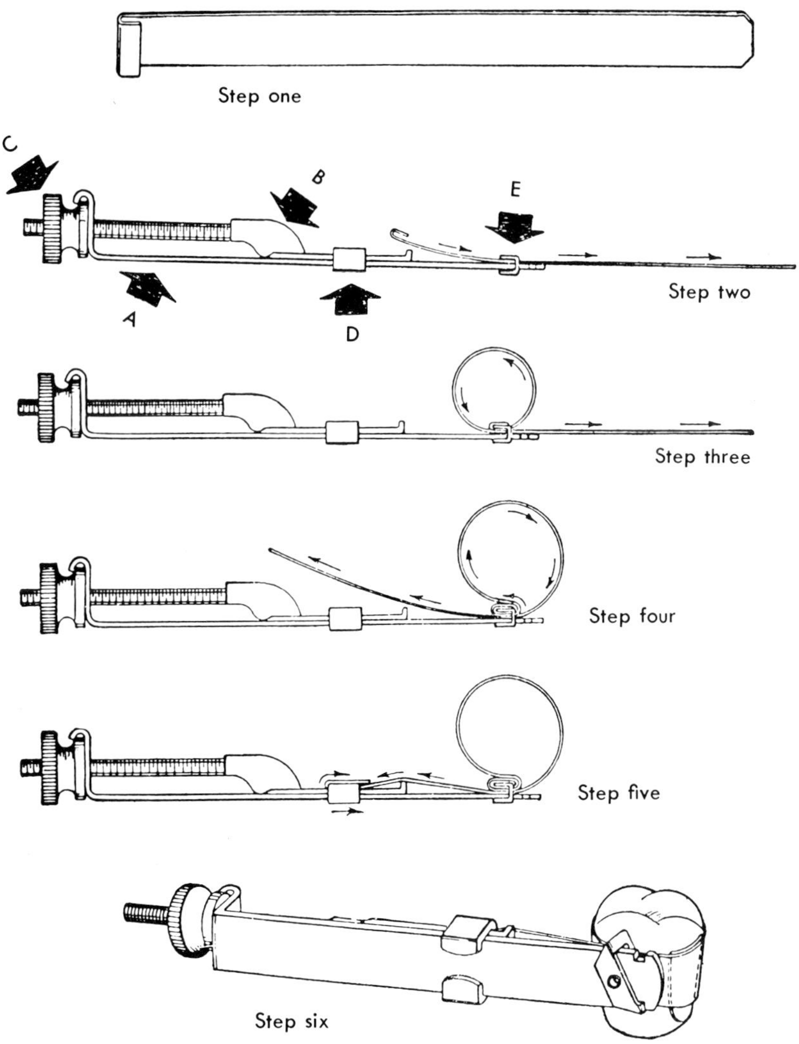

Fig. 20-5. Siqueland adjustable matrix.

part of a two-surface intracoronal retainer is contiguous to an edentulous space and the other proximal surface is in contact with its adjacent tooth, that part of the band touching the contact point is trimmed away, so that its gingival margin lies occlusally from the contact point; this ordinarily leaves a band in this area not more than 1 to 2 mm. wide (Fig. 20-4).

It is recommended that the rivet be placed on the labial or buccal aspects of the band and the overlap face toward the mesial surface; this arrangement facilitates access to the lap and to the rivets.

After the matrix has been fitted, it is carefully examined so that no rough or sharp edges are left at the gingival periphery to lacerate the soft tissues and so that a sufficient clearance exists between the inner surfaces of the band and the prepared tooth. The inside of the band is then lubricated lightly with a thin oil prior to being filled with softened inlay wax.

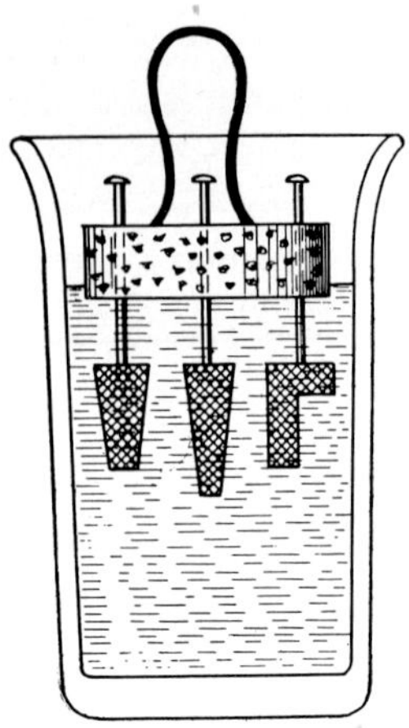

Fig. 20-6. Wax placed in water bath for 10 minutes at correct temperature will bring it to its proper working condition.

Manipulation of inlay wax

The manipulation of inlay wax is the next step in obtaining an accurate wax pattern of the retainer. This is an important procedure and one fraught with innumerable pitfalls. No attempt is made here to discuss in detail the chemical components and manufacture of inlay wax, since available texts dealing with dental materials[3, 4] cover this subject adequately; yet an effort will be made to point out those physical factors and manipulative procedures of immediate concern in daily practice.

Wax has a definite thermal response to temperature changes. A combination of different kinds of waxes formulated for a specific use but undergoing different temperature changes at various stages of its manipulation presents problems of controlling its thermal expansion, contraction, flow, elasticity, plasticity, and ductility.

Recognizing the requirements of inlay waxes used in dentistry, the American Dental Association Research Commission of the National Bureau of Standards has formulated Specification No. 4 for dental inlay waxes, Type I to be used for the direct wax pattern method, and Type II wax to be used in the indirect method of forming a wax pattern.

The standard inlay waxes may be used, provided they meet the requirements and specifications for this material as determined by the American Dental Association Research Commission of the National Bureau of Standards:

(1) The color shall be such as to facilitate the carving of patterns to contrast with the hard and soft tissues of the mouth; (2) the materials shall soften without becoming flaky; (3) the materials shall trim to a fine margin without appreciable chipping or flaking; (4) the materials shall be capable of being melted and vaporized without leaving solid residues other than carbon.

Since it is necessary to soften inlay wax to a consistency that will enable its being adapted accurately to the walls and angles of the preparation, the method used in softening wax is an important item. Wax may be softened by dry heat over a Bunsen burner or in an electric heating chamber; likewise, it may be brought to a workable consistency by submerging it for a few minutes only in water heated to 120 to 125° F. While the open flame may give satisfactory results, there is danger of volatilizing some of the ingredients of the wax if it is overheated, thus changing its physical properties. A preferable method is one where the wax is held at a constant temperature of 120 to 125° F. for a slightly longer time, thus ensuring that the entire mass is thoroughly plastic and workable. A warm water bath is simple and most efficient for this purpose. A simple device for quickly warming the wax to the desired temperature (104 to 113° F.) may be made by piercing a layer of cork with pins and allowing the pointed ends of the pins to extend about ¼ inch beyond the surface of the cork. Cones of inlay wax are then stuck to the pin points, after which the cork and wax cones are turned over face down and kept submerged for 10 minutes in a container of water of the proper temperature (Fig. 20-6). Wax warmed in this manner is thoroughly softened and of the proper degree of plasticity for immediate use. It should not, however, be kept submerged in warm water longer than 10 minutes.

Those waxes that require a temperature higher than 125° F. to make them workable should not be used; neither should those whose percentage of flow at mouth temperature exceeds 1 percent. Good inlay waxes are those that may be carved and removed from the tooth at mouth temperature without distortion. At no time should a wax pattern be chilled with ice water while it is in the tooth because: first, the excess stresses set up in the wax; and second, it has been demonstrated that, even if chilled, the wax pattern quickly returns to mouth temperature before it is removed from the tooth.

Once the wax pattern has been made and removed from the tooth, it should be invested immediately. Wax patterns allowed to lie around for a considerable length of time before being invested are likely to distort because of the reaction of wax to the slightest temperature changes and because of the continued release of stresses within the wax pattern with the lapse of time.

Phillips and Biggs[5] have demonstrated that all wax patterns, regardless of how they are manipulated, contain a certain degree of internal stresses. These are induced by (1) the contraction of the wax upon cooling from 120 to 125° F. to tooth temperature; (2) by altering the form of the wax by pressure; and (3) by the usual custom of adding molten wax to correct margins and contour.

Most patterns that are not invested immediately upon their removal from the cavity show harmful distortion after 30 minutes. The longer the pattern is allowed to stand at room temperature, the greater will be the amount of distortion taking place. This will be more so if the room temperature is high. This distortion is due to the release of the internal stresses. If permitted to stand for a sufficiently long time, most of the stresses will be released and the pattern will be ruined, so far as accuracy of fit is concerned.

If patterns must be left to the end of the day before investing, then provision should be made to maintain the patterns at a low temperature. If kept at 36° F., the distortion, even after several hours, is negligible. It has been observed that when wax is manipulated at a higher temperature, say 125° F., less internal stress is evident and a smaller degree of distortion takes place in a stored pattern. For the same reason, once the wax pattern has been formed, no hot instruments should be applied to it; neither should additions of wax be made to the finished wax pattern in any considerable amounts. If done, internal stresses result which, when released, cause a distorted pattern and casting.

Use of lubricant

Usually it is not necessary to treat the prepared tooth prior to making the wax pattern, saliva being a sufficient lubricant to prevent adhesion between the wax and smooth walls of a preparation. Where a lubricant is desired, the cavity walls are wiped with a semidry pellet of cotton and light lubricant. This is then followed by thoroughly wiping the walls with a dry pellet before the wax is applied. After the wax pattern has been completed and removed from the tooth, any lubricant remaining on the inside of the pattern is removed by using a sable hair brush and washing the wax with a solution consisting of equal parts of green soap and hydrogen peroxide; this is followed by a thorough washing with plain water. The water and cleansing solution should be at room temperature. Better still, the cavity may be wiped out with a pellet of cotton moistened with a silicone type of lubricant.

DESIGN OF TOOTH FORM AND OCCLUSION—EVERITT PAYNE METHOD

A knowledge of the individual characteristics of coronal form is of extreme importance in reproducing properly located and properly shaped proximal contacts and concavities. The ability to reproduce the coronal shape of a tooth with proper contour so as to afford maximum self cleansing, proper tissue stimulation and protection, and good esthetics is all part of good crown and fixed partial prosthodontics. It is also impossible to obtain good functional occlusion without a knowledge of the occlusal characteristics of each tooth. A knowledge of individual tooth form must be complemented with an understanding of occlusal function and occlusal tooth-to-tooth relationship and with a practical and workable technic to give this proper relationship. The following is such a technic.

"Reproduction of Tooth Form" is a technic of functional anatomic waxing based on a relatively new approach to the technical problem of obtaining good functional occlusion.* This technic has been clinically tested for many years by researchers at the University of Southern California, where the method was first taught by Dr. Everitt Payne, who developed the technic. Many who have taken courses from Dr. Payne, with Dr. Thomas, or with the Ney study group have found it to be a technic which, with a little practice, is rapid in practical application and much easier to master than the older methods of carving. In this technic we are reproducing tooth form in the same manner as nature does with calcium deposits. The advantages of this technic are that it embodies a natural tooth-to-tooth and cusp-to-cusp relationship and deals with the complete occlusal problem rather than just individual tooth form.

This method should give a better understanding of occlusal function and an easier method of waxing-in this function with a minimum amount of correction after the waxings are cast.[6]

Planning and preparations

While the principles of this technic may be applied to any number of units of fixed prosthesis, the steps for the waxing of complete upper and lower arches are only considered in outline form.

As with any technic, planning is of the utmost importance. Therefore, the case is planned with the use of x-rays and properly mounted study casts before preparation is started. At this time the desired vertical is established and proper vertical space is maintained between preparations to allow for the desired curve of occlusion or curve of Spee (Fig. 20-7, *A* and *B*).

This technic should be performed one step at a time. After a little practice the steps may be combined and the procedure will become routine and fast. With practice it has proved to be faster than the old

*Courtesy Dr. Everitt Payne and Keith Smith, Ney Co., Hartford, Connecticut (1962).

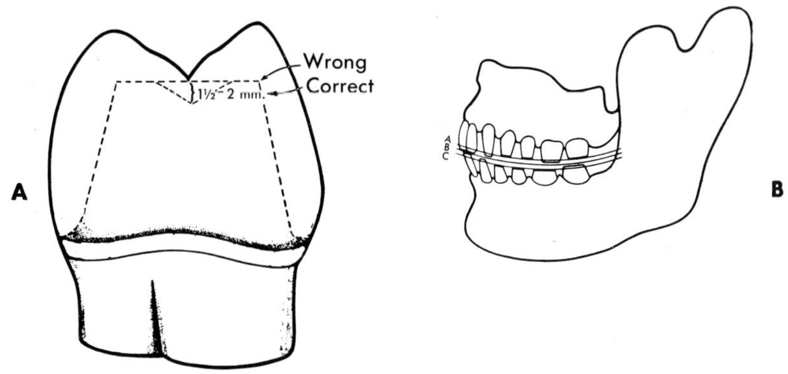

Fig. 20-7. A, Enough space should be allowed for sufficient thickness of wax to duplicate desired coronal and occlusal contour. **B,** Preparations should conform to lines A and C so that correct occlusal curve can be maintained along line B. Preparations extending beyond lines A and C will make it difficult to reproduce proper occlusion and still maintain good curve.

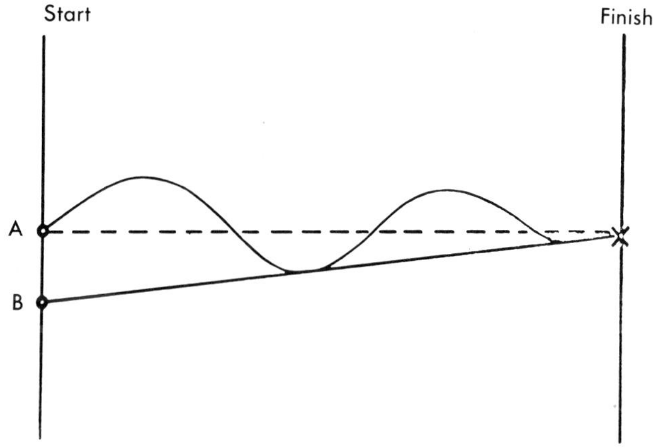

Fog. 20-8. Completion of process by former methods indicated by line A.

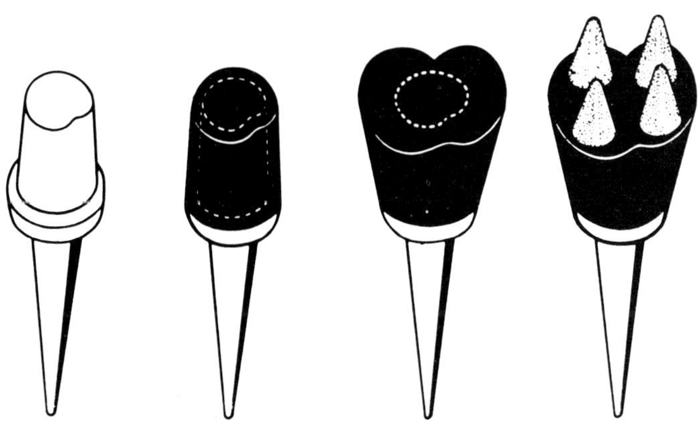

Fig. 20-9. Lubricated dies, with sufficient clearance for cusp heights.

method of building up wax, cutting away, building up again, and so on until completed as shown by line A in Fig. 20-8.

With this technic only the ivory cusp wax is placed where it remains until completed, as shown in line B. On a practical case the dies would be lubricated and the waxing would be built up from margins to the height of the occlusal fossa, leaving enough clearance between preparations for cusp heights (cones) (Fig. 20-9).

Materials

Special materials for the Everitt Payne technic include a No. 23 sickle explorer used as a wax spatula. This allows one to carry small droplets of the various colors of wax to the desired areas and results in a more natural refinement of the waxings. The degree of perfection that one can obtain in duplicating the occlusal relationships of the natural dentition depends not only on how well the waxing is done but also on how accurately the various colors are distributed in order to have the restored morphology of the tooth duplicate its various occlusal interrelationships during normal functional movements.

Four colors of waxes are employed—ivory, red, green, and blue—in the following locations:

1. Mandibular cusp cones (ivory wax)
2. Maxillary buccal cusp cones (ivory wax)
3. Buccal ridges of the mandibular buccal cusps (red wax)
4. Lingual ridges of the maxillary buccal cusps (red wax)
5. Mesial and distal cusp ridges of the maxillary and mandibular buccal cusps (green wax)
6. Maxillary lingual cusp cones (ivory wax)
7. Mesial and distal ridges of the maxillary lingual cusps (green wax)

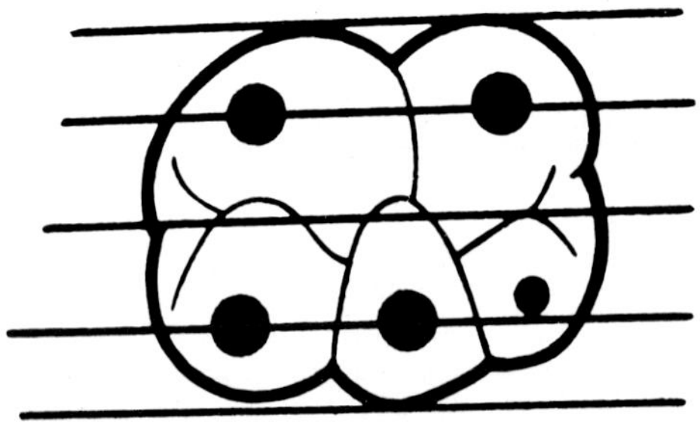

Fig. 20-10. Division into quarters of buccolingual width.

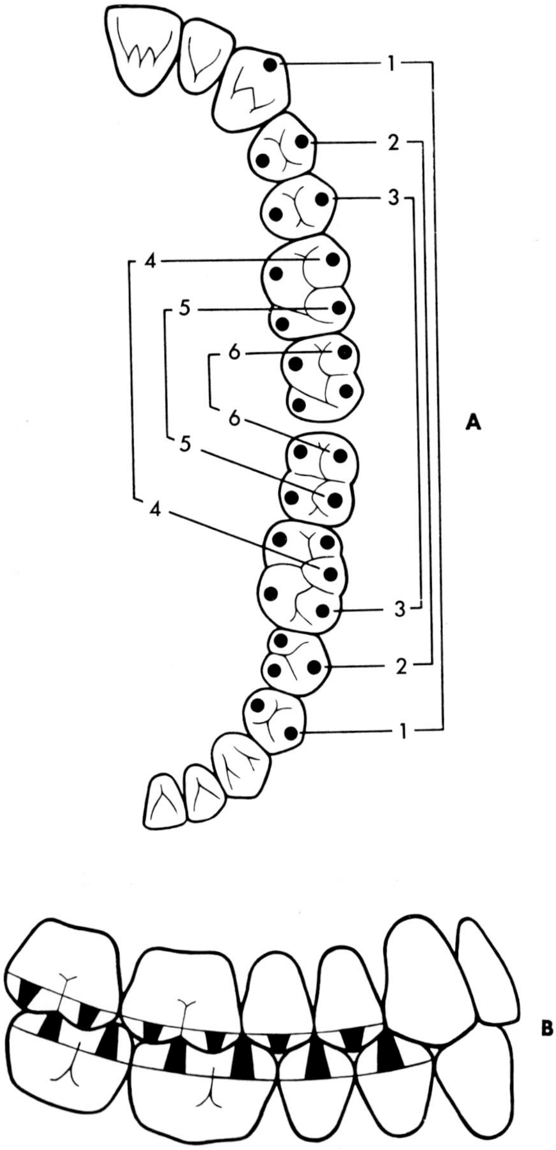

Fig. 20-11. A and B, Tips of cusp will fall along interproximal lines and buccal grooves on molars.

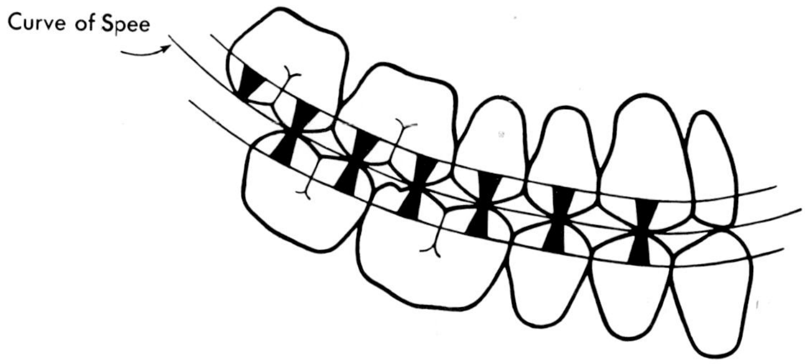

Fig. 20-12. Curve of Spee obtained by dividing vertical space.

8. Buccal and lingual cusp ridges of the maxillary lingual cusps (red wax)
9. Mesial and distal marginal ridges of the maxillary teeth (blue wax)
10. Lingual ridges of the mandibular buccal cusps (red wax)
11. Lingual cusp cones of the mandibular teeth and the distobuccal cusp of the mandibular first molar (ivory wax)
12. Buccal and lingual ridges of the mandibular lingual cusps (red wax)
13. Mesial and distal ridges of the mandibular lingual cusps (green wax)

Step 1. (1) To obtain buccolingual position of cusp tips, the buccolingual width of the tooth is divided into quarters (Fig. 20-10). Buccal cusps are located on first buccal quarter line. (Lingual cusp will fall on first lingual quarter line.) (2) To obtain mesiodistal position of cusp tips, place models in centric. Tips of cusp will fall along interproximal lines and buccal grooves on molars (Fig. 20-11, *A* and *B*). Ivory-colored wax is used for mandibular and maxillary cusps. (3) The occlusal curve (curve of Spee) is obtained by dividing vertical space to allow sufficient cusp height for upper and lower (Fig. 20-12). (4) Wax the cone tips of the upper and lower buccal cusps tip to tip in the lateral-protrusive relation. Shaded areas on the upper and lower arches indicate the cone tips of cusp tips of the teeth being developed. These tips must be protected in

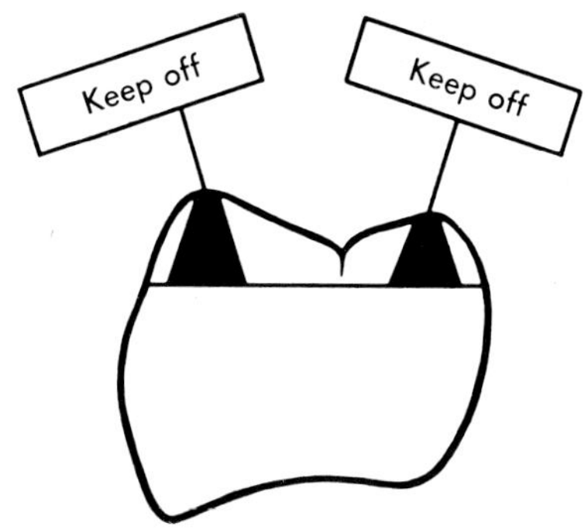

Fig. 20-13. Cone tips of cusp tips of teeth being developed must be protected. Ivory-colored wax is used.

all subsequent steps of waxing (Fig. 20-13).

Step 2. Determine height of upper lingual cusps so that they do not interfere in balancing relation: (1) the tip of the lingual cusp of the upper first bicuspid with the tip of the buccal cusp of the lower second bicuspid; (2) the tip of the lingual cusp of the upper second bicuspid with the tip of the mesiobuccal cusp of the lower first molar; (3) the tip of the mesiolingual cusp of the upper first molar with the distal and distobuccal cusp of the lower first molar; (4) the tip of the distolingual cusp of the upper first molar with the mesiobuccal cusp of the lower second molar; and (5) the tip of the mesiolingual cusp of the upper second molar with the distobuccal cusp of the lower second molar (Fig. 20-14).

The heights of the lower lingual cusps

are formed so as not to collide with the upper lingual cusps as they move through the working range in lateral excursion, as well as all other functional ranges.

Step 3. Wax the upper and lower inner and outer aspects: (Fig. 20-15, *A* and *B*). (1) Add wax to finish properly contour of upper buccal outer aspect and lower lingual outer aspect. Since these areas are nonfunctional there are no controlling factors. (2) Build up first upper inner aspect of buccal cusp and then outer aspect of lower buccal cusp; adding wax to one and then the other, and work them through all excursions. (3) Repeat method of building up upper lingual outer aspect and lower lingual inner aspect. (4) Repeat step 3 in

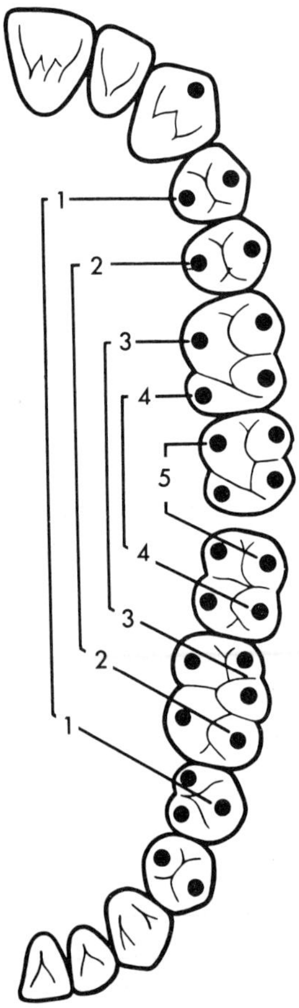

Fig. 20-14. Heights of upper lingual cusps must not interfere in balancing relation.

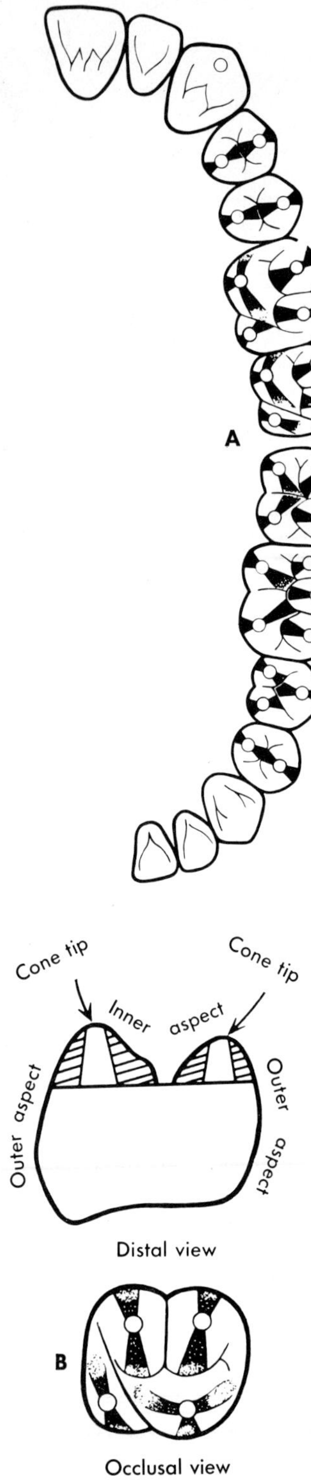

Fig. 20-15. A and **B,** Waxing upper and lower, inner and outer aspects.

building up upper lingual inner aspect and lower buccal inner aspect. Follow the proper angle of inner and outer aspect.

Step 4. The distal slope of the upper buccal cusps will determine the mesial slope of the lower buccal cusps as they pass through the protrusive, lateral, and lateral protrusive ranges (Fig. 20-16, *A* and *B*). In forming the mesial and distal slopes of the lower first molar, they must be waxed so as not to interfere with the upper mesiolingual cusp of the first molar. In the balancing to centric range, the mesiolingual cusp of upper first molar passes through the sulcus between the distal and the distobuccal cusp of the lower first molar (Fig. 20-17). In the protrusive to centric range, the mesiolingual cusp of the upper first molar passes over the distal cusp of the lower first molar. Therefore, all of these areas must be waxed up together while going through all functional ranges.

Step 5. Add wax to the mesial slope of the upper buccal cusps and move them

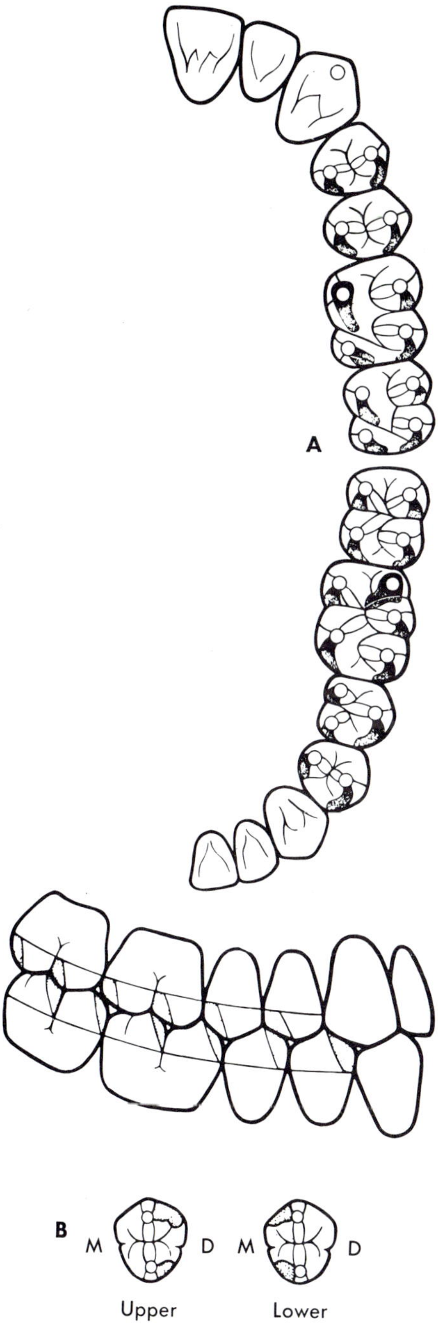

Fig. 20-16. A and **B,** See text.

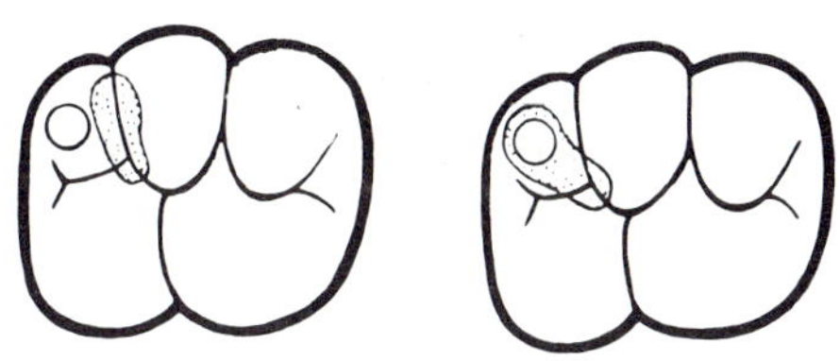

Fig. 20-17. See text.

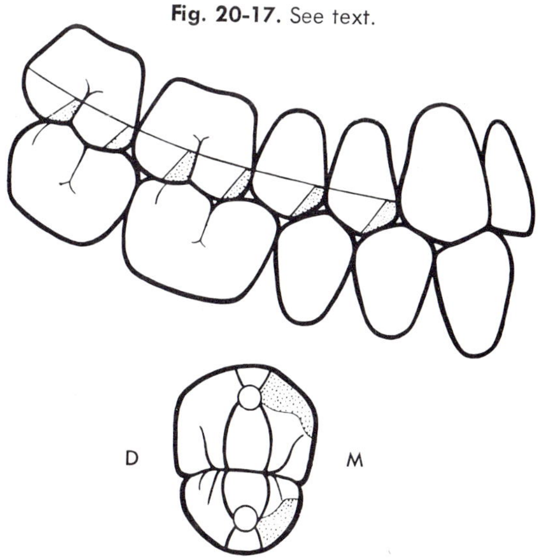

Figs. 20-18 and **20-19.** Add wax to mesial slope of upper buccal cusps and move them from working to centric against newly formed distal slope of lower buccal cusps.

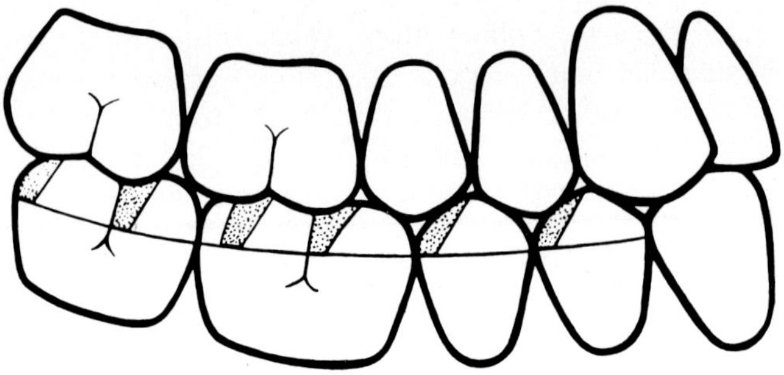

Fig. 20-19

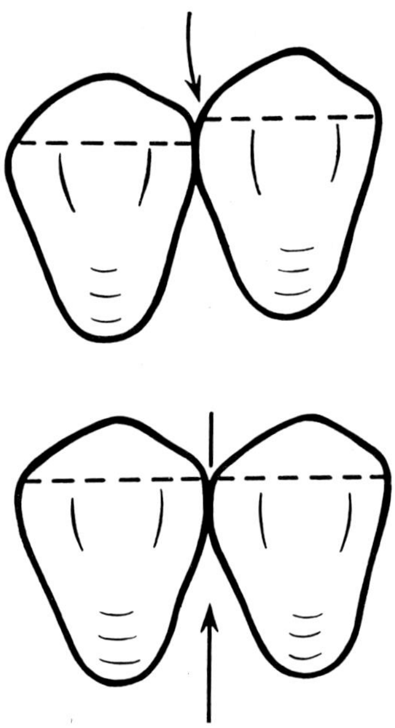

Fig. 20-20. Even interproximal heights maintained.

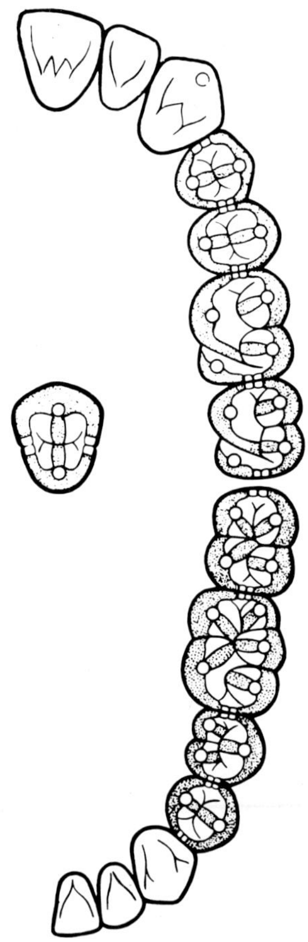

Fig. 20-21. See text.

from working to centric against the newly formed distal slope of the lower buccal cusps (Fig. 20-18). Add wax and build up the distal slope of the lower buccal cusps to the base of the previously waxed mesial slope of the adjacent cuspids (Fig. 20-19). Maintain even heights at proximals, as shown in Fig. 20-20.

Step 6. After the cusps have been formed to articulate in all positions, the marginal ridge areas are waxed in, making sure that the contact with opposing cusps are in centric only and do not interfere in functional movements (Fig. 20-21).

Step 7. To complete the wax-up, the

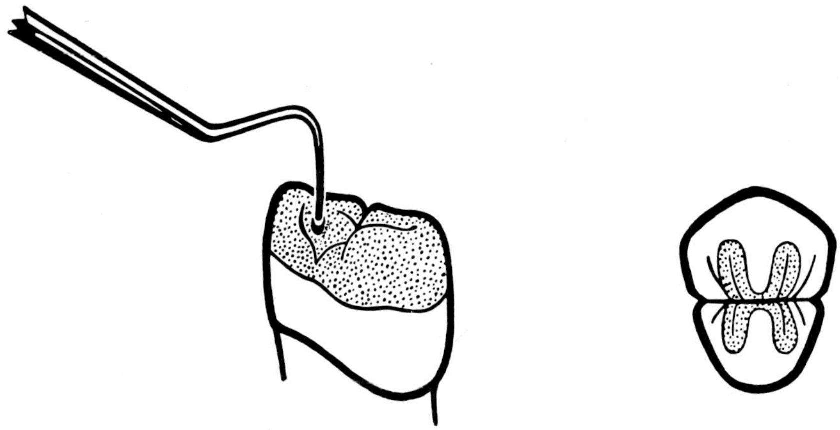

Fig. 20-22. Fossae waxed in.

fossae are waxed in (Fig. 20-22). To ensure that the contact between the upper and lower is not interfering or is too broad, zinc stearate powder is brushed on the wax and the articulated models are then moved through all functional ranges. After fabricating and refining wax patterns to the envelope of motion or to the dictates of the anatomic articulator, we now want to establish proper ball-point occlusal contacts.

The mandible in its terminal position should arc, bringing all teeth into a balanced contact. The lingual cusps of all maxillary bicuspids and molars should fit into the distal and central fossae of each opposing member in the mandibular arch. The buccal cusps of the lower bicuspids and molars should fit into the central fossae of the maxillary teeth.

The ideal is to have the upper cuspid act as a protector of the occlusion in extreme lateral excursions. We do not want broad flat contacts of occlusal surfaces in lateral excursions but seek to utilize the shearing action between the oblique, transverse, and marginal ridges of the posterior teeth as chewing strokes are made to and from lateral and protrusive positions of the mandible. For additional information on the philosophy of occlusal rehabilitation and functional waxing technics, the reader is referred to the works of Huffman and others,[6] McCollum,[7] Stuart,[8] Thomas,[9] and Granger.[10]

Forming the wax pattern by direct method in the mouth*

Prior to placing the softened wax inside the matrix, the inner surface of the band is lubricated very lightly. The matrix is then filled with softened inlay wax and forced to place on the prepared tooth. While doing so, pressure is maintained with the finger or thumb held over the top of the matrix, so that the softened wax is carried to the gingival margins, into the angles, and against the walls of the preparation. If an adjustable matrix is used, the slight slack in the matrix is taken up by tightening the screw on the matrix holder; this brings the wax into intimate contact with all surfaces and margins of the preparation. The wax is held under pressure until it no longer flows.

Using the high points made by the opposing teeth as indices, the occlusal surface is carved in the hardened wax to its proper anatomy both in centric relation and in eccentric paths of contact. If the wax pattern is for an anterior tooth, the correct thickness of wax on the lingual surface is

*See Chapter 22 for indirect method.

thus established, and the excess is trimmed away.

After the occlusal surfaces have been trimmed and carved to their correct anatomic form, the matrix is carefully removed. If a seamless band or a soldered copper matrix is used, the matrix is cut through with a sharp instrument on the buccal or the labial surface. If the riveted type of matrix is employed, a flat instrument is inserted into the flap, and the band is opened by disengaging the small flanges of the rivet joint. If an adjustable matrix is used, the band is loosened slightly by releasing the grip of the matrix holder. In any case care must be exercised not to distort the wax pattern while peeling away the matrix from the wax.

Any wax that has been forced beyond the gingival margin of the metal matrix, either on the lingual or the proximal surfaces, is removed with a sharp explorer or suitable trimming instrument before the matrix is cut open and removed.

Upon removal of the matrix, the wax pattern is retained firmly in position in the tooth, while the excess marginal wax is shaped to the desired contour. In trimming the surplus wax from the margins of the cavity, the carving instrument is so manipulated that the surplus is cut from the wax pattern toward the tooth margin. In doing so, however, the straight-edged cutting blade is held in constant contact with the tooth surface so that the plane of the wax surface is even with the margin of the tooth. Similarly, when carving the occlusal anatomy, it is advisable to have the cutting blade of the instrument in contact at all times with the occlusal planes of the tooth. The set of Hollenback wax-carving instruments is ideal for this purpose. Some prefer to leave a marginal excess of wax that is later polished off in the finished casting. This, however, is a questionable technic.

After the wax pattern has been carved and verified for correct contour, occlusion, and gingival fit, the margins of the pattern may be wiped against the tooth by means of a cotton pellet soaked in water not exceeding 100° F. At no time should a wax solvent be used to smooth the surface of a wax pattern; if chloroform or other similar solvents are employed, the sharp marginal edges of the wax pattern will be lost, with a subsequent defective and ill-fitting casting.

Attaching sprue pin

A simple wax pattern is never removed from the tooth with a sharp explorer. Preferably, a hollow sprue pin may be attached to the pattern while it is still in the cavity; this then serves as a handle to remove the wax pattern.

Where the pattern is thin, instead of applying the heated sprue pin directly to the wax pattern with a possible resultant distortion, it is safer to add a small bead of "sticky" wax to the open end of the pin where the sprue pin is to be attached to the wax pattern (Fig. 20-23). The sprue pin is heated and the "sticky" wax spreads as a thin film on its surface; it is then attached to the bead of wax previously added to the wax pattern. If the sprue pin is of the correct temperature, the molten wax on it will unite with that of the wax pattern, causing little if any disturbance of the thermal equilibrium of the wax pattern.

The sprue pin should be placed in the greatest bulk of the pattern and slanted at such an angle that when the molten metal enters the mold in the investment, it will fill it with the least amount of turbulence.

In those patterns involving two or more surfaces, better results are obtained by using the double or staple-shaped sprue pin instead of the single one. Fig. 20-23 shows the possible distortions of the wax pattern that may result from the improper placement of the sprue pin or improper removal of the pattern from the tooth. When used, the staple sprue pin is of a width that permits the two arms of the

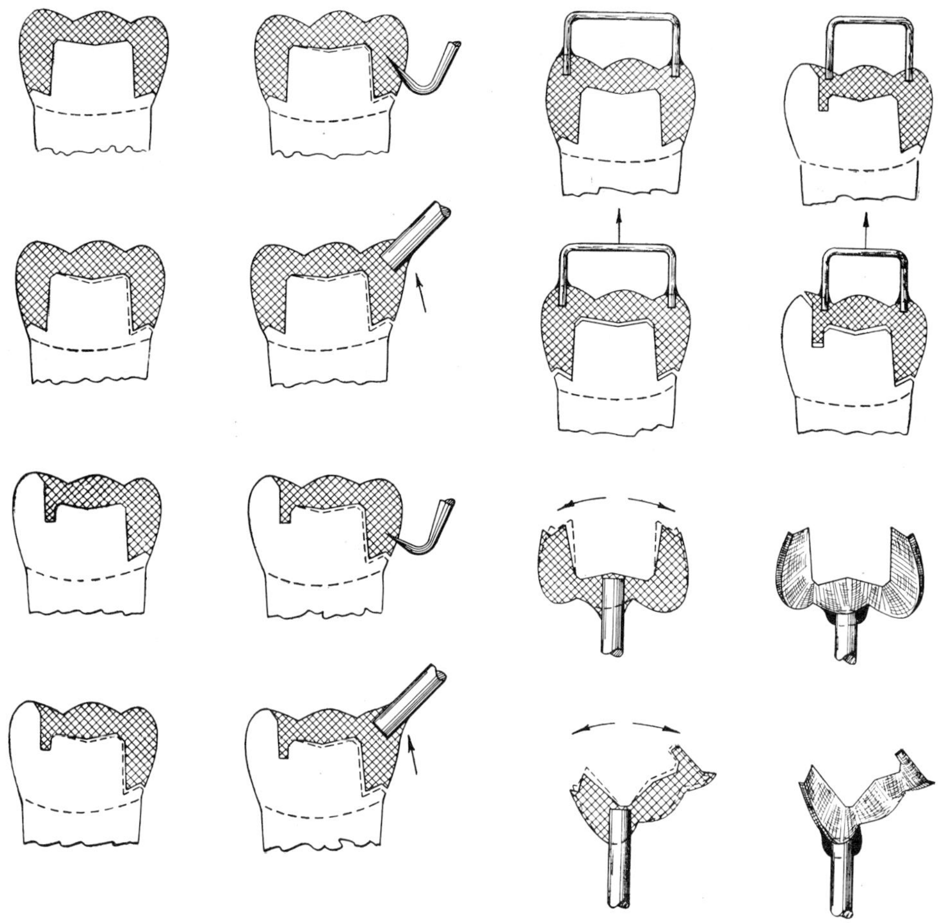

Fig. 20-23. Incorrect application of sprue pin to wax pattern may cause its distortion. (After R. E. Sturdevant.)

staple to be attached to the proximal areas of the wax pattern and in a line parallel to the axis of the preparation (Fig. 20-24).

An equalized traction is thus exerted on the wax pattern, permitting its removal without distortion.

Experience has shown that the size and the length of the sprue pin bear a definite relationship to the success obtained in casting. The diameters of sprue pins generally used are: 16 g., approximately 1 mm., utilized for small inlays only; 14 g., approximately 1.5 mm., used for larger inlays and with a staple shape; 12 g., approximately 2 mm., used mostly in large-type inlays.

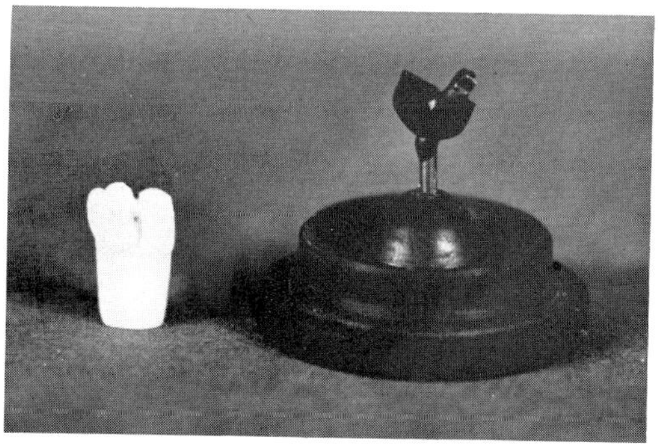

Fig. 20-24. Wax pattern attached to sprue pin and mounted in casting ring base.

In selecting the sprue pin its length should be such that when the wax pattern is mounted and in the casting ring, the pattern is approximately ¼ inch away from the bottom of the ring (Fig. 20-24). If the pattern is mounted higher so that it is in the center of the ring, the extra thickness of investment between the wax pattern mold and the bottom of the ring will inhibit the rapid exit of the gases when molten metal is cast into the mold. This creates a back pressure that is frequently responsible for rounded margins, porosity, and voids in the castings.

Another factor to be considered is the method by which the casting is to be made, namely, air pressure or centrifugal force. If air pressure is used, then the sprue pin is of a smaller diameter, 16 gauge, to prevent the molten gold from running down the sprue during the melting of the gold in the investment crucible of the ring. If centrifugal force is employed, then the larger gauges may be safely used, 14 gauge to 12 gauge.

Use of reservoir

When the sprue pin is placed in the sprue base, the attached wax pattern should not be more than ¼ inch from the base. Before mounting the wax pattern and the sprue pin in the base or crucible former, a small piece of wax is attached to the sprue pin about $\frac{1}{16}$ inch away from the pattern. This serves as a reservoir for molten gold when the casting is made (Fig. 20-25). It is known that, when molten gold enters the mold, solidification of the metal occurs from the outer walls inwardly; the crystal growth occurs at the expense of the residual molten metal within the mold. If additional molten metal is available during the solidification process so that the crystals can continue to form until the entire mold is filled, the casting will be solid throughout. If, however, the available supply of molten gold is limited only to the amount initially entering the mold, the solidified crystals, as they approach the center of the casting, will lack sufficient molten metal to complete their development to fill the entire mold; this latter condition results in voids and porous areas in the casting. Such a casting usually results if no reservoir is used, especially if a sigle sprue pin is used and one that is of a small gauge and excessively long. A reservoir acts as a feeder of molten metal to the casting until it is fully solidified. The size of the reservoir should be equal in volume to that of the wax pattern.

Treatment of wax pattern

If oil or debris is present on the wax pattern, it is washed off with a solution consisting of equal parts of hydrogen peroxide and liquid green soap and is rinsed in room temperature water. Next, the pattern is dried and carefully painted with one of the wetting agents to break down the surface tension. The wax pattern is again dried; when the investment is applied it will flow smoothly and adhere to the treated wax pattern.

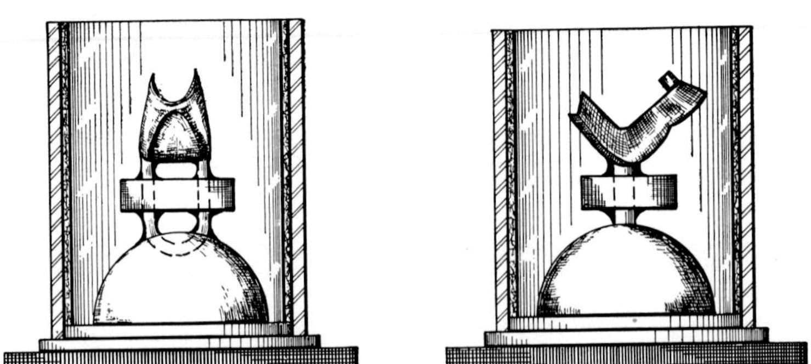

Fig. 20-25. Wax added to sprue pin to furnish reservoir for molten gold.

Investing

A crucible former (Fig. 20-25) and ring are selected of such size that, when invested, the wax pattern will be surrounded by at least ¼ inch of investment material and will also be that distance from the open end of the ring (Fig. 20-26). A dry asbestos liner is placed inside of the casting ring. Preferably, the ends of the strip should meet evenly inside the ring and be cut ⅛ inch short at each end of the ring. After the strip is adapted to the inner wall of the ring it is dipped in water and laid aside while the investment is being mixed. It should not be touched any more as this might compress the asbestos and reduce its space for the needed setting and thermal expansions later.

The purpose of the asbestos liner is: first, to allow an effective setting and thermal expansion to take place; second, to serve as an insulator against the loss of heat during the casting process; third, to permit a more free thermal and hygroscopic expansion of the investment material; and finally, to facilitate the removal of the investment from the ring after the casting has been made.

Compensating for shrinkage. Recognizing the general information prevalent today relative to investing and casting technics, a brief résumé of some of the salient factors still may be desirable. The aim of any casting technic is to produce a casting from the wax pattern that will fit the cavity snugly without grinding or swaging and that may be placed with finger pressure. Such a casting should have its surfaces smooth, nonporous, and free from nodules or blisters. A successful casting must also reproduce the wax pattern as formed within the tooth cavity or on a stone die without any appreciable dimensional change. It is known that a contraction of the gold alloy occurs in solidifying and in cooling to room temperature. Coleman[11] established the linear casting shrinkage of gold and its alloys as 1.25 percent, ±0.1 percent. Shell[10] reported a shrinkage of approximately 1.7 percent; Scheu[12] found that a compensation value of 1.55 percent was necessary to secure precision results. More recently, Hollenback[13] has reported that there is a casting shrinkage ranging upward from 1.35 percent for gold alloys to 1.65 percent for pure gold. Intermediate percentages of shrinkage for gold alloys vary according to the composition of the alloys.

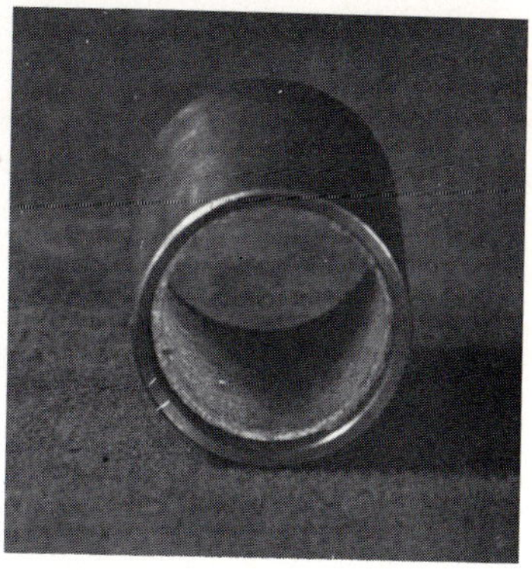

Fig. 20-26. Casting ring lined with asbestos.

Therefore, any technic to be successful must compensate for these shrinkages in addition to the shrinkage that took place in the wax pattern when it was removed from the tooth to room temperature. Several methods have been employed to compensate for these shrinkages: namely, (1) the thermal expansion of the wax pattern; (2) the thermal expansion of the investment; (3) the setting and hygroscopic expansion of the investment.

Because of the inherent dangers associated with the thermal expansion of the wax pattern, this technic has been largely discarded today.

Expansion of casting investments

The selection of a proper dental casting investment depends largely upon the type of casting to be made and the amount of expansion desired and whether the expansion is to be obtained mainly by thermal means or by a combination of hydroscopic and thermal expansion. A.D.A. Specifications for Inlay Casting Investment specify No. 1 type for the thermal and No. 2 type for the hydroscopic method.

The total thermal expansion of a casting investment occurs in two phases. However, it is possible to eliminate the wax pattern from the investment at a relatively low temperature. When this is done the molten gold alloy is cast into an investment mold whose walls are hard and smooth. This is possible by the hygroscopic inlay casting technic as originally advocated by Hollenback.

Where a wax pattern has been mounted on the sprue former, the pin is inserted into the opening in the center of the rubber crucible former (Fig. 20-24).

Inlay casting investments usually consist of two main ingredients—the binding agent, which is either plaster of Paris or some form of Hydrocal, and the thermal expanding ingredient, usually some form of silica (SiO_2) such as crystobalite or quartz. By utilizing normal setting and high thermal expansions it is possible to compensate for shrinkages of up to 1.65 percent. However, to obtain such a high percentage of thermal expansion it is necessary to heat the investment to temperatures of 1300 to 1400° F.

At these high temperatures, the binding material, Hydrocal, loses most of its water of crystallization, resulting in the reduction of its binding power. When this occurs, the inner walls of the mold in the investment may become rough and powdery, resulting in rough castings. Yet it is necessary in the high thermal expansion technic to employ high temperatures, (1) to obtain the necessary thermal expansion, and (2) to eliminate the wax pattern.

Setting expansion. The first phase is the "setting expansion," usually 0.3 percent. This takes place when the initial crystallization and setting of the binding agent have occurred (Fig. 20-27).

Thermal expansion. The second is the

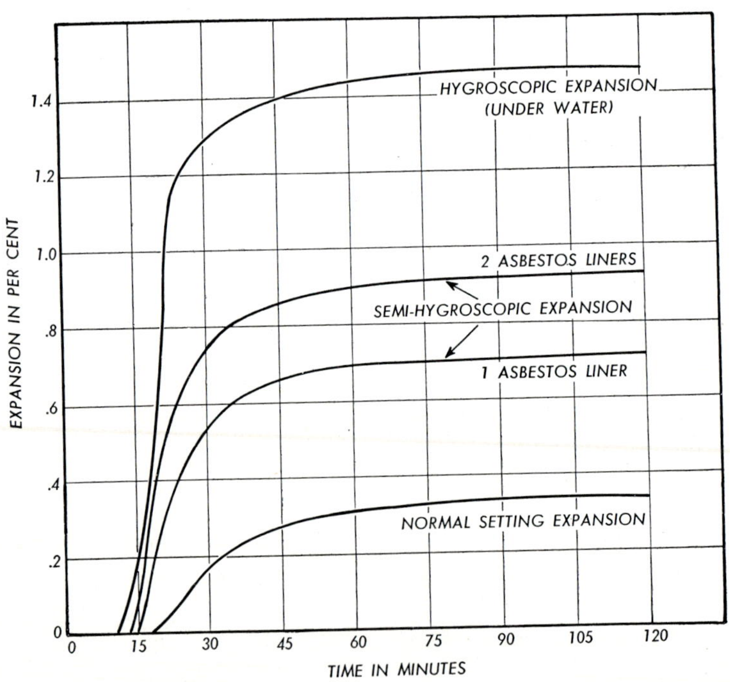

Fig. 20-27. Setting expansion of Beauty Cast Investment. (Courtesy Whip-Mix Corporation.

"thermal expansion," which may reach as high as 1.5 percent; this takes place when the investment is subjected to high heat. By taking advantage of one or both of these expansions in a casting investment, it is possible to compensate for the 1.25 percent or more shrinkage of gold alloy. To what extent the normal "setting expansion" of an investment may be utilized is uncertain; however, it is probable that the usable amount of effective expansion is considerably less than the maximum indicated by the manufacturers of dental investments; hence more dependence is placed upon the available "thermal expansion."

Dental casting investments vary in their "thermal expansion" from 1 to 1.5 percent (Fig. 20-28). The chart of physical properties that accompanies present-day casting investments indicates the percentage of expansion that may be obtained from the investment when it is heated to certain temperatures. This chart presupposes, however, that the correct water-investment ratio has been used in the mix. Increasing

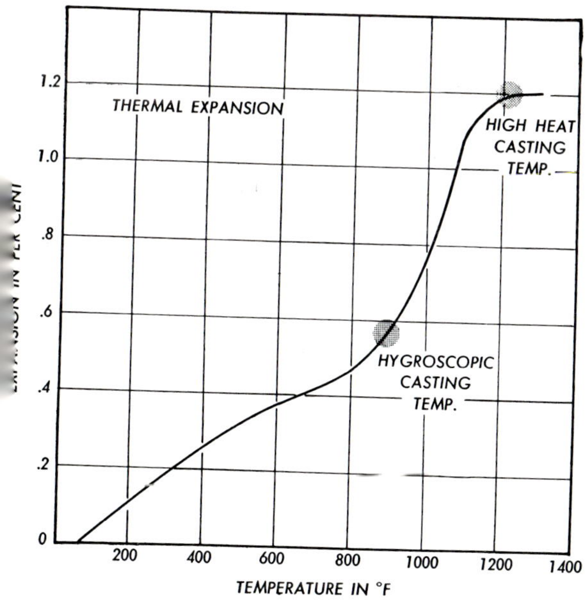

Fig. 20-28. Thermal expansion of Beauty Cast Investment. (Courtesy Whip-Mix Corporation.)

the water content of a mix usually decreases the relative thermal expansion of the investment.

In the high thermal expanding investments much of the initial expansion takes place by the time the investment is heated to 400° C. or 752° F. From this point on there is a gradual but less marked increase in expansion (to 1.0 to 1.3 percent) as the temperature of the investment is raised. The curve gradually flattens into a plateau when a temperature of 700° C. (1292° F.) to 800° C. (1472° F.) is reached.

Since it is rather difficult to control the exact temperature of the mold and because a temperature drop occurs in the mold from the time it is removed from the furnace until it is cast, it is desirable to heat the investment slightly higher than the correct casting temperature, so that in cooling there will be only a negligible loss of expansion in the investment.

Water-investment ratio. Every manufacturer of a dental casting investment furnishes the proper water-investment ratio for his product; this should be adhered to strictly. Increasing the water content beyond the specified proportions not only reduces the amount of available expansion, but also may cause cracks to develop in the investment and form so-called blisters on the surfaces of the casting. Most of the investments prescribe a ratio of 28 to 34 ml. of water to 100 Gm. of the investment. Since the average inlay ring may be filled with 50 Gm. of investment, the amount of water used will vary from 14 to 17 ml., depending upon the product used.

Extremes in temperature of the water used should be avoided, room temperature, between 70 and 85° F., being preferable. In those sections of the country where the water has a high or a variable chemical content, it is advisable to use distilled water to ensure constantly uniform results.

Since the setting time of the investment

is affected by particles of set plaster of Paris or old investment, it is essential that all the utensils used, such as plaster bowls, spatulas, or mechanical mixers, be absolutely clean. The initial and final setting time of the investment should be known to the dentist so that he may adapt his investing technic to the time available to him for this purpose.

Mixing investment. After the wax pattern has been attached to the sprue pin, to which a reservoir has also been added, the entire assembly is mounted on the sprue base (Fig. 20-25), which later also forms the crucible in the investment. A casting ring is selected of such size that when the wax pattern is invested it will be surrounded by at least ¼ inch of investment material and it will also be the same distance from the open end of the ring when seated on the sprue base. A dry asbestos liner is placed inside the ring so that the ends meet evenly and do not overlap. A speck of sticky wax will attach the liner to the ring. As previously stated, the asbestos liner allows the investment to expand later, during initial and thermal expansions.

There are several methods of mixing investment: (1) by hand with a spatula and rubber bowl; (2) mechanical hand-spatulator; and (3) mixing and investing in vacuum. The water is poured into a clean bowl or spatulator, into which the investment is then slowly sifted. The mechanical spatulator of the hand type is preferred to mixing by hand with a spatula and bowl, since a thorough mix may be obtained with it in a shorter time. The spatulation requires 40 to 60 seconds and takes approximately 100 to 120 turns of the blade. Too rapid spatulation is not desirable, since air bubbles may be incorporated in the mix. By increasing the length of time of spatulation, the setting time is hastened. If the spatulation has been done by hand with a spatula and rubber bowl, it is well to place a piece of glass across the top of the rubber bowl and holding both together, the bottom of the rubber bowl is pushed in, forcing out some air, after which the glass is held firmly against the rim of the rubber bowl which is then tapped gently on the laboratory bench for a few seconds; this creates a slight vacuum within the bowl, which draws to the surface any trapped air bubbles within the investment. Mixing investment in vacuum will be discussed more fully later. The mixing of investment in vacuum was reported by Coleman[11] at the Bureau of Standards in 1928.

Hand investing of wax pattern. The next step is investing the wax pattern or imbedding it with the investment material. The purpose of investing the pattern in a high-heat refractory material is to produce a mold into which molten gold alloy can be cast to reproduce an exact replica of the pattern. The investment forming the mold should not distort the fragile wax pattern when it is imbedded in it. The investment must be capable of expanding sufficiently to compensate for the shrinkages that take place in the metal when cooling from its solidification temperature to room temperature, in addition to the slight shrinkage of the wax pattern when removed from mouth temperature to room temperature. The investment must tolerate a degree of heat sufficient to eliminate the wax completely without leaving a residue and still leave a hard, smooth surface. However, it must be sufficiently porous to permit air to escape from the mold when the molten metal is cast into it. It must be able to withstand the impact force and high temperature of the molten metal entering the mold without cracking or powdering. It must not change the chemical composition of the alloy. Finally, the casting should be easily removed and cleaned. For these reasons one must understand and respect the physical properties and the proper manipulation of dental casting investments.

To secure a casting that has smooth surfaces and is free from blisters and nodules, it is necessary first, that all lubricants and debris be removed from the wax pattern; second, that the investment covers all angles and surfaces of the wax pattern, care being taken to avoid trapping air bubbles or leaving areas not covered by the investment. These are more readily attained by first painting the entire wax pattern with a wetting agent to reduce surface tension.

The initial application of the investment to the wax pattern is best made with a small sable or camel's-hair brush. The cavity side of the wax pattern is first covered with the investment. A small amount of the investment is taken up with the damp brush and applied to the inner surface of the pattern at the gingival margin. With a gentle, vibrating motion of the brush, the investment is gently pushed ahead of the bristles until it reaches the floor of the pattern. Care must be exercised at this stage of the procedure that no air bubbles are trapped in the angle formed between the pulpal and axial walls of the wax pattern. Additional small amounts of investment are carried to the wax pattern until the entire inner surfaces are covered, carrying a slight excess beyond the margins. If any doubt exists as to the presence of air bubbles clinging to the inner angles of the wax pattern, all the investment is blown off until only a thin film remains. This will disclose whether the pattern is completely covered and whether any air bubbles were trapped during the operation. If not, additional investment is immediately reapplied with the camel's-hair brush to the wax pattern until it is entirely covered with investment. Although the brush is used, at no time should it be used with a scrubbing motion. After the pattern has been covered to a depth of ¼ inch, the sprue pin and the reservoir should also be carefully painted and covered with investment. This is done to avoid trapping air between the wax pattern and the reservoir. The time required to perform this initial investing should not exceed 1½ to 2 minutes.

The partially invested wax pattern seated in the base is now ready to be invested within the inlay ring. The wet asbestos-lined ring is next placed on the crucible-forming base. Quickly, some of the investment remaining in the mixing bowl is taken up with a spatula, carried to the ring, and gently slid off the spatula with the finger, down the inside of the ring. The investment is carefully worked to the bottom of the ring with the brush; this is repeated until the entire ring is gradually filled and the wax pattern is embedded in the investment. At no time should the base or the ring be tapped or vibrated, as this may draw air bubbles and free water to the surface of the wax pattern, resulting in nodules and blisters in the casting. Another method employed to invest the painted pattern is to place the ring on a glass slab and fill it with the inlay investment remaining in the bowl; then, holding the crucible former and the painted pattern in an inverted position above the ring, the covered wax pattern on the base is settled gently into the soft investment until the crucible-forming base is seated on the ring.

It is well to let the investment set for one-half to one hour after investing the pattern. After the expiration of this time, the final set of the investment usually has occurred; the crucible-forming base and the sprue pin may then be removed. A sharp twist will dislodge the base from the ring and the sprue pin and the excess investment is trimmed from the inside of the ring to a depth of about ¹⁄₁₆ inch. All loose particles of investment are removed.

The sprue pin, protruding beyond the investment, is now grasped with a pair of soldering pliers that have been heated to a cherry red. Sufficient heat is thus transferred to the sprue pin so that its attachment to the wax pattern is loosened, whereupon it may be withdrawn from the investment with a slow half-turn. In doing this, the invested ring is held in an inverted position, so that, when the sprue pin is removed, any loosened pieces of investment are kept from dropping down the sprue hole. If a sharp, thin edge of the investment remains at the opening of the sprue hole, it should be beveled or countersunk to prevent its breaking off during the casting process and being carried into the mold. This trimming is also done with the ring held in an inverted position.

Satisfactory results may be obtained by placing the invested wax pattern in an inverted position, with the sprue hole down, in an oven maintained at a constant temperature of 300° F. (Figs. 20-29 and 20-30). The ring is kept at this temperature for 30 minutes. No harm results either to the mold or to the investment material if it is left in the low-temperature furnace for a longer period of time than 30 minutes.

When the investment mold has been completely dried and heated uniformly throughout, the ring is then inverted and heated to a temperature of 1200° F. or 700° C. The invested ring is now placed with the sprue hole up, so that any gases of volatilization may escape freely through the opening. The invested ring is kept in the high temperature furnace for 30 to 45 minutes, or longer if unavoidable. Thirty minutes at the high temperature usually

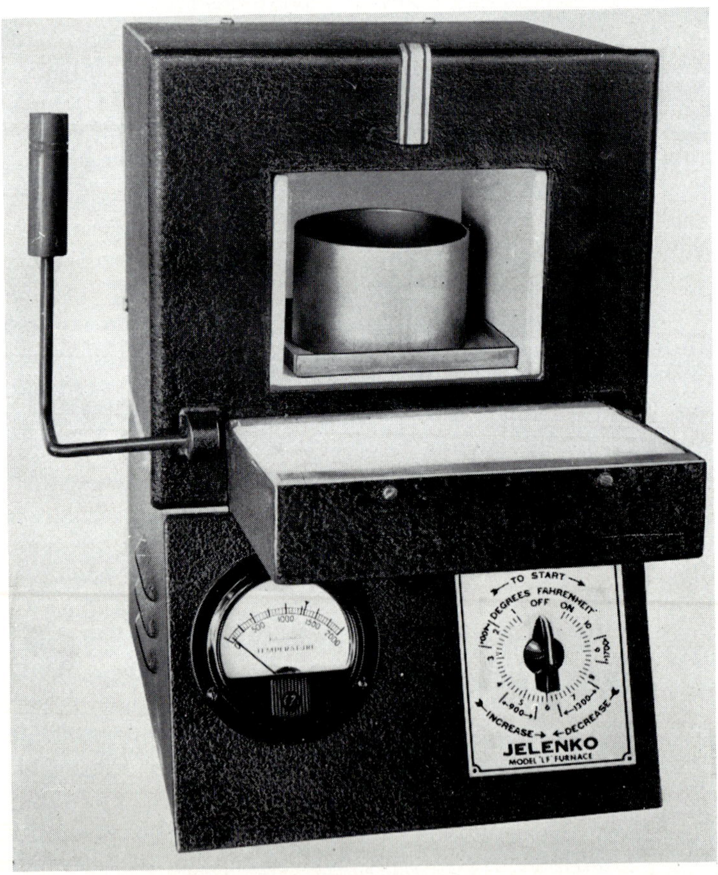

Fig. 20-29. Controlled temperature oven for elimination of invested wax patterns. (Courtesy J. F. Jelenko & Co., Inc.)

suffices for all normal-sized wax patterns. More time may be necessary for the larger patterns to make certain that no wax residue is left in the mold.

During the heating at low temperature, all the moisture is eliminated from the investment; too, some of the wax has flowed out through the sprue hole, while that which remains in the mold gradually permeates the walls of the investment. A certain amount of thermal expansion, approximately 0.2 percent, also has occurred at this low temperature.

Placing the invested ring at first in a low-temperature furnace permits the investment to dry and expand gradually. If a cold ring and investment are placed immediately in a hot furnace, the ring will expand more rapidly than the investment; the outer portion of the investment being exposed to the high heat first expands a greater amount than the inner portion, hence cracks develop in the peripheral part of the investment, producing fin-like metal extensions on the surface of the casting.

There is another danger associated with heating the invested ring too rapidly; the entire investment may explode due to the steam generated by heating it too rapidly. Steam so generated may also result in a rough casting due to particles of investment being blown off the sides of the mold.

Where a furnace with temperature control and pyrometer readings is not available, the correct temperature may be judged by observing the color of the heated investment. This usually attains a

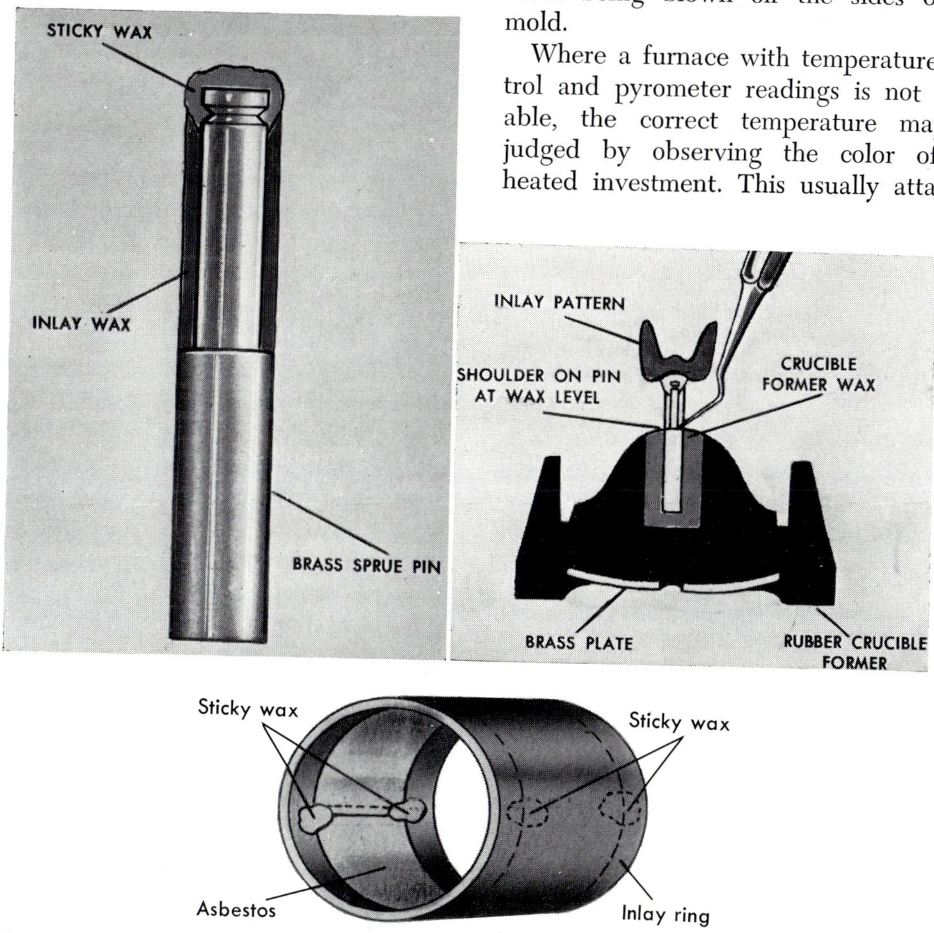

Fig. 20-30. Sprue pin, rubber base, and ring used in Vac-U-Spat method. (Courtesy Whip-Mix Corporation.)

temperature of 1200 to 1300° F. when the sprue hole shows a cherry red color when viewed in a shadow.

It is now ready for casting.

Vacuum—hygroscopic expansion technic. The other, more generally used method of investing a wax pattern and compensating for casting shrinkages is the one in which the mixing of the investment and the investing of the wax pattern are done in a vacuum. The method utilizes the hygroscopic setting expansion of the investment to compensate for a large percentage of the shrinkage of the gold alloy. By definition, the hygroscopic expansion phenomenon occurs whenever a mixed mass of dental casting investment, while undergoing the setting process, is brought into intimate contact with water by submersion or by the controlled addition of water; maximum expansion results if this is done as soon as possible after the mix has been poured into the casting ring. The wax pattern may be eliminated from the investment mold by means of boiling water, and, finally, the casting is made in a mold heated to 850-900° F.

Mixing-investing—hydroscopic method. While thermal expansion is also utilized, it is done only at low temperatures. Castings made by this method are extremely smooth and accurate. The method may be modified to give castings of any degree of tight or loose fit. The technic is simple although exact; it requires some special equipment.

Ordinarily, the effective setting expansion of an inlay investment is 0.3 to 0.35 percent. By immersing the inlay base and ring in water immediately after the wax pattern is invested, and before the initial set has taken place, a phenomenon known as hygroscopic expansion of the investment occurs, resulting in an expansion that varies from 1.0 to 2.6 percent, depending upon (1) the type of investment used, (2) the temperature of the water bath, (3) the water-powder ratio used, (4) the time that elapses before placing the ring in the water bath after investing the wax pattern, and (5) the length of time that the invested ring is left in the water bath. Scheu[12] first called attention to this phenomenon.

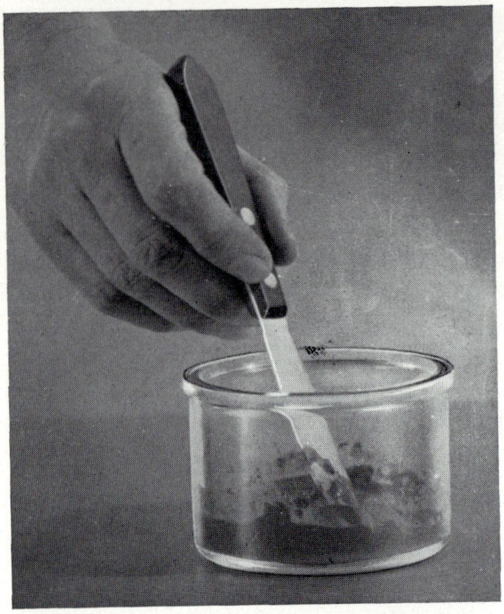

Fig. 20-31. Initial puddling manually before mechanically mixing the investment under vacuum. (Courtesy Whip-Mix Corporation.)

Although the exact mechanism of hygroscopic setting expansion has not been determined, the investigations by Mahler and Moffitt point toward the premise that "hygroscopic expansion is simply normal setting expansion under the influence of water brought into intimate contact with the gypsum material during the setting process and that the basic mechanism for both hygroscopic and normal setting expansion is the growth of gypsum crystals from suprasaturated solutions. To continue, the only difference between the two expansions would then be the influence of this additionally supplied water and it would appear that the only procedure needed to define the mechanism of hygroscopic expansion would be a determination of exactly how this added water influences the normal setting expansion. . . ."[14]

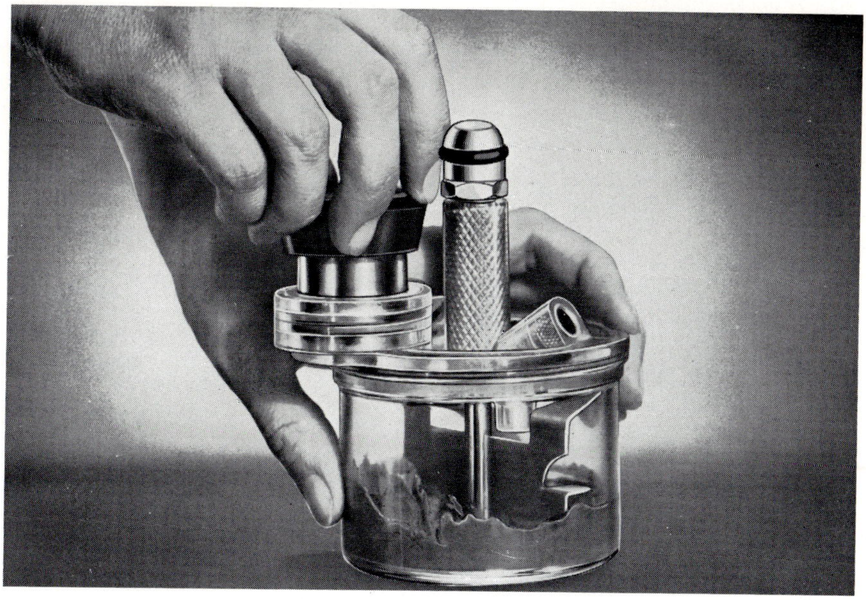

Fig. 20-32. Vacuum mixing and investing equipment. (Courtesy Whip-Mix Corporation.)

It has been demonstrated that one factor which significantly affects the actual amount of setting expansion is the nature and magnitude of forces which oppose the force of the growing gypsum crystals. Examples of this effect are the increase in expansion of a setting gypsum material in the direction of the open ends of a solid unlined ring and also the increase in expansion which occurs when intercrystalline bonding forces are reduced as a result of the addition of inert materials in dental casting investments.

Vacuum method: mixing and investing. As in preceding technics, it is necessary to mount the pattern on a sprue pin; this is then inserted in a rubber crucible former and base. The mounted wax pattern is cleaned as described previously (Figs. 20-24 and 20-25).

In order to obtain the desired amounts of setting and thermal expansion, the correct water investment ratio must also have been employed.

After the inlay ring has been lined with dry asbestos liner and then moistened (Figs. 20-25 and 20-30), it is positioned properly on the rubber crucible former. The correct amount of water, 15 ml. to 50 Gm. of investment (Beauty Cast), is measured. First, the water is poured into the plastic bowl, then the investment is sifted in and thoroughly incorporated with the water by means of hand spatulation so that no dry powder is visible (Fig. 20-31).

It will be observed that the upper portion of the assembly (Fig. 20-32) consists of the mixing blade, the receptacle for the inlay ring, and a tapered opening for the vacuum hose. When the investment and water have been puddled sufficiently in the plastic bowl, the upper portion is seated as shown in Fig. 20-32. The inlay ring with the rubber sprue former and its mounted wax pattern are now gently twisted into the round receptacle on the left side of the cover.

The vacuum hose is next attached to the opening on the right side of the lid (Fig. 20-33). The vacuum is activated either by means of the vacuum pump or by the water aspirator (Fig. 20-34).

It will be observed that the inverted ring and base must be held firmly in position until the vacuum is activated (Fig. 20-33). Once a vacuum has been created inside of the mixing bowl, the inlay ring with its rubber base will be held firmly against the lid by the vacuum (Fig. 20-35, A).

When the gauge shows a working vacuum of 28 inches, it is held for 20 seconds. It is important that the vacuum *valve* in the lid be held in an *upright position* in order not to suck the investment into the vacuum hose (Fig. 20-35, A).

The motor is turned on low speed, 1,750 rpm, and let run for 20 seconds.

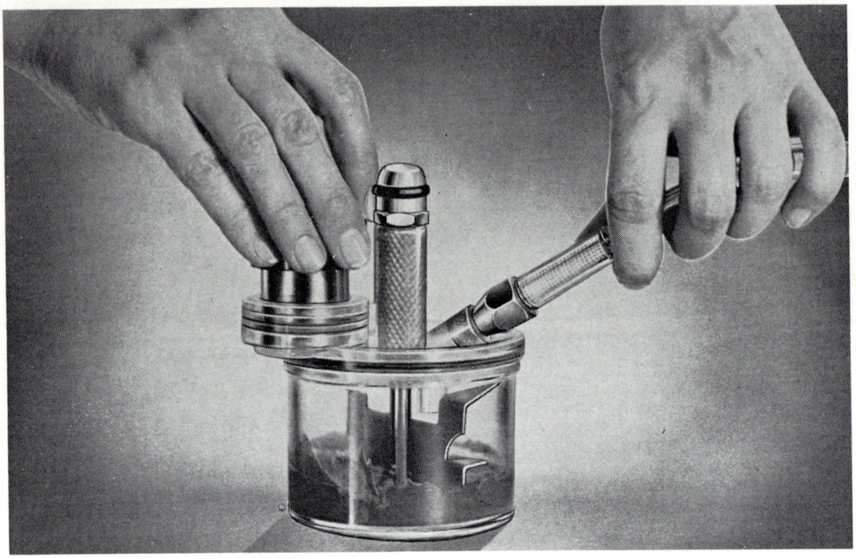

Fig. 20-33. Vacuum hose attached to mixing bowl with inlay ring, base, and mounted wax pattern in position. (Courtesy Whip-Mix Corporation.)

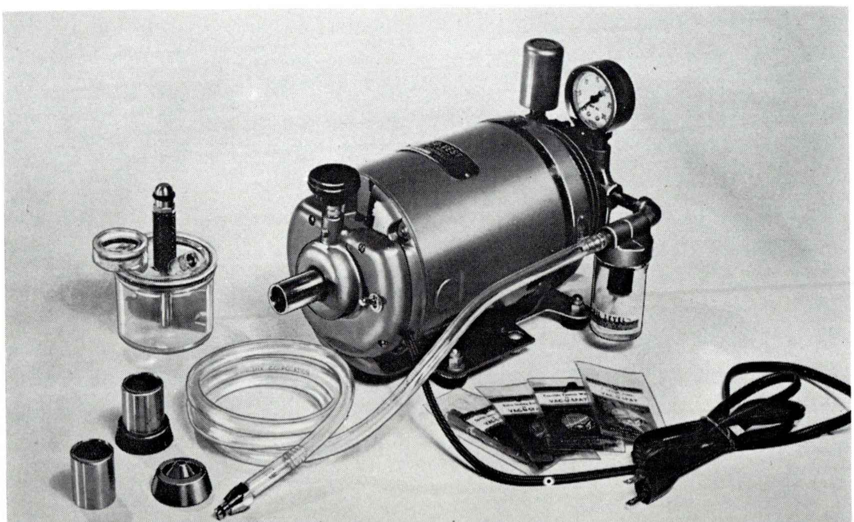

Fig. 20-34. Vac-U-Spat mixer, vibrator, and vacuum pump. (Courtesy Whip-Mix Corporation.)

A

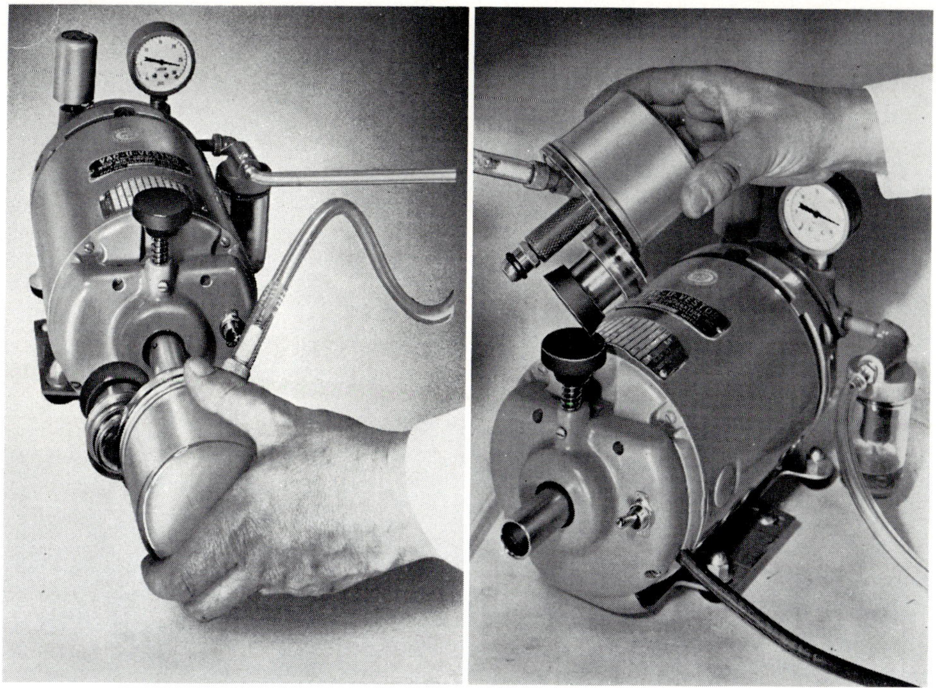

B

Fig. 20-35. A, Mixing investment under vacuum. **B,** Vibrating investment into ring, still under vacuum. (Courtesy Whip-Mix Corporation.)

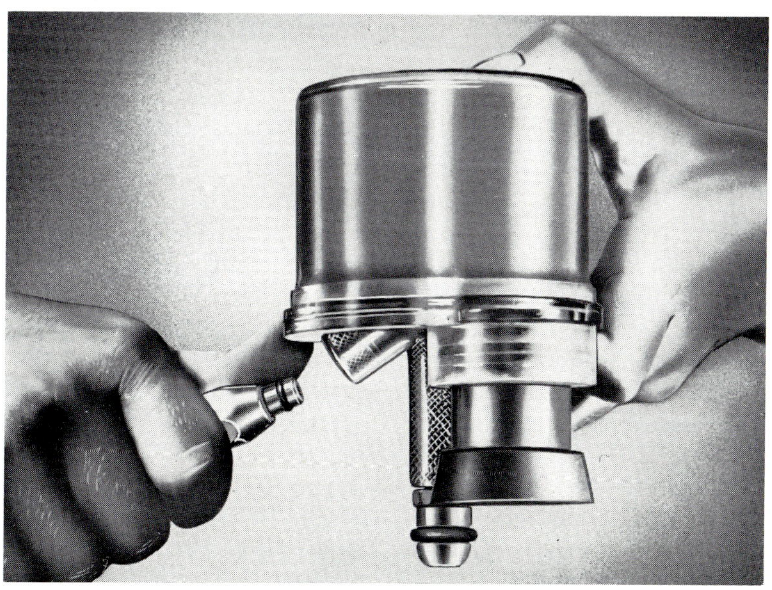

Fig. 20-36. Breaking vacuum. (Courtesy Whip-Mix Corporation.)

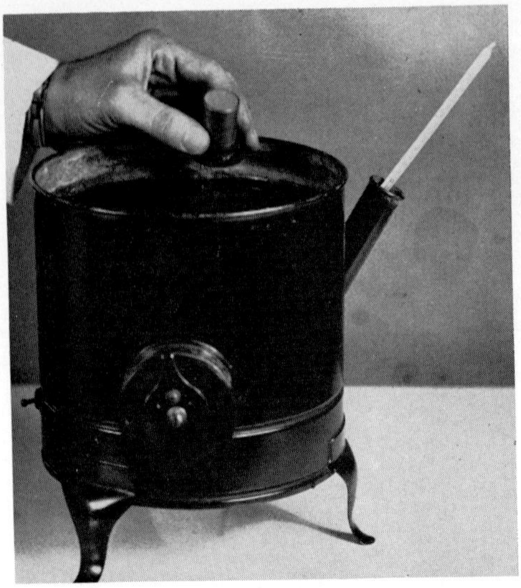

Fig. 20-37. Invested wax pattern and ring with attached rubber base submerged in water bath to obtain hygroscopic expansion of investment.

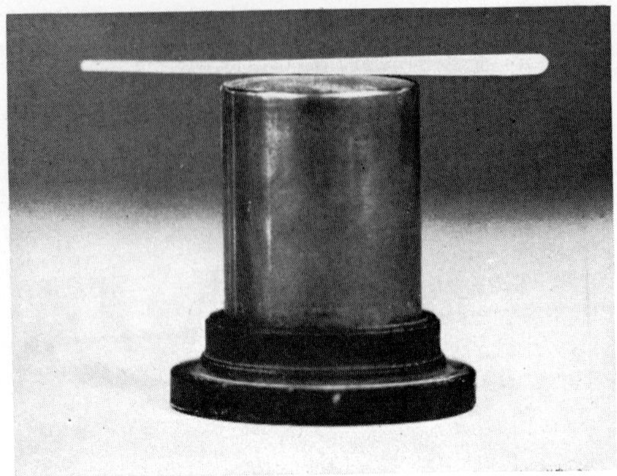

Fig. 20-38. Expansion of investment beyond end of ring following hygroscopic expansion is trimmed off.

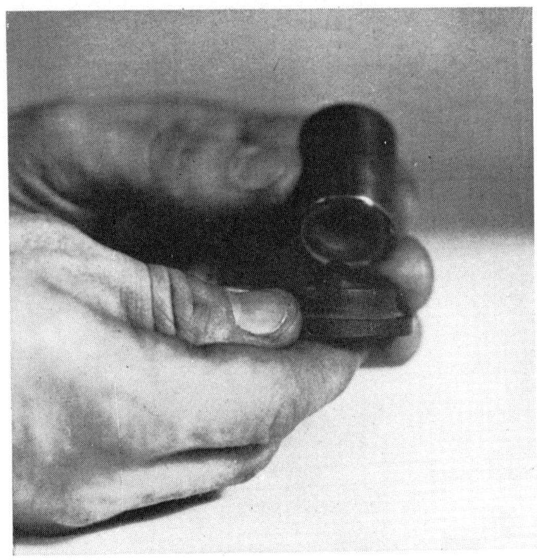

Fig. 20-39. Separating rubber base from ring after wax has been eliminated.

At the expiration of this time the mixer is withdrawn from the driving mandrel of the motor *without breaking the vacuum.*

The bowl and ring assembly are next inverted as shown in Fig. 20-35, *B*, lightly rested on the vibrator platform at the angle shown, and vibrated for about 10 seconds or until the ring is filled with investment; this may be seen since the lid of the bowl on which the ring rests is made of clear plastic. *It should be noted that the vacuum opening is held at a higher level than the hole in the lid through which the investment enters the inlay ring.*

After the inlay ring has been filled and removed from the vibrator platform, it is held firmly against the lid and the vacuum hose is released from the opening in the lid—*not before.* Now it is necessary to hold the ring and the rubber curcible former together since the vacuum is broken (Fig. 20-36).

Holding the mixer as shown (Fig. 20-36), the filled inlay ring and base are carefully removed from the mixer-top seal by gently twisting and pulling downward. Immediately the invested ring and base assembly is submerged in a water bath of 98.6 to 100° F. and left there for at least 30 minutes (Fig. 20-37).

The investment in the top of the inlay ring is in direct contact with the water. It is during this period that the setting of the investment and the phenomenon of hygroscopic expansion occur. Expansion beyond 2 percent can be obtained if desired (Fig. 20-38). After the ring base assembly is removed from the water bath, the base is separated from the ring (Fig.

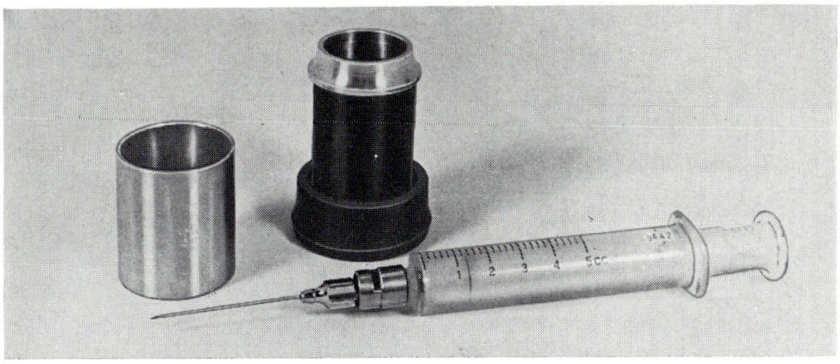

Fig. 20-40. Equipment used in controlled water addition technic. (Courtesy Whip-Mix Corporation.)

20-39) and a sprue pin is withdrawn; the investment, which has expanded beyond the open edge of the ring, is trimmed off (Fig. 20-38).

The ring is ready for placement in a furnace heated to 300° F., to eliminate the moisture from the investment, to melt the wax pattern and allow it to flow out through the sprue hole, and, finally, to allow complete thermal expansion of the investment to take place.

Controlled water added technic. A modification of the hygroscopic technic developed by Peyton showed that "the amount of hygroscopic expansion which occurs when a specific amount of water is brought into intimate contact with a dental casting investment during setting is directly related to or defined by this amount of water."[15]

In this method the metal asbestos-lined ring is not used; instead, a flexible expandable rubber ring is used as shown in Fig. 20-40. In addition, a flexible sprue base that fits the rubber ring, a metallic sleeve to encompass the rubber ring, and a narrow metallic ring to provide additional room for the water that is to be added to the investment after the ring is filled are also required. Since the water is added in very small increments, a hypodermic syringe is usually used for this purpose.

When the sprued wax pattern is mounted on the rubber base and the rubber ring is repositioned around it, the investment is mixed and placed into the ring by either the hand mechanical procedure or the vacuum investing procedure.

If vacuum is used, the supporting metal tubing must be placed around the ring prior to investing, but must be removed immediately afterward. If this metal ring were allowed to remain permanently around the flexible ring, the expansion would be restricted and proper compensation would not be effected. The flexible ring having been filled, the level of investment is struck off flush with the top of the ring. The narrow metal reservoir ring is placed in position, and the required amount of water is carefully added. The exact amount of water to be added is given in the manufacturer's instructions for the investment being used. After 45 minutes the flexible ring, reservoir ring, sprue base, and sprue pin are removed, thereby leaving the cylinder investment formed by the inside of the rubber ring. The wax is then eliminated by placing the investment mold into an oven heated to 300° F., where it remains for at least 30 minutes.

Wax elimination: oven temperature

In comparing the water added method with the customary abestos-lined, metallic-ring technic, it is obvious that the investment of the former method must be of maximum strength to withstand both high temperatures of burning out the wax and the impact of the molten metal forced into the mold not having an outer, reinforcing metallic ring. For this reason it is better to let the invested pattern set for 1 hour before placing it in the oven.

The invested inlay pattern is placed in the oven in an inverted position with the sprue hole down, in an oven maintained at a temperature of 300° F. for 30 minutes. This allows the bulk of the wax to melt and flow out through the sprue opening, leaving only a thin film of wax to be later volatilized at a higher temperature. The cylinder of investment is now placed with the sprue hole up, so that any gases of volatilization may escape freely through the opening. Failure to remove all vestiges of wax may result in poor margins of the casting. It is important also that the gases can escape easily, or a thin layer of carbon may be formed over the walls of the mold thus impairing the margins of the casting.

The temperature of the oven is allowed to rise to 1200°, or to 1300° F. if the "high-heat" method of expansion and mold temperature is desired; or it is only raised to 700° to 900° F. if the "low-heat" method of wax elimination is used. The "low-heat" temperatures are generally used if the hygroscopic method is used, due to the fact that usually 1.3 to 1.4 percent of hygroscopic expansion has already been obtained, and only a small percentage of thermal expansion, 0.4 to 0.8 percent, is needed. This amount of expansion is obtainable between 700° and 900° F. However, to assure complete elimination of the wax it is recommended that all hygroscopic investments be held between 700° and 900° F. for a full 60 minutes. Likewise, for the "high-heat" method, the Type I *thermal* inlay casting investment is used, whereas the Type II *hygroscopic* investment is used for the "low-heat" technic (A.D.A. Specification No. 2 for dental inlay casting investments). For a more comprehensive understanding of the phenomena involved in hygroscopic expansion of dental casting investments, the reader is referred to the standard textbooks on dental materials.[3-5]

Casting

After the invested ring is removed from the furnace, the casting should be made within 1 minute or less. If a longer time is taken, the ring, if asbestos lined, will cool approximately 50° F. per minute; without the asbestos liner, it cools approximately 100° F. per minute.

To expedite the casting operation, it is advisable to preheat the ingot of gold that is to be used in casting; this may be done on a charcoal block with a reducing, blowpipe flame. When the gold on the charcoal block has been brought up to a molten state, the flame is laid aside, the invested ring removed from the furnace and placed in the casting machine, and the preheated nugget of gold immediately placed in the crucible. The reducing flame of the blowpipe is again applied, the gold melted, and the casting made. In this way very little time elapses between the removal of the ring from the furnace and the actual casting of the inlay. Later a method will be given for melting gold in an electrically heated muffle, where the exact temperature of the melt is under the control of the dentist.

Casting golds. In selecting the gold alloys for casting bridge retainers, it is a protection to the dentist to use only those alloys which meet the specifications for dental inlay casting golds as formulated by the Research Commission of the American Dental Association at the Bureau of Standards. Specification 5 classifies the inlay casting golds into four groups: soft, medium, hard, and extra hard, also designated as Types A, B, C, and D gold alloys. The hard or Type C alloys are usually used for bridge retainers. Type C golds are those that contain at least

78 percent of the gold and platinum group metals and have a Brinell hardness number ranging from 90 to 140, a maximum elongation of approximately 12 percent, and a yield of 27,000 pounds per square inch as a minimum requirement. This type of gold alloy has a minimum fusing range of approximately 1650° F. The very hard Type D casting gold is frequently used in the thinner types of retainers, such as the three-quarter extracoronal restorations; it is also used when the bridge span is longer than usual.

Type C golds differ from the Type A primarily in that they are capable of being hardened by heat treatment. This property of the alloy exists because its composition is such that its chemical formula and its physical properties may undergo definite changes under controlled heat treatment while the metal is in a solid state. This property is not possessed by alloys consisting almost entirely of pure gold.

The fact that a Type C gold alloy does not have a definite solidification point, but instead a solidification range, makes it easier to obtain an accurate and sharp casting with such an alloy than with pure gold, which freezes at a definite temperature. Enough of the alloy should be used to fill both the inlay mold and the reservoir and still leave a residual button equal in volume to the casting.

While it is best to use a new batch of alloy for each casting, reservoirs and residual buttons from previous castings may be remelted and used again, provided they are thoroughly cleaned of all investment. When remelting gold alloy, it is advisable to add some new metal to that previously used. After a metal has been recast several times, it may become sluggish in the molten state or the castings may come out coarse and pitted; in such event it is quite probable that some of the basic ingredients of the alloy have been destroyed and its original composition considerably altered. This may occur if the alloy originally contained zinc as one of its ingredients and if an oxidizing flame was used.[3-5]

Melting the gold alloy. One of the important precautions to observe when melting gold alloy is to adjust the flame so that the tip of the reducing cone comes in contact with the metal. This part of the flame not only prevents oxidation of the metal, but also is the hottest portion; consequently, it reduces the alloy to a molten state in the shortest possible time.

It is well to keep the molten alloy well fluxed.

The temperature and the condition of the gold at the time it is cast into the mold are very important. When gold alloy is melted, it passes through several characteristic stages. If the casting is made in a centrifugal machine, the crucible is sometimes lined with asbestos before the alloy is placed in it. The alloy should be placed on the side of the crucible rather than in its deepest part; by placing it on the side, the reducing flame is enabled to melt it more quickly, and, when melted, it flows to the bottom of the crucible. At this initial stage of fluidity, however, the molten alloy is fairly sluggish and of a light orange color. A casting made at this stage is likely to result in an incomplete casting or one having rounded margins.

The flame is continued, therefore, until the button of gold is changed to a lighter hue and appears to be spinning under the flame. While it is fairly safe to cast at this stage of fluidity, when using the higher fusing casting golds, it is suggested that the flame be applied for several seconds longer, when the gold will be in a very fluid state and have a light hue. It may then be cast.

If at any time the molten alloy is covered with a thin film of oxidation, this may be readily removed by applying a flux. Although illuminating gas and air is the melting agent most frequently used, other combinations may also be employed, such

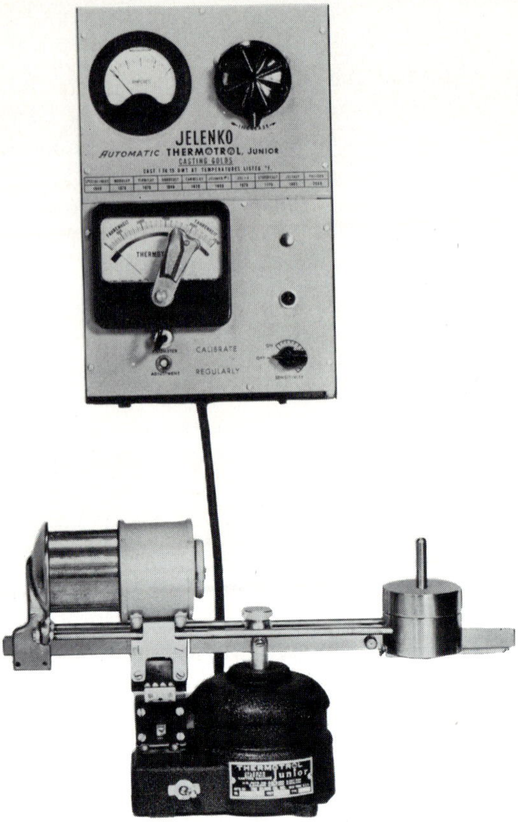

Fig. 20-41. Automatically controlled electric casting machine.

as oxygen and hydrogen gas and air, and illuminating gas and oxygen. If the latter types are employed, care must be exercised not to overheat the molten gold. To eliminate these undesirable possibilities, a simple, efficient and accurate method of melting gold alloys under definite temperature control is the one using an electric muffle (Fig. 20-41).

One of the cardinal rules to be observed in making a casting if a blow-torch is used is to keep the flame on the molten gold until the very instant that the casting is made; if the flame is withdrawn before the molten metal is on its way into the mold, the possibility exists of chilling the metal to a point where an imperfect or rounded casting is the result.

To summarize, these are the possible pitfalls in the melting of the gold alloy: (1) underheating the melt; (2) overheating; (3) using an oxidizing flame; (4) chilling metal before it is cast into mold; and (5) inability to cast at a predetermined casting temperature.

If the alloy is below its proper casting temperature, the casting will have rounded, indefinite margins. If overheated 300° or 400° F. above the upper limit of its melting range, the casting will cool more slowly through its melting range, since a greater amount of residual heat must be dissipated by radiation. Thus, slower cooling of the casting will give it a coarse-grained structure with little strength and little ductility. Each alloy has its most favorable casting temperature, usually 150° F. above the upper limit of its melting range. Since all reliable gold alloy manufacturers give the melting ranges of their alloys, it is a simple matter to determine the best casting temperature for each type of alloy. The Thermotrol casting machine enables the dentist to melt and cast the alloy at the exact temperature desired.

Another advantage of melting gold by electricity is that the gold is contained in a carbon crucible within the muffle in a reducing atmosphere; hence there is little danger of oxidizing the metal.

Because the alloy is maintained at its proper temperature until the instant of casting there is no opportunity for chilling the metal. There is also the practical advantage of no noise or hot blow pipe atmosphere in the laboratory procedure.

Other methods used in casting. Castings are made today either by the air pressure method or with the centrifugal types of casting machines. While some centrifugal casting machines are operated manually, most of those used today are actuated by a spring that is first wound then released to develop the centrifugal force necessary to force the molten metal into the mold. The machines are so designed that three to six turns of the casting arm wind the

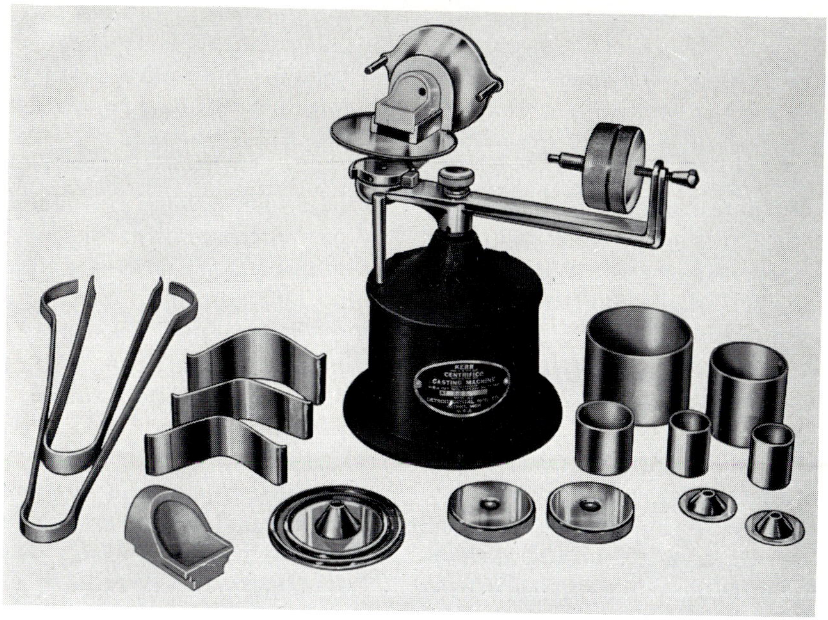

Fig. 20-42. Another type of casting machine and equipment. (Courtesy Kerr Manufacturing Co.)

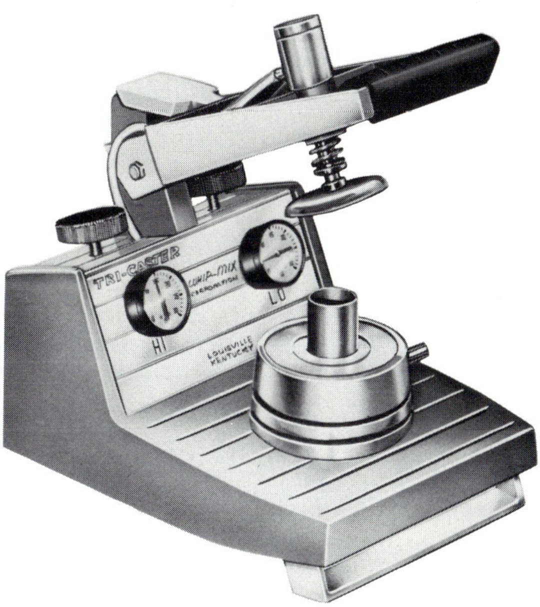

Fig. 20-43. Whip-Mix Tri-Caster.

spring sufficiently to develop the necessary casting force (Fig. 20-42).

Casting by suction alone is rarely done today because of the difficulty of maintaining a complete seal between the base of the inlay ring and the suction machine. The combination of suction and pressure is one of the recent improved methods of casting (Fig. 20-43).

Recovering the casting. After the casting has been made, it is well to leave it in the investment until the solidified gold has lost its red glow; this usually occurs in about 1 minute. The entire ring, investment, and casting may now be quenched in water. In doing so, several things are accomplished; first, it leaves the alloy in a quenched or softened condition; second, the casting will have a finer grained structure; and third, the reaction caused by the heated investment coming in contact with the cold water will facilitate the removal of the casting since the investment will be disintegrated to a large extent by this procedure. While this may be done with small castings, it is not recommended for larger ones, such as removable partial dentures.

After quenching, the casting is recovered and thoroughly scrubbed with a stiff brush; this removes any particles of investment still adhering to it. When it is difficult to remove all the investment, the casting is placed in a 40 or 50 percent solution of hydrochloric or sulfuric acid and brought to a boil. This usually cleans the casting of all investment and any surface oxides. Hydrofluoric acid is sometimes used to remove the investment. After the casting has been boiled in acid, it is neutralized in a solution of bicarbonate of soda, washed in water, and dried.

Examining the casting. Before placing the casting on the prepared tooth, it should be carefully examined with a magnifying glass to see that all surfaces are smooth and dense and that no nodules or blisters are present, especially on the cavity side of the casting. Occasionally, a small nodule may be present on an outer surface which does not come in contact with the tooth structure; this may be readily removed with a sharp instrument and still make the casting usable. The inner angles and surfaces should be particularly examined for slight imperfections, for, if present and left undiscovered, they will prevent the perfect seating of the casting within its cavity.

Another condition that frequently develops is a casting with rounded margins or a deficiency of metal in a thin area. This defect is usually the result of one of three causes: first, the alloy was not sufficiently heated before casting; second, the wax pattern was not burned out at a sufficiently high temperature; and third, insufficient casting force was used.

Castings may have all their margins sharp with the exception of one or two places; in such cases the deficiencies are sharply notched. This type of defect is the result of a piece of investment falling into the mold and lodging where the notch occurs, thus excluding the molten metal from that area. If a piece of loose investment in the mold lodges in the region of the occlusal or proximal surfaces, the casting will disclose a void having the shape of the particle of investment. This explains why the ring should be held in an inverted position when the sprue pin is removed from the investment prior to its burning out.

Where a casting is porous, particularly in the region of the sprue, the cause may be attributed to: first, the lack of a reservoir; second, the use of a sprue pin that is too long; or third, a sprue pin whose gauge is too small in diameter. If such porosity is found in the occlusal portion of a three-surface intracoronal retainer, it is quite likely that it will necessitate remaking the casting.

Ryge and others[16] classified porosities into internal and external types. The internal types. The internal porosites are caused by (1) cooling and solidification; i.e., (a) localized shrinkage, (b) subsurface porosity, (c) microporosity; (2) porosities caused by gas; i.e., (a) pinhole porosity, (b) gas inclusions.

The external porosities are: (a) those due to incomplete burnout and (b) those due to insufficient casting pressure or foreign particles.

Fortunately, most castings produced are satisfactory. When such a casting is obtained, it is placed in the tooth to verify its fit. For this initial trial, some prefer to leave the reservoir attached to the casting to act as a handle to facilitate the placing and the removal of the casting from the tooth. Others remove the residual button and the reservoir, leaving a small section of the sprue by which the casting may be readily manipulated.

Before the advent of controlled expansion in casting investments, one of the most serious difficulties was the shrinkage of the castings, resulting in too tight a fit. With the development of the expanding type of casting investments, both thermal and hygroscopic, the tendency to overexpand sometimes results in castings that fit too loosely on the tooth. While such expansion enables the dentist to seat the retainer easily in the prepared tooth, the retentive qualities of the casting are greatly reduced. Hence, in crown and bridge prosthesis an effort is made to make castings which, while fitting snugly, yet may be carried completely to place with finger pressure.

On the other hand, a casting which fits too tightly and which must be driven to place with considerable force is very prone to have unfavorable biologic reactions in the pulp, caused by the great pressure which the compressive power of the casting exerts on the dentin of the prepared cavity walls. Many teeth that develop tenderness and soreness following the placement of bridge retainers on vital teeth may trace the cause to castings that fit too tightly.

To avoid such a condition, some suggest etching the inner surfaces of the cast retainer with aqua regia to within 1 mm. of its margins. Others recommend the grinding of the inner surfaces with stones. While either method may be helpful, it should not be necessary to resort to these procedures, when by a properly controlled casting technic a retainer of the correct degree of expansion can be constructed.

After the fit of the casting has been verified in relation to the surfaces of the cavity walls, the margins, and the contour, it should also be checked in its relationship to the remaining natural teeth, i.e., its proximal, occlusal, and gingival tissue relationships.

Fitting the casting. All cutting, carving, and finishing of the gold casting should be done while the gold is in a softened condition, i.e., after the casting has been heated to 1300° F. and quenched. Such treatment of the Types C and D casting gold makes it soft, workable, and possessed of a high percentage of elongation. If much cutting of the metal is done, it may be necessary to reheat and requench the casting more than once in order to maintain its workable qualities.

Bridge retainers should receive a semifinal finish and polish before a final impression is taken for the bridge. It is not advisable, however, to finish the margins of the filling at this time; this operation is left for the final finishing operation after cementation.

Where a casting is to be set individually, such as a single complete or partial veneer crown, it is given its final polish and then hardened by suitable heat treatment. Following its heat treatment, the individual restoration is then cemented. In fixed partial denture prosthesis, however, the heat-treating process is deferred until the entire bridge is completed and polished, and just before cementation of the porcelain facings or crowns.

SELECTED REFERENCES

1. Hollenback, G. M.: The cast gold inlay, Int. Dent. J. 1:67, 1951.
2. Smith, D., and Potter, H. R.: Practical bridgework, Los Angeles, 1928, University of California Press.
3. Peyton, F. A., and others: Restorative dental materials, ed. 3, St. Louis, 1968, The C. V. Mosby Co.
4. Skinner, E. W., ad Phillips, R. W.: The science of dental materials, ed. 6, Philadelphia, 1967, W. B. Saunders Co.
5. Phillips, R. W., and Biggs, D. H.: Distortion of wax patterns as influenced by storage time, storage temperature and temperature of wax manipulation, J.A.D.A. 41:28-37, 1950.
6. Huffman, R. W., Regenos, J. W., and Taylor, R. R.: Principles of occlusion, Columbus, Ohio, 1969, H & R Press.
7. McCollum, B. B.: Fundamentals involved in prescribing restorative dental remedies, a research report, South Pasadena, California, 1955, Scientific Press.
8. Stuart, C. E.: Why dental restorations should have cusps, J. South. California Dent. Ass. 27:198, 1959.
9. Thomas, P. K.: Full mouth waxing technique for rehabilitation, San Francisco, 1967, University of California Press.
10. Granger, E. R.: Practical procedures in oral rehabilitation, Philadelphia, 1962, J. B. Lippincott Co.
11. Coleman, R. L.: Physical properties of dental materials, Bull. D. Res. 1:867, 1928.
12. Scheu, C. N.: Precision casting utilizing the

hygroscopic action of plaster in investments in making expended molds, J.A.D.A. **20**:1205, 1933.

13. Hollenback, G. M.: Thermal expansion of pattern wax, J. South. California Dent. Ass. **28**:6, 1960.
14. Mahler, D. B., and Moffitt, R. E.: Further evidence of the hygroscopic expansion of dental gypsum materials, J. Dent. Res. **37**: 95, 1958.
15. Peyton, F. A., and others: Controlled water-addition techniques for hygroscopic expansion of dental casting investments, J.A.D.A. **52**:155, 1956.
16. Ryge, G., and others: Porosities in dental gold castings, J. Dent. Res. **54**:746, 1957.

GENERAL REFERENCES

Aplin, A. W., Sorenson, F. M., and Cantwell, K. R.: Method for measuring temperature changes in the tooth during restorative procedures, J. Dent. Res. **42**:925-933, 1963.

Asano, K., The depth of the gingival sulcus, II: J. Tokyo Dent. College Soc. **67**:40, 1967.

Asgar, K., Mahler, D. B., and Peyton, F. A.: Hygroscopic technique for inlay casting using controlled water addition, J. Prosth. Dent. **5**: 711, 1955.

Asgar, K.: Effects of different investments on the sulfide contamination of the imbedded metals in casting procedure, J. Dent. Res. **40**:767, 1961.

Asgar, K., and Peyton, F. A.: Pits on inner surfaces of cast gold crowns, J. Prosth. Dent. **9**:448, 1959.

Asher, H. H.: Galvanoplasty in dentistry, D. Digest **42**:300, 1936.

Barone, J. J., Huff, R. L., and Dickson, G.: Surface roughness of gold casting, D. Progress **1**:78, 1961.

Bartelle, A.: Technic for direct wax patterns of three-quarter crowns, J.A.D.A. **42**:138, 1951.

Bassett, R. W., and Stauts, B. M.: Evaluation of electrochemical milling (stripping) versus etching with aqua regia, J. Southern California D. A. **34**:478, 1966.

Behrend, D. A.: Temporary protective restorations in crown and bridge work, Aust. Dent. J. **12**(5):411-416, 1967.

Bharucha, D. P.: Improved types of casting sprues, J. All India D. A. **29**:132, 1956.

de Boer, J. G.: An inlay is as good as its margin's fit, Nederl. T. Tandheelk. **74**(5):347-353, 1967.

Braden, M.: Heat conduction in teeth and the effect of lining materials, J. Dent. Res. **43**: 315-322, 1964.

Brown, M. H.: Impression procedures for restorative dentistry, Dent. Clin. N. Amer. pp. 147-161, March, 1967.

Braasch, W. F.: Preparation and wax patterns for single and multiple inlays, North-West Dent. **40**:3, 1961.

Brumfield, R. C.: Dental gold structures, New York, 1949, J. F. Jelenko & Co.

Cannistraci, A. J.: A new approach to impression taking for crown and bridge, Dent. Clin. N. Amer., pp. 33-42, March, 1965.

Charbeneau, G. T.: Some effects of cavity roughness on adaptation of gold castings, J. Dent. Res. **37**:95, 1958.

Chong, J. A., Chong, M. P., and Docking, A. R.: The surface of gypsum cast in alginate impressions, D. Pract. **16**:107, 1965.

Christensen, G. J.: The effect of water swaging on stress and strain in dental-wax patterns, J. Dent. Res. **44**:930-934, 1965.

Christensen, G. J.: Marginal fit of gold inlay castings, J. Prosth. Dent. **16**:297, 1966.

Cohn, L. A.: The gold thimble-acrylic resin pattern: an improved technique in prosthodontics, J. Prosth. Dent. **15**:1076-1093, 1965.

Council on Dental Materials and Devices: New American Dental Association specification No. 21 adopted, J.A.D.A. **78**(3):577-579, 1969.

Courtade, G. L.: Pin pointers, I: new instruments, J. Prosth. Dent. **16**:4, 1966.

Courtade, G. L.: Pin pointers, II: venting and cross pinning, J. Prosth. Dent. **16**:5, 1966.

Craig, R. G., Eick, J. D., and Peyton, F. A.: The properties of natural waxes used in dentistry, J. Dent. Res. **44**:1308-1316, 1965.

Craig, R. G., Eick, J. D., and Peyton, F. A.: Strength properties of waxes at various temperatures and their practical application, J. Dent. Res. **46**:300, 1967.

Custer, F., and Diemer, R.: Porosities in dental gold castings: effects in sprue size, investment manipulation, venting and casting pressure, J. Missouri Dent. Ass. **47**(8):10-15, 1967.

Earnshaw, R.: The effect of restrictive stress on the setting expansion of gypsum bonded investments, Aust. J. Dent. **9**:169-176, 1964.

Earnshaw, R., and Marks, B. I.: The measurement of setting time of gypsum products, Aust. J. Dent. **9**:17-26, 1964.

Freimark, J.: Waxing procedures for crown and bridge work, Cereb. Palsy Rev. **1**:3-5, 1966.

Fusayama, T., and others: Distortion of castings due to reheating in investment, Bull. Tokyo Med. Dent. Univ. **12**:373-377, 1965.

Henry, R. W., and Phillips, R. W.: Influence of particle size of stone on surface detail of casts, J. Prosth. Dent. **11**:169, 1961; J. Oral Surg., Anes. & Hosp. D. Serv. **19**:63, 1961.

Henry, R. W., and Phillips, R. W.: Reproducing surface detail with electroplated impressions, D. Progress **2**:29, 1961.

Henschel, C. J.: Direct gold inlay, Oral Hyg. **52**: 37, 1962.

Herrick, P. W.: Hygroscopic with control water added technic, Chron. Omaha Dist. D. Soc. **23**:272, 1960.

Higashiguchi, S.: Studies on precision dental casting, with special reference to technics for depressing the setting expansion of an investment, J. Osaka Odont. Soc. **31**(1):1-16, 1968.

Hollenback, G. M., and others: An evaluation of the accuracy of the one-piece cast partial denture, J. S. California Dent. Ass. **41**:496-500, 1965.

Hollenback, G. M., and Smith, D. D.: A further investigation of the physical properties of hard gypsums, J. S. California Dent. Ass. **43**: 221-227, 1967.

Hosoda, H.: The effects of various lining technics on longitudinal expansion of dental casting investments, J. S. California Dent. Ass. **33**:428-433, 1965.

Jones, D. W., and Wilson, H. J.: Variables affecting the thermal expansion of refractory investments, Brit. Dent. J. **125**(6):249-255, 1968.

Jørgensen, K. D.: The hygroscopic setting expansion of gypsum, Acta Odont. Scand. **18**: 461-477, 1960.

Kahl, R. E.: Simplified method for precision castings, Dental Digest, **73**:404, 1967.

Krikos, A.: Self-curing resins in constructing patterns for small castings, J. Prosth. Dent. **20** (3):235, 1968.

Kusner, W., and Michman, I.: Setting expansion of plaster of Paris, J. Dent. Res. **46**(4):661-665, 1967.

Kusner, W.: Final expansion of plaster, J. Dent. Res. **47**:694, 1968.

Linkow, L. I.: Copper plating of impressions, J. Prosth. Dent. **16**:1116, 1966.

Lorey, R. E., Asgar, K., and Peyton, F. A.: Multiunit bridge castings utilizing the water added hygroscopic investing technic, I.A.D.R. Abstract M31 40th general meeting, St. Louis, Mo., March, 1962.

Mahler, D. B., and Ady, A. B.: An explanation for the hygroscopic setting expansion of dental gypsum products, J. Dent. Res. **39**:578-589, 1960.

Mahler, D. B., and Asgarzadeh, K.: The volumetric contraction of dental gypsum materials on setting, J. Dent. Res. **32**:354-361, 1953.

Mahler, D. B., and Ady, A. B.: The effect of the water bath in hygroscopic casting techniques, J. Prosth. Dent. **15**:1115, 1965.

Mahler, D. B., and Ady, A. B.: The influence of various factors on the effective setting expansion of casting investments, J. Prosth. Dent. **13**:365-373, 1963.

Marcum, J. S.: The tissue response to different crown marginal depths, S. Carolina Dent. J. **26**:13-20, 1968.

Mason, H. J.: Sprue size adjustment in dental castings, theory of control of heatflow, North-West Dent. **40**:291, 1961.

Meyer, F. S.: Shrinkage in cast gold inlays, D. Cosmos **54**:758-764, 1912.

Mumford, G., and Phillips, R. W.: Dimensional change in wax patterns during setting of gypsum investments, J. Dent. Res. **37**:351-358, 1958.

Ohashi, M., and Paffenbarger, G. C.: Melting, flow, and thermal expansion characteristics of some dental and commercial waxes, J.A.D.A. **72**:1141-1150, 1966.

Ohashi, M., Stanford, J. W., and Paffenbarger, G. C.: Pertinent data on some physical properties of different investments used in the casting of gold alloys, J. Nihon University **9**(3): 121, 1967.

Overberger, J. E., and Samay, H. J.: Strength properties of dental stone, West Virginia Dent. J. **42**:23-28, 1968.

Paffenbarger, G. C.: New developments in dental materials—a world wide survey, Int. Dent. J. **15**(3):356-358, 1965.

Peyton, F. A.: Significance of dental materials science to the practice of dentistry, J. Dent. Educ. **30**:268-277, 1966.

Peyton, F. A., and Craig, R. G.: Compatibility of duplicating compounds and casting investments, J. Prosth. Dent. **12**:1111, 1962.

Phillips, R. W.: Recent improvements in dental materials that the operative dentist should know, J.A.D.A. **73**:84-90, 1966.

Powers, J. M., Craig, R. G., and Peyton, F. A.: Calorimetric analysis of commercial and dental waxes, J. Dent. Res. **48**:1165, 1969.

Rogers, O. W., and Armstrong, B. W.: Electroforming a gold matrix for indirect inlays, J. Prosth. Dent. **11**:959, 1961.

Sahs, E. A., and Wick, J. H.: Determining the accuracy of inlays by mercury micro-measurement, D. Progress, **3**:26, 1963.

Scheu, C. H.: A new precision casting technic, J.A.D.A. **19**:630-633, 1932.

Shaheen, H. M.: Behavior of the casting investment in the mold cavity and its effect on the wax pattern during setting, Egypt Dent. J. **13** (2):3-21, 1967.

Shell, J. S.: The effect of longitudinal restrictive force on hygroscopic expansion, J. Dent. Res. **40**:287-293, 1961.

Shell, J. S., and others: Amount of compensation for casting shrinkage required at different mold temperatures, J. S. California Dent. Ass. **33**:517-519, 1965.

Shell, J. S., and others: Setting and thermal investment expansion in longitudinal and transverse directions, J. S. California Dent. Ass. **41**: 511-514, 1965.

Skinner, E. W., and Degni, F.: Hygroscopic expansion of dental investments, J.A.D.A. **54**: 603-608, 1957.

Skinner, E. W., and others: Influence of the asbestos liner and size of the casting ring on the mold setting expansion, I.A.D.R. **40**:91, 1962 (abst.).

Smith, D. C., Earnshaw, R., and McCrorie, J. W.: Some properties of modelling and baseplate waxes, Brit. Dent. J. **118**:437-442, 1965.

Smyd, E. S.: Factors which influence casting accuracy: a universal casting technic, J.A.D.A. **36**:160-172, 1948.

Souder, W., and Sweeney, W. T.: Tentative specifications for dental casting investments, J.A.D.A. **17**:780, 1930.

Stibbs, G. D.: Mechanical separators, Ferrier design, J. Prosth. Dent. **17**:603, 1967.

Sturdevant, C. M.: Impressions for direct inlays, J.A.D.A. **54**:360, 1957.

Suno, Y. G., Smith, D. C., and Skinner, E. W.: Effect of accelerators and retarders on the setting and crystal structure of plaster, J. D. Res. **40**:765, 1961.

Taggart, W. H.: A new method of making gold inlays, D. Cosmos **49**:1120, 1907.

Taggart, W. H.: Cast gold inlays—a clinical demonstration and lectures, D. Items Interest **29**: 949, 1907.

Teteruck, W. R., and Mumford, G.: The fit of certain dental casting alloys using different investing materials and techniques, J. Prosth. Dent. **16**(5):910-927, 1966.

Tuccillo, J. J., and Nielsen, J. P.: Sprue design for cast gold alloys, Dental Laboratory Review, June-July, 1964.

Tuccillo, J. J.: The influence of investment on casting fit, Thermotrol Technician **21**:1967.

Van Aken, J.: Distortions of inlay wax patterns caused by investment setting or expansion, D. Abst. **7**:266, 1962.

Van Horn, C. S.: Concerning casting methods and casting devices, D. Cosmos **52**:664, 1910.

Van Horn, C. S.: Standardizing the investing process and simplifying the casting process, D. Cosmos **53**:1109-1119, 1911.

Waerhaug, J.: Histologic considerations which govern where the margins of restorations should be located in relation to the gingiva, Dent. Clin. N. Amer., pp. 161-176, March, 1960.

Wagner, A. W., Burkhart, J. W., and Fayle, H. E., Jr.: Contouring abutment teeth with cast gold inlays for removable partial dentures, J. Prosth. Dent. **20**:330, 1968.

Chapter 21

Construction of retainers: indirect method–materials, equipment, and procedures (hydrocolloids)

HYDROCOLLOIDS—REVERSIBLE AND IRREVERSIBLE

Although great accuracy is obtained in the construction of inlays, crowns, and bridges by the use of the direct method at the chair, the accompanying fatigue and time consumed on the part of both the dentist and the patient resulted in a search for a method that would enable the dentist to reduce his chair time, to increase the number of patient appointments, and to delegate most of the laboratory work to the technician.

In the indirect method the wax pattern is not made directly on the prepared tooth in the mouth but on a die made of stone, metal, or a refractory material. Customarily the dies are removable from the working cast. Many men have contributed to the development of the technics and materials presently used in this method.

Die fabricated in elastic impression materials

The dies may be made of amalgam, of one of the Hydrocal stones, of electrodeposited metal, or of a high thermal refractive investment material.

THE DIFFERENCES BETWEEN MAKING A WAX PATTERN DIRECTLY ON THE TOOTH AND INDIRECTLY ON DIES

Tooth

Body temperature changes to room temperature on removal from tooth.

There is moisture content of tooth tissue.

There is difficulty of access to the cavity and to contour the wax pattern.

Usually there is need for a matrix to confine the wax in intracoronal patterns.

Lubricant is usually saliva.

Type I inlay wax is used.

There is need for more total expansion.

Die

Types of impression materials that can be used to take impression:

A. Hydrocolloid
   1. Stone die: Class 2 dental stone used
   2. Ceramic investment die with refractory bond
   3. Colloidal metal powder with stone or polymer binder
   4. Amalgam
   5. Electroforming
      a. copper
      b. silver
   6. The porous materials are Nos. 1 and 2, the nonporous are Nos. 3, 4, and 5

Type II inlay casting wax is used for the indirect method

Because the pattern is made out of the mouth there is no necessity for compensating for the contraction of wax from body to room temperature, 0.3 to 0.5°.

It is necessary to use some form of artificial lubricant on the die.

The pattern will require less total expansion than one made in the mouth.

No need for a matrix in the intracoronal preparations.

There is ease of access.

The wax pattern may be easily reproduced on the die if a casting failure occurs.

It is possible to verify the fit of the casting on the die before trial is made in the mouth.

Saves time at the chair in waxing directly on the tooth.

Initial trimming and adjusting of the occlusal and contact areas may be made on the die and working model.

Saves the number of patient appointments required.

It is possible to use two types of wax in making the wax pattern by placing the softer and the hard regular wax in those areas of the wax pattern which will respond to the initial and the hydroscopic setting expansion, which takes place in the pattern when invested. (Regular blue wax or the softer green wax may be used.)

Metal dies

Amalgam:

The impression of the prepared tooth must be taken in an inelastic impression material (Electrodeposited die: copper, silver).

Metal dies are good conductors of heat, therefore wax cools rapidly and contracts.

It is advisable to warm the die slightly before applying the wax so as to reduce the internal stresses in the wax.

The instruments used should also be slightly warmed during the carving process.

The die must be thoroughly lubricated before waxing.

DISADVANTAGES OF THE INDIRECT METHOD

There are more steps involved in the indirect method than in the direct. The impression material involved in taking the impression offers many possible pitfalls; the material used in constructing the die also offers many possible errors in manipulation; and, finally, the wax used in constructing the wax pattern offers the same problems as those found in the direct method.

The development of the indirect method passed through several stages—first, employing modeling compound, Dietrich's impression material, and similar products. This gradually led to the development of other elastic impression materials and technics that are at present being used extensively by the dental profession. The materials most generally used are the reversible hydrocolloids of the agar-agar type, the irreversible hydrocolloids of the alginate type, the mercaptan rubber base type, and, finally, the silicone base type.

One of the earliest methods utilized modeling compound that was heated and placed within a copper band to take an impression of a cavity or of a complete crown preparation. Silver or copper amalgam was mixed and packed into the impression. When the amalgam set completely after 12 to 24 hours, it was removed from the impression, softened in warm water, and was trimmed to the desired shape so that it could be made removable from the working cast. The wax pattern was made on the lubricated amalgam die, inserted in the cast, and its fit verified. The complete procedure also takes place when a removable die is utilized to construct a complete porcelain veneer crown. The same method, with slight modifications, is usable for other types of crowns and for intracoronal and extracoronal bridge retainers.

The main objections to the use of an amalgam die are: the time elapsing from taking the impression to having a workable die (usually 12 to 24 hours); the difficulty sometimes encountered in removing the compound impression from the tooth if any undercuts exist or if some compound flowed into the interproximal space at the cervical level; and the possible danger of irritating the pulp if the material was overheated and applied to the vital prepared tooth. Some operators cite as an objection the additional cost of the amalgam used. Attention should also be called to the fact that amalgam cannot be used successfully in elastic impressions because amalgam must be placed and condensed against firm, resisting surfaces of tooth tissue, a metal matrix, or other rigid material.

That the indirect technic is being used more generally in dentistry is due primarily to the development of materials that can accurately reproduce all areas and types of preparations and retain their dimensional accuracy upon removal from the mouth.

As materials were improved, so were the technics in their use. Special trays were designed to replace those using modeling compound; brushes and syringes were substituted to cover the prepared abutments with the hydrocolloid. These helped to expedite the technic at the chair and enabled the dentist to have complete control of the time and temperature factors, which are so important in the indirect technic for complete accuracy.

HYDROCOLLOID IMPRESSION MATERIALS

All methods and materials used today have their indications and contraindications. While it is true that most restorations can be constructed by the indirect method, those dentists who have for years utilized the direct method can make a wax pattern directly in the mouth in a fraction of the time that it takes to prepare the materials and trays, take the impressions, and pour up the models in order to make the pattern indirectly. Even when a technician is immediately available, it is still a matter of judgment whether to make a single, simple wax pattern in the mouth directly or indirectly.

The hydrocolloid is by definition "a colloid with water as the dispersion medium." There are two general types of hydrocolloids that may be used in the indirect technic: (1) the reversible or agar-agar type and (2) the irreversible or alginate type.

The agar-agar type of hydrocolloid is obtained from certain types of seaweed, and has a gelation temperature at or above mouth temperature.

The irreversible hydrocolloid is some form of soluble alginate. An alginate is a salt of alginic acid that is extracted from marine kelp. Sodium or potassium alginate may be used.

The difference between the two types of hydrocolloids lies in the method by which the gel is formed in the mouth.

The reversible hydrocolloid (agar-agar type) is heated in water and is changed to a sol or liquid condition. In this condition it is placed in a tray and carried to the mouth, whereupon the sol is changed to a gel by circulating cold water through the tray. When the entire mass within the tray has cooled sufficiently until it gels, the tray with hydrocolloid is then removed from the mouth; it contains an accurate impression of the teeth and the adjacent tissues.

The irreversible hydrocolloid (alginate type) consists of a soluble alginate dissolved in water; it is mixed in a bowl to form an insoluble gel. To give the material sufficient working time, retarders are usually incorporated in it. The mix is similarly placed in a tray and carried to the mouth. After a few minutes, a chemical reaction takes place, forming a gel that takes an accurate impression of the teeth and the adjacent tissues. The insoluble gel so formed is a calcium alginate.

This type of hydrocolloid was used in 1925 by A. Poller[1] of Vienna and subsequently by E. H. Golden in 1932.[2] Since their introduction, the materials and technic have received the attention of many dentists and researchers; at the present time both types of hydrocolloids are capable of producing casts with a high degree of accuracy.

As with other materials used in dentistry, the elastic impression material is not a panacea. It has its advantages and disadvantages.

Among the advantages the following may be listed:

1. In mouth reconstruction all the abutment preparations may be accurately reproduced with their proper relationships to each other in the arch.
2. Its use conserves the patient's time.

3. It conserves the dentist's time at the chair and also much of his nervous energy.
4. Dental service is rendered to the patient in a shorter length of time.
5. A high degree of accuracy is possible because each operation may be checked back on the model during the construction process.
6. Present-day equipment and materials have been highly improved, simplifying the technic greatly.
7. The technic, if meticulously followed, is a relatively simple one.
8. Use of the hydrocolloids enables the dentist to utilize the services of a good technician to the fullest extent.
9. It is possible to establish the contact areas between restorations beforehand.
10. The major waxing and the finishing of the restoration may be accomplished beforehand.
11. Use of the material enables one to record accurately in the impression any undercuts and dovetails.

Among the disadvantages the following may be listed:

1. The technic is not foolproof, but because of its relative simplicity, there is a danger that it might be abused by the careless operator.
2. A certain degree of care and skill is necessary in its use.
3. The stone dies ordinarily used in the technic are more fragile than those made of amalgam or electroformed metals.
4. To use this technic to its greatest advantage, it is usually necessary to have an assistant or a technician available to pour the dies or the model immediately or within a period of 30 minutes.
5. If the dentist must do this himself at the sacrifice of chair time, it is not usually economical for him to do so.
6. There is the possibility of injuring the gingival tissues, including the periodontal membrane, when the gum is retracted.
7. There is the possibility of burning the soft tissues of the patient if the operator is careless or if he does not have the proper equipment.

Research shows that it is possible to obtain accurate results by the use of the alginate impression materials. Because of the greater number of variables in the alginate materials and their manipulation, it has been the experience of most dentists using the indirect method to prefer the agar-agar, reversible type of hydrocolloids and the rubber type. The following technic will refer to the reversible, agar-agar type of hydrocolloid.

REVERSIBLE (AGAR-AGAR) IMPRESSION MATERIAL

Although the composition of the reversible hydrocolloids is not printed on the package containing the material, most of the products consist of the following approximate composition: 80 percent water, 15 percent agar-agar, 5 percent thermoplastics, inert materials, chemicals, antiseptics, and so on. The physical properties of hydrocolloids produced by different manufacturers vary because the seaweed from which the agar is obtained may be from different species and from different parts of the world. Therefore, it is important to acquaint oneself with the physical properties and phenomena that accompany the use of the specific material used and to follow the instructions given by the manufacturer since these are based on the results of extensive experiments conducted in their research departments.

To use the reversible hydrocolloid successfully, it must be liquefied at or slightly below the boiling point of water; subsequently it must be applied to the oral tissues at a temperature not harmful to the tissues. It must be capable of becoming a stiff gel at a lowered temperature within

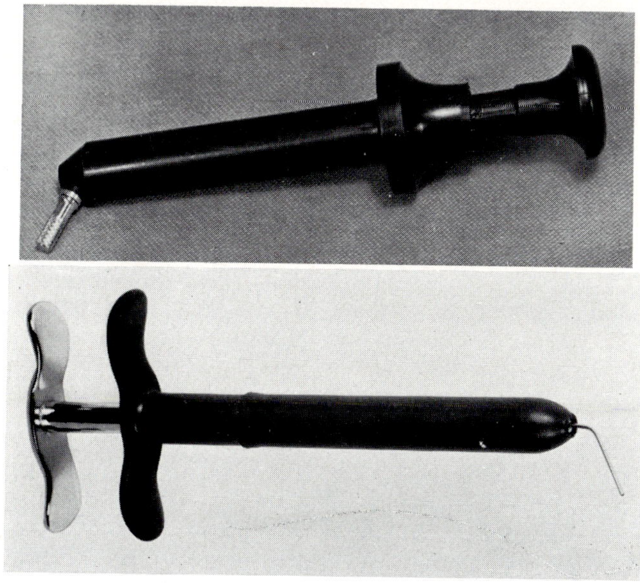

Fig. 21-1. Small syringes used to inject hydrocolloid in cavity preparation. (Courtesy Dr. M. J. Thompson.)

a reasonable length of time; it must give an accurate impression without distortion.

The indirect technic, employing reversible hydrocolloid, involves ten distinct phases of procedure:

1. Liquefying the material by boiling for a least 8 minutes.
2. Storing the boiled material in the syringes or tubes at a temperature of 150° to 155° F. and holding it at this temperature until ready for use.
3. Lowering the temperature of the tray material by placing it in the tempering chamber at a temperature between 102° and 115° F. and holding that temperature between 5 and 15 minutes.
4. Injecting the fluid hydrocolloid through the needle in the small syringe into the prepared teeth.
5. Filling, tempering, and placing the tray in the mouth after scraping off the top layer of hydrocolloid that was exposed to the water.

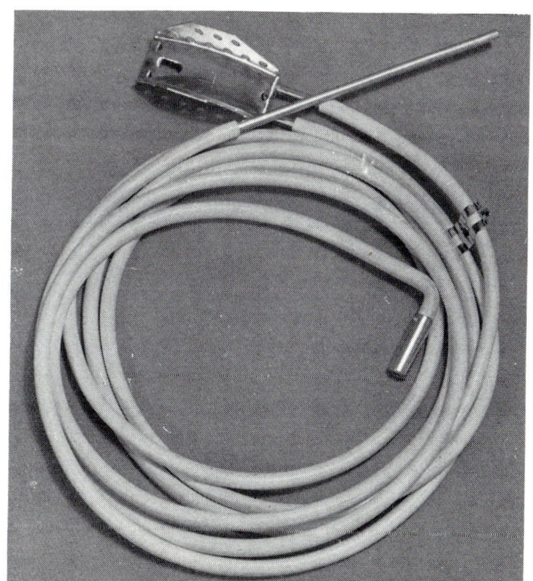

Fig. 21-2. Thompson water-cooled perforated tray. (Courtesy Dr. M. J. Thompson.)

6. Changing the sol into a gel by the circulation of 50 to 60° F. water through the tray.
7. Treatment of the impression after removal from the mouth.
8. Pouring the stone dies and the master model.
9. Waxing and casting the units of the restoration.
10. Assembling and finishing the restoration.

Although it is possible to obtain satisfactory results with the hydrocolloid material without equipment designed for this purpose, it will prove economical to utilize the special equipment developed for this technic. The specially designed small syringes (Fig. 21-1) for injecting the material into the cavity preparation will facilitate this step in the procedure. Water-cooled trays of different designs (Figs. 21-2 and 21-3) are also available in the par-

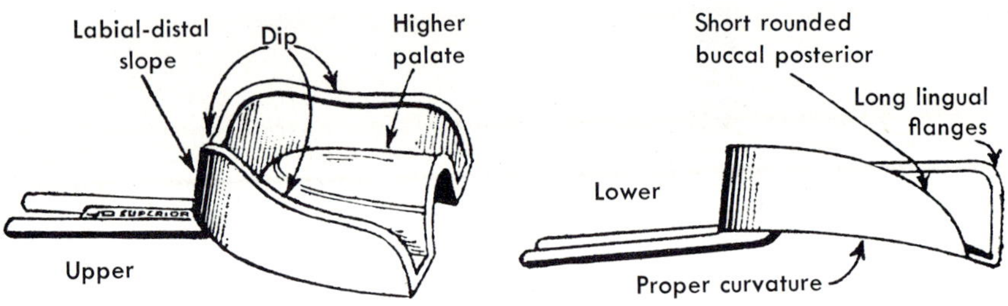

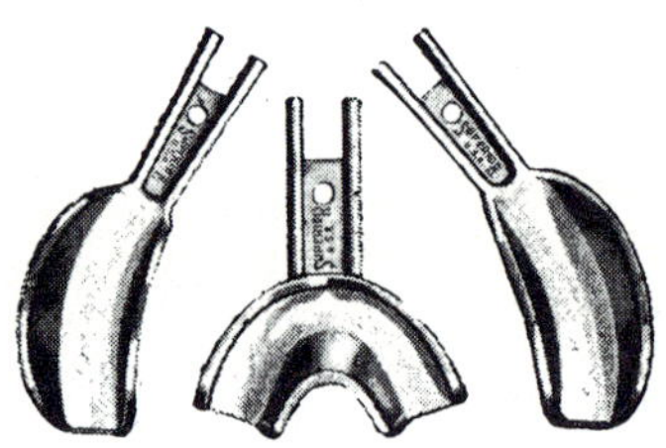

Fig. 21-3. Superior water-cooled rim-lock trays. (Courtesy Blue Island Specialty Co.)

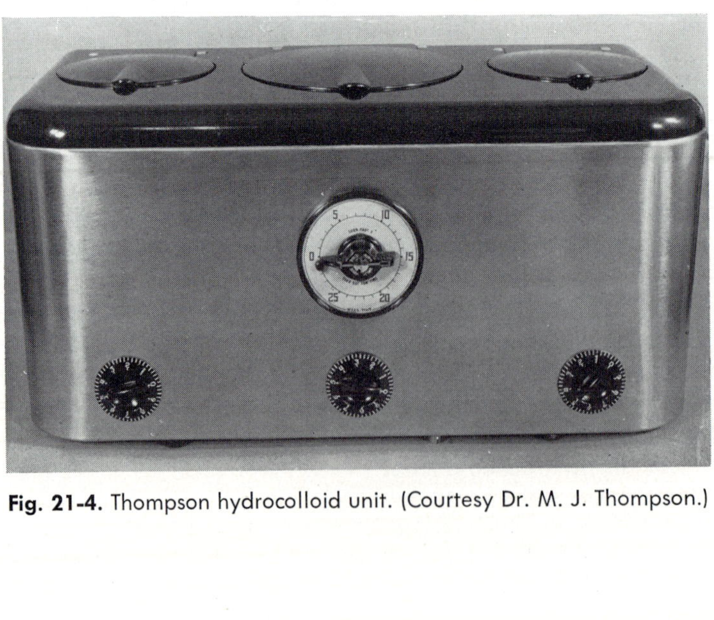

Fig. 21-4. Thompson hydrocolloid unit. (Courtesy Dr. M. J. Thompson.)

tial and the complete arch sizes. Finally, there are available conditioners (Figs. 21-4 and 21-5) that are thermostatically controlled so that the three temperatures necessary for boiling, tempering, and storing of the material are accurately maintained. For anyone contemplating the use of this technic, such equipment is indispensable from the standpoint of convenience and economy of operation.

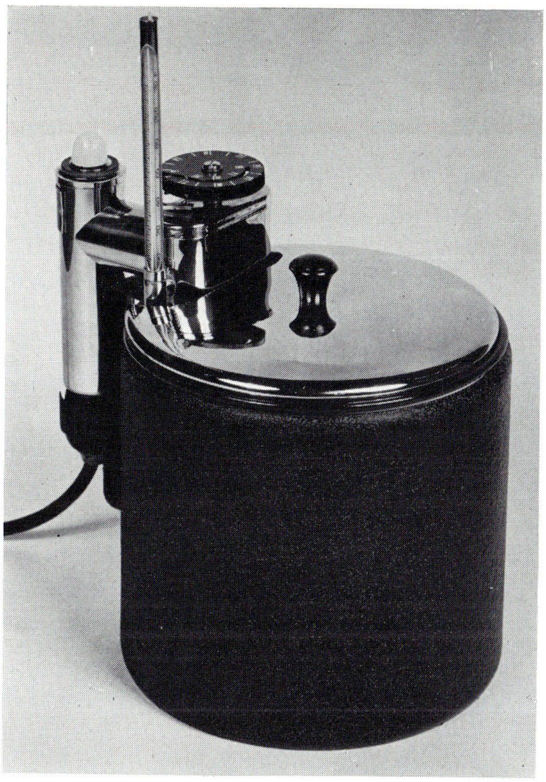

Fig. 21-5. Kerr's hydrocolloid unit. (Courtesy Kerr Manufacturing Co.)

The hydrocolloid is usually supplied in two sizes: (1) in large metal tubes, which are used for filling the impression tray after the material has been liquified (Fig. 21-6, *A*), and (2) smaller sticks in jars, which may be placed in the small syringes for boiling and conditioning prior to injection into the prepared cavity (Fig. 21-6, *B*).

The conditioning of the hydrocolloid may be divided into three steps: (1) liquefaction, (2) storage, and (3) tempering.

Liquefaction. The first step is the proper liquefaction of the gelled material as it comes from the manufacturer in the sealed tubes or in the syringes (Figs. 21-7 to 21-10). A minimum of 8 minutes boiling time is indicated for fresh materials. Whenever unused hydrocolloid is allowed to gel and is later reboiled, it will require the addition of several minutes to the original 8 minutes ordinarily required for fresh material. Boiling for a reasonable length of time beyond eight minutes will cause no harm to the hydrocolloid.

At high altitudes where the boiling point

A

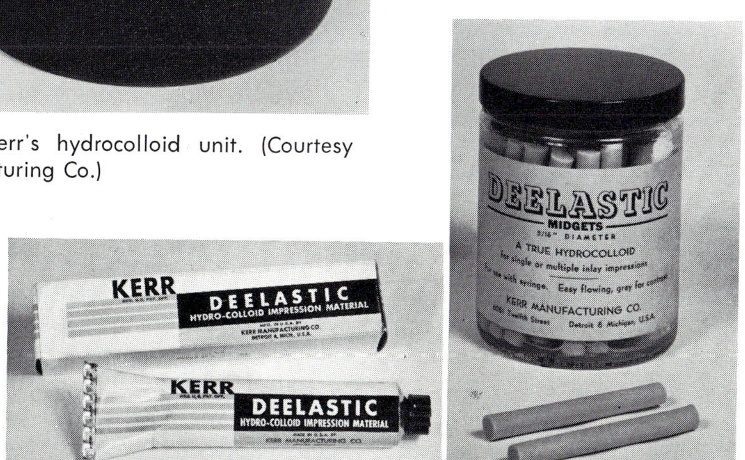

B

Fig. 21-6. Hydrocolloid packaged either in collapsible tubes or jars. (Courtesy Kerr Manufacturing Co.)

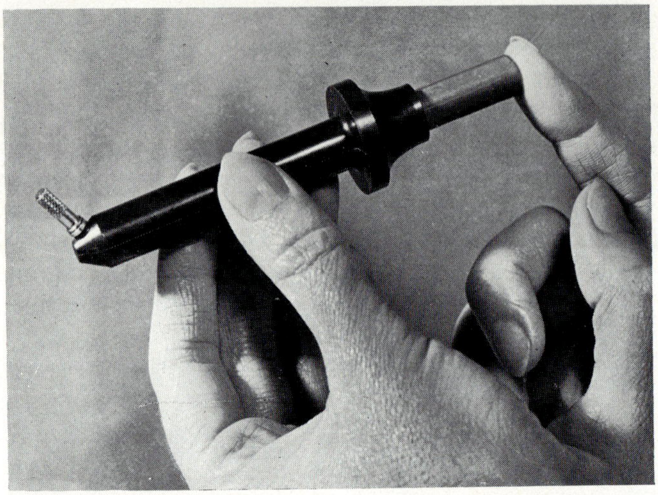

Fig. 21-7. Filling small syringe. (Courtesy Dr. M. J. Thompson.)

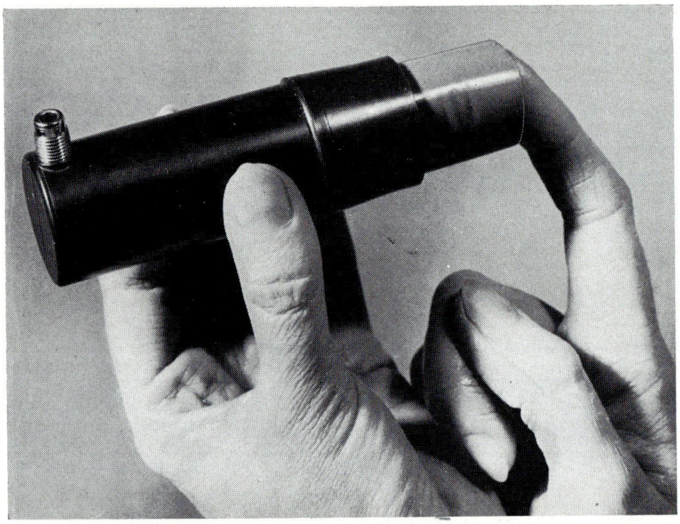

Fig. 21-8. Filling large syringe. (Courtesy Dr. M. J. Thompson.)

of water is reduced below 212° F., it may be necessary to use pressure cookers in order to liquefy the material.

Storage. Once the material has been liquefied, either in the syringes or in the manufacturer's tube, it may be placed in the storage chamber at a temperature of 145 to 150° F. until ready for use (Fig. 21-11). When an automatic conditioner is used, the material may be boiled at the beginning of the day and stored at 145 to 150° F. It will then be ready for use at all times. The storage temperature should not be allowed to drop below 145 to 150° F. because it may start to gel and be too stiff to be flowed easily into the prepared teeth. When the material is boiled and is to be used immediately, it should be placed in the tempering bath of 150° F. and kept at this temperature

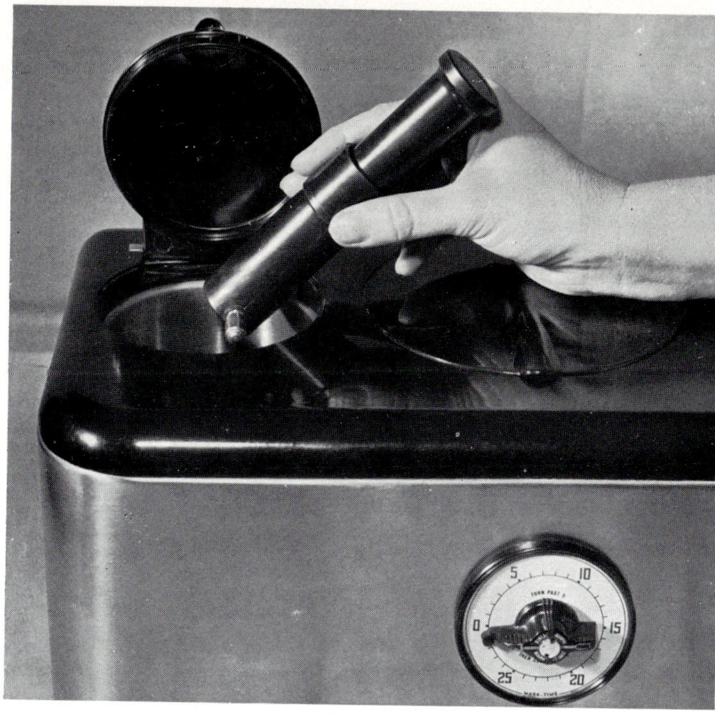

Fig. 21-9. Inserting large syringe into boiling compartment. (Courtesy Dr. M. J. Thompson.)

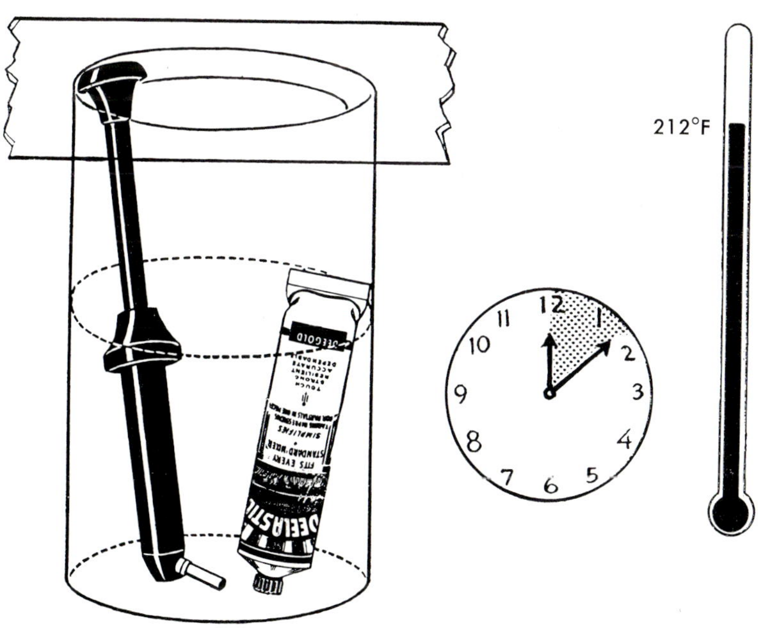

Fig. 21-10. Syringe with stick inserted and tube of Deelastic in compartment of boiling water (8 minutes). (Courtesy Handy and Harmon Co.)

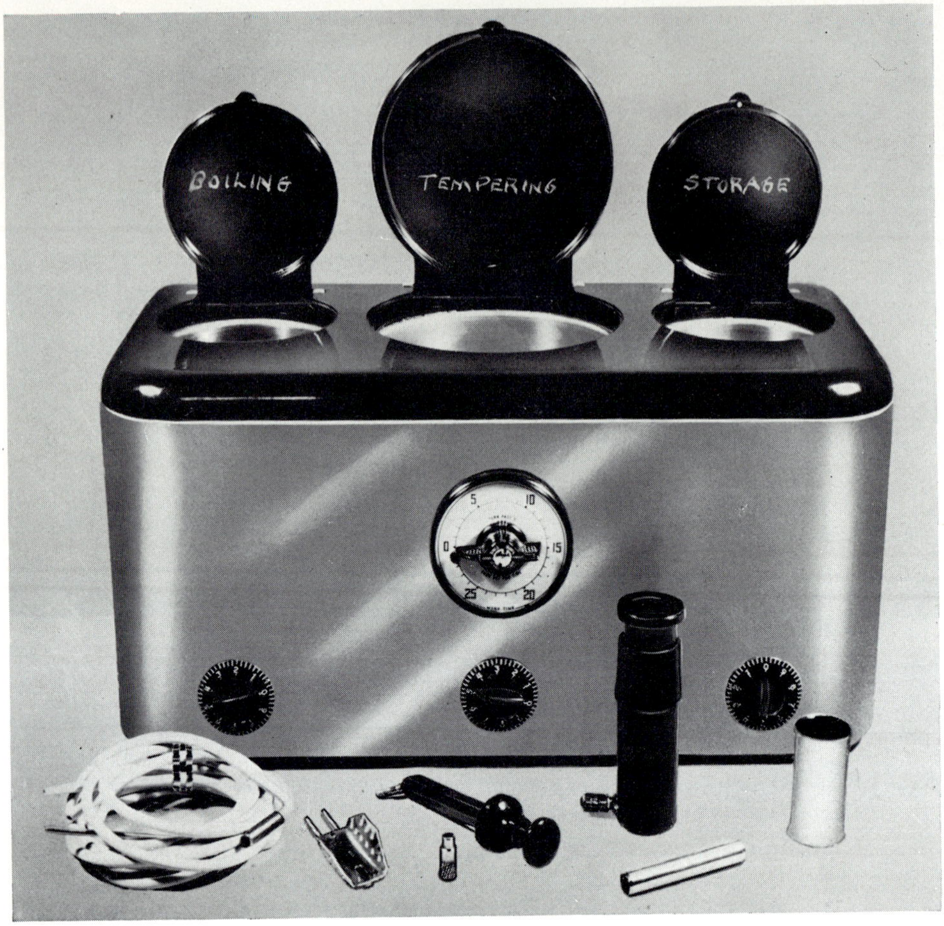

Fig. 21-11. Hydrocolloid conditioner with accessory equipment. (Courtesy Dr. M. J. Thompson.)

for at least 8 minutes to bring the temperature down from the boiling point.

The hydrocolloid in the small syringe is kept in the storage bath at a temperature of 150° F. until ready for injection in the tooth. The material in the larger syringe is used for filling the tray; it must be additionally cooled later in the tray by being tempered to 102 to 115° F. before insertion of the tray into the mouth.

Tempering. The third step involves the tempering of the hydrocolloid in the tray (Figs. 21-12 and 21-13). Although the hydrocolloid from the small syringe is injected at a temperature of 145 to 150° F. directly into the cavity preparation, the material in the filled tray must be cooled to a lower temperature before inserting it into the mouth.

The tempering of the impression tray material causes a partial gelation and stiffening of the mass of material; also, it is more comfortable thermally to the tissues. If the hydrocolloid in the tray were placed in the mouth at a temperature of 150° F., not only would it be uncomfortable to the tissues but it would be so liquid that it would flow out of the impression tray and away from the teeth and tissues. Tempering of the tray material is accomplished by various combinations of time and temperature.

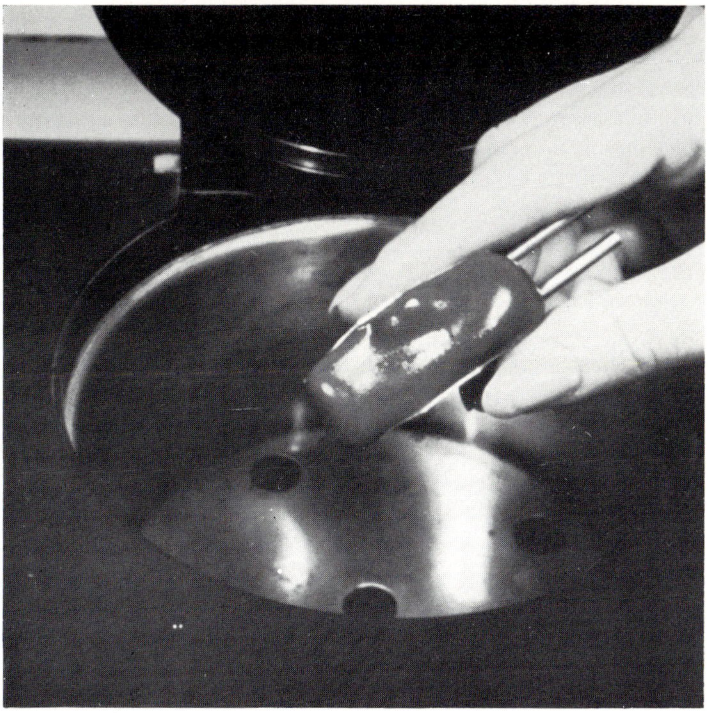

Fig. 21-12. Inserting impression tray and hydrocolloid in tempering chamber. (Courtesy Dr. M. J. Thompson.)

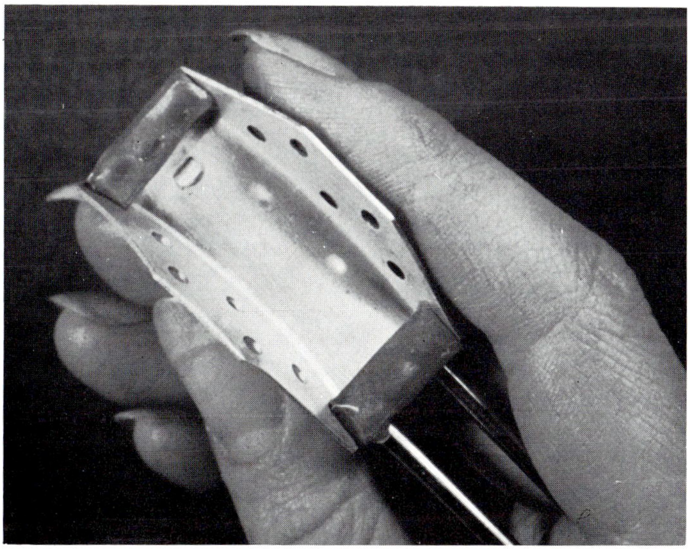

Fig. 21-13. One type of impression tray for taking hydrocolloid impressions. (Courtesy Dr. M. J. Thompson.)

Tempering of the tray hydrocolloid is accomplished by lowering its temperature to 102 to 115° F. This will depend upon the length of time that the tray and the material are allowed to remain in the tempering bath. The following time-temperature schedule for tempering is suggested:

115° F.—5 to 15 minutes
110° F.—5 to 10 minutes
105° F.—5 minutes
102° F.—2 minutes

If 102° F. is used, the filled tray should not be left in the tempering bath longer than 2 minutes; if 105° F. is used, then 5 minutes; if 110° F., then 5 to 10 minutes; if 115° F. is used, it may be left up to 15 minutes before being placed in the mouth. It must be remembered that gelation depends on coordinating the two factors of time and temperature.

In an investigation by Thompson[3] it was found that a hydrocolloid-filled tray placed in a water bath of 102° F. dropped in temperature from 140° to 107° F. in 3 minutes. Care must be exercised not to place the tray of material in a low temperature for too long a period of time because the gelation may progress so far that the material becomes too stiff for use. Therefore, it is necessary for the dentist to so time himself that his operation at the chair and the application of the hydrocolloid to the prepared teeth from the small syringe will consume the number of minutes required for tempering of the tray material at a selected temperature. Once a satisfactory time-temperature schedule has been established, it may be followed as routine procedure.

Certain procedures are required prior to filling the tray with hydrocolloid and placing it in the tempering bath.

If a ready-made tray is to be utilized for taking the impression (Fig. 21-13), it should be sufficiently large to allow for at least ¼ inch thickness of impresison material, so that if undercuts are present there will be sufficient bulk of impression material to allow it to pass over these without permanent distortion. Likewise, the tray should be long enough so that the impression extends beyond the prepared teeth and includes at least one or two teeth in either direction.

In order to prevent the tray from being carried to close to the occlusal surface of

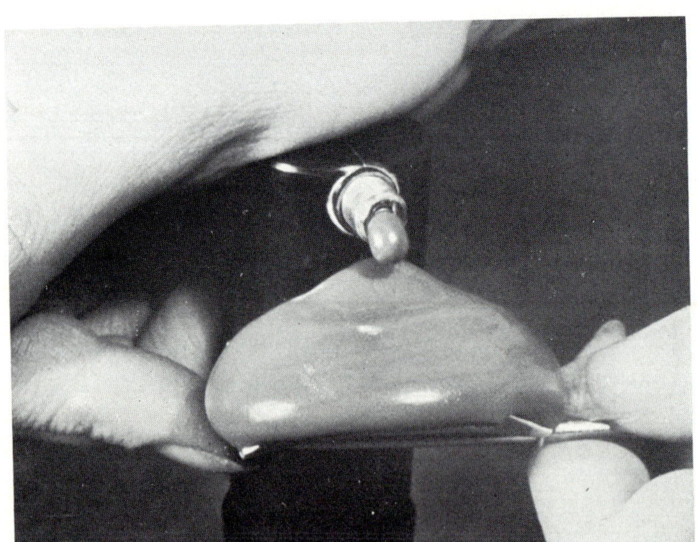

Fig. 21-14. Filling impression tray with hydrocolloid prior to placing it in tempering chamber. (Courtesy Dr. M. J. Thompson.)

the teeth, a small amount of modeling compound is placed at either end of the tray beyond the prepared teeth; these "stops" assure a sufficient thickness of the hydrocolloid material in the finished impression over the occlusal area of the prepared teeth.

When filling the tray with hydrocolloid, folding or incorporating air bubbles into the material must be avoided. This is done by placing the nozzle of the tube or syringe in the bottom of the tray and squeezing out the necessary amount of material until the tray has been slightly overfilled (Fig. 21-14). The filled tray is immediately placed in the tempering bath and kept there for the proper length of time, usually 5 to 15 minutes, and at the selected temperature. This is done by the dental assistant. It is during this time that the dentist retracts the gum and injects the hydrocolloid into the cavity preparations from the small syringe.

Retraction of gingival tissue

For successful results, it is essential that the cavity be properly prepared and finished with no undercuts present. The tooth must be clean and dry, without saliva or blood on any of its surfaces or margins. The margins of the cavity must be fully exposed. This is especially true in the gingival region because the hydrocolloid will not displace moisture or gum tissue.

There are several methods available for gum retraction[3-6] and for exposing the gingival margins (Fig. 21-15). (See also Chapter 20.)

As is well known, the depth of the gingival crevice usually varies with the age of the patient. In the younger patient, there is usually less depth to the crevice; consequently, more difficulty may be experienced in retracting the gum tissue in order to expose the cavity margins. There are other instances in the adult and older patients, in which the crevice is unusually deep and is surrounded by a pendulous gingiva that is soft, inflamed, and bleeds easily.

Because all margins of a prepared tooth must be completely exposed and the cavity dry, varying gum conditions must be recognized, and a suitable method for the retraction of the tissues must be decided upon.

The several methods available for the retraction of tissues have been described in Chapter 20. It is known that the hydrocolloid impression materials, whether of the agar-agar type or of the alginate type, will not displace soft tissues or fluids of the oral cavity; hence the necessity for gum retraction. Any technic of tissue retraction must normally be conservative so as not to cause detachment of the tissues from the tooth or injury that may ultimately result in permanent tissue recession.

Extreme precaution in retraction of the gum tissue is especially important when done on anterior teeth. Injury to the soft gingival tissues, whether by traumatic or chemical means, will result in shrinkage after the gum heals. In placing the cervical margin of a preparation beneath the crest of the gum tissue, similar precautions should be taken. The method whereby the rubber dam and clamp are utilized to depress the gum tissue while lowering the cervical margin beneath the gingival crest is an excellent precaution. Cotton thread or wrapping cord is usually used to distend and retract the gum tissues; this also should be done carefully so as not to detach the membrane from the tooth.

Thompson[3] has indicated the following drugs and methods to be useful for gingival retraction. The first one utilized styptics: either zinc chloride 8 percent, ferric subsulfate (Monsel's powder), tannic acid 20 percent (full strength), or alum 40 percent (full strength).

Thread or wrapping cord of the proper thickness is usually impregnated with the drug and then dried. These are later used

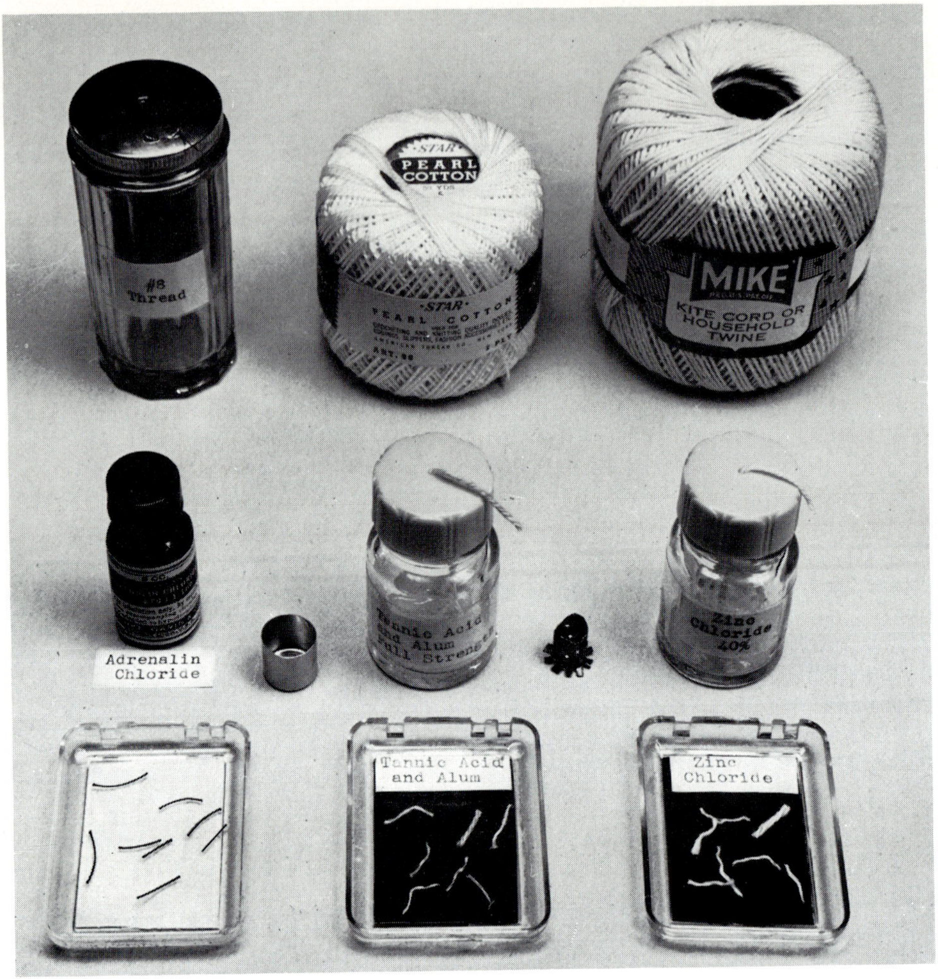

Fig. 21-15. Materials for gingival retraction. **Top, left to right,** Sewing thread (sterilized) in dispenser, cotton crochet thread (medium gauge), kite cord (household twine). **Center,** Adrenalin chloride (1%), aluminum cap, dispenser for cord impregnated with crystals of tannic acid and alum, prepared copper band (with ears projecting), dispenser for cord impregnated with crystals of zinc chloride (40%). **Bottom,** Lengths of plain thread (Nos. 8 to 22), short fibers impregnated with crystals of tannic acid and alum, short fibers impregnated with crystals of zinc chloride. (Courtesy Dr. M. J. Thompson.)

either in single strands or wrapped around the tooth (Fig. 21-16). When carried into the gingival crevice, the cord not only retracts the gum tissue but the exudate of the gingiva dissolves the drug and its styptic action is utilized to keep the area dry.

If there is no bleeding or seepage, untreated wrapping cord may be used to distend the tissue. When this is done, a vasoconstrictor such as Adrenalin chloride (epinephrine) 1 percent or ephedrine sulfate 3 percent may be applied to the cord after it has been tucked into the crevice in order to obtain the vasoconstrictor action of the drug.

Thompson[3] suggested that where a loop is formed with the cord a single knot be utilized, and that after the cord has been gently pressed into the crevice a drop of warm wax be added on the knot to hold

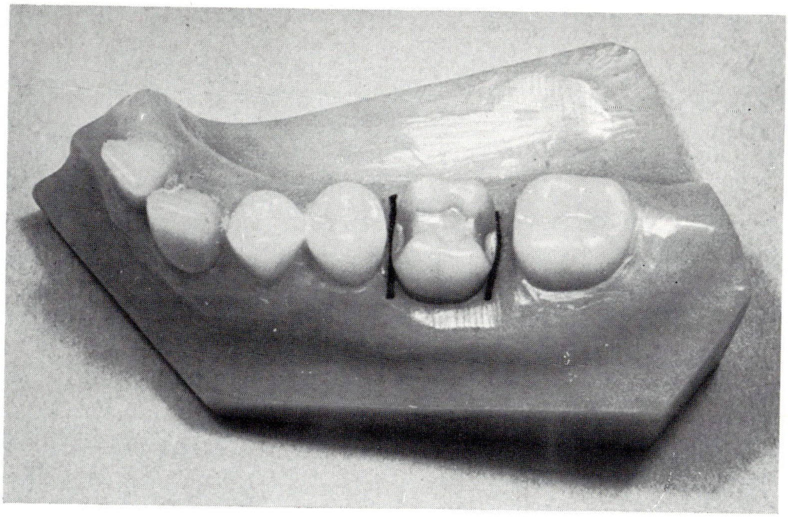

Fig. 21-16. Vasoconstrictors, styptics, or caustic chemicals may be used to clear cavity margin by alleviating seepage or hemorrhage before taking hydrocolloid impression. Application is facilitated by packing crevice with short lengths of cotton thread or string impregnated with chemical of choice. Plain thread in short lengths is also used to depress gingival tissue. (Courtesy Dr. M. J. Thompson.)

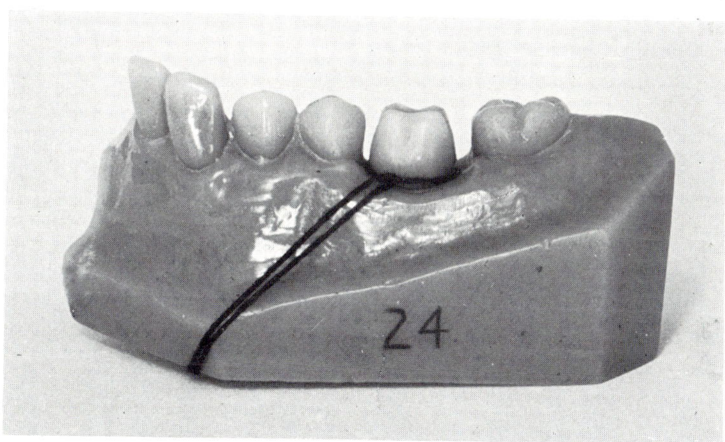

Fig. 21-17. Gingival crevice may be opened up or retracted mechanically with cotton thread or string. Bleeding or seepage is stopped with styptic before application of thread. (Courtesy Dr. M. J. Thompson.)

the loop taut around the tooth (Fig. 21-17); still, the knot will yield sufficiently if it is necessary to press it further into the crevice.

Some operators remove the cord prior to taking the hydrocolloid impression; others take the impression with the cord in place. If the stronger drugs are utilized, it is inadvisable to let these remain during the impression taking. It is suggested that the treated cord be removed, the tissue washed, dried, and a dry piece of cord replaced into the crevice. If seepage persists, a pellet of cotton dampened with epinephrine may be applied or alum-impregnated cord may be placed for a few minutes.

Some conditions require the removal of

A B

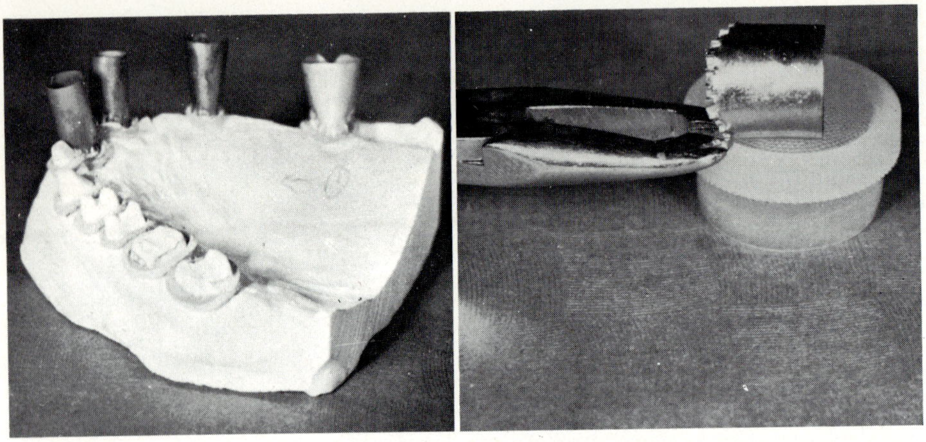

Fig. 21-18. A, Adapting copper bands to parallel curvature of gingivae at cervical plane of abutments. **B,** Crimping gingival margin of festooned copper band using Pagenkopf pliers.

hypertrophied gum tissues or those which cannot be retracted successfully by conservative means. For this purpose, chemical cautery is utilized by using cord impregnated with 40 percent zinc chloride; alternatively, sodium sulfide or potassium hydroxide may be used to cauterize undesirable gingival tissue. Caution is necessary because of the danger of excess tissue destruction. Chemical cautery is also indicated when it is desirable to increase the clinical length of a submerged crown. Following the impression, the tissue should be treated with a mild antiseptic and covered with a pack of zincoxide–eugenol, if chemical cautery is used. Such a protection for several days will allow the damaged tissue to heal.

Still another method of radical retraction, if it can be called such, is by means of surgery wherein the tissue is removed either by the knife or by electrosurgery as recommended by Malone.[5] The usual surgical precautions should be observed and should be followed with the pack previously mentioned, if needed.

Failure in properly placing the cotton thread or cord to obtain gingival retraction is largely the cause of disappointment in the use of the indirect method.

To overcome the difficulty of retracting the gum and exposing the gingival margin, particularly in three-quarter and complete crown preparations, a technic has been devised by Pagenkopf[6] that simplifies this step. He described his technic as follows:

> Select a copper band just a little larger than the greater circumference of the tooth and carefully festoon it [Fig. 21-18, *A*]. Then, with a pinking-crimping pliers, pink and crimp this gingival edge [Fig. 21-18, *B*]. This may also be done with a Joe Dandy disc. The occlusal portion of this band is closed with temporary stopping. Then select a washer, stamped out of buckskin, chamois, or felt; saturate it with astringent and hemostat [Fig. 21-19, *A*]. Of the many on the market, I have found aluminum sulfate, the styptic pencil used for cuts while shaving, to give the best results. Place the band over the preparation and apply pressure with the pinked and crimped edge of the band until it forces the washer beyond the gingival line [Fig. 21-19, *B*]. Continuous pressure may be exerted by having the patient apply force on the band with his opposing teeth. The pinked and crimped bands prevent the washer from slipping either inside or outside of the band and defeating its purpose. This is left for about ten minutes after which time the impression can be taken.*

Those using this technic can attest to its simplicity and effectiveness.

Greene[4] has reported a new method of

*From Pagenkopf, A. A.: Hydrocolloid method: if not—why not?, North-West Dent. 34:93, 1955

A 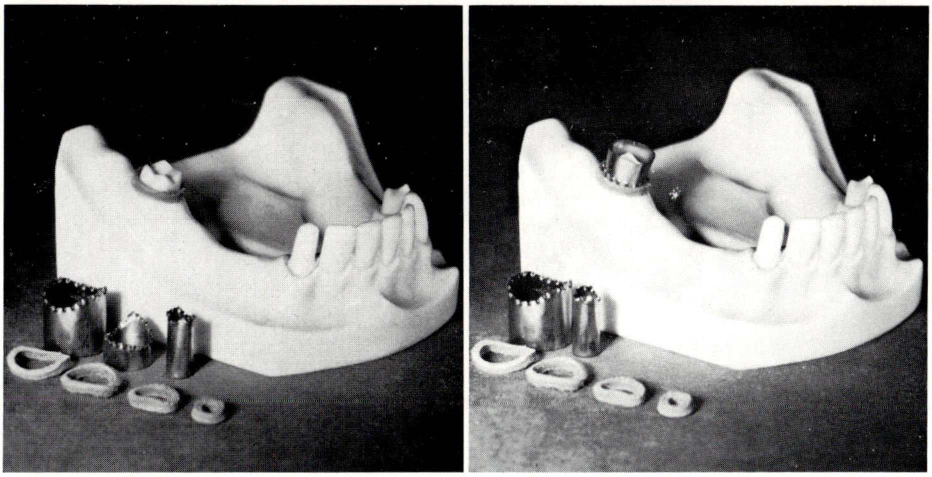 B

Fig. 21-19. A, Festooned, crimped bands and chamois washers used in Pagenkopf technic. **B,** Chamois washer carried into gingival crevice of molar by means of crimped band, thereby distending gingiva.

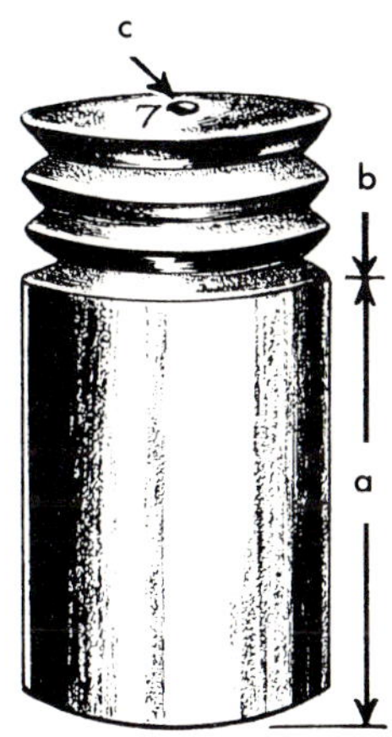

Fig. 21-20. Compressomatic aluminous cap. (Courtesy L. L. Greene and N. A. Greene.)

taking an impression either of an individual tooth preparation or of multiple impressions of abutments prepared for a fixed prosthesis. A newly designed aluminum collapsible impression cap has been designed (Fig. 21-20) which consists of a smooth body part, a series of compressible corrugations, and a series of vent holes (Compressomatic).

The usual steps in fitting a cap for an impression are followed: (1) a proper size of cap is selected, usually slightly larger than the circumference of the abutment; (2) the open end of the cap is trimmed to parallel the curvature of the crest of the gingiva; (3) the length of the cap is adjusted so that the first bellow acts as an occlusal stop (Fig. 21-21); (4) vent holes are established in the buccal and lingual smooth surfaces of the cap, and in the occlusal portion of the cap; (5) the cap is finally filled with heavy body rubber-type impression material so that a slight excess of the impression material may ooze out of the hole vents.

The filled cap is placed on the prepared abutment tooth and is carried slightly beyond the cervical level of the preparation, at which time the first bellow acts as a stop to prevent the edge of the cap from injuring the subgingival tissues.

With the body of the cap held firmly, pressure is applied with the tip of the finger to the occlusal surface of the cap (Fig. 21-22). This compresses the bellows, forcing some of the material beyond the gingival margin of the band subgingivally, ensuring a sharp impression of the cervical chamfer or shoulder. Overdisplacement of the gingival tissue is avoided by the escape of excess impression material through the

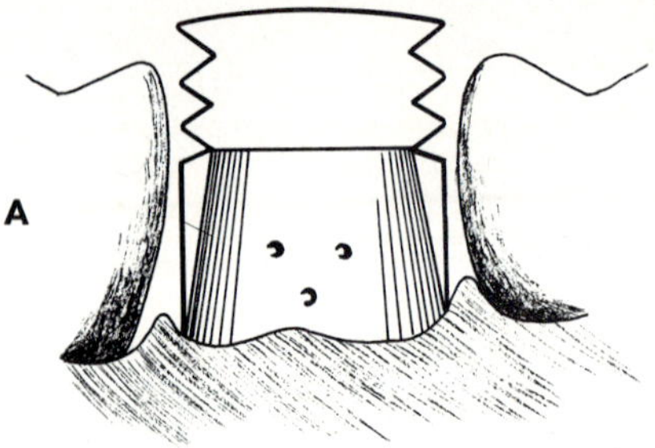

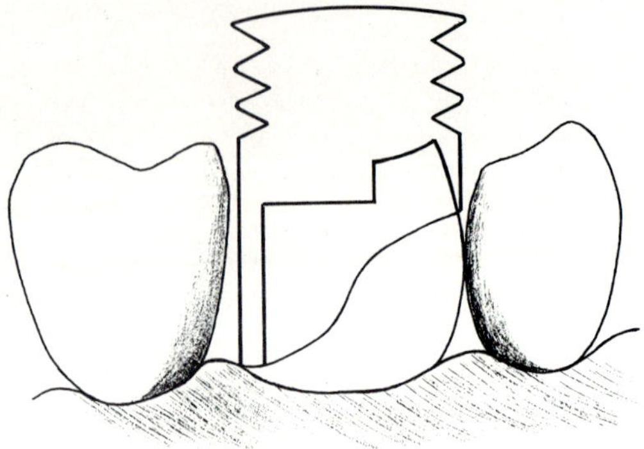

Fig. 21-21. A, Compressomatic cap fitted to curvature of gingiva prior to filling with impression material for complete crown preparation. **B,** Cap trimmed for intracoronal impression. (Courtesy L. L. Greene and N. A. Greene.)

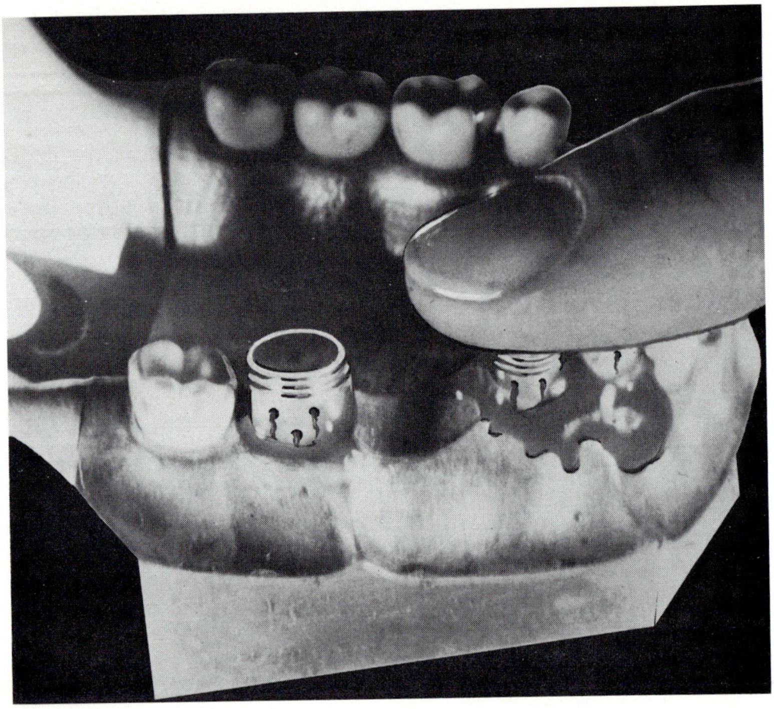

Fig. 21-22. Left, Filled cap in position over prepared tooth. **Right,** Bellows of cap compressed while placing impression material into gingival crevice. (Courtesy L. L. Greene and N. A. Greene.)

buccal and lingual vent holes. The same procedure is followed on any remaining abutment preparations (Fig. 21-23).

With the several impression caps in position on the prepared teeth, an impression in heavy body material is taken in a tray to include all of the teeth in the quadrant; however, a complete arch impression is preferred.

When the impression material has completely set, the tray with impression cap is removed, and the several impression caps will be imbedded within it (Fig. 21-24). The dies and the working models are

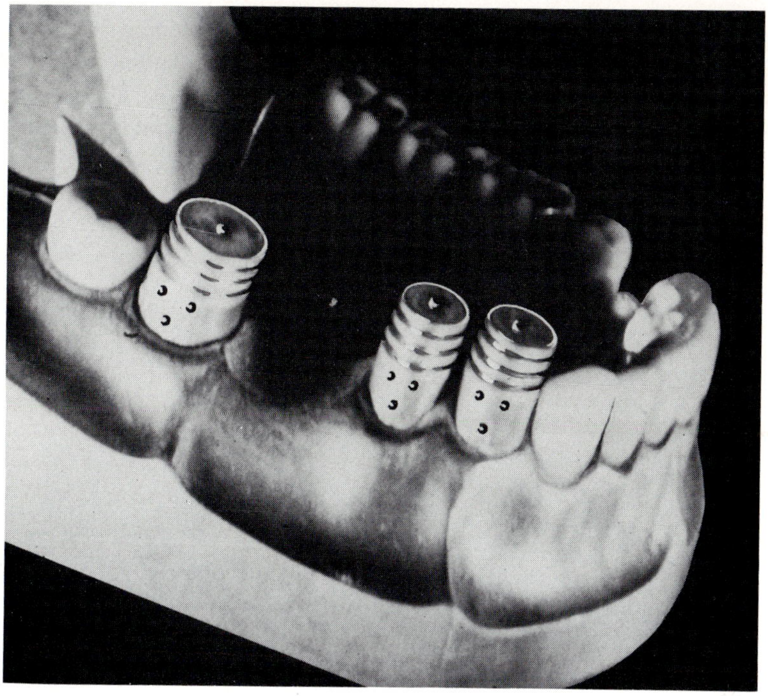

Fig. 21-23. Multiple caps and individual impressions can be taken and left in place for unilateral impression in tray. (Courtesy L. L. Greene and N. A. Greene.)

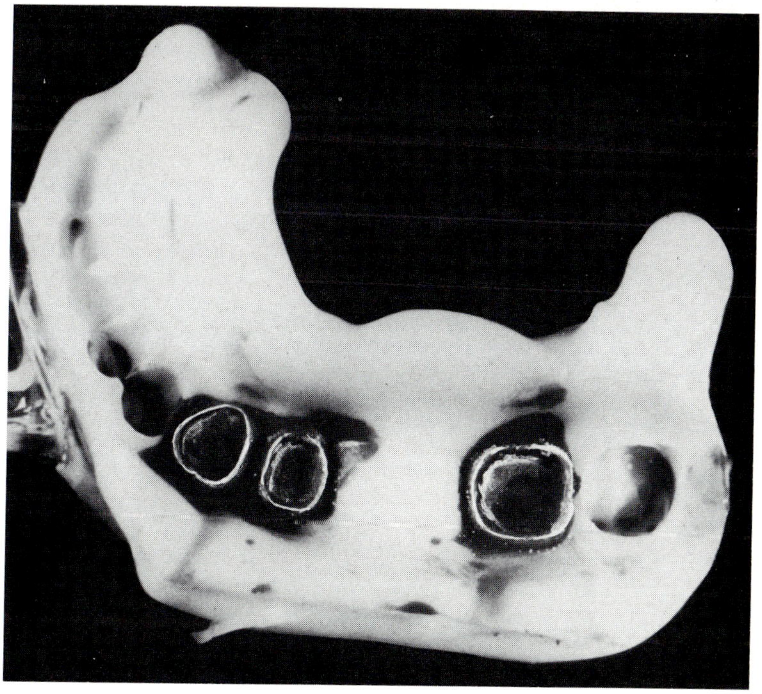

Fig. 21-24. Tray impression removed with impression caps imbedded. (Courtesy L. L. Greene and N. A. Greene.)

then fabricated by any of the customary technics employing removable stone or electroformed metal dies; the working model is then poured in stone.

Injection of hydrocolloid material

The next phase of the technic is the injection of the hydrocolloid material into the prepared cavities. The temperature of the material in the small syringe has dropped from 212° F. to between 145 and 150° F., after having been left in the storage bath for 8 minutes. While this temperature may seem a little high for the direct application of the hydrocolloid to a tooth with a vital pulp, when the material

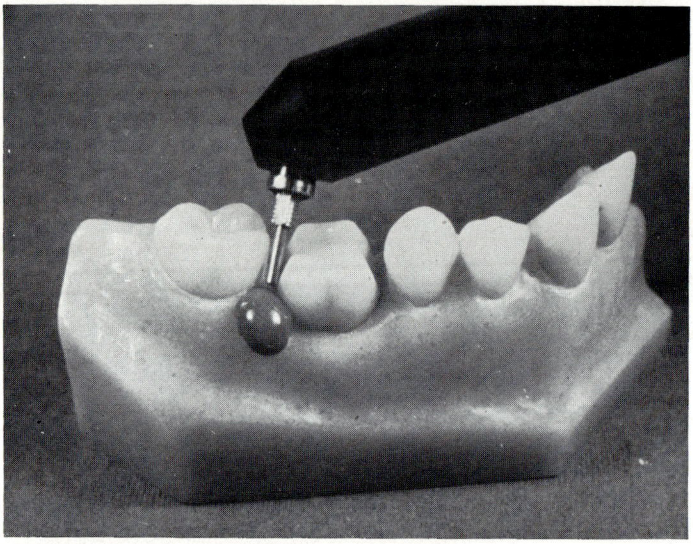

Fig. 21-25. Location of initial injection of hydrocolloid in gingival interproximal area. (Courtesy Dr. M. J. Thompson.)

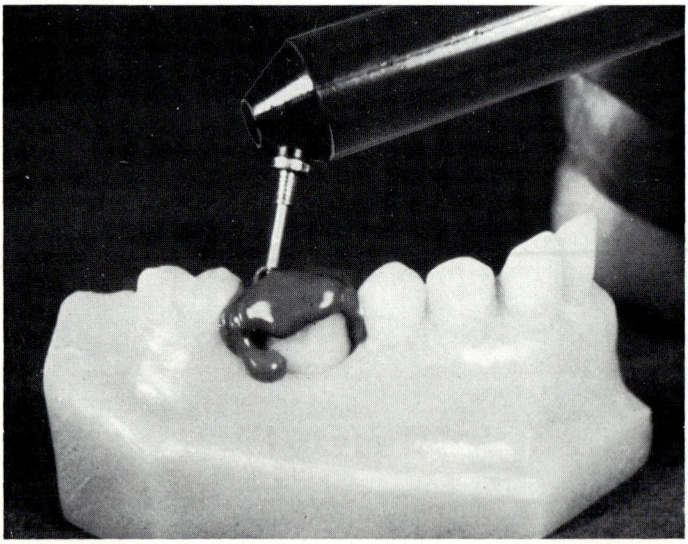

Fig. 21-26. Covering occlusal surface and rest of tooth after initial gingival application of hydrocolloid. (Courtesy Dr. M. J. Thompson.)

flows through the needle, its temperature has dropped from 10 to 15° F. when it comes in contact with the tooth.

Several gauges of needles are used; the 19-gauge needle is used for the usual types of preparations; the 21-gauge needle is employed in the pinledge types of preparations.

The gum tissue having been retracted and the cavity preparations dried so that no saliva or blood is present, the syringe is removed from the 140 to 150° F. storage chamber, carried to the mouth, the needle is placed alongside the prepared tooth, and a small amount of material is extruded on the gum. This is done for the purpose of clearing the needle of any trapped air or water that may have found its way into it. The point of the needle is next brought into contact with the gingival floor on the distal surface of the most posterior abutment and the hydrocolloid extruded (Fig. 21-25); the needle is then raised occlusally to the pulpal floor and down into the mesial, all the time keeping the point of the needle in contact with tooth structure and within the mass of hydrocolloid already extruded (Fig. 21-26). If the material has been properly liquefied and stored, it will flow easily out of the needle and flatten out without forming any folds. At no time should the needle be withdrawn from the mass of material and reinserted; such a procedure will cause air bubbles to form within the extruded hydrocolloid. When withdrawing the needle from the covered abutment, it should be withdrawn from the occlusal portion of the mass of hydrocolloid and not from the proximal aspect.

After the posterior tooth is entirely covered with the material, the anterior tooth is covered likewise (Fig. 21-27). A globule of impression material is expressed on the labial surface of a tooth on the opposite side of the arch to serve later as a guide to the complete gelation of the material in the tray.

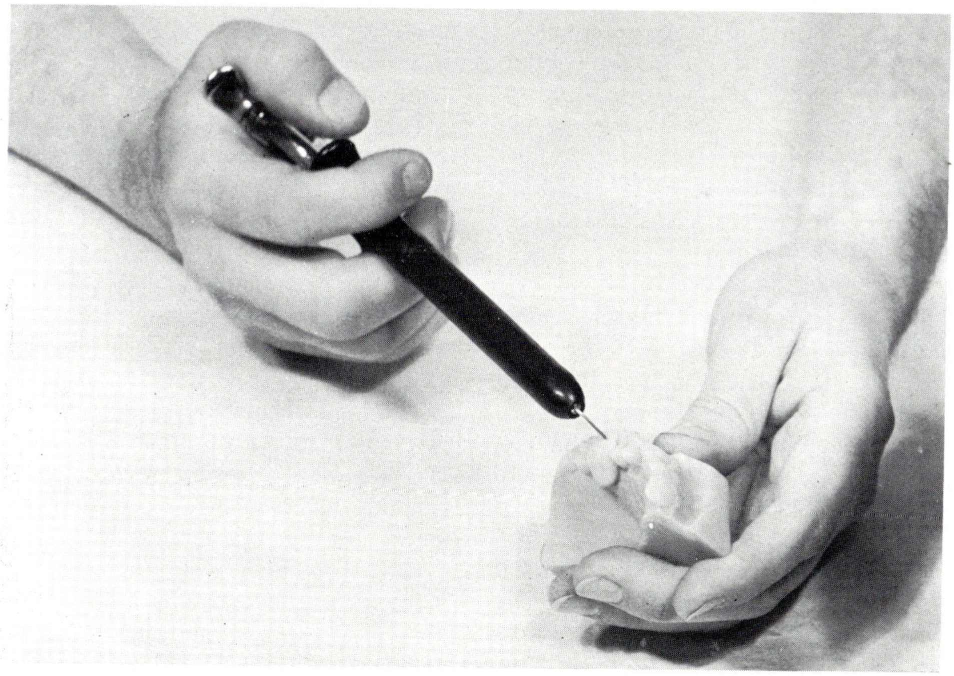

Fig. 21-27. Remaining prepared abutments are covered in similar manner with hydrocolloid, demonstrated on model. (Courtesy Kerr Manufacturing Co.)

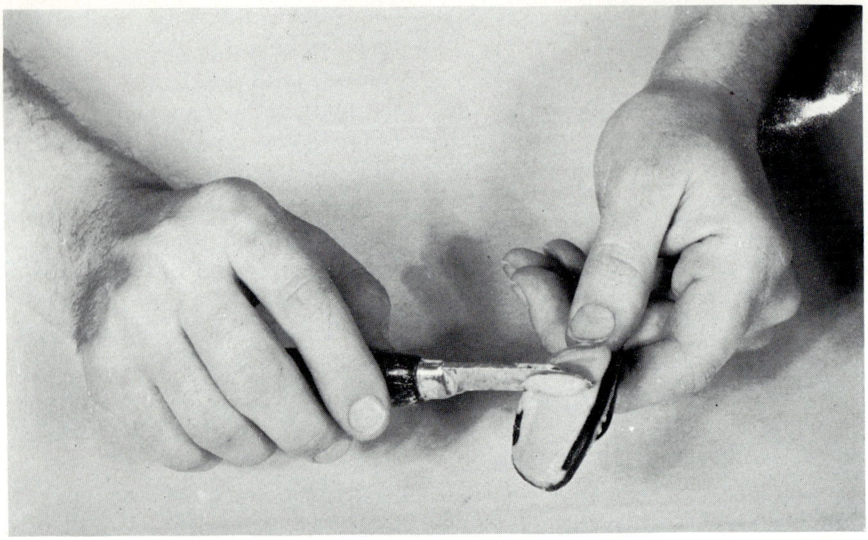

Fig. 21-28. Shaving off top layer of hydrocolloid after removing tray from tempering compartment, prior to taking impression. (Courtesy Kerr Manufacturing Co.)

This initial application of the hydrocolloid to the abutment teeth must be carried out with relative rapidity so as not to allow the material to cool to the point of gelation. Should gelation occur, the hydrocolloid in the tray will not adhere to that in the tooth when the impression is taken; in addition, the gelled hydrocolloid covering the teeth cannot be compressed against the teeth to secure all the details of the cavity preparation.

Positioning the tray

While the dentist is applying the hydrocolloid with the small syringe to the abutment teeth, the assistant removes the filled tray from the tempering compartment, attaches the water tubing to the tray handle, and with a sharp knife shaves off the top layer of hydrocolloid, which was exposed to water (Fig. 21-28). This gives a fresh surface of hydrocolloid that is undiluted and that will adhere to the soft hydrocolloid covering the abutment teeth.

The hydrocolloid in the tray has been tempered to a temperature varying from 102 to 115° F.; the preferable temperature is nearer 115° F. than 102° F. The tray is carefully centered over the prepared teeth and slowly carried to position (Fig. 21-29). The stops previously placed in the tray act as a guide in positioning the tray, confine the hydrocolloid in the tray, and also assure a correct amount of hydrocolloid between the bottom of the tray and the occlusal surfaces of the prepared teeth. After the tray is positioned properly, it is held steadily without any further vertical or lateral movements. Water is now permitted to pass through the rubber tubing and circulate through the tray for 5 to 7 minutes, cooling the material to the point of gelation. It is not advisable to use ice water for this purpose. It is recommended that tap water of approximately 50 to 60° F. be used. Ice water produces a certain amount of distortion in the impression, besides causing discomfort to the patient. Different products vary in their composition and in their gelation time. A safe rule to follow before removing the impression is to hold it in position for 3 minutes after initial gelation has taken place. The total cooling time will vary, depending upon

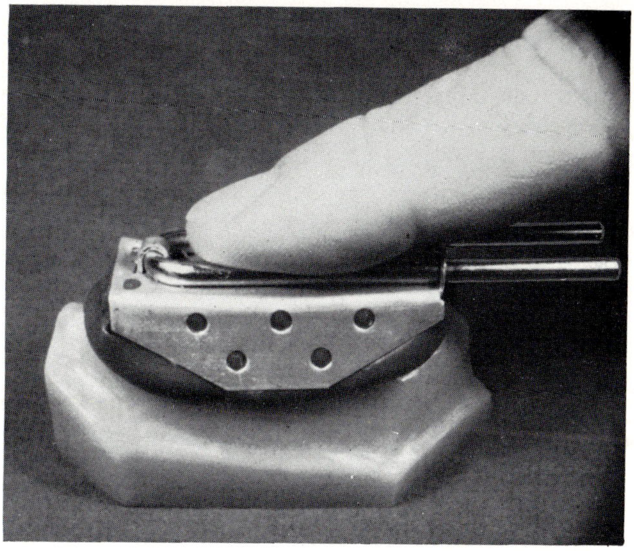

Fig. 21-29. Tray and properly tempered hydrocolloid are positioned over covered abutments and held in place without any movement until complete gelation of hydrocolloid has taken place in water-cooled tray. (Courtesy Dr. M. J. Thompson.)

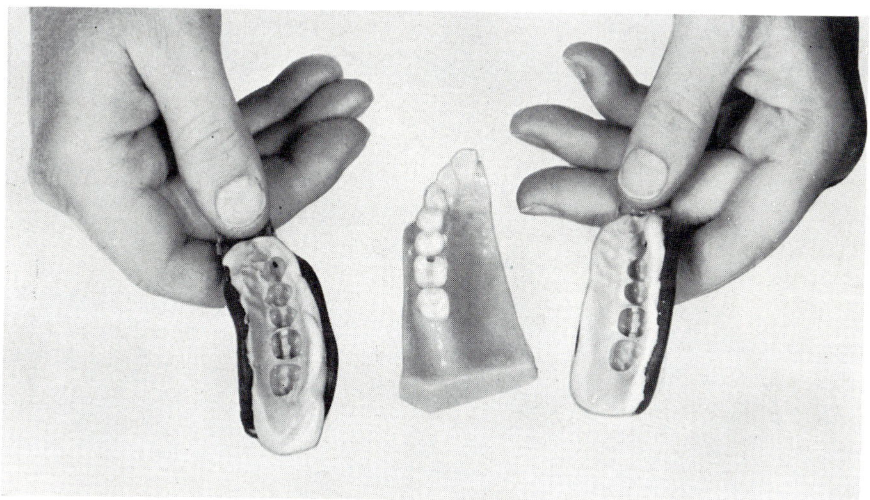

Fig. 21-30. Upon removal from mouth, impressions are examined for accuracy and sharpness of detail. (Courtesy Kerr Manufacturing Co.)

the volume of hydrocolloid contained in the impression tray. The labial globule will serve as a guide.

Removal and treatment of impression

The removal of the tray impression is one of the most critical procedures in the entire technic. The tray should not be removed by its handle; instead the fingers should be placed under the rim of the tray and any hydrocolloid covering the rim; then with a sharp, straight pull away from the teeth, the impression is dislodged with a quick motion. At no time should the impression be teased out or removed with a rocking motion. Such movement will distort the impression. Investigations have disclosed that the hydrocolloid gel can resist fracture better with a sudden deformation than if the impression is withdrawn slowly from undercut and irregular surfaces. If the tray and hydrocolloid separate in the removal of the impression, it should be discarded.

Upon its removal, the impression is examined for sharpness and accuracy of detail, also for the presence of any air voids within the material or signs of dragging and tearing (Fig. 21-30).

At this time, a complete impression of the opposing arch is taken in hydrocolloid; also the necessary registrations to orient the casts properly to each other on the articulator.

Pouring cast in stone and completion

If the impression with the prepared teeth is satisfactory, it is air dried but not desiccated, and poured in stone.

Some hydrocolloid materials (agar-agar type, reversible) do not require any other treatment prior to pouring the stone; others (the alginate type, irreversible) require the immersion of the impression in a 2 percent solution of potassium sulfate for 2 to 5 minutes (Fig. 21-31), following which the impression is removed from the solution and air dried, and the stone is poured (Fig. 21-32).

Those having extensive experience in the use of the hydrocolloids recommend that impressions be poured immediately. If not poured within 15 to 30 minutes none of the hydrocolloids will give an accurate model or die.

If the alginate impression is exposed to air it will shrink; if it is immersed in water for any length of time beyond 5 minutes it will imbibe water and expand. Since the hydrocolloid is locked in the perforations

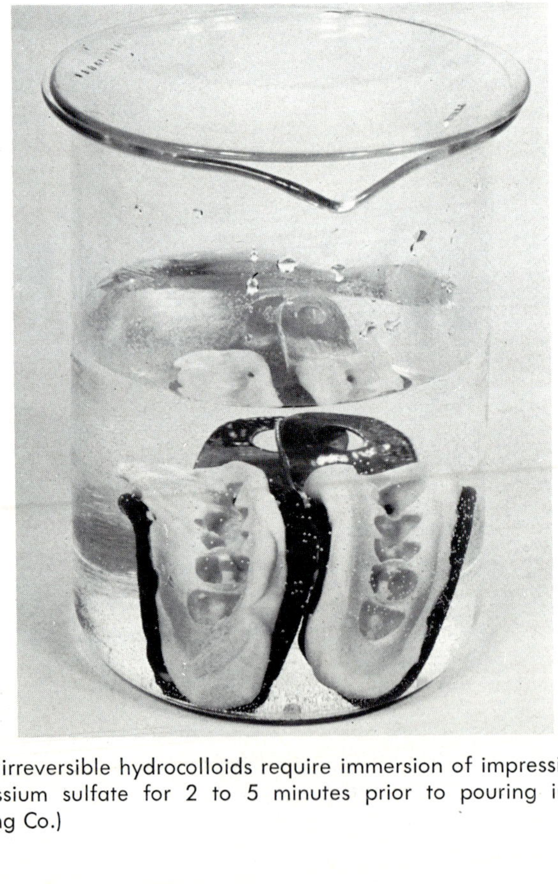

Fig. 21-31. Some irreversible hydrocolloids require immersion of impressions in a 2 percent solution of potassium sulfate for 2 to 5 minutes prior to pouring in stone. (Courtesy Kerr Manufacturing Co.)

of the tray, the shrinkage of the material will be toward the walls of the tray, and the model and the dies of the prepared teeth will be larger than the original preparations. If the impression is allowed to remain in water and expand, the dies of the prepared teeth will be smaller than the original preparations. Hence the importance of pouring the impression immediately.

Thompson,[3] Phillips and Ito,[7] and others have found that placing the poured impression in a 2 percent potassium sulfate solution for a few minutes accelerates the setting time of the stone; also it gives a smoother and a harder surface to the stone than if the impression were left in water (Fig. 21-33).

Where circumstances prevent the immediate pouring of the impression, Phillips and Ito[7] recommend that it be maintained in an atmosphere of 100 percent humidity but not beyond 30 minutes.

Some employ the procedure of immersing an impression in water for 30 to 60 minutes on the assumption that any shrinkage that might have taken place in the impression from the time it was taken to when it is poured would be compensated for by the expansion of the hydrocolloid from its imbibition of water. True, expansion takes place, but it does not parallel the amount or direction of the contraction that took place; a distorted model or dies result.

Although regular dental stones have been used to pour the dies and working models, improved stones have more recently been made available for this purpose. The research of Peyton and associ-

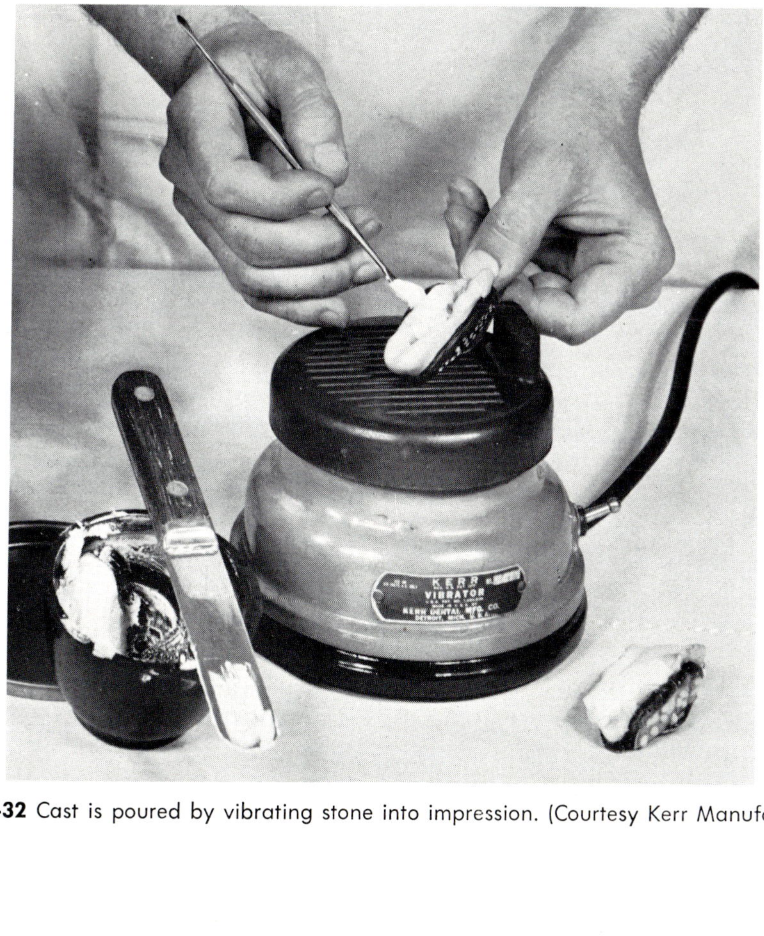

Fig. 21-32 Cast is poured by vibrating stone into impression. (Courtesy Kerr Manufacturing Co.)

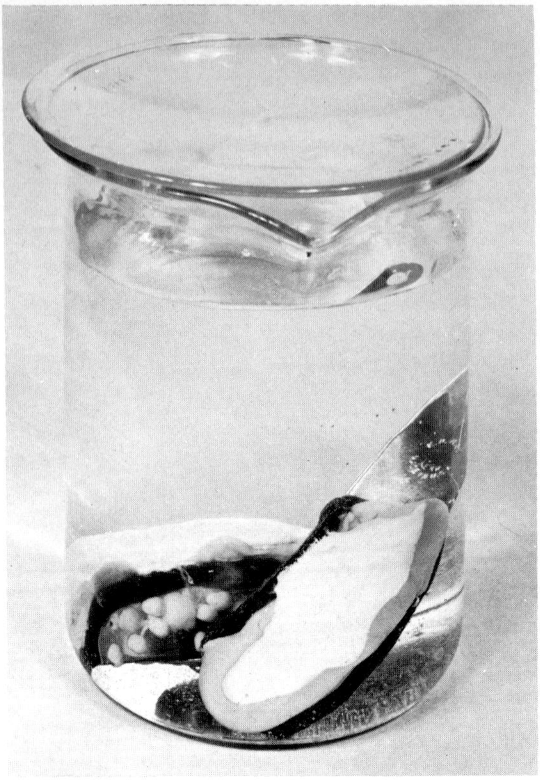

Fig. 21-33. Poured cast and impression placed in potassium sulfate solution to accelerate setting time and increase surface hardness of stone cast. (Courtesy Kerr Manufacturing Co.)

ates,[8] Hosoda,[13] and others has shown that these improved stones are superior in their resistance to abrasion and in hardness. These stones have been specially prepared for the indirect technic; they possess a minimum amount of setting expansion and a superior surface smoothness.

Requirements for the die materials

1. To be able to reproduce a positive die of the negative impression accurately.
2. To be dimensionally stable.
3. To have a minimum response to thermal change either in expanding or contracting.
4. To be able to reproduce in fine detail and accurately.
5. To have a hard, smooth surface.
6. To have edge strength against a shearing force.
7. To have a contrasting color with the inlay wax that is to be carved on it.
8. The die should be fabricated within a reasonable length of time for withdrawal from the impression. The instrument and materials used should not be complicated or dangerous to the technician.

When using stones for this purpose, it is essential that the water-powder ratio indicated by the manufacturer be used. A deviation from the recommended water-powder ratio will result in an uncontrolled setting expansion of the material. Although it is possible to obtain a good mix of stone by the usual methods of spatulation, stone mixed in a vacuum has given improved results. Another precaution to be taken is to eliminate all excess potassium sulfate solution or water from the impression. There is less likelihood of trapping air in the model if the stone is vibrated mildly into the impression. Phillips and Ito[7] have shown that the rate at which stone is flowed into the impression has a very significant effect upon the surface of the die, likewise the amount of vibration that accompanies the flowing of the stone into the impression. It has been found that if the stone is added in large quantities and is accompanied by excessive vibration, there is a tendency to entrap air bubbles and produce nodules in the finished die. It is important to fill the impression by placing small increments of stone in one section of the impression and allowing the stone to flow into other parts of the impression from this initial point of application.

Immersing the poured die in a 2 percent potassium sulfate solution for 10 to 15 minutes will improve it. After the stone die has been poured it should be allowed to harden for at least 1 hour before separating it from the impression.

If possible, the dies or model should not be worked on for 24 hours since they reach their maximum strength and hardness at the end of this time. The investigations of Peyton[8] indicated that the dry crushing strengths of stone are greater than the wet and that oil immersion treatment of dies made of stone apparently decreases their crushing strength.

The final structure of a stone die is composed of interlocking crystals between which are the pores containing the excess water required for mixing.

It has been found that water saturated with powder made from an old stone cast accelerates the setting time of a new stone mix but it does not affect its expansion. The dry strength of plaster and stone is twice that of wet stone or plaster. Increased hardness, smoothness, and strength in stone may be obtained in using a putty-like consistency of mix. Class II stones, which are hemihydrate, are used for dies.

To avoid the formation of air bubbles in mixing stone, it is advisable to sift in the powder slowly and to spatulate it mechanically under vacuum.

If the technic is such that it is necessary to replace a die into a rubber impression prior to pouring the working cast, it is advisable to soak the die for a few minutes in the water saturated with the stone powder prior to lubricating the root extension.

There are several methods available in making the dies and models used in the indirect technics. Many men have contributed to the development of these methods; consequently it is difficult to give credit to each one individually; however, their specific contributions may be found in the bibliography at the end of the chapter.

The first method requires two separate impressions. Into the first impression, individual dies are poured using one of the improved stones (Fig. 21-34). These dies are subsequently used for making and finishing the wax patterns for the individual prepared teeth. The second impression is used to pour a solid, master model of stone (Fig. 21-35). On this, wax patterns are fitted to determine correct occlusion and contact points (Fig. 21-36); after the castings are made, the model is also used for the construction and positioning of the pontics (Fig. 21-37). The component parts of the bridge are later assembled on the model and by means of a plaster index are removed and soldered. The bridge is then replaced on the master model to verify its fit, then finished (Fig. 21-38).

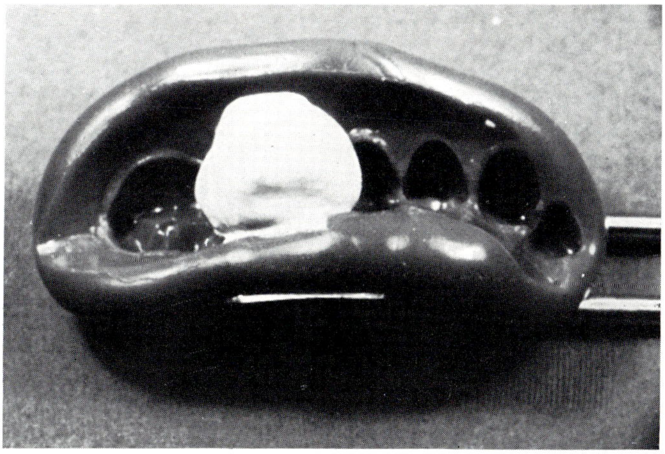

Fig. 21-34. Stone poured to make individual dies of prepared abutments. (Courtesy Dr. M. J. Thompson.)

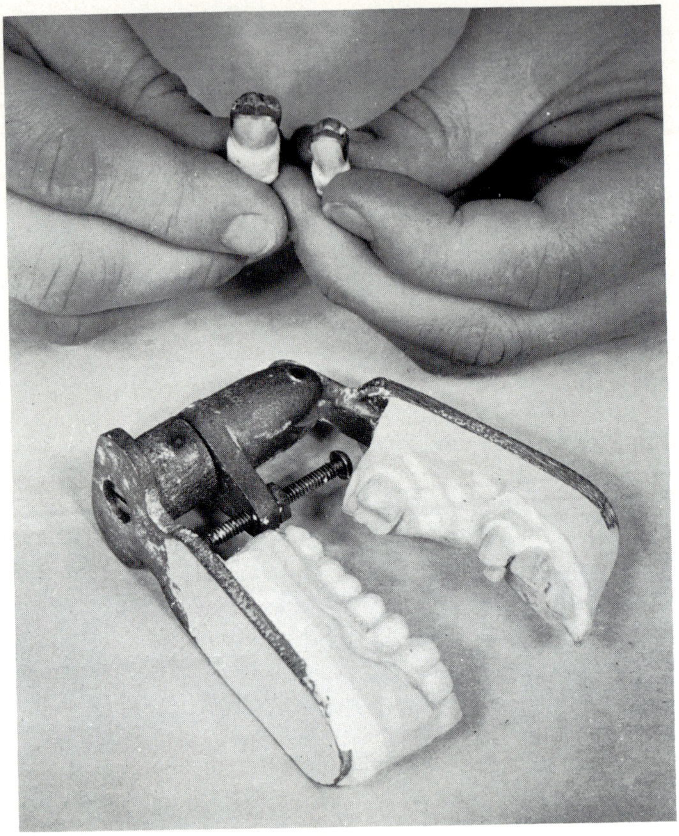

Fig. 21-35. Above, Two individual stone dies which were poured in first impression. **Below,** Solid master model mounted in articulator. (Courtesy Kerr Manufacturing Co.)

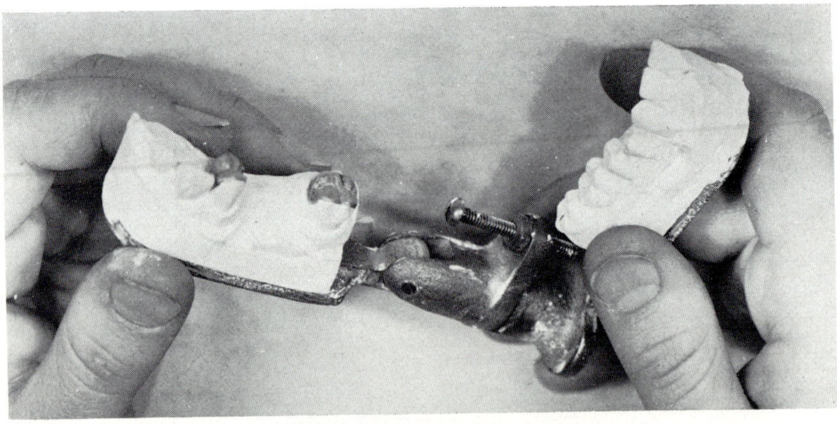

Fig. 21-36. Wax patterns are first fitted on master model for occlusion, contour, and proximal contacts. They are then removed and placed on their respective individual dies for final marginal adaptation. (Courtesy Kerr Manufacturing Co.)

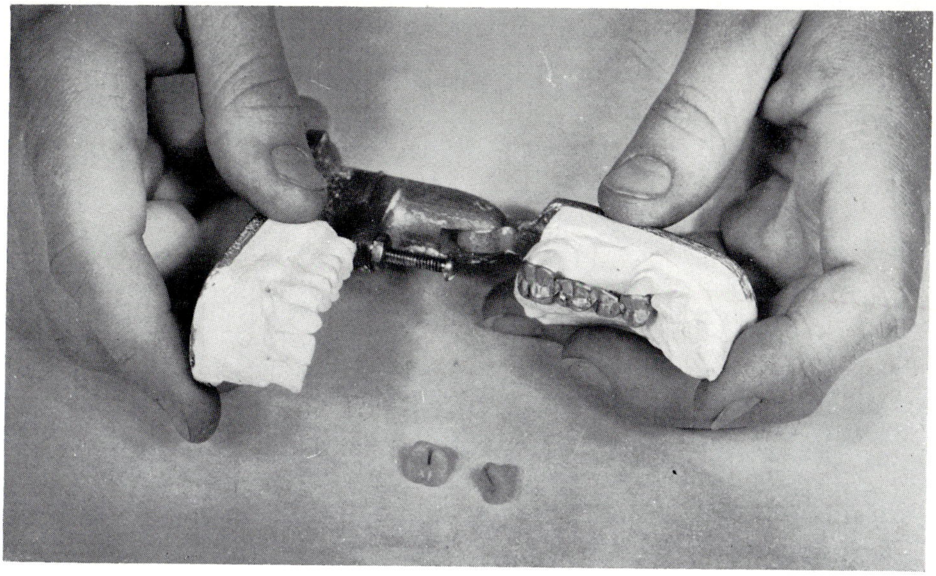

Fig. 21-37. Cast retainers are placed on prepared abutments of master model, and pontics are constructed. (Courtesy Kerr Manufacturing Co.)

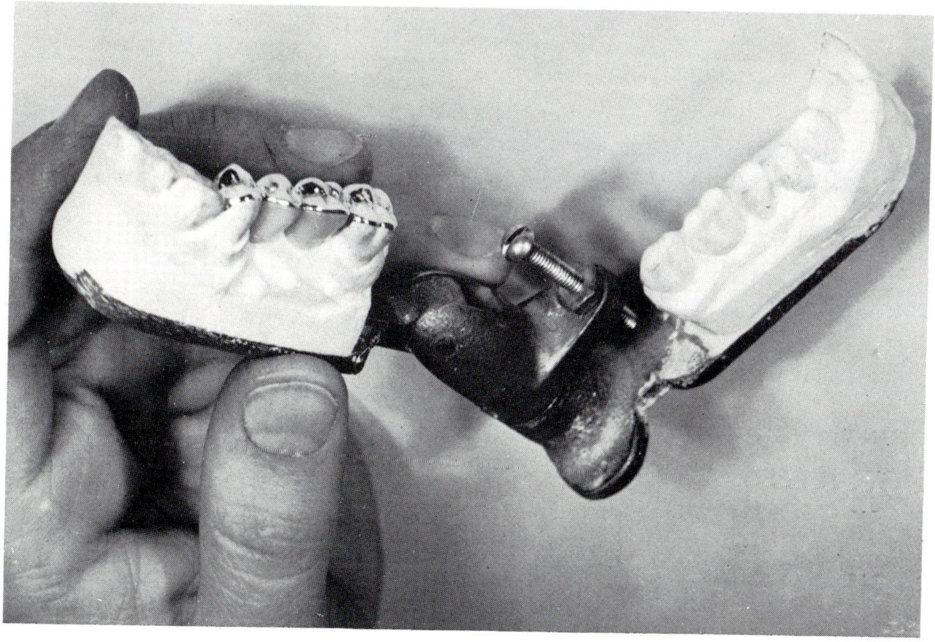

Fig. 21-38. Pontics and retainers are assembled, removed for soldering, and finished on master model. (Courtesy Kerr Manufacturing Co.)

The second method employs one master impression. Into the impressions of the prepared teeth, individual stone dies are poured and allowed to set in an atmosphere of 100 percent humidity. In pouring the individual dies, an excess of stone is heaped up in the shape of a cone, approximately ¾ inch in height (Fig. 21-39, *A*). This excess is later shaped to a tapered root form. At the end of 30 minutes, the individual stone dies have set, whereupon they are removed from the impression. The root ends are now tapered, lubricated, and replaced in their respective positions in the master impression. A new batch of stone is mixed and poured into the impression enveloping the lubricated root extensions of the dies. After setting, the master stone model is removed from the impression; the individual dies of the prepared teeth are removable and may be replaced accurately in their respective sockets (Fig. 21-39, *B*). By this method the individual dies are utilized to construct the wax patterns, and also to establish the correct occlusion and contact relationships.

A third method is suggested. After the individual dies have set for 30 minutes in an atmosphere of 100 percent humidity,

A

B

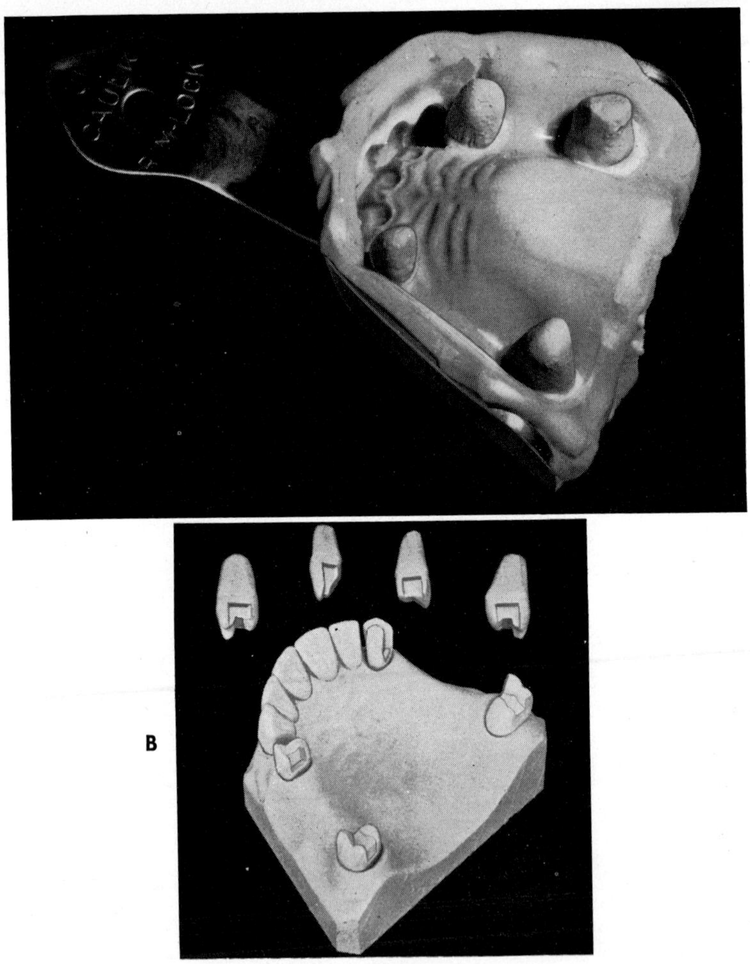

Fig. 21-39. Individual stone dies and working cast made from one impression. (Courtesy J. M. Ney Co.)

they are carefully removed from the impression, trimmed, and laid aside. A new batch of stone is then poured into the entire impression, giving a solid master model that contains replicas of the prepared abutments.

The individual dies are used for the final adaptation and marginal finish of the wax patterns; the master model is used for the initial adaptation of the wax pattern, for determining occlusion and contacts, and for the completion of the bridge as described in the first method.

The fourth method employs one impression in which a master model is made with individual, removable stone dies. This method differs from the preceding one in this respect: after the individual dies are poured, they are not removed from the master impression. Once the individual stone dies have been poured they remain in the impression until the remainder of the model is poured. The technic is as follows: first, the improved stone is poured into each abutment preparation, but before the stone has set a Ney Universal

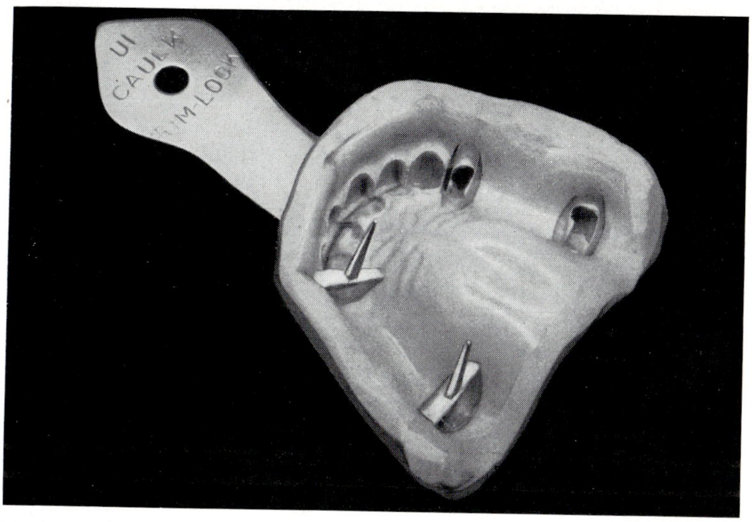

Fig. 21-40. Use of Ney Universal dowel in conjunction with removable stone dies. (Courtesy J. M. Ney Co.)

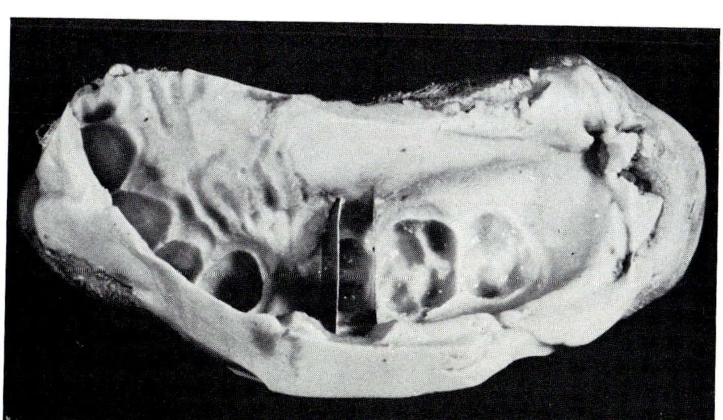

Fig. 21-41. Use of steel matrix strips in impression in forming removable stone dies. (Courtesy Dr. H. D. Kimball.)

dowel pin is inserted into each of the dies (Fig. 21-40). Where two or more dies are poured, an effort should be made to parallel the dowel pins with each other. Kimball[9] and J. M. Ney Co.[10] have suggested the use of steel matrix strips, 0.002 inch thick, inserted mesially and distally of the abutment impression area and extending from the buccal to the lingual area (Fig. 21-41). These strips are inserted at a slightly converging angle apically so that a tapered die of the prepared abutment is formed when stone is poured between them (Fig. 21-42). The entire impression with the individual stone dies containing the dowel pins is now placed in a humidor of 100 percent humidity until the stone has thoroughly set. This usually requires 20 to 30 minutes. The impression is then removed from the humidor, the dowels and

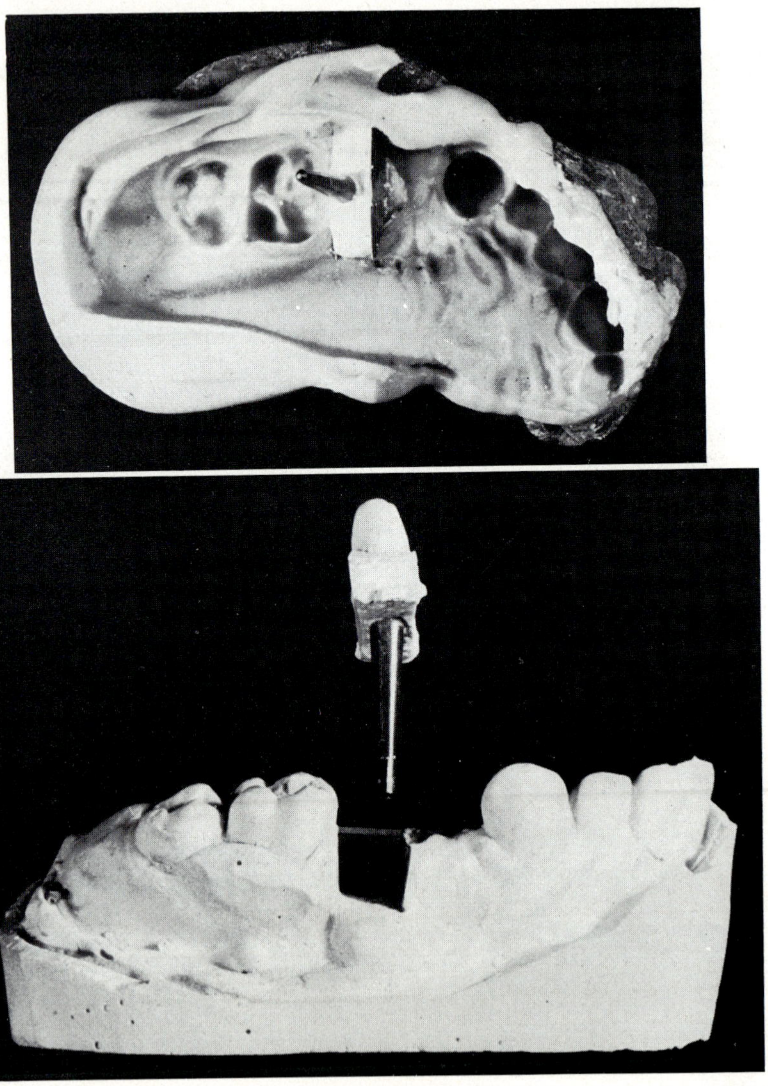

Fig. 21-42. Tapered base stone die with dowel, after cast is poured, may be readily removed and replaced accurately. (Courtesy Dr. H. D. Kimball.)

the exposed bases of the stone dies are lubricated, and the entire impression is poured in stone.

Again the poured impression is placed in 100 percent humidity and allowed to set for 30 minutes. At the end of this time, the stone model is removed from the impression. We now have a master model containing two or more removable stone dies. These dies are maintained in their correct position and relationship in the master model by the dowel pins and the slightly tapered stone bases (Fig. 21-43).

Another method is described in Chapter 28.

Wax pattern fabrication on dies

Three steps are involved in making the wax pattern if separate dies have been constructed, and a solid master model is also available that contains the abutment preparations. Step 1 consists of forming the wax pattern on the individual stone die. The pattern may be made by the dipping process or by confining softened wax within a matrix and conforming it over the lubricated die. When the pattern has been contoured to its proper anatomy on the individual die it is transferred to the articulated master model in order to verify contact areas and occlusion. Points of interference on the master model that may prevent the seating of the pattern may be trimmed away so that the pattern may be fully seated and the occlusal and axial surfaces corrected. The pattern is then rechecked for marginal fit on the individual die.

To allow for polishing and adjusting the contact areas on the castings, Thompson[3] suggested that a small bead of melted wax be added to the wax pattern in the area of the contacts, and immediately upon its congealing, the pattern is seated, thereby compressing the soft wax in the contact areas. When the pattern is removed from the master model and transferred to the individual die for final finishing of the margins, the compressed contact area wax expands slightly, giving a plus contact in the casting. This is caused by the release of stresses of compression.

A wax pattern is prepared for each of the dies, invested, and cast.

The castings having been made, they are cleaned and fitted on the individual dies. Each casting is finished and polished to within 1 mm. of its margins.

The finished castings are now transferred to the master model, which may (1) be solid, (2) contain removable dies, or (3) consist of sections assembled on a keyed plastic or metal plate. The pontics are then constructed and united with the

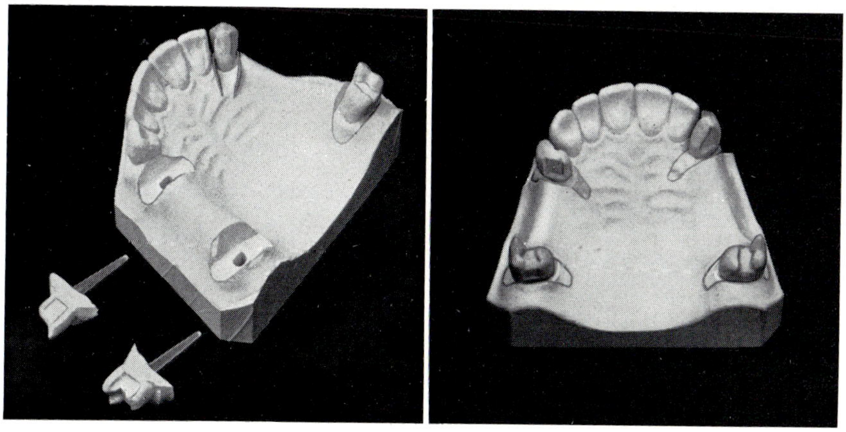

Fig. 21-43. Similar method to Fig. 21-42, using Ney Universal dowels. (Courtesy J. M. Ney Co.)

cast retainers, using the stone index technic. The bridge is finished before the patient arrives for the second sitting.

The hydrocolloid indirect technic makes it possible to prepare all the abutments and take the impressions at one of the patient's visits and at the second visit to cement the finished bridge. Only the final polishing of the margins needs to be done after the bridge is cemented in place.

One word of caution is offered. Unless each step in the technic is performed with meticulous care and the materials manipulated properly, the results will not be satisfactory. The rapid development and acceptance of this technic by a large segment of the dental profession testifies to its merits and possibilities. For a more detailed and comprehensive discussion of registering and mounting casts and working models in an articulator, see Chapters 28, 29, and 34.

LIMITATIONS OF IRREVERSIBLE (ALGINATE) IMPRESSION MATERIAL

Laboratory experiments indicate that the alginate impression material is as accurate as the reversible type.[11] However, its limitation as an impression material for cavity, crown, and bridge impressions lies in the fact that it has a comparatively short working time. This does not allow sufficient time for the operator to fill the cavity with the syringe and the tray, and still have time left to carry the tray into position while the material is in its sol condition. As a result, there frequently is a lack of union between the material covering the tooth and that in the tray.

Efforts have been made to increase the setting time of the alginate material by utilizing ice water and chilling the plaster bowl and spatula.

If an alginate hydrocolloid is selected for cavity and bridge impressions, then a type of material must be used that has the necessary viscosity without changing the water-powder ratio as recommended by the manufacturer. Such a material should possess a gelation time of 6 to 8 minutes at room temperature.

It has also been found that when alginate hydrocolloid is applied to a dry surface there is adhesion of the material to the tooth; consequently, a better impression is obtained when the surface is not completely dried. However, although the surface must not be desiccated, there should not be any free saliva in the cavity when the impression is taken.

To prevent the impression material from adhering to the teeth, Rudd[12] recommends the application of a nondrying silicone material to the tooth surfaces. He incorporates the silicone into a prophylactic compound to clean the teeth prior to taking the impression. The cleaning paste consists of 50 Gm. of silicone compound,* 50 drops oil of peppermint (USP), 20 drops liquid petrolatum, and 40 Gm. fine flour of pumice.

After brushing the teeth lightly with the compound, the mouth is flushed with water and thoroughly dried; then it is coated with a cotton applicator with the liquid silicone and excess is displaced with air. The mouth now is ready to have the impression taken.

Generally, it has been found that the reversible hydrocolloids are more suitable for the indirect technic in operative and crown and bridge restorations, whereas the alginates find greater use for impressions involving removable partial dentures and as a wash for complete dentures.

If alginate hydrocolloid is used for cavity impressions, then the same precautions and methods of tissue retraction are employed as for the reversible hydrocolloid.

Any type of hydrocolloid impression material is stretched and stressed upon removal over undercuts. Stresses, when released, may cause discrepancies in the finished dies or casts; these are found to be more nearly negligible in removable

*Dow Corning Silicone 555.

partial denture casts than in dies of prepared cavities.

Attempts have been made to combine the two types of hydrocolloid in one impression; since there is no union between the two materials, other than a mechanical one, there is danger of a distorted die or cast.

Because the change from the sol to the gel is the result of a chemical reaction and is not dependent upon change in temperature, it is not necessary to use a water-cooled tray; however, in order to lock the gelled material securely within the tray it is necessary to use a perforated tray or a rim-lock type. If the gelled material should be displaced accidentally from the tray, the impression will give a distorted cast, and such an impression should not be used.

As with the reversible hydrocolloids, the alginate impression should not be left standing in the air, since it will lose moisture and contract; nor should it be stored in water, as it will imbibe water and become distorted. If it must be stored for a short time, it should be kept in an environment of 100 percent relative humidity.

The successful use of the alginate hydrocolloid depends upon the correct lapse of time between its spatulation and placement in the mouth. It is well to make a preliminary mix using water at 70° F., and to determine the initial and final set of a new batch of hydrocolloids. Most of the alginates on the market today have an initial set of 2 to 3 minutes and a final-set period of 3 to 4 minutes, a total of 5 to 7 minutes. The time of final gelation is usually measured from the beginning of the mix until the final set has occurred. Once the gelation has started it must not be disturbed, since a distortion will result.

It must be remembered that the alginate hydrocolloid is of relatively recent manufacture. Investigation has shown[3] that materials stored for 1 month at 65° C. were unsuitable for dental use, were unreliable as to their setting time, and had decreased in compressive strength. As the temperature was lowered to 50° C., deterioration also took place but more slowly. When the material was stored at a temperature of 37° C., it showed no deleterious effects. Consequently, if a large supply of the material is to be stored, it should be kept at low temperatures. This may answer some of the unexplainable dimensional instability of alginates that has been observed even when all other variables have been constant.

Whether to place the alginate impression in a fixing solution or not depends largely on the product used. Some manufacturers advocate and furnish a fixing solution with their material, but the more recent types of hydrocolloids do not require this additional treatment. If the fixing solution is advocated by the manufacturer, it should definitely be used since it will hasten the setting and prevent any surface softening of the stone die or cast.

Some dentists recommend that, after the stone die or cast has been poured into the impression, both be placed back into the fixing solution, usually a sulfate. In any event, the impression should never be left exposed to air for any length of time; neither should it be exposed to tap water longer than required to wash off any debris or saliva. If the impression is immersed in a hardening or fixing solution, 10 minutes should be enough for the surface layer of the gel to obtain a sufficient hardening effect.

As with the reversible hydrocolloid, the stone cast or die should not be removed from the impression before 1 hour. This is true even though the hydrocolloid requires the use of a hardening solution prior to pouring the cast. Also, it has been found inadvisable to place the poured cast and impression in tap water while it is setting; the resultant cast will have an inferior surface.

SELECTED REFERENCES

1. Poller, A.: Improved material for moulding articles of all kinds, more particularly parts of living bodies: British Patent No. 252112, Sept. 4, 1925.
2. Golden, E. H.: A study of impression and model materials for facial casts, M.S. Thesis, Northwestern University Dental School, 1932.
3. Thompson, M. J.: Exposing the cavity margin for hydrocolloid impression, J. South. California D. A. **19**:17, 1951.
4. Greene, L. L., and Greene, N. A.: Use of compressible dental impression cups with elastic materials, Dent. Dig. **74**(2):62-66, 1968.
5. Malone, W. F., and Manning, J. L.: Electrosurgery in restorative dentistry, J. Prosth. Dent. **20**:417, 1968.
6. Pagenkopf, A. A.: Hydrocolloid method: if not—why not? Northwest Dent. **34**:93, 1955.
7. Phillips, R. W., and Ito, F. J.: Factors influencing the accuracy of reversible hydrocolloid impressions, J.A.D.A. **43**:1, 1951.
8. Peyton, F. A., Leibold, J. P., and Ridgley, G. V.: Surface hardness, compressive strength, and abrasion resistance of indirect die stones, J. Prosth. Dent. **2**:381, 1952.
9. Kimball, H. D.: Hydrocolloid in restorative operative dentistry, D. Digest **55**:64, 1959.
10. Ney, J. M.: The Ney Chayes technic, Hartford, Connecticut, 1952, The J. M. Ney Co.
11. Skinner, E. W., and Pomés, C. E.: Dimensional stability of alginate impression materials, J.A.D.A. **33**:1253, 1946.
12. Rudd, K. D.: Accurate alginate impressions, J. Prosth. Dent. In press.
13. Hosoda, H., and others: Measurement and reinforcement of the superficial hardness of indirect stone models, J. Dent. Res. **41**:752, 1962.

GENERAL REFERENCES

Alexander, J. M.: Separating medium for alginate impressions, Brit. Dent. J. **120**:436, 1966.

Anderson, J. N.: Flow and elasticity in alginates, Dent. Progress, **1**:63-70, 1960.

Baker, C. R.: Adapting root forms to working dies, J. Prosth. Dent. **11**:929, 1961.

Bartlett, J. A.: Tissue management preceding the elastic impression, Detroit D. Bul. **30**:6-7, 1961.

Bassett, R. W., Vander Heide, J. D., and Smith, D. D.: Clinically oriented tests comparing accuracy of elastic impression materials, J. Southern California Dent. Ass. **37**:2, 1969.

Benfield, J. W., and Lyons, G. V.: Precision dies from elastic impressions, J. Prosth. Dent. **12**: 737-752, 1962.

Benfield, J. W., and Lyons, G. V.: Precision dies from elastic impressions, J. Prosth. Dent. **12**: 737, 1962.

Berman, M. H.: Technique of the copper band-compound impression, D. Digest **68**:272, 320, 364, 1962.

Block, P.: Indirect-direct method for constructing crowns to fit existing partial dentures, Dent. Dig. **71**:394-398, 1965.

Braden, M.: Characterization of the rupture properties of impression materials, Dent. Pract. **14**: 67-71, 1963.

Bull, A. W., and Brinsden, G. I.: Gingival tissue retraction for the elastic impression materials, Aust. Dent. J. **12**(4):310-313, 1967.

Christy, J. M., and Pipko, D. J.: A simplified method of indexing working dies, J. Prosth. Dent. **19**:160, 1968.

Council on Dental Research: American Dental Association Specification No. 18 for dental hydrocolloidal impression materials—alginate type, J.A.D.A. **67**:758-764, 1963.

Donnison, J. A., and Docking, A. R.: Alginate impression materials, Aust. Dent. J. **5**:280-281, 1960.

Ellis, F. N.: Direct-indirect technique for individual gold crowns, J. Prosth. Dent. **10**:545, 1960.

Federation Dentaire Internationale: Commission on Dental Materials, Instruments, Equipment and Therapeutics, Specification No. 9 for alginate impression material, Int. Dent. J. **16**:429-436, 1966.

Fellman, S.: Electrosurgical preparation of gingival marginal tissue for fixed prosthodontics, J. Prosth. Dent. **17**:583-589, 1967.

Fusayama, T., and Nakazato, M.: The designs of stock trays and the retention of irreversible hydrocolloid impressions, J. Prosth. Dent. **21**: 136, 1969.

Gogerty, J. H., Strand, H. A., Ogilvie, A. I., and Dille, J. M.: Vasopressor effects of topical epinephrine in certain dental procedures, Oral Surg. **10**:614-622, 1961.

Hamilton, A. I., and Kramer, I. R. H.: Cavity preparation with and without waterspray, Brit. Dent. J. **123**:281, 1967.

Harrison, J. D.: Effect of retraction materials on the gingival sulcus epithelium, J. Prosth. Dent. **11**:514, 1961.

Henry, R. W., and Phillips, R. W.: Influence of particle size of stone on surface detail of casts, J. Prosth. Dent. **11**:169, 1961.

Hosoda, H., and Fusayama, T.: Distortion of irreversible hydrocolloid and mercaptan rubber-base impressions, J. Prosth. Dent. **11**:318, 1961.

Jelenko, J. F., & Co., Inc.: Crown and bridge construction using hydrocolloid impressions, ed. 2, New York, 1956, The Company.

Kelly, W. J.: Symposium of electro-surgery, A.D.A. Conference, October, 1967, Washington, D. C.

Killebrew, R. H.: Direct-indirect technique for multiple inlays and fixed bridges, D. Digest **67**:271, 1961.

Klug, R. G.: Gingival tissue regeneration following electrical retraction, J. Prosth. Dent. **16**:955-962, 1966.

Krug, R. S., and Markley, M. R.: Cast restorations with gold-foil-like margins, J. Prosth. Dent. **22**:55-67, 1969.

LaForgia, A.: Mechanical-chemical and electrosurgical tissue retraction for fixed prosthesis, J. Prosth. Dent. **14**:1107-1114, 1964.

LaForgia, A.: Cordless tissue retraction for impressions for fixed prosthesis, J. Prosth. Dent. **17**(4):379-386, 1967.

Leer, J. H., and Gilmore, H. W.: Management of gingival tissue during indirect impression procedures, J.A.D.A. **75**:924-928, 1967.

Linkow, L. I.: Oral rehabilitation technique utilizing copper band impressions, J. Prosth. Dent. **11**:716, 1961.

Lisgarten, M. A.: Electron microscopic features of the newly formed epithelial attachment after gingival surgery, J. Periodont. Res. **2**:46-52, 1967.

MacPherson, G. W., Craig, R. G., and Peyton, F. A.: Mechanical properties of hydrocolloid and rubber impression materials, J. Dent. Res. **46**(4):714-721, 1967.

Marcum, J. S.: The effect of crown marginal depth upon gingival tissue, J. Prosth. Dent. **17**:479-487, 1967.

Markley, M. R., and Krug, R. S.: Silverplating rubber base material for superior dies and casts, J. Prosth. Dent. **22**:103-110, 1969.

Maves, T. W.: Recent experiments demonstrating wax distortion on all wax patterns when heat is applied, J.A.D.A. **19**:606, 1932.

Miller, I. F., and Feinberg, E.: Electronic surgery, N. Y. J. Dent. **32**:172-175, 1962.

Moffa, J. P.: Standardized hydrocolloid indirect inlay technique, J. Prosth. Dent. **13**:143-155, 1963.

Oringer, M. J.: Electrosurgery in dentistry, Philadelphia, 1962, W. B. Saunders Co.

Pelzman, D., and Salber, S.: Dental assistants' role in the hydrocolloid technic, D. Assistant **29**:11, 1960.

Peyton, F. A., and Craig, R. G.: Compatibility of duplicating compounds and casting investments, J. Prosth. Dent. **12**:1111, 1962.

Pogue, W. L., and Harrison, J. D.: Absorption of epinephrine during tissue retraction, J. Prosth. Dent. **18**:242, 1967.

Pollock, S.: Gingivoplasty technique using rotary diamond stones at ultra speed, Dent. Clin. N. Amer., pp. 99-110, March, 1964.

Pope, J. W., Gargiulo, A. W., Staffileno, H., and Levy, S.: Effects of electrosurgery in wound healing in dogs, Pedodontics **6**:30-37, 1968.

Reither, W.: Gingival retraction using approved medicaments other than epinephrine-derivatives, Zahnaerztl Welt. **67**(6):214-216, 1966.

Rinne, V. W.: Effects of various treatments on the surface hardness of stone die materials, J. Nebraska D. A. **36**:14, 1960.

Rogers, O. W.: Electrodeposited copper individual impression trays, J. Prosth. Dent. **16**:19-25, 1966.

Rubinstein, J.: Displacement of tissue in elastic impression procedure, D. Digest **67**:21, 1961.

Scully, B. R.: Paralleling dowel pins for removable dies, J. Prosth. Dent. **20**:157, 1968.

Shippee, R. W.: Accuracy of impressions made with elastic impression materials, J. Prosth. Dent. **10**:381, 1960.

Smith, D. C., and Fairhurst, C. W.: Effect of hydrocolloid impression materials on the surface of dental stone, J. D. Res. **41**:1103, 1962.

Stark, M. M., Nicholson, R. S., Scott, H. E., and Hill, B.: The detection of C-14 labeled epinephrine in the blood stream of a Rhesus monkey following gingival retraction, I.A.D.R., March, 1966, p. 118.

Stern, A. J., and Vernon, H. M.: Development of a new tool in restorative dentistry, J. Prosth. Dent. **21**:536, 1969.

Storer, R., and Skinner, E. W.: Evaluation of gypsum cast and die materials, I.A.D.R. **40**:90, 1962.

Sturdevant, C. M.: Gold castings by the hygroscopic technic: advantages and disadvantages, J. North Carolina D. Soc. **39**:93, 1956.

Thayer, K. E., and Sawyer, J. D.: Gingival retraction agents, reaction in dogs, Iowa D. J. **8**:382-385, 1963.

Thompson, M. J.: Reversible hydrocolloid impression material: its treatment and use in operative and prosthetic dentistry, J.A.D.A. **39**:708, 1949.

Thompson, M. J.: Hydrocolloid—its treatment and application in securing consistent accurate models for indirect inlays and fixed bridges, Bull. Oklahoma D. A. **38**:7-24, 1949.

Thompson, M. J.: Hydrocolloid: its role in restorative dentistry, Dent. Clin. N. Amer., pp. 101-105, March, 1959.

Toreskog, S., Phillips, R. W., and Schnell, R.

J.: Properties of die materials: a comparative study, J. Prosth. Dent. **16**:119, 1966.

Tylman, S. D.: Reversible and irreversible hydrocolloid impression materials, Dent. Clin. N. Amer., Nov., 1958, p. 713.

Van Horn, C. S.: Eliminating variables in the making of cast gold inlays, D. Cosmos **67**:159, 1925.

Wiland, L.: Elastic impressions and split remounting plates, J. Prosth. Dent. **16**:445-450, 1966.

Wilson, H. J.: Elastomeric impression materials, Brit. Dent. J. **121**(6):277-283, 1966.

Wilson, H. J.: Elastomeric impression materials, part 2: the set materials, Brit. Dent. J. **121**: 322-328, 1966.

Wilson, H. J., and Smith, D. C.: The bonding of alginate impression materials to impression tray, Brit. Dent. J. **115**:291-294, 1963.

Woycheshin, F. F.: Evaluation of the drugs used for gingival retraction, J. Prosth. Dent. **14**:769, 1964.

Chapter 22

Construction of retainers: indirect method–materials, equipment, and procedures (mercaptan–silicone base)

In addition to the reversible and the irreversible hydrocolloid impression materials, two new types have more recently been made available to the profession that offer certain advantages over the hydrocolloid types. The advantages and the reasons for the rapid, general acceptance of the so-called rubber and silicone types are, first, less equipment is required than in the reversible hydrocolloid method and, second, the critical time-element is not so involved from the moment the impression is removed from the mouth until the die or the cast is poured. Finally, there is the added advantage that the stone cast or die is less likely to have a porous or dimensionally distorted surface.

Both types of these newer materials may be used either for individual tooth impressions or for bridges and removable partial dentures. They are also used in connection with complete denture construction.

The additional advantage of the mercaptan base or silicone-type impression materials is the ease with which impressions may be electroplated either with copper or silver. The technic for silver electroplating these materials will be given later in detail.

The mercaptan base material, usually referred to as "Thiokol" rubber impression material, is, according to Skinner,[1] a polyfunctional mercaptan which, when mixed with a chemical accelerator such as lead peroxide and sulfur, is polymerized, or as is sometimes stated "vulcanized," to form a rubber-like material.

The material as supplied by the manufacturer comes in two separate tubes; one contains the base material in a paste form, while the other, in similar form, contains the accelerator. The pastes usually come in two different colors to enable the dentist, when he makes the mix, to see whether both ingredients have been thoroughly incorporated into each other; a complete mixture is a prerequisite for developing the desirable physical properties in the impression material. The correct proportions of the base material and the accelerator are usually specified by the manufacturer—likewise, the correct length of time used in making the complete mix.

The chemistry of self-curing silicone impression material, according to Shell,[2] consists basically of three ingredients: (1) an organopolysiloxane containing terminal silicone-bound hydroxyl groups—usually the methopolysiloxane is used; (2) an alkyl silicate, usually ethyl silicate; and

(3) a metallo-organic compound of lead, tin, or zirconium, combined usually in the tin octoate form. These three ingredients in combination with suitable fillers cause the fluid mixture to change into a firm, elastic solid, possessing the necessary desirable physical properties of strength, elasticity, elongation, and hardness. In the early types of silicone materials, trouble was experienced with the formation of small pits and pockmarks on the surface of the stone die due to gas developed during the setting process. This difficulty has been eliminated with the present-day silicone impression materials.

To explain the physical properties that accompany the use of the rubber or silicone types of impression materials, Shell[2] indicated that primarily they consist of chain-like molecules arranged in a coiled position; when the material is stretched, the molecules uncoil without breaking, and when the tension is released, they recoil. He stated further that, "compared with metals, rubber types of materials have a low modulus of elasticity and a low elastic limit when measured in pounds, but a high elongation (measured in inches) below the elastic limit. Rubbers are capable of sustaining large deformations without rupture or permanent elongation; therefore, they return to their original dimensions when the stress is removed. This is a most important property for elastic impression materials which are used in dental impressions. They must be capable of stretching around undercuts and returning to their original shape if accurate dies are to be obtained."[2]

PHYSICAL AND MECHANICAL PROPERTIES OF IMPRESSION MATERIALS

The setting time of the mercaptan and the silicone impression materials is influenced both by the proportions of the base material and by the accelerator used in the mix. For the mercaptan types, usually equal lengths of the base material and the catalyst are placed on the mixing pad; both are then thoroughly spatulated for ½ to 1 minute so that no differentiation exists between the color of the base material and that of the accelerator. This is absolutely essential in order to get optimum results. The viscosity of the syringe type of mercaptan impression material is less than that used in the tray; it is of a softer consistency. This is also true of the silicone materials.

The silicone impression materials may also come entirely in paste form, but frequently the base material is a paste, while the accelerator is a liquid. When the materials are in paste form, usually equal amounts of each are used in the mix. Where the base materials for both the syringe and the tray come in paste form but the accelerator for each is a liquid, then the manufacturer's instructions relative to the correct amount of liquid to use must be strictly followed. A separate tube of the liquid accelerator is furnished for the base material, and a separate tube for the syringe material, each of a different color.

In mixing the mercaptan or the silicone impression materials, a period of 45 to 60 seconds is utilized. Because the syringe impression material has a longer setting time than the tray material, the syringe type is mixed first and the syringe is filled; then the tray material is mixed and the tray is filled.

The temperature at which a mix is made affects the setting time of the mercaptan material more than it does the silicone type.[3] A higher room temperature will accelerate the setting time of the mercaptan types; the addition of a drop of water to the mix will do the same, but it may result in a tacky impression and one that may distort easily when the stone is poured into it. The addition of one or two drops of oleic acid will retard the setting time of the mercaptan material.

The length of time elapsing after the

tray mix has been made on the pad and before the impression is seated in the mouth is critical. If seating the impression tray in the mouth is delayed to the point where a setting of the material has started, there is the possibility of stresses developing in the material that will result in a distorted die.

The time required for the various materials to set completely will vary with different products. It is recommended that a minimum of 10 minutes be allowed from the time that the mix is started until the impression is removed from the mouth. Another practical and simple method is the following: after the prepared teeth have been covered with the syringe material, a small amount of the material is placed gingivally against the labial surfaces of the lower incisors and is allowed to remain there. The impression tray is then carried to place. Later, a round blunt instrument is used to test the degree of set of the labial material at 1 minute intervals. When the tackiness of the material has disappeared, the tray is left in position for an additional 5 to 7 minutes, after which the impression tray may be removed. This procedure assures us that the softer, injection type of material has set.

Impressions of elastic material, whether of the mercaptan or silicone types, should not be distorted when withdrawn from the prepared cavities or undercuts; for this reason a maximum period of time should be allowed for the material to set. Up to the present, it has been difficult for investigators to determine the exact amount of distortion of the impression when it is drawn over undercuts. Because of this difficulty, some manufacturers and investigators use the Shore Durometer, which measures a combination of the stiffness and elasticity of the material. A measure of the stiffness of the material by this method is obtained by determining the deformation effect of added weight on the surface of a rubber cylinder and then plotting a stress-strain diagram. Shell[2] has reported the comparative Shore Durometer readings on the silicone and mercaptan rubbers as shown in Table 22-1.

Table 22-1. Comparative Shore Durometer readings*

R & R Silicone		*Mercaptan rubbers*		
Fast set—more catalyst	*Slow set—less catalyst*	*Heavy base*	*Regular base*	*Light base*
51	49	54	39	28

*From Shell, J. S.: Chemistry of RTV silicones, Bulletin No. 9, Toledo, Ohio, 1959, Ransom & Randolph Co.

Because of the greater tensile strength, tear strength, and compressive strength of the tray type of material it is superimposed on and confines the syringe type of material, which covers the tooth preparation.

When permitted to set properly, the improved, present-day mercaptan and silicone materials exhibit excellent elastic properties and dimensional stability after their removal from the mouth.

One of the reasons for the general acceptance of these materials by the profession is that they do not change as rapidly dimensionally as the hydrocolloid impression materials upon their removal from the mouth. The hydrocolloids, both the alginate and the agar-agar types, exhibited marked dimensional changes unless the impressions were poured within 15 minutes after their removal from the mouth. Any changes of the mercaptan and silicone impression materials, when they do occur, take place very slowly and are relatively stable even after a period of half an hour. Nevertheless, it is recommended that the mercaptan and silicone impressions be poured immediately or within a period not exceeding 30 minutes.

Because neither the mercaptan nor the silicone impression materials adhere to the tray, it is necessary to apply an adhesive to the tray, even if it is perforated, so as to attach the impression material securely to the tray. By utilizing the adhesive between the tray and the impression material, another function is served; namely, the bonding of the impression material to the tray slightly inhibits the contraction of the materials. The dimensional stability of the mercaptan and silicone materials is superior to that of the hydrocolloid types.

The amount of impression material used in the impression has a significant bearing on the accuracy of the stone die. It has been found that the greater the bulk of material used, the greater the dimensional distortion of the die. Therefore, the tray should be so conformed to the teeth and tissues that there will be a uniform thickness of from 2 mm. to 4 mm. of the material in the impression. Tests have shown that where severe undercuts exist there is a greater possibility of distortion in the impression than when parallelism is approached. The consensus at present is that greater accuracy is possible with the mercaptan types of materials than with the silicone types, because the latter are more recent in development and there still exist more variations in the product. In time, no doubt, the silicones will be developed to the same degree of accuracy and dependability as the mercaptan types. One other disadvantage, up to the present, of the silicones has been their short shelf life.

IMPRESSION TECHNIC USING MERCAPTAN RUBBER BASE IMPRESSION MATERIAL

Constructing the tray

Prior to starting the preparation on the abutment teeth it is advisable to make a custom tray of self-curing resin on the study models (Fig. 22-1). This may be done some time prior to the arrival of the patient. The tray for the side where the bridge is to be placed is made so that there will be approximately from 2 to 4 mm. of space between its inner surface and the teeth and tissues. The trays should have occlusal stops so that a space of 2 to 4 mm. is also maintained between the occlusal surfaces of the prepared teeth and the tray. Although a ready-made metal tray may be used, usually an excessive amount of the impression material will be required; this may result in a greater amount of distortion after the impression material has set. Preferably, two such individualized acrylic trays should be made; the second one is utilized later in the construction of a temporary acrylic bridge.

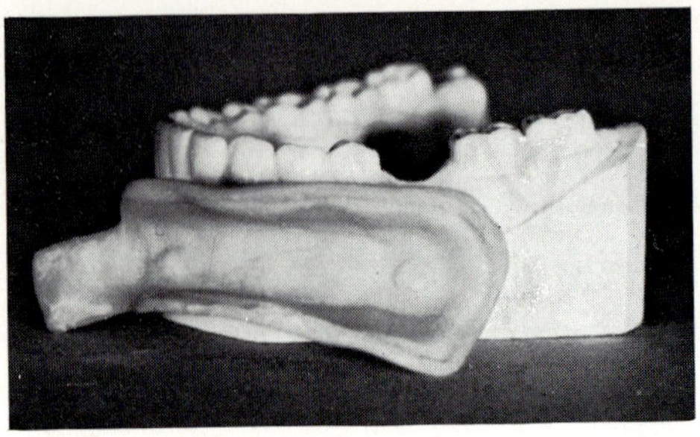

Fig. 22-1. Custom tray, made of self-curing resin, with occlusal stops.

When the preparations of the abutment teeth have been completed, the gingivae are retracted and the seepage is controlled by the methods described in Chapter 21.

In the meantime, the assistant has prepared the following materials and equipment for taking the impression with the mercaptan type of impression material: one syringe of the type shown in Fig. 22-2; a heavy mixing spatula (Fig. 22-3); a package of the heavy-bodied base and catalyst; a package of the light-bodied base and catalyst. In addition there should be two mixing pads, spatulas, and one dappen dish; also, a packet of small gauze squares that are used to wipe off the excess impression material from the sleeve of the syringe (Fig. 22-4). It is important that the syringe be properly assembled and that the plastic tip be positioned correctly so that there will be no leakage (Fig. 22-5). The rubber-ring washer on the plunger of the syringe is lightly lubri-

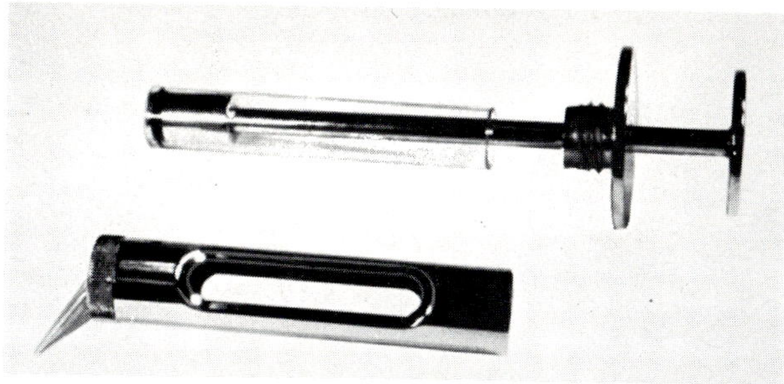

Fig. 22-2. Type of syringe used for light-type impression material, either mercaptan or silicone. (Courtesy Kerr Manufacturing Co.)

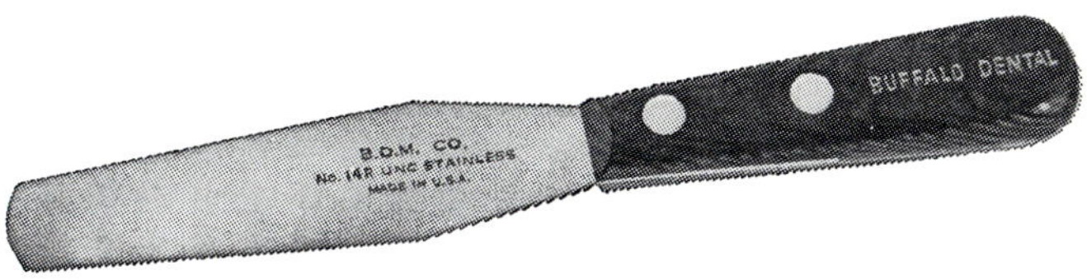

Fig. 22-3. A heavier type of mixing spatula, 14R. (Courtesy Novocol Chemical Mfg. Co.)

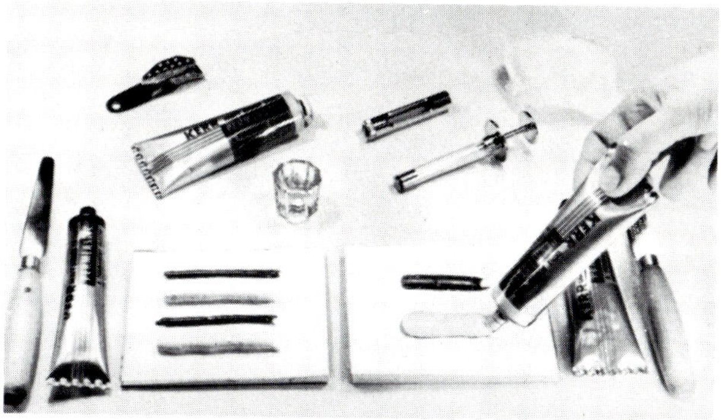

Fig. 22-4. Mercaptan impression materials, light and heavy, with complete armamentarium for their use. (Courtesy Kerr Manufacturing Co.)

cated to ensure a sufficient vacuum to draw the impression material up into the plastic sleeve.

If a metal tray is used, it is necessary to coat the inside of the tray with the adhesive material that is permitted to dry (Fig. 22-6). If an individualized, plastic tray has been made, adhesive must also be applied to the inside of the tray.

Two paper mixing pads are usually supplied with the impression material. However, better results are obtained if the mixing of the material is done on plate-glass slabs or sheets of stainless steel. Considerable pressure with the spatula is applied during the mixing of the two ingredients of the impression material, and frequently the paper will wrinkle under the force of mixing.

As shown in Fig. 22-4, the two spatulas, the two pads, the syringe, the dappen dish, and the impression tray are arranged and

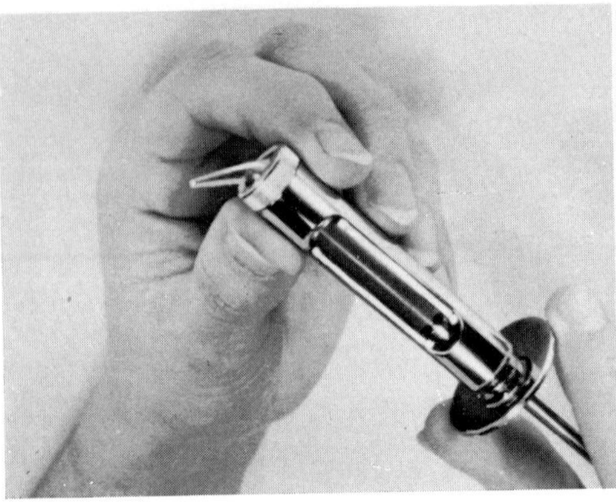

Fig. 22-5

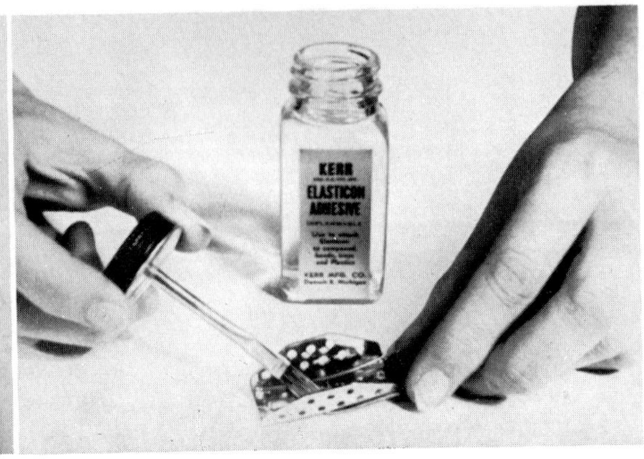

Fig. 22-6

Fig. 22-5. Assembled syringe for use with light-bodied impression material. (Courtesy Kerr Manufacturing Co.)
Fig. 22-6. Adhesive applied to inside of metal tray in order to bind impression material to tray. (Courtesy Kerr Manufacturing Co.)

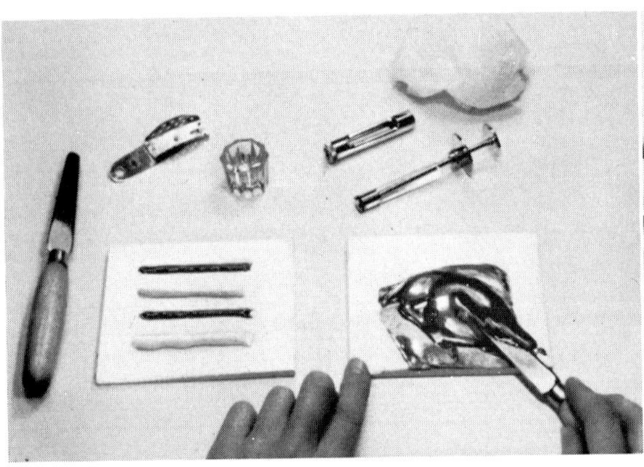

Fig. 22-7

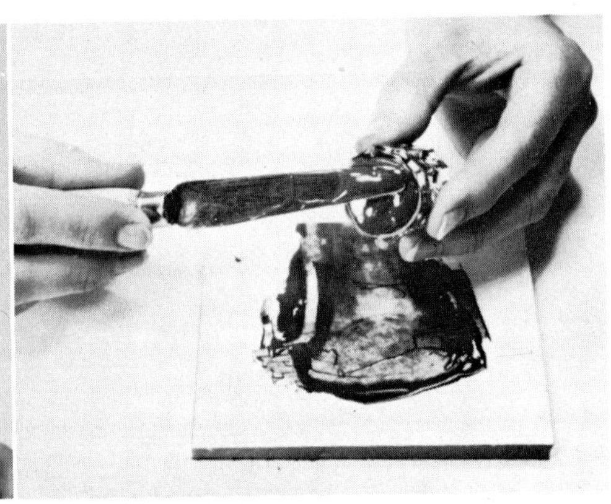

Fig. 22-8

Fig. 22-7. Mixing light-bodied mercaptan impression material to be used in syringe. (Courtesy Kerr Manufacturing Co.)
Fig. 22-8. Light-bodied impression material is placed in dappen dish. (Courtesy Kerr Manufacturing Co.)

the heavy-bodied material with its catalyst is proportioned on the slab on the left side and the light-bodied impression material is proportioned on the right. An inch and one-half to two inches is usually sufficient for the light-bodied syringe material, whereas six inches of the base and of the catalyst are required for the impression tray, depending upon the area to be covered; sometimes twice or three times this amount will be required to fill the tray.

In Fig. 22-7 the light-bodied base and catalyst are being spatulated thoroughly for approximately 45 to 60 seconds. When there is no streaking of color in the mix-

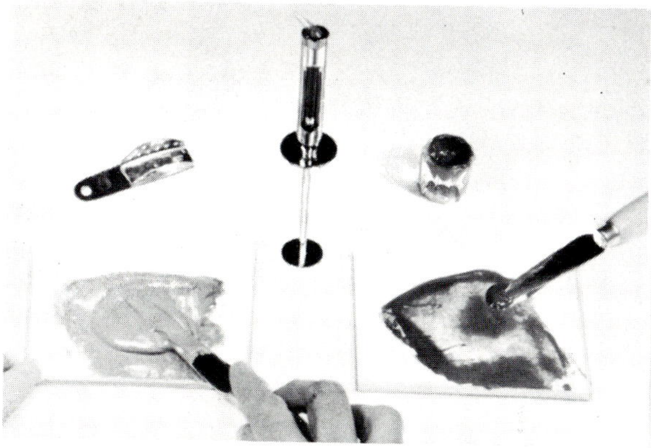

Fig. 22-9

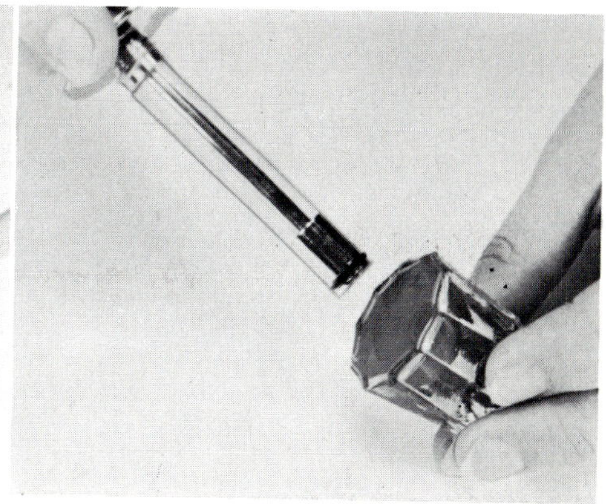

Fig. 22-10

Fig. 22-9. Syringe is filled, while tray material is mixed on left. (Courtesy Kerr Manufacturing Co.)
Fig. 22-10. Light-bodied impression material about to be drawn up into plastic sleeve. (Courtesy Kerr Manufacturing Co.)

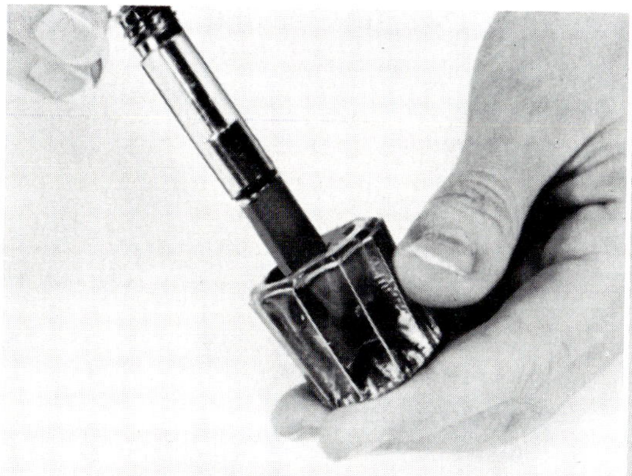

Fig. 22-11

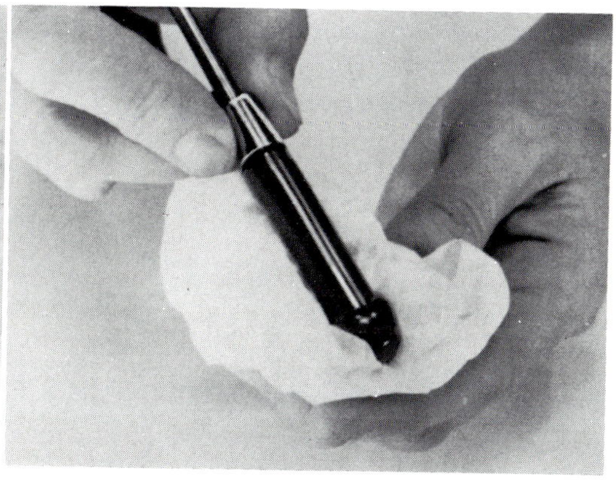

Fig. 22-12

Fig. 22-11. Light-bodied material being drawn into plastic sleeve by slowly withdrawing plunger. (Courtesy Kerr Manufacturing Co.)
Fig. 22-12. Wiping off excess material from outer surface of plastic sleeve prior to screwing on plastic tip. (Courtesy Kerr manufacturing Co.)

ture, it is gathered up with the spatula and transferred to the dappen dish as shown in Figs. 22-8 and 22-9.

In order to suck the impression material into the plastic sleeve of the syringe it is necessary first to remove the plastic tip. With the plunger inserted to the very end of the plastic sleeve, it is brought in contact with the impression material in the dappen dish (Fig. 22-10); at the same time the plunger is withdrawn slowly, sucking impression material into the plastic sleeve (Fig. 22-11).

With a small square of gauze, the excess material on the outside end of the plastic sleeve is wiped off (Fig. 22-12).

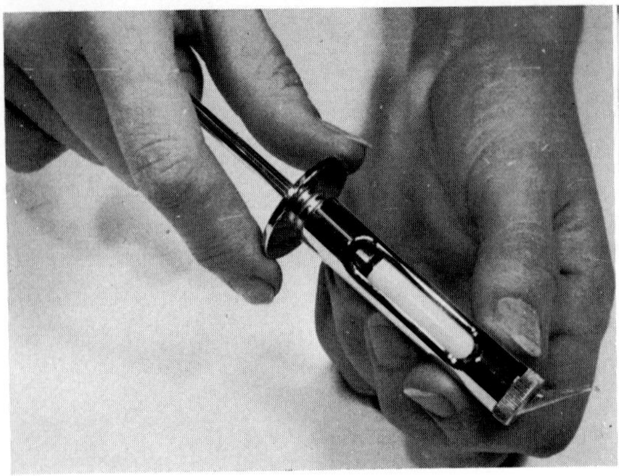

Fig. 22-13

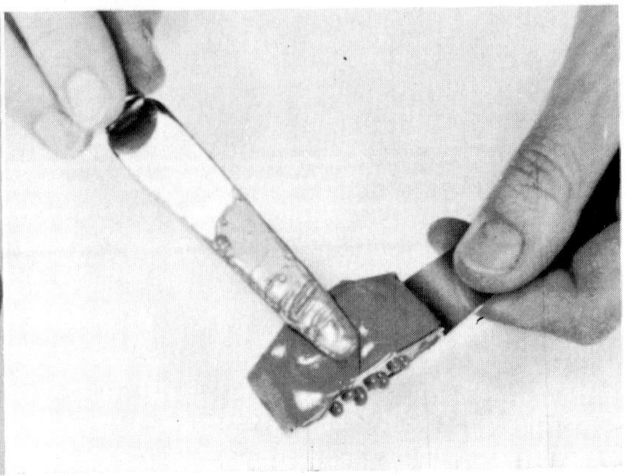

Fig. 22-14

Fig. 22-13. Plastic sleeve filled with impression material is inserted into metal barrel and plastic tip is attached to metal barrel with metal locking disk. (Courtesy Kerr Manufacturing Co.)
Fig. 22-14. Tray is filled with heavy-bodied mercaptan impression material. (Courtesy Kerr Manufacturing Co.)

The filled plastic sleeve with its plunger is inserted into the metal barrel of the syringe, the plastic tip is screwed tightly to the end of the metal barrel of the syringe (Fig. 22-13), and at the upper end of the syringe, the locking-metal-disk is screwed down as far as possible. This secures the plastic sleeve filled with impression materials so that there is no leakage possible.

If an assistant is available at the chair, she can now start mixing the heavy-bodied impression material for approximately 1 minute, after which the tray is filled. If no assistant is available, the syringe, filled with the light-bodied material, is set aside upright as shown in Fig. 22-8, and the dentist makes a mix of the heavy-bodied base and catalyst and fills the tray, as shown in Fig. 22-14. It is possible for one person to make both mixes because the light-bodied impression material has a longer setting time.

When the gingival packing has been removed and the abutment teeth dried, the light-bodied impression material is injected into and over the preparations employing the same technic as was used with hydrocolloid, i.e., the plastic tip is first carried into the gingival area where a small amount of the material is expressed against the gingival floor (Fig. 22-15); then with continued pressure more material is extruded until it flows out buccally and lingually. Maintaining contact with the prepared tooth, the plastic tip is carried over the occlusal area and to the other side and finally over all other surfaces; care is exercised not to incorporate any air bubbles. All of the prepared abutments are overfilled, after which a small globule of the light-bodied material is placed in an anterior area on a tooth not involved in the impression. This later provides a means of checking the set of the material (Fig. 22-16).

Immediately after the abutments are covered, the filled tray is seated to place with a gradual rocking motion (Fig. 22-17).

Holding the tray in position firmly but without excessive pressure, the impression is allowed to set for approximately 10 minutes from the beginning of the syringe mix. If, however, there is any doubt as to the set, it is advisable to take a round blunt

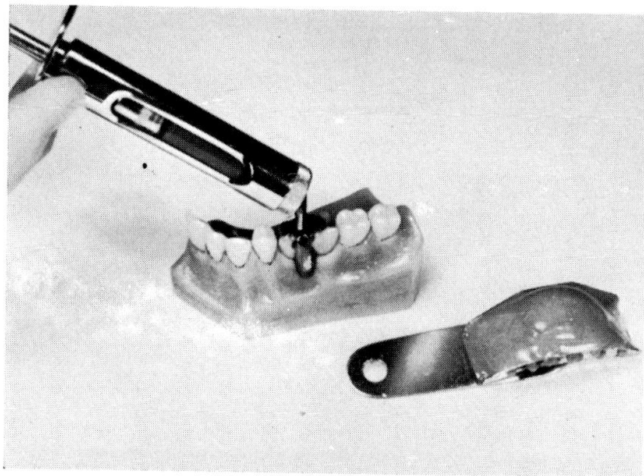

Fig. 22-15

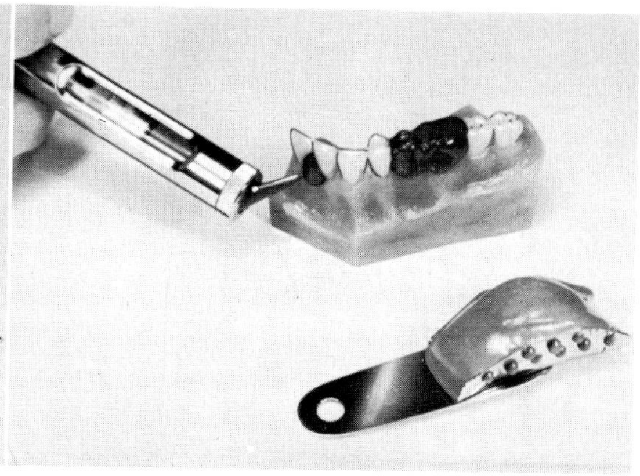

Fig. 22-16

Fig. 22-15. Initial application of syringe material in gingival interproximal area. (Courtesy Kerr Manufacturing Co.)
Fig. 22-16. After abutment teeth are covered with light-bodied material, small amount is extruded anteriorly in area not be be included in tray impression. This serves as index of degree of set of material. (Courtesy Kerr Manufacturing Co.)

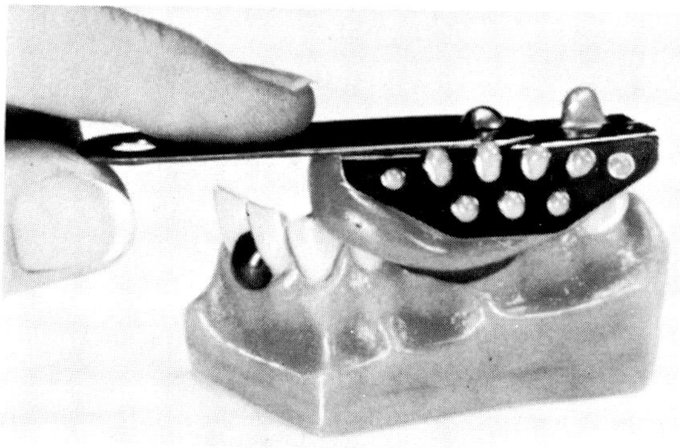

Fig. 22-17

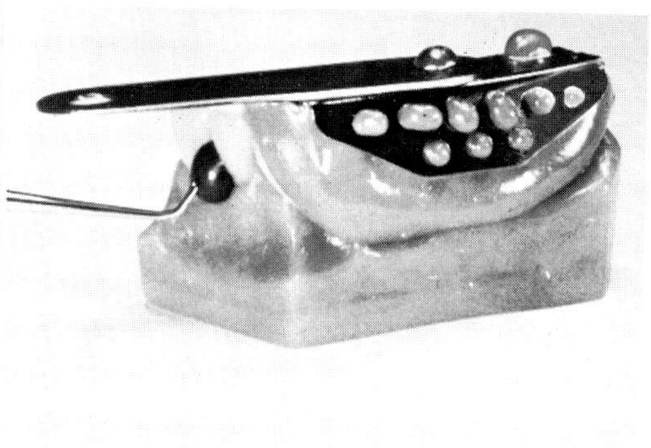

Fig. 22-18

Fig. 22-17. Seating impression tray filled with heavy-bodied mercaptan material over abutment teeth covered with light-bodied material. (Courtesy Kerr Manufacturing Co.)
Fig. 22-18. Testing set of impression material by pressing blunt instrument against button of light-bodied material. (Courtesy Kerr Manufacturing Co.)

instrument and press it against the small button of impression material that was placed in the anterior region of the mouth (Fig. 22-18). When no imprint remains in the material upon the removal of the instrument, it may be assumed that the syringe mix has set and that it is safe to remove the tray from the mouth.

In using the heavy-bodied material over the light-bodied, a compressive force is exerted on the thinner material, forcing it into close contact with all the angles and surfaces of the preparation. Too much time must not elapse between the covering of the teeth with the light syringe material and the seating of the tray with the heavier material, otherwise there will be an imperfect coalescence of the two materials. Furthermore, the material in the tray must still be in its fluid state when

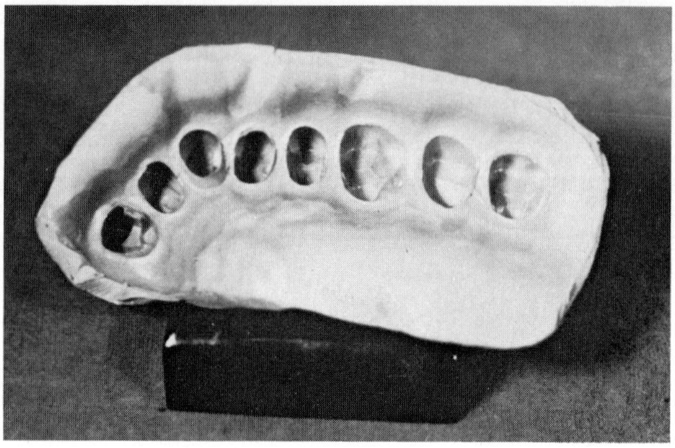

Fig. 22-19. Impression taken of inlay preparation. (Courtesy Kerr Manufacturing Co.)

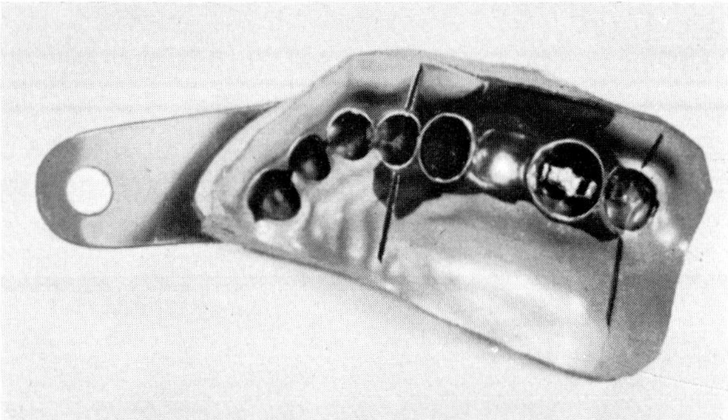

Fig. 22-20. Impression of abutments prepared for bridge. (Courtesy Kerr Manufacturing Co.)

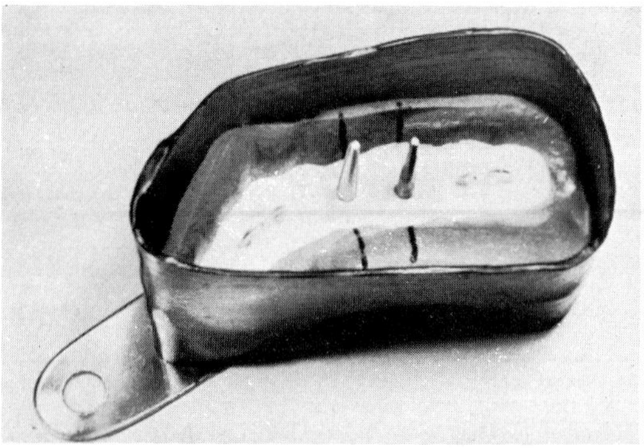

Fig. 22-21

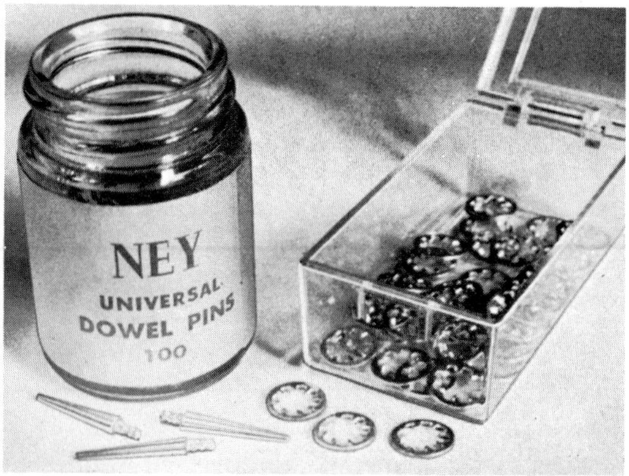

Fig. 22-22

Fig. 22-21. Removable stone dies with Ney's dowels in position; edentulous space is filled with stone, and lock washer is inserted for locking it later to master cast. (Courtesy Kerr Manufacturing Co.)
Fig. 22-22. Ney's dowel pins and lock washers. (Courtesy Kerr Manufacturing Co.)

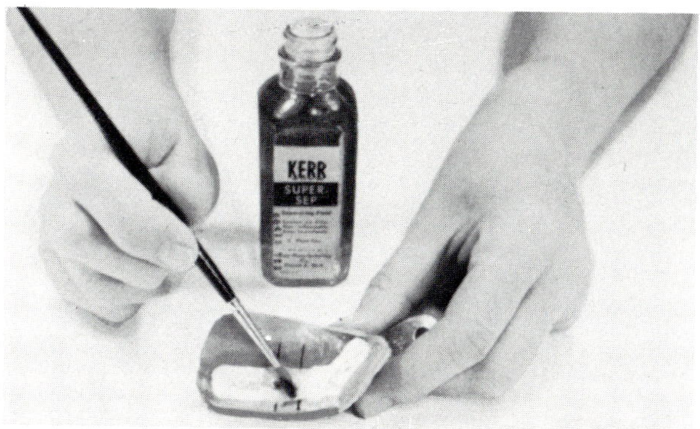

Fig. 22-23. Two removable die bases with dowels and initial stone poured into edentulous area (Fig. 22-21) are lubricated with separating medium. (Courtesy Kerr Manufacturing Co.)

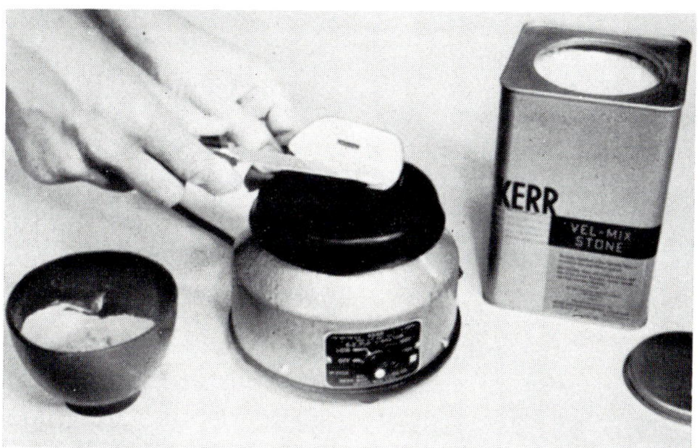

Fig. 22-24. Vel-Mix stone is poured to complete working cast. (Courtesy Kerr Manufacturing Co.)

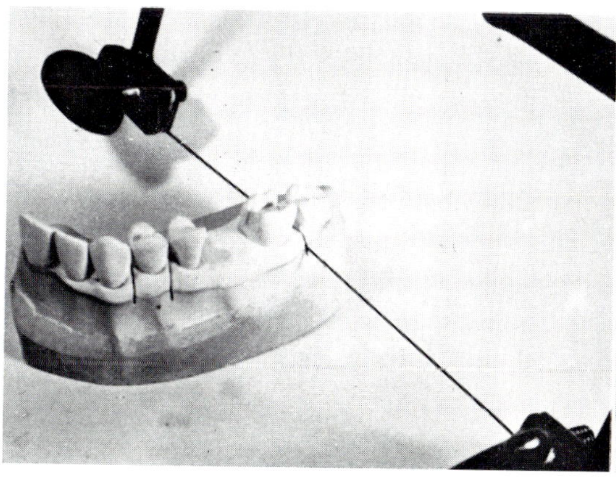

Fig. 22-25

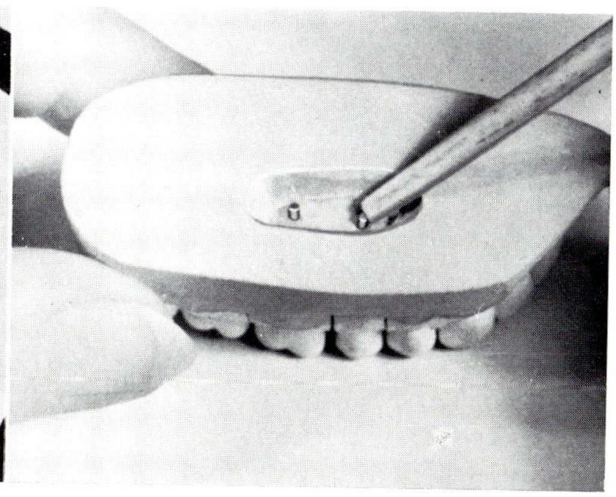

Fig. 22-26

Fig. 22-25. Saw cuts are made alongside abutment teeth to depth reaching level of second Vel-Mix pouring; this permits removal of doweled dies. (Courtesy Kerr Manufacturing Co.)

Fig. 22-26. By pressing on exposed ends of dowels, dies are dislodged occlusally. (Courtesy Kerr Manufacturing Co.)

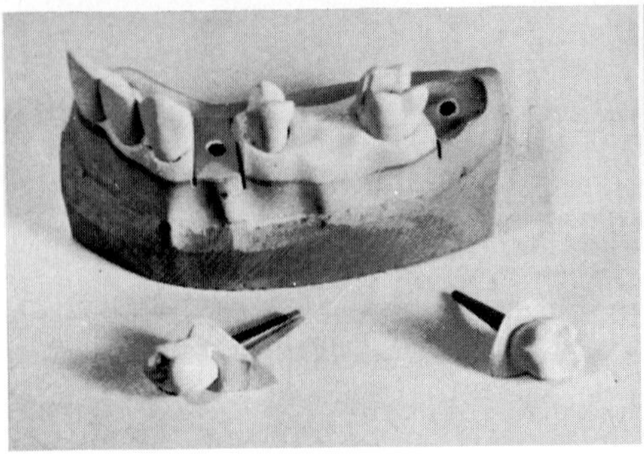

Fig. 22-27

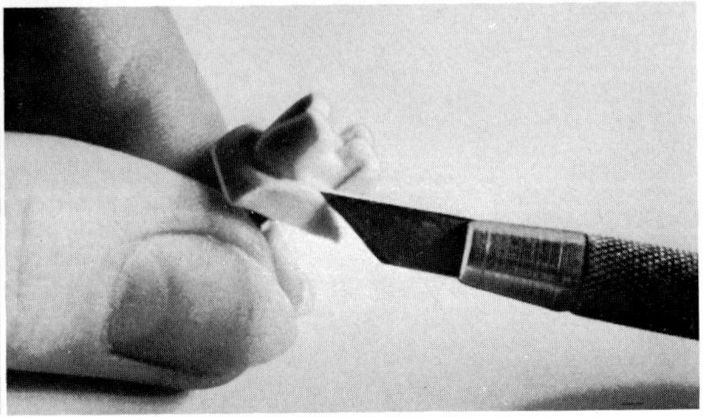

Fig. 22-28

Fig. 22-27. If desired, two teeth adjacent to prepared abutments may be made removable, leaving abutments united in solid section. (Courtesy Kerr Manufacturing Co.)

Fig. 22-28. When abutment dies are made removable, gingival margins of preparation are made accessible by trimming away any interfering excess stone. (Courtesy Kerr Manufacturing Co.)

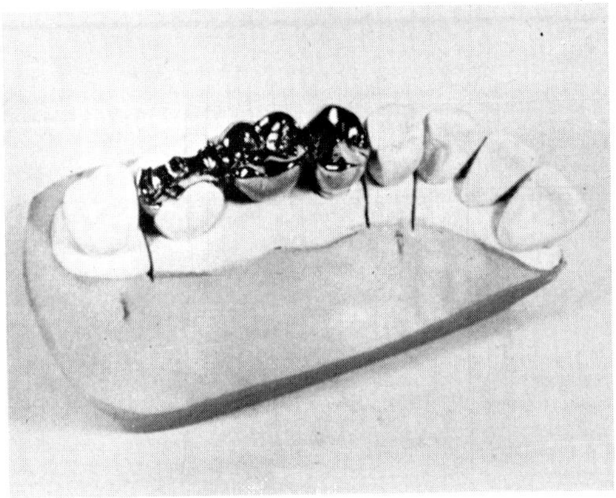

Fig. 22-29. Complete castings and bridge on cast. (Courtesy Kerr Manufacturing Co.)

seated, because, once it has started to set, the stress produced in the partially set impression will result in distortion of the impression.

As with the hydrocolloid impressions, the mercaptan impression must be withdrawn vertically from the teeth with a snaplike motion, without any rolling or rocking action.

The impression should be rinsed and blown dry before constructing the stone die as shown in Fig. 22-19 for inlay casting and in Fig. 22-20 for a bridge cast. Figs. 22-21 to 22-29 show the pouring and completing of the working model and dies in stone.

The dies and models may now be poured in Vel-Mix stone or they may be electroplated by the silver electroplating technic. The construction of stone dies and casts by various technics has been described in Chapter 21; later in this chapter the construction of dies and casts by the silver electroplating method is described.

Individual impressions in bands

There are situations in which it is deemed advisable to take individual impressions of the prepared abutments in aluminum or copper bands. If there are several abutments, the impressions may be made one or two at a time and allowed to set; they are not removed until later when an impression is taken of the entire arch with the individual band impressions left in place. When the entire arch impression is removed from the arch it will be found that the individual band impressions will come away with the complete mercaptan impression, maintaining their correct relationship with the other teeth and tissues. This technic is particularly advisable when complete-coverage abutments are prepared.

A 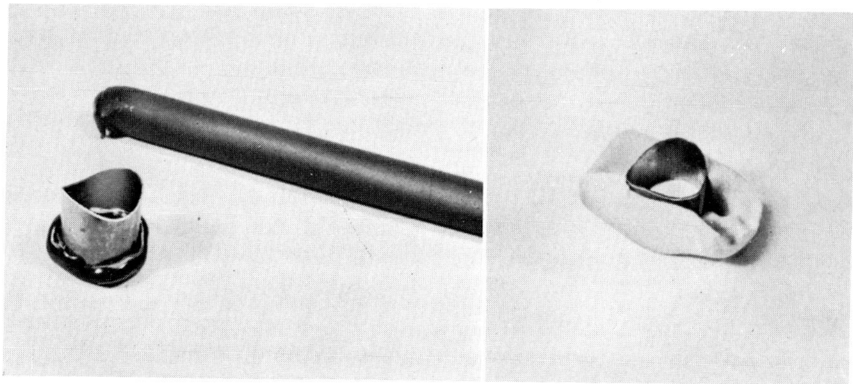 B

Fig. 22-30. A, Preparing band for single tooth impression. **B,** Re-enforcings and closing occlusal end of band to be used for single impression. (Courtesy Kerr Manufacturing Co.)

A 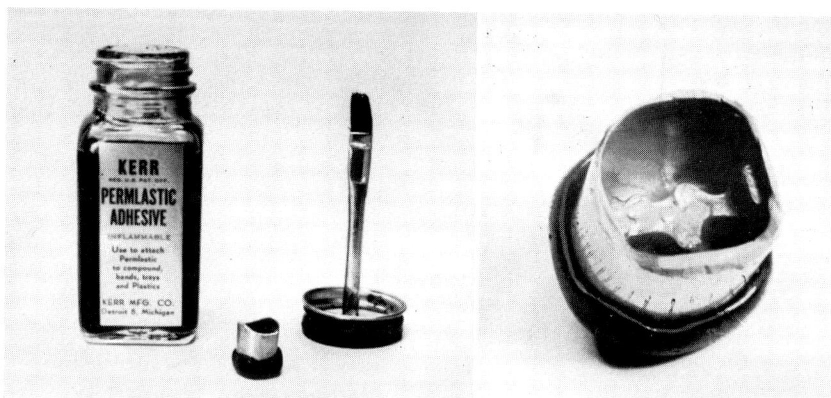 B

Fig. 22-31. A, Inside of band and occlusal stop painted with adhesive. **B,** Modeling compound used to close occlusal end of band before taking impression in mercaptan impression material. (Courtesy Kerr Manufacturing Co.)

The detailed technic is as follows:

1. Select a band that has not been annealed and one that is slightly larger than usually used, so that it will permit an inner-wall thickness of the impression material of about 3 mm. covering all surfaces of the preparation (Fig. 22-30, *A*).

2. If an open-end copper band is used instead of a shell, it is then necessary to attach a stop of compound or of self-curing resin to the occlusal end of the open band in order to reinforce it and to prevent its distortion upon withdrawal of the impression (Fig. 22-30, *B*). It also serves another purpose in that it confines the impression material and compresses it against the preparation.

3. The inside of the band and the compound or resin stop that shows on the inside is coated lightly with the adhesive cement (Fig. 22-31, *A*). This is then allowed to dry thoroughly. If no adhesive is available, then the band should be perforated and roughened on the inside with a mounted stone.

4. The prepared tooth is dried thoroughly and covered completely and subgingivally with the light-bodied material in the syringe.

5. Immediately, the band full of the

heavy-bodied material is carried to place gingivally over the covered tooth with a rocking motion and held without movement until it is thoroughly set. Since the light-bodied material requires a longer time to set than the heavy-bodied, the small button of light-bodied material placed anteriorly will serve as a guide (Fig. 22-18); when no indentation remains upon the withdrawal of a blunt instrument from its surface, the light- and the heavy-bodied materials within the band are set. Usually the total time from the beginning of the mix of the light-bodied material is approximately 10 minutes.

This procedure is followed on the several individual prepared abutments, after which the complete arch impression is taken for the bridge.

The same technic is followed where an individual impression is desired for a single crown.

In order to attach securely the modeling compound or acrylic-resin occlusal stops to the copper band, Hudson[4] recommended that cuts 1 or 2 mm. long be made around the band at its occlusal end (Fig. 22-31, *B*). Each section of the cut band is then turned outward and downward on the outside of the band; these are then engaged by the compound or the resin, locking the stop securely to the band. When individual impressions are to be removed, there is less danger of separating the occlusal stop from the band.

Proper orientation of the copper band with respect to the long axis of the abutment is important in order to avoid an uneven distribution of the rubber base material around the tooth. If this is not done there will be distortion, because the rubber-base impression materials shrink slightly during their set and since the material is held by the adhesive to the inside of the band, the slight contraction would give an oversized stone die. This is also one reason why an individualized custom-made acrylic tray is preferable to a stock metal tray because of the more even distribution of the impression material and its better orientation to the arch.

If an individual band impression is to be removed, this also should be done with a straight pull, gripping the band only by the reinforced occlusal stop of resin, because if the band is thin and distorted there will be a simultaneous distortion of the impression.

After the impression, whether of single or compound type, has been removed from the mouth, it is rinsed and dried so there are no particles of debris, blood, or saliva apparent. The impression is then poured in stone or silver electroplated.

In addition to the use of Type II, densite stone, and electroformed copper or silver dies, it is possible to fabricate individual dies of Steele's Copper-Die investment.

STEELE'S COPPER-DIE

Copper-Die is a material used in making dies for crown and bridges. It can also be used at other times when dies are required and for sectional models. It comes in powder and liquid form; included is a liquid silicone release agent that is applied to the impression, or mold, and that enhances the release of the finished die.

When mixed properly, Copper-Die will flow under vibration into the impression without the use of a centrifuge. However, a centrifuge may be used. It may be used in rubber base, silicone, and compound impression materials. It should *not* be used in hydrocolloid or alginate impression materials, as the moisture present adversely affects the setting and surface hardness of Copper-Die. The setting time of Copper-Die can be regulated within reason. With the application of heat (not to exceed 150° F.), the dies can be ready for use in 20 minutes. It will bench-harden, at room temperature, in 4 hours.

A recent development in die materials is the Ceramco high-temperature refractory die material; its uses, preparations, and manipulation are discussed in Chapter 26.

SILICONE ELASTIC IMPRESSION MATERIALS

Technic for mixing and taking the impression

Some of the advantages of the silicone impression materials over the mercaptan types are their more pleasant odor, color, and greater ease of manipulation. Although silicone fluids are water repellent, they will wet other surfaces readily because of their low surface tension. Hence, they adapt themselves to every surface detail with a minimum of external pressure.[2]

In order to more easily distinguish the tray material from the syringe material, the liquid of each is of a different color. The particular material described here uses the red liquid for the tray material and the yellow for the syringe.

Proportions

The following instructions refer to Kerr's Elasticon tray material and Syringe Elasticon.

For the Elasticon tray material the proportions are 1 inch of base material to 2 drops of the red accelerator. For individual copper band impressions, they are 3 drops accelerator to 1½ inches of base; for small unilateral trays, 12 drops of accelerator to 6 inches of base (Fig. 22-32, *left*).

For Syringe Elasticon the proportions are 1 drop accelerator, yellow liquid, to 1 inch of syringe base material. Usually it requires 4 drops of the yellow accelerator to 4 inches of the syringe base material (Fig. 22-32, *right*).

It will be noted that the mixing pads are marked off in 1-inch spaces to facilitate the measurement of the paste impression material. To ensure the uniform size of the drops of the accelerator, the tube should be held in a vertical position when dispensing it drop by drop on the pad. Likewise the accelerator liquid should not be brought in contact with the base until the beginning of the mix.

Tray elasticon base

The selection of the tray or copper band is similar to that described when using the mercaptan impression material. Likewise, an adhesive is painted on the inside of the tray or the band and permitted to dry before the application of the impression material (Fig. 22-33). For a small unilateral bridge impression, 6 inches

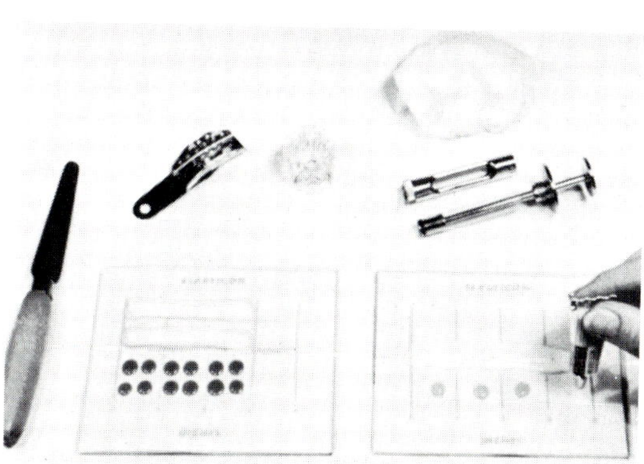

Fig. 22-32. Elasticon impression materials for tray, **left,** and for syringe, **right.** (Courtesy Kerr Manufacturing Co.)

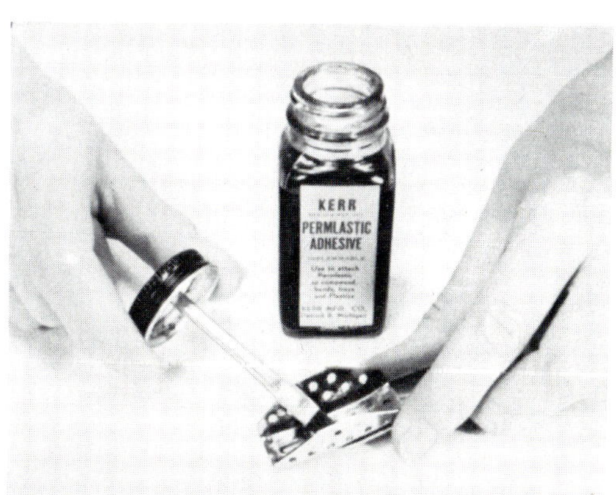

Fig. 22-33. Painting inside of tray with Elasticon adhesive. (Courtesy Kerr Manufacturing Co.)

of the tray paste material is extruded on the mixing pad. Place twelve drops of the red accelerator on an area of the pad apart from the base material.

Mixing

Using a second pad, 4 inches of the syringe base material is extruded on the pad and immediately 4 drops of the yellow accelerator is dropped directly on the material and mixed at once for a maximum of 30 seconds (Fig. 22-34). To facilitate mixing, it is advisable to start by holding the blade of the spatula at a 45° angle quickly to incorporate the liquid into the paste. At the end of 5 or 10 seconds the blade is lowered in a horizontal position and the mix spatulated to completion so

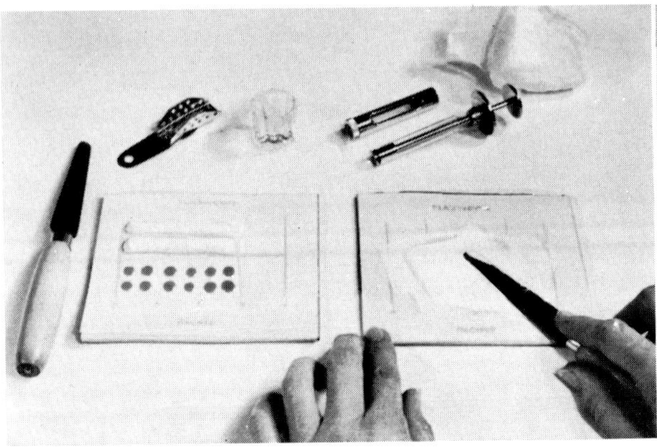

Fig. 22-34

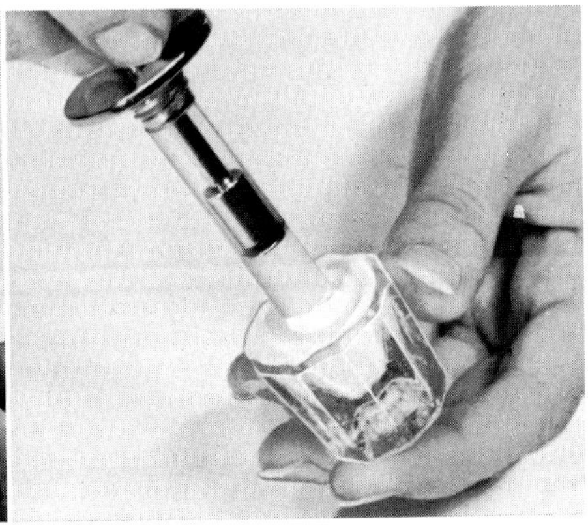

Fig. 22-35

Fig. 22-34. Mixing syringe Elasticon impression material. (Courtesy Kerr Manufacturing Co.)

Fig. 22-35. Loading syringe from dappen dish with Elasticon syringe impression material. (Courtesy Kerr Manufacturing Co.)

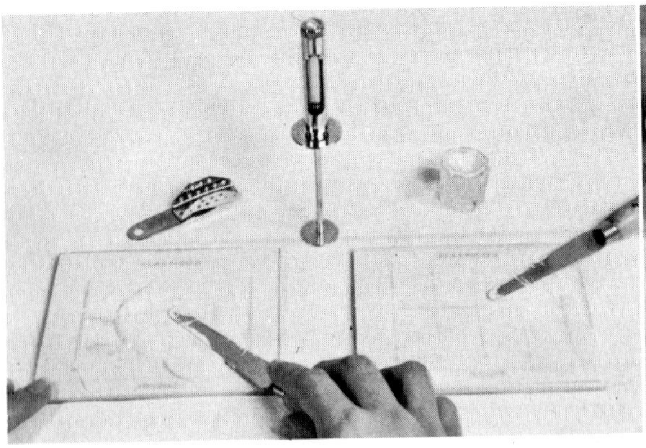

Fig. 22-36

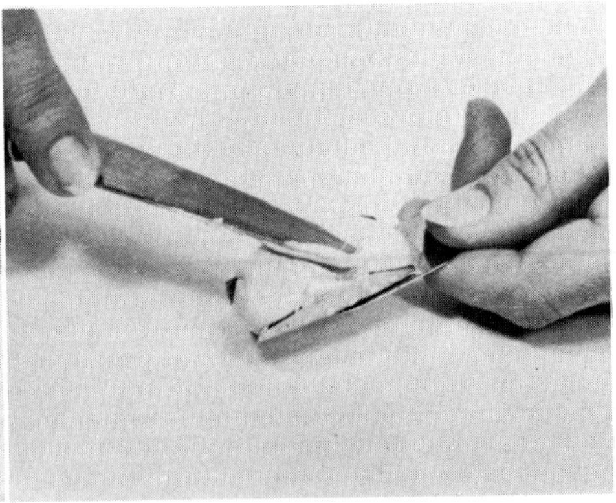

Fig. 22-37

Fig. 22-36. Filled syringe is set upright while Elasticon base material is mixed. (Courtesy Kerr Manufacturing Co.)

Fig. 22-37. Filling impression tray with Elasticon base material. (Courtesy Kerr Manufacturing Co.)

that no streaks of the mixing fluid show; instead there must be a homogenous, light-yellow mixture. The material is now quickly gathered from the mixing pad and carried to a dappen dish as shown in Fig. 22-35. The syringe is quickly loaded with the mix and momentarily set aside. The entire time consumed from the beginning of the mixing to the loading of the syringe should not exceed one and one-half minutes. The same method of filling the syringe is used as was employed with the mercaptan rubber as illustrated in Fig. 22-11.

Next, the tray material consisting of 6 inches of the base and 12 drops of the red accelerator is mixed for forty-five seconds on a separate pad and with a separate spatula (Fig. 22-36), after which it is gathered with the spatula and the tray filled, the tray having been previously coated with the adhesive (Fig. 22-37). The filled tray is momentarily set aside.

The prepared teeth are now dried and overfilled with the syringe silicone material, also the material is carried into the subgingival crevices (Fig. 22-38). A small amount of the syringe material is placed between the teeth in an anterior area not involved in the impression (Fig. 22-39). This is to serve as a check for the set of the material before removing the impression.

Immediately after the prepared teeth

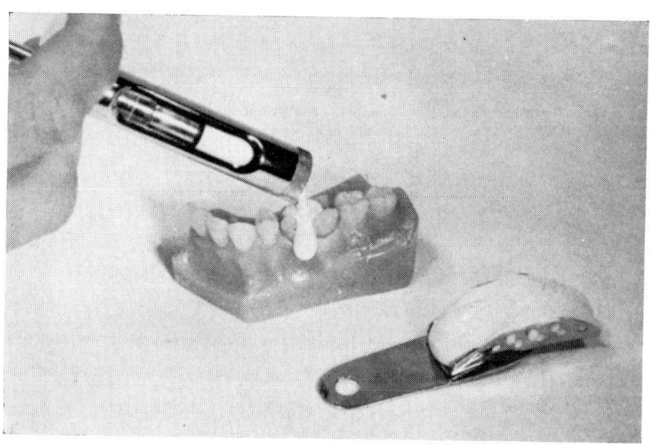

Fig. 22-38. Initial placement of syringe Elasticon in gingival interproximal area. (Courtesy Kerr Manufacturing Co.)

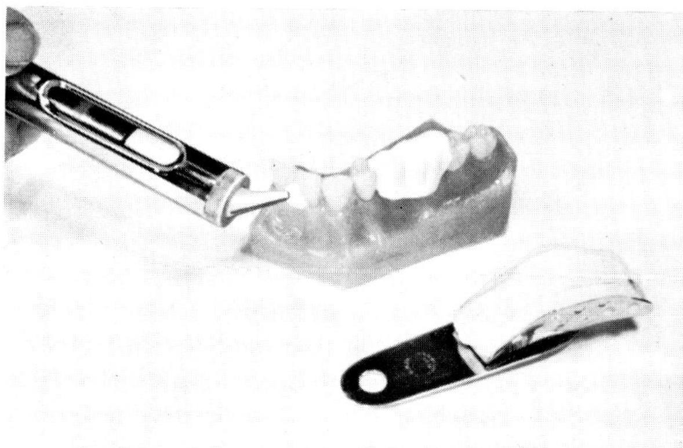

Fig. 22-39. Abutments are covered and tray filled with Elasticon base material ready for impression. (Courtesy Kerr Manufacturing Co.)

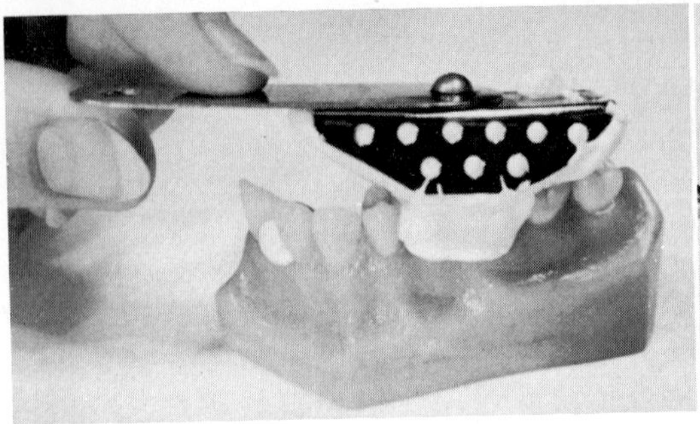

Fig. 22-40

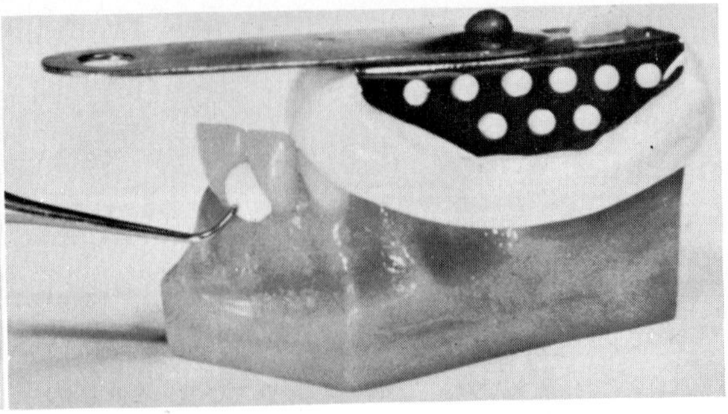

Fig. 22-41

Fig. 22-40. Lowering filled impression tray over covered abutments. (Courtesy Kerr Manufacturing Co.)
Fig. 22-41. Testing for set of impression material. (Courtesy Kerr Manufacturing Co.)

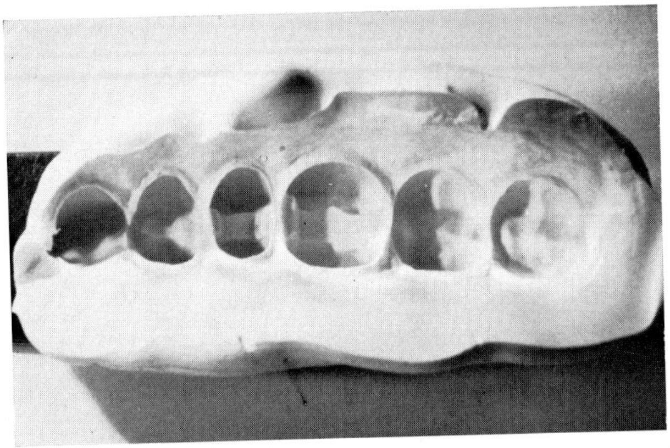

Fig. 22-42. Silicone impression of teeth prepared for individual fillings. (Courtesy Kerr Manufacturing Co.)

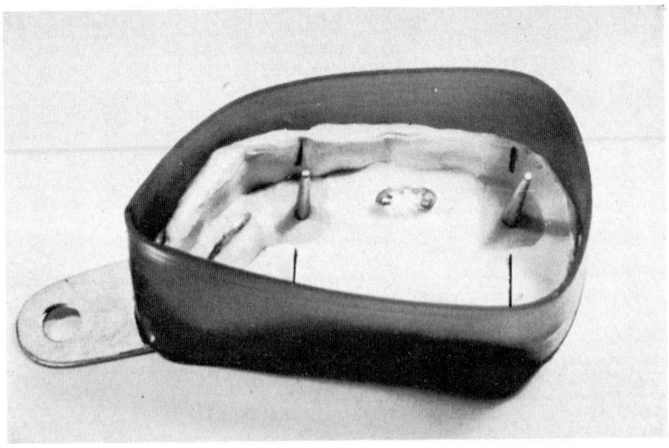

Fig. 22-43. Ney's dowels and lock washers placed in initial pour of stone. (Courtesy Kerr Manufacturing Co.)

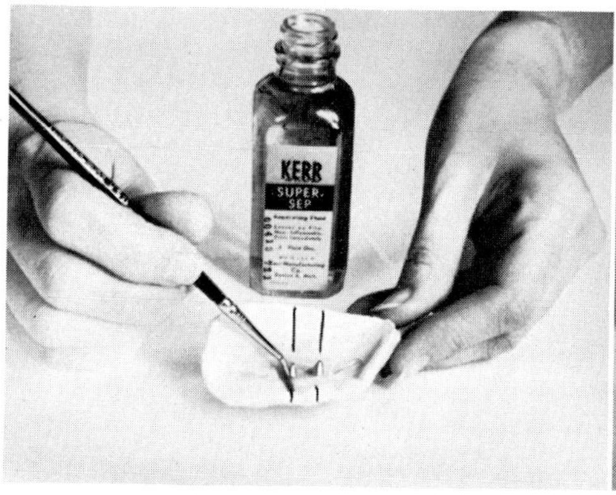

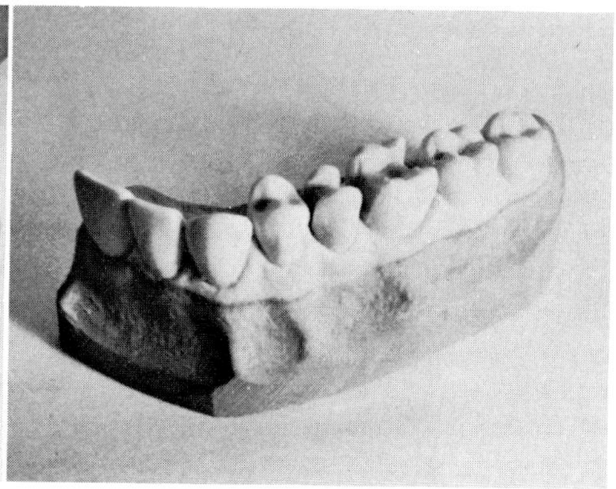

Fig. 22-44

Fig. 22-45

Fig. 22-44. Applying separating medium to set stone. (Courtesy Kerr Manufacturing Co.)
Fig. 22-45. Completed stone working casts showing dividing plane between first and second pourings of stone. (Courtesy Kerr Manufacturing Co.)

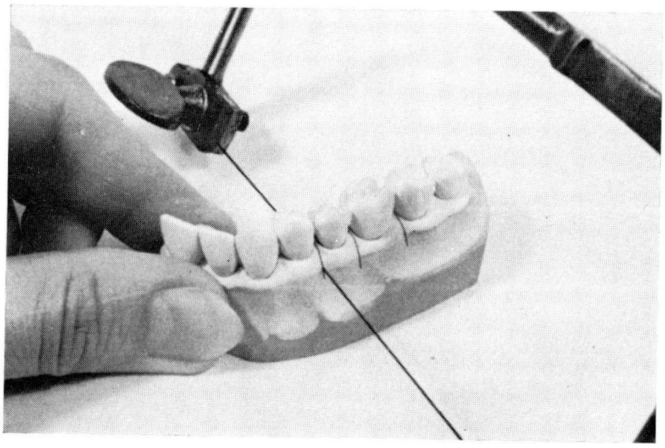

Fig. 22-46. Cutting between prepared teeth. (Courtesy Kerr Manufacturing Co.)

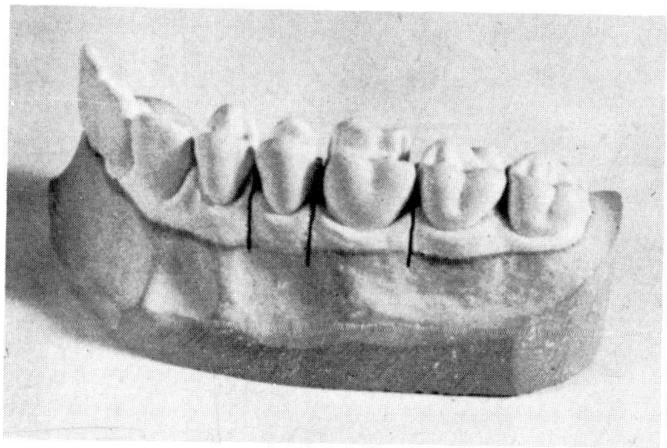

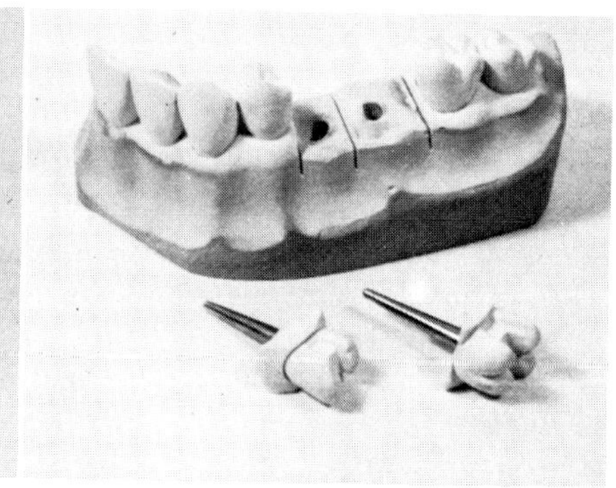

Fig. 22-47

Fig. 22-48

Fig. 22-47. Interproximal saw cuts completed between prepared teeth below junction of first and second pourings of stone. (Courtesy Kerr Manufacturing Co.)
Fig. 22-48. Two stone dies removed from working cast. (Courtesy Kerr Manufacturing Co.)

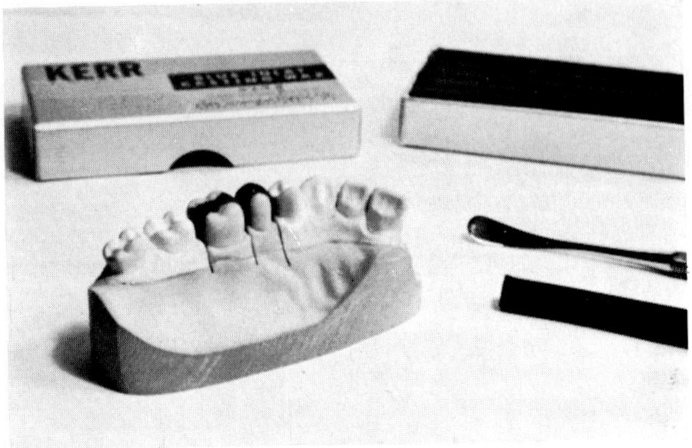

Fig. 22-49. Wax patterns prepared on stone dies. (Courtesy Kerr Manufacturing Co.)

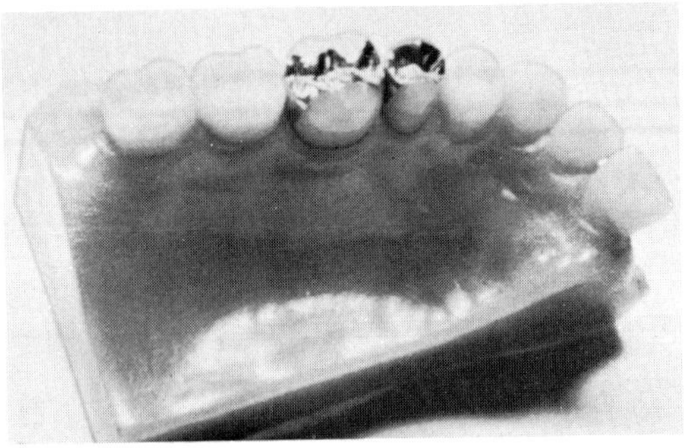

Fig. 22-50. Finished inlays in prepared teeth in model. (Courtesy Kerr Manufacturing Co.)

have been covered with the syringe material, the tray is carried to place with a rocking movement and held gently without movement until it is set (Fig. 22-40).

Usually the set occurs at the end of 10 minutes from the beginning of the syringe mix. However, by pressing a blunt instrument against the small button of material placed on the anterior teeth, completeness of the set can be determined if no indentation remains when the instrument is withdrawn (Fig. 22-41).

When set, the impression is removed vertically with a straight pull without any rocking motion. It is rinsed, dried, and examined to see that all angles and surfaces of the preparation are accurately reproduced (Fig. 22-42). The impression is then ready to be poured in stone or it may be silver electroplated. Figs. 22-43 to 22-50 show the steps in constructing inlays by this method, utilizing two removable dies.

Cleaning the syringe

A clean syringe is essential to the successful use of the mercaptan and the silicone impression materials. If care is taken to seat the plastic tip properly and to wipe away the excess material from the plastic sleeve after filling, and if the locking disk is tightened securely, very little care is needed to keep the syringe clean and ready for reuse. To clean the syringe after use, the remaining material must be completely set. To accelerate the set of the material remaining in the syringe, it can be placed in warm water not exceeding 120° F., for a minute of two. The plastic sleeve in the syringe should not be placed in water of a higher temperature nor for a longer time than 1 or 2 minutes, because it may swell and not fit the metal barrel of the syringe.

After the injection of the material over the prepared teeth has been completed, a small bead of the material is left at the end of the plastic tip; it is left there until it sets. Subsequently, when the syringe is to be cleaned the little bead of impression material at the end of the plastic tip is gently rolled and pulled outwardly, causing it to detach from the inner surface of the tip. If one is careful, this detachment may extend a considerable distance up into the cone-shaped tip; eventually it will break and pull away from the mass within the tip. The syringe is dissembled by unscrewing the large locking disk and withdrawing the plunger. If the inside of the plastic sleeve was previously covered with a thin film of petrolatum, the material remaining within the tube withdraws in one piece, including any portion inside the plastic tip. The inside of the plastic sleeve is cleaned by passing the slightly lubricated brush through the sleeve several times. Caution must be taken not to use an excess of the lubricant as it may interfere with the working qualities of the impression material.

While the plastic tips are intended to be disposable, they are sometimes reused after being placed in a cold disinfectant solution. All metal parts of the syringe can be sterilized by any conventional method.

Electroformed dies and casts

Although stone dies and casts have proved satisfactory in the past, many dentists prefer the use of metal electroformed dies. The silicone impressions may be electroplated with copper or silver; the mercaptan impressions are best suited to silverplating.

There are several reasons why dies electroformed in silicone or mercaptan impressions are preferred to stone dies. First, they are stronger; second, they have a better marginal definition; third, it is much easier to wax a pattern and rewax several times if necessary; fourth, in finishing a casting there is less danger of injuring the margins of a die or a model; fifth, there is less danger of damaging the die in trying on the casting; sixth, the problem of expansion or contraction of the stone material is not present; seventh, undercuts in the preparation are more easily detected on the silver die; eighth, when making a repair of a pontic, a silver die facilitates the spot grinding of porcelain; ninth, a complete occlusal counter-cast made of silver prevents the wear of its cusps during the construction of an appliance in the opposing arch; and tenth, high spots in the occlusion are easily detected without the use of carbon paper.

The electroforming method may be used for individual teeth prepared for inlays or crowns; likewise, it may be employed for casts used in constructing fixed and removable partial dentures.

Silver electroplating. The equipment needed for dies and working casts made by the silver electroplating method follows.

Equipment necessary. The equipment needed for silver electroplating is similar to that employed for copper electroplating; the exception is that: (1) a silver in place of a copper anode is used, also a solution of silver cyanide is employed instead of copper sulfate—the anode is of pure silver, of a size and weight suitable to the size, shape, and volume of the liquid in the tank; (2) the ammeter must register in milliamperes and is so adjusted that the current may be delivered within a range of 0 to 500 milliamperes; (3) a plating tank of glass, hard rubber, or some type of plastic is needed that will not react to the cyanide solution, a 1- or 2-quart container sufficing for the average dental office—the container should have a well-fitting cover to prevent the evaporation of the solution; (4) a cathode suspension holder of the single or multiple type is needed, also an anode holder, preferably one made of stainless steel; (5) the silver cyanide solution may be bought prepared in concentrated form, which is then diluted with distilled water in the proportions recommended by the manufacturer. Usually a freshly made solution should be permitted to stand for at least a day before it is used. For those wishing to make their own solution, the following formula has been recommended by Hudson: silver cyanide, 4 ounces; potassium cyanide, 7½ ounces; potassium carbonate, 6 ounces; 1 gallon of distilled water.[4] It will be found that, from time to time, the level of the solution may be lowered due to evaporation; when this occurs it is necessary to add distilled water to restore the proper level. If much plating is done, it may be necessary to filter it to remove debris particles or other impurities.

Cyanide compounds are extremely poisonous, especially if brought in contact with acid. *If a copper sulfate solution bath is used in the same room where the cyanide solution is kept, they should be kept far apart from each other.* Hands should be thoroughly washed if contact with the plating solution occurs.

Additional equipment needed includes a bottle of metallizing powder of pure silver, a bottle of Kerr's masking lacquer, and sable brushes No. 000, No. 1, No. 3. This completes the list of items necessary for electroforming silver dies.

Temperature of plating solution. It is not advisable to heat the cyanide solution, because there is danger from the fumes that might be formed. The solution should be maintained at a room temperature of approximately 77 to 80° F. If the solution has been thoroughly mixed, there is no necessity for continuous agitation of the liquid during the plating process.

Cleaning the impression for plating. It is always advisable to clean an impression before electroplating it, to get rid of any blood, saliva, or any loose tooth particles present. This may be done with running water and a medium-sized sable brush. A slight amount of liquid detergent such as Kerr's debubblizer may be added to the water to facilitate the cleansing process. After this has been done, the impression is thoroughly dried with a stream of air.

Electroforming the impression. There are two types of impressions: one is the individual tooth, the other a section of or a complete arch.

A copper-band impression of an individual tooth. The following are the steps in the treatment of a copper band impression of an individual tooth for silverplating.

1. After the copper-band impression is removed from the mouth, it is washed and dried; the outer surfaces of the band are covered with a thin sheet of wax or Kerr's adhesive cement. If a compound or an acrylic stop has been used to close the occlusal end of the band, this is also covered with wax or adhesive cement.
2. Attach the copper band to the cathode holder so that there is intimate contact between the margin of the band and the metal portion of the cathode holder. An insulated copper wire is sometimes used in place of a cathode holder.
3. With a sable brush, silver powder is applied and burnished over and into the tooth impression. Care must be taken that all of the surfaces in the impression are completely covered with powder; any excess, loose powder should be blown out.
4. A sheet of wax (Kerr's 30-gauge green) is wrapped around the band and extended just slightly beyond the gingival end of the band.
5. Using a medicine dropper, the silver-burnished impression is filled with the silver cyanide solution taken from the tank.
6. The copper-band impression attached to the cathode holder is placed in the tank solution; the open end of the band impression should face the silver anode suspended in the solution at the other end of the tank. Trapping air in the impression when it is submerged in the solution must be avoided.
7. The electric current is turned on and the milliammeter knob is adjusted so that the current does not exceed 50 milliam-

peres (ma.). At the end of 5 to 10 minutes the impression is examined to see that all surfaces have the initial silver deposit. If bare spots appear, the impression is removed and dried, the spots are reburnished with silver powder using a sable brush. The impression is refilled with the cyanide solution and replaced in the tank.

If no unplated areas are exposed at the end of 30 minutes, the current is raised to 70 ma., where it remains for 4 to 6 hours, 6 being preferable. This will give a layer of silver approximately 0.004 inch in thickness. If too high a current density is initially employed, the deposited silver will look gray and will be accompanied by a bubbling of the solution; such a deposit is also very brittle.

8. When the plating of the impression is completed, it is removed from the solution, rinsed, and dried. The die may now be filled and completed with Vel-Mix stone, acrylic resin, or a low-fusing metal alloy.

9. When the metal, resin, or stone has hardened, the copper band is slit and peeled away. The silver die can now be easily pulled out of the impression with a rolling motion.

10. The gingival area and the root portions of the die may now be trimmed to the desired shape to facilitate making the wax pattern.

A tray impression of multiple tooth preparations. The steps for taking a tray impression of multiple tooth preparations are as follows.

1. The impression is cleaned in the manner described for the copper-band impression (Figs. 22-51 and 22-52).

2. If a metal tray is used to take the impression, the edge of the tray is brought in intimate contact with the cathode holder or the wire. The rest of the exposed tray is covered with wax or adhesive cement. If a plastic tray is used, a hole is drilled through the tray and impression material in the palatal area. A copper wire is then inserted and twisted securely through the hole; this wire later attaches the tray and impression to the cathode holder (Figs. 22-53 and 22-54).

3. The next step is masking the impression for a sectional-area plating. All portions of the impression not to be plated are covered with four or five coats of Kerr's Permlastic plate mask, each of which is permitted to dry completely. The prepared abutment teeth, their two adjacent teeth, and the edentulous ridge areas to

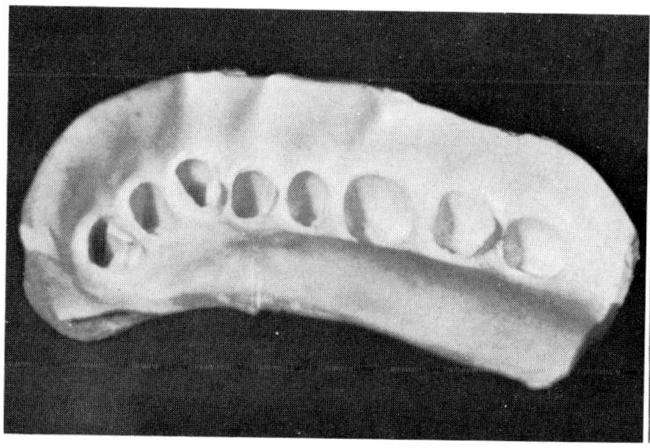

Fig. 22-51

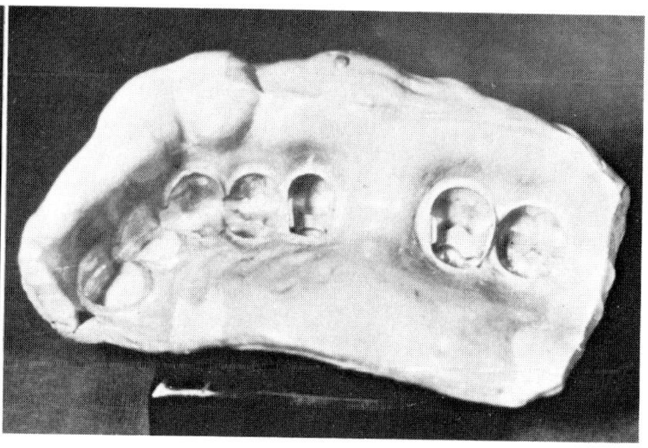

Fig. 22-52

Fig. 22-51. Impression of teeth prepared for individual fillings and crowns. (Courtesy Kerr Manufacturing Co.)

Fig. 22-52. Impression of abutments prepared for bridge retainers. (Courtesy Kerr Manufacturing Co.)

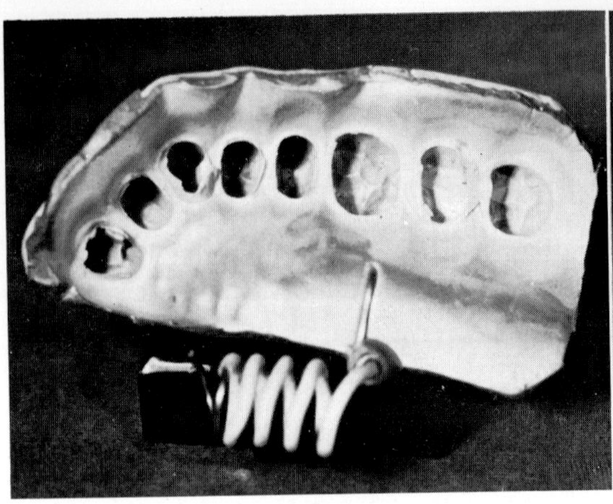

Fig. 22-53

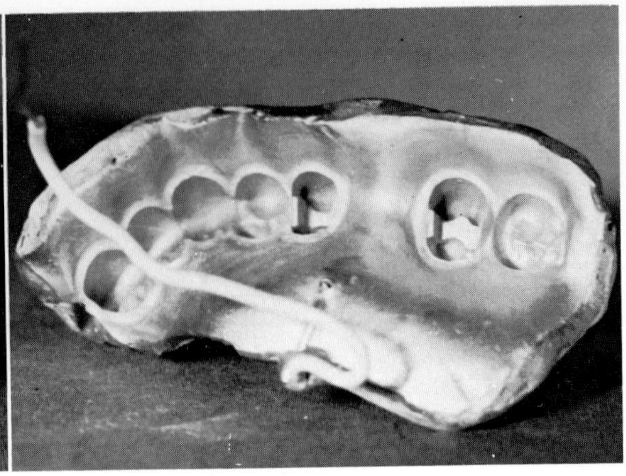

Fig. 22-54

Fig. 22-53. Copper wire attached to plastic impression tray with individual preparations. Other end of wire gripped in cathode holder. (Courtesy Kerr Manufacturing Co.)
Fig. 22-54. Same method as used in Fig. 22-53 to prepare tray for electroplating bridge impression. (Courtesy Kerr Manufacturing Co.)

A

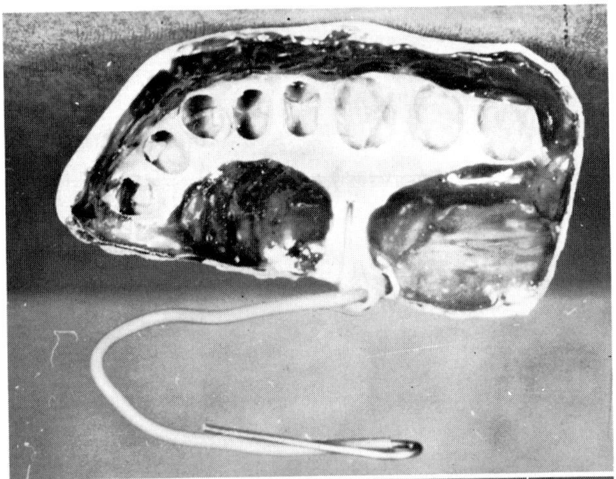

B

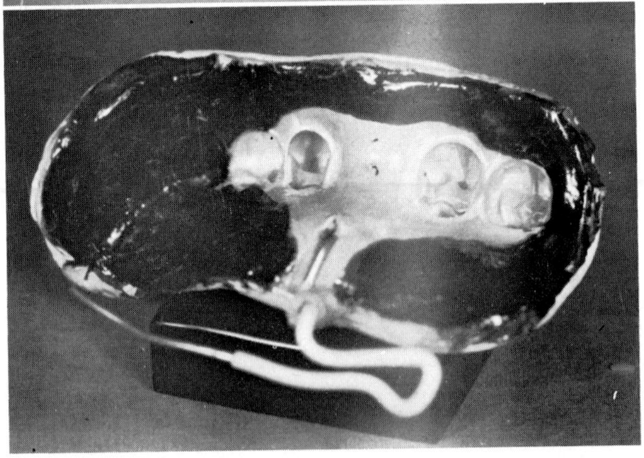

Fig. 22-55. Areas of impressions not to be plated are covered with several coats of plate mask. **A,** Impression with several individual preparations. **B,** Impression with two preparations for retainers and edentulous ridge area. (Courtesy Kerr Manufacturing Co.)

be plated are left free of the masking material (Fig. 22-55).

4. The teeth and edentulous ridge area that have been left exposed are dusted with the silver metallizing powder and burnished in with a sable brush. The silver powdered surface must be extended to make contact with the cathode holder or wire (Fig. 22-56). Since those areas to be plated have been metallized with powder, the dried plate mask material may now be peeled off; silver will be electroformed only in areas burnished with the silver powder.

5. With a medicine dropper, the impression is filled with some plating solution, care being taken not to trap air in the deeper portions of the impression.

6. The tray that is attached to the cathode holder is lowered into the cyanide solution and the milliammeter is set at approximately 140 ma. The amount of milliamperes to use is calculated as follows: Allow 10 ma. per tooth to be plated, with an additional 10 ma. for each additional area, comparable to the area of a tooth surface. Thus, four teeth to be plated require 40 ma.; the edentulous ridge and palatal areas may equal the surface area of ten teeth; this adds an additional 100 ma.; therefore, the initial current setting would be 140 ma. After 5 to 10 minutes in the solution, a uniform, clean, white layer of silver should be deposited on the metallized portion of the impression. If all desired surfaces are covered by the

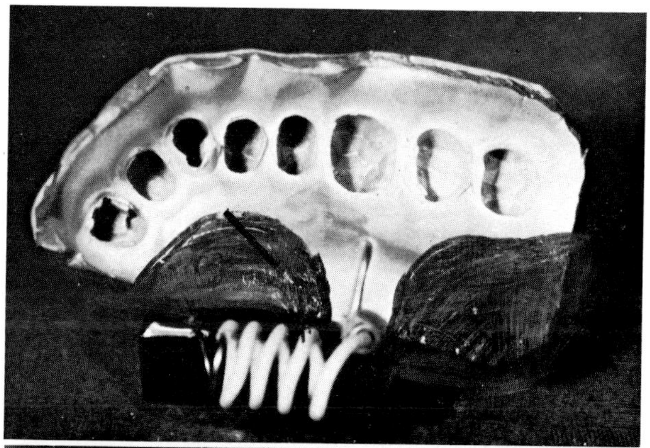

A

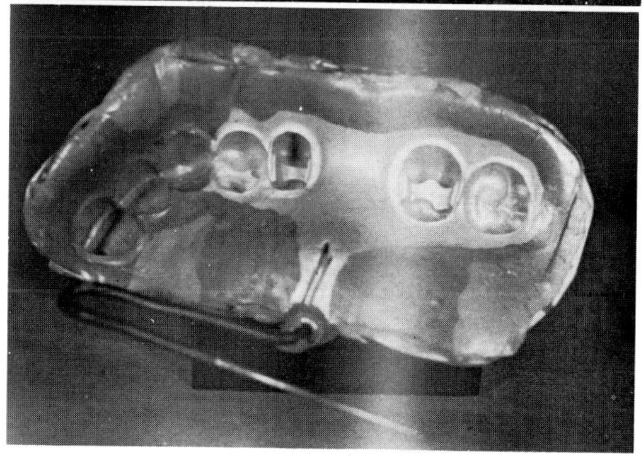

B

Fig. 22-56. Teeth and tissue areas not covered with plate mask are brushed with colloidal silver powder, then burnished with brush. (Courtesy Kerr Manufacturing Co.)

silver deposit, the tray, still attached to the cathode holder, is retured to the solution at this milliamperage for 3 hours.

At the end of this time, the current is increased to 280 ma. and the impression is left in the solution for 6 to 8 hours. Too early removal from the solution will result in a thin deposit of silver that will strip easily from the filled cast, because it will lack sufficient bulk to be engaged later by the stone or the low-fusing metal.

7. When the plating has been completed, the impression tray is removed from the solution, rinsed in water, and dried (Fig. 22-57). If the plate mask material has not been previously removed, this is done now.

8. Vel-Mix stone or low-fusing metal is poured into the impression to the level of the gingival line of the teeth; dowel pins are placed parallel to each other into each abutment tooth. If low-fusing metal is used, a solution of equal parts glycerin, water, and hydrocholoric acid is first painted into each plated depression. Two or more lock washers are also placed to provide the necessary anchorage between

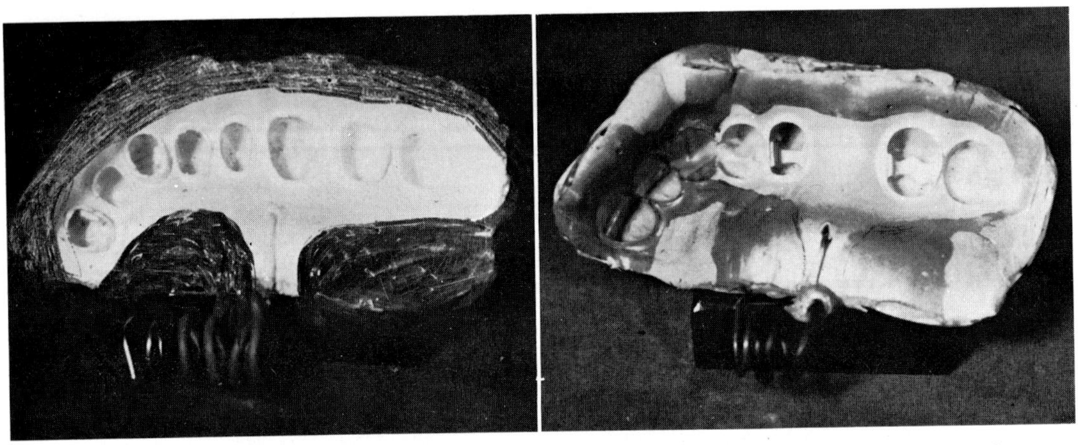

Fig. 22-57. Completed plating of individual tooth and abutment preparation types of impressions. (Courtesy Kerr Manufacturing Co.)

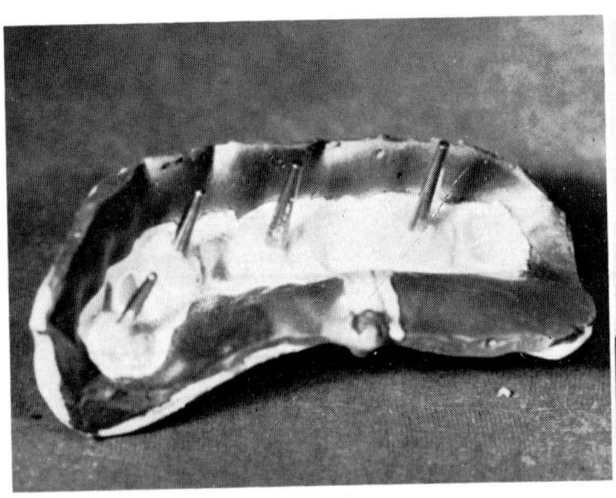

Fig. 22-58

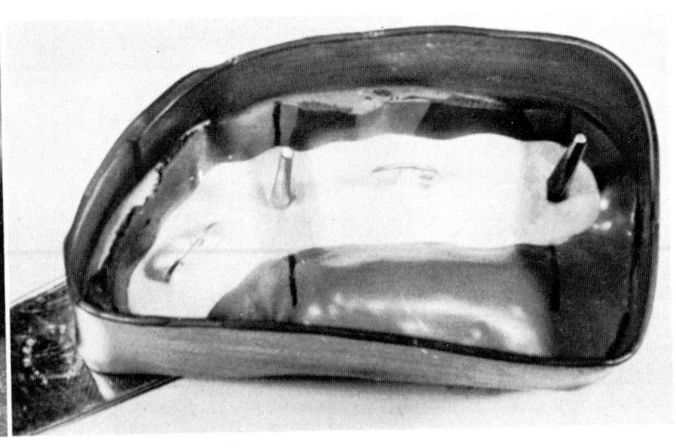

Fig. 22-59

Fig. 22-58. Stone poured and Ney dowels placed in first portion of working cast for individual restorations impression tray A. (Courtesy Kerr Manufacturing Co.)

Fig. 22-59. Friction washers and dowels placed in stone poured into silver-plated impression of abutment teeth impression tray B. (Courtesy Kerr Manufacturing Co.)

the first pour of stone or metal and the second pour of stone (Figs. 22-58 and 22-59).

9. After the first pour of stone has set, one or more coats of lubricants are applied over the areas where the dies are to be removable; a piece of utility wax is placed across the ends of the dowel pins. A second mix of the Vel-Mix stone is poured into the impression to complete the cast.

10. When the stone has set, the cast is removed from the impression. The two prepared abutments, their adjacent teeth, as well as the edentulous ridge and palate areas consist of electroformed silver, while the rest of the cast is stone.

11. With a 2/0-gauge saw blade, vertical cuts are made on either side of the prepared abutments, starting at the gingival area and converging apically. The cuts are carried to the level of the first pour of stone or metal. Two horizontal cuts on the buccal and lingual areas are made next with a knife-edged stone through the thickness of the silver plate, also at the level of the first pour of stone (Figs. 22-60 and 22-61).

12. By removing the utility wax from the ends of the dowel pins, the silver electroformed abutment teeth may now be tapped free from the cast. Any interfering silver in the proximal areas may be carefully trimmed to permit easy access to the gingival margin of the die for waxing purposes.

13. After the retainers are cast, they are placed on the silver dies held in their correct positions in the cast by means of the dowel pins. The pontics and the bridge may now be completed (Figs. 22-62 to 22-64).

Alternate methods. For those desiring a solid, fixed position of the two abutments, two methods are available. In the first, dowel pins are placed into the two teeth *adjacent to* the prepared abutments and not into the abutments as was previously

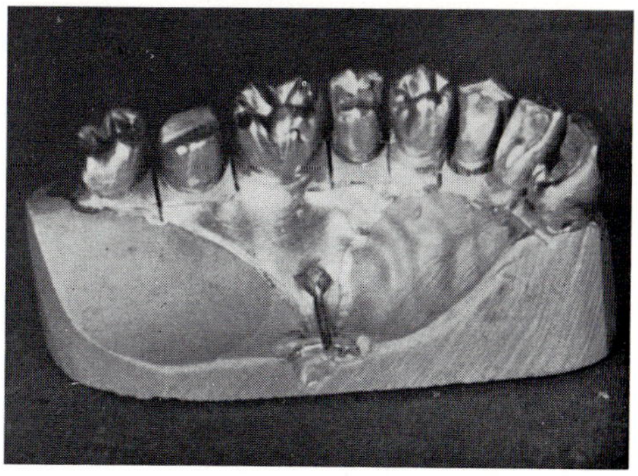

Fig. 22-60. Saw cuts made through electroplated portion of cast A to level of second stone pour. Prepared teeth are removable; others are locked to second stone pour by washers. (Courtesy Kerr Manufacturing Co.)

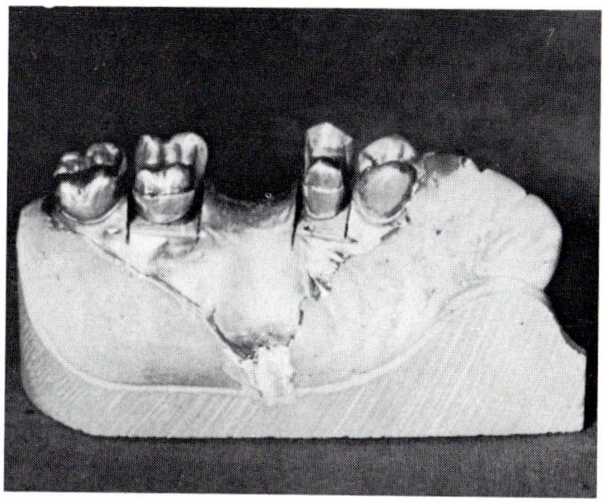

Fig. 22-61. Vertical and horizontal cuts made through silver plate (cast B) permit removal of abutment silver-plated dies which are attached to Ney's dowels. (Courtesy Kerr Manufacturing Co.)

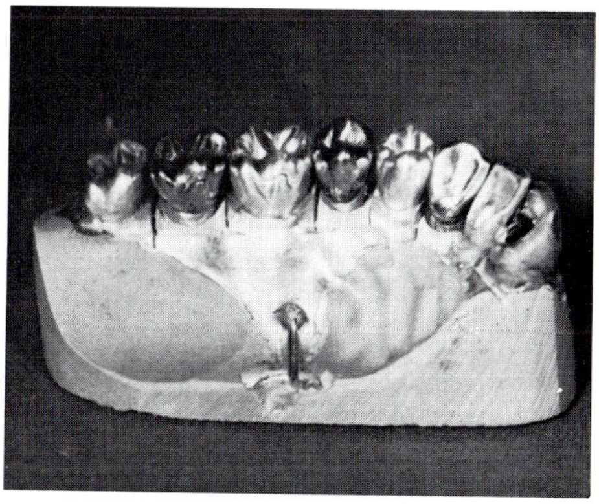

Fig. 22-62. Wax pontic aligned between two finished bridge retainers seated in silver-plated dies (cast B). (Courtesy Kerr Manufacturing Co.)

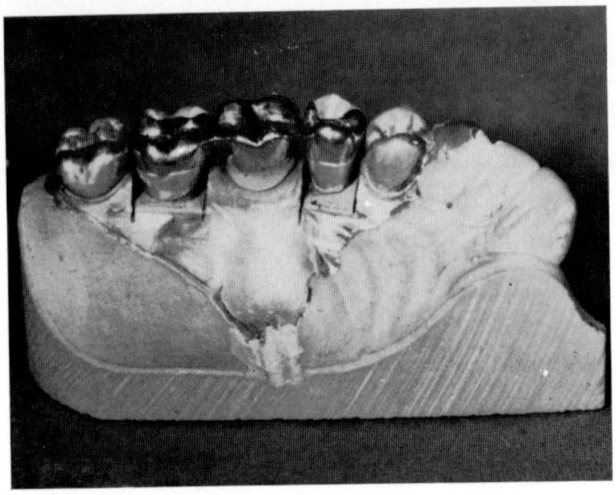

Fig. 22-63. Completed bridge on cast B, buccal view. (Courtesy Kerr Manufacturing Co.)

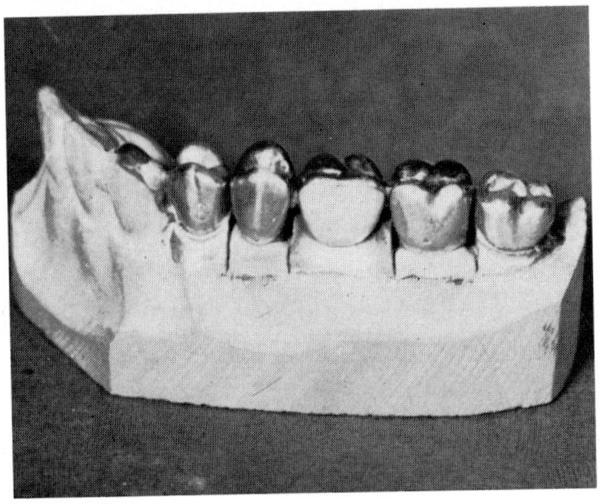

Fig. 22-64. Lingual view of Fig. 22-63. (Courtesy Kerr Manufacturing Co.)

done in Step 8; these are subsequently removable, while the remainder of the cast is a solid unit. This type of cast affords excellent access on the proximal surface of the abutment die, which faces the removable die, but the access is more restricted on the proximal surface facing the edentulous space.

In the second method no dowel pins are used and *all the teeth and soft tissues in the impression are metallized* with silver powder and electroformed (Fig. 22-65). The area to be plated usually is so large that 150 ma. are required for the initial 3 hours of plating; this is followed by 6 to 8 hours at 300 ma. After the plated impression has been removed from the solution it is dried and poured in Vel-Mix stone. When the stone has set, the casts are carefully withdrawn from the impressions and the axial walls of the stone base are slightly tapered. These are then lubricated and seated into a stiff mix of stone (Fig. 22-66). After the stone matrix has set, the cast is withdrawn and two vertical cuts are made in it with a saw blade as follows: one-third the distance from the gingival area toward the base; then one-third the distance from the base toward the middle of the cast. The middle third is then cracked by prying it apart with a knife. The vertical cuts are made, one mesial to the anterior abut-

A

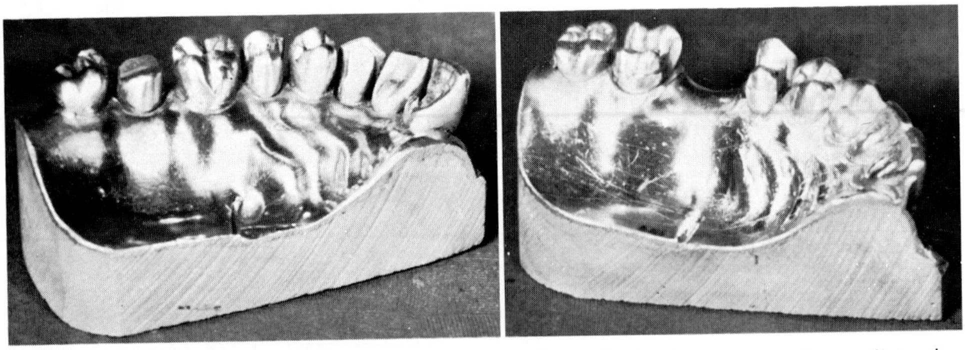

B

Fig. 22-65. Second method of constructing electroformed silver casts reproduces all teeth and soft tissue surfaces in impression. **A,** Individual preparations on second molar, second bicuspid, cuspid, and central incisor. **B,** Second molar and second bicuspid abutments prepared. (Courtesy Kerr Manufacturing Co.)

ment, the other distal to the posterior abutment (Fig. 22-65, *B*). The three sections may now be replaced in the stone matrix, each maintaining its proper relation interproximally (Figs. 22-68 and 22-69).

Copper electroplating. While the technic and procedure for copper electroforming dies and working casts are similar to those employed for constructing them of silver, there are certain differences in the details of procedure and materials used. A copper anode is used instead of silver and a solution of copper sulfate is employed as the electrolite, employing the following formula recommended by Phillips and Dettman:

Copper sulfate, anhydrous	225-250 Gm.
Sulfuric acid, concentrated	75 ml.
Phenol	10 ml.
Ethyl alcohol	25-50 ml.
Distilled water	1,000 ml.[5]

Although copper plating may be utilized with some of the newer silicone elastic impression materials, it is usually associated with the use of modeling com-

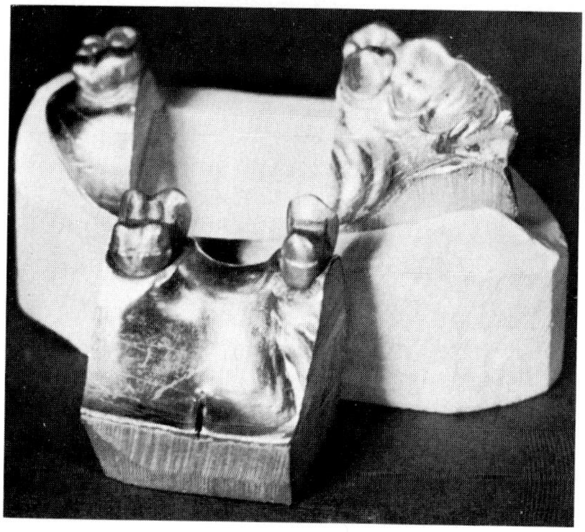

Fig. 22-67. Silver dies are held rigidly in center section of working cast, permitting no individual movement of dies. (Courtesy Kerr Manufacturing Co.)

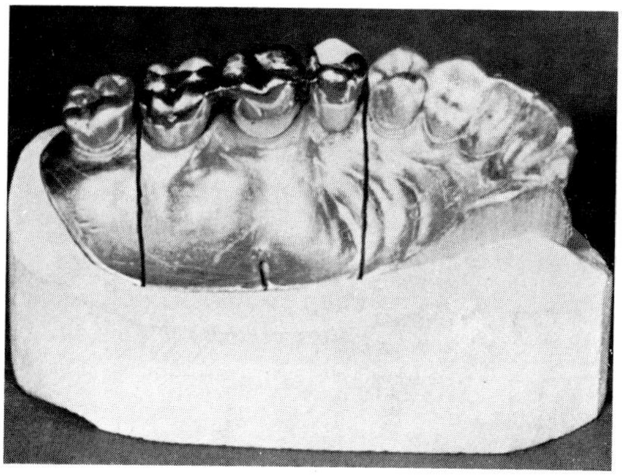

Fig. 22-68. Lingual view of finished bridge on electroformed silver casts. (Courtesy Kerr Manufacturing Co.)

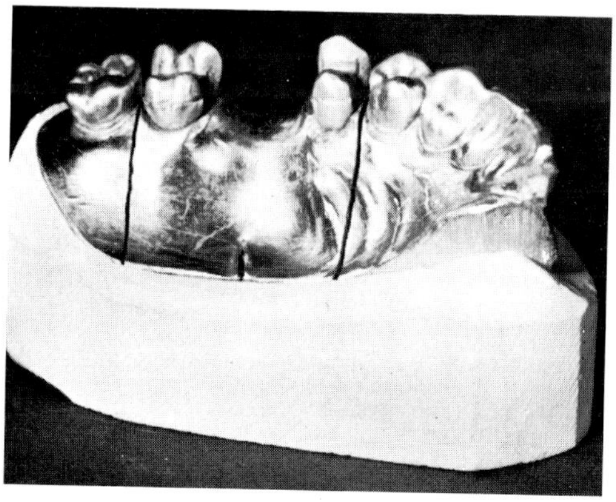

Fig. 22-66. Stone base of finished silver cast (Fig. 22-65, *B*) is tapered, lubricated, and seated into stone matrix. After stone matrix has set, tapered section may be removed and replaced as needed. Vertical cuts are made through silver cast, and sections are separated and reassembled in stone matrix. Individual preparations as in Fig. 22-65, *A*, may be similarly made removable from cast. (Courtesy Kerr Manufacturing Co.)

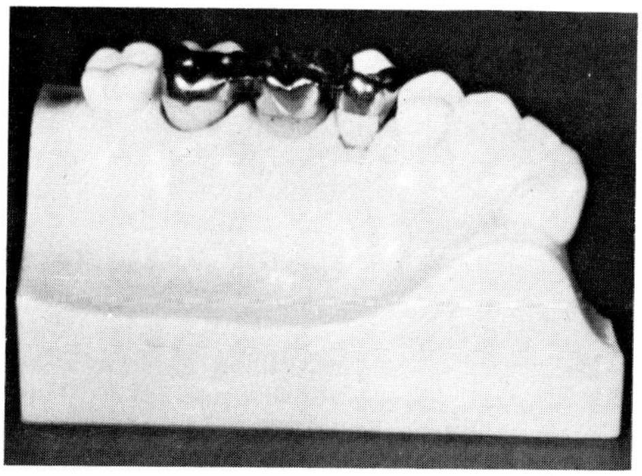

Fig. 22-69. Same bridge as in Fig. 22-68, placed on model used to take original impressions.

pound for impression purposes. In order to facilitate the deposition of the copper on the surface of the impression, it is first necessary to metallize the surface with a microscopic layer of copper to which subsequently the electrode deposition of copper is made.

To accomplish this initial deposition, the usual method employed is that of burnishing metallic powder to the surface of the impression, which is previously moistened either with an aqueous or oil solution. A more recent development is the silver film technic described by Phillips and Dettman, wherein a silver film two millionths of an inch thick can be deposited on the surface of the impression by chemically reducing an aqueous solution of silver nitrate. In the first group of materials used may be listed Aqua-Dag, Silbryte, Silverizer (which is a mixture of very fine silver powder dispersed in a bottle of thin volatile liquid), and bronzing powder burnished to a surface previously covered with a thin layer of oil of bitter almonds.

The plating solution should be contained in a one- or two-quart glass container. The electroplating equipment should have a range of 0 to 1,000 ma. in addition to the usual cathode and anode suspension holders, both single and multiple types.

The amount and rate of current application is similar to that recommended in constructing silver dies, namely, 10 ma. per tooth or tooth-surface-area involved in a tray impression, as described previously in this chapter.

Here again it must be pointed out that if a copper sulfate solution bath is used in the same room where the cyanide silver solution is kept, they should be kept far apart from each other, and the solutions should be distinctly marked on the jar.

In the use of the powders or powder/liquid combinations, extreme care must be observed in order not to leave any excess or unwanted powder particles in the impression, because the finished die would be deficient in sharpness and accuracy in those areas where the powder remained. Therefore all excess must be carefully burnished or blown out to avoid this possibility.

Although good results may be obtained by the use of the powder/liquid method, the investigations of Phillips and Dettman[5] indicate that the precipitation of a silver film proved to be a better method.

The silver film method recommended by the investigators is as follows:

> A silver film, approximately 2 millionths of an inch thick,* can be deposited evenly over the surface of an impression by the chemical reduction of an aqueous solution of silver nitrate. . . .
>
> The impression to be metallized was first lightly painted with the sensitizing solution to ensure coverage and then immersed in this solution for several minutes. The composition of this solution is:
>
> | | |
> |---|---|
> | Hydrochloric acid, concentrated | 1.5 ml. |
> | Stannous chloride | 1.0 Gm. |
> | Distilled water | 100.0 ml. |
>
> Although the exact mechanism is not known, apparently the stannous chloride tends to wet the surface more easily or actually gives the surface an affinity for the silver ion.†
>
> The impression was then removed, rinsed *gently* with tap water, and placed in another cup or beaker. A small amount of the reducing agent, sufficient to cover the impression, was poured into this vessel. The composition of this solution is:
>
> | | |
> |---|---|
> | Pyrogallic acid, crystals | 3.4 Gm. |
> | Citric acid, granular | 0.7 Gm. |
> | Distilled water | 100.0 ml. |
>
> • • •
>
> There are a number of complex immediate compounds found in the reaction of pyrogallol and silver nitrate, but the net result is the precipitation of silver film.‡ The solution turned black in color, and after setting for five or ten minutes,

*Radio Corporation of America, Engineering Division, Indianapolis, Indiana; Personal communication.

†Ellis, R.: Electro-deposition and its application in dentistry, issued by the Canadian Dental Research Foundation, Toronto, Canada, 1943.

‡Conant, J. B.: Chemistry of organic compounds, New York, 1933, The Macmillan Company, p. 408.

it turned to a lighter brown color. The solution was then poured out and tap water is used to rinse the metallized impression. Examination of the impression after drying with a blast of compressed air showed that a light grayish silver film evenly covered the entire impression. Occasionally there were voids in a small and deep impression. These were easily covered by repeating the process.

Surface tension difficulties are practically nil; therefore, no wetting agent needs to be used. The dry impression is merely immersed in the plating bath and agitated back and forth a few times to remove any entrapped air bubbles. The copper deposit entirely covers the impression in approximately 30 seconds. The electrical conductivity of this film is obviously high.*

To construct an opposing, complete, occluding arch in silver, all of the exposed impression material in the tray is metallized with silver powder, after which it is electroformed using the correct time and milliamperage determined on the same basis as previously.

Contrary to the apparent complexity of the technique, it is extremely simple to use and does not require particular proficiency on the part of the technician.

The sensitizing solution may be used indefinitely and seems to have unlimited shelf life. However, the reducing and silver nitrate solutions do deteriorate. Storing these two solutions in dark bottles helps stability. The solutions which were used in this work produced excellent results after being stored for several months, even though there was some darkening of the reducer and some silver oxide precipitated into silver nitrate solution. The solutions are not explosive as are ammoniacal silvering soltuions.†

*Frankel, C. B.: A scientific approach to the solution of practical problems encountered in electroforming copper dies, J.A.D.A. **32**:1130, 1952.
†Blum, W., and Hogaboom, G. B.: Principles of electroplating and electroforming, ed. 3, New York, 1949, McGraw-Hill Book Co., Inc.

SELECTED REFERENCES

1. Skinner, E. W.: Properties and manipulation of mercaptan base and silicone base impression materials, Dent. Clin. N. Amer., Nov., 1958, p. 685.
2. Shell, J. S.: Chemistry of RTV silicones, Bulletin No. 9, Toledo, Ohio, 1959, Ransom & Randolph Co.
3. Myers, G. E., Wepfer, G. G., and Peyton, F. A.: The Thiokol rubber base impression materials, J. Prosth. Dent. **8**:330, 1958.
4. Hudson, W. C.: Clinical uses of rubber impression materials and electroforming of casts and dies in pure silver, J. Prosth. Dent. **8**: 107, 1958.
5. Phillips, H. A., and Dettman, F. J.: A study of some variables associated with copper-plating of dental impressions, J. Prosth. Dent. **6**:101, 1956.

GENERAL REFERENCES

Addicks, L.: Silver in industry, New York, 1940, Reinhold Publishing Corp.

Azaria, H.: Simplified method for copper or silver plating rubber base and silicone dental impressions, D. Digest **68**:315, 322, 1962.

Blum, W., and Hogaboom, G. B.: Principles of electroplating and electroforming, ed. 3, New York, 1949, McGraw-Hill Book Co., Inc.

Braden, M.: Characterization of the setting process in dental polysulfide rubbers, J. Dent. Res. **45**:1065, 1966.

Brotman, I. N.: Copper tube, acrylic resin, and Thiokol rubber-base impressions for full veneer preparations, J. Prosth. Dent. **9**:635, 1959.

Dubir, J. T.: Premedication and gingival retraction for the Thiokol "mercaptan" rubber base impression technique, J. Dist. Columbia D. Soc. **35**:4, 1960.

Duxbury, J. H.: The versatility of the rubber-base impression, J. Prosth. Dent. **13**:489, 1963.

Eastman, R. F.: Individual copper band rubber base impressions for inlays and crowns, J.A.D.A. **59**:966, 1959.

Fairhurst, C. W., and others: Elastic properties of rubber base impression materials, J. Prosth. Dent. **6**:534, 1956.

Feuerstein, R. M.: Physical properties and use of rubber-base impression material, J. Prosth. Dent. **10**:179, 1960.

Gilmore, W. H., Schnell, R. J., and Phillips, R. W.: Factors influencing the accuracy of silicone impression materials, J. Prosth. Dent. **9**: 304, 1959.

Harris, L. W.: Mixing Thiokol rubber impression materials, J. Prosth. Dent. **10**:386, 1960.

Henry, R. W., and Phillips, R. W.: Reproducing surface detail with electroplated impressions, D. Progress **2**:29, 1961.

Herrick, P. W.: Use of mercaptan rubber impression material, Iowa D. J. **45**:307, 1959.

Hoppenstand, D. C.: Production of silver surfaces on dental casts, J. Prosth. Dent. **10**:733, 1960.

Joram, P. R., Grogan, H. T., and Pruzansky, S.: Flexible rubber molds for accurate multiple reproduction of plaster casts, J. Prosth. Dent. **8**:100, 1958.

LaForgia, A.: Rubber-base impressions for fixed prosthesis, J. Prosth. Dent. **11**:735, 1961.

Loveday, J.: Gold plating without the use of electricity, D. Technician **11**:79, 1958.

Lund, M. R., and Shryock, E. F.: Castings made directly to refractory dies, J. Prosth. Dent. **18** (3):251-256, 1967.

McLean, J. W.: Physical properties influencing the accuracy of silicone and Thiokol impression materials, Brit. D. J. **110**:85, 1961.

Miller, N., and Myers, G. E.: Silicone impression materials, J. Prosth. Dent. **12**:951, 1962.

Miller, W. A. C., Jr., Hansen, W. C., Dickson, G., and Sweeney, W. T.: Physical properties of synthetic-rubber-base dental impression materials, J.A.D.A. **60**:211, 1960.

Myers, G. E., and Peyton, F. A.: Clinical and physical studies of the silicone rubber impression materials, J. Prosth. Dent. **9**:315, 1959.

Myers, G. E., and Stockman, D. G.: Factors that affect the accuracy and dimensional stability of the mercaptan rubber-base impression materials, J. Prosth. Dent. **10**:525, 1960.

Phillips, R. W.: Physical properties and manipulation of rubber base impression materials, J. Indiana Dent. Assn. **47**:105-108, 1968.

Schnell, R. J., and Phillips, R. W.: Dimensional stability of rubber base impressions and certain other factors affecting accuracy, J.A.D.A. **57**:39, 1958.

Skinner, E. W.: The properties and manipulation of mercaptan base and silicone base impression materials, Dent. Clin. N. Amer., p. 685, Nov., 1958.

Sturdevant, C. M.: Mercaptan rubber impression technique for single and multiple restorations, Dent. Clin. N. Amer., 699-711, 1958.

Wayne, J. V.: New techniques and materials in crown and bridge prosthetics, Georgetown D. J. **27**:25, 1961.

Yoder, J. L., and Thayer, K. E.: Rubber-base impression technique for fixed partial dentures, J. Prosth. Dent. **12**:339, 1962.

Chapter 23

Tooth preparation and construction of complete metal crowns without dowels: posterior and anterior class II, type I

POSTERIOR TEETH

The complete veneer metal crown employed today has undergone considerable change and development since its introduction by W. N. Morrison in 1869. Originally the Morrison crown consisted of two pieces of gold plate, an axial band, and a swaged occlusal cap soldered together. By the skillful manipulation of contouring pliers, the band was shaped to restore the axial contour of the tooth, while the occlusal portion was swaged between a die and a counterdie to reproduce the occlusal anatomy. Because the finished crown reproduced the tooth form by means of a thin shell of gold, it was also known as a "gold shell" crown.

In the past, teeth requiring crowns were usually first devitalized. Since this was the accepted procedure during the latter part of the nineteenth century, most of the gold crowns were placed on teeth from which the pulps had been removed. Because a certain percentage of treated teeth ultimately fail, the loss of crowned treated teeth was not attributed to poor root filling technic, but to the fact that the tooth was crowned. Although it is probable that some of the failures were directly attributable to improper preparations and incorrectly fitted and contoured gold crowns that caused the death of the pulp, as well as gingival inflammation and infection, it is evident, from our present knowledge of what constitutes a properly constructed metal crown, that it did not deserve the condemnation heaped upon it in the early part of this century.

Unfortunately, the mistaken ideas have permeated the medical profession as well as the laity that a crown constructed of metal is dangerous to the health of a patient, and that it is not used in the better type of dental health service. While it is true that the metal crown is not universally adaptable, still, where indicated and when properly prepared, the complete metal crown is a safe and useful type of restoration.

Although it is occasionally constructed of platinum and its alloys, more generally it is made of gold and its alloys.

INDICATIONS

The complete metal crown may be used as an individual restoration or it may serve as a bridge retainer. As with other crowns, the gold crown is used only when a tooth cannot be restored by means of fillings. It must always be kept in mind that the complete crown is the last resort in the reclamation of a carious or fractured tooth. On the other hand, there are indications for the placement of a complete gold crown, even when the tooth could be repaired with fillings. For example, there are teeth so weakened and undermined by caries that the placement of a complete veneer crown affords the best protection against possible fracture of the remaining tooth structure. In mouths in which caries is very active, it frequently serves a preventive purpose to place a complete crown instead of extensive intracoronal fillings.

Where a tooth is used to retain a clasp for a removable partial denture in a mouth that is susceptible to caries, it is wise to place a complete veneer crown, both for retentive and preventive purposes. Many natural teeth carrying clasps would remain useful for a longer period of time if first they were covered with a complete metal crown, made of either metal or porcelain and metal.

Where it is impossible to correct the alignment or occlusion in malposed teeth with fillings, the complete gold crown may be employed. When it is necessary to use a noncarious tooth for a bridge abutment, ordinarily some type of intracoronal or extracoronal retainer is preferred. If, however, the gingivoclusal height of the tooth is relatively short, there may be considerable difficulty in getting sufficient retention with the inlay or the partial veneer retainers, in which event the complete crown is indicated.

Although a gold crown may be constructed on both vital and pulpless anterior or posterior teeth, it is primarily indicated on the posterior teeth. When used anteriorly to the second bicuspid, the esthetic requirements are fulfilled by placing a porcelain or acrylic resin veneer in the buccal or labial surface of the crown. Unless so modified, the complete veneer metal crown is rarely, if ever, used in the anterior teeth.

REQUIREMENTS

The first requirement of the complete metal crown, as with other preparations, is that of pulp conservation. This implies that every precaution will be taken during the preparation of the tooth for the crown and after it has been completed and cemented.

To be a satisfactory restoration, the complete metal crown, as Orton[1] so ably expressed it over five decades ago, "must be one that will exactly reproduce in all its essential details that particular tooth which it is intended to replace, bearing in mind the age of the patient and the variation from the normal which it may be necessary to reproduce in order to have the crown in harmony with its environment."*

This implies not only the axial and occlusal contours of the individual tooth, but also those relationships that exist between the restored tooth and its adjacent and opposing teeth, i.e., correct contact areas, proximal embrasures, occlusal wear, and proper functional coordination with the other teeth.

Where it is possible to place any one of several types of crowns, that one should be selected which does not require an undue or excessive sacrifice of tooth tissue. The indiscriminate or deep cutting of the tooth, besides being unnecessary, usually results in the degeneration or death of the pulp.

An acceptable gold crown requires that its gingival margin be correctly adapted to the tooth and placed in its proper relationship to the gingival tissues. The previous discussion dealing with the correct placement of the gingival margin also applies to the complete veneer metal crown; the gingival termination of the crown should never be extended so far rootwise

*From Orton, F. H.: Absence of standards in crown work, D. Items Int. 39:345, 1917.

that it will cause a recession of the gingival tissues or result in their detachment. It is found in younger patients that the gingival margin of the crown terminates at or slightly above the crest of the gum tissue, whereas in older patients it is lowered beneath the crest and terminates in the gingival crevice. There is very little likelihood of causing irritation either to the pulp or to the investing gingival tissues, if care is exercised in the amount and the area of the tooth tissue removed and if the contour and fit are proper.

The requirements of an acceptable gold crown also demand that the materials used in its construction be intrinsically strong enough to withstand the forces and wear of mastication to which the crown will be submitted. Therefore, gold or its alloys must be carefully selected for the purpose they are intended to serve. This presupposes that the fineness of the gold alloy will be such as to prevent tarnish or corrosion from oral secretions. The advantages of the complete metal crown are that it is inherently strong and that it may be so constructed that it exerts great retentive powers, being dislodged with difficulty. This is accomplished by properly preparing the occlusal and axial surfaces of the tooth as explained in Chapter 11. Another advantage of this type of crown is its general adaptability to posterior as well as anterior teeth, when used with the porcelain or acrylic resin veneer facing. Its construction does not demand unusual skill, since it can be well made by anyone possessing average skill.

Although this type of crown was formerly used almost exclusively on pulpless teeth, with the improved present-day technic it is possible to restore badly decayed teeth and at the same time to preserve their vitality.

DISADVANTAGES

One of the chief disadvantages of the gold crown is that it lacks the esthetic requirements; hence, when made entirely of metal, it is limited to the posterior teeth. The preparation of a tooth for the reception of a gold crown is generally regarded as a simple task, particularly with the advent of the high speed cutting technics; in reality, it is one of the most meticulous operations that the dentist is called upon to perform. Unfortunately, an ill-fitting crown placed on an improperly prepared tooth often stays in place for many years before the resultant serious harm to the investing tissues and the pulp is discovered. This, more than anything else, has been the cause of the ill repute into which the gold crown has fallen.

Although the complete gold crown should be placed where indicated, its promiscuous use should be discouraged because of the difficulty of reestablishing the correct axial contours and the correct gingival continuity of the axial surfaces once they have been removed or altered. In addition to this there is the possibility of not obtaining an accurate gingival peripheral fit. If these obstacles are not overcome, they will result in the irritation, inflammation, and possibly the infection of the gingival tissues.

Another disadvantage of this type of crown lies in the difficulty of recognizing and locating incipient caries starting at the gingival margin of the crown; this sometimes penetrates underneath the crown and remains undiscovered until the damage done is irreparable.

Ante[2] estimates that a complete crown preparation requires the removal of one-sixth of the tooth tissues from the axial walls and one-fourth from the occlusal; this should be avoided, if at all possible, by using some other type of restoration. One should not be entirely deterred, however, from using the complete gold crown, since in some types of extensive intracoronal retainers large amounts of tooth tissue are also removed and in regions that lie even more closely to the pulp.

DIFFICULTY IN CEMENTING CROWN

A situation which may at times prove serious is the trouble encountered while cementing the crown on the tooth. The cement frequently prevents the proper seating of the crown, resulting in an improper occlusal relationship and gingival fit; this may cause the ultimate destruction of the tooth. This problem may be controlled: first, by mixing the cement to a proper consistency; second, by establishing sluiceways on the inner surfaces of the crown through which the cement more easily may escape gingivally; or third, by cutting a small hole with a machinist's small drill, size 82, through the occlusal surface of the wax crown which is later filled in the cast crown, either with gold foil or with clasp metal wire of the correct diameter, finished flush with the surface of the crown.

PREPARATION OF CARIOUS TOOTH

Teeth that have been affected by extensive caries are usually restored with gold crowns. When vital teeth have small cavities, the decayed portion is removed to determine the depth and the extent of the cavity, after which it is filled with cement. Where caries is extensive, resulting in a large cavity, first, it is well to obtain a roentgenograph of the tooth to learn the extent of the decay, second, the pulp should be tested to determine its vitality, and, third, if there is any question of exposing or involving the pulp during the removal of the decay, the rubber dam should be first applied. Having taken these precautions, it is safe to proceed with the removal of all decayed tooth tissue. At times, it is not necessary to remove all undermined enamel, since in the finished preparation the entire coronal portion of the tooth is covered by the gold crown.

After the decay has been removed, preferably with a rubber dam in place, the cavity is dried, coated with a very thin film of cavity lining, and filled with cement. Where the walls of the cavity lie close to the pulp, it is advisable first to use a layer of thymolized calcium hydroxide, after which the cement is placed. Where the pulp is hypersensitive or the tooth tender, it is prudent to wait several days or even weeks until the tooth responds normally.

Where one or more of the axial surfaces of a vital tooth have been destroyed by caries that extends gingivally far below the crest of the gum tissue and where a complete metal crown must be placed, the gingival deficiency is not restored with cement, but with a metal filling. In teeth having vital pulps, the metallic filling should be a gold alloy and not amalgam. The crown is placed later after the remainder of the tooth has been suitably prepared.

USE OF PULPLESS TOOTH

At times a gold crown is placed on a tooth where little of the crown portion remains and where it is necessary to remove the pulp and fill the root canals. When such a tooth is used, it is necessary that its missing coronal portion be rebuilt to afford the necessary contour and retention to the crown. One or more threaded dowels, the so-called screw post, may be placed in one or more of the filled root canals, and amalgam may be built around the threaded dowels, restoring the lost crown portion of the tooth.

When the threaded dowels are screwed into the root canal, a matrix is fitted and trimmed to proper occlusal height; it confines the amalgam while it is condensed against the threaded dowels. The matrix is left in place until the patient's next appointment, at which time it is removed, leaving the amalgam in position. This, with the remaining tooth tissue, is prepared as though the entire coronal portion were of natural tooth structure.

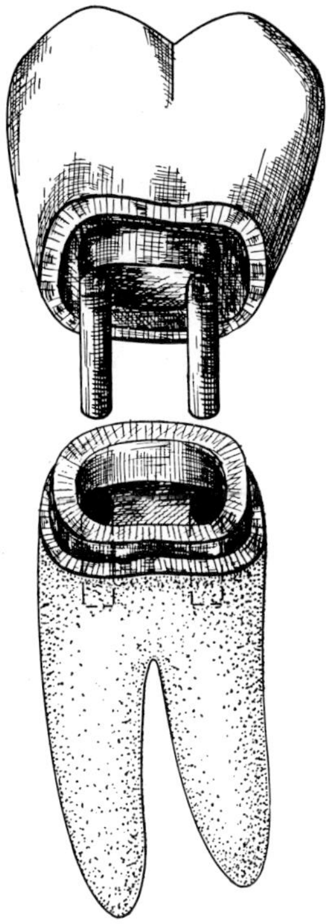

Fig. 23-1. Dowels cast as integral part of crown.

WHEN TO USE DOWELS

Occasionally, it is more expedient to cast the entire coronal portion in gold; such a crown depends entirely for its retention upon two or more dowels placed in the root canals (Fig. 23-1). Here, the remaining portion of the tooth is prepared with a gingival shoulder encircling a slightly raised plateau of tooth structure; this is similar to the preparation made for a cast core, complete porcelain veneer crown. This latter type of complete gold crown is satisfactory as an individual restoration, but it is contraindicated as a bridge retainer.

At other times, one or more dowels without threads are fitted into the root canals, and the missing portion of the crown of the tooth is built up in wax and cast. After the casting has been cemented to place, the preparation of the tooth is completed.

When one dowel is used, it must be sufficient gauge and must extend sufficiently far into the pulp canal to resist the

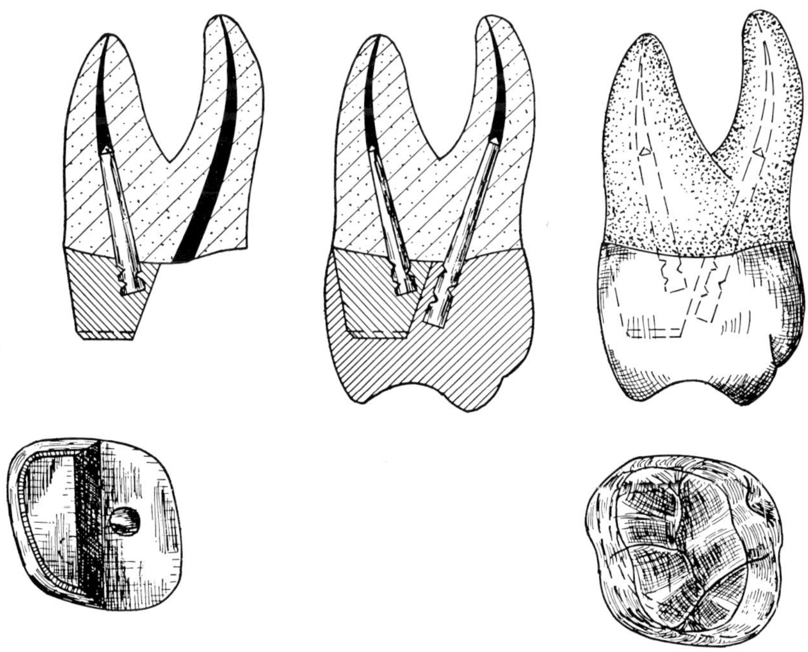

Fig. 23-2. Complete gold crown cast in two parts and employing two dowels. (After C. Rodgers.)

forces of shear and displacement. When two dowels are used, these are paralleled with each other in order to permit their withdrawal and subsequent cementation.

Fig. 23-2 illustrates a technic whereby a casting with a dowel restores part of the axial contour of the crown, while at the same time it is partially covered by the remainder of the cast crown, which completes the contour of the tooth.

TYPES OF COMPLETE CAST METAL CROWNS WITHOUT DOWELS

The complete cast metal crown may be one of the following categories: (1) cast, (2) swaged, (3) swaged-cast combination, and (4) the metal plus fired porcelain to metal or the acrylic resin combination.

Each of these may be further subdivided into the shoulder and the shoulderless types and may be used either on the posterior or the anterior teeth.

While it is possible to make a satisfactory gold crown restoration by the swaged or the so-called "shell crown" method, yet, the certainty and the comparative simplicity with which accurate results may be obtained by the cast or the combination swaged-cast types of crowns have caused the two-piece shell crown to be largely discarded. Not that the method of construction is wrong per se, but a large percentage of gold shell crowns constructed in the past were improperly made and constituted a menace instead of an asset to the health of the patient.

Advantages of the cast type of crown

Dressel[3] enumerated the merits of the all cast type of complete crown as compared to the all swaged plate crown, by stating that the former is: (1) a stronger and sturdier crown; (2) proper contact areas may be established; (3) proper embrasures and interproximal spaces may be established; (4) proper buccal and lingual anatomical form may be obtained, assuring proper alignment with the approximating teeth; (5) better gingival adaptation may be obtained; and (6) a better occlusion."* (See Figs. 13-42 and 13-43.)

As previously stated, the complete veneer metal crown, while primarily a restoration for posterior teeth, may be placed on the anterior teeth when used in combination with porcelain or acrylic resin veneer facings in the labial surface.

PREPARATION OF TOOTH

In the preparation of a tooth for a complete cast metal crown, it is not necessary to remove all the enamel from the tooth; only enough is removed to allow a thickness of gold on the occlusal sufficient for strength and wear; while on the axial surfaces, enough is removed to permit the gingival margin of the crown to draw occlusally without encountering any overhanging tooth structure. The complete veneer gold crown possesses an inherent strength which is lacking in the complete veneer porcelain crown; consequently, the metal crown may be made less bulky and still will withstand the forces that will be imposed upon it.

The preparation of a tooth for a complete cast metal crown may be accomplished in five steps. While a relatively difficult procedure, if undertaken in a haphazard manner, it is comparatively simple if the steps are executed in proper sequence and with the proper instruments. It must be kept in mind that: (1) the finished preparation has axial walls that are nearly parallel, with but a slight gingivoclusal convergence; (2) the coronal portion has the general shape of a frustum of a cone with its base situated at or slightly below the crest of the gum tissue; and (3) its occlusal surface, where possible, reproduces the natural anatomy of the tooth, but at a level 1.5 to 2 mm. below the normal occlusal plane. Although many technics and instrumentations have been

*From Dressel, R. P.: Principles of fixed bridge construction, D. Cosmos **72**:565, 1930.

A

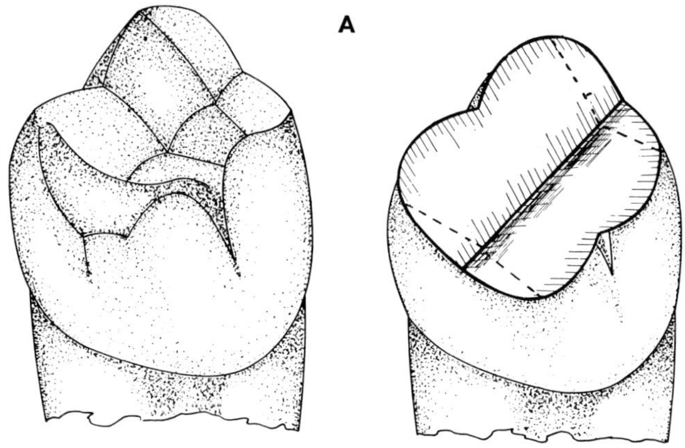

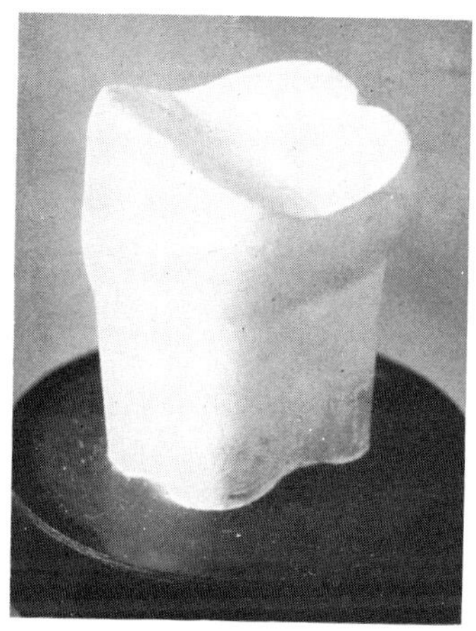

B

Fig. 23-3. A, Step 1 in preparation: occlusal reduction. **B,** Model showing Step 1 in pulpless tooth.

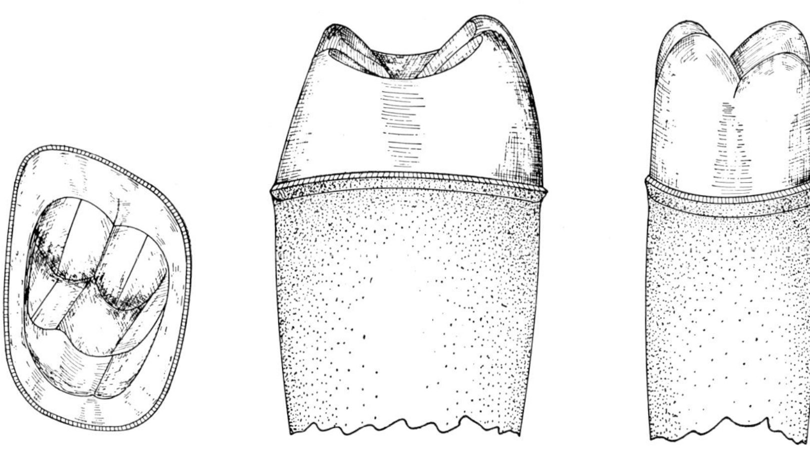

Fig. 23-4. In teeth with vital pulps, occlusal anatomy is maintained.

A

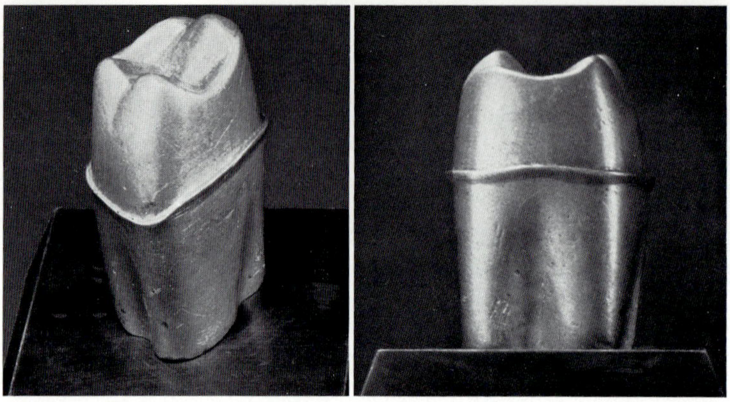

B

Fig. 23-5. A, Occlusal anatomy maintained in teeth with vital pulps. **B,** Proximal view of tooth shown in **A.**

A

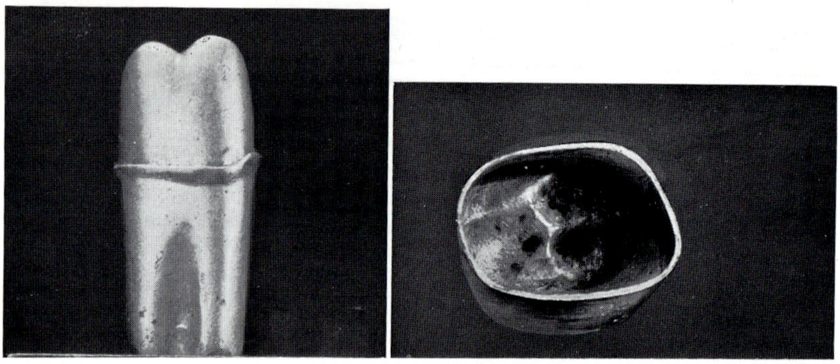

B

Fig. 23-6. A, Buccal view of tooth shown in Fig. 23-5, A. **B,** Inner surface of cast gold crown showing occlusal anatomy of preparation.

developed, the following is found to be quite satisfactory.

Reduction of occlusal surface. The first step consists of the reduction of the occlusal surface. This is accomplished by removing enough of the tooth with a wheel-shaped stone (Densco 2J) so that a uniform space 1.5 to 2 mm. deep is established in this area for gold in the finished crown (Fig. 23-3, *A* and *B*).

If the tooth has a vital pulp, the occlusal surface is reduced uniformly throughout, maintaining the normal inclined planes, fissures, and cusps, but at a lower level (Figs. 23-4 to 23-6). If the preparation is made on a pulpless tooth that has a considerable amount of its coronal tissue destroyed by caries, the occlusal surface may be prepared in two planes, a buccal and a lingual, as shown in Figs. 23-3, 23-7, and 23-8.

The latter type of occlusal preparation is contraindicated on a tooth with a vital pulp, since the planes would come too close to the pulpal horns of the tooth, with the possibility of exposing them.

By another technic, the initial cut is made on the occlusal surface with a thin, knife-edged diamond stone (Densco 1-V) through the mesial marginal ridge to a depth of 1 to 1.5 mm. The cut stops at the level of the point of contact with the adjacent tooth and is made buccolingually; it establishes the proximal height of the preparation on the mesial surface.

Using the same stone, a similar cut is

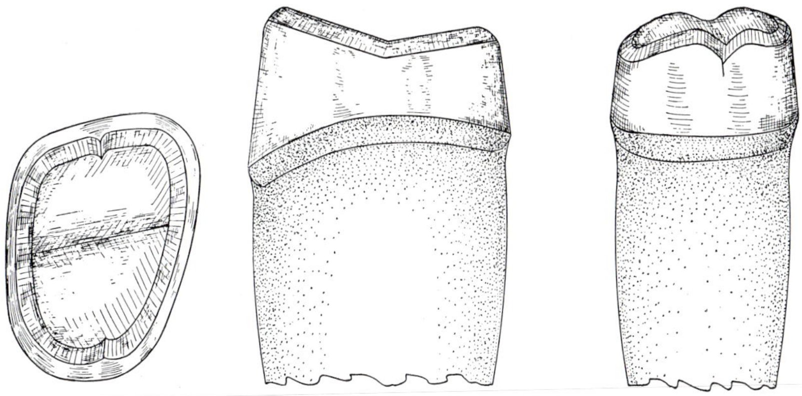

Fig. 23-7. Occlusal surface having buccal and lingual plane—may be used on pulpless tooth.

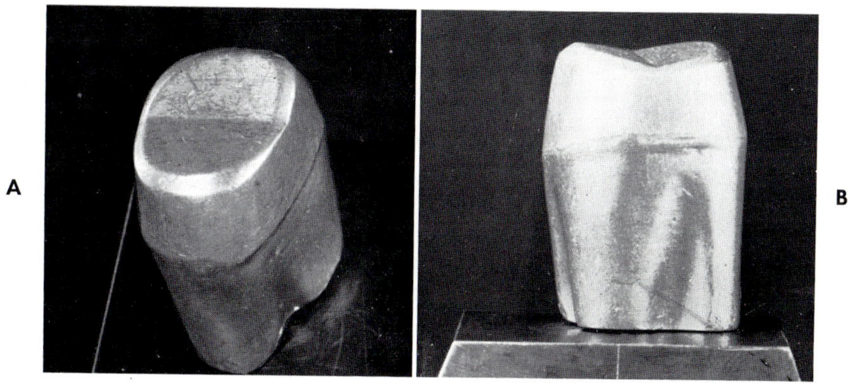

Fig. 23-8. A, Same occlusal surface as shown in Fig. 23-7. **B,** Proximal view.

made in a buccolingual direction through the distal margingal ridge.

The initial two cuts are then united mesiodistally by means of a groove 1 mm. in depth, cut with the same stone. The groove is not cut in a straight line, but it is curved to follow the direction taken by the occlusal groove. In an upper molar supplementary grooves 1 mm. in depth are made through the distolingual and through the buccal grooves.

It is now a simple matter to lower the inclined buccal and lingual planes of the occlusal surface to the desired level by using small, mounted, wheel-shaped stone (Densco 2½J), inverted cone stones (Densco 7½K and 8½K), and cylinder-shaped stone (Densco 5E) (Fig. 23-9).

Reduction of proximal surfaces. The next step is the reduction of the proximal surfaces (Figs. 23-10 and 23-11). A ⅝-inch diamond conical disk (Densco 4-O) is placed on the occlusal surface approximately 1 mm. from the distal contact point, and the edge of the disk is directed rootwise in such a way that, when the disk emerges gingivally, it will leave a proximal cut whose plane is nearly parallel to the long axis of the crown. No shoulder is formed at the gingival margin. In young patients whose epithelial attachment is still in contact with the enamel of the tooth, this margin will usually terminate at or slightly above the crest of the gingiva; in older patients it may be placed below the crest of the gum, terminating in the gingival crevice (Fig. 23-11, *A*).

Another cut, using a ⅝-inch straight

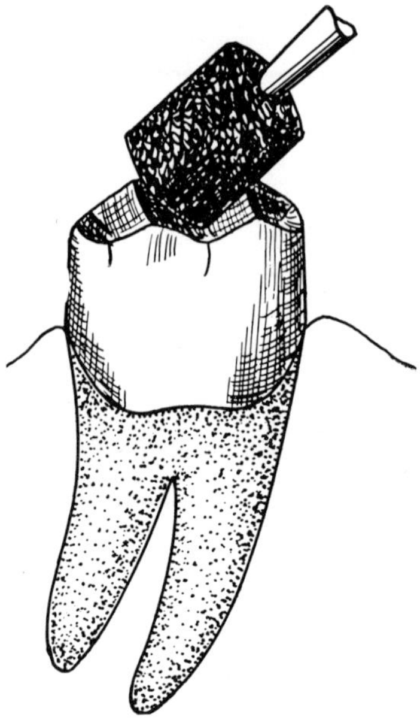

Fig. 23-9. Establishing occlusal inclined surfaces and grooves with small mounted stones. (After D. Smith.)

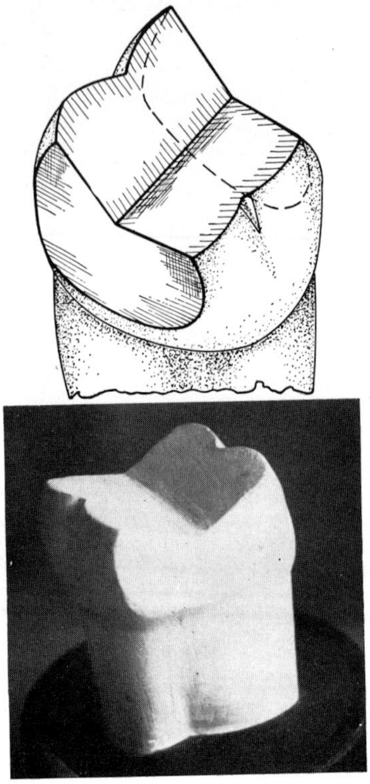

Fig. 23-10. Second step includes reduction of two proximal surfaces on pulpless tooth.

disk (Densco 4TP), is made on the opposite proximal surface. Although maximum retention requires that these walls be as near to parallelism as possible, it is necessary to converge them slightly gingivoclusally (Fig. 23-11, *B*).

Reduction of buccal and lingual surfaces. The next step consists of reducing the buccal and lingual surfaces (Fig. 23-12). As a preliminary procedure, it is advisable to cut with a small, mounted knife-edged stone (Densco 1V) a groove 1 mm. in depth, extending from the crest of the gum tissue to the occlusal surface. This cut is made in the buccal and in the distolingual grooves of an upper first molar; it starts shallow at the gingival surface and is gradually deepened to 1 mm. as it approaches the occlusal surface.

With mounted, wheel-shaped stone (Densco 2½J) and safe-end tapering stone (Densco 2DS) the buccal and the lingual surfaces are reduced so that their planes are almost parallel to the axis of the crown (Fig. 23-13). These planes extend from the occlusal surface gingivally, terminating at or slightly below the crest of the gum tissue, depending upon the height of the epithelial attachment. Here, likewise, no shoulder is formed at the gingival margin.

In reducing the buccal and lingual surfaces, the stone is carried mesiodistally with a light sweeping motion, while the amount of tooth tissue removed is governed largely by the groove previously cut, which serves as a depth gauge.

When preparing upper molars or bicuspids, it is imperative that a sufficient amount of the lingual surface be removed in the occlusal one-third region; likewise, in the lower bicuspids or molars sufficient tooth tissue must be removed from the

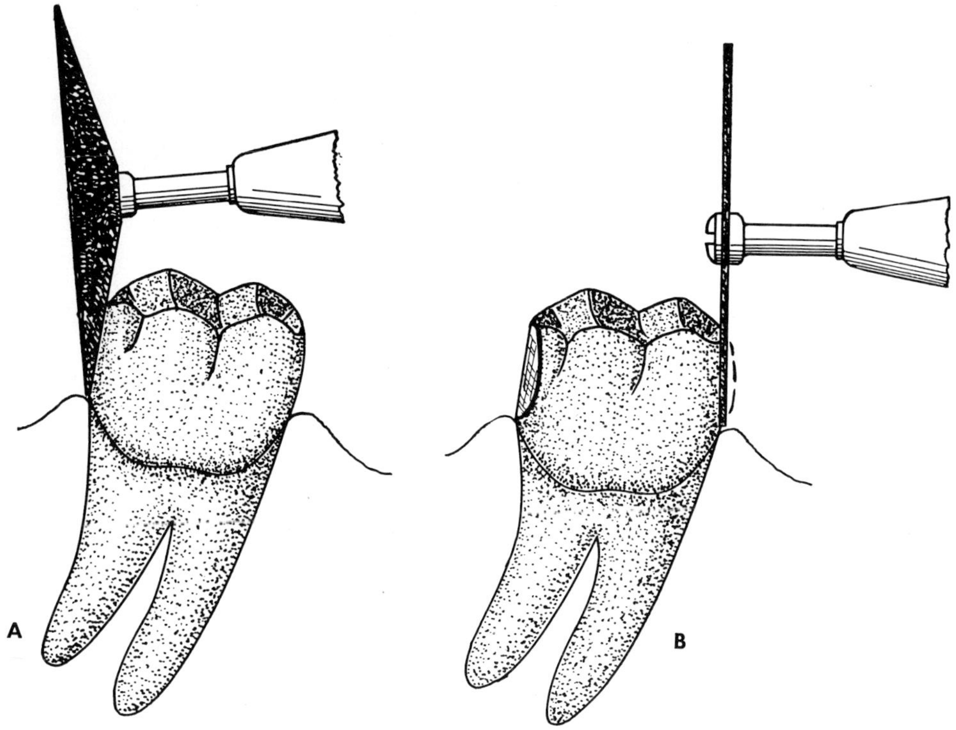

Fig. 23-11. Instrumentation in cutting of distal and mesial surfaces of tooth with vital pulp. (After D. Smith.)

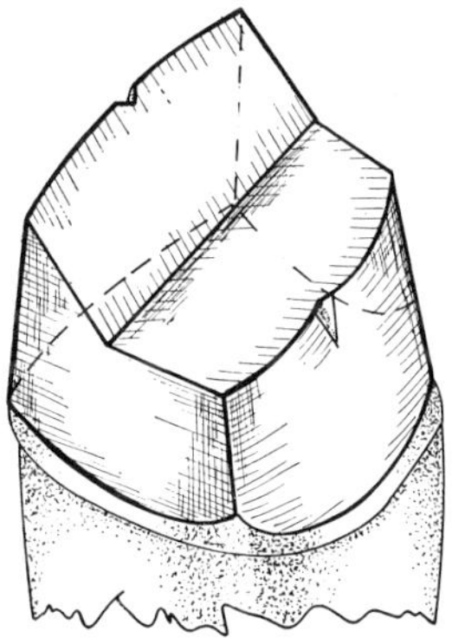

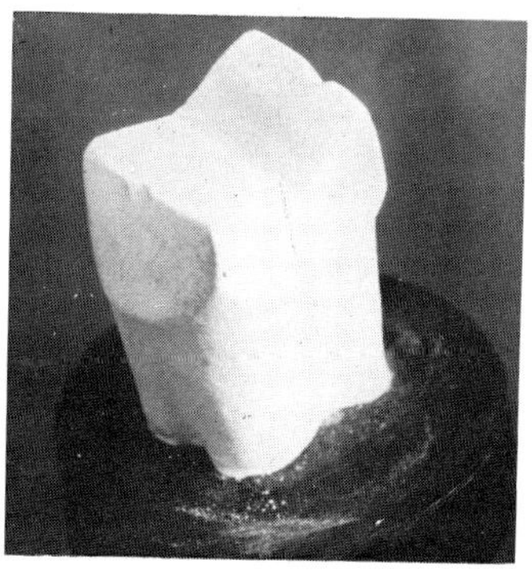

Fig. 23-12. Reduction of buccal and lingual surfaces of pulpless tooth.

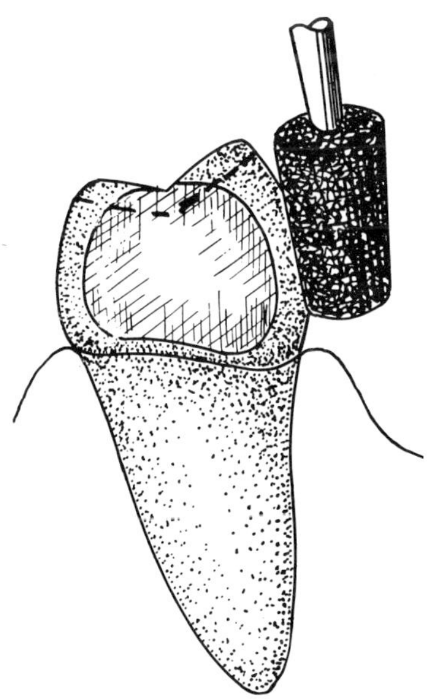

Fig. 23-13. Instrumentation for removal of buccal and lingual surfaces. (After D. Smith.)

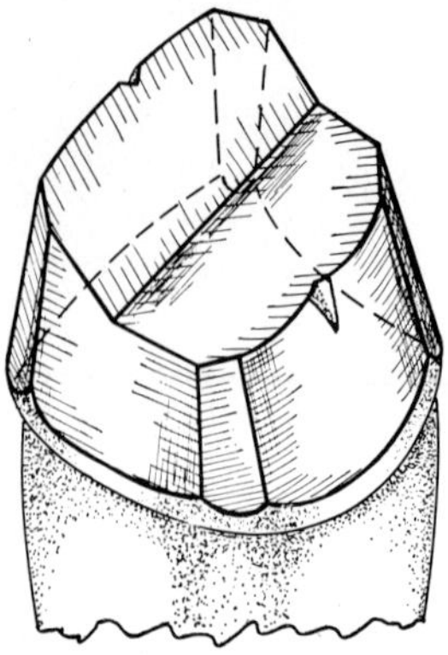

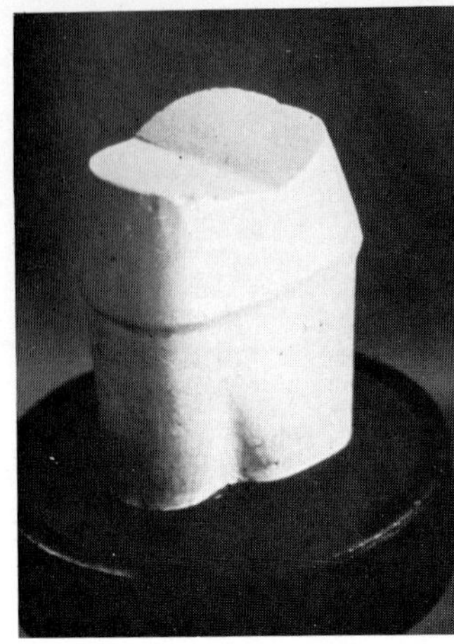

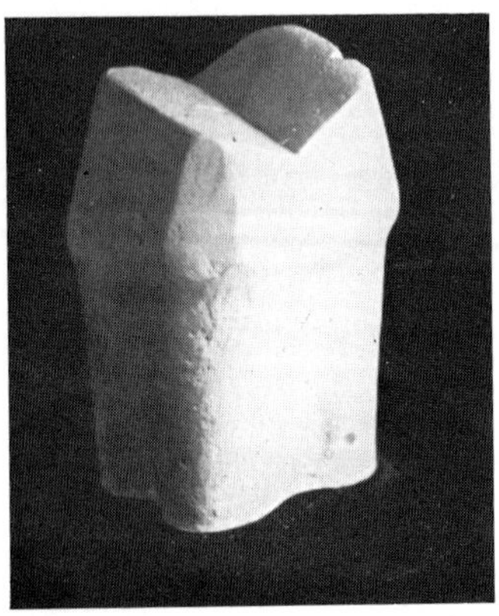

Fig. 23-14. Rounding axial line angles.

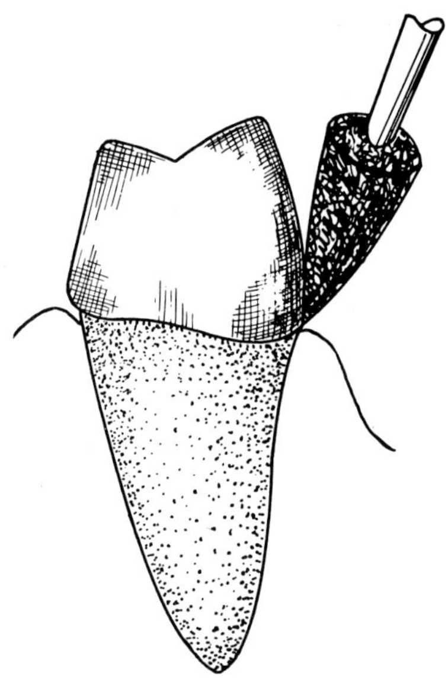

Fig. 23-15. Instrumentation for step shown in Fig. 23-14. (After D. Smith.)

occlusal one-third of the buccal surface; this precaution is necessary in order that a sufficient space be established for gold and the proper contouring of the finished crown. Failure to do this will result in a crown that does not have the necessary amount of metal or one that is contoured too wide buccolingually in the occlusal third region.

Reduction of axial angles. The corners or line angles between the proximal and the buccal and lingual surfaces (Fig. 23-14) are next rounded so that these surfaces blend into each other without any sharp angles, which might interfere with the subsequent fitting of the axial band or the making of the casting (Fig. 23-15). This operation is best performed by the use of small mounted concave or convex inverted cone diamond stones (Densco 7½K and 8½K), and tapering stone (Densco 1½A) (Fig. 23-15).

Occlusoaxial bevel. If any sharp angles remain between the axial walls and the occlusal surface (Fig. 23-16, *A*), these are removed by establishing a bevel extending around the entire occlusal periphery (Figs. 23-16, *B*, and 23-17). This is accomplished with a mounted, cylinder-shaped diamond stone (Densco 5E) (Fig. 23-17). The pur-

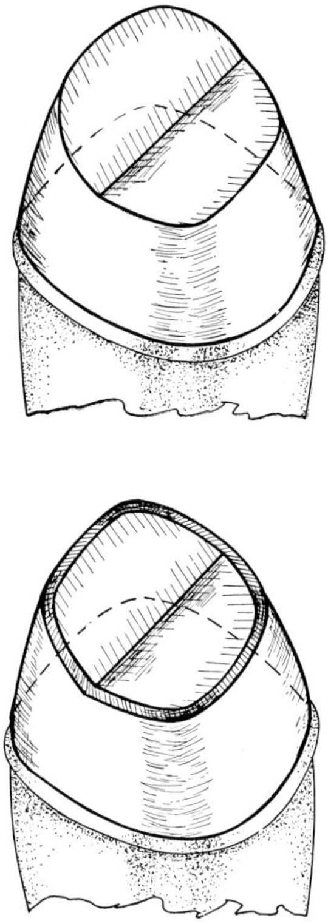

Fig. 23-16. Finishing of occlusoaxial line angle by cutting of bevel.

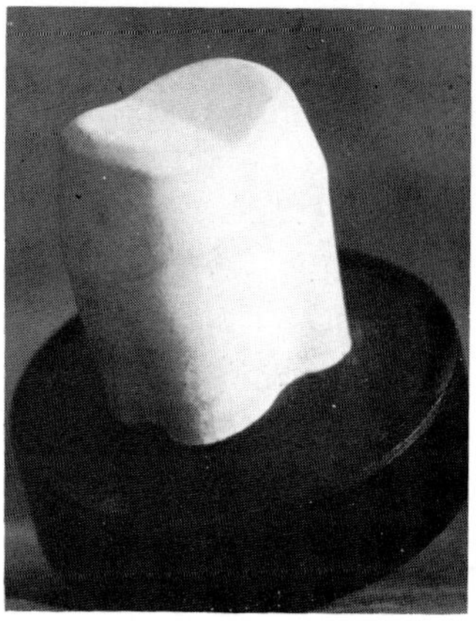

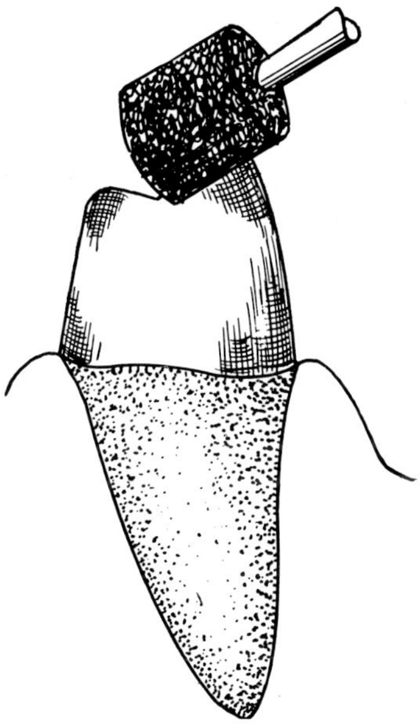

Fig. 23-17. Instrumentation for placing axi-occlusal bevel on occlusal surface.

pose of this bevel or cove is to facilitate: (1) swaging of the axial band over the occlusal surface, if a swaged type of crown is used; (2) obtaining an accurate wax pattern and gold casting by eliminating the sharp angle; and (3) obtaining a casting capable of resisting greater forces of distortion than when a sharp angle existed between two surfaces.

Finishing the shoulderless preparation at the gingival margin

The entire preparation is now polished with fine diamond points, disks, and cocoa butter, making certain that all undercuts have been eliminated and that the axial surfaces taper slightly from the base of the preparation at the cervical margin to the occlusal surface.

It can be seen from this description that no effort is made to remove all the enamel, either from the proximal or the occlusal surfaces. On the contrary, only enough is taken off to provide sufficient space for the metal and to assure the removal of overhanging tooth tissue that lies occlusally of the cervical margin. This preparation again calls attention to the fact that in most instances in which the gum tissues and their relationship to the tooth are normal, it is not necessary to remove all the enamel lying in the gingival crevice. However, it is still necessary to have the base of the preparation lie between the crest of the gingiva and the bottom of the gingival crevice. This will assure having the base of the finished crown beneath the crest of the gum tissue.

Another technic to lower the base of the preparation below the crest of the gingiva is the one suggested by Selberg.[4] (See Chapter 21.)

The shoulderless type of preparation is usually used when a thin gauge axial gold band is fitted accurately to the cervical base of the preparation, to the correct contour of the gingiva, and to its correct position in the depth of the sulcus. When the band is used the contour of the crown and its occlusion is subsequently built on it in wax and cast in metal.

The shoulderless type of preparation presents a serious difficulty in waxing directly to the prepared tooth. The alternative method is to construct a die of amalgam or stone upon which to do the waxing. In the majority of instances a shoulder preparation is preferred when dies of stone can be poured into an elastic material impression of the preparation. The shoulder preparation is used mostly when insufficient tooth structure remains or when the vision or access to the tooth prohibits making a good shoulder or chamfer margin.

METHODS OF CONSTRUCTING POSTERIOR METAL CROWNS

The swaged-cast shoulderless type

Because of the marked improvements made in casting technics, the principle of the swaged crown may be successfully combined with the casting process. In the swaged-cast combination type of complete veneer crown, an axial band is first fitted accurately to the axial surfaces of the preparation, following which the occlusal portion and the axial contour of the crown are restorted with a casting. The two parts are then united with solder at the cervical area to complete the crown.

Wire measurement. The first step in constructing this type of crown is to obtain the measurement of the prepared tooth for the axial band (Fig. 23-18). A piece of 34-gauge annealed iron wire is formed into a loop and held in a dentimeter or a broach holder. This is applied to the tooth preparation at a level corresponding to the highest point of the gum tissue; here, the wire is twisted until it is brought in snug contact with the tooth around its entire periphery. The wire measurement should not be curved to parallel the curvature of the gum tissue; neither should it be placed beneath the crest of the gingivae. This measurement is taken to determine the correct length to which the band is cut. Any difficulty in removing the wire mea-

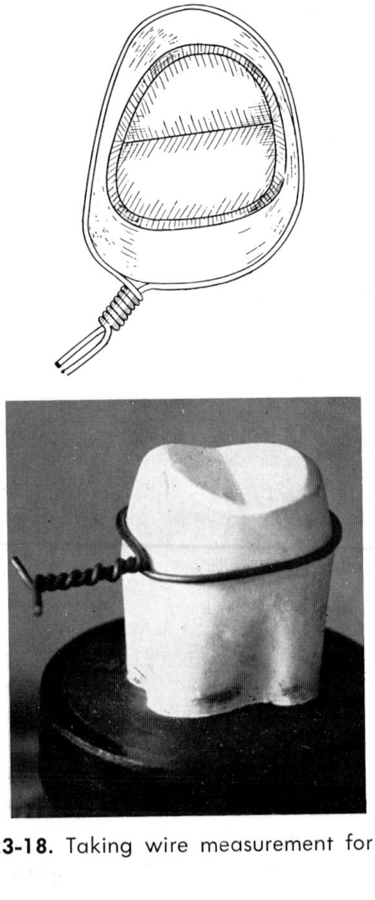

Fig. 23-18. Taking wire measurement for axial band.

surement occlusally indicates that undercuts exist, and these should be removed before any further work is done.

Height of band. The height of the band is determined either with calipers or by inserting a tapering piece of cardboard alongside the prepared tooth. To this measurement is added half the distance of the greatest occlusal diameter of the tooth.

Construction of axial band. The loop wire is now cut and the ends straightened (Fig. 23-19). The wire measurement is marked off on 24-carat gold plate, 36- or 34-gauge, and a band of the proper length is cut. It may be cut straight at both ends, or it may have these on a slight diagonal; however, one side is kept the same length as the original wire measurement. Usually the ends are left straight, except in those instances in which the occlusal circumference of the crown is greatly reduced in proportion to the gingival periphery. Twenty-four carat gold, 36- or 34-gauge plate is used because of the ease with which it may be fitted and contoured accurately to the prepared tooth.

The two ends of the band, having been filed flat, are brought together, forming a band that is nearly cylindrical in form or tapering occlusally to a slight degree (Fig. 23-20, *A*).

Flux is applied to the two edges of the band, and a small piece of 22-carat gold solder is laid across the two ends. Only enough solder should be used to fill the space between the two ends of the bands.

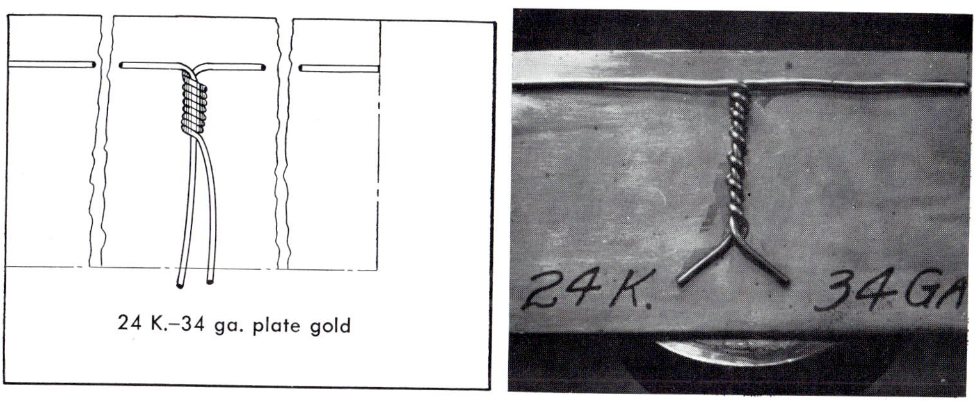

Fig. 23-19. Taking wire measurement and transferring it to gold plate.

A

B

C

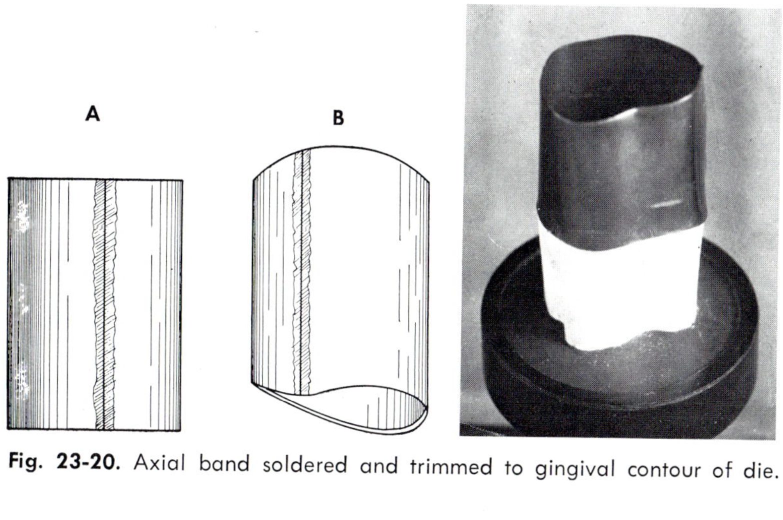

Fig. 23-20. Axial band soldered and trimmed to gingival contour of die.

The solder is placed on the inside of the band. With soldering pliers on the side opposite the joint, the band is held in a Bunsen flame and slowly heated until the solder flows, uniting the two ends. If difficulty is experienced in keeping the two ends of the band in contact during the soldering operation, a loop of wire is placed on the outside of the band and gently twisted until the two ends are brought in close contact.

Fitting the band. The gold band is now placed on the amalgam die, the soldered joint facing one of the proximal surfaces; if the band is slightly cone shaped, the wider end corresponding to the wire measurement is placed cervically. The gingival margin of the gold band is then fitted to the die so that the periphery of the band parallels and lies in close contact with the line marking the base of the crown preparation (Fig. 23-20, *B* and *C*). In other words, the gingival margin of the band stops where the axial walls of the prepared tooth reach their maximum flare; this may be below or above the crest of the gum tissue.

The gingival periphery of the gold band is then beveled with a fine file, placing the edge of the sharp bevel in contact with the prepared tooth.

The band is again replaced on the amalgam die and carried to its correct position. If it is found that it does not extend sufficiently cervically, slight pressure applied on the occlusal end of the band will stretch and seat it farther gingivally. This stretching may also be obtained by means of pliers. If, after contouring the gingival margin, it is found that the band is too large, the excess is best taken up by cutting out a small piece of the band and resoldering it. Trying to reduce the excess with contouring pliers is rarely successful.

Adapting band to axial and occlusal surfaces. The next step consists in adapting the band to the axial surfaces of the prepared tooth and in forming the occlusal cap. This may be done in two ways. The first method consists in cutting out triangular pieces of gold from the occlusal extension of the band (Fig. 23-21, *A*). These cuts, usually four or more in number, are situated at the proximolingual and buccal line angles and are extended gingivally one-third to two-thirds the height of the band.

The slotted band is then returned to the die, after which the proximal, buccal, and lingual segments of the band are burnished against the axial surfaces of the preparation. The more nearly parallel the axial

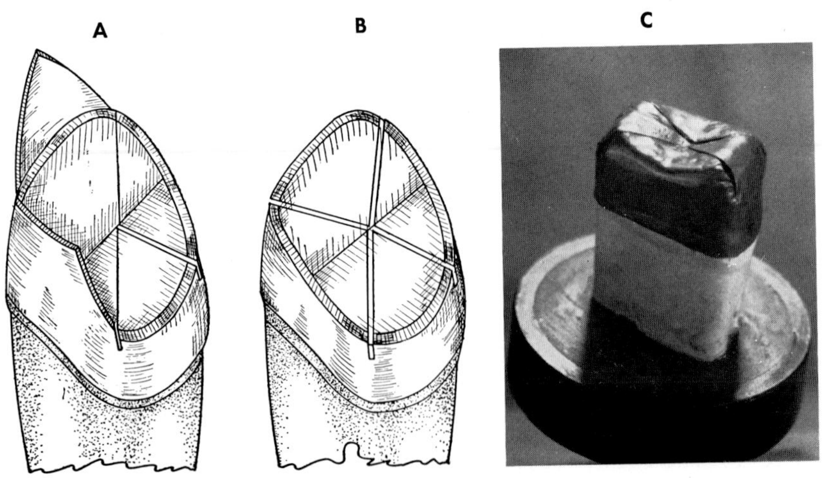

Fig. 23-21. Adapting band to occlusal and axial surfaces.

walls are, the less necessary it is to make the triangular cuts deep; in fact, those teeth having nearly parallel walls require very little removal of band material on the occlusal portion.

The final step in completing the cap is to bend the four occlusal extensions of the band toward the occlusal center of the tooth and to burnish them to conform to the occlusal anatomy of the preparation (Fig. 23-21, *B* and *C*). Where these extensions overlap, they are trimmed so that their margins approximate each other, while at the same time the entire occlusal surface is covered with gold; it is not necessary to solder these margins on the occlusal surface.

Occasionally, the contour of the axial surfaces converges occlusally to such a degree that it is impossible to obtain an accurate adaptation of the band by cutting out only four pieces. In such event, a series of axial slits is made, resulting in many narrow, long segments of the band on each surface. These are then closely adapted to the axial surfaces by overlapping their edges. The excess thickness of overlapping gold plate on the occlusal surface is then removed so that only one layer covers this area. This completes the cap.

The other method of completing the cap is as follows: after the axial band has been properly fitted at the gingival margin and axially, that portion of the band extending beyond the occlusal surface of the preparation is now trimmed to the height of the occlusal plane; a piece of 34-gauge, 24-carat plate is swaged to the occlusal surface of the amalgam die, waxed to the band, removed, and soldered to it, thus completing the cap.

At this point the finished cap is tried on the prepared tooth in the patient's mouth in order to verify the accuracy of the gingival fit and the correct length of the band. This procedure is very important since the ultimate fit and service rendered to the patient depend largely upon it.

Waxing the contour of the crown. If satisfactory, the cap is removed from the tooth and replaced on the amalgam die. The next step consists of developing the occlusal and axial contours of the crown in inlay wax. A thin film of sticky wax is first melted on the band so that the film covers the upper axial as well as the occlusal surfaces. Care must be exercised in doing this that none of the wax flows on the inside of the band. A small amount of softened inlay wax is then applied to the outer surfaces of the band and attached with a hot spatula. This prevents the inlay wax, when it is chilled, from breaking away from the smooth gold band.

The occlusal portion of the gold band is then covered with more thoroughly warmed inlay wax, and the opposing cast is brought into occlusion, first in centric and then in lateral and protrusive relationships; the wax is chilled and the excess removed with a sharp instrument.

The axial contour is completed by adding more inlay wax, after which the crown is carefully examined for correct inclination of occlusal planes and the position and height of the cusps. The characteristic contours of the proximal surfaces must also be accurately reproduced with properly formed and positioned contact areas (Fig. 23-22).

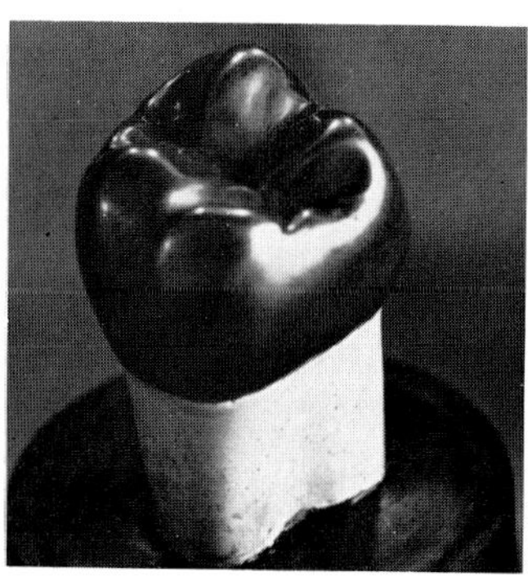

Fig. 23-22. Contour of crown waxed to cover entire band to its cervical margin.

To obtain the correct degree of interproximal contact between the proximal surfaces of the cast crown and its adjacent teeth, a small bead of inlay wax is added to each contact area of the wax crown and allowed to congeal. The wax crown is now gently positioned over the prepared tooth, and the excess of newly added, semihardened wax in the contact area is compressed. When the crown is removed for investing, the stresses of compression developed in the wax at the contact areas manifest themselves by expanding slightly, thus giving a plus contact contour in the finished cast crown.

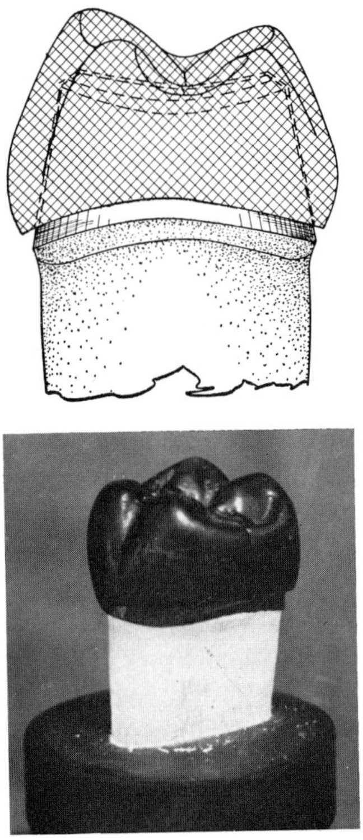

Fig. 23-23. Crown contoured in casting wax and 1.5 mm. of wax cut away at gingival margin, exposing axial gold band.

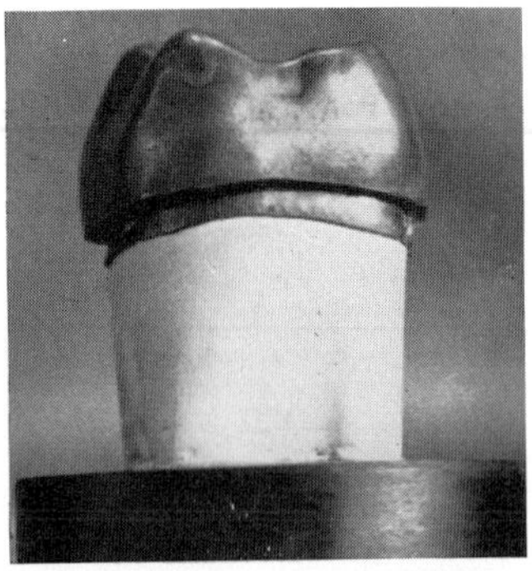

Fig. 23-24. Cast crown having cervical 1.5 mm. of axial band exposed for reburnishing, if necessary.

After this, the waxed crown and band are held on the prepared tooth, and the occlusion and contour are verified in the mouth. The patient should be asked to move his mandible into centric, lateral, and protrusive positions and through the various masticatory movements. Once the correctness of these relationships has been established, the waxed crown and band are removed from the tooth and prepared for investing and casting.

Cutting away gingival wax. Before attaching the crown to the sprue former, a collar of inlay wax 1 to 1.5 mm. in width is removed from the gingival periphery of the crown, leaving this much of the 24-carat, 36- or 34-gauge band material exposed. The wax is cut away at right angles to the band so that it ends as a sharp, flat gingival wall (Fig. 23-23).

This is done for the following reasons: (1) it eliminates the difficulty or possibility of the gold casting being short at the gingival margin; (2) after the casting has been made, it enables the dentist to replace the casting on the natural tooth, to reexamine and reburnish, if necessary, the exposed part of the band to the tooth.

Spruing. While one large sprue former is usually sufficient, it is advisable at times to place two or more supplementary ones; these should be placed so that the metal will flow in the direction of the waxed contour instead of being directed at right angles against the gold cap. The technic of investing and casting is given in Chapter 20.

Because of the cuplike form of the crown mold, and the presence of the metal cap, there is greater difficulty for the hot gases in the mold to escape through the investment. A back pressure develops causing incomplete castings or pinholes, extending back into the sprue rod. This difficulty may also arise in the full cast crown that does not employ the gold cap.

To eliminate this difficulty, it is suggested that a vent be formed to allow the gases to escape. An asbestos rope, 10-gauge, is dipped in wax and cooled. A piece of asbestos ¾ inch long is attached at one end to the outer surface of the wax crown and the other end is attached to the crucible former. The crown is then invested and burned out. The wax in the asbestos cord is also eliminated, leaving a porous vent for the escape of the gases from the mold; at the same time the asbestos prevents the molten gold from entering the vent.

When casting against metal, it is advisable to use sprues of 14- to 12-gauge; the distance between the pattern and the base should not exceed ¼ inch, and better results are obtained if a deoxidizing casting investment is used.

Readapting gingival margin. After the casting has been completed and recovered from the investment material, the crown is cleaned, boiled in acid, and washed; it is then placed on the *prepared tooth* to be given its final gingival adapatation. With a fine, sharp explorer, the gingival margin of the band is examined for the accuracy of its fit. Since 1 to 1.5 mm. of the 24-carat, 36- or 34-gauge band material is not covered by the casting, it is a simple matter to reburnish and refit any portion of the periphery with a small burnisher (Fig. 23-24).

Soldering the peripheral margin. If the crown fits accurately, it is removed, carefully washed, and dried; the inner surface of the band is painted with a small amount of antiflux, after which it is filled with a crown and bridge investment. The end of a slate pencil may be embedded in the investment, to serve later as a handle during the soldering of the periphery of the crown.

After the investment has hardened, the exposed gingival part of the band is fluxed and the entire mass gently heated to a

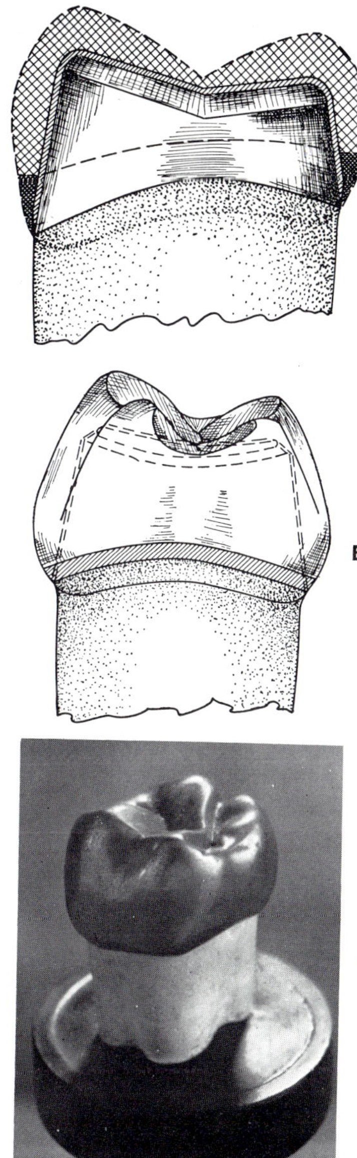

A

B

C

Fig. 23-25. A and **B,** Cross section of crown showing relative positions occupied by axial band, cast gold crown, and gingival portion consisting of 20-carat gold solder. **C,** Finished cast crown.

cherry red color. Strips of 20-carat solder are applied between the gingival margins of the band and the casting, and the solder is melted around the entire periphery. Additional pieces are added until the gingival contour is fully developed (Fig. 23-25, A).

The crown is then finished and polished and tried on the natural tooth for final approval (Fig. 23-25, *B* and *C*).

MODIFIED TYPE: CAST OCCLUSAL SURFACE

A modification of this type of crown is sometimes made where only the occlusal portion of the crown is cast to a fully contoured axial band. In this method, however, the band material consists of 29-gauge, 22-carat gold plate.

After the wire measurement is taken, the band is cut as before, both ends being cut straight or slightly slanting; in the latter the cuts slant outward from the measurement of the wire. When the ends of the band are soldered, the smaller opening of the band now becomes the gingival portion, while the wider or the flaring part extends occlusally (Fig. 23-26).

After the smaller end has been properly festooned and conformed to the gingival margin of the preparation, the occlusal end of the band is trimmed so that it extends about 0.5 mm. beyond the occlusal plane of the preparation; at the same time, it is trimmed so that it does not interfere with the closure of the opposing teeth.

With suitable contouring pliers the axial surfaces of the band are contoured to reproduce their correct tooth form, proper interproximal spaces, and correct contact areas (Fig. 23-27, A).

The band is then removed from the die and carried to the prepared tooth in the mouth where final verification of fit and contour is made. If satisfactory, the band is removed, cleaned, and dried, and a small amount of flux is applied to the occlusal edge of the band, which is fixed

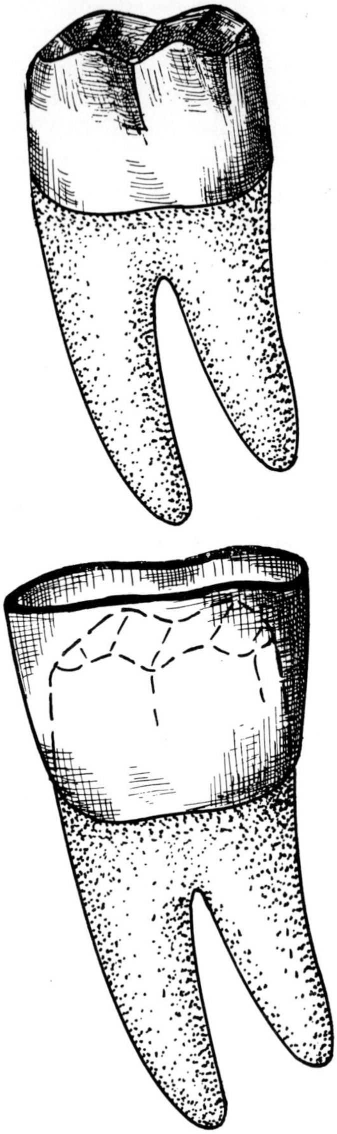

Fig. 23-26. Finished shoulderless preparation with flaring axial band, 29-gauge, 22-carat plate.

in a Bunsen flame by bringing the band to a cherry red color.

A small piece of 27-gauge pink casting wax is placed over the occlusal opening of the band and its edge attached with a hot spatula (Fig. 23-27, *B*). The gold band with the wax cap is now covered with softened inlay wax, after which the patient is instructed to close into centric and

A

B

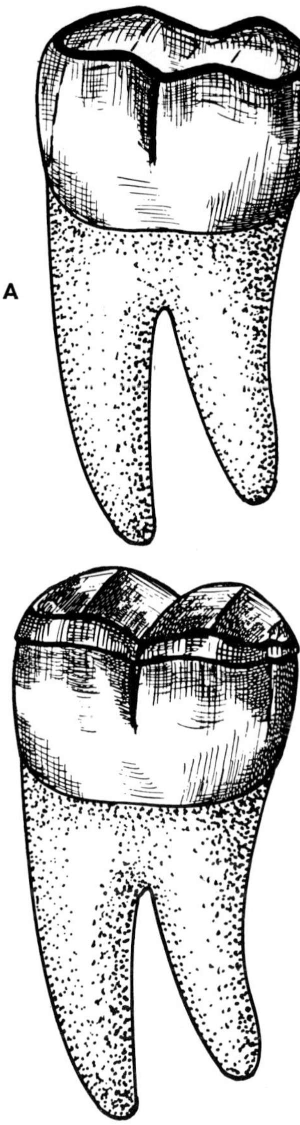

Fig. 23-27. A, Axial band contoured. **B,** Occlusal surface restored in casting wax.

then into the various lateral and protrusive occlusal relationships.

When the wax is chilled, the occlusal anatomy is completed and the band with the waxed occlusal portion is removed from the prepared tooth, invested, and cast (Fig. 23-28, *A*).

After the crown has been cleaned and pickled in acid, a small piece of solder

A

B

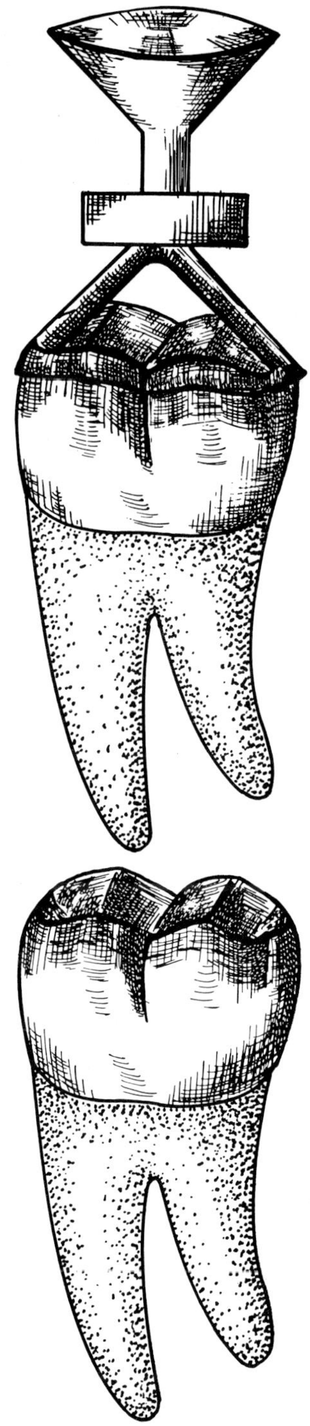

Fig. 23-28. A, Occlusal portion of crown cast in gold directly to axial band. **B,** Finished crown.

is flowed on the inside of the crown at the junction of the casting with the occlusal margin of the axial band (Fig. 23-28, *B*). Occasionally, it is also necessary to flow solder on the outer surface at the junction of the casting and the band, in which event 22-carat solder is used.

ALL-CAST TYPE OF CROWN

The third type of complete veneer metal crown, from many considerations the most satisfactory, is the all-cast type, which does not employ an axial band.

Although it may be constructed by the direct technic, this crown is usually made by the indirect method, with only one intermediary step checked directly in the mouth. This step involves verifying the fit and contour of the wax crown before it is cast (Fig. 23-29).

Preparation of tooth: shoulder and shoulderless types

The preparation for this type of crown may be either of the shoulder type (Figs. 23-30 to 23-32) or of the shoulderless type (Figs. 23-33 and 23-34). If the shoulder type of preparation is employed, no further modification or treatment of the amalgam die is necessary; if, however, the

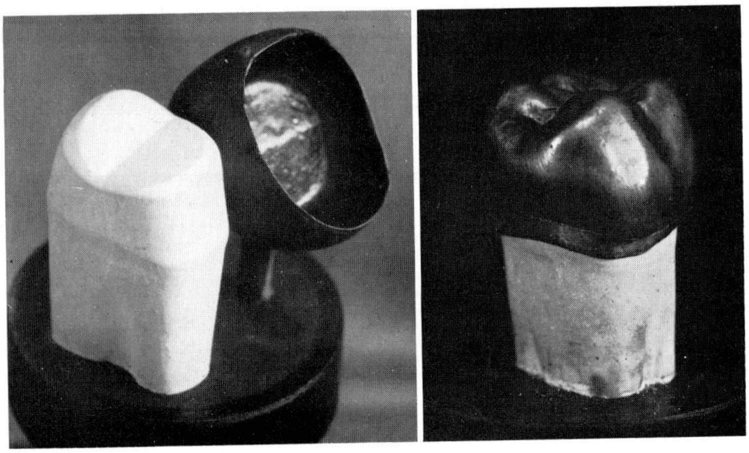

Fig. 23-29. Shoulderless type of complete veneer cast metal crown without axial band.

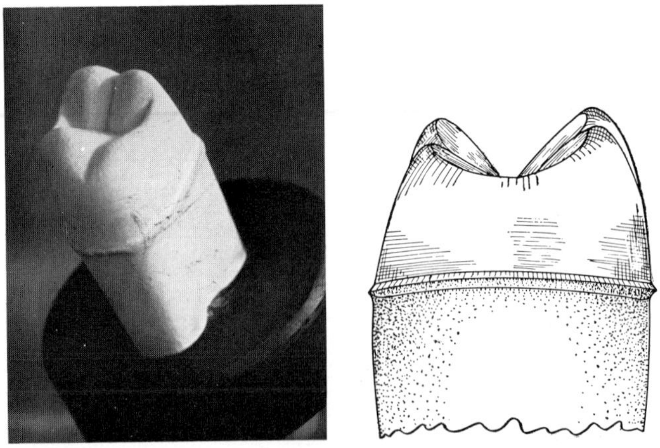

Fig. 23-30. Shoulder type of preparation for molar crown on vital tooth.

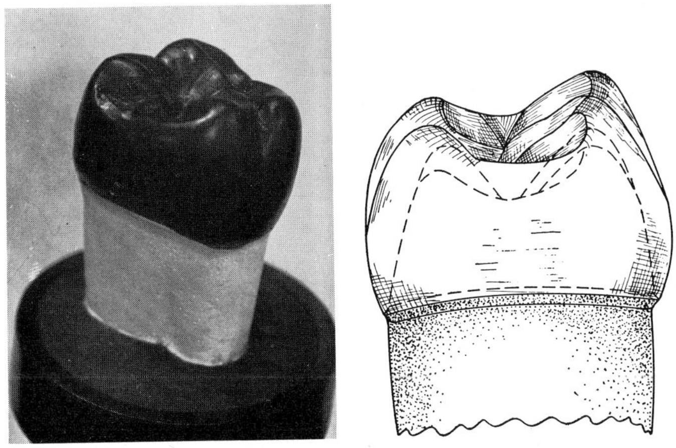

Fig. 23-31. Shoulder type of preparation with crown built entirely of wax.

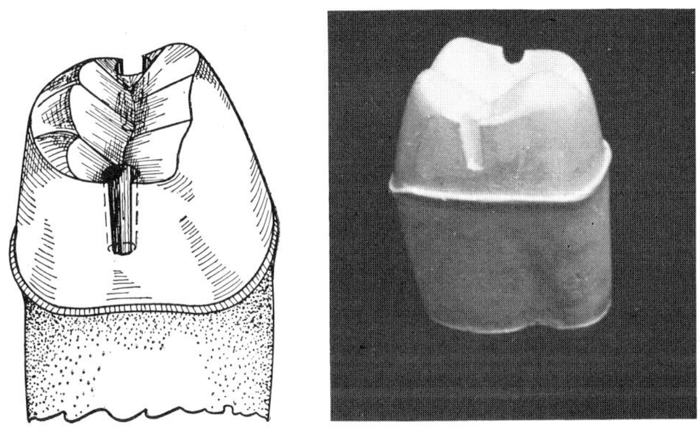

Fig. 23-32. Shoulder type of preparation modified by preparing two proximal keyways for additional resistance to displacement.

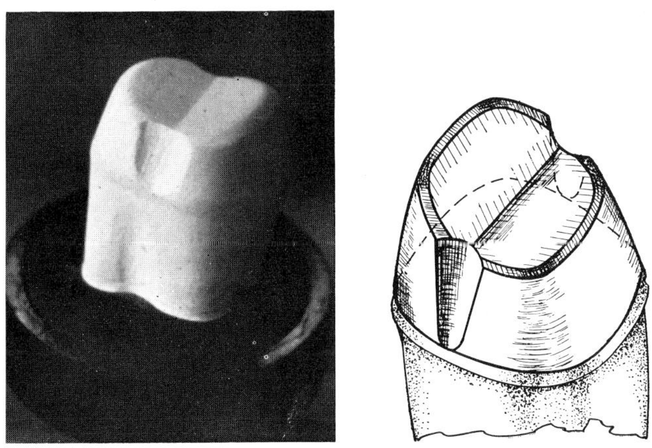

Fig. 23-33. Proximal shallow keyways placed in shoulderless type of preparation on pulpless tooth.

shoulderless type of preparation is employed (Fig. 23-34, *A* and *B*), the amalgam die is removed from the working model and notched around its entire periphery, 0.5 mm. below the finish line of the preparation (Fig. 23-35). This is done so that when the wax pattern of the crown is carved it is easier to follow the curvature of the gingival margin; it also affords a better edge against which to finish the wax pattern and casting.

The amalgam die is then thoroughly lubricated with a thin oil and returned to the working model. In order to confine the soft inlay wax and adapt it accurately to the amalgam die, a copper matrix band is employed. The same copper band may be used in which the modeling compound impression was taken of the prepared tooth, or, if this has been destroyed, another band is fitted to the die so that it conforms to the gingival contour of the preparation and extends as high occlusally as the occlusal plane. It should be made certain that the band will not interfere when the opposing cast of the working model is brought into occlusion.

Waxing the crown

The copper band is then removed from the amalgam die, slightly lubricated on its inner surface, and filled with softened inlay wax. In order to facilitate the flow of the softened wax against the amalgam die, the die should be slightly warmed, so that when it comes in contact with the wax it will not harden before it is carried to the gingival margin.

The band, filled with softened wax, is centered over the die, and, with the finger applied to the occlusal surface, both wax and band are pressed down until the gingival margin of the band has passed beyond the gingival finishing line on the amalgam die. The opposing teeth are then brought into centric occlusion; with the wax still soft, the mandibular cast is moved into lateral and protrusive relationships. After the wax is hard, it is carved to occlusion within the confines of the copper band; then, carefully, the band, wax, and the amalgam die are lifted from the working model.

The copper band is carefully cut through with a vulcocarbo disk on that side hav-

A

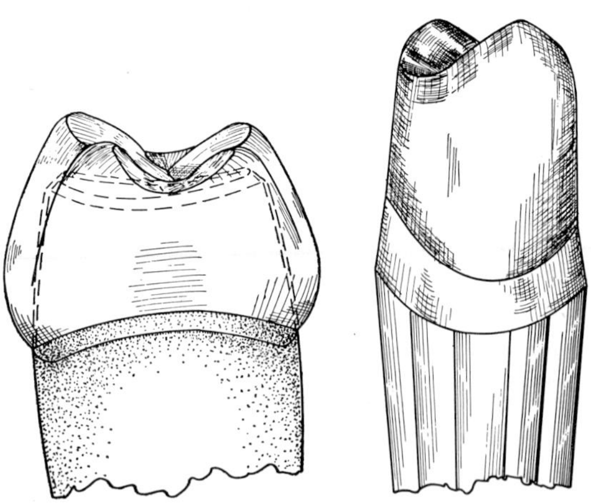

B

Fig. 23-34

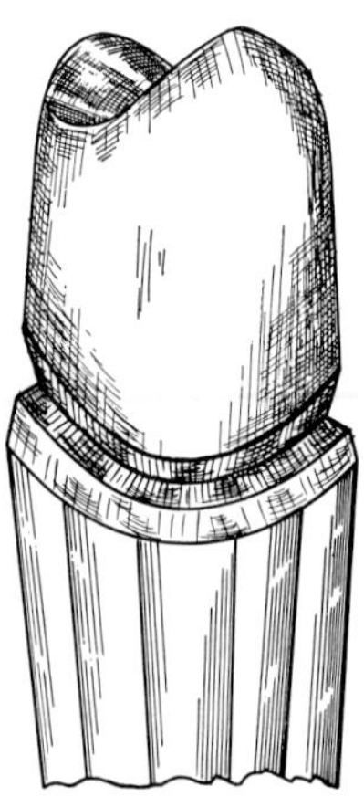

Fig. 23-35

Fig. 23-34. A, Cross section of cast crown on shoulderless preparation. **B,** Amalgam die of shoulderless preparation for all-cast bicuspid gold crown.
Fig. 23-35. Notching of amalgam die prior to contouring crown in casting wax. (Suggested by D. Smith.)

ing the greatest bulk of inlay wax. Care is exercised not to cut through the wax, so as not to mutilate the amalgam die. The band is then carefully peeled away from the wax, allowing the excess of wax to extend rootwise beyond the finishing line on the amalgam die. Before removing this excess wax, more is carefully added to the axial and the occlusal surfaces. The waxed crown and die are returned to the working model where the complete axial contour and occlusion are developed.

After this, the die and crown are removed from the working model and the wax extending beyond the gingival finishing line is carefully cut away with a sharp lance, the notch acting as a guide to the gingival curvature (Fig. 23-36, *A*). In trimming away this gingival surplus, it is advisable to leave the wax slightly in excess of what will be desired in the finished crown. This excess will later make it possible to give the finished gold crown the necessary buccal and lingual cervical area convexities.

In starting, a wax crown may be built up on the lubricated die by dipping it in molten wax several times until the desired thickness of wax has been obtained. The contour is then completed with wax added with a hot spatula.

After the final contour and polish, the waxed crown is removed from the die and prepared for investing and casting.

Before doing so, however, it is advisable to transfer it to the prepared tooth in the mouth and to verify the occlusal relationship, contour, contact points, and gingival adaptation. Although this final fitting has certain advantages, care must be exercised not to distort the wax pattern in doing so.

Should there be any difficulty in seating the wax crown on the natural tooth, it is suggested that it be first submerged for 1 minute in water of 95° F.

Finishing and cementing crown

If found satisfactory, the wax crown is removed from the tooth and the mesiobuccal angle is perforated with a size 82 machinist's drill, even with the occlusal surface of the prepared tooth; the wax crown is sprued, cleansed of all lubricant, invested, and cast. When removed from the casting investment, it is thoroughly cleansed, boiled in acid, and examined for any possible imperfections in casting.

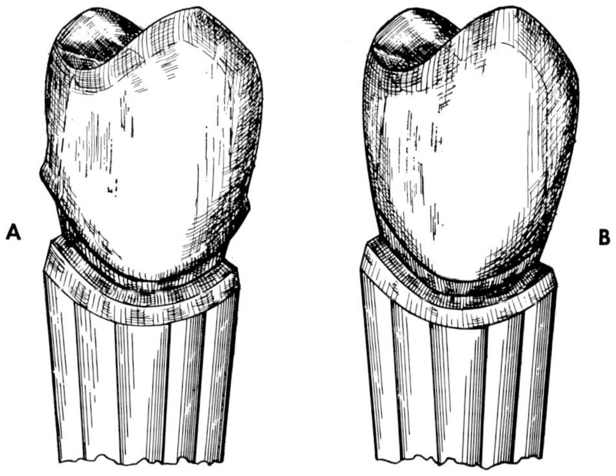

Fig. 23-36. A, Waxed crown on amalgam die. Note surplus wax at gingival margin. **B,** Cast gold crown finished on amalgam die. Excess gold at gingival margin permits establishing correct gingival contour.

If none exists, the casting is placed on the amalgam die, where the major part of the finishing is done. The excess of gold around the gingival periphery may also be contoured at this time, care being taken to maintain the proper gingival convexity at the buccal and lingual surfaces (Fig. 23-36, *B*). The crown is then given its final polish for final trial on the prepared tooth.

When the patient returns, the temporary crown is removed, and the cast gold crown is tried for gingival fit, correct contact areas, contour, and occlusion in centric, lateral, and protrusive relationships. If satisfactory, it is cemented. The opening in the mesiobuccal angle is then filled with gold foil or with a piece of clasp metal wire.

In teeth prepared with a shoulder or chamfer, it is not necessary to notch the die, since the outer angle of the chamfer or shoulder furnishes a definite finishing line to which the wax is trimmed.

HOLLENBACK CAST SHOULDER CROWNS USING PORCELAIN VENEER FACING

While the complete cast crown fulfills all mechanical requirements, unfortunately its use is largely confined to the posterior region, unless it is modified to meet the esthetic requirements by using a porcelain veneer facing. This modification is occasionally employed in the molars and the second bicuspids, although it is more frequently used in the first bicuspids and the anterior teeth. When the porcelain veneer is used, the tooth preparation is usually modified by establishing a shoulder on the labial or buccal surfaces. This modification allows additional space for the thickness of porcelain.

This type of crown is usually designated as the Hollenback crown. In several respects it is similar to the preparation of a tooth for a complete porcelain veneer crown. (See Chapter 24.) The four points of difference are the following: (1) the labial shoulder is usually wider than that for a complete porcelain veneer crown; (2) the lingual margin, which extends half the distance labially on each proximal surface, is prepared as a chamfer instead of a shoulder; (3) less of the lingual surface is removed from the tooth; and (4) slightly more of the labial surface is removed because of the deeper labial shoulder and the need for more space to accommodate the porcelain facing.

It is obvious that *this type of crown can be employed only on older patients because of the danger of pulp exposure in younger patients.* It may be used as an individual restoration or as a retainer for a bridge. Usually it is employed in short-bite cases and for patients with a strong musculature.

The steps in the preparation of an upper central incisor are as follows:

1. The incisal plane is reduced 1.5 to 2 mm. with a mounted diamond stone (Densco 2J), so that a suitable thickness of gold will protect the incisal part of the porcelain facing (Fig. 23-37, *B* and *C*).
2. The reduction of the two proximal surfaces is accomplished with a ¾ inch diamond disk (Densco 4TP). The cut is started on the incisal plane about 2 mm. from the proximal surface and the disk directed gingivally so that when the cut is made through the body of the tooth, the proximal plane will emerge at or slightly below the crest of the gingiva, without making a shoulder. The other proximal surface is similarly treated.
3. The removal of the enamel from the labial surface is accomplished in the same manner as was done for the complete porcelain veneer crown described in Chapter 24.
4. In preparing the lingual surface, it is necessary to remove only enough of the enamel surface to allow for 0.5 mm. of gold in the finished casting (Fig. 23-37, *B* and *C*). All the enamel is not removed as was done for the complete porcelain

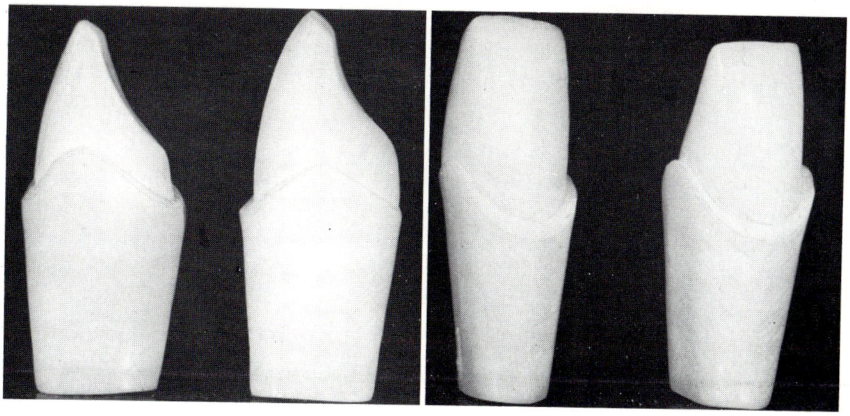

A B C D

Fig. 23-37. A and **D,** Complete porcelain veneer crown has 0.5 to 1.5 mm. uniform width of shoulder prepared on all surfaces. Lingual surface reduced 1.0 mm. **B** and **C,** Hollenback cast shoulder crown preparation for porcelain veneer facing has labial shoulder 0.75 to 1.5 mm. wide and lingual cervical chamfer 0.5 mm. wide. Lingual surface reduced 0.5 to 1.0 mm.

A

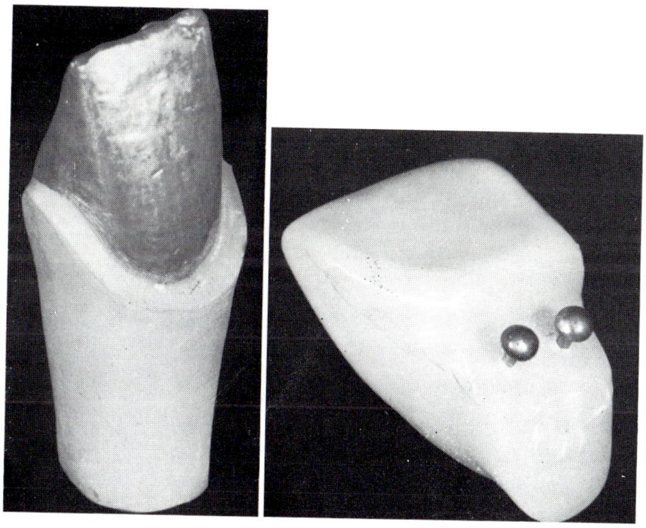

B

Fig. 23-38. A, Platinum matrix used with cast crowns employing porcelain veneer facing. **B,** Denture tooth used to grind porcelain veneer.

veneer crown (Fig. 23-37, *A* to *D*). The lingual reduction is made with a diamond stone (Densco 2½J).

5. Three seamless copper bands are fitted to the gingival curvature of the gingiva. One is used for the compound impression of the finished preparation from which the amalgam die is made, one to construct the acrylic resin temporary crown, and the third to make a cement or stone die on which the low fusing metal transfer crown is made.

6. The rubber dam and clamp are applied to the tooth prior to preparing the shoulder on the labial side and the chamfer on the lingual side. This depresses the gingiva and exposes the cervical part of the tooth lying in the gingival crevice.

This is the area in which the shoulder and the chamfer will terminate. The labial shoulder is cut as previously described, except that its width is 0.75 to 1.5 mm. (Fig. 23-37, *C*). The lingual surface terminates in a chamfer and is prepared as described in Chapter 17.

The labial shoulder meets and is confluent with the chamfer midway on the proximal surfaces; this differs from the complete veneer crown, in which the shoulder continues around the lingual surface.

7. Two impressions of the finished preparation are secured in modeling compound. One is used to make the amalgam die on which the crown is constructed; the other to make a cement or silicate die on which the low fusing metal transfer crown is made to be used when the impressions for the working model are taken. The third copper band is used later to make the temporary acrylic crown.

8. A platinum matrix, 0.0005 inch, is made with a tinner's joint on the lingual or proximal surfaces. The gingival margin of the matrix does not cover the shoulder; it terminates at the inner angle of the shoulder; it gives rigidity to the waxed crown, especially the labial portion (Fig. 23-38, *A*).

9. A denture tooth is selected of the proper color, type, width, and slightly longer incisogingivally. The extra length is desirable to allow for the grinding and fitting of the facing to the gingival shoulder (Fig. 23-38, *B*). The pins are dissolved by boiling in aqua regia (Fig. 23-39, *A*).

10. With diamond stones (Densco 2½J and ½MW), the lingual surface of the denture tooth is hollow ground mesiodistally, forming a concave channel extending from the gingival margin to within 1 mm. of the incisal plane (Fig. 23-39, *B*). The width and depth of this concave surface are determined by the width and convexity of the labial surface of the amalgam die of the prepared tooth. Although the convexity of the die and the concavity in the porcelain tooth should fit into each other accurately, enough additional porcelain must be ground away to leave a small intervening space for the waxing of the crown.

At this time, care must also be taken to establish the correct mesiodistal alignment as well as the labiolingual relationship of the porcelain tooth to the adjacent teeth.

The gingival margin of the porcelain facing is ground to contact evenly the labial shoulder of the preparation. The facing is ground at the gingival end when shortening its gingivoincisal length. When the proper length has been established, an additional 0.3 mm. is removed at the gingival end to allow room for wax, and later gold, between the porcelain and the

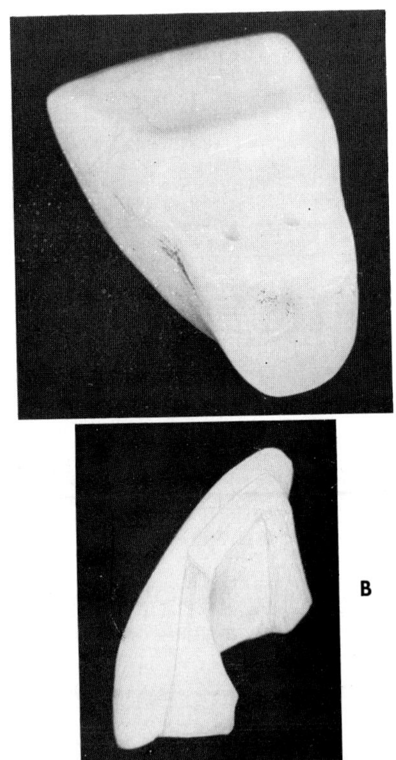

A

B

Fig. 23-39. A, Pins removed from denture porcelain tooth. **B,** Finished porcelain facing ready to be waxed on platinum matrix.

shoulder. The incisal plane of the porcelain facing is prepared with a modified groove (Fig. 23-39, *B*) to furnish a sufficient thickness of gold for protection against fracture. All ground surfaces are polished.

11. The proximal surfaces of the porcelain facing are next prepared (1) so that the line where the gold and porcelain meet on the proximal surfaces will not be seen when the tooth is viewed from the labial surface and (2) so that two tapering wings or flanges of porcelain will extend lingually into the mesial and distal portions of the cast crown so that a staple-like retention is secured (Fig. 23-39, *B*).

In order to conserve as great a bulk of porcelain as possible, the lines establishing the labial limits of the gold on the proximal surfaces are cut very shallow, 0.2 mm. in the incisogingival direction. From this shallow groove the porcelain is tapered lingually. The shallower the initial grooves are cut, the stronger and less liable to fracture will be the porcelain flanges. When all the ground porcelain surfaces have been polished they are lightly lubricated.

12. A small bead of red carding wax is attached to the labial surface of the platinum matrix, which is in position on the die. The facing is carefully pressed against the soft wax and properly aligned, care being taken that a 0.3 mm. space exists at the gingival area between the facing and the shoulder (Fig. 23-40, *A*). Melted inlay wax is now placed between the facing and the platinum matrix and between the porcelain and the lubricated die at the shoulder. The proximal and lingual contours are completed in inlay wax.

13. A piece of sticky wax is attached to the labial surface of the facing; after the wax hardens the facing is withdrawn labially and laid aside (Figs. 23-40, *B* and 23-41, *A*).

14. The waxed crown with its platinum matrix remaining inside (Fig. 23-41, *B*) is sprued, cleaned, invested, and cast. It is important that the casting be smooth and that it be accurate dimensionally (Fig. 23-42, *A* and *B*). If it is not, the porcelain facing will not fit properly, and the flange-like porcelain extensions may be fractured. The casting should be thoroughly cleaned

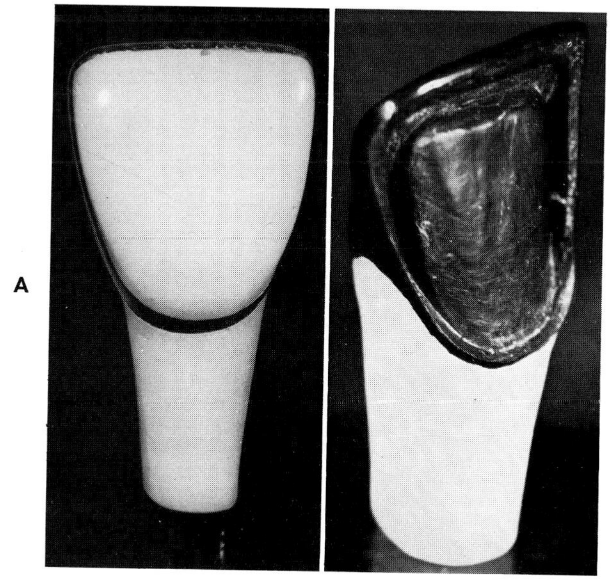

Fig. 23-40. A, Veneer facing waxed into contoured crown. **B,** Facing removed to show recesses in wax into which lateral extensions of porcelain facing extend.

A 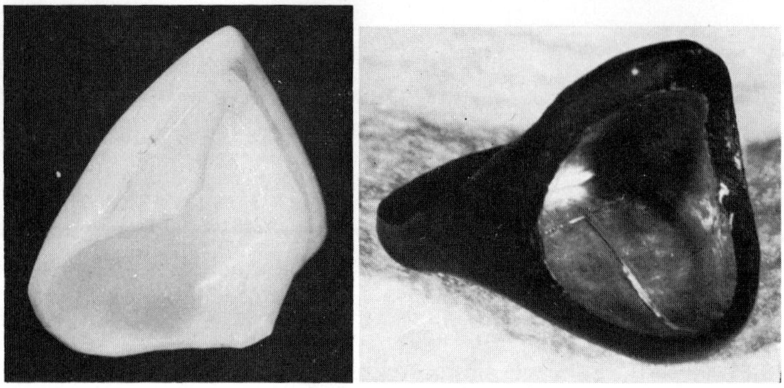 B

Fig. 23-41. A, Lingual aspect of prepared porcelain veneer facing. **B,** Inner view of waxed crown showing platinum matrix, which is left in crown when it is cast.

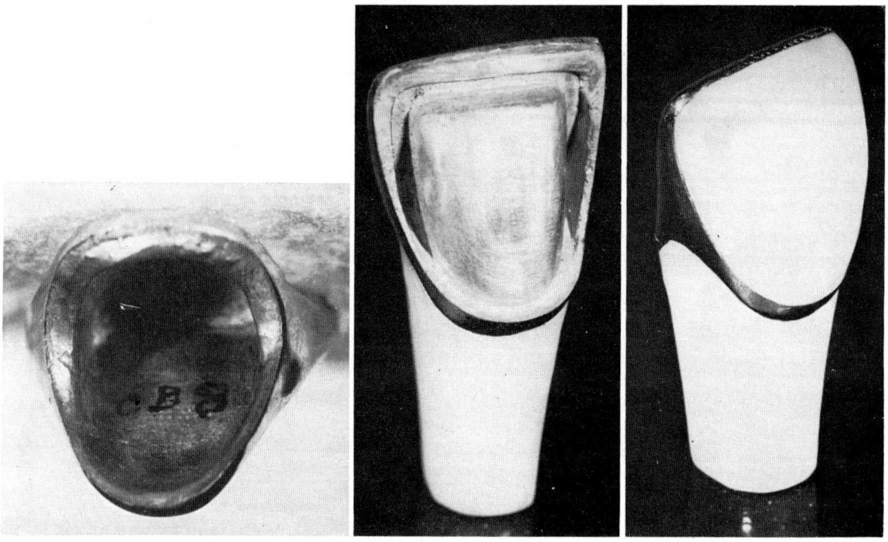

A B C

Fig. 23-42. A and **B,** Cervical and labial views of cast metal crown. **C,** Porcelain veneer cemented into cast crown.

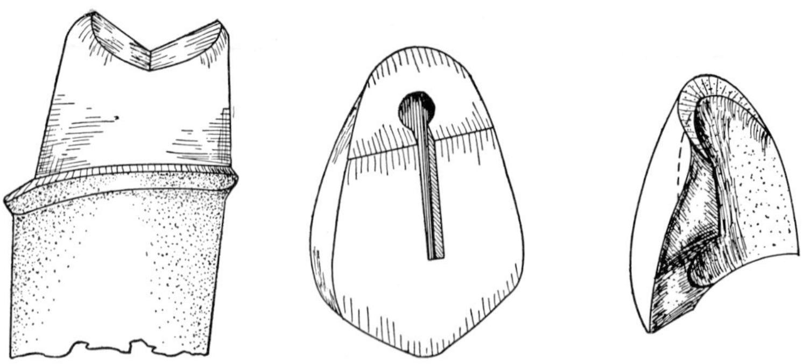

Fig. 23-43. All-cast shoulder crown with Steele facing used as veneer. Proximal flanges on proximal surfaces of facing aid in retention of facing in crown.

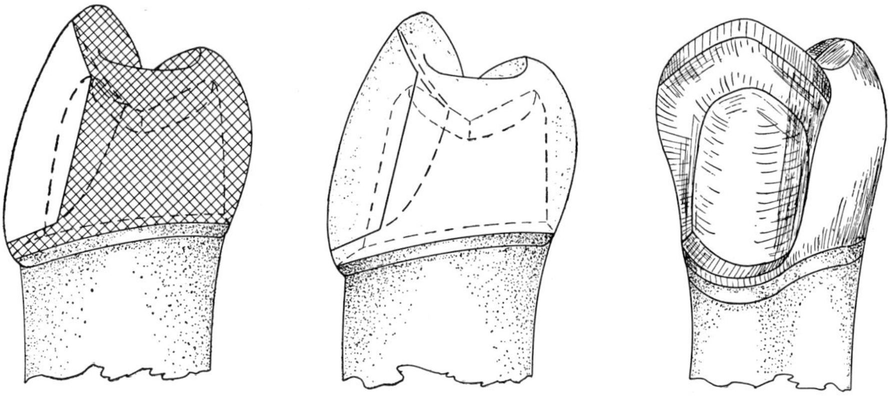

Fig. 23-44. Cross section and finished crown shown in Fig. 23-43.

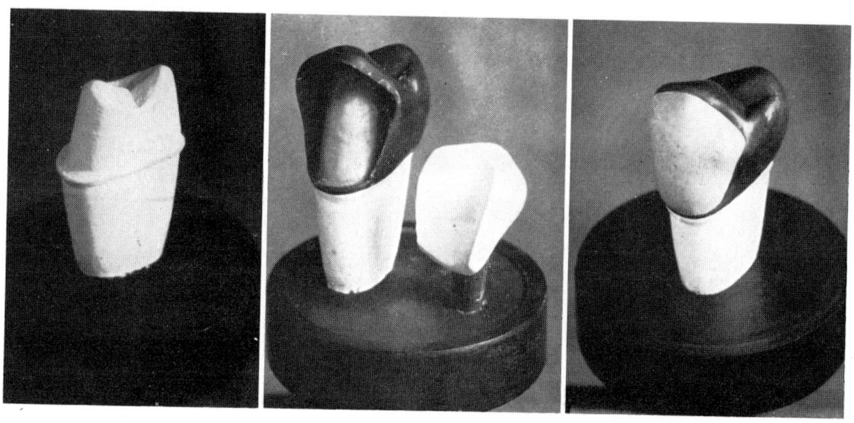

Fig. 23-45. All-cast shoulder crown, using Trubyte denture tooth for porcelain veneer.

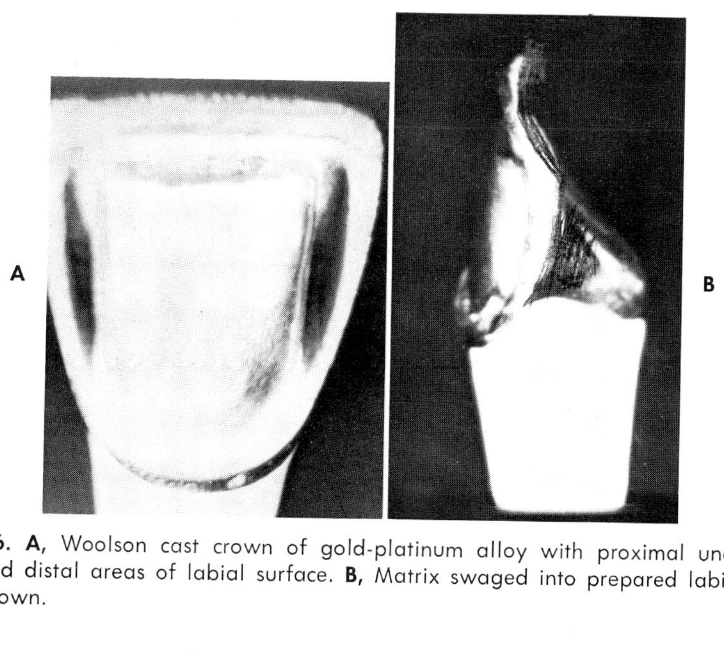

Fig. 23-46. A, Woolson cast crown of gold-platinum alloy with proximal undercuts in mesial and distal areas of labial surface. **B,** Matrix swaged into prepared labial surface of cast crown.

A

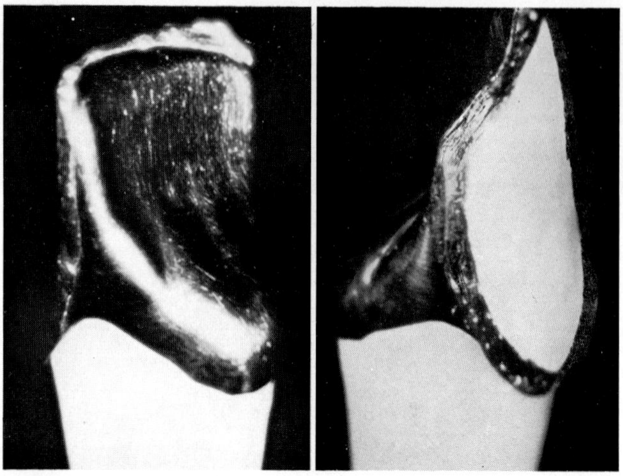

B

Fig. 23-47. A, Adapted matrix extended beyond border of veneer labial outline. **B,** Opaque coat and first layer of porcelain applied to matrix.

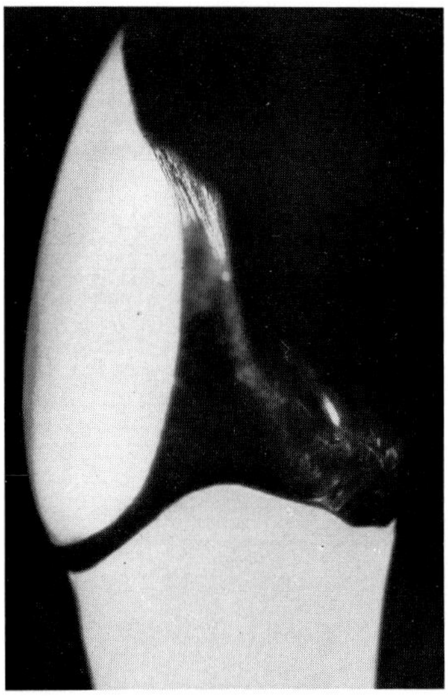

Fig. 23-48. Finished crown with porcelain veneer fired directly into cast crown.

of all investment before trying to fit the porcelain facing. When this has been done, the crown is polished and the facing cemented (Fig. 23-42, *C*). The final finish is given to the margins between the gold and porcelain. The crown is now ready to be cemented on the prepared tooth. Such a crown is highly esthetic and strong.

Figs. 23-43 to 23-45 show the same method applied to a posterior tooth.

FIRED PORCELAIN VENEER FACING TYPE

An early effort to overcome the difficulty which arises when porcelain is fired to metal was that of Woolson presented in 1940 at the Washington State Meeting. He realized that porcelains fired to gold alloys developed cracks after firing due to the different coefficients of contraction and expansion of the two materials. He reasoned if he could interpose a slip plane so each could manifest its own physical laws of contraction and expansion, the difficulty of porcelain checking would be solved. This he did by the following technic.[5]

A wax pattern for the gold crown is made in the usual manner. It is shaped as an open faced crown with a thin layer of wax covering the die, back of the opening and an ample undercut for locking the porcelain veneer in position. The crown is cast in an alloy of 24 karat C.P. gold and 10 per cent platinum, melting point 2069° F. [Fig. 23-46, *A*]. The recessed face of the casting should be thin and roughened, and the margins of the recess well undercut.

A 50 g. matrix of 96 parts gold and 4 parts platinum is swaged into the recessed face of the casting [Fig. 23-46, *B*]. The matrix must be well adapted, and extended 1 mm. beyond the labial margins [Fig. 23-47, *A*].

The margins only of the matrix are covered with Apco 1875° F. porcelain; this is baked in a porcelain furnace to 1775° F. [Fig. 23-47, *B*].

The thin coat of Apco opaque porcelain can be fired at 1775° F. if necessary. The contour of the facing is built up in subsequent firings. Generally, three bakes are needed to complete the facings All pieces of the restoration can be removed from the furnace while it is at the firing temperature without danger.

The use of 24 karat gold plate between the casting and the porcelain seems to be the secret of success.

After the porcelain is baked, the crown can be soldered to by the ordinary investing and soldering technique. The restoration may be used as an abutment for fixed bridgework or for a precision attachment in removable partial dentures.*

Fig. 23-48 shows the finished crown.

*From Woolson, A. H.: Restorations made of porcelain baked on gold, J. Prosth. Dent. **5**:65, 1955.

SELECTED REFERENCES

1. Orton, F. H.: Absence of standards in crown work, Dent. Items Int. **39**:345, 1917.
2. Ante, I. H.: The gold crown as you make it, Australian D. J. **10**:1, 1938.
3. Dressel, R. P.: Principles of fixed bridge construction, D. Cosmos **72**:565, 730, 853, 941, 1173, 1272, 1930; **73**:130, 253, 342, 1931.
4. Selberg, A.: Cast gold crowns, J. Tennessee D. A. **29**:21, 1949.
5. Woolson, A. H.: Restorations made of porcelain baked on gold, J. Prosth. Dent. **5**:65, 1955.

GENERAL REFERENCES

Aeziman, H. T.: Fabrication of full gold crowns under previously constructed partial dentures, North-West Dent. **40**:334, 1961.

Asgar, K., and Peyton, F. A.: Pits on inner surfaces of cast gold crowns, J. Prosth. Dent. **9**: 448, 1959.

Asgar, K., and others: Effect of the investment material and mold temperature on the quality of the union achieved during gold casting to embedded attachment metals, I.A.D.R. **40**:93, 1962.

Baker, C. R.: Banded-cast metal crowns, J.A.D.A. **56**:522, 1958.

Baker, C. R.: Adapting root forms to working dies, J. Prosth. Dent. **11**:929, 1961.

Barishman, H.: Impression making for complete crown restorations, J.A.D.A. **61**:161, 1960.

Beeson, P. E.: The use of acrylic resins as an aid in the development of patterns for two types of crowns, J. Prosth. Dent. **13**:493, 1963.

Berman, H., and Lustig, L. P.: Primary substructures and removable telescopic superstructures in dental reconstruction, J. Prosth. Dent. **10**: 724, 1960.

Carter, R.: Electrolytic action in the presence of gold crowns placed over amalgam restorations: case report, Australian Dent. J. **10**:317-319, 1965.

Craig, R. G., El-Ebrashi, M. K., and Peyton, F. A.: Experimental stress analysis of dental restoration, I: two-dimensional photoelastic stress analysis of crowns, J. Prosth. Dent. **17**(3): 292-302, 1967.

Ewing, J. E.: Construction of accurate full crown restorations for an existing clasp by using a direct metal pattern technique, J. Prosth. Dent. **15**:889, 1965.

Ewing, J. E.: Direct metal pattern technique for full crown restorations, J.A.D.A. **63**:822, 1963.

Ewing, J. E., and Bentman, D.: Porcelain-veneered full-crown restorations made with cadmium patterns, J. Prosth. Dent. **18**(2):140-150, 1967.

Gordon, T.: Telescope reconstruction an approach to oral rehabilitation, J.A.D.A. **72**:97-105, 1966.

Henschel, C. J.: Double cast crowns, Oral Hyg. **52**:37, 1962.

Herlands, R. E., Lucca, J. J., and Morris, M. L.: Forms, contours, and extensions of full coverage restorations in occlusal reconstruction, Dent. Clin. N. Amer., pp. 147-162, March, 1962.

Herrick, P. W., and others: Investigation of hygroscopic investment (control water added) for casting multi-unit bridges, J. Dent. Res. **40**:774, 1961.

Herrick, P. W., and others: One-piece casting or multi-unit bridges, D. Progress **2**:93, 1962.

Hausman, M.: Occlusal reconstruction using transitional crowns, J. Prosth. Dent. **11**:278, 1961.

Hirshberg, S. M.: Compatible temporary tooth health and gingival protection, J. Prosth. Dent. **18**:151, 1967.

Isaacson, G. O.: Telescope crown retainers for removable partial dentures, J. Prosth. Dent. **21**:458-465, 1969.

Killebrew, R. H.: Crown construction for broken down partial denture abutments, J. Prosth. Dent. **11**:93, 1961.

Kovaleski, J.: Technic for casting gold to gold and for repairing dentures, D. Abst. **6**:342, 1961.

Kuratli, J.: Restoration of broken down vital teeth for fixed partial denture abutments, J. Prosth. Dent. **8**:504, 1958.

Lavine, S.: Construction of cast-gold crowns and

fixed partial dentures by use of gold bands, J. Prosth. Dent. **10**:959, 1960.

Leff, A.: Evaluation of high speed in full-coverage preparations, J. Prosth. Dent. **10**:314, 1960.

Lewis, R. M., and Owen, M. M.: Mathematical solution of a problem in full crown construction, J.A.D.A. **59**:943, 1959.

Lyon, D. M., Cowger, G. T., Woychesin, F. F., and Miller, C. B.: Porcelain fused to gold—evaluation and esthetics, J. Prosth. Dent. **10**: 319, 1960.

McCabe, D. J., and Rinne, V. W.: Treatment of carious teeth: disadvantage of full coverage, Dent. Clin. N. Amer., p. 639, Nov., 1960.

Malson, T. S.: Anatomic cast crown reproduction, J. Prosth. Dent. **9**:106, 1959.

Marcum, J. S.: The effect of crown marginal depth upon gingival tissue, J. Prosth. Dent. **17**: 479, 1967.

Miller, I. F., and Feinberg, E.: Full coverage restorations, J. Prosth. Dent. **12**:317-325, 1962.

Miller, I. F., and Belsky, M. W.: The full shoulder preparation for periodontal health, Dent. Clin. N. Amer. pp. 83-102, March, 1963.

Modjeski, P. J.: Cavity preparation pertaining to fixed partial dentures, Illinois D. J. **16**:408, 1947.

Raucher, F.: Systematic approach to full crown preparations using high speed instruments, New York D. J. **27**:284, 1961.

Schweitzer, J. M.: Gold copings for problematic teeth, J. Prosth. Dent. **10**:163, 1960.

Segat, L.: Restoration of non-vital teeth, J. Michigan D. A. **44**:254, 1962.

Selberg, A.: Full cast crown technique, J. Prosth. Dent. **7**:102, 1957.

Strickland, W. D., and Sturdevant, C. M.: Porosity in the full cast crown, J.A.D.A. **58**:69, 1959.

Swartz, M. L., and Phillips, R. W.: Study of adaptation of veneers to cast gold crowns, J. Prosth. Dent. **7**:817, 1957.

Thielemann, K., and Thielemann, E.: (A) Band-crown-bridge-retainer blended with porcelain for vital front teeth; (B) semi-crown-bridges on jacket-crowns (porcelain jacket-crowns), Internat. D. J. **7**:569, 1957.

Tylman, S. D.: Ultrasonic techniques for crown and bridge retainers, J. Prosth. Dent. **8**:167, 1958.

Wagman, S. S.: Tissue management for full cast veneer crowns, J. Prosth. Dent. **15**:106-117, 1965.

Weinberg, L. A.: Double casting of metal to metal in full coverage, J.A.D.A. **63**:821, 1961.

Wheeler, R. C.: Restoration of gingival or cervical margins in full crowns, D. Cosmos **73**:238, 1931.

Chapter 24

Tooth preparation for complete porcelain veneer crowns: anterior and posterior teeth—class II, type I

The complete porcelain veneer crown, more generally referred to as the porcelain jacket crown, has been in use for over 65 years. Clark[1] reported that Charles H. Land described and presented the present type of veneer crown to the dental profession in 1902. It was not until 1916, however, that a definite technic and instrumentation were presented by Schneider[2] and it has been since without any great modifications. That this crown has been increasingly used during the intervening years with success and has gradually received universal acceptance is a tribute to the genius of the men who conceived and developed its full possibilities.

ADVANTAGES AND DISADVANTAGES

The complete porcelain veneer crown as used today attributes its success to the fact that it meets nearly all the requirements of a successful dental restoration. If placed where indicated and if the tooth is properly prepared, it is one of the best restorations available to the dentist for maintaining a normal, vital pulp. In addition to this the porcelain veneer crown meets the most exacting esthetic requirements; by its use, it is possible not only to simulate the remaining natural teeth, but also to reproduce any of the characteristic markings or peculiarities of the individual dentition.

Clinical evidence indicates that properly fired and contoured porcelain is the most acceptable to the investing soft tissues of any of the materials used in restorative dentistry. This compatibility with the soft tissues places the porcelain veneer crown in the foremost rank among dental restorations.

Because porcelain powder can be built to any desired contour and carved to meet the existing occlusion in the mouth, it can be adapted to any functional relationships.

The technic developed for the construction of a porcelain veneer crown assures a total freedom from gingival irritation due to the accuracy with which the crown may be adapted to the prepared tooth.

This type of crown is primarily indicated on teeth with vital pulps; its physical properties are such that it is an excellent insulator and protects the pulp against thermal shock.

The porcelain veneer crown may be used as an individual restoration or as a bridge retainer. It may be placed on teeth having vital pulps and on those from which the pulps have been removed.

While its use requires enough remaining tooth structure for a strong foundation, it is possible to rebuild a foundation for a badly broken-down tooth with castings without removing the pulp.

Opposed to its advantages, there are

some disadvantages and difficulties incident to its use. The first is the inherent weakness of the material itself. Fused porcelain is friable and is susceptible to fracture much more so than restorations made of gold alloys. However, if porcelain is placed so that it is supported properly by underlying tooth tissue or metal, it is capable of withstanding enormous forces.

Another of its difficulties, and perhaps the most serious to the general practitioner, relates to the selection and reproduction of color of the natural teeth. Seemingly difficult at first, the color problem in porcelain is not an insurmountable one; in fact it is within the province of most men to master it by diligent study and intelligent experimentation.

A third objection sometimes cited is the exactness of the technic that this type of work demands and the possible strain that a patient undergoes when receiving this type of service. This objection is groundless, for the technic is no more difficult to master than the placing of a gold foil filling or making a cast inlay.

INDICATIONS

The complete porcelain veneer crown may be used either on vital or pulpless teeth; when used on the latter, the teeth have usually been discolored following the death or removal of the pulp. A frequent indication for the complete porcelain veneer crown is a tooth having large proximal cavities in which the labial enamel surface is involved or in which a bad discoloration shows through the silicate fillings. Teeth whose incisal angles have been accidentally fractured or broken off without exposing the pulp may also be restored with this type of restoration. Where a tooth is malformed, the so-called peg lateral, the complete veneer porcelain crown is an ideal method of restoring it to normal tooth form. Cases of dystrophy, excessive attrition, rotation, hypoplastic enamel, or those teeth in lateral displacement all, at times, may be corrected by the use of complete veneer porcelain crowns.

The question is sometimes raised: "Where is this type of crown indicated?" Although the bicuspids and molars may be suitably restored with the complete porcelain veneer crown, the six anterior teeth and the first bicuspids are the ones most frequently restored by this method due to the esthetic demands of their position in the arch. When used on posterior teeth, the veneer crown may also be expected to give satisfactory service under the most severe conditions.

As stated previously, crown and fixed partial prosthesis is a service for patients primarily between the ages of 20 and 55 years. Under certain conditions, however, a complete porcelain veneer crown may be placed on patients younger than 20 years of age. When so used, the cervical shoulder should not be placed beneath the crest of the gum tissue. Gottlieb and Orban[3] have demonstrated histologically the presence of an enamel cuticle or epithelial attachment that extends from the crest of the gingiva onto the surface of the enamel (see Plate 3). In removing the enamel subgingivally in young patients, this attachment is destroyed, producing a trauma to the soft tissues, which very frequently ends in a pathologic condition. With those patients in their early twenties, extreme care should be taken to determine (1) the presence and (2) the depth of the gingival crevice. Following this, the decision may be made (a) whether a procelain veneer crown is indicated, (b) whether it is to be of the shoulder or the chamfer type, and (c) to what depth, if any, the shoulder should be lowered into the gingival crevice.

REQUIREMENTS

In considering the placement of a complete veneer porcelain crown, it is essential: first, that a sufficient amount of tooth structure be left, after the preparation has

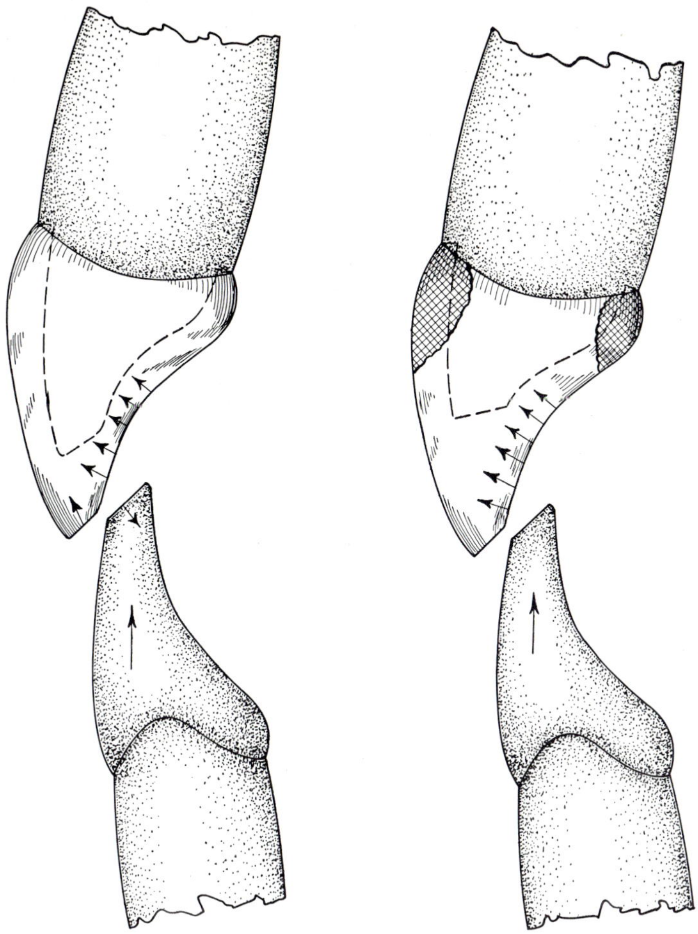

Fig. 24-1. Forces applied to tooth properly prepared, **left,** and to one improperly prepared, **right,** causing fractures of crown in gingival area.

been completed, to withstand the forces to which the crown will be subjected; second, that the finished preparation have planes at right angles to these forces; and third, that there be a sufficient amount of tooth structure left to protect and maintain the normality of the pulp. There is one additional requirement; namely, the finished preparation is, in general, a miniature reproduction of the tooth that is being restored. In the case of young patients not only is all of the enamel not removed from the anatomic crown, but at times some of the enamel covering the clinical crown is also left intact.

In the central and lateral incisors and cuspids it is also necessary that the preparation be sufficiently long to eliminate the danger of crescent-shaped fractures at the gingival margin (Fig. 24-1) and that the mesiodistal width of the preparation be sufficient to prevent fracture from torsional forces (Fig. 24-2).

In young children whose anterior teeth have been fractured or injured by accident and the pulp not exposed, it is advisable to defer extreme or radical types of preparations and to resort to some temporary means of treatment until the pulp and the investing tissues present more favorable conditions for permanent restorations. Usually a temporary crown of acrylic

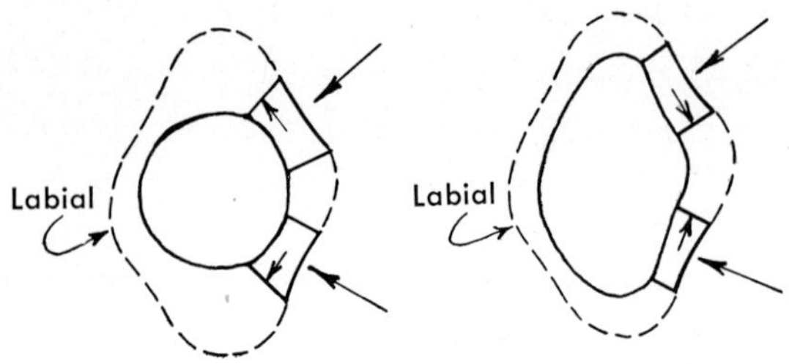

Fig. 24-2. Improper mesiodistal contour of tooth prepared for porcelain veneer crown. (Courtesy H. Conod.)

resin is placed on the tooth with very little, if any, shoulder preparation.

ROENTGENOGRAPHS AND STUDY CASTS

Before undertaking porcelain veneer restorations, either in young or older patients, it is advisable that roentgenographs be made; where more than one tooth is involved, it is good practice to construct complete study casts. This procedure will disclose the condition of the alveolar bone, the size and the position of the pulp, and, frequently, the presence and location of unusual pulpal horn extensions.

USE OF WARM WATER AND ANESTHETICS

The removal of enamel from a tooth is likely to cause some pain to the patient. To lessen its intensity, some dentists use either a local, infiltration, or block anesthesia; when an anesthetic is not employed, a constant stream of warm water of about 115° F. applied to the tooth while it is being cut is helpful. Recent experiments suggest the possibility of using very cold water as an obtunding agent. With either method, the use of cocoa butter is suggested as a lubricant for all abrasive cutting instruments such as stones and disks that come in contact with tooth tissue. As previously explained, the cocoa butter and water not only increase the cutting efficiency of the stones and disks, but also reduce the frictional heat generated during the cutting process. Since the pain in cutting teeth is largely due to the heat produced by the rapidly revolving stone, cocoa butter and hot water reduce this discomfort to a minimum. It is possible by the use of anesthetics to eliminate all pain, but, at the same time, all the danger signals are removed which warn one of possible operating dangers, because the anesthetized patient is unable to warn the dentist when the pulp is approached too closely or if too much heat is being generated. Many dead pulps under restorations had their incipiency in the degenerative changes initiated during operations performed many years previously. In spite of apparently normal responses to thermal and electrical tests, many pulps so injured never return to their normal condition and eventually die.

TYPES OF PREPARATIONS

There are two general types of preparations made for the complete veneer porcelain crown; one is shoulderless, the other is with a shoulder.

Shoulderless preparation

It has been claimed by Both[4] that the shoulderless type of preparation is made on a tooth when it is so narrow at its cervical diameter that the vitality of the pulp may be endangered by cutting a shoulder. He also stated that: "The shoulderless preparation is indicated for mandibular incisors, many maxillary lateral incisors, first maxillary bicuspids with bifurcated roots, and many molars, as well as teeth from which the gingival tissue has receded beyond the enamel matrix. Trauma is greatly reduced by the elimination of the shoulder preparation." A different viewpoint is expressed by Wheeler,[5] who stated:

> A crown or inlay can be feather-edged and burnished but a porcelain jacket crown must be shouldered to obtain the above relationship.
>
> Porcelain cannot be manipulated after firing; therefore, the margins and fit depend upon the adaptation of the matrix to the model of the

preparation itself. Thus we see that a shoulder or step must be used to give us a finish line in adapting our matrix.

Porcelain cannot be finished to a feather-edge. Even with the utmost care in finishing, magnification will show a saw edge and this edge, besides being rough, will have small bubbles along it and a sort of intermittent glaze. This is a veritable roost for bacteria and in my own experience the gum tissue is less likely to tolerate it than a gold margin of the same apparent roughness.*

Ewing[6] pointed out that there arise in practice many unusual conditions in which the dentist must compromise between the shoulder and the shoulderless types, sometimes because of mechanical problems, at other times because of biologic considerations.

The Both type of crown. Because certain difficulties are present in finishing a complete veneer porcelain crown of the shoulderless type, without leaving sharp edges of porcelain to act as irritants to the investing tissues, technics have been developed for those teeth in which the shoulderless type of preparation is employed and the restoration still possesses the desirable features of a complete veneer porcelain crown. Fig. 24-3 is a cross section of such a restoration; the gingival margin of the crown is constructed of metal and can therefore be accurately finished; the rest of the crown, incisally or occlusally, is built of porcelain.

The following technic for this preparation is given by Both.[4]

(1) The tooth is first carefully prepared. A preparation is made which resembles in outline the original tooth, with its incisal edge, its lingual and labial surfaces following the original shape of the tooth, whether the tooth is prepared with or without a shoulder. (2) The fitted copper band is then marked with a clear scratch on its gingival collar to the exact outline of the gingival tissue, which thereby shows how far the copper band extends under the free margin. These markings are carefully preserved during laboratory procedure. (3) It is absolutely indispensable to take a plaster impression for the shoulderless jacket crown, because it enables the technician to know the exact position of the gingival tissue. (4) It is also advisable to make some kind of an accurate fusible metal coping which is placed on the prepared tooth before taking a plaster impression, in order to seat the amalgam die more accurately into the impression. (5) The amalgam die is accurately seated in the plaster model. (6) A casting wax collar is constructed around the die. (7) In this wax collar a shoulder is carved just below the gingiva, the wax being extended incisally in a thin layer for a sufficient distance to form an accurate and definite seat for the resultant casting. (8) This wax may be cast in gold or in a platinum-group alloy [see

*From Wheeler, R. C.: Restoration of the gingival or cervical margins in full crowns, D. Cosmos 73:238, 1931.

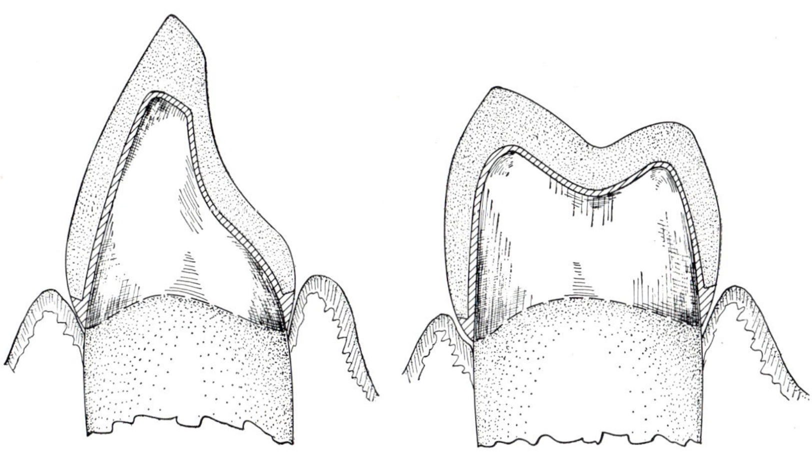

Fig. 24-3. Shoulder type of porcelain veneer crown used with shoulderless metal casting.

Chapter 35]. If cast in gold, most of the labial and lingual surfaces of the prepared tooth may be left uncovered. (9) After the wax pattern with its carved shoulder has been cast and has been replaced upon the shoulderless amalgam die, the jacket crown is constructed, the shoulder now supplied by the metal casting being employed. (10) If the casting is of platinum-group alloy, no additional matrix need be made, because the jacket may be baked directly on the casting. A platinum matrix is made for a gold casting. Although the gold casting necessitates the making of a platinum matrix, it has the advantage of being smaller in that it need not cover the entire preparation on the tooth.*

Because formerly it was relatively difficult to obtain an accurately fitting platinum casting with standard equipment and materials and because the gold casting does not require that the labial surface of the tooth be covered with metal, the gold type was usually used.

Shoulder preparation

The more generally accepted procedure is the shoulder type of preparation, except possibly where the tooth is abnormal in form; even here some sort of a finishing line or chamfer is preferred.

Since the shoulder type of preparation is usually employed, it entails a study of the relationships existing between the enamel and the investing soft tissues, so that a decision may be made whether part or all of the enamel in the gingival area is to be removed and at which level the shoulder is to be placed with reference to the gingival crevice. (See Plate 2.)

As previously stated, in younger patients and those in their early twenties, the presence of a high epithelial attachment and the absence of a gingival crevice contraindicate the removal of the enamel below the crest of the gingiva. This should be left to a later period in the patient's life, usually beyond middle age.

Where, however, the epithelial attachment lies below the cementoenamel junction and a definite gingival crevice exists, it is safe to remove all the enamel lying in the gingival area, but with great care.

Position of shoulder. Where the first condition exists, the gingival shoulder of the preparation is placed at or above the crest of the gum tissue; if the clinical examination discloses a slight gingival crevice, it may be advisable to construct a retractor or to use a rubber dam and clamp to push the tissues back slightly and thus enable the dentist to prepare the shoulder just below the gingival crest.

Where, however, the epithelial attachment has receded and is attached only to the cementum, it will usually be found that there is present also a gingival crevice of varying depth. In such an environment the shoulder is placed in the subgingival crevice slightly below the gingival crest.

Where the gum tissues have receded excessively, the shoulder is placed at a level of the cementoenamel junction.

In the first instance, i.e., in the younger patients, the shoulder is cut almost entirely within the enamel of the crown; in the second instance, since the enamel is removed, the entire shoulder is cut in dentin. It is evident that the latter type of preparation comes closer to the pulp and may be used with safety only in older patients whose pulp chamber is completely formed and usually protected by formations of secondary dentin.

Width and angle of shoulder. The width and the angle of the shoulder are important considerations. The width of a shoulder in a vital tooth may vary from the merest chamfer of 0.3 mm. on some of the smaller anterior teeth to 0.5 or 1.0 mm. on the molars. As a general rule the shoulder width does not exceed 0.5 mm.

The angle of a shoulder may vary by being an acute or a right angle. An obtuse angle is similar to a chamfer bevel and hence may be considered as a modified shoulder preparation.

The question of whether the angle of

*From Both, H. S.: Newer methods in preparing vital teeth for porcelain jacket crowns, D. Digest 43:481, 1937.

the shoulder is an acute or a right angle is largely one of relativity. A tooth properly prepared for a complete veneer porcelain crown has its axial surfaces slightly converging incisally or occlusally; in other words, its axial planes converge toward the axis of the tooth. If the bur, either No. 56 or 957, used to cut the shoulder is held parallel to the axial surface of the tooth, the end of the bur will cut a gingival plane that will be at right angles to the axial wall of the tooth. This same plane, however, when related to the long axis of the tooth, forms an acute angle (Fig. 24-4). It may be said, therefore, that *the plane at the gingival shoulder is placed at right angles to the axial surfaces.* An acute axial angle may be made with specially designed instruments, but this is not necessary.

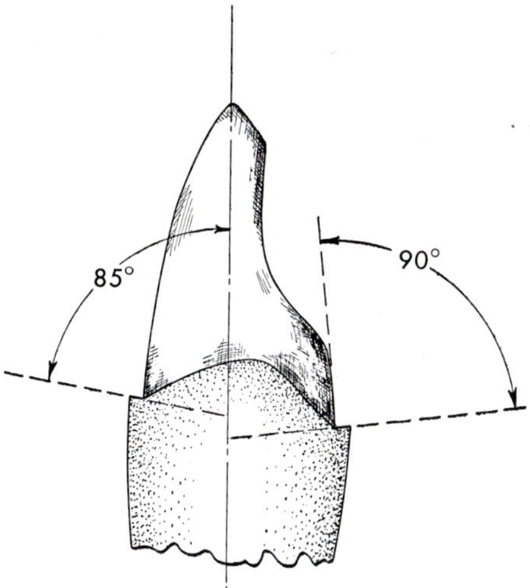

Fig. 24-4. Plane of shoulder made at right angle to axial surface of tooth.

Removal of occlusal and incisal enamel. The finished preparations for the upper and lower posterior teeth do not necessarily require the removal of all of the enamel from the occlusal area. Only a sufficient amount is removed to create space for enough porcelain to give the necessary strength to the crown; usually 2 mm. of occlusal reduction is sufficient for this purpose. In cutting down the occlusal surfaces, every effort should be made to reproduce in a general way the normal morphology of the tooth but at a lower level.

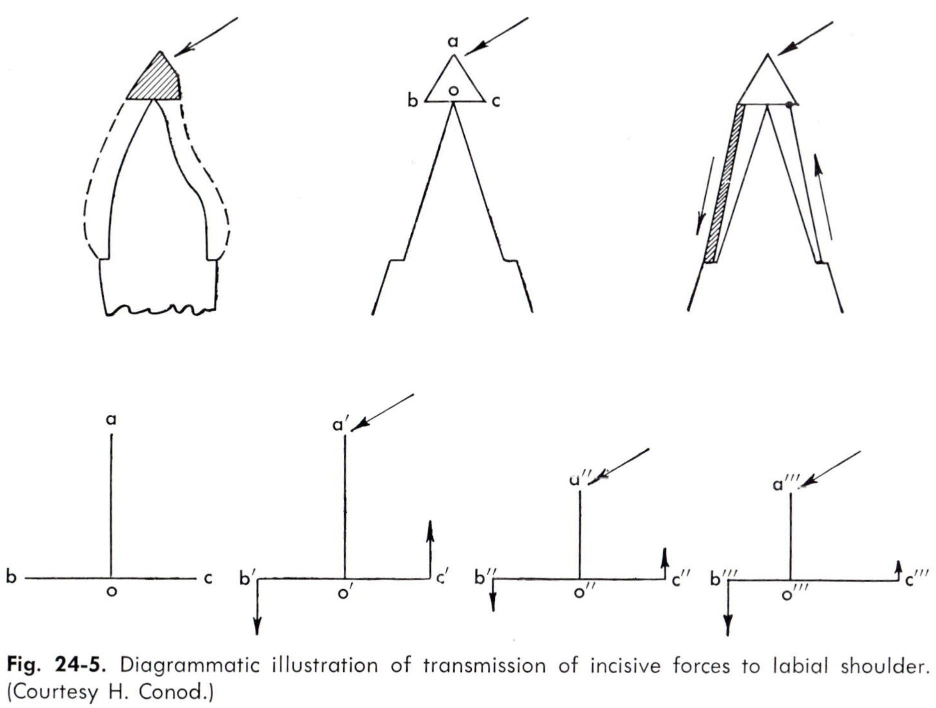

Fig. 24-5. Diagrammatic illustration of transmission of incisive forces to labial shoulder. (Courtesy H. Conod.)

In the preparation of an anterior tooth, rarely, if ever, is more than 1.5 to 2 mm. of the incisal length reduced. If more than this amount is taken off, a section of porcelain in the finished veneer crown will be left entirely unsupported, which condition will cause the crown to fracture when lingual force is applied to the incisal part of the crown (Figs. 24-1 and 24-5, A). In keeping with the rule that planes are placed at right angles to applied forces, the incisal plane of the upper anterior teeth slopes lingually, while that of the lower teeth slopes labially.

Fundamentals of preparation. Conod[7] and Grubb[8] call our attention to certain fundamentals in the preparation of teeth for porcelain veneer crowns. Figs. 24-5 to 24-11 are based on Conod's work as reported by him in 1937; they help to emphasize the importance of recognizing and applying certain rules of mechanics and physics to the proper preparation of teeth for complete porcelain veneer crowns.

Anterior teeth. In Fig. 24-5 the shaded, incisal portion of the crown is represented diagrammatically in the middle figure by the triangle *abc* balanced on the incisal edge, point *o*. If force is applied at a point *a*, in a linguolabial direction, angle *b* will be forced gingivally and will press downward against the labial shoulder, while point *c* will rise incisally and pull away from the lingual shoulder. The labial pressure is resisted by (1) the shoulder preparation and (2) the adhesion or friction between the length of the inner surface of the crown and the labial surface of the preparation.

In studying the lower series of drawings, it is seen that if the lever *a″-o″* is shortened, the forces at *b″* and *c″* are likewise reduced; if, however, *a′-o′* is legthened, the forces at *b′* and *c′* are increased. If the line *b″-o″* is shortened by moving *o‴* toward *b‴*, the force is increased at *b‴* and traction is lessened at *c‴*.

Therefore, the incisal edge of the tooth preparation *o* should be as close as possible to the incisal edge *a* of the porcelain crown; also the incisal edge *a* should be brought labially to shorten the line *b‴-o‴*. The force at the gingival is then absorbed by a properly prepared angle between the shoulder and the labial wall of the preparation (Fig. 24-6, *A* and *D*). If improperly prepared, the forces shown in Fig. 24-6, *B*, cause labial fractures, *C* (*c* and *d*).

Fig. 24-7 illustrates cross sections through the plane *a-b* showing the correct, *B*, and the incorrect, *C*, *D*, *E*, mesiodistal contours of the lingual surface of preparations for complete veneer porcelain crowns. It can be readily seen that *D* and *E* lack planes set at right angles to the applied forces, hence the porcelain fractures;

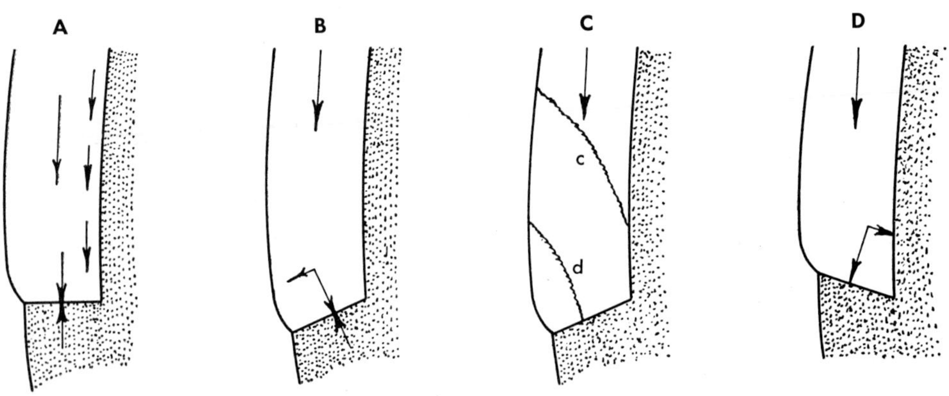

Fig. 24-6. Acute or right angle is preferred to obtuse angle of shoulder in relation to axial surface of preparation. (Courtesy H. Conod.)

in *C* the exaggerated contour sets up lines of cleavage. Conod points to three areas of the lingual surface requiring special consideration (Fig. 24-8). The area *A-B*, represented by the horizontal hatching, indicates the position of centric occlusion. Area *B-C*, the vertical hatching, comes in contact with the opposing teeth during active functional occlusion. Both these areas are so situated that they are supported by suitably prepared walls of tooth structure and hence can resist the forces to which they are subjected.

Area *D-C*, oblique hatching, also repre-

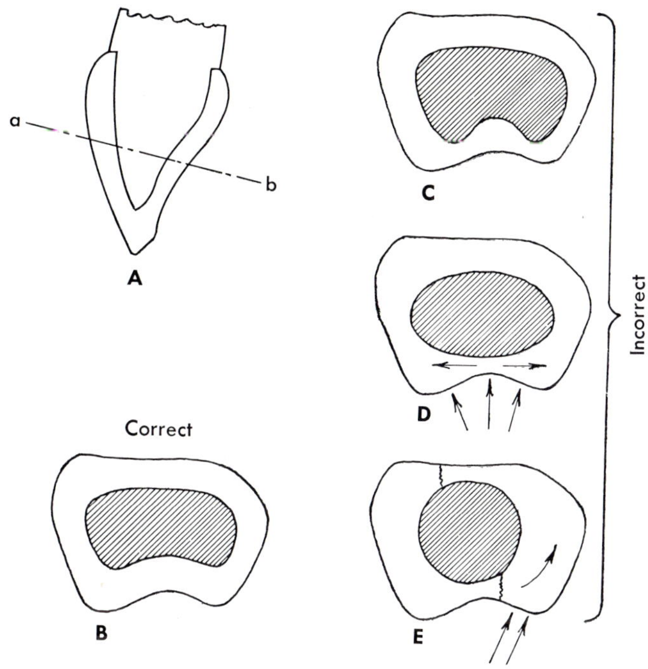

Fig. 24-7. Correct and incorrect mesiodistal contours of lingual surfaces of upper incisors. (Courtesy H. Conod.)

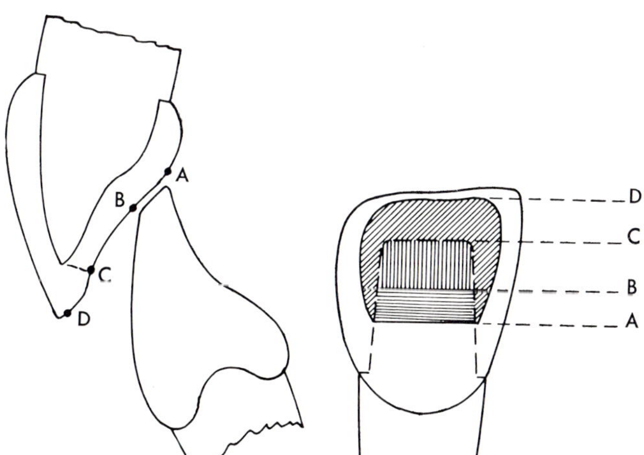

Fig. 24-8. In area **A** to **C**, porcelain is supported by underlying tooth tissue; in area **C** to **D** it is not. (Courtesy H. Conod.)

sents actively functioning surfaces, but these are not supported by underlying, supporting walls of dentin because the porcelain extends incisally and proximally beyond the tooth preparation. To reduce the danger of fracture from excessive vertical-compressive and lateral-torsional forces, it is suggested that this unsupported area be relieved of full surface contact with the opposing teeth.

Posterior teeth. The same general principles hold true in the preparation of the posterior teeth for complete porcelain veneer crowns. In Fig. 24-9, A, it is evident that the force developed between *b* and *d* is likely to fracture the unsupported porcelain cusps *d;* therefore, it is advisable to relieve these cusps as indicated by the dotted lines in *B*.

Another problem presents itself when

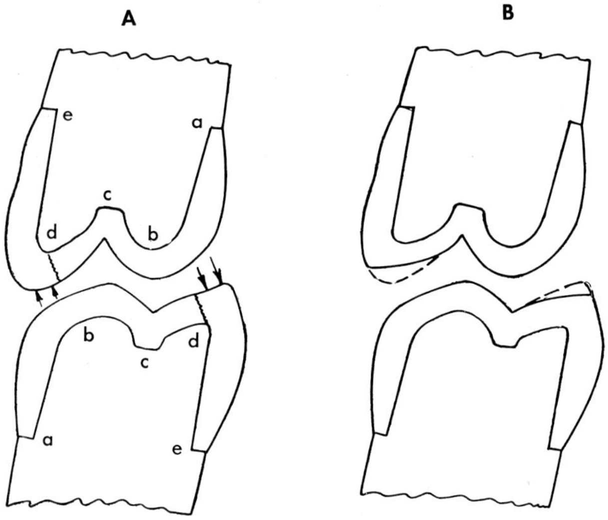

Fig. 24-9. Posterior preparations require underlying tooth tissue support for porcelain veneer crown. (Courtesy H. Conod.)

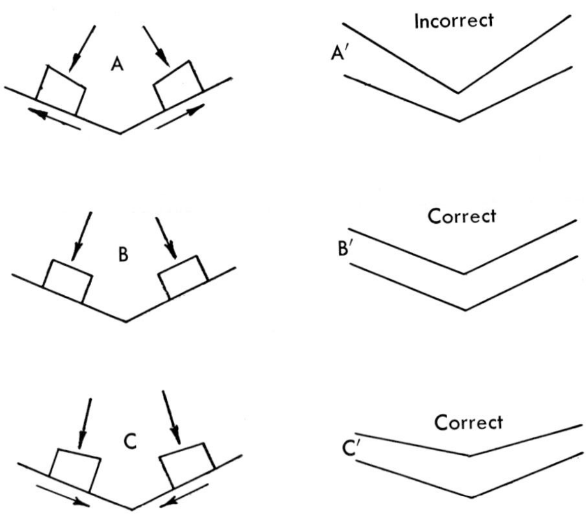

Fig. 24-10. Correct angulation at which occlusal planes should be prepared in tooth. (Courtesy H. Conod.)

the lingual cusp (Fig. 24-9, *A, b*) of the upper molar occludes with the lingual *d* and buccal *b* inclined occlusal planes of the lower molar. If the angle formed by the buccal and lingual planes of the occlusal surfaces of the porcelain crown is more acute than the angle formed by the underlying occlusal planes of the prepared tooth (Fig. 24-10, *A* and *A′*), the tendency is to separate the porcelain segments (Fig. 24-9, A, *b-c* and *c-d*) and cause the crown to fracture at *c*.

If the angles of the planes of the two surfaces parallel each other (Fig. 24-10, *B* and *B′*), they are then in equilibrium.

If the occlusal planes of the prepared tooth meet at a more acute angle than those of the porcelain crown, the tendency is to force the porcelain toward the center of the tooth (Fig. 24-10, *C* and *C′*).

Although it may seem that the last reaction (Fig. 24-10, *C* and *C′*) is not objectionable, Conod shows that, when these segments of porcelain are forced toward the middle of the tooth, they have a tendency to mount the adjacent inclined planes (Fig. 24-11, *A* and *B*). To counteract this tendency, he suggests cutting a wall to act as a stop to each segment as shown in *C*. To simplify the operative procedure and furthermore to allow sufficient depth in the porcelain to carve occlusal grooves, he suggests uniting both stop walls in *C* in a rounded channel *D*, which extends the full mesiodistal width of the tooth. This method then allows room for carving occlusal anatomical grooves as in *F*, without developing areas of weakness, as in *E*.

Types of preparations. Oppice[9] has classified the types of preparations for complete veneer porcelain crowns.

(1) Teeth containing vital pulps:
   a. With the gingival tissues attached to the enamel as well as the cementum;
   b. with the gingival tissues attached to the cementum only.
(2) Pulpless teeth:
   a. requiring a full core;
   b. requiring a partial core.*

To these may be added:
(3) Teeth to serve as bridge abutments.
(4) Special preparations for shoulderless and platinum group-alloyed reinforced crowns.

Steps of preparation (normal tooth). The technic and the instrumentation first

*From Oppice, H. W.: A résumé of ideas on porcelain jacket crown preparations, J.A.D.A. **21**: 1030, 1934.

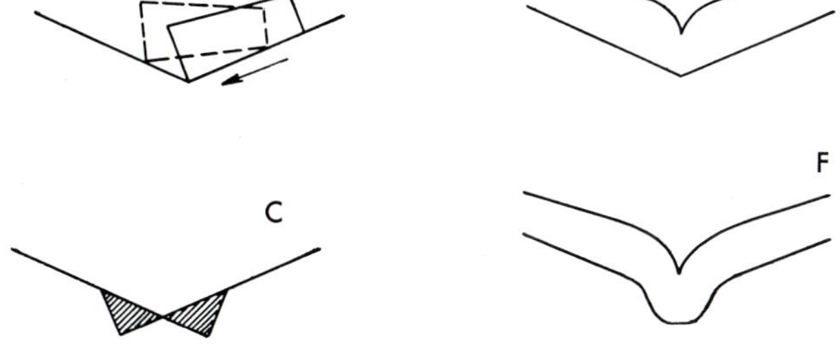

Fig. 24-11. Supplementary resistance to displacement or fracture of posterior porcelain veneer crown is obtained by preparing occlusal stops. (Courtesy H. Conod.)

to be considered are for normally contoured and positioned teeth containing vital pulps. The first step is the reduction of the incisal edge on an upper anterior tooth.

Incisal reduction. With a stone (Densco 2J), the incisal surface is reduced 1.5 to 2 mm.; this much clearance is allowed between the incisal plane and the opposing teeth. This plane is inclined at an angle of approximately 45°, and it is cut mostly at the expense of the lingual plate of enamel (Fig. 24-12). In the lower anterior teeth the incisal plane is inclined toward the labial surface (Figs. 24-31 and 24-32).

After the incisal plane is cut to the proper depth, the dentin will be visible between the labial and lingual enamel plates (Figs. 24-12 and 24-13).

Proximal surface reduction. The next step is the removal of the enamel on the proximal surfaces. For this, a safe-sided diamond disk ½ inch in diameter (Densco 3T-P) is used; it is coated with cocoa butter and sprayed with a stream of warm water during the cutting operation (Fig. 24-14, *A*). While revolving rapidly, the

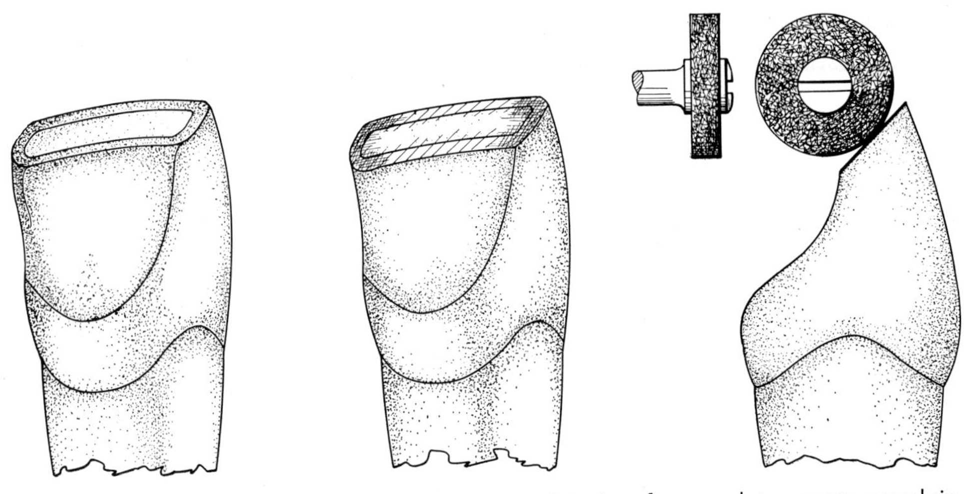

Fig. 24-12. Initial step in preparing upper central incisor for complete veneer porcelain crown.

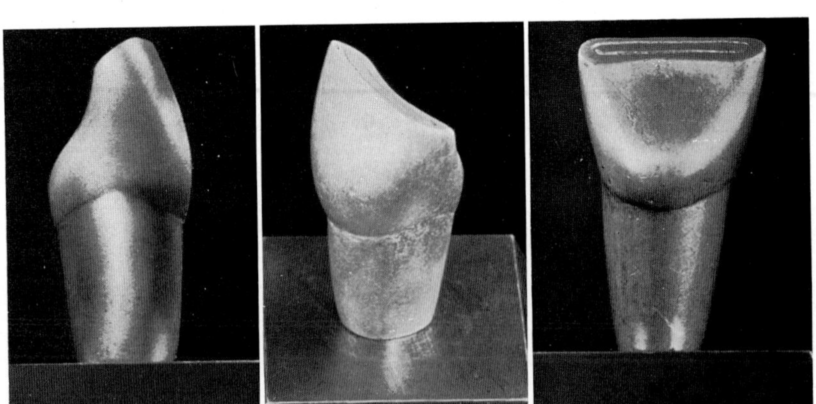

Fig. 24-13. Other views of incisal reduction of upper central incisor.

edge of the disk is placed on the incisal plane approximately 1 to 1.5 mm. from the proximal surface (Fig. 24-14, *B*); the disk is then inclined toward the tooth axis and sighted toward the gingival edge in such a direction, in the case of younger patients, that, when the cut is completed, the disk will emerge gingivally at the crest of the gingival tissues (Fig. 24-14, *C*). If it is an older patient and the gingival epithelium is attached entirely to the cementum, the cut will end gingivally, slightly beneath the crest of the gum tissue. The depth to which it is carried into the gingival crevice depends entirely upon the depth of the gingival crevice. An effort is usually made to locate it midway between the crest of the gingiva and the bottom of the crevice. The same operation is repeated on the opposite proximal surface (Fig. 24-14, *D*).

It should be noted that these proximal cuts, whether for young patients or for older ones, do not end in a shoulder.

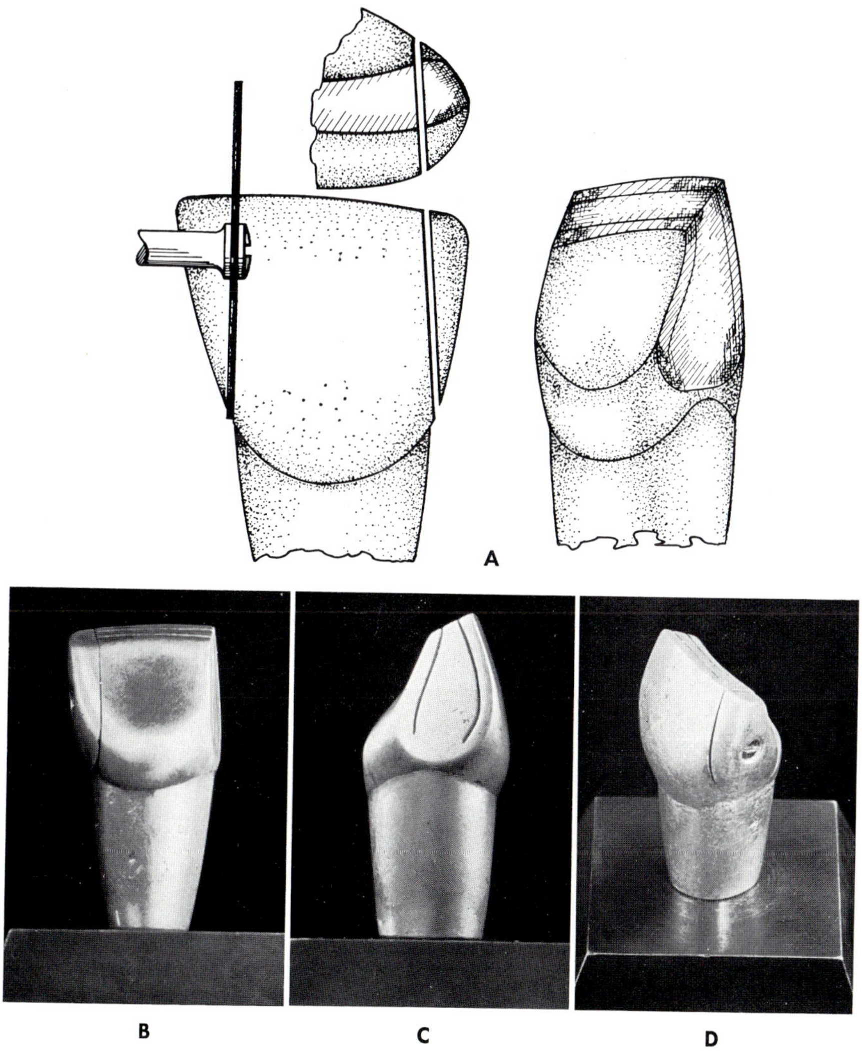

Fig. 24-14. Starting point, direction, and termination of proximal cuts; note no shoulder at gingival end of cut.

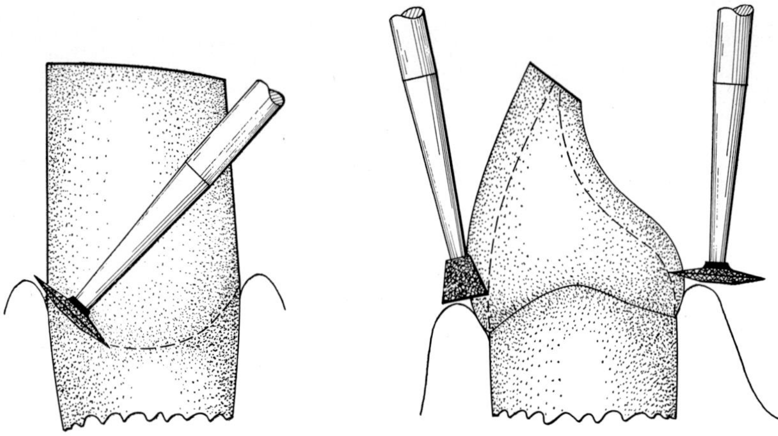

Fig. 24-15. Establishing depth of enamel cut at height of gingiva on labial and lingual surfaces.

Since the depth of the gingival crevice varies not only in different teeth but also in different regions of the same tooth, it is advisable to examine the crevice of each tooth about to be prepared for a complete veneer jacket crown. This may be done by using a flat, thin periodontal membrane explorer.

Removal of labial enamel. The removal of the labial plate of enamel is the next step. With a small knife-edged stone (Densco 1-V), or an inverted cone stone (Densco ½K), a narrow groove is cut in the labial surface extending from the mesial to the distal proximal cuts; this groove is cut parallel to the gingival curvature of the soft tissues and is placed level with the crest of the gingiva. In making this cut, an attempt is made to penetrate only the thickness of the enamel, which rarely exceeds 0.5 mm. in this region; the bottom of the cut should terminate at the dentinoenamel junction (Fig. 24-15). This groove marks the approximate position of the labial shoulder in those patients still having an attachment of the enamel cuticle to the enamel and whose gingival crevice is practically zero in depth.

The balance of the labial enamel may be removed by using mounted diamond stones, or, better, by a series of grooving, splitting, and planing of the enamel. The latter method is found to be the least painful and most easily controlled. Using a ⅛ inch knife-edged diamond disk, or a mounted, knife-edged stone (Densco 4Q), the edge of the stone is placed on the incisal edge of the labial enamel plate. While revolving rapidly, it is brought from the incisal to the gingival groove, cutting through the thickness of the enamel to the dentinoenamel junction (Fig. 24-16, *A*). By placing this cut 1 mm. from the proximal surface, a knife-edged blade of enamel is left standing between the labial cut and the proximal surface (Fig. 24-16, *B*). If this cut is properly made, i.e., if the bottom of the groove lies at the dentinoenamel junction in its entire length incisogingivally, the deepest part of the groove will be parallel with the incisogingival curvature of the labial surface (Fig. 24-16, *C*). If this cut is made in a straight line, too much of the dentin will be cut into and the finished preparation on the labial dentin surface will come too close to the pulp. By using cocoa butter on the stone and a stream of warm water during the cutting operations, very little pain will be felt because the cutting of enamel stops at the dentinoenamel junction. By inserting the blade of a No. 12-5-6 hatchet, or a No.

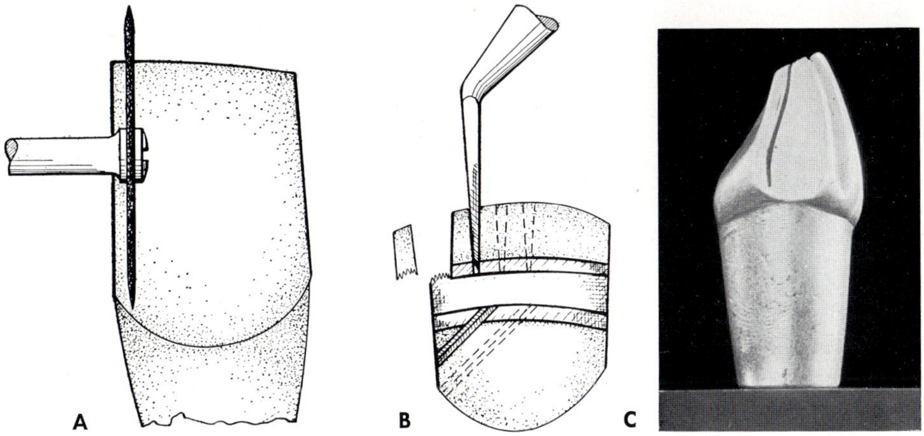

Fig. 24-16. Removal of labial enamel is done in successive steps of grooving, splitting, and planing away of enamel.

20 straight chisel into the groove and by using the remaining enamel wall as a fulcrum, the thin strip of enamel is easily broken off at the dentinoenamel junction, if the remaining enamel strip is not left too wide. The prying is started at the incisal edge and is carried gingivally to the gingival groove. This operation is followed by planing the exposed dentin wall with a No. 15 or 20 straight chisel to remove any remaining enamel. By following this procedure, the dentist is certain of having removed all the enamel within this limited strip area before proceeding to another.

Successive grooving and stripping of the enamel is continued until the entire labial plate is removed, except that portion lying in the subgingival area. These cuts are made one at a time, and the enamel is removed after each cut before another is made. If the entire surface were to be grooved at one time, there would be no fulcrum available against which to pry.

The advantage of this method of removing the labial enamel plate, compared to the immediate and exclusive use of a tapered cylinder (Densco 4-DS) diamond stone, moved mesiodistally over the enamel surface, is that, with the latter method, it is difficult to recognize the thickness of the enamel plate still remaining between the curved interface of enamel and the dentin. As a result, a flat labial plane may be created.

Where the successive grooving and splitting away of the enamel appears to be too time consuming and tedious, then the other safe method is to cut a guide-groove in the mesiodistal labial center from the incisal plane to the gingival crest (Fig. 24-16). If the bottom of the groove lies at the dentinoenamel interface in its entire incisogingival distance, the deepest part of the groove will be parallel with the curvature of the labial surface. One reason for pulp pathology developing under porcelain veneer crowns, and more so under the porcelain fused to metal crowns, is cutting a flat plane incisogingivally that dangerously approximates the pulp. Hence the importance of a pilot guideline cut through the enamel.

Removal of lingual enamel. The lingual plate of enamel is removed in a similar manner (Fig. 24-17, *A* and *B*) except that, where the access is difficult, the grooves are sometimes cut diagonally (Fig. 24-17, *C*). When it is not necessary to remove all the lingual enamel, the required reduction may be made with the tapering diamond stone (Densco 2DS) and the wheel stones (Densco 1J) and stone (Densco

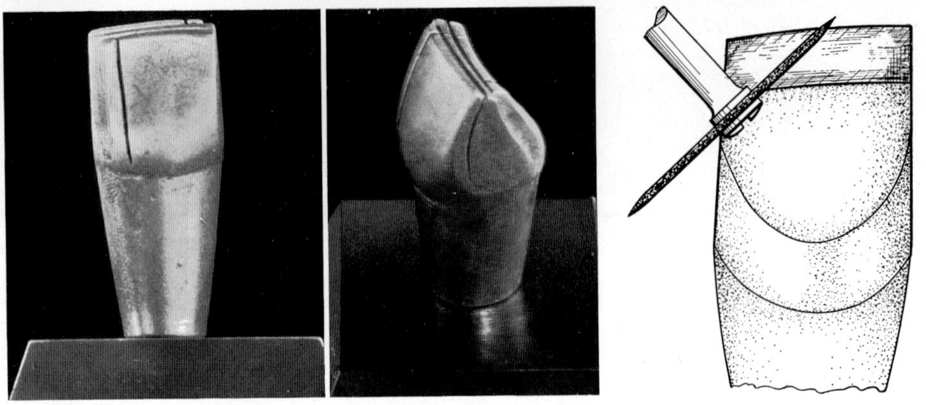

A B C

Fig. 24-17. Principle of enamel removal on lingual surface is similar to that done on labial surface. Occasionally grooves are cut diagonally through enamel.

6BX). In use, these stones are started at the gingival groove and drawn toward the incisal plane.

The enamel remaining on the proximolabial and the proximolingual angles of the tooth is removed by using a ½ inch cup-shaped diamond disk, or an inverted cone, stones (Densco 7½ K or 8½K) in a contra-angle handpiece. With the present high speeds and the available carbide burs and diamond stones, the tendency sometimes prevails to cut laterally and vertically across the surfaces of the enamel without any orderly procedure. This makes it difficult to determine if all of the required enamel has been removed and also if the dentin is being cut too deeply.

Removal of subgingival enamel. If the preparation is for a tooth whose epithelial attachment lies below the cementoenamel junction, a condition which usually exists in older patients, the next procedure involves the removal of the two segments of enamel lying in the labial and the lingual subgingival areas (Fig. 24-18, *A* to *E*).

It will be recalled that the direction of the enamel rods in this region inclines rootwise at an angle of 6 to 12° from the horizontal plane. Because of this direction of the enamel rods, the enamel may be readily removed with enamel cleavers. The cleavers (Fig. 24-18, *B*) are shaped very much like Black's pull scalers, except that they are made heavier and stronger due to the heavier pressure used in their manipulation. The instruments are so designed that they come in pairs of rights and lefts, and the shanks are so shaped that access may be gained to any surface of the tooth. Their cutting blades are beveled obliquely, so that one end of the blade terminates in an acute angle, while the other is obtuse.

In use, the instrument is employed with the palm-and-thumb grasp, so that great lateral pressure may be exerted yet be under complete control. The cleaver is carried subgingivally with the acute angle of the cutting blade in contact with the collar of enamel. Considerable lateral pressure is then exerted against the tooth as the instrument is drawn incisally. The pressure with the acute angle of the blade causes fracture lines to develop in the enamel. Very frequently parts of the enamel break away during this procedure. This operation is repeated and fracture lines are made 1 mm. apart, extending from the mesial to the distal proximal surfaces.

The cleaver is now turned so that its straight cutting edge engages the enamel at the cementoenamel line (Fig. 24-18, *B*); again lateral pressure is applied as the

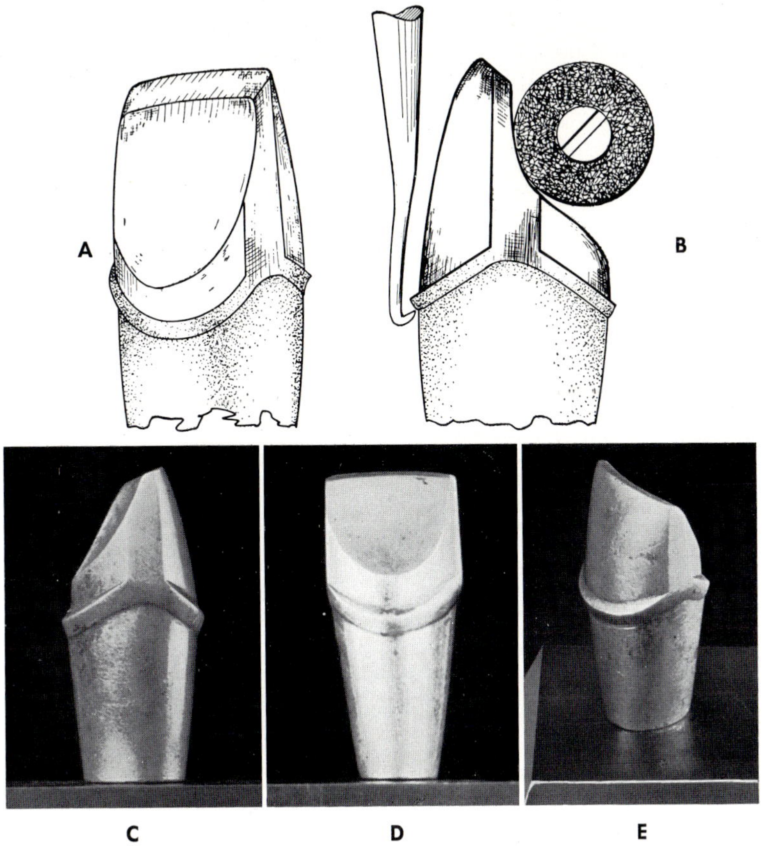

Fig. 24-18. Various views of upper central incisor prepared to point where only subgingival enamel remains on labial and lingual surfaces. **B,** application of enamel cleaver to remove enamel, also cutting lingual enamel, if necessary, to create sufficient space for porcelain.

cleaver is drawn incisally. Because the cutting edge of the blade is applied along cleavage planes of the enamel and because of the fracture lines developed, the enamel is easily removed.

Extreme caution must be taken not to gouge deep grooves with the cleavers in the dentin or to lacerate or tear the gingival tissues from the cementum. It may prove desirable first to use a gum retractor of metal or gutta-percha for a period of 24 hours. At the expiration of this time, the gingival tissues will be retracted. This step is unnecessary; however, if the operator is careful of his instrumentation he may remove this strip of enamel with a (Densco 1½A) cone diamond stone. Some dentists prefer to place the rubber dam and clamp at this point to complete the preparation and take the band impressions.

The same procedure is followed in the removal of the subgingival segment of enamel on the lingual surface. If grooves should accidentally be cut in dentin with the cleavers, these may be smoothed with small files or stones (Densco 1½A).

That portion of the lingual surface lying between the incisal plane and the top of the cingulum is now checked for sufficient clearance between the preparation and the opposing teeth. Usually the removal of the lingual plate of enamel accomplishes this, but, if necessary, some of the dentin may be removed by using the mounted, wheel-shaped stone (Densco 2J). Attention at this time should be called to the fact that the lingual surfaces of the central and lateral incisors are concave gingivoincisally and slightly so mesiodistally (Fig. 24-24), whereas the cuspid tooth is prepared with two planes, a mesial and a distal, which rise to meet in the central ridge (Fig. 24-27). Similarly, it should be noted that the incisal planes of the central and lateral incisors lie in one plane mesiodistally, whereas the cuspid has a mesial and a distal incisal slope.

The preparation of the coronal portion at this time should leave no sharp points

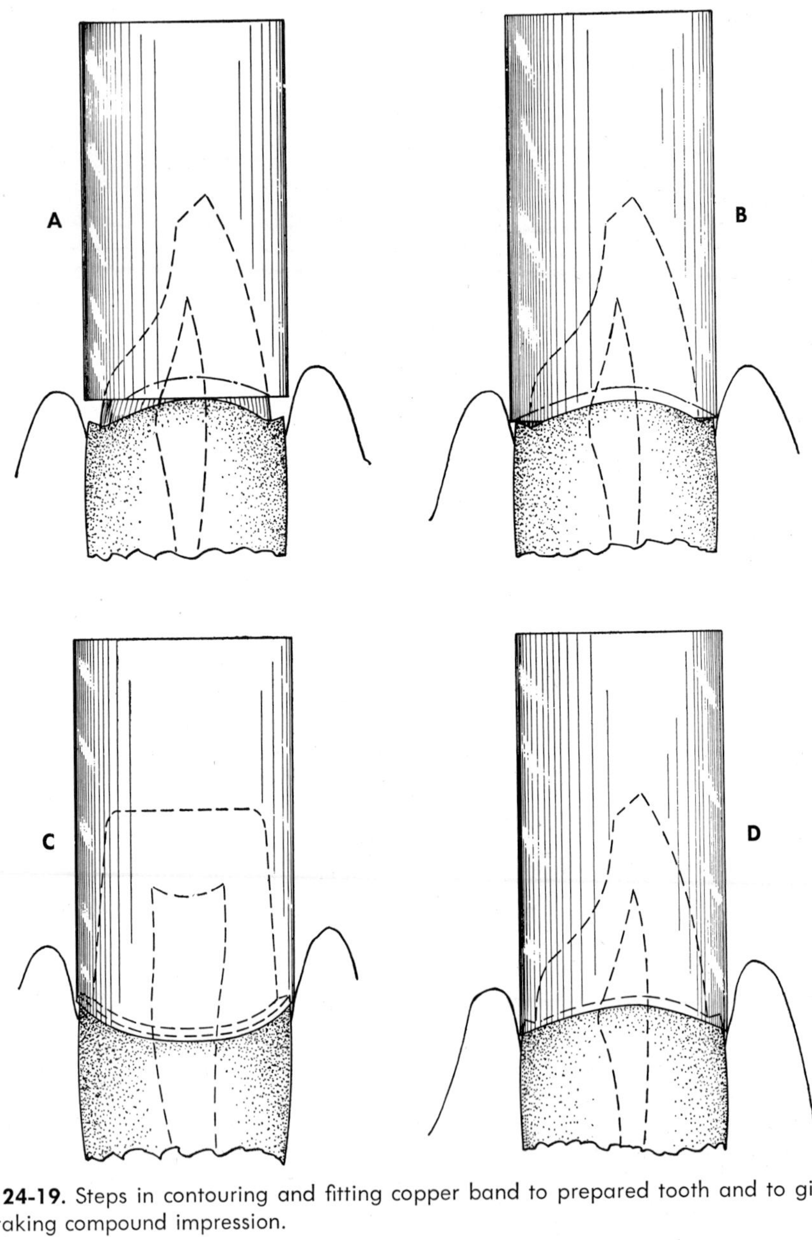

Fig. 24-19. Steps in contouring and fitting copper band to prepared tooth and to gingivae for taking compound impression.

or axial line angles. It should also be noted that no attempt has been made up to this stage of the preparation to cut a shoulder. It will facilitate fitting the copper band if the band is fitted over a tooth that is still cone-shaped instead of having a ledge or shoulder interfering (Fig. 24-22).

Fitting copper band. If one plans to use the copper band–modeling compound technic to take the impression of the finished preparation, then it is advisable first to *fit the band before the shoulder is prepared.* If desired, however, another technic may be used. The shoulder is immediately prepared and the gingival tissues are retracted and a quadrant impression is taken in a tray using the rubber type impression material with the injection syringe. This is then followed by a tray impression which, when removed, is poured in densite stone from which a working cast with removable dies will be made. If, however, the individual modeling compound and copper band technic is to be used, the next step is the selection and preparation of a copper matrix band in which the impression of the prepared tooth will be taken. For this, a wire measurement of the tooth is taken slightly beneath the crest of the gum tissue. Two copper bands of the same circumference are then selected or made. If made from copper matrix material, the technic previously described is followed. Usually, however, the manufactured seamless copper bands are used for this purpose (Fig. 24-19, *A*). These are made in sizes varying in diameter up to ½ inch and in lengths of ½ to ¾ inch. A band open at both ends is preferable to the thimble type, which is closed at one end. Bands of 34-gauge copper are preferred to the heavier gauges, since they can be adapted and fitted more readily to the prepared tooth. After a band of the proper size has been selected, it is conformed to the peripheral outline of the tooth. The gingival outline of the band is next trimmed to parallel the curvature of the gingival tissues according to the technic already described (Fig. 24-19, *B*). When the gingival margin of the band parallels exactly the crest of the gum tissue, it is then carried beneath the crest of the gum, so that the edge of the band extends slightly more than half the distance toward the bottom of the crevice, this distance having been determined previously by the use of the flat periodontal explorer. The band is held at this level while sharp lines are marked on its labial and lingual surfaces even with the crest of the gum tissue (Figs. 24-19, *C*, and 24-20, *A*). In teeth that are round or oval, it is well to place some identification mark

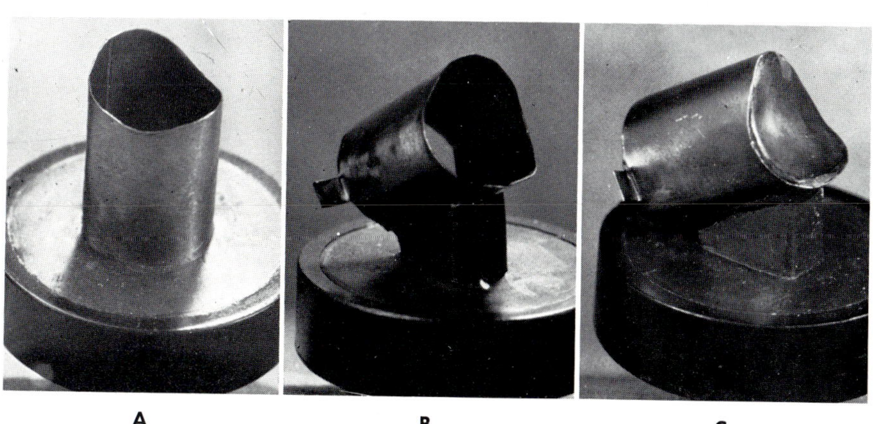

Fig. 24-20. Properly fitted copper bands, **A** and **B,** and copper band filled with modeling compound, **C.** Note wings bent over incisal edge of bands in **B** and **C.**

on the labial surface of the band so that later when the impression is taken in modeling compound there will be no possibility of mistaking the labial for the lingual surface (Fig. 24-19, *D*). To prevent carrying the copper band too far gingivally, two wings are sometimes bent over to rest on the incisal edges of the adjacent teeth (Fig. 24-20, *B*).

Since the gingival margin of the copper band must pass beyond the outer angle of the prepared gingival shoulder to obtain an accurate impression of it, it is necessary that the circumference of the band be slightly larger than that of the prepared tooth (Fig. 24-19, *D*). It should not be too large, however, for in taking the impression it may catch some of the gingival tissues between the shoulder and the margin of the band and thus prevent an accurate impression.

After two such bands have been properly fitted and contoured to the tooth, they are removed, filled with modeling compound, and laid aside (Fig. 24-20, *C*). The filling of the bands with compound at this time is a precautionary measure, since this will prevent their distortion if they should drop to the floor or have some heavy object accidentally laid on them; the hardened compound inside will prevent distortion of the band.

Cutting gingival shoulder. The next step is cutting or completing the gingival shoulder in the tooth. The technic will be described first for completing the shoulder on a tooth whose gingival tissues are still attached to its enamel. This usually occurs in young patients. In such teeth the shoulder has already been prepared on the labial and lingual surfaces (Fig. 24-15). It is now only necessary to unite these by continuing the shoulder through the proximal surfaces. Since no attempt is made in these teeth to lower the shoulder below the crest of the gum tissue, and since the access and visibility are good, a ⅝ or ½ inch knife-edged perforated diamond disk (Densco 4TPS) is held against the proximal surface. By tilting the disk incisally so that it inclines axially about 2° from the vertical plane, a shoulder is cut at the gingival, uniting the labial and lingual shoulders. In carrying this cut from the lingual to the labial surfaces, or vice versa, care should be taken that the plane of the shoulder parallels the *level of the crest* of the gingival tissues (Fig. 24-21). If the proximal shoulder is cut in a straight line labiolingually, it is very likely not only that the gingival tissues will be detached from the enamel, but also that the fibers of the periodontal membrane will be severed. The width of the shoulder rarely exceeds 0.5 to 0.75 mm. The completion of the shoulder at the labioproximal and the linguoproximal angles is completed with cup-shaped, knife-edged diamond disks (Densco 7½K and 8½K).

With the smallest, cylinder-shaped stone (Densco 6E), a No. 6-2-6 hoe of Black's set of cutting instruments, and the spiral fissure bur (No. 557-S), the plane of the shoulder is squared and placed at right angles to the axial surfaces of the preparation. Where the direction of the enamel rods demands it, the enamel portion of the gingival shoulder is planed with a binangle

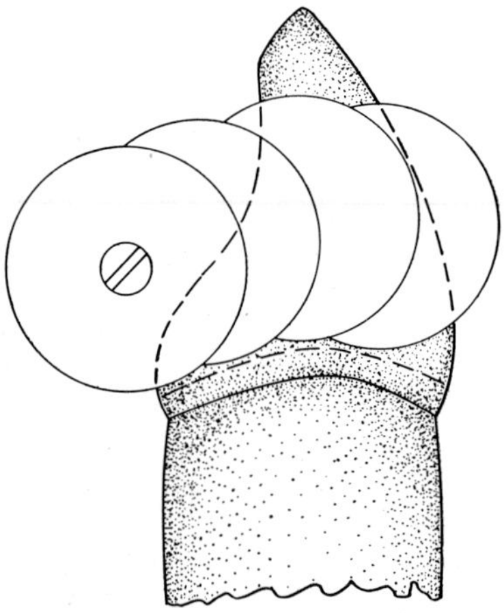

Fig. 24-21. Proximal shoulder is placed parallel to crest curvature of interproximal gum tissue.

chisel (No. 15) or the No. 8-3-6 hoe, so that no unsupported enamel rods remain.

Where the gingival enamel is entirely removed (Fig. 24-22), the cutting of the shoulder involves a different technic. In this case, since all the enamel has been removed, the shoulder is prepared entirely within dentin; likewise, the plane of the shoulder lies slightly below the level of the gingival crest.

Here also the shoulder rarely exceeds a width of 0.5 to 0.75 mm.; likewise, the plane of the shoulder is cut at right angles to the axial surfaces of the preparation and is usually located midway between the crest of the gum tissue and the bottom of the gingival crevice.

The shoulder should never be placed so far rootwise as to encroach upon the attachment of the soft tissues to the cementum. If this is done, there will not be sufficient room left for the copper band containing the compound to pass rootwise beyond the margin of the shoulder without detaching or causing injury to the periodontal membrane fibers while taking the impression.

If all the enamel has been removed, the shoulder is readily cut with a No. 56 or 57 plain fissure bur. Holding the handpiece with the palm-and-thumb grasp for upper anterior teeth, the bur is applied with slight pressure to the labial surface near one of the proximal cuts. The bur is so held that its axial surface parallels the plane of the labial surface (Fig. 24-23, *A*, left). The end of the bur is held on the *same level* with the crest of the gum tissue. Held in this position, the revolving bur is now moved back and forth from the mesial to the distal proximal cuts, slowly cutting into the dentin as increased pressure is applied to it. Gradually the bur cuts to its full diameter into the dentin. It should be observed that the bur is not initially sunk to its full width into the dentin, but that this is accomplished gradually with a planing motion from side to side. It is also to be noted that the shoulder parallels the curvature of the free gum margin. When possible, the labial shoulder is extended into the proximal surfaces lingually, past the labioproximal angles, as far as can be conveniently done.

The same procedure is duplicated in cutting the shoulder on the lingual surface; here the lingual shoulder is extended around the linguoproximal angles into the proximal surfaces, uniting with the labial and proximal cuts. To facilitate cutting the lingual shoulder on upper teeth, the patient should be so positioned in the chair that this region is easy of access. After the shoulder encircles the tooth, the next

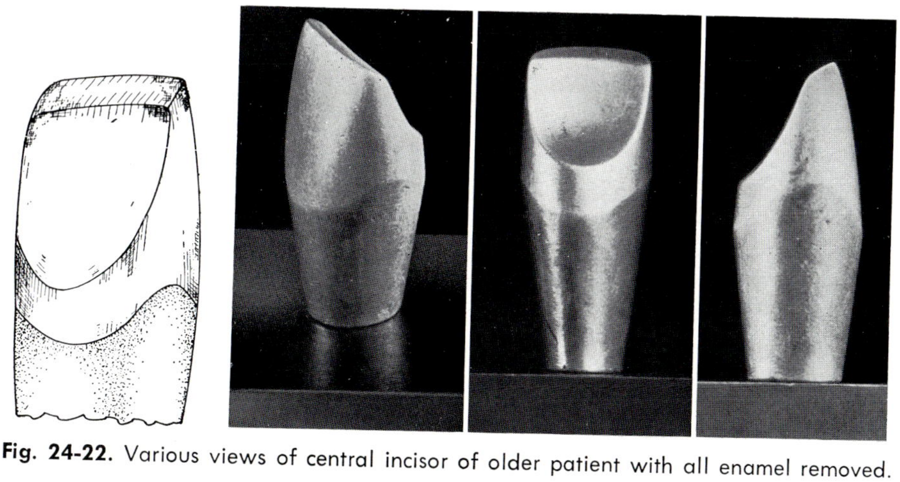

Fig. 24-22. Various views of central incisor of older patient with all enamel removed.

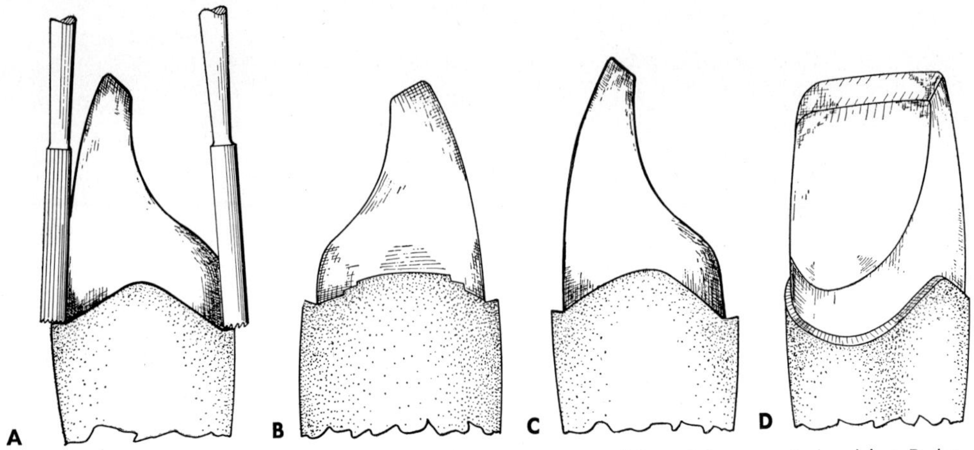

Fig. 24-23. A, Use of plain fissure, **left,** and end cutting burs, **right,** to cut shoulder. **B,** Improperly prepared shoulder having steps instead of continuous plane. **C** and **D,** Sharp line angles where axial surfaces meet incisal and lingual surfaces are rounded and polished with disks.

procedure involves *lowering its level* beneath the crest of the gum tissue, if desired. This may be done with the No. 900 end-cutting bur (Fig. 24-23, A, right), or the No. 56 fissure bur (Fig. 24-23, A, left) previously used. If high speeds are used, great care must be taken to avoid overcutting. In the preparation of the shoulder it is wiser to use speeds in the 25,000 to 50,000 rpm range.

The No. 900 end-cutting bur, because its axial surface blades are smooth, may be used without danger of undercutting the axial walls of the preparation. The No. 56 fissure bur may also be safely used to drop the plane of the shoulder subgingivally, since it was moved into the dentin to its full diameter when the shoulder was cut; the periphery of the bur, therefore, is confined within the circumference of the tooth structure. In using the No. 56 bur, care must be exercised not to widen the shoulder more; hence only the end of the bur is used when lowering the shoulder.

After the shoulder has been lowered into the gingival crevice, sometimes there exists a series of steps at different levels, instead of a smooth, continuous plane (Fig. 24-23, *B*). These may be planed perfectly smooth by using a No. 6-2-6 or a No. 8-3-6 hoe, or special files.

The preparation is then carefully examined for any possible undercuts of the axial surfaces, particularly in the region of the gingival shoulder. If any are found, they may be readily removed by using the flat Krause files or the No. 20 straight chisel.

The preparation is given a final polish by disking with fine sandpaper disks and cocoa butter (Fig. 24-23, *C* and *D*).

Finished preparation. The finished preparation should be a miniature reproduction of the original tooth with certain modifications, namely: (1) a gingival shoulder located at or below the crest of the gum tissue (Fig. 24-24, *A*); (2) an incisal plane placed approximately at a 45° angle to meet the forces of mastication at right angles (Fig. 24-24, *B*); (3) a lingual surface on the central and lateral slightly concave mesiodistally and gingivoincisally, and extending from the incisal plane to the crest of the cingulum (Fig. 24-24, *C*); (4) the gingival third region of the lingual surface is changed from a convexity to an axial wall converging incisally (Fig. 24-24, *C*); (5) all axial surfaces converging slightly toward the axis of the prepara-

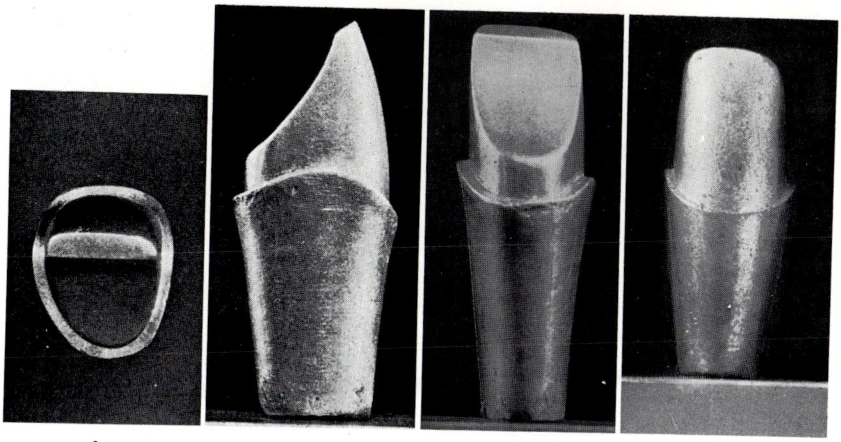

A B C D

Fig. 24-24. Various views of finished upper central incisor prepared for porcelain veneer crown.

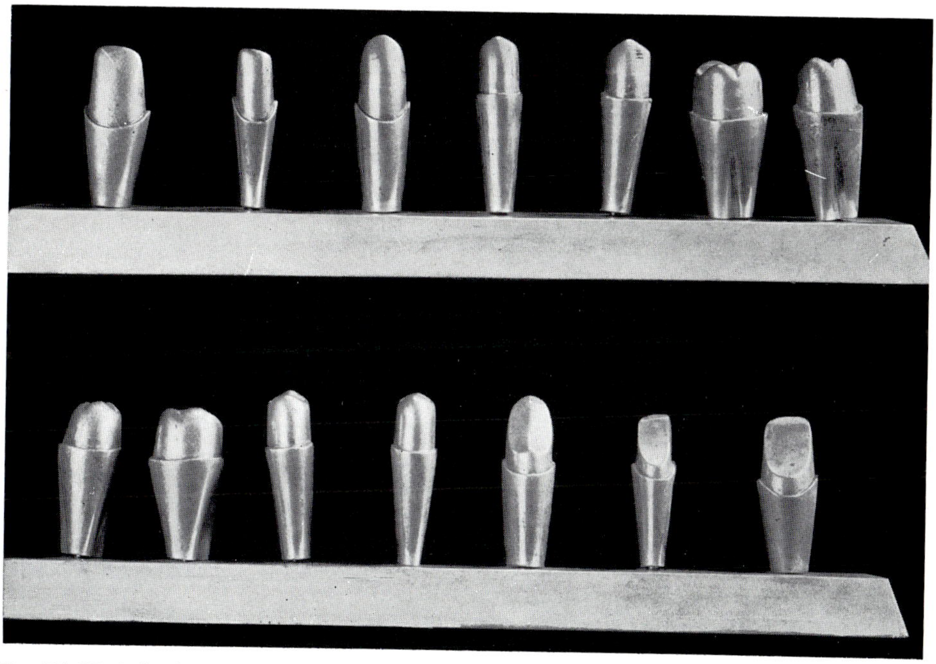

Fig. 24-25. Labial and buccal views of finished preparations for upper teeth, **above,** and lingual views of same, **below.**

tion (Fig. 24-24, *B* to *D*); (6) a labial surface that is convex mesiodistally and gingivoincisally (Fig. 24-24, *D*); (7) sufficient clearance lingually and incisally to allow for a sufficient amount of porcelain between the preparation and the opposing tooth, a minimum of 1 mm.

The next step is securing the impression of the prepared tooth as described in Chapter 26.

Fig. 24-25 shows the labial and lingual views of upper preparations for complete veneer porcelain crowns.

Photographs of models of teeth are as

follows: prepared for upper lateral incisors (Fig. 24-26), cuspids (Fig. 24-27), bicuspids (Fig. 24-28), and molars (Fig. 24-29). Fig. 24-30 is a comparative illustration of upper and lower preparations.

Figs. 24-31 to 24-35 show the labial and lingual views of lower teeth.

Cast core modified preparations. The previous discussion considered the preparation of a normal tooth that had sufficient remaining coronal structure to withstand the forces of mastication and that permitted the preparation of properly placed planes to meet the functional forces at right angles.

Fig. 24-36, *A*, shows the lingual, and 24-36, *B*, the labial views of modified preparations. Fig. 24-37 shows views of the end-to-end bite, Fig. 24-38, views of a shoulderless preparation on lower incisor, and Fig. 24-39, views of a preparation for a cast core.

A complete veneer porcelain crown is sometimes indicated on those teeth excessively destroyed by caries or accident and where but a small amount of tooth structure is left. Where the removal of proximal decay leaves the tooth in such a weakend condition that the remaining dentin cannot furnish sufficient resistance to the applied forces, the incisal two-thirds of the crown is cut away after the pulp has been removed and the root canal filled. A stone (Densco 5J), ⅛ inch in diameter and ¹⁄₁₆ inch wide, is used for cutting down the tooth. In such cases it is general-

Text continued on p. 525.

A B
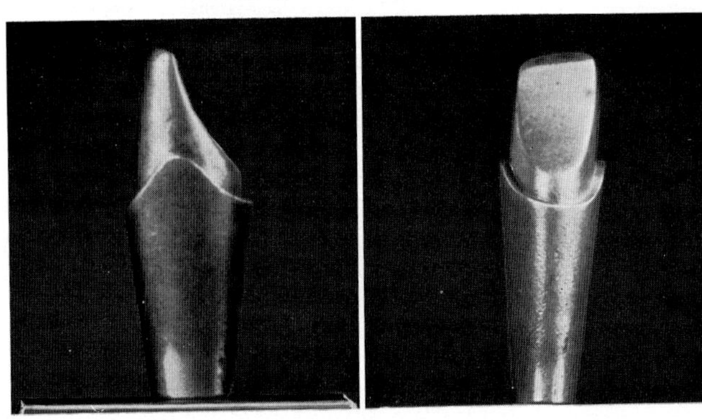

Fig. 24-26. Upper lateral incisor preparations.

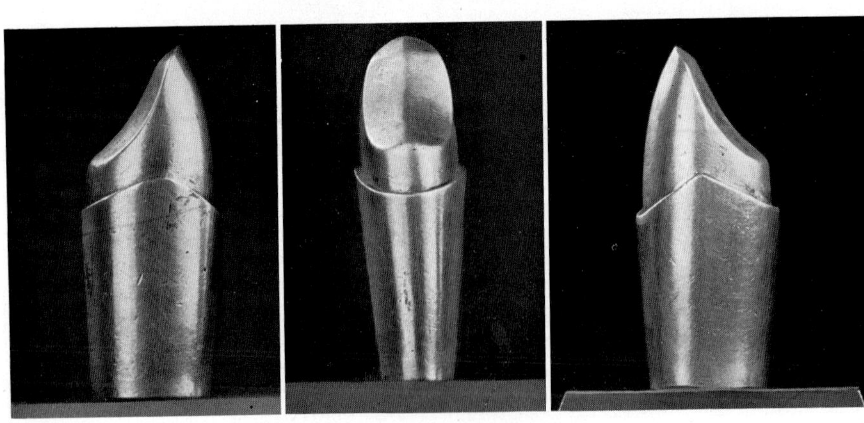
A B C

Fig. 24-27. Upper cuspid.

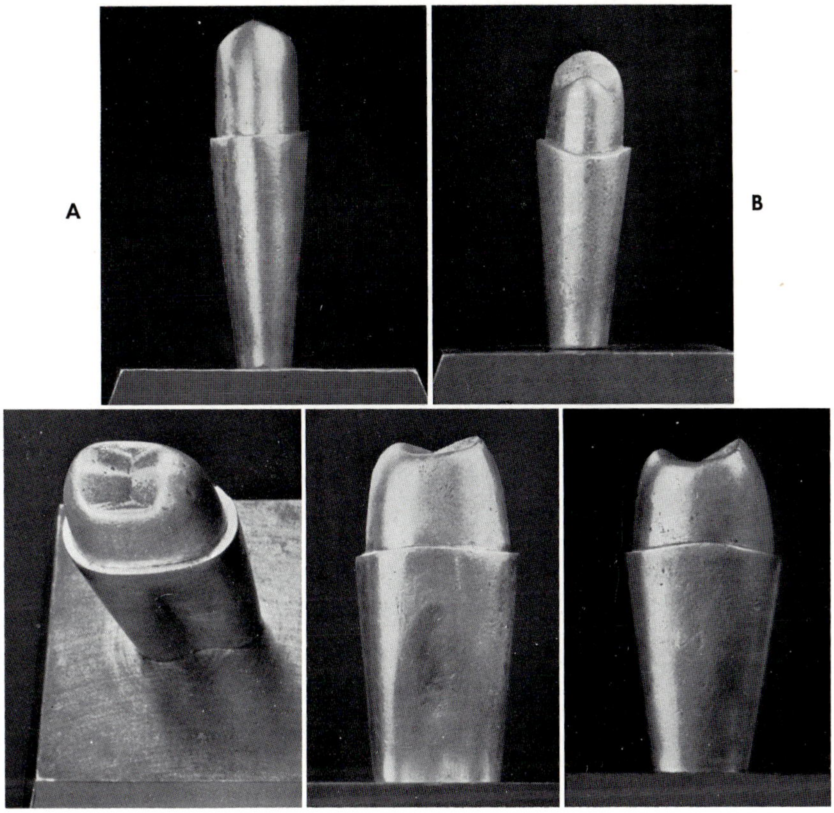

A B

C D E

Fig. 24-28. A and **B,** Upper first bicuspid. **C** to **E,** Upper second bicuspid.

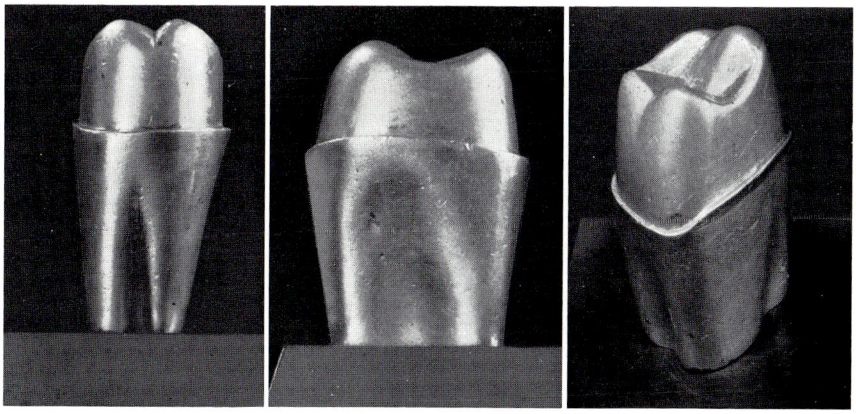

A B C

Fig. 24-29. Upper molar preparations.

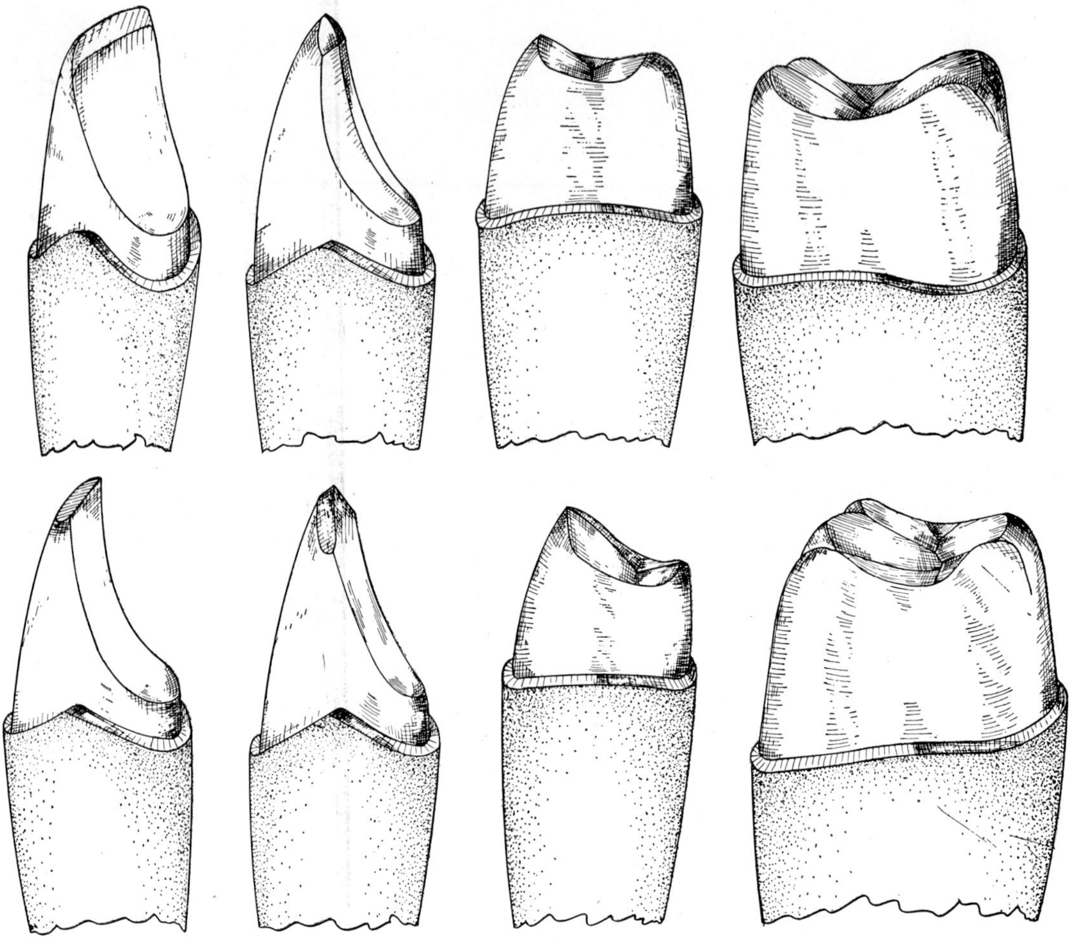

Fig. 24-30. Comparative study of upper and lower preparations. Note placement of incisal planes on upper anterior teeth compared to those on lower anterior teeth, also two incisal and two lingual planes on cuspids compared to one on incisors.

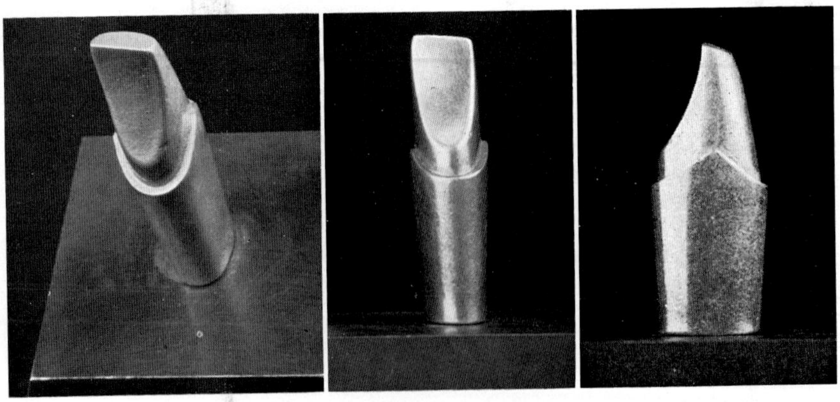

Fig. 24-31. Three views of lower central incisor preparation for porcelain veneer crown.

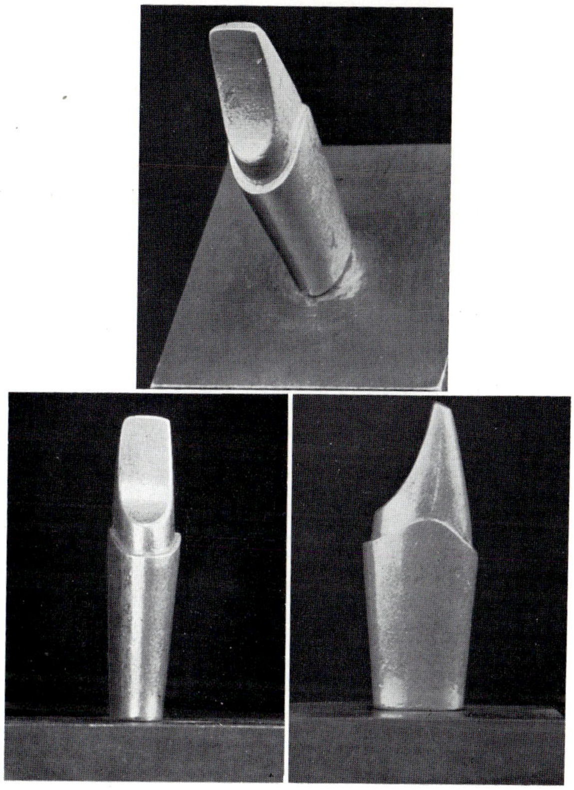

Fig. 24-32. Lingual and proximal views of lower lateral incisor preparations for porcelain veneer crowns.

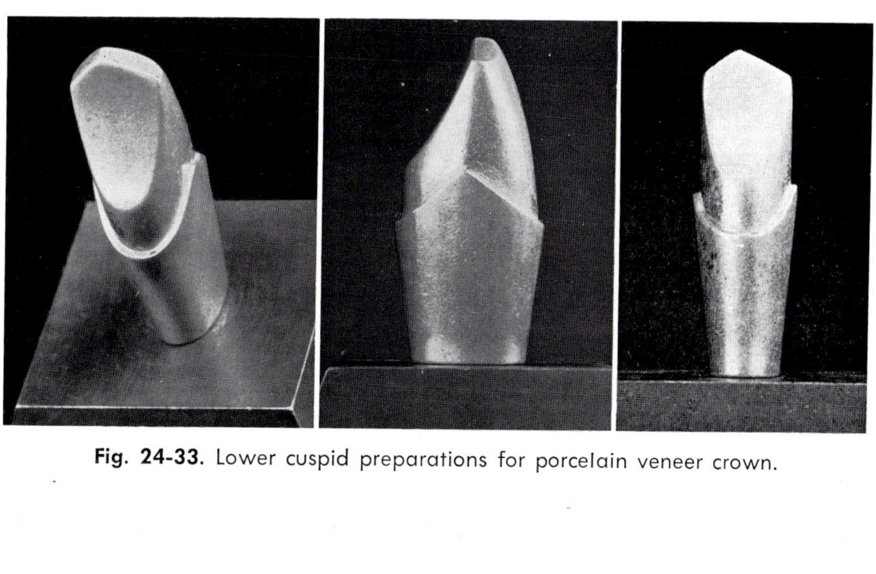

Fig. 24-33. Lower cuspid preparations for porcelain veneer crown.

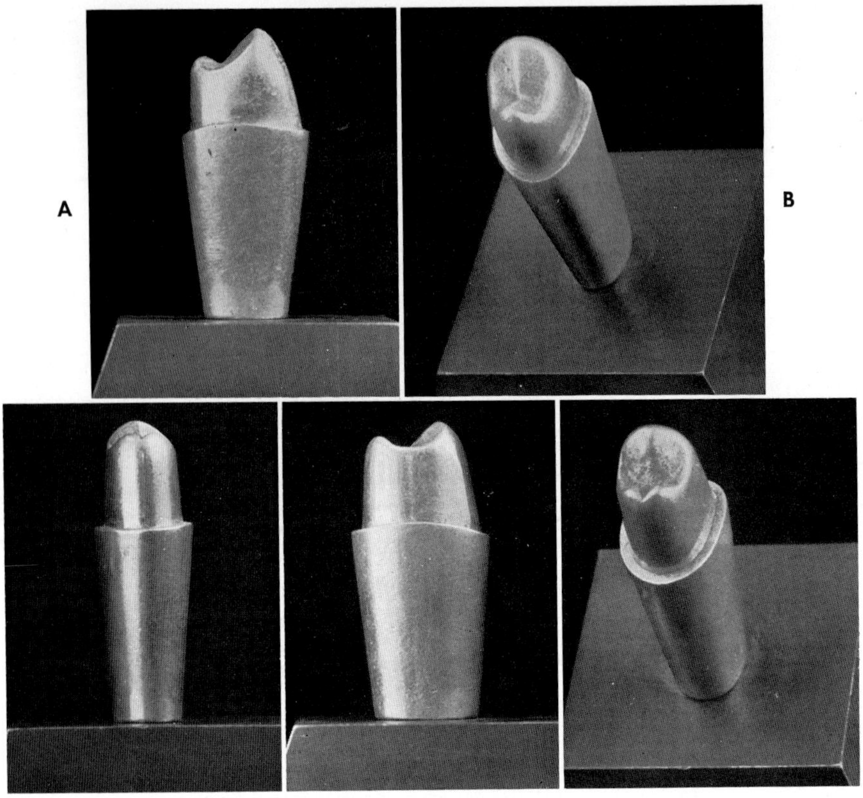

A B

C D E

Fig. 24-34. A and **B,** Lower first bicuspid preparations for porcelain veneer crown. **C** to **E,** Lower second bicuspid preparations for porcelain veneer crown.

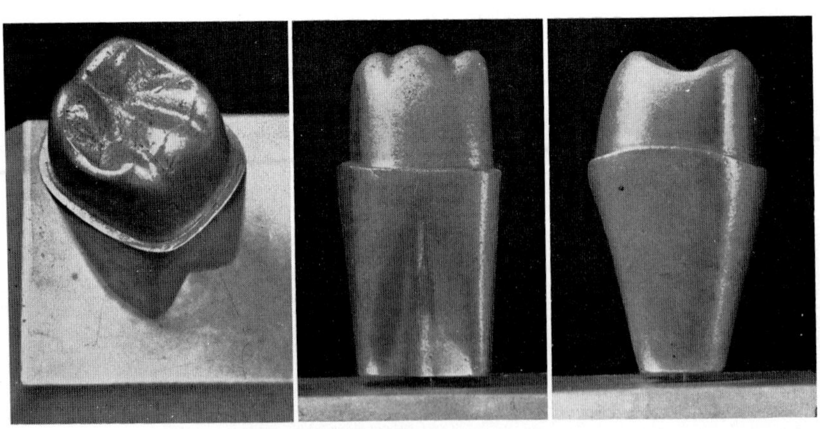

A B C

Fig. 24-35. A to **C,** Lower first molar preparations for porcelain veneer crown. **D** to **F,** Lower second molar preparations for porcelain veneer crown.

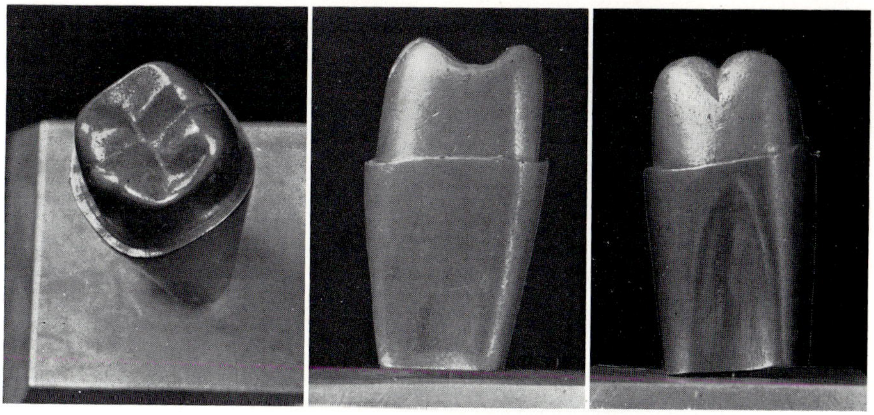

D E F

Fig. 24-35, cont'd. For legend see opposite page.

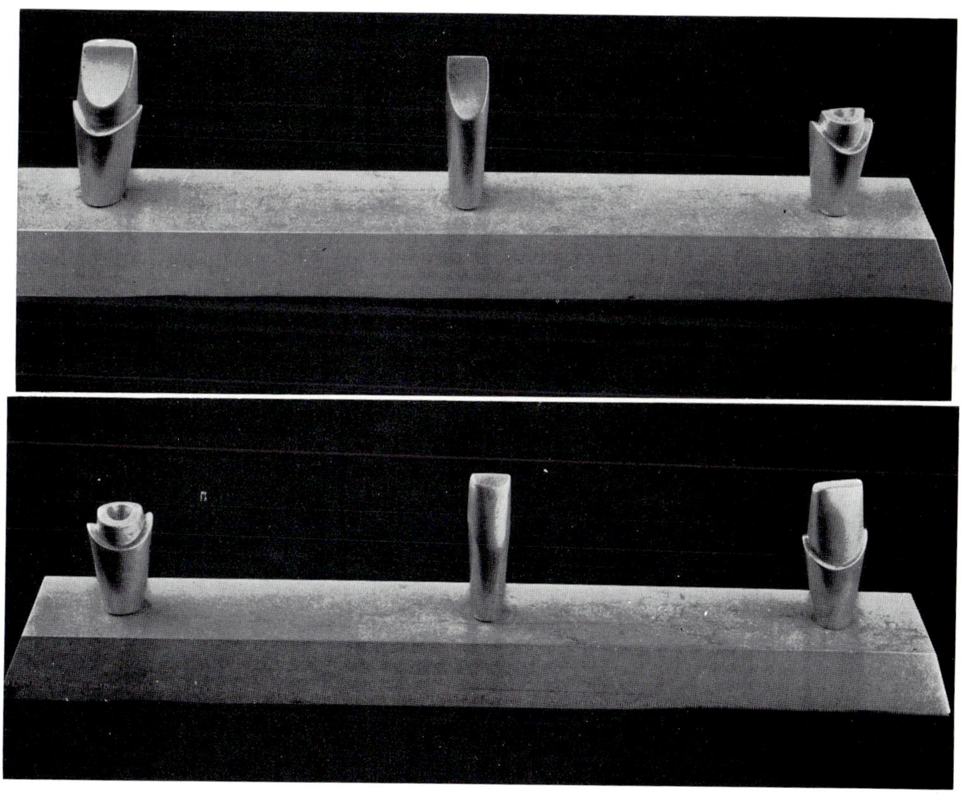

A

B

Fig. 24-36. A, Left to **right:** lingual view of normal preparation for upper central; lingual view of shoulderless lower central; lingual view of upper central preparation for a cast core with dowel. **B, Left** to **right:** lower labial view of upper central for cast core with dowel; labial view of shoulderless lower central preparation; labial view of preparation with cast gold core in place.

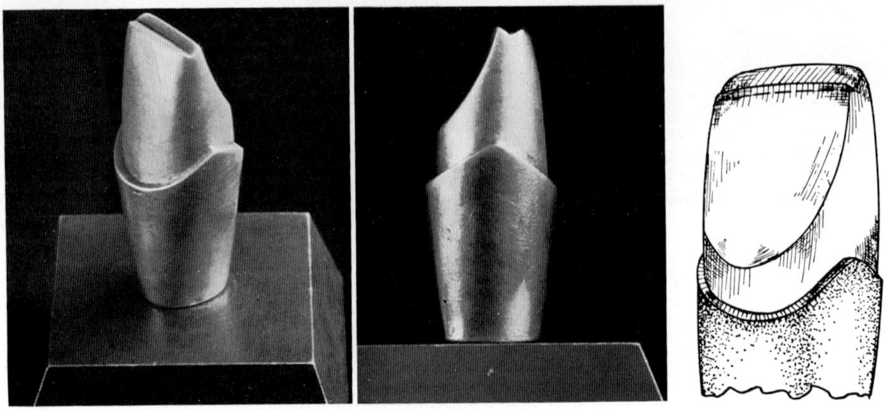

Fig. 24-37. Preparation for end-to-end bite on upper central.

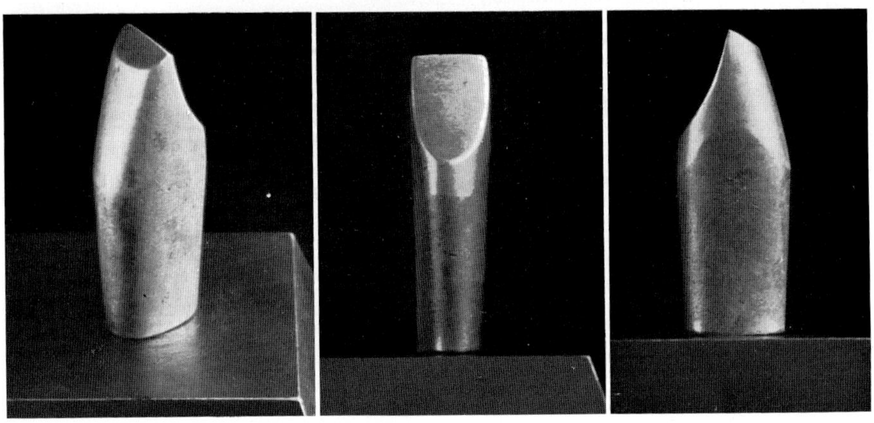

Fig. 24-38. Shoulderless preparation for lower central incisor.

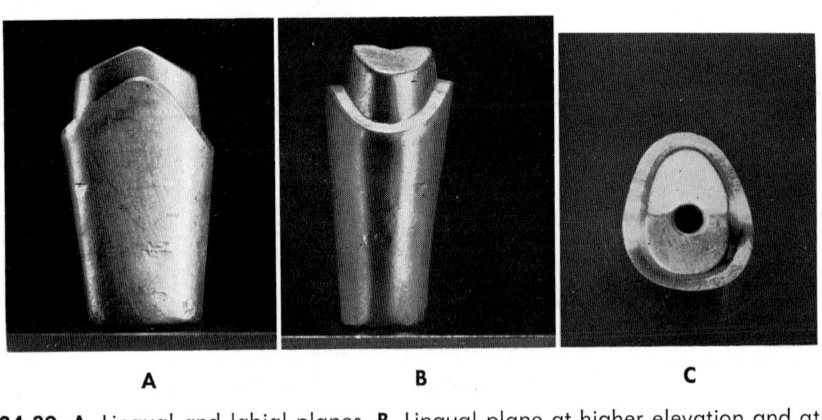

Fig. 24-39. A, Lingual and labial planes. **B,** Lingual plane at higher elevation and at more acute angle. **C,** Top view: upper plane, lingual; lower plane, labial.

ly found that the gingival tissues have receded and are attached below the cemento-enamel line; therefore, the shoulder is readily prepared below the crest of the gum tissue. The cervical enamel on the labial, lingual, and proximal surfaces of the remaining portion of the crown is removed in the manner described earlier in the chapter. This leaves an extension of dentin incisally of 3 to 4 mm. in height along the gingival crest. A wire measurement is taken and two copper bands are fitted as previously described. Following this, a shoulder is cut as before, carrying it below the crest of the gingival tissues. This shoulder, however, is made twice the normal width, i.e., it is at least 1 mm. wide. As explained later, half this width is encircled by the cast core.

The preparation is completed with a root facer or stone (Densco 2J) to develop two planes. One plane slopes gingivally and labially from the root canal, terminating slightly above the crest of the gingiva. The other plane slopes lingually from the root canal, but at a slightly less acute angle, and ends 2 to 3 mm. above the crest of the gingiva (Fig. 24-39). The opening to the root canal is countersunk with a No. 9 or 10 round bur.

Reaming and enlarging root canal. The next step involves reaming out, at low speed, the gutta-percha and enlarging the root canal to receive a dowel of the proper length and gauge. The initial cut into the gutta-percha root filling is made with a No. ½ round bur, which is lowered from 1 to 2 mm. in the center of the filling material (Fig. 24-40, *A*). This cut is then enlarged to the same depth with a No. 3 round bur (Fig. 24-40, *B*). Finally a No. 6 round bur is used to enlarge the canal to a diameter large enough to accommodate the correct gauge of dowel (Fig. 24-41, *A*). In making this enlargement most of the gutta-percha in this area is removed as well as a part of the dentin walls of the root canal.

The three steps of the cutting process and instrumentation are repeated, carrying the enlargement of the canal to the second and lower level; finally, by repeating the procedure, the canal is enlarged to the correct size and depth, as shown in Fig. 24-41, *B*.

By using the smaller size bur first, it follows the path of least resistance in cutting, i.e., it follows the gutta-percha, thus avoiding the possibility of a lateral root perforation. After the initial enlargement the gutta-percha is easily visible for further cutting operations. The correctness of the enlargement is verified by trying the dowel in the enlarged root canal. Under no circumstances should the long, large dowel reamers be used, especially with the high-speed handpieces because of the danger of root perforation.

Fitting dowel. Clasp metal wire of 14-gauge is used for dowels in upper central incisors and cuspids; the lateral usually requires a 16-gauge dowel. Where two dowels are used, as in the upper first bicuspid, 18-gauge wire is frequently employed.

The *depth* to which a dowel extends into the root canal corresponds to the gingivoincisal height of the crown. To this length is added a 4 or 5 mm. incisal extension of the dowel to which the core is cast.

Although a slight taper is permissible in a dowel, it is preferable to leave the wire with parallel sides, except at its apical end, where it is beveled 45°. If this end of the dowel is left flat instead of beveled, it acts as a plunger when cemented to place, thereby hindering the escape of the cement from the canal and preventing the complete seating of the casting. That portion of the dowel which extends incisally beyond the root face is roughened or notched to give a better mechanical retention to the casting of the core.

Impression technic. A copper band, fitted as shown in Figs. 24-19 and 24-

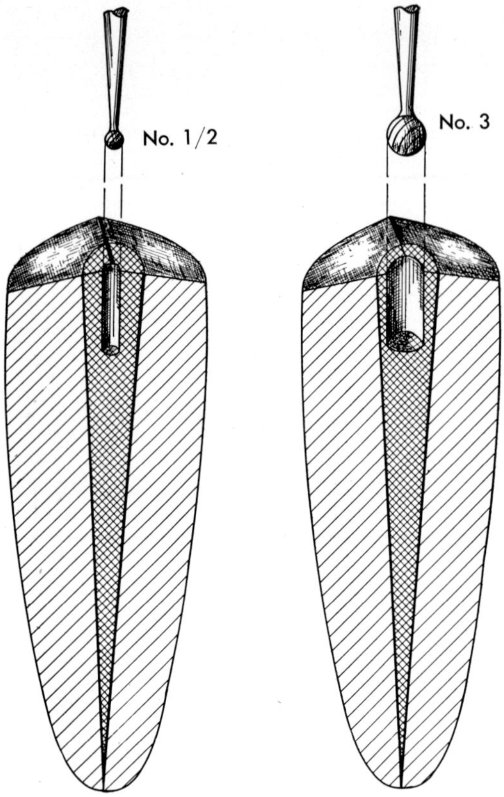

A B

Fig. 24-40. First and second steps in enlarging filled root canal to receive metal dowel for cast core.

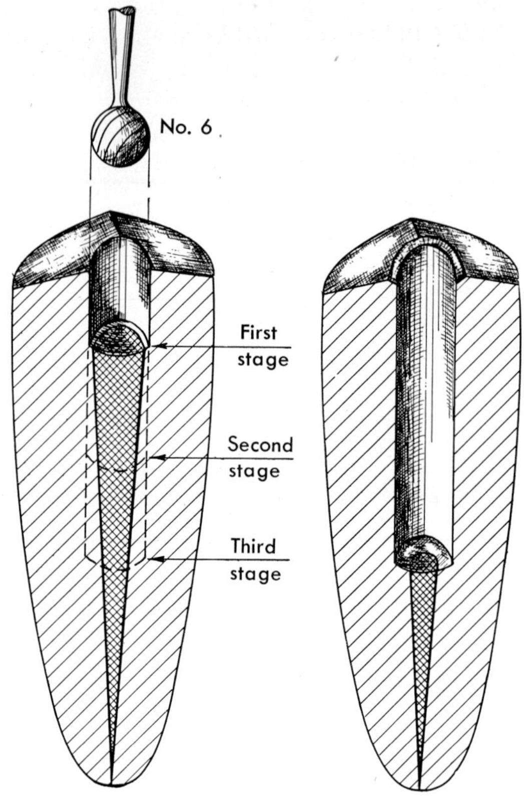

A B

Fig. 24-41. Third and final stage in preparing filled root canal to receive metal dowel.

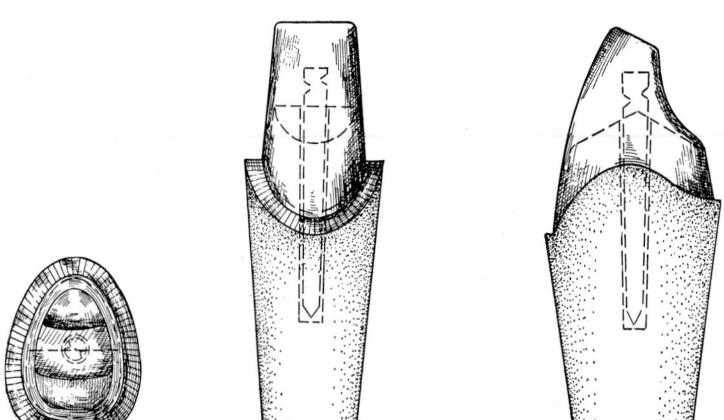

Fig. 24-42. Cast core encircles plateau portion of preparation, occupies half width of shoulder.

20, filled with modeling compound, is now warmed, and the impression is taken of the root preparation with the dowel in place. After the compound is cooled with water to room temperature, it is withdrawn, carrying the dowel with it. The band and impression are encircled with wax and the exposed portion of the dowel is painted with Steele's antiflux or a thin layer of cavity varnish. Amalgam is then packed into the impression around the dowel and extended at least ¼ inch beyond the incisal end of the dowel. It is allowed to set completely.

Amalgam die and core. The amalgam die, when removed from the impression, not only is an exact reproduction of the prepared root, but also holds the dowel in its correct relationship. By grasping the incisal extension of the dowel with flat-nosed pliers and slightly turning the dowel first to the right and then to the left, it will loosen; it may then be readily withdrawn from the amalgam die. After it has been cleaned in acid, the dowel is lubricated and replaced in the die that has also been lubricated; the coronal portion of a typical complete veneer crown preparation is then carved in inlay wax. The gingival portion of this core not only contacts the two planes of the root face, but it encircles the axial surfaces of the preparation and ends gingivally, occupying half the width of the shoulder (Fig. 24-42). A core constructed in this manner not only takes advantage of the retention furnished by the dowel, but also receives the additional support furnished by the bulk of cast metal encircling the axial surfaces of the preparation. This encirclement of the tooth also minimizes the possibility of root fracture. The casting is approximately 0.5 mm. in width at the shoulder, still leaving a 0.5 mm. shoulder in the natural tooth over which the complete porcelain veneer crown is fitted.

After the cast core has been polished and cemented to place, it is regarded in all subsequent procedures as if it were a preparation of a vital tooth. The subsequent procedures involve taking an impression of the cemented core to completing the veneer crown.

Cast core as bridge retainer. A modified form of the cast core in conjunction with a partial veneer porcelain crown permits its use as a bridge retainer.[10] Where so employed, the proximal portion of the core

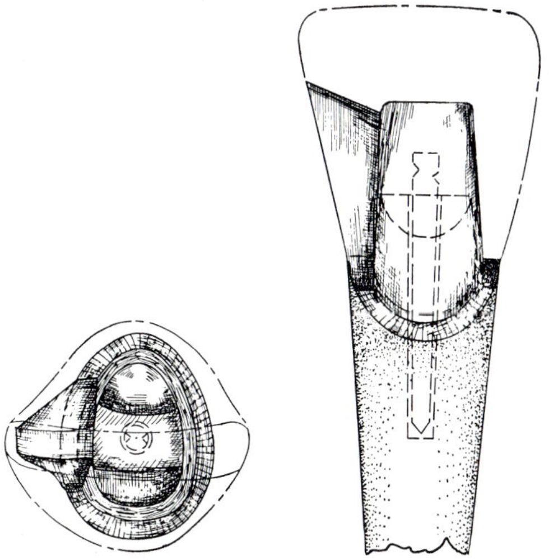

Fig. 24-43. Cast core with proximal wing used as bridge retainer.

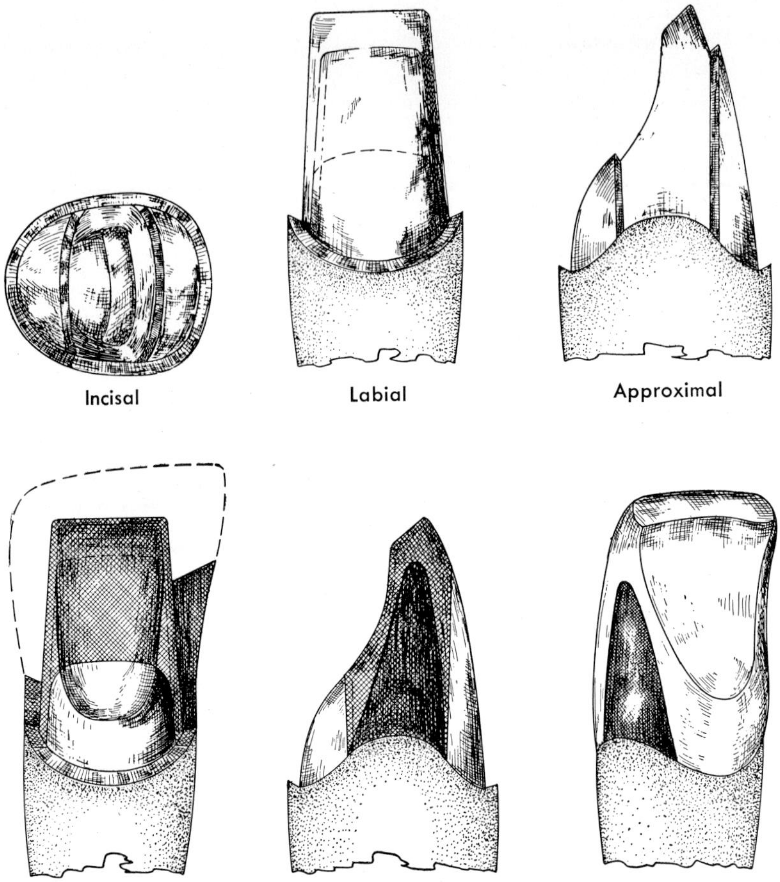

Fig. 24-44. Other methods of constructing cast core without using metal dowel in root canal. (After Tofflemire.)

contiguous to the edentulous space is fully contoured gingivoincisally to the height of the contact area (Fig. 24-43). The shoulder is complete covered by the core from the linguoproximal to the labioproximal angles of the preparation. The plane of the shoulder rises from the gingivolabial angle until it reaches the contact area; then it descends lingually until at the gingivolingual angle it merges with the shoulder of the natural tooth.

When cast, this proximal wing of gold constitutes the area to which the pontic is soldered. After the bridge is cemented, the procelain veneer crown is placed over the remaining core, eliminating the display of all metal.

Core for vital tooth. Fig. 24-44 shows a modification of this principle applied to a tooth with a vital pulp and having sufficient tooth structure; this method is suggested by Tofflemire.[10] The extracoronal partial veneer principle is applied here; portions of the labial and lingual surfaces are left uncovered. By adding the proximal wing extension, this type of casting may be used as a bridge retainer in conjunction with the porcelain veneer crown; it may also be used without the proximal wing to lengthen the preparation incisally on short teeth to furnish the necessary support to the veneer crown in its incisal third. It is especially valuable for this purpose.

SELECTED REFERENCES

1. Clark, B. E.: Requirements of the jacket crown, J.A.D.A. **26**:355, 1939.
2. Schneider, A. E.: The preparation of a tooth for a porcelain veneer crown, Chicago, 1916.
3. Gottlieb, B., and Orban, B.: Biology and pathology of the tooth and supporting mechanism, New York, 1938, The Macmillan Co.
4. Both, H. S.: Newer methods in preparing vital teeth for porcelain jacket crowns, D. Digest **43**:481, 1937.
5. Wheeler, R. C.: Restoration of the gingival or cervical margins in full crowns, D. Cosmos **73**:238, 1931.
6. Ewing, J. E.: Atypical porcelain jacket crown preparations, J. Prosth. Dent. **2**:865, 1952.
7. Conod, H.: Etude sur la statique de la couronne jaquette, Rev. mensuelle Suisse d'Odontol. **47**:485, 1937.
8. Grubb, H. D.: Basic procedures essential for successful porcelain restorations, Read at Dental Centenary, Baltimore, March, 1940.
9. Oppice, H. W.: A résumé of ideas on porcelain jacket crown preparations, J.A.D.A. **21**: 1030, 1934.
10. Tofflemire, B. F.: A new abutment preparation and attachment for anterior fixed bridgework, D. Cosmos **75**:1139, 1933.

GENERAL REFERENCES

Argue, J. E.: The porcelain jacket crown, J.A.D.A. **26**:1472, 1939.

Avary, H.: Porcelain jacket crowns, J.A.D.A. **15**: 601, 1928.

Back, P.: Porcelain jacket crown preparation, D. Survey **12**:38, 1936.

Bartels, J. C.: Dental ceramics, J. Prosth. Dent. **11**:537, 1961.

Bartels, J. C.: Preparation of the anterior teeth for porcelain jacket crowns, J. South. California D. A. **30**:199,1962.

Bastian, C. C.: Porcelain jacket crowns, D. J. Australia **43**:288, 1939.

Both, H. S.: Less operative trauma in preparing vital teeth for jacket crowns, New York J. Dent. **9**:154, 1939.

Doner, F. H.: The molded porcelain jacket crown, D. Cosmos **78**:16, 1936.

Ewing, J. E.: Beautiful but glum—porcelain jacket crowns, J. Prosth. Dent. **4**:94, 1954.

Feinschneider, I. L.: Ceramique en art dentaire, J. Canad. D. A. **27**:829, 1961.

Felcher, F. R.: Shoulderless lingual reinforced jacket crown, D. Digest **45**:226, 1939.

Gill, J. R.: Construction of the porcelain veneer crown, J.A.D.A. **27**:1844, 1940.

Holland, M. W.: Improved method for securing the impression and die for porcelain jacket crown construction, Dent. Clin. N. Amer., March, 1959, pp. 125-131.

Hovestad, J. E.: Modern achievement in dental ceramics, D. Survey **7**:36, 1931.

Jordan, H. A.: Restorative ceramics, Quart. Nat. D. A. **18**:15, 1959.

Lehman, M. L., and Hampson, E. L.: Study of strain patterns in jacket crowns on anterior teeth resulting from different tooth preparations, Brit. D. J. **113**:337, 1962.

Lund, M. R., and Bonlie, D. R.: Baked porcelain restorations without the use of the platinum matrix, I.A.D.R. **40**:94, 1962 (abst.).

Moulton, G. H.: Porcelain veneer crown, North-West Dent. **38**:363, 1959.

Nuttall, E. B.: Factors influencing success of porcelain jacket restorations, J. Prosth. Dent. **11**:743, 1961.

Pilkington, E. L.: Porcelain jacket crowns, D. Cosmos **72**:1259, 1930.

Pruden, W. H., II: Porcelain veneer crown, J. Prosth. Dent. **10**:955, 1960.

Richard, E. L., and Brodtmann, N. V.: Cast copings for jacket crowns, J. Prosth. Dent. **12**: 129, 1962.

Sayre, L. D.: Porcelain jacket crowns, Florida D. J. **4**:2, 1933.

Sayre, L. D.: Physics and mechanics involved in serviceable porcelain jacket crown restorations, J.A.D.A. **31**:3, 1942.

Sayre, L. D.: Operative and laboratory procedures in the construction of porcelain jacket crowns, J. D. Soc. New York **8**:17, 1942.

Thompson, G. A.: A new preparation for jacket crowns, J. Minnesota State D. A. **10**:29, 1931-1932.

Vehe, W. D.: A consideration of the porcelain veneer crown from the standpoint of the general practitioner, Illinois D. J. **1**:453, 1931-1932.

Vehe, W. D.: Tooth preparation for porcelain veneer crown, Minneapolis Dist. D. J. **23**:23, 1939.

Viverito, J. A.: Porcelain restorations for hypoplastic enamel, D. Cosmos **78**:1080, 1936.

Walton, C. B., and Leven, M. M.: A preliminary report of photoelastic tests of strain patterns within jacket crowns, J.A.D.A. **50**:44-48, 1955.

Wheeler, R. C.: A comparison of periodontal attachment levels: anteroposteriorly, D. Digest **41**:261, 1935.

Wheeler, R. C.: Etiology, treatment and prevention of chronic gingival irritation around porcelain jacket crowns, J.A.D.A. **25**:1742, 1938.

Wheeler, R. C.: Dental anatomy and physiology, ed. 4, Philadelphia, 1968, W. B. Saunders Co.

Chapter 25

Color: principles, selection, and reproduction in crowns and fixed partial prosthodontics—materials, equipment, and application

PRINCIPLES AND THEORIES

Every dentist strives toward the ideal in facial art when he replaces lost teeth with crowns or fixed partial dentures. Although the requirements of function and comfort are important in a restoration, the fact cannot be minimized that the esthetic values are also extremely desirable. Psychologically, the esthetic factors are of considerable consequence because of the reactions they produce in the individual. Many patients who have avoided social contacts because of the appearance of their dentures, either natural or artificial, have returned to their normal social and business relationships after rehabilitation of their mouths through prosthetic means.

Normal facial expression, correct occlusion, and proper mastication are frequently concomitant with and dependent upon the restoration of the esthetic factors.

Art or, more specifically, facial art, has been defined in many ways. As it applies to partial denture prosthesis, it possesses certain fundamentals whose objectives are to restore lost form, function, and appearance, without, at the same time, disclosing the presence of restorations or the means used in the attainment of those objectives.

The concept and the development of the esthetics of teeth have found some unusual methods of expression. The use of war paint and cosmetics was common practice throughout the ages; the placing of jewels in ears and rings in the nose is likewise known and recorded. Even the mutilation of different parts of the body was thought to contribute something to the esthetic qualities of the individual; as witness the flat heads of some Indian tribes, the bound feet of Chinese women, and the coloring, filing, or even the knocking out of teeth by many of the African tribes. From this primitive and distorted idea of facial art, the concept has gradually passed through a process of evolution to a higher plane and to a better appreciation of the fundamentals of true facial art.

FUNDAMENTALS OF FACIAL ART

First among these fundamentals may be listed harmony, as expressed through likeness in contour and color of the eyes, hair, skin, and teeth; also, the harmony of texture, direction of axes, etc.; second, interest, as created by sufficient variety in shape, color, texture, and contours. Then there is the fundamental of proportion, the proportion of form and size of the teeth themselves, the dentures as a whole, and the relationships that exist between the forms of the teeth, the face, and the head. The fundamentals of balance, both symmetric and asymmetric, are found in the occlusion. The fundamental of exactness, as related to restorative dentistry, applies to the restoration of the correct anatomy, position, and dental relationships.

Another fundamental of facial art is an understanding of the light factors, both artificial and natural, and the physical changes that they produce in the color effects, and the subjective, physiologic variations or contrasts developed in each individual. The last important fundamental is that of color. This involves not only its composition and analysis, but also the relevance of these factors to the restoration of esthetic values in dentistry.

Fundamentals of color (hue)

In order to select and reproduce colors in porcelain restorations, either crowns, bridges, or inlays, it is essential that the dentist be familiar with the theory, classification, and phenomena of color. Although it is true that some men are possessed of an inherent sense of color harmony, the majority may acquire this faculty only by intense study and experimentation.

A knowledge of color may be gained in two general ways: one is by observation and association, i.e., a person may by constant contact with objects of beauty and color acquire an intuitive color sense. This method, however, is a slow process and uncertain in its creative esthetic possibility. The other way is to study the theory, application, and phenomena of color and light. This will acquaint the student with the laws and principles of color, which, once understood, enable him to perceive, match, and reproduce the color effect of natural teeth with confidence and success. The fascination of the work increases as progress is made.

Color defined. The term "color," as ordinarily applied, is the sensation or impression produced by the number and character of light rays striking the retina. The effect of light is the result of light waves, just as the effect of sound is the result of sound vibrations striking the eardrum. It is impossible to tabulate directions for using color without an understanding of the physical laws of light, which explain some of the color phenomena with which the dentist must contend in prosthetic restorations.

Physical laws of light and color. If the texture and composition of all objects were so similar that all the rays of light would be reflected from the object to the eye, everything would be white. Since this is not so, it is concluded that various objects differ both in texture and composition to such a degree that they absorb certain rays and reflect others. These different rays travel at varying speeds. A demonstration of this fact may be obtained by passing a single ray of white light through a prism, which will break up the white light into a brilliant strip of a variety of colors, among which are a pure blue, a pure red, and a pure yellow, with the intermediary gradations. This is known as the spectrum (Plate 5).

If an object absorbs all the color rays except the blue, which it reflects, it is designated as a blue object or blue effect.

Substances through which one can see other objects clearly are called *transparent*, but those through which vision is impossible are designated as *opaque*. When a substance transmits some light but not enough for vision, it is *translucent*. When a beam of light strikes a smooth body lying in its path, a large part of the light which falls upon it from one direction is sent off in some other direction by *reflection*. If the surface of the object is rough, the light which falls upon it is scattered in all directions and gives *diffused reflection*. Some of the light incident upon the object will sometimes penetrate it;

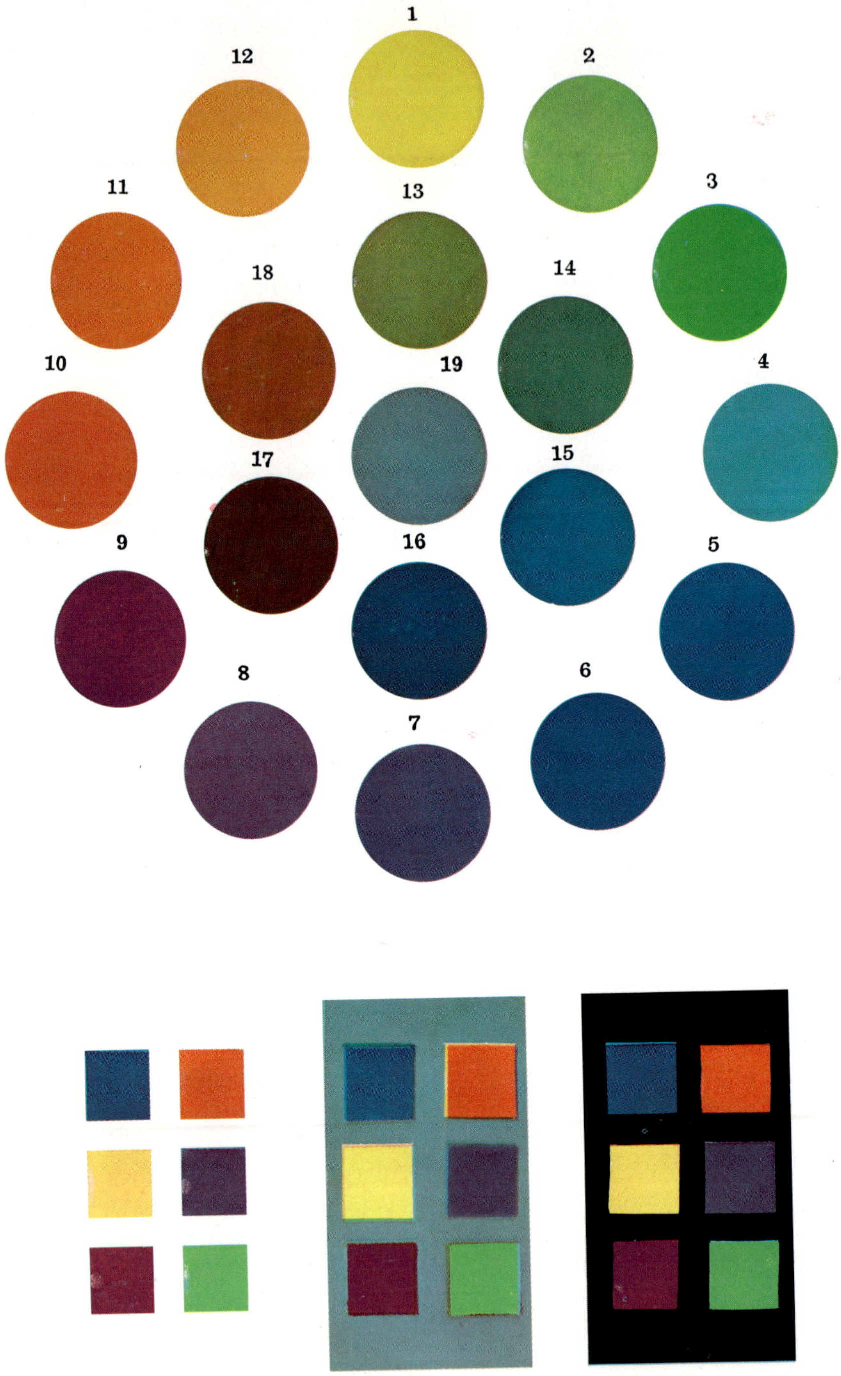

Plate 5. Spectrum, **above,** and effects on color by simultaneous contrasts, **below. 1,** yellow; **2,** yellow green; **3,** green; **4,** blue green; **5,** blue; **6,** blue violet; **7,** violet; **8,** red violet; **9,** red; **10,** red orange; **11,** orange; **12,** yellow orange; **13,** gray yellow; **14,** gray green; **15,** gray blue; **16,** gray violet; **17,** gray red; **18,** gray orange; **19,** neutral gray.

the rays which pass through it are said to be *transmitted.* This process of transmission is always accompanied by some loss of light; light which is lost in this way is said to be *absorbed.* When all the rays are absorbed, the object is *opaque.*[1]

Any classification of colors is arbitrary to a certain degree[2] (Plate 5). Men will dispute whether the primary colors are red, yellow, and blue, or red, green, and violet-blue. The first group is classified according to pigments, while the other is classified according to lights. The dentist is not interested so much in a color system that attempts to establish one particular classification as he is in a method whereby he more easily can select porcelains of certain colors or combinations of colors and by their proper manipulation reproduce the color *effects* found in the natural teeth.

The problem does not deal with the various pigments alone; if it did there would be very little difficulty inasmuch as porcelains are available in various colors, shades, and tints. The colors at the dentist's disposal possess certain qualities, which, if utilized, enable him more nearly to simulate Nature.

Color constants. Just as a certain musical sound or a combination of sounds may produce an agreeable or a disagreeable sensation, so also may a certain color or a certain combination of colors produce analogous effects. Every color or hue has three qualities called color constants: (1) color tone, or the quality by which, for example, bluish-red differs from orange-red; (2) color luminosity (chroma), by which, for example, light red differs from dark red; (3) color purity (value), by which, for example, a pure or spectral red differs from a broken or grayish-red. (Webster.) To the dentist it is of importance to know that the most luminous colors or hues are yellow first, and orange next, while the least luminous are blue and violet (see lower portion of Plate 5). Teeth, therefore, that have a predominance of gray and dark brown present a lifeless appearance, while those predominating in yellow or orange appear vital and translucent. In one the rays are mostly absorbed; in the other they are transmitted and reflected. By the addition of certain hues to others, the luminosity or translucency can be increased or decreased. The addition of red to brown or yellow increases its luminosity; similarly, its removal decreases it. The removal of a pulp, no doubt, has some effect on the luminosity of a tooth. Since yellow and orange possess this highly desired characteristic of luminosity, these hues should be used as the foundation for most inlays and crowns.

Next in importance to yellow with its red modifications is the blue hue. This may vary in shade toward the variations with red or toward the greenish tints. It has its importance in the incisal and the occlusal regions. The tints of greenish hue are the more luminous inasmuch as green is a combination of blue with yellow. Although green is rarely used as a pure color, except for staining purposes, its addition to grays of a bluish tendency tends to intensify the grays. Brown made more brilliant by the addition of yellow is indicated as a base color for either inlays or crowns for older patients or those with stained teeth. Whenever it is desired to dull a color, such as yellow, the slight addition of gray will accomplish the result (Plate 4). Certain colors, known as advancing colors, have a feeling of warmth about them, while others, called the receding colors, have a cold, bleak reaction. Who has not, at one time or another, studied a painting and felt that something was lacking? The slight addition of a color would change the entire effect; the following is an example of this.

A picture depicts an evening scene on the shores of a bay. Projecting out into the water, on a small promontory, squats a fisherman's hut. The artist beautifully portrays fleecy clouds floating in the moonlit sky, the trees nodding in the evening breezes, and tied to the pier a small boat riding the undulating waves. Everything seems to lend to the scene an atmosphere of peace and calm, and yet something is lacking. One dip of the brush, a few strokes, and an inanimate scene is transformed into one radiating with life; it is simple; the dark windows of the hut are painted with orange color. At once there is life in the hut, life in the picture. This helps to explain why yellow and orange are referred to as "warm colors."

Again, it is noticed upon viewing distant mountain ranges that the general effect is one of a bluish haze. The outline of the mountains is visible, but there is no definite differentiation of color until one comes nearer, when not only the different colors, but also the various tones of colors can be distinguished. These phenomena are more noticable if there is no sunshine.

Color contrast and harmony. In addition to the effect produced by adding one color to another, there is the effect produced by contrasting one color with another (Plate 4). If red, yellow, and blue are used as the basis for the color scheme, three secondary colors are obtained by combining two of these primary colors. Red and yellow produce orange; yellow and blue produce green; while blue and red produce violet. The secondary colors likewise may be combined to form tertiary combinations, and these may again form others. With such a variety of colors to contend with, it is reasonable to suppose that certain combinations will harmonize while others will clash.

The interest of the dentist is mainly in those colors that harmonize. Color harmony may be of two kinds, harmony of analogy and of contrast. This phase of the color problem is also of special importance to the complete denture prosthetist, who must harmonize the artificial dentures with the predominating colors of each patient. When there are two tones of one color, such as orange and red, there is harmony of analogy because there is a common ingredient in both, i.e., red. However, it is possible to have harmony with neither color having a common ingredient. This is a harmony of contrast exemplified by the colors of red and green, red being a primary and green a combination of the other two primaries, yellow and blue. Another factor of importance to the dentist is the type of light available and the effect of the different colored lights on color selection and reproduction. A light may come from a concentrated source, as from a focused lamp, or it may come from a large luminous body, such as the sun. The former type of light will cast a sharp, well-defined shadow of an object, while the latter type of light, such as daylight, will cast a shadow of an indefinite, fading outline. This may explain some of the phenomena that confront a dentist in his practice. A porcelain inlay viewed in daylight always looks better than under a focused light, because with the latter the shadows are sharper.

Effect of light on color. In addition to the intensity of the light it is advisable to determine the *color* of the *light used* at the time a color is selected. Normal daylight varies in its hue, depending on the time of day. The early morning rays are of a pinkish tint; the sun at high noon sends white rays; while near the horizon it emits rays of an orange-red hue. A cloudy day usually casts purplish rays. The light from a skylight is bluish white, while that from an electric arc varies from white to bluish white and violet. An incandescent lamp of normal brilliancy gives yellow light, but, when the voltage is low, it turns orange.

In selecting colors, therefore, the type of light and the time of day must be taken into account. There is also a change in the color effect when the rays of one color fall upon another. This fact should call attention to the influence that the color of the curtains and walls may have on color determination and selection.

Simultaneous contrast. Another effect which must be taken into consideration during color selection is that obtained by simultaneous contrast (Plate 5). As will be observed, some colors show to better advantage on a black background; others show better on a gray, while all look good on white. The juxtaposition of black has the effect of intensifying the luminosity of the colors; gray subdues and neutralizes them; while white deepens their tone. The practical value of this principle is evident when determining the tone of a basic color in a natural tooth.

Color in natural teeth

The next consideration is the color value found in natural teeth. It is essential that a thorough study of the predominating colors be made before any attempt is made at matching with shade guides. The color of natural teeth is not uniformly of a single hue or purity value. Even in the same individual there exists a marked difference of intensity not only between the different teeth, but even in the same tooth, where there is a variation of tint, shade, or intensity. It is of utmost importance to be able to discern color *pigmentation* and color *effect,* as well as their mutual interdependence. While it is true that the pigment of a tooth determines its basic color, there are other factors involved: the thickness and density of dentin; the thickness and distribution of enamel; the pulp size and proximity to labial surface; environment darkness, depth of oral cavity, the color and mobility of the lips; abrasion; stains; external surface texture and contour; position in arch; intensity and color of light falling upon the tooth.

Upon careful study of natural teeth one is able to distinguish the following basic colors: yellow, orange, and yellows with a greenish or a brownish tinge; in the enamel or overlying colors there may be blue or gray with a mirage effect toward the yellow. The color of the incisal enamel is not due to pigmentation so much as it is to the reaction of a translucent substance to light, subject to the laws of physics.

Selection of color for prosthetic restorations

Color distribution in teeth. The first consideration in the selection of colors is the variation of hues in the various sections of the tooth. The gingival third is usually some tone of orange or yellow; the incisal one-third is either a blue or a gray; while the middle section may be an overlapping of both colors. The distribution of these colors is not always uniform, at least the color effects are not. For this reason it is advisable to draw a diagram of the tooth (Fig. 25-1, *A*) and divide it into squares, noting how far the gingival color extends incisally on the labial and on the labioproximal line angles; this record will assist one later when applying the porcelain.

Determination of color. A difficulty usually encountered in color perception is the interference from surrounding colors. To eliminate this influence, a piece of neutral gray paper with an opening cut in it should be placed over the teeth. The colors may then be more accurately determined. Many dentists have had failures in the selection of colors for inlays because they determined the shade in the same manner that they make a selection for a complete porcelain crown or a denture, i.e., from a standard tooth guide without first determining the basic and the overlying colors. Others have had difficulty because they selected a basic color and proceeded to bake the inlay with the one color. This will usually result in partial success only, because the color of a natural tooth varies from the gingival to

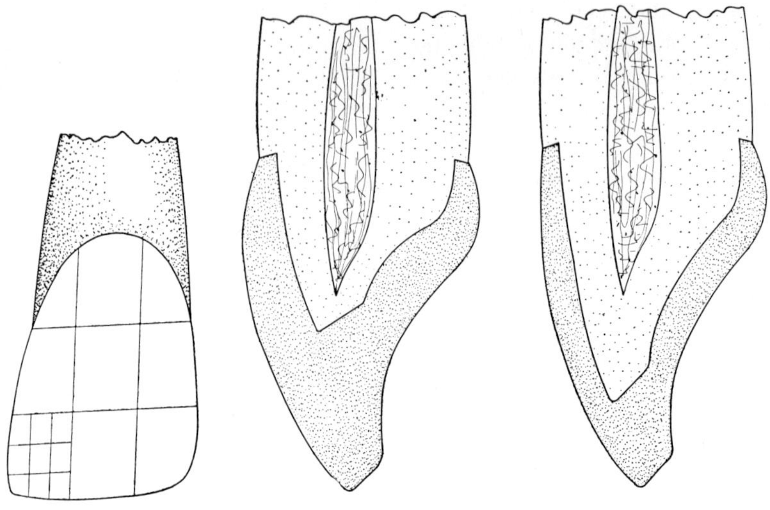

Fig. 25-1. A, Chart to indicate selection of color and its intensity and distribution. **B,** Although correct lines of body and enamels are same, color effect will be different because of variation in thickness of labial surfaces of porcelain.

the incisal areas. It is well to remember also that in different locations on the labial or buccal the thickness of the enamel varies. In other words, a labial inlay in the gingival region would be simulated by a thin *overlying* color of blue or yellowish gray and a *deep layer* of basic color. Inasmuch as dentin is slightly translucent and its surface, microscopically, is not smooth (Fig. 4-1), the underlying porcelain color must present an unglazed surface of the same characteristic texture. Similarly, a labial inlay in the incisal half of a tooth could have a thinner but more intense layer of basic color with a thicker overlying enamel color. Again, a similar inlay in a bicuspid would need an intensified enamel-colored porcelain, inasmuch as the enamel in a natural bicuspid is very thick in the occlusal half.

For the same reasons, when selecting colors for a jacket crown, it is necessary to determine the basic hue and its distribution and intensity of tone. This latter condition can be determined through a study of the effects produced by firing porcelains of certain hues in varying thicknesses. To illustrate: look through one sheet of amber-colored glass; it has a certain hue, a certain luminosity. By superimposing another similar sheet of glass and looking through both, the hue remains pure, but its effect is a deeper tone; a third sheet will further accentuate the effect. The same is true of porcelains. The basic hue may be correct, but, unless it is applied and fired in the proper thickness, the depth of the hue will not harmonize with the tooth. As a rule, it is necessary to intensify the basic hue of a porcelain veneer crown. The dentin of a natural tooth has normal fullness, which gives the effect of a certain luminosity. Were it possible to set the finished porcelain crown without interposing cement, the object would be to reproduce the natural tone of the basic hue; as it is, the cement not only excludes the color of the dentin, but it also absorbs much of the transmitted light striking the crown.

Effect of tooth preparation on color. The gingivoincisal length of the tooth preparation in relation to the gingivoincisal length of the finished crown also has an influence on color selection and reproduction (Fig. 25-2, *B*).

Effect of light on color. Frequently the dentist determines and selects the proper color, but does not analyze the effect of light upon it. If the tooth has an irregular or a marked surface, it may influence the dentist in selecting a porcelain of a darker shade. It is well in selecting colors to view the tooth from all angles in order to study the reflection of light, the influence of the lips in excluding light, the position of the lips in repose and in laughter. It is necessary to obtain a close view, as well as one several feet distant. If there exists any doubt as to the proper color to use or the proper thickness of the various colors, veneer shade guides of several combinations and thicknesses should be constructed. These, when fired and tabulated, will prove of great help for subsequent doubtful cases. Such an individualized, custom-made shade guide will prove extremely valuable not only in the selection and reproduction of tooth colors in the complete porcelain veneer crown, but even more so in color determination for porcelain fused to metal crowns. They can be constructed quickly and, in time, constitute a valuable color guide.

Enamel color. It is doubtful whether enamel possesses any color pigment. Even in those cases in which it appears quite blue or gray, upon illuminating it from the lingual aspect, it is found to be quite translucent, even bordering on transparency. The depth of the oral cavity and the width of the lip line have an important bearing on the incisal color effect. It is probable that the size, arrangement, and shape of the enamel rods may also have some bearing on the color effect.

REPRODUCING COLORS IN PORCELAIN

The dentist should not only have an understanding of color and be able to recognize its various qualities, but should also be able to reproduce the needed color in porcelain. As stated previously, colors are produced by various mesmeric pigmented porcelains or by superimposing one pigmented layer of porcelain upon another. By increasing or decreasing the thickness of different layers, various effects may be produced with two pigments. If the overlying layer is too thin, it becomes translucent to a degree that the basic color reflection destroys the effect of the enamel color; if the basic color is too deep it also may affect the desired color scheme.

For reproducing the desired color in inlays, several ways have been suggested and used. Some dentists apply the various shades in layers; others build the inlay in sections; some mix their colors before applying; while still others use one basic color and control the desired shade by the color of cement used. The layer method is preferable. By its use the location and amount can be accurately controlled and the natural gradations of hue obtained. Each tone will maintain its individuality and yet they will blend into a harmonious blend.

Influence of cement on color

The influence of cement on the color of porcelain is greater in the inlay than in the crown. When light is incident upon the surface of an inlay, its angle of reflection may permit its transmission. Should the direction be such as to encounter cement, a shadow results. A transparent cement would help solve to a degree this difficulty; recent efforts along this line are encouraging, but they are still in the experimental stages.

Although the color of cement influences that of the crown, its effect is not very pronounced, except when the labial wall of porcelain is too thin or too thick (Fig. 25-2). The reproduction of colors in the porcelain veneer (jacket) crown is dependent upon several factors. One of the important ones is a correct tooth prepara-

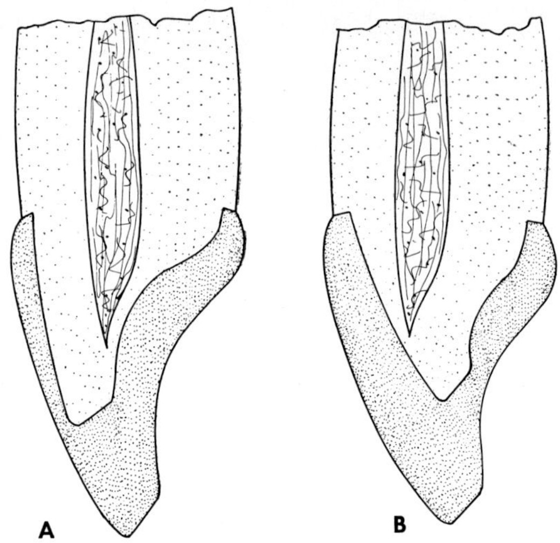

Fig. 25-2. Cement color will show through crown on left; thick layer of porcelain on right crown will produce different color effect.

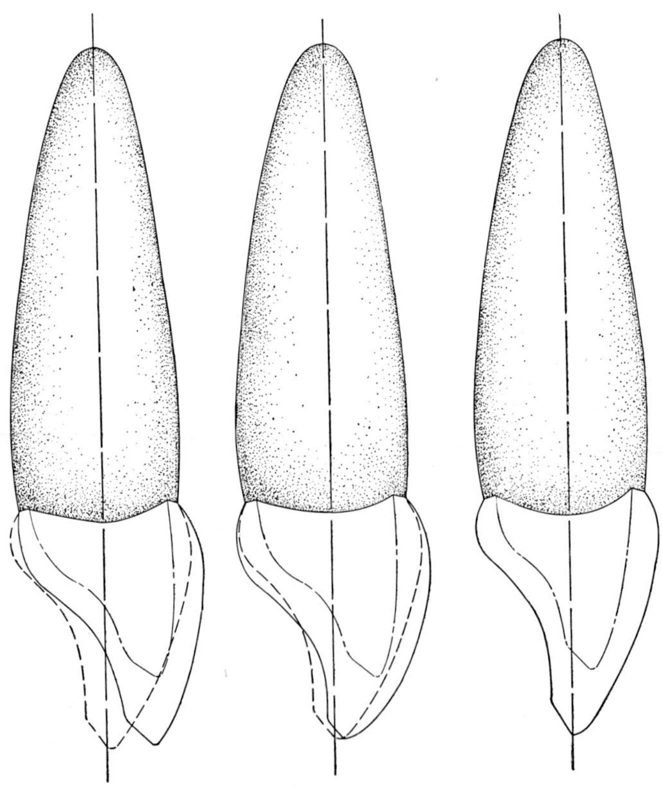

Fig. 25-3. Crowns on left were built too far labially due to improper preparation of teeth; crown on right, labial contour in proper alignment with proximating teeth.

tion (Fig. 25-3); another is the proper distribution of the basic and the overlying porcelains, generally known as the gingival or body colors and the incisal or enamel colors.

Distribution of porcelain

In addition to correct distribution of colors, the thicknesses of the two pigmented porcelains must be in proper proportion. The natural tooth color effects are usually reproduced in a crown: first, by placing a layer of the predominating body color porcelain in the gingival third; and second, by restoring the incisal third usually in one color, the enamel. These two colors, one extending incisally and the other gingivally, overlap each other in the middle third of the tooth and give the desired blended color effect of a natural tooth (Fig. 25-4, *A*). When it is necessary to shorten the incisal length of a finished crown, the shaded color effect area appears to locate incisally.

Surface texture of porcelain

The texture of the porcelain surface influences the shade of a porcelain veneer (jacket) crown. Given two crowns of identical hues, distribution, and degree of firing, it is a simple matter to deepen the hue value of one by placing grooves or facets in its labial surface; this may be done with stones or a diamond point and by refiring the restoration.

Position and shape of tooth

A tooth in the anterior part of the mouth appears lighter than one in the bicuspid or molar region, due to the angle of the reflected light. The degree of mesiodistal convexity also influences the color effect.

There are times when three colors of porcelain are used, in which event the distribution may be made as shown in Fig. 25-4, *B*. The intermediate zone consists of a mixture of the gingival and incisal porcelains.

Use of stains and stained porcelain

In a crown having the correct basic gingival and incisal colors, the color of the facing or the tooth may be modified in two ways: first, by the use of stains; second, by the use of stained porcelain. The former is a true mineral stain, while the latter is porcelain of a modified composition and a lower fusing range than that with which the crown was built, except that a pigment has been added to it to

A

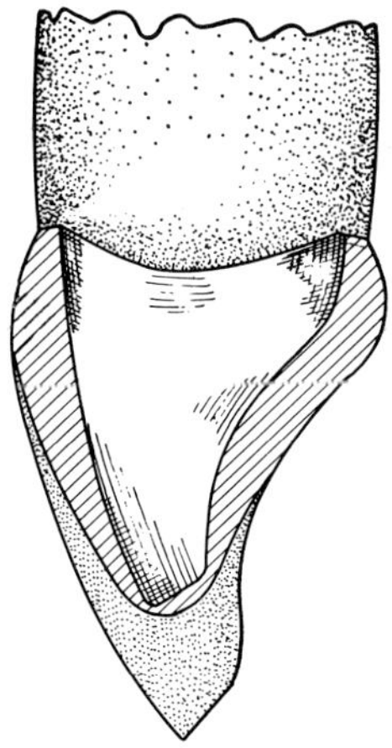

B

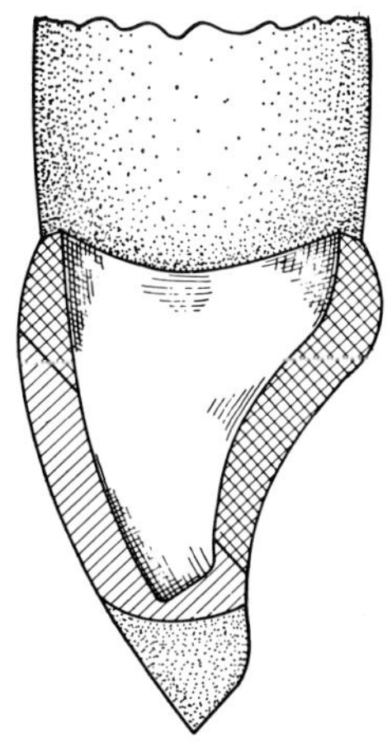

Fig. 25-4. A, Usual distribution of body and enamel-colored porcelain. **B,** Three colors of porcelain may be distributed as shown.

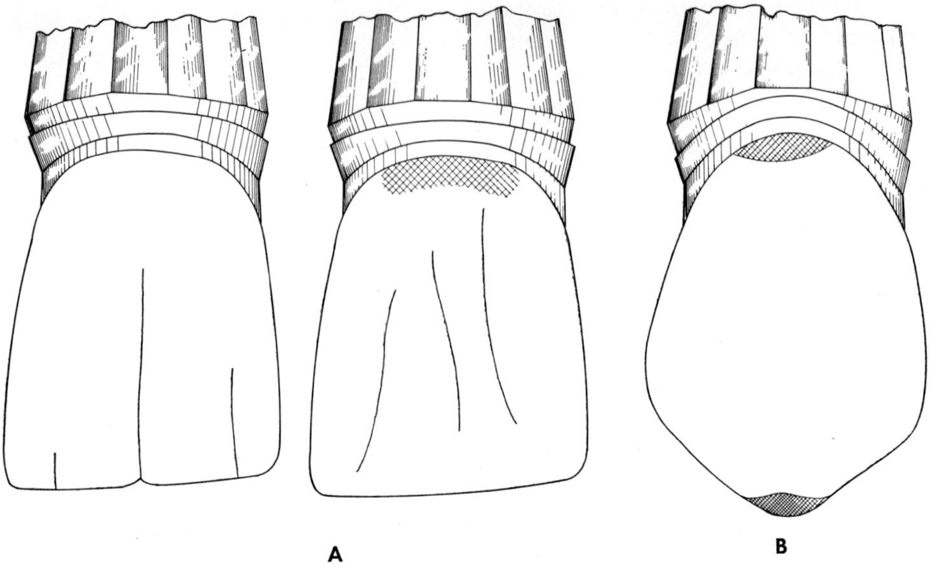

Fig. 25-5. A, Enamel checks and fissures simulated by using stains or stained porcelain. **B,** Enamel defects and stains simulated by using stained or translucent porcelain.

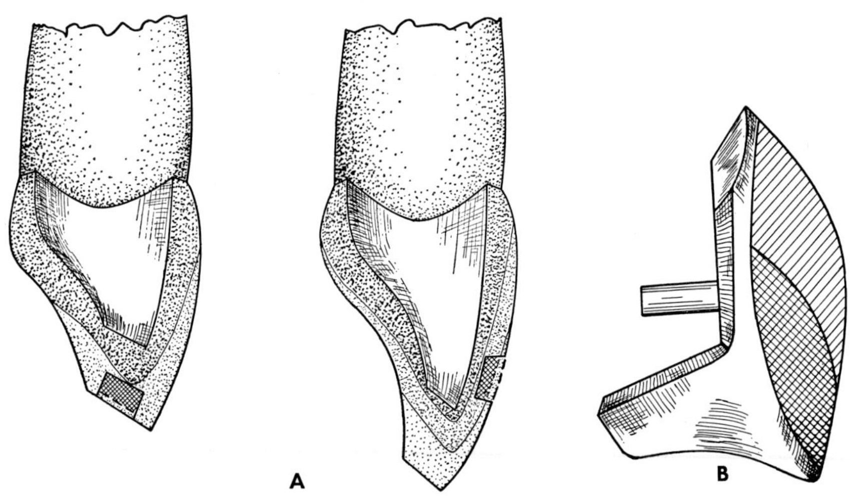

Fig. 25-6. A, Method of preparing crowns for application of stained porcelain to incisal or labial surfaces. **B,** Method used to change or modify shade of a porcelain pontic.

give the desired depth of stain. The judicious use of stains or stained porcelains will result in artistic effects not attainable in any other manner. Teeth may be darkened or lightened; labioenamel checks, cervical stains (Fig. 25-5, *A*), or incisal stains may also be effectively reproduced (Fig. 25-5, *B*). The pale bluish effect may also be obtained by the proper application of stains at the incisal (Fig. 25-5, *B*).

Although similar results may be obtained by using stained porcelain, certain preliminary procedures are necessary.

To reproduce an enamel check, a pencil line of the desired length and depth is scratched on the labial surface of the crown or facing with a diamond point. The scratch is filled with a small amount of lower fusing stained porcelain, the excess being carefully brushed away, and the added porcelain is fired to a glaze.

To reproduce a dark stained surface frequently seen along the incisal edge of the anterior teeth, a groove is first cut mesiodistally into the incisal surface of the porcelain crown to the desired width and to a depth of about 0.25 mm. This is filled with the stained porcelain of the desired color and glazed (Fig. 25-6, *A*). To obtain a more natural effect, stained porcelain is usually covered with a thin layer of the incisal colored porcelain; after glazing the effect is more natural since the stain appears embedded in dentin rather that superficially applied.

The use of mineral stains is contraindicated on the incisal edge or on those surfaces that may be exposed to attrition; in such locations mineral stains are worn away in a relatively short time.

If neither mineral stains nor the stained porcelains are available for modifying or changing the color of a facing or crown, the labial surface is ground down until only a basic layer of porcelain remains. Using this as a foundation, new porcelains, usually of a lower fusing range but of the proper basic and incisal colors, are applied and fused; in this way a new color is developed in the facing or crown (Fig. 25-6, *B*).

Restoring glazed surface

Whenever it is necessary to grind a facing or a porcelain crown to alter its contour, it is imperative that the surface be reglazed in order that its true color effect be restored and that a hygienic surface be assured.

A glaze may be restored to a ground porcelain surface in one of three ways: First, the facing or crown, having been thoroughly cleansed, may be replaced in the muffle and brought to a glaze temperature. The danger of such a procedure lies in the possibility of the porcelain restoration rounding its margins, thus losing its fit. Furthermore, by subjecting a facing or crown to a second glazing temperature, the color of the porcelain is likely to be diluted.

A second method for restoring the glaze surface of a porcelain crown consists in the application of a thin layer of porcelain, which will glaze at a lower temperature than the crown or facing, thus eliminating the possibility of rounded edges or color changes.

The third method, usually employed, is the application of dental glazes. Whereas the lower fusing porcelain used in the second method is of the same color as the facing or the crown, dental glazes are transparent and colorless. A dental glaze also fuses at a lower temperature than the porcelain surface to which it is applied. While a glaze is used as a thin film and without any effect on the color, low-fusing porcelain must usually be applied in bulk and hence may alter the shade of the facing or crowns. To be satisfactory, a dental glaze must have approximately the same coefficient of expansion and contraction as the porcelain to which it is applied; otherwise, the surface will appear crazed upon cooling.

In every instance in which a crown surface is to be reglazed by any one of the three methods, certain precautions must be taken: first, that the surface is absolutely clean of all debris; second, that the surface has been first polished smooth; and third, that all the little pores and openings in the porcelain crown or facing first have been filled with compatible dry porcelain powder or glaze before the final glazing is done.

Grinding porcelain. One precaution should be observed in grinding porcelain with an abrasive stone; contamination of the porcelain with grinding debris should be avoided. This may be done by using only new, clean stones for the grinding. When the grinding is performed dry, it should be done under a blast of compressed air so that all loose particles may be immediately blown clear of the porcelain. The other and better method of avoiding contamination is to hold the porcelain and the stone under water while grinding. "Grinding semiwet" will produce a paste consisting of particles of porcelain, abrasive crystals, and the bonding material of the stone; once this paste works into the pores of the porcelain, it is almost impossible to remove it, except in an ultrasonic cleaning device.

Glazing technic. Several manufactured glazes are available to the dental profession. Each is satisfactory, provided the instructions of the manufacturer are carefully observed.[3] (See Chapters 26 and 35.)

Additional methods of altering the contour or the color of teeth, together with additional technics for reglazing, may be found in the standard texts.[4, 5]

Usually it is simpler to match the correct color in manufactured bridge facings than in crowns built up entirely from porcelain powders. Manufactured bridge facings are available that correspond to the colors found in the shade guides of the manufacturer. When using such facings, it is only ncessary that the dentist be able to recognize the basic gingival and incisal predominating colors in the natural teeth and to relate them correctly with the colors in the shade guide. If this is accurately done, very little color difficulty should be experienced. Certain precautions, however, must be observed relative to the backing, soldering, or cementing of the facings; if disregarded, a color modification may occur to alter the original selection of the facing.

When using manufactured teeth, either for crown or bridge restorations, their selection should be correct from the standpoint not only of color but also of size and form. A size should be selected that requires very little grinding or modification for its use; the form should correspond with the characteristic type of the arch and face of the patient.

The technic and procedures involved in the application and firing of porcelain are discussed more fully in Chapter 34, which deals with the construction of porcelain veneer crowns.

At this time attention is called to the relationship that exists between optical illusions and restorative dentistry, whether it be a single porcelain veneer crown or a unit of a fixed partial denture. Blancheri[6] offers the following excellent observations and illustrations in explaining this relationship.

Visual perception is the response of the eye to the following factors:

1. Light
2. Movement
3. Outline form
4. Surface form
5. Color

The eye is, first of all, sensitive to light but tires (fatigues) very rapidly to continued stimulus. Light reflection is of importance but is more properly discussed under surface form.

Sensitivity to movement of an object is next in order but is of little significance in this discussion.

The eye is very sensitive to outline form. This is easily understood by remembering how easily a silhouette is recognized. Surely each of us has had the experience of watching a carnival artist cut out black paper silhouettes which were immediately recognized. The value of this principle was understood by military authorities in the recent conflict when thousands of airplane pilots and observers were trained to recognize aircraft by silhouette alone. This is a principle which has been relatively neglected in dentistry and yet is particularly true regarding teeth, as perception of outline form is differentiation of very unlike things: that is, the tooth, relatively white in color, surrounded gingivally by the gingival tissue, interproximally by the dark and usually stained interproximal contacts, and incisally by the shadow of the oral cavity. This shadow is very important in talking and smiling. It silhouettes the incisal edges.

The eye is understandably less sensitive to surface form of teeth as it involves the delicacy of binocular perspective of minute variations. However, surface form must not be disregarded as it its easily controlled and is responsible for light reflection. Control of light reflection is one of our most valuable tools, especially when enamel offers such an excellent reflecting surface.

Finally, the eye is less sensitive to color than is commonly supposed, particularly to the infinite and minute color variations found in teeth. This is stated, not to minimize the importance of correctly matching shades, but instead to emphasize other relatively neglected factors. It must also be remembered in selecting shades that the eye fatigues very rapidly to color stimulus. First impressions are more accurate. It is much better to compare shade samples with teeth in five second glances than to compare steadily for sixty or even thirty seconds.

Not only is the eye sensitive to stimuli but it is also suceptible to trickery. We are well aware of the trickery practiced by the sleight-of-hand artist; we are less aware of the trickery of lines and angles. [This is demonstrated in Figs. 25-7 to 25-9.]

The main principles to be learned from these examples [Figs. 25-7 to 25-9] are that vertical lines accent height—horizontal lines accent width—shadows add depth—angles influence the lines they intersect. Also remember that curved surfaces are softer, more pleasing than harsh angles.

In applying these principles to everyday dental problems, let us first consider the problem of restoring a missing central where the space is

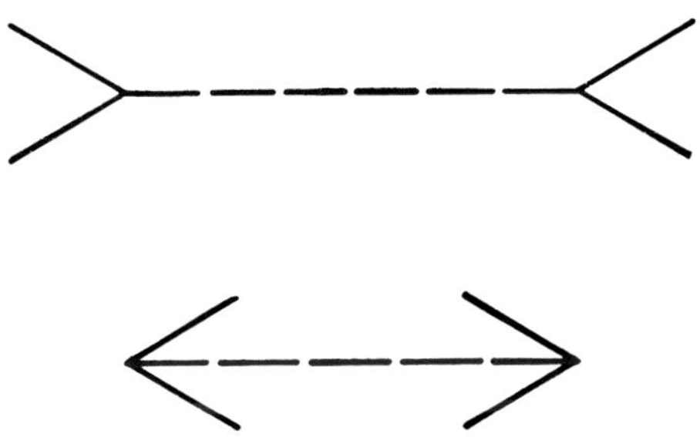

A

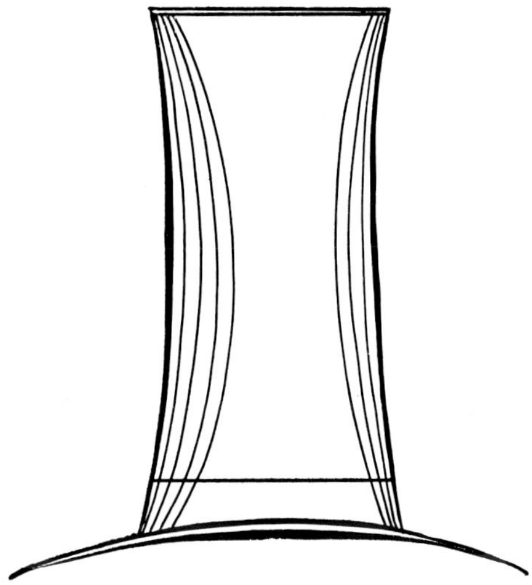

B

Fig. 25-7. A, Both horizontal lines are same length. **B,** Brim of hat is as wide as hat is tall. (Courtesy R. L. Blancheri.)

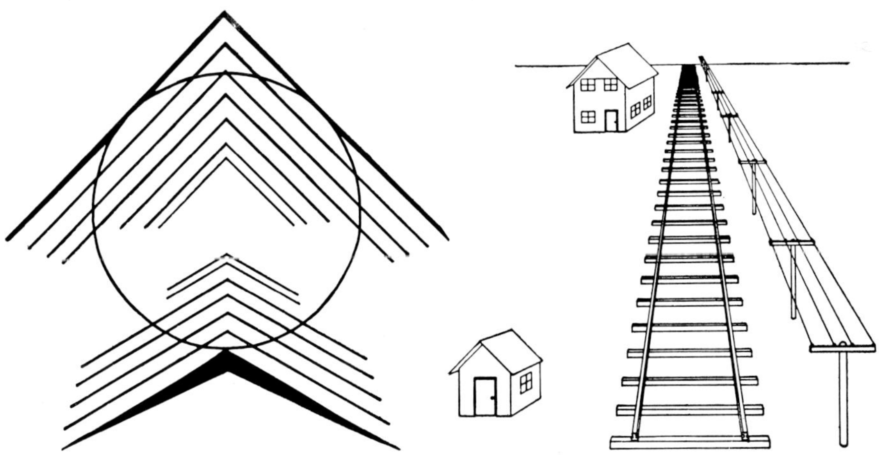

A B

Fig. 25-8. A, Circle is true circle. **B,** Both houses are exactly same size. (Courtesy R. L. Blancheri.)

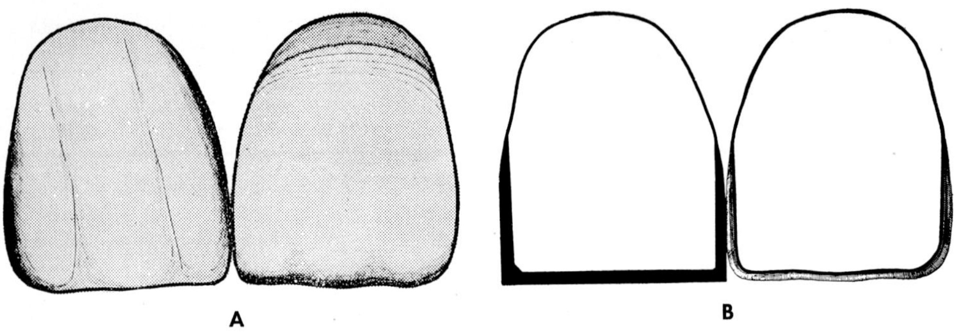

Fig. 25-9. A, Both teeth are same width and length. **B,** Careful contouring of partial veneer preparation minimizes objectionable display of gold. (Courtesy R. L. Blancheri.)

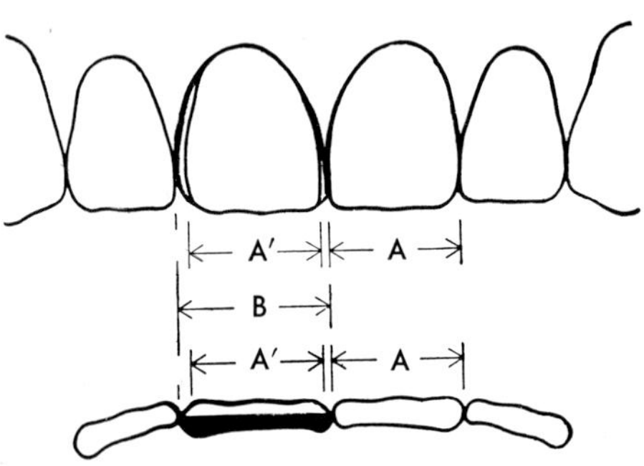

Fig. 25-10. A, Width of remaining central incisor. **A′,** Superimposed pattern of remaining central incisor. **B,** Space originally available. (Courtesy R. L. Blancheri.)

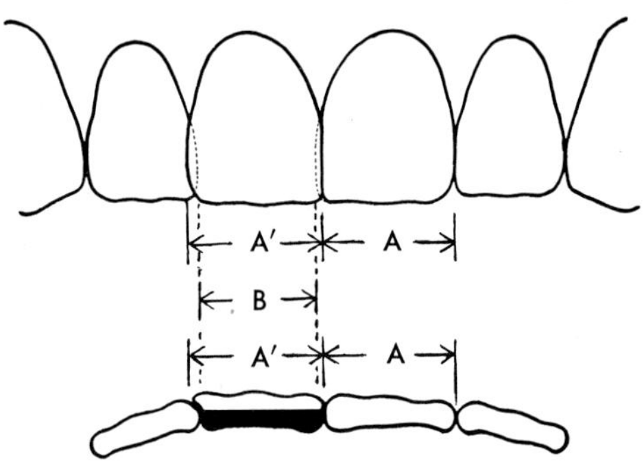

Fig. 25-11. A, Final width of remaining central incisor. **A′,** Superimposed pattern of remaining central incisor. **B,** Space to be filled (total width of porcelain). (Courtesy R. L. Blancheri.)

wider, narrower, or longer than the remaining central. If the space is wider [Fig. 25-10] a very practical solution is to use a replacement wide enough to fill the space. The porcelain is kept as thick labio-lingually as possible and the contact point is kept as far lingually as possible. On the labial surface, we will mentally superimpose the labial outline form of the remaining central and by grinding the mesial and distal surfaces (mostly on the distal surface) we will taper the facing from the contact area to the superimposed labial outline form. The new mesial and distal surfaces formed by grinding should be glazed and stained to lend depth. By greying these edges they appear indistinct and fade away. Also, remembering that darker shades appear smaller and lighter shades appear larger, it would be wise to use a shade slightly darker than the natural central. At the time of grinding the mesial and distal surfaces to shape the new outline form, the labial surface form of the remaining central is closely copied, with particular attention being paid to duplicating any ridges and depressions that will reflect light. It is not the presence of these ridges and grooves per se that gives individual character to a tooth; it is the individual pattern of light reflection that determines tooth character.

To reverse the application, let us assume the same missing tooth but with a space narrower than the remaining central [Fig. 25-11]. First the remaining tooth may be narrowed by slightly reducing the mesial surface. A facing wider than the space is chosen and the labial outline form and surface form of the remaining central is duplicated as nearly as possible, again keeping in mind factors of light reflection. The mesial and distal surfaces are then ground from the lingual labially, taking care to not alter the labial outline, until the facing fits the space, resorting to overlapping if necessary.

Where excessive ridge resorption presents the problem of requiring a facing much longer than the tooth to be matched [Fig. 25-12, A], it is again desirable to superimpose the outline form of the remaining central and grind in a very definite

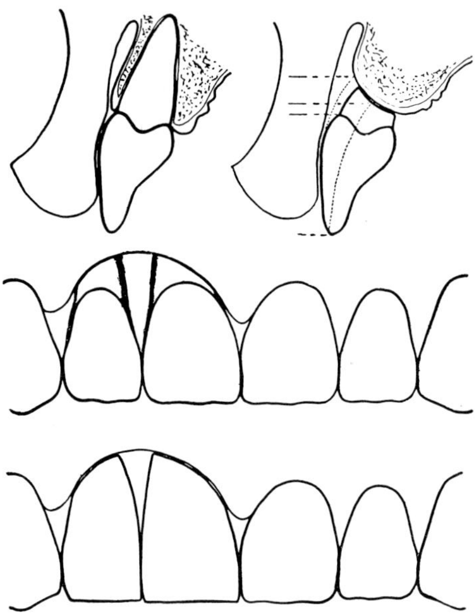

Fig. 25-12. Excessive resorption of ridge necessitating longer crown or facing. Normal outline form superimposed. Cementoenamel line ground. (Courtesy R. L. Blancheri.)

cemento-enamel junction line [Fig. 25-12, *B*]. Again copy the surface form as closely as possible, also keeping in mind the correct position in the arch. The root position may then be sloped back to contact the ridge [Fig. 25-12, *A*], glazed and stained a yellowish color to simulate an area of gingival recession. A faint deepening of the color toward the apex of the root form, as well as a definite demarcation line at the cemento-enamel junction, heightens the illusion. I prefer this method to the addition of any type of pink stain or material in an attempt to match gum tissue.

The same principles are applied to restoring bicuspids except, that instead of superimposing the labial outline form, the portion of the buccal surface between the mesio-buccal line angle and the buccal height of contour is copied [Figs. 25-13 and 25-14].

Let us assume an upper right second bicuspid is missing and the space is wider than the first bicuspid [Fig. 25-13]. A replacement is chosen which is wide enough to fill the entire space and by grinding the distal half of the buccal surface, the height of buccal contour is moved mesially until the mesial half of the buccal surface approximates that of the first bicuspid.

Assuming the same missing tooth but with a space too narrow for a full pontic, the same prin-

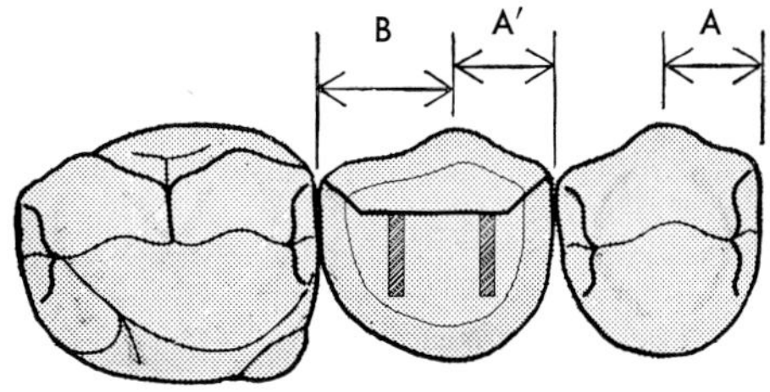

Fig. 25-13. A, Width of first bicuspid from mesial surface to height of buccal contour. **A′,** Width of pontic from mesial surface to height of buccal contour. **B,** Width of distal half of pontic (wider than mesial half). (Courtesy R. L. Blancheri.)

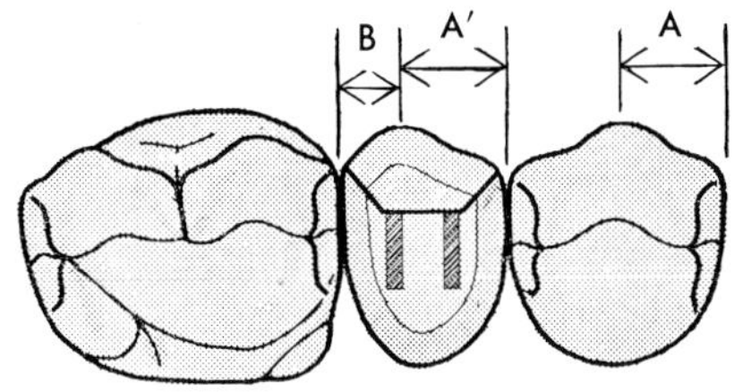

Fig. 25-14. A, Width of first bicuspid from mesial surface to height of buccal contour. **A′,** Width of pontic from mesial surface to height of buccal contour. **B,** Width of distal half of pontic (narrower than mesial half). (Courtesy R. L. Blancheri.)

ciple is applied [Fig. 25-14]. A pontic is chosen and ground so the buccal form from the mesiobuccal angle to the height of buccal contour approximates that of the first bicuspid. This leaves the distal half much narrower than the mesial half but, inasmuch as this distal plane is not visible during average mouth movements, the total effect is very favorable.

These basic applications can be altered to suit practically any variation found in the mouth.*

*From Blancheri, R. L.: Optical illusions and cosmetic grinding, Rev. de Assoc. Dent. Mexicana 8:103, 1950.

SELECTED REFERENCES

1. Crew, H.: General physics, ed. 3, New York, 1918, The Macmillan Co., chap. 12.
2. Snow, B. E., and Froehlich, H. B.: The theory and practice of color, Chicago, 1920, The Prang Co., p. 20.
3. Columbus Dental Mfg. Co.: The art of staining and glazing artificial teeth, Columbus, Ohio, 1936.
4. Peyton, F. A., and others: Restorative dental

materials, ed. 3, St. Louis, 1968, The C. V. Mosby Co.
5. Skinner, E. W., and Phillips, R. W.: The science of dental materials, Philadelphia, 1967, W. B. Saunders Co.
6. Blancheri, R. L.: Optical illusions and cosmetic grinding, Rev. de Assoc. Dent. Mexicana **8**:103, 1950.

GENERAL REFERENCES

Berger, C. C.: Control of color of crowns for pulpless anterior teeth, J. Prosth. Dent. **19**(1): 58-59, 1968.

Gill, J. R.: Color selection—its distribution and interpretation, J.A.D.A. **40**:539, 1950.

Heilbrun, G.: Problem of taking shades, Illinois D. J. **31**:249, 1962.

Katz, S. R.: Aesthetics in ceramics, J. Canadian Dent. Assn. **32**(4):224-230, 1966.

Pilkington, E. L.: Natural effects in porcelain, J.A.D.A. **17**:1290, 1930.

Pincus, C. L.: Esthetic variations in jacket crowns involving periodontal and other deformities, New York J. Dent. **24**:132, 1954.

Saklad, M. J.: Esthetic factors in selection of tooth form and color, Dent. Clin. N. Amer., March, 1959, pp. 231-252.

Tashjian, H. H.: Color problem in jacket crowns, J.A.D.A. **50**:193, 1955.

Thomas, J. E., Lacroix, R., and Villemot, J.: Color in ceramics, Ann. Odontostomat. **24**(5): 209-214, 1967.

Weinberg, L. A.: Esthetics and the gingivae in full coverage, J. Prosth. Dent. **10**:737, 1960.

Wheeler, R. C.: Complete crown form and the periodontium, J. Prosth. Dent. **11**:722, 1961.

Yock, D. H.: Porcelain jacket veneer crown preparation, Iowa D. J. **43**:267, 1957.

Chapter 26

Construction of complete porcelain veneer crowns, securing impression of preparation, constructing dies, and firing porcelain

IMPRESSION, DIE CONSTRUCTION

Securing impression of preparation. (This sequence follows Chapter 24.) After a shoulder has been developed, either in the natural tooth or by means of a supplementary casting, the impression in modeling compound and the copper band or a rubber base impression is taken as previously described.

An impression of the prepared coronal portion is then secured in one of the two copper bands which previously were fitted and filled with modeling compound. The compound is heated until it is thoroughly softened; then it is quickly dipped in hot water and centered over the preparation (Fig. 26-1, *A*).

The copper band is held lightly between the thumb and middle finger, leaving the index finger free. With the incisal end open, the band is carried rootwise until the gingival margin of the band passes the outer angle of the shoulder. While the band is being lowered over the preparation, the excess compound in the band is displaced through the open incisal end (Fig. 26-1, *B*). When the margin of the band passes the outer angle of the shoulder, the index finger is pressed against the modeling compound at the incisal end of the band. The band is then carried apically until the gingival marks previously placed and denoting the height of the crest of the gum margin are brought level with the gingival crest (Fig. 26-1, *C*).

The modeling compound is air-cooled to room temperature or is cooled with water and then is removed from the prepared tooth in a line parallel with the long axis of the preparation. At no time should the impression be rocked to facilitate its removal, as this will produce a distorted impression and die. The impression should be dried and examined for a possible undercut, an irregular or imperfect shoulder, or any other defects. If present, these should be corrected on the tooth and another impression taken. If the impression is accurate and satisfactory, it is dried and laid aside temporarily. This is Impression 1 (Fig. 26-1, *C*) and may be used for the construction of a temporary die; artificial stone or silicate cement is mixed and packed into it; such a die is available for use within 10 or 15 minutes (Fig. 26-2, *A* and *B*).

While the first die is hardening, the second copper band, which was previously fitted and filled with compound, is used to secure Impression 2 for the permanent amalgam die (Fig. 26-3).

At the same time, the shade of the

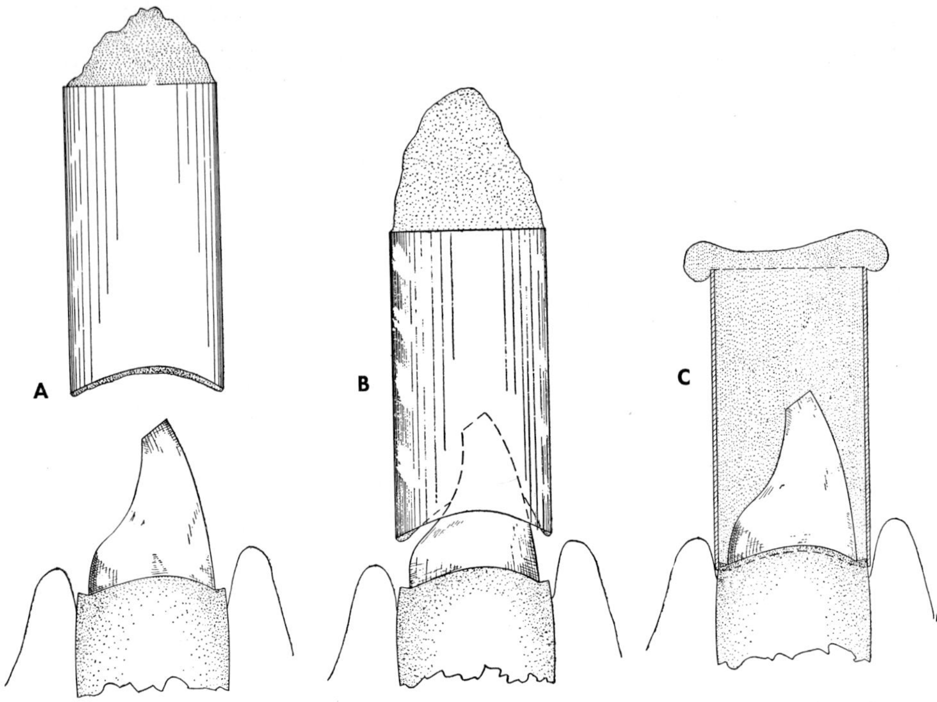

Fig. 26-1. Steps in securing modeling compound impressions of prepared tooth.

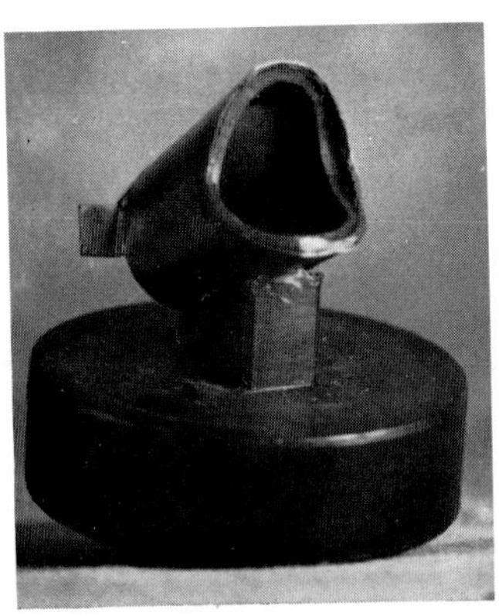

Fig. 26-2. First impression used for construction of permanent amalgam die.

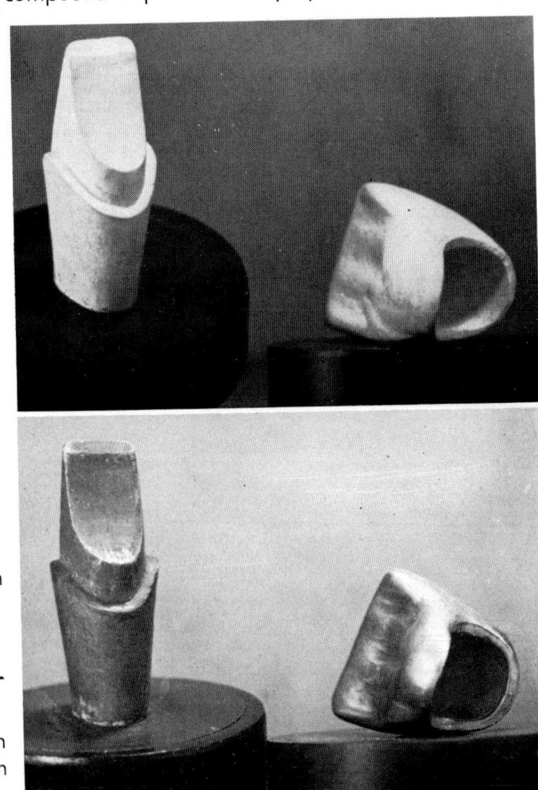

Fig. 26-3. A, Temporary acrylic resin crown made on cement die. **B,** Permanent amalgam die and low-fusing metal transfer crown.

tooth may be selected and a plaster, hydrocolloid, or rubber impression taken of the opposing arch.

The cement die made from Impression 1 is carefully removed from the band by immersing the impression in warm water (Fig. 26-3, *A*). Two matrices of 40-gauge tin foil are constructed on this die, using the technic described in Figs. 26-15 to 26-17. The gingival margins of each matrix are finished flush with the outer angle of the gingival shoulder.

One of the tin foil matrices is used to construct a temporary resin crown, which the patient wears during the interval in which the permanent crown is being constructed (Fig. 26-3, *A*). The temporary crown may be made either of silicate cement, low-fusing metal, or acrylic resin. Whichever material is used, the crown is finished flush with the outer angle of the gingival shoulder and then cemented on the prepared tooth with zinc-oxide–eugenol before the patient is dismissed.

On the second tin foil matrix, a low-fusing *transfer* metal crown is constructed with flat proximal surfaces and no contacts; this is used at the time the wax bite and the plaster impression are taken (Fig. 26-3, *B*).

This transfer metal crown comes away in the plaster impression and is used to seat the permanent amalgam die, which is later made from Impression 2. Since the development and improvement in the impression materials, technics have been presented in the literature that dispense with the individual modeling compound impression.

Taking impression and wax registration. The following technic, if carefully followed, will secure the proper relationship between the amalgam die and the adjoining and opposing teeth. The transfer

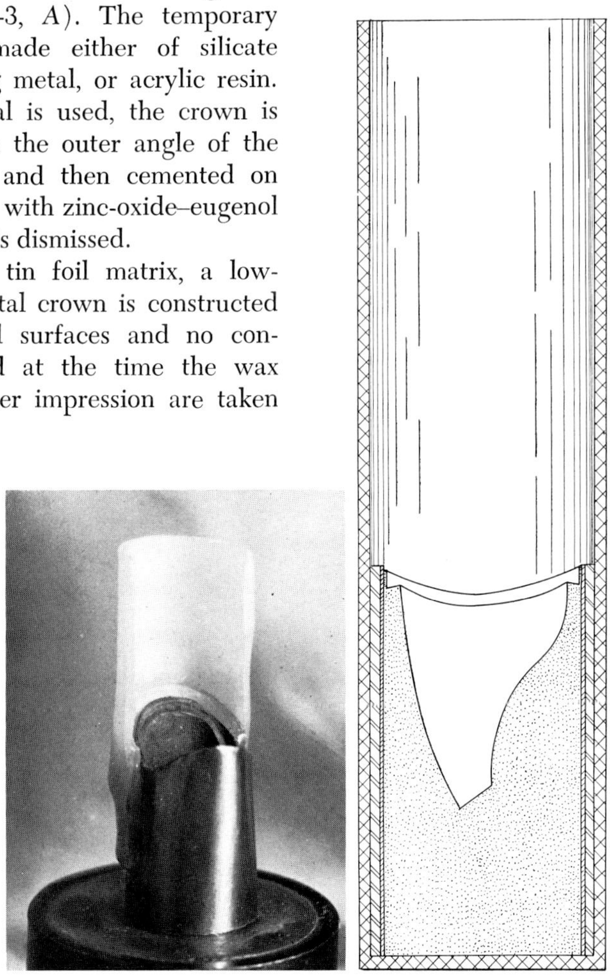

Fig. 26-4. Steps in preparing modeling compound impression to construct amalgam die. **A,** First layer of wax; **B,** second layer encircles first.

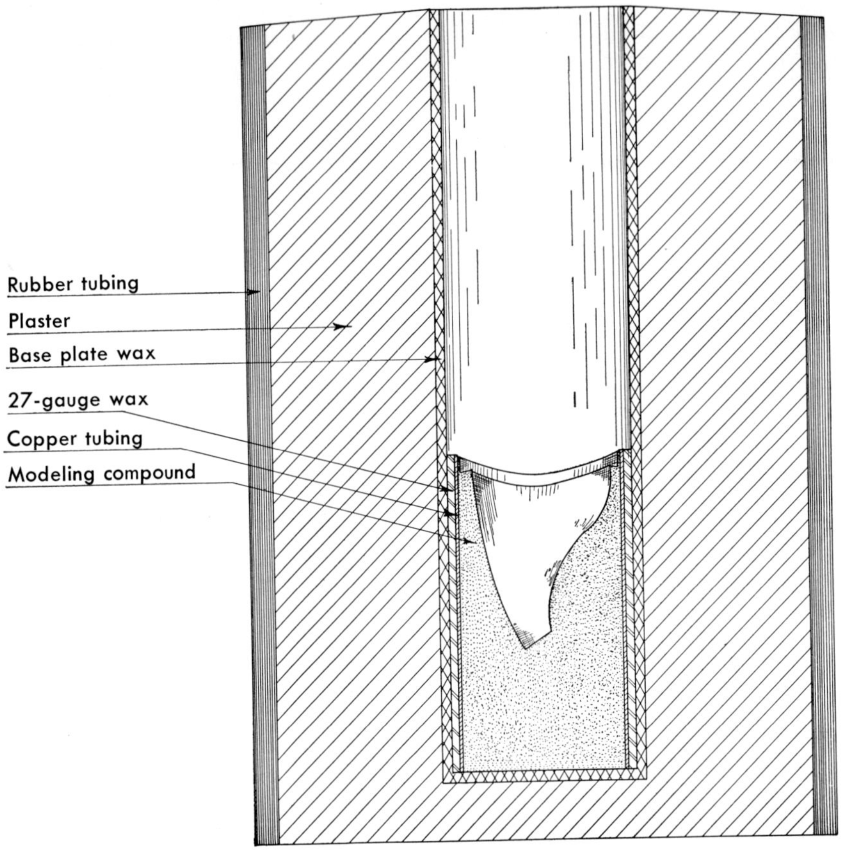

Fig. 26-5. Prepared impression embedded in wax bands and plaster before packing amalgam die.

crown of low-fusing metal is placed on the prepared tooth and the opposing arches are brought together to make certain that there is no occlusal interference.

A wax bite is then taken to record the mere imprints of the occlusal surfaces of the opposing arches. For this purpose, two pieces of pink base-plate wax are used; a piece of 40-gauge tin foil is placed between the two wax sheets, which are then thoroughly warmed and placed in the mouth; the bite is secured. By interposing the tin foil, the teeth are prevented from biting through the tin foil, since it is stretched over the cusps and into the fossae without tearing. Some dentists prefer to use a piece of gauze in place of the tin foil. An alternative method is the use of the Kerr Bite-Frame and Registration paste.

A plaster of Paris impression is then taken while the transfer metallic crown is in position on the prepared tooth. After the impression is removed and reassembled, the transfer metal crown is replaced in its correct position within the impression; it is then ready to receive the permanent amalgam die.

Construction of the amalgam die. Fig. 26-2 shows the copper band and impression removed and the excess compound trimmed from the incisal and gingival peripheries.

Before the impression is packed with amalgam, it is necessary to first wrap wax rootwise about ¾ inch beyond the band to permit the building of an amalgam root (Fig. 26-4, *B*).

The first layer of 27-gauge wax is

wrapped around the band, ending flush with its gingival margin. This, in turn, is encircled with one thickness of pink baseplate wax extending ¾ inch beyond the band (Fig. 26-4, *B*).

The doubly wrapped impression is now embedded in plaster held within a rubber tubing as shown in Fig. 26-5. Care must be exercised when embedding the impression to prevent the soft plaster from flowing inside the impression.

After the plaster has *set and cooled*, the impression is packed with amalgam.

Since the embedded compound impression lies at a low level, care must be exercised that no air is trapped in packing the amalgam and that it is well condensed against all surfaces and angles of the impression.

If silver amalgam is used, the die may be removed within 3 hours; copper amalgam should be permitted to set for at least 24 hours.

When sufficiently set, the impression, die, and plaster are removed from the rubber ring, and the plaster is cut away from the wax ring with its enclosed die. After removing the wax cylinders, the modeling compound is softened in warm water and separated from the die. The recovered amalgam die is shown in Fig. 26-6, *A*. In order that the die may be readily removed and replaced in its correct position in the working model, it is necessary that the root portion of the die be shaped so that it tapers apically. This should not be made cone-shaped, but should consist of a series of planes as illustrated in Fig. 26-6, *B*. It is also advisable to cut a key at the end of the root as shown in the illustration.

In order to facilitate the withdrawal later of the swaged platinum matrix from the die, that portion of the die lying apically of the gingival shoulder is trimmed in such a way that the first millimeter of the die has parallel walls, followed by a slight divergence extending 2 to 3 mm., after which the remaining portion of the root is given its tapered form. When the platinum matrix extends beyond the shoulder of such a die, the tendency for locking is eliminated and it may be easily removed.

The tapered amalgam die is then placed in the low-fusing metal crown embedded in the plaster impression of the upper arch.

If the technic has been carefully followed to this point, the die should seat exactly and in its correct relationship with the adjacent teeth.

When it is not feasible to take individual modeling compound impressions to construct amalgam dies, it is possible to use the rubber type impressions and to make removable dies of stone, metal, or

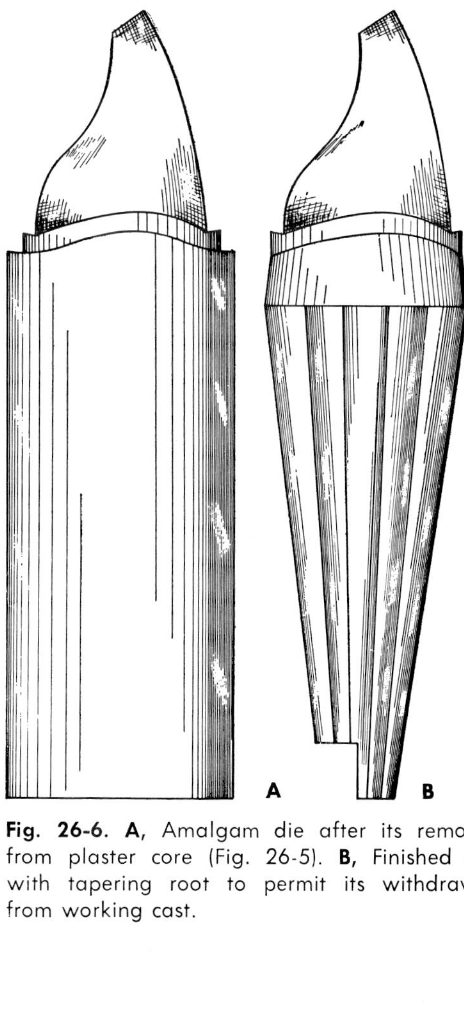

Fig. 26-6. A, Amalgam die after its removal from plaster core (Fig. 26-5). **B,** Finished die with tapering root to permit its withdrawal from working cast.

a high refractory investment. These dies are then made with dowels so that they can be readily removed from the working model.

Construction of the working model. A stone model is then made from the plaster impression containing the metal crown and the amalgam die. Preliminary to this, however, the two teeth in the impression, adjacent to the low-fusing metal crown, are first packed with amalgam so that they will retain their contour and contacts during the construction and baking of the porcelain crown.

Other technics suggest making the adjacent teeth also of low-fusing metal instead of amalgam. Either serves the purpose well and is better than if they were made entirely of plaster or artificial stone. For a more complete discussion of types and methods of constructing working models, see Chapters 28, 29, and 36.

After the adjacent teeth have been filled with amalgam or low-fusing metal, the balance of the impression, having been treated with a separating medium, is completed in artificial stone. To assure the easy removal of the amalgam die of the prepared tooth from the model, the root portion of the die should be thoroughly lubricated or have a tin matrix cone swaged around it before the artificial stone is poured.

An impression of the opposing arch is taken in plaster, hydrocolloid, or a rubber type impression material from which an occluding model is made either of low-fusing metal, artificial stone, or silver electroplated.

After separating the models, both upper and lower, they are related in the tin foil wax bite and mounted in an articulator.

When a single anterior tooth is restored, at least the six anterior teeth, as well as the two bicuspids on either side, should be included in the sectional impression; the lower impression should be similarly inclusive. When a bicuspid or a molar tooth is restored, it is advisable to include the entire upper and lower arches, as models made from such impressions enable the dentist more easily to construct a porcelain crown with cusps of proper height and of correctly inclined occlusal planes.

When the models have been mounted on the articulator, the wax registration is carefully removed after it has been softened in warm water. The temporary metal crown, having served its purpose, is also removed, leaving the amalgam die in its correct position and relationship in the working model.

The apical end of the amalgam die is located in the cast and a small opening is made through the labial or buccal surface, exposing the end of the die. By placing a blunt instrument underneath it, the die may be easily raised out of the model and carefully cleaned. The matrix is next adapted or swaged to the die.

MATRIX CONSTRUCTION

It is advisable for students and beginners to familiarize themselves with the technic of matrix construction by fabricating one or more matrices, using No. 40 tin foil instead of platinum. After the

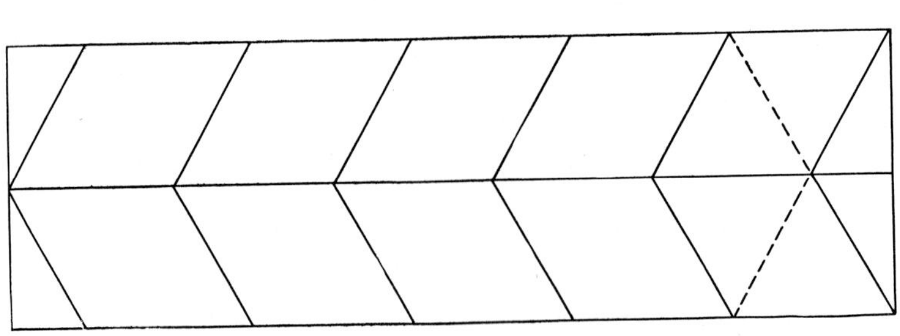

Fig. 26-7. Platinum foil cut into diamond shape to obtain maximum number of matrices.

details of construction have been mastered, a platinum matrix is made for the amalgam die using 0.001 in. platinum foil.

Before cutting the pattern for the matrix, it is necessary to decide where the tinner's joint is to be located. While generally placed on the lingual surface (Fig. 26-7 to 26-14), there are times when it is more desirable on the proximal surface (Figs. 26-15 to 26-17).

The technic first described places the joint on the lingual surface. A piece of platinum foil 0.001 inch thick is cut to a pattern made by opening up one of the experimental tin foil matrices. Another method is to cut the matrix material in diamond-shaped strips. A 1 dwt. piece of 0.001-inch foil will usually give nine or ten such pieces (Fig. 26-7).

Fig. 26-8, *A*, shows the first step in which a triangular piece of matrix is placed against the labial surface of the amalgam die with an extension of 2 to 3 mm. beyond the incisal and a similar extension beyond the gingival shoulder.

The matrix is next adapted roughly to the labial surface with the fingers at the time it is burnished to the gingival shoulder with burnishers (Fig. 26-8, *B*). Held in this position, two triangular pieces are

A

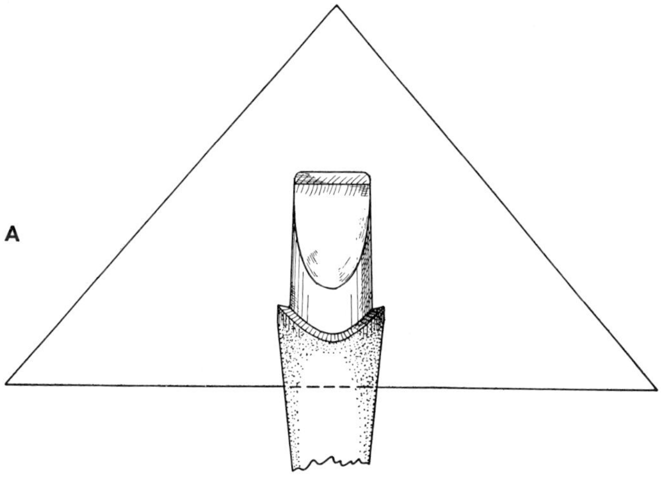

B

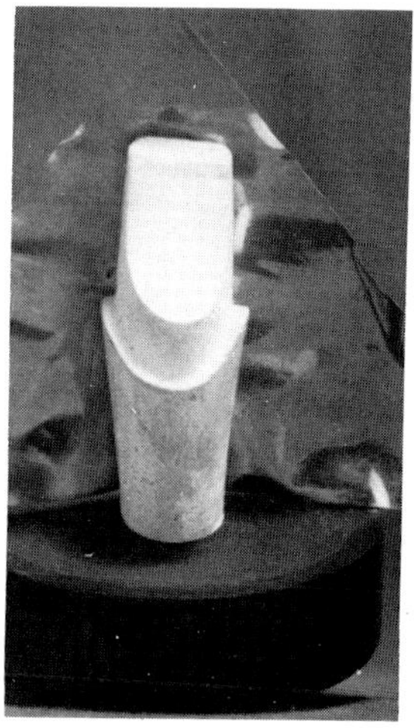

Fig. 26-8. First step in adapting platinum foil to amalgam die against labial surface.

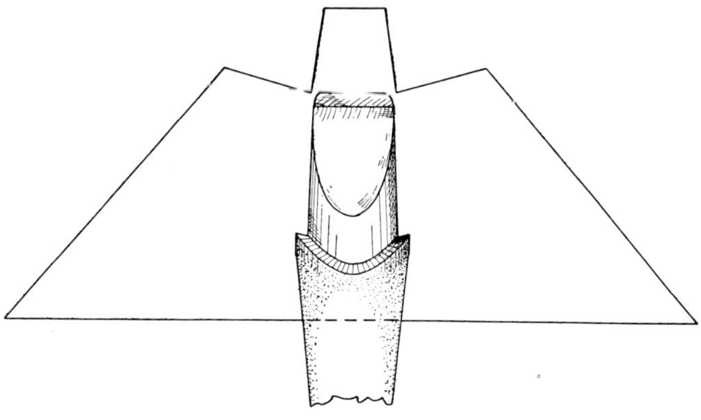

Fig. 26-9. Triangular pieces cut away at incisal edge of platinum.

removed mesially and distally at the incisal angles of the preparation as shown in Fig. 26-9.

The central portion of the matrix is then burnished over the incisal plane and extended 1 mm. onto the lingual surface, as shown in Fig. 26-10.

The two wings of the matrix are next brought around the proximal surfaces and carried into the lingual surface; these are first roughly adapted to the die with the fingers and then burnished more closely so that the matrix conforms exactly to the shoulder and to the axial and lingual surfaces.

When the two wings meet at the center of the lingual surface, they are bent at right angles to this surface, as shown in Fig. 26-11, *A*. The edges projecting at right angles to the lingual surface are now trimmed to a length of 2 mm. (Fig. 26-11, *B* and *C*).

Next, one of the extensions is reduced one-half, along its entire length, as shown in Fig. 26-12, *A* to *C*.

The longer extension is then folded over the shorter one as shown in Fig. 26-13, *B*. This step may be readily accomplished using the beaks of a pair of cotton pliers. Fig. 26-13, *B* is a cross-section view of the joint at this stage of its construction.

Before a finished porcelain crown is

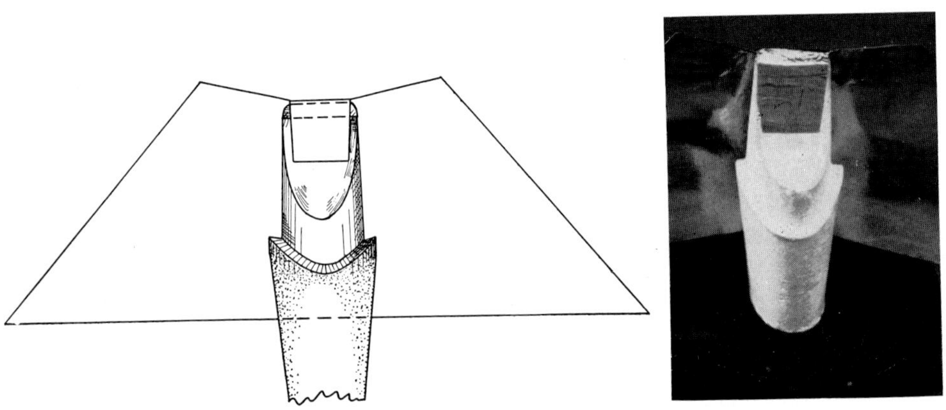

Fig. 26-10. Incisal extension of platinum matrix burnished over incisal plane of amalgam die and against lingual surface.

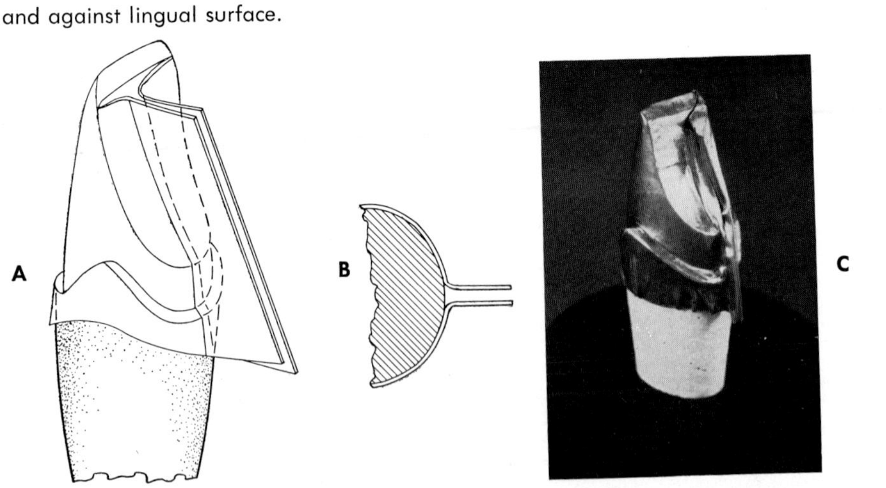

Fig. 26-11. Platinum matrix brought around two proximal surfaces meeting in center of lingual surface; excess platinum is bent lingually at right angles to lingual surface.

cemented permanently, the platinum matrix is always removed. If this matrix is of uniform thickness throughout, the crown will settle this distance uniformly and no marginal discrepancy will exist. However, it will be noted that the thickness of the matrix is uniform at all points, except where the tinner's joint is made on the lingual surface; here there is an excess of 0.003 inch extending the entire length of the joint, from incisal plane to cervical edge.

After the matrix is removed from the inner surface of the completed veneer crown, a channel 0.003 inch deep remains in the inner surface of the crown; it starts at the incisal plane and terminates at the outer angle of the gingival shoulder. If such a crown is cemented on the prepared tooth, there is a perfect marginal fit around the entire gingival periphery except in the space previously occupied by the tinner's joint, where there would exist a 0.003 inch deficiency filled with cement. The rest of the 0.003 inch channel on the inside of the porcelain tooth does not matter, since it is confined within the peripheral outline of the tooth.

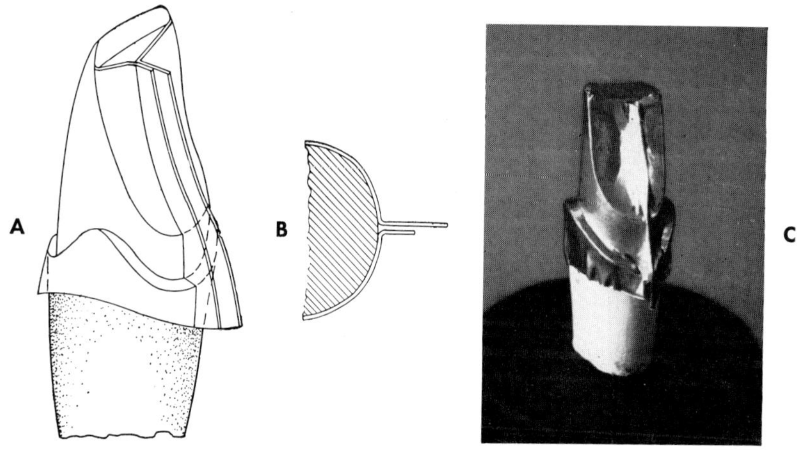

Fig. 26-12. One of lingual extensions is reduced one-half its width.

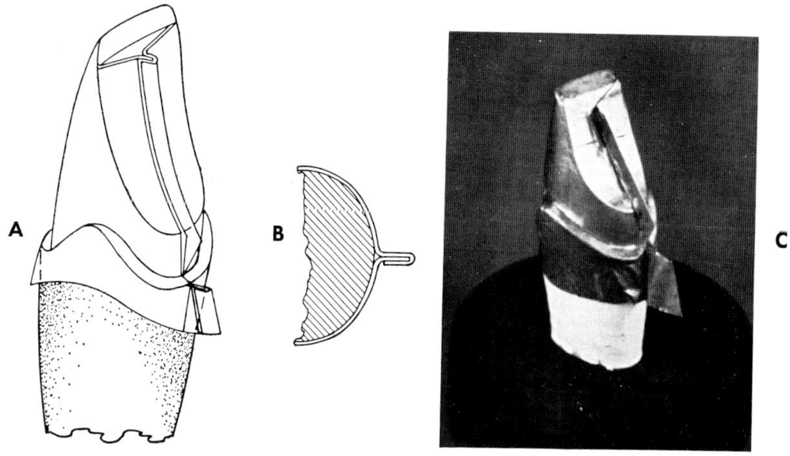

Fig. 26-13. A and **C,** Triangular section cut away at gingival shoulder. To obtain tinner's joint, longer extension of platinum is folded over shorter extension **(B).**

Lingual relief of tinner's joint

To prevent the deficiency of porcelain at this point, two methods may be used to eliminate the three extra thicknesses of foil in that part of the tinner's joint covering the shoulder area. The first method is to remove the three thicknesses of matrix by carefully cutting them away with a small, inverted cone (Densco ½K). The removal of three thicknesses extends only from the inner to the outer angle of the shoulder. By removing this excess, a uniform thickness of 0.001 inch is now established around the entire plane of the gingival shoulder. That portion of the matrix extending apically of the shoulder, called the apron of the matrix, retains its typical tinner's joint as does that part extending incisally from the inner angle of the shoulder.

The same result may be accomplished by cutting away a small triangular piece of the tinner's joint that lies over the shoulder of the preparation. A horizontal cut is made through the three thicknesses of the tinner's joint; this cut is placed at the level of the plane of the shoulder and is brought to the inner angle of the shoulder. Another cut is made incisogingivally, ending in the inner angle of the shoulder; this removes the triangular piece of tinner's joint (Fig. 26-13, *A* and *C*). When the final bend of the joint is made, as in Fig. 26-14, *B*, it is done in two sections; one extends from the inner angle of the shoulder to the incisal edge, while the other extends from the outer angle of the shoulder apically (Fig. 26-14, *A* and *C*), leaving only one thickness of matrix covering the shoulder.

Proximal tinner's joint. Where a normal amount of tooth structure cannot be removed from the lingual surface of the tooth, the tinner's joint is placed on the proximal surface. The same general technic is followed with the exception that the first adaptation is made on one proximal surface and the joint is completed on the opposite proximal side. Figs. 26-15 and 26-16, *A* show the rough adaptation of the matrix to the proximal, labial, and lingual surfaces, bringing the two ends of the matrix together around to the opposite proximal surface. Fig. 26-16, *B*, shows the matrix trimmed, leaving an extension to cover the incisal plane. Fig. 26-17, A, presents the incisal portion of the matrix burnished to the incisal plane and the

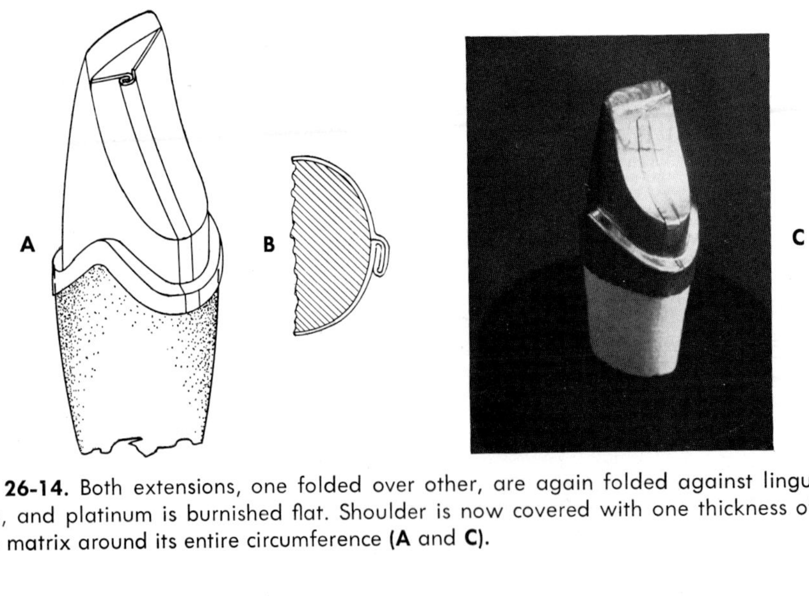

Fig. 26-14. Both extensions, one folded over other, are again folded against lingual surface, and platinum is burnished flat. Shoulder is now covered with one thickness of platinum matrix around its entire circumference (**A** and **C**).

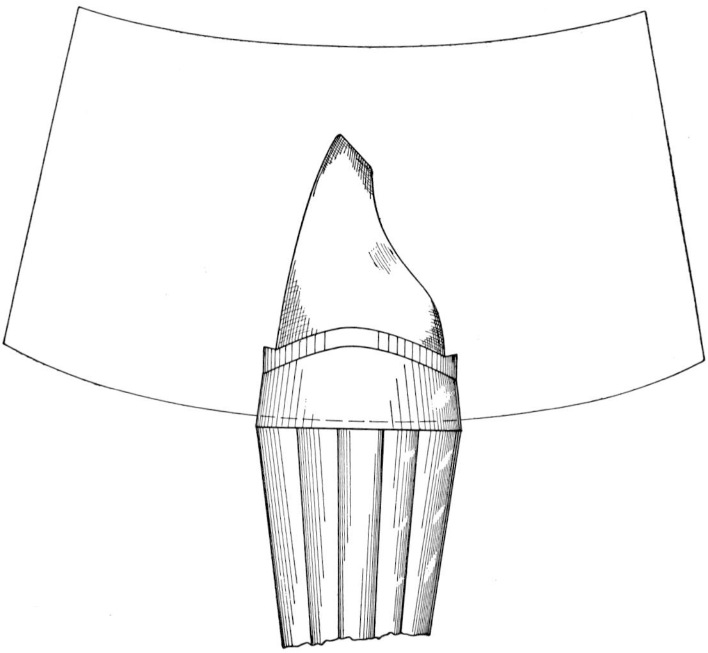

Fig. 26-15. Application of platinum matrix to proximal surface when tinner's joint is to be made on opposite proximal surface of die.

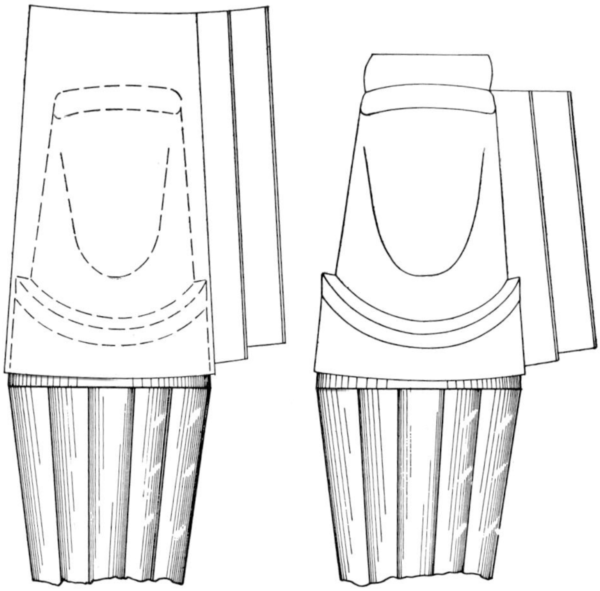

A **B**

Fig. 26-16. A, One extension is reduced one-half on opposite proximal surface. **B,** Excess platinum is reduced at incisal edge, leaving incisal flap.

first step of the tinner's joint completed. Fig. 26-17, *B*, illustrates the completed matrix, and Fig. 26-17, *C*, shows the matrix with the tinner's joint reduced at the shoulder.

It will be observed that the illustrations showing the tinner's joint on the lingual surface have the apron trimmed to conform to the curvature of the shoulder, whereas those with the tinner's joint on the proximal surface have the apron trimmed to a horizontal plane. If the die has been properly shaped, the latter method of trimming the apron is preferred, since it is less likely to distort during the firing of the crown. The curved apron is likely to cause the crown to roll over on the tray unless it is supported. Fig. 26-18 shows labial and lingual views of matrices for an upper central incisor, bicuspid, and molar.

It is the custom of some dentists to swage the platinum matrix to the die for its final adaptation. While not necessary, there is no objection to this procedure, if carefully done.

After being swaged to the amalgam die, it is occasionally found that the matrix cannot be removed, or it is removed with great difficulty. When this happens, the entire outer surface of the platinum matrix is covered with sticky wax; this is allowed to cool and it is then attached to a stick of wax. The matrix may then be readily dislodged with a slight incisal pull. It should be replaced and removed from the die several times, after which the wax is burned clean from the matrix.

After cleaning, the platinum matrix is placed on a tray and into the muffle of the electric furnace where it is brought to 2400° F., after which it is removed and allowed to cool (Fig. 26-19).

The matrix is then placed on the amalgam die, which is replaced in the working model.

Relief to allow for porcelain shrinkage

Inasmuch as porcelain shrinks during the firing process from 8 to 20 percent, the latter being the more frequent, it is necessary to compensate for this shrinkage in order to have an accurate fit of the finished crown at the shoulder. There are five ways to prepare for this shrinkage: first, by painting the platinum shoulder and apron

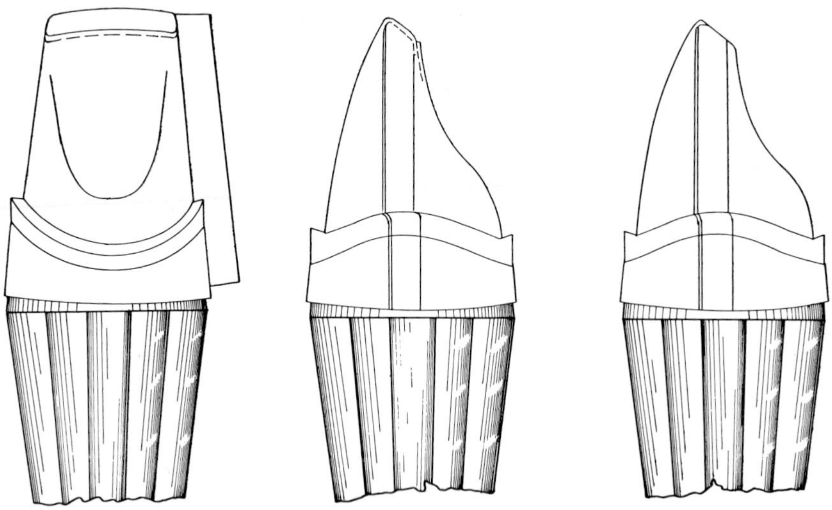

Fig. 26-17. A, Incisal flap folded under lingual platinum matrix. **B** and **C,** Finished platinum matrices.

with shellac; second, by melting a thin film of inlay wax in the same location. Both of these materials will burn out clean during the firing of porcelain and leave a space between the platinum shoulder and the fired porcelain; this prevents the shrinking porcelain from pulling the platinum matrix away from its original shoulder position. The resulting space then permits the reburnishing of the platinum to the shoulder on the die. The third method of compensating for the shrinkage is to "ditch" the porcelain powder around the shoulder to uncover the platinum matrix in this area before the crown is given its first firing. The fourth method consists of making a vertical cut through the porcelain powder and in extending it from the incisal plane to the gingival shoulder. This causes the porcelain to shrink proximally and labially. The opening is later filled before the second firing, The fifth method takes advantage of the fact that porcelain shrinks in the direction of its greatest bulk. No provision is made for the fired porcelain pulling away from the shoulder matrix. Instead, a 1 mm. collar of porcelain is first applied to the shoulder area of the matrix extending it slightly onto the apron; also a thin layer 2 or 3 mm. is extended incisally. When fired, the porcelain shrinks down toward the shoulder matrix. The subsequent firings do not pull the fused porcelain away from the shoulder level.

CHARACTERISTICS OF PORCELAIN

Before describing the application of porcelain and its firing, it is well to review very briefly some of its characteristics and physical phenomena. More complete and detailed information may be obtained from any of the standard textbooks dealing with dental materials, particularly those by Peyton[1] and by Skinner-Phillips.[2] Most porcelains consist of feldspars, quartz, and glass; in addition to this, they contain a metallic oxide which imparts the color to

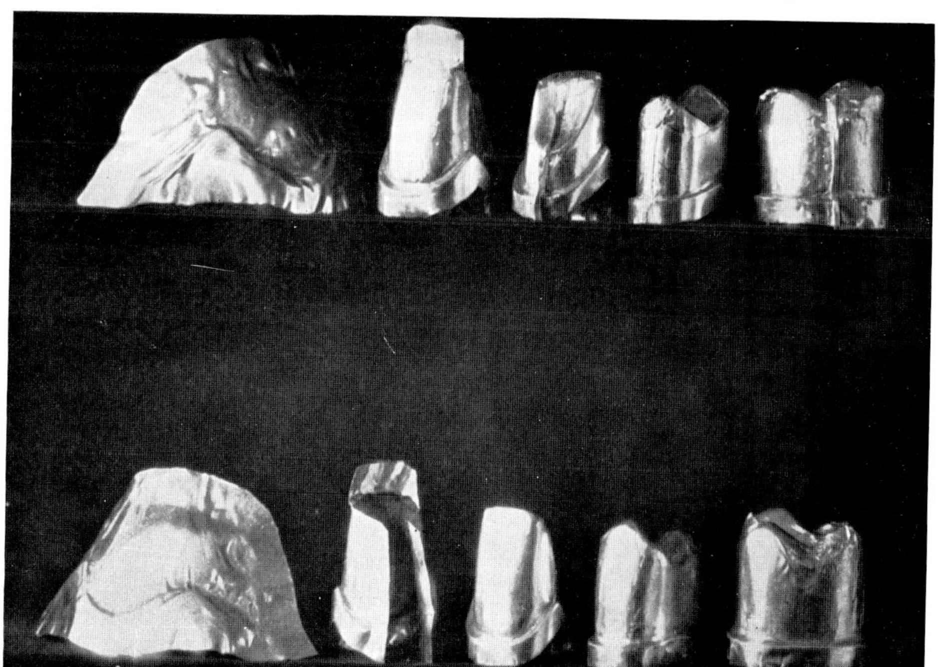

Fig. 26-18. Labial and lingual aspects of matrices for anterior and posterior platinum matrices for porcelain veneer crowns.

the porcelain.[1] For a discussion of the new alumina reinforced porcelain and its uses, see Chapter 36.

Porcelain when mixed with distilled water does not react chemically, but, when subjected to varying degrees of temperature, it undergoes a pyrochemical reaction. On the basis of their firing temperatures, dental porcelains are designated as low firing, having a range of 1600 to 1850° F.; medium firing, 2000 to 2200° F.; and the high firing, 2300 to 2500° F.

Although porcelain meets the highest esthetic demands and is insoluble in mouth fluids, its inherent strength is less than that of gold alloys; likewise, its shrinkage frequently presents a serious problem in restorative work. Because it is possible to obtain an impervious surface with glazed porcelain, it is the most compatible of materials when placed in contact with oral tissues.

Porcelain is mixed with distilled water and kept in a damp condition during the entire period of its manipulation. It should be neither too dry nor too wet, but of a plasticity that will permit its being applied, carved, and burnished without falling apart. Since the amount of shrinkage in porcelain depends to a large extent upon the compactness with which the particles of porcelain are rearranged, every effort is made to remove air spaces and excess moisture from the porcelain during its application to the platinum matrix. A cardinal point in the manipulation of porcelain is the requirement that porcelain be kept free of all traces of dirt and foreign particles.

Low-fusing porcelain

Low-fusing porcelains are not usually used in the construction of porcelain crowns or bridges; their main use lies in modifying contours or adding contact areas to previously glazed porcelain restorations made of medium- or high-firing porcelains. Some question the solubility of the low-fusing type of porcelain in the oral fluids.

Medium-fusing porcelain

The medium-fusing porcelain is of special value in the construction of porcelain pontics. It may also be used for constructing porcelain inlays, crowns, and fixed partial dentures.

High-fusing porcelain

The high-fusing porcelains are indicated for the alumina reinforced types of restorations and as a foundation for the medium-firing porcelains. This is also true in the construction of metal-reinforced porcelain bridges. High-firing porcelain possesses high qualities of strength, color, and translucency.

METHODS OF APPLYING PORCELAIN

Although five or more methods have been suggested for the application of porcelain, three methods are in general use: (1) the vibration, (2) the spatulation, and (3) the capillary attraction methods.

In the vibration method the wet porcelain is applied to the platinum matrix; by vibrating the die on which the matrix rests, with a serrated porcelain instrument, the porcelain powder settles to place as a closely packed mass; the excess moisture rises to the surface and is removed with clean blotting paper or a linen napkin. It is carved and burnished to shape, after which more porcelain is added and the process repeated until the entire crown is built to contour.

In the spatulation method moist porcelain of a consistency drier than that used for the vibration method is applied to the platinum matrix with a porcelain spatula where it is spatulated and burnished to place, bringing the excess water to the surface from which it is absorbed with blotting paper or a clean linen napkin. In using the spatulation method, the spatula blade is always stroked toward the gingival shoulder, especially in the initial stages of building the crown.

The capillary attraction method depends on the ability which a dry powder, paper, or cloth possesses to withdraw excess water from a wet mass by capillary attraction, thus condensing the mass of porcelain powder by pulling the porcelain particles toward a central point. Thoroughly moistened porcelain powder is painted on the platinum matrix with a small sable hair brush, until the entire surface of the matrix is covered with a very thin layer. One surface of this thin layer of porcelain is touched to some dry porcelain powder placed on a slab; immediately the excess moisture is absorbed from the layer of porcelain covering the platinum matrix. This leaves the entire matrix covered with a very thin veneer of porcelain powder. The dry porcelain powder, paper, or cloth serves the same purpose as the blotting paper does in the other two methods.

A second application of the wet porcelain is made, but this time only to one side of the matrix; it is then touched to the dry absorbent, but on the side opposite from that to which the last application of porcelain was made. Since the excess water is drawn to the opposite side of the matrix to which it was applied, the porcelain particles are packed tightly against the platinum matrix. This process is continued until the entire contour of the crown is developed.

Whichever one of the three methods is employed to contour the crown fully, a large sable or camel's hair brush is finally used with a whipping motion to compress further the porcelain particles and to bring to the surface any excess moisture, whereupon it may be absorbed. This whipping action also smooths the surfaces of the porcelain before the crown is placed in the muffle.

DRYING THE PORCELAIN CROWN

A freshly built crown, no matter how thoroughly condensed or how carefully dried, still contains a certain amount of moisture which must be entirely removed before the crown can be safely placed in the hot muffle. This is best done by first allowing the porcelain crown to dry, either on top of the muffle, in front of the open muffle, or in the drying chamber found on the newer types of porcelain furnaces. If the crown is placed in the muffle while moist, there is danger of its being blown apart by the steam generated within the porcelain.

FIRING PORCELAIN IN AIR OR VACUUM

Whether done in an environment of atmosphere or in a vacuum, in firing porcelain there are two general considerations: (1) the temperature attained, and (2) the temperature together with the length of time it is maintained. In the first method the temperature in the muffle is increased uniformly until the firing stage specified by the manufacturer is reached, whereupon the current is turned off; the restoration will be found fired to the desired degree of vitrification. In the second method the temperature is raised to a specified degree within a definite length of time; this degree of temperature is below that usually designated by the manufacturer as the firing point of the porcelain. The porcelain crown is kept in the muffle at this lower temperature for a measured length of time, whereupon it undergoes the desired degree of vitrification. (See Chapter 35 for detailed schedules for firing several types of porcelains.)

Either method gives satisfactory results once the dentist has learned (1) the characteristics peculiar to the porcelain he is using, (2) the peculiarities of his furnace, and (3) the electric current available to him.

Whatever method is used, it will be found that a better pyrochemical reaction will be obtained in the porcelain if sufficient time is given during the firing process.

Generally speaking, the pyrochemical reactions begin in high-firing porcelains after a temperature of 1200 to 1400° F.

has been reached. At this point, complete dehydration has occurred, while oxidation of organic materials continues to 1600° F.

When a restoration is subjected to continued or repeated firing, the pyrochemical reaction finally reaches a stage where complete vitrification occurs. If carried beyond this point, an overglazing of the porcelain occurs accompanied by loss of color and loss of contour of the mass with a glassy surface appearance; finally, the porcelain becomes weak and full of bubbles.

Number of firings required

Most porcelain restorations require three firings. The first firing, also known as the "biscuit" or "underglaze" bake, occurs about 100° F. below the specified fusing stage of the porcelain. The greater shrinkage occurs during this firing, which gives a slightly granular appearance to the porcelain surface.

The second firing is also brought to a bisque or underglazed stage; it likewise occurs at a temperature 100° F. below the glazing point of the porcelain.

The final firing or "glaze" occurs when complete vitrification of the porcelain has been effected, either at the temperature designated by the manufacturer or at a slightly lower temperature, but held for a specified added length of time.

After this stage of vitrification has occurred, the current is turned off and the furnace and crown are cooled slowly to 1200° F., after which it is removed from the muffle and placed under a pyrex dish to cool to room temperature. This anneals the porcelain and decreases the

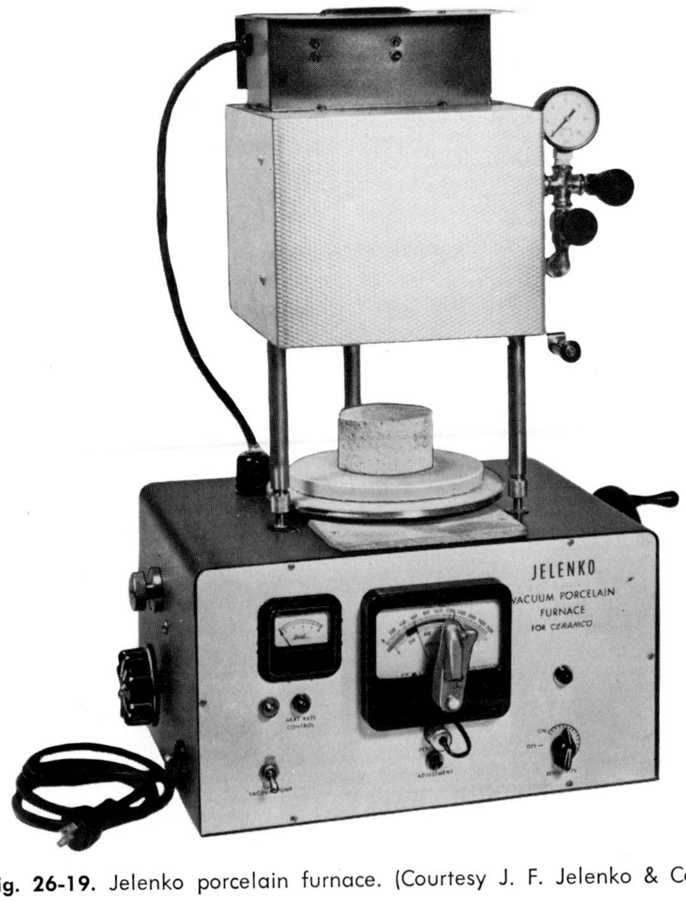

Fig. 26-19. Jelenko porcelain furnace. (Courtesy J. F. Jelenko & Co.)

possibility of checks developing due to internal stresses, which are likely to develop when porcelain is cooled too rapidly.

If necessary to remove the crown from the muffle immediately after it has been glazed, it should be placed in the annealing tray under the muffle or under a heated Pyrex dish where it may be permitted to cool slowly to room temperature.

The degree of final vitrification or glaze will be determined largely by the type of surface desired in the finished crown. An attempt should be made to obtain a surface comparable to that of natural enamel, rather than one having a shiny, glassy appearance.

Porcelain furnace

A dental porcelain furnace consists of three parts: (1) the rheostat with its resistance coils controls the amount of current permitted to enter the muffle; (2) the muffle is the heating element containing a platinum wire coil, usually contained within an insulated fireclay shell; (3) the thermocouple and pyrometer indicate the degree of heat within the muffle chamber (Fig. 26-19).

Operation of the furnace. It is very important to observe carefully the directions for operating an electric dental furnace. This is particularly true of the newer types of furnaces, which are capable of firing porcelain either under atmospheric conditions or in a vacuum. Functionally, dental porcelain furnaces perform similarly but they differ slightly in design of muffles.

The Jelenko furnace (Fig. 26-19) has a vertical round muffle unit with an elevator lift shaft, whereas the Ney furnace (Fig. 26-20) has the conventional horizontal muffle, rectangular in shape.

Detailed instructions for the operation of each of these furnaces will not be considered here since these are usually furnished with the furnace.

Calibrating porcelain furnace

Recognizing correct temperature control, the ceramist must constantly be aware of

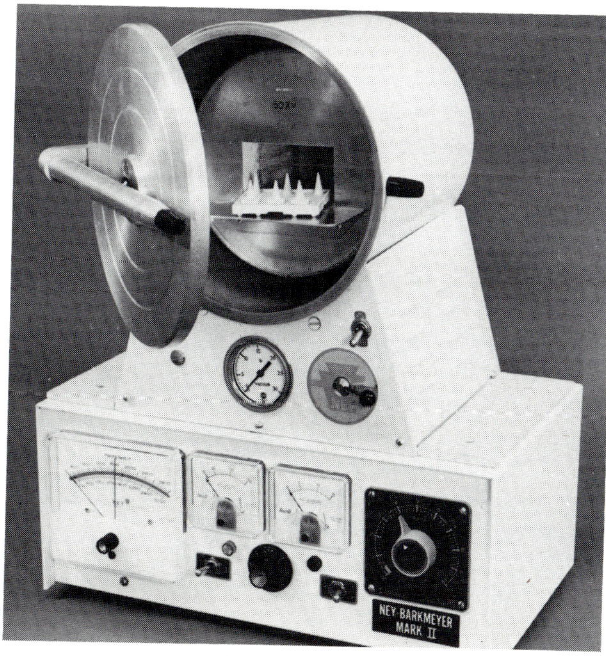

Fig. 26-20. Ney porcelain furnace. (Courtesy J. M. Ney Co.)

a possible variation in pyrometers and thermocouples. A simple test for checking the accuracy of the muffle temperature is to place a small strip of pure gold plate on the firing tray, bending a part of the plate in a vertical position. This is then inserted into the muffle directly under the thermocouple. The muffle door is closed and the heat is allowed to rise slowly on the first step of the rheostat. After the pyrometer reading reaches 1700° F. the rheostat is adjusted in position so that this temperature will be held for 2 minutes. The muffle door is opened quickly to see if the end of the gold plate is still upstanding. If so, the door is closed and the temperature is raised to 1720° F. and again held for 2 minutes, after which it is again examined. This is repeated at 2-minute intervals until the gold melts (gold has a melting point of 1945° F.). If, however, the pyrometer reads 1845° F. when the gold melts the reading of the muffle temperature is 100° F. too low and the pyrometer should be adjusted to 1945° F.

With the muffle properly adjusted to temperature reading one can then confidently follow the instructions issued by the manufacturer.

Air-fired porcelain often has innumerable small voids or bubbles beneath the outer thin glazed surface of the crown that is being baked. It has been found[3-5] that an air-fired porcelain crown contains by volume 94 percent porcelain and 6 percent air, the latter in the form of bubbles or voids. If the glazed surface is ground through, these voids are encountered. These minute pores are found throughout the mass of porcelain; they not only affect the strength of the porcelain but also make it difficult to reproduce the natural tooth color in the porcelain crown because they reflect and diffuse light in such a way as to give the crown an unnatural color effect. Furthermore, a ground surface cannot be brought back to the smooth original surface without again reglazing it.

Complete consideration of the porcelain mix, the use of the proper grain size of porcelain material, and reduction in amount of plasticizer used are all helpful in reducing the size and quantity of the air voids. However, even these factors are contingent upon whether the crown is fired under atmospheric conditions or under vacuum. Better translucency is obtained with large grain size materials in air firing whereas smaller grain size gives better translucency when the crown is vacuum fired.

DUPLICATING COLORS

Generally, the color of a shade guide is reproduced by applying the gingival or basic color to the gingival portion of the crown and the incisal or enamel color to the incisal portion of the crown; the two blend by overlapping in the middle section of the crown (Fig. 25-4, *A*).

Each manufacturer of porcelain has developed a chart which indicates what colors and proportions of porcelains are to be used in order to duplicate the shade selected on his own shade guide.

In order to reproduce the color of the shade guide that matches the natural tooth, it is only necessary to refer to the chart the manufacturers supply; this chart indicates the numbers of the gingival and the incisal colors that are to be used to duplicate the color of the natural tooth. Occasionally, several colors are used to reproduce either the incisal or the gingival shades of the crown (Fig. 25-4, *B*).

The proper shade having been determined and the correct porcelain powders selected, the next step is the application of the porcelain to the platinum matrix and the firing of the crown.

APPLICATION OF PORCELAIN IN CONSTRUCTING CROWNS

To simplify the description of the method employed, a complete veneer porcelain crown will be constructed for an upper central incisor. It is assumed that two porcelain colors have been selected, a gingival and an incisal. A small amount of each is placed in a Dappen dish and a sufficient amount of distilled water is added until the entire mass of porcelain powder has been saturated. The excess water is then absorbed with a clean napkin, leaving the porcelain in a plastic, workable condition. The correct amount of moisture in the porcelain may be recognized when the granular surface becomes moist if it is gently patted with the porcelain instrument.

First application

For the first application of porcelain, the amalgam die with its platinum matrix with wax over the shoulder (Fig. 26-21, *A*) is removed from the working model and the gingival color is distributed and applied to the matrix. This may be done by any one of the three methods previously mentioned. After the gingival contour has been fully developed in the gingival color, the porcelain is carried incisally until the entire matrix is covered. It will be noted, however, that, as it approaches the incisal plane, the thickness of the porcelain diminishes until it barely covers the incisal region (Fig. 26-21, *B*).

The amalgam die, matrix, and the first application of porcelain are now placed back in the working model. The incisal color is added, while the gingival porcelain is still moist. The crown is built with the incisal porcelain to its full contour and occlusion. Although the incisal portion of the crown consists almost entirely of enamel color, it is carried cervically on the labial area so that it overlaps the gingival porcelain in the middle third of the crown.

The porcelain ends at the shoulder and does not extend beyond the thin layer of shellac or inlay wax which covers the shoulder. The crown is smoothed with a whipping motion of the sable brush and is removed with the die from the working model.

Upon its removal from the model, the mesial and distal contact areas of the crown require the addition of small amounts of porcelain in these areas. This should be done before it is placed in the muffle.

A porcelain crown shrinks from 10 to 20 percent during firing; therefore, it is advisable to build the incisal edge 1 to 2 mm. beyond that of the adjoining teeth. To compensate for the mesiodistal shrinkage of the crown, experience has shown that if the crown is overbuilt mesiodistally so that it touches the labioproximal and linguoproximal surface angles of the ad-

A

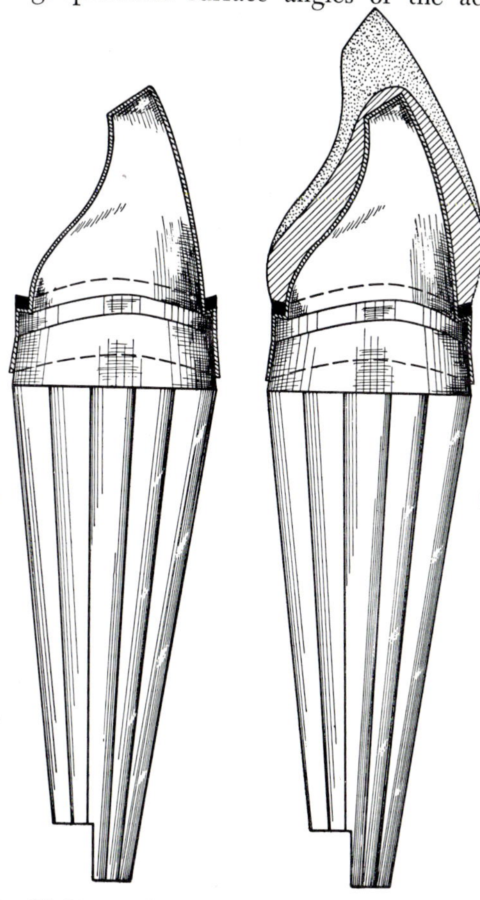

B

Fig. 26-21. A, Shellac or wax applied to shoulder area of matrix to permit fired porcelain to shrink without pulling matrix away from shoulder. **B,** Body and enamel colors applied to platinum matrix in correct amounts and distribution.

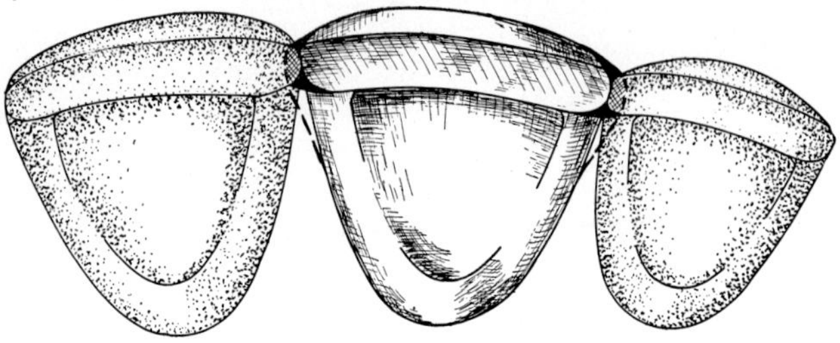

Fig. 26-22. Extending mesiodistal contour of crown to compensate for shrinkage of crown during firing.

joining teeth and if the resultant concavity is filled in with porcelain after the crown has been removed from the model, this additional contour will give the crown, after its first firing, the correct mesiodistal width. Fig. 26-22 illustrates the proximal overextensions and the areas to be filled in before the first firing is made.

The crown is now removed from the amalgam die and placed on a muffle tray covered with silex granules. The tray and crown are placed on top of the muffle or in front of the open muffle and allowed to dry.

Before inserting the crown and tray into the muffle, a final inspection of the furnace should be made to see that the pyrometer is registering correctly and that the temperature of the furnace is the desired degree.

When using muffles with exposed wires, the current is first disconnected, after which the tray and the crown are carefully inserted. The muffle door should be left open until all discoloration of the porcelain has disappeared and the smoke generated by the shellac or inlay wax around the shoulder of the crown has escaped. The muffle door is then closed and the firing of the porcelain is done according to the schedules given previously.

When the desired degree of vitrification has been attained, the movable lever on the rheostat is returned to zero, and the electric current is turned off. The furnace door is opened diagonally about ⅛ inch and the temperature allowed to drop to 1500° F.

The tray with the crown is then carefully removed with furnace tongs and placed in the annealing chamber beneath the muffle, or it may be covered with a Pyrex dish and be permitted to cool to room temperature.

Second application

When cool, the crown is returned to the amalgam die, where the platinum matrix is reburnished to the gingival shoulder and porcelain is packed into the gingival space formed where the inlay wax was burned out (Fig. 26-23, *A*).

Since the gingival space is frequently very narow, it is sometimes difficult to pack porcelain into this narrow space without at the same time trapping air. To eliminate this difficulty, it is advisable first to fill this gingival opening with distilled water and then to place a small amount of porcelain into the water-filled space. Since the water has displaced all the air in the crevice, it now also acts as a vehicle for carrying the porcelain particles into the deepest portions of the gingival space. The excess water is then absorbed, leaving the porcelain solidly packed in the crevice. Since some shrinkage of the porcelain will occur again in this area, the porcelain is applied to cover the surface of the apron also, resulting in a convex gingival addition of porcelain (Fig. 26-23, *B*). During the second firing, this excess porcelain acts as a reservoir, supplying additional porcelain to that in the gingival area as it shrinks during the firing process. Because of its location, the porcelain added to the

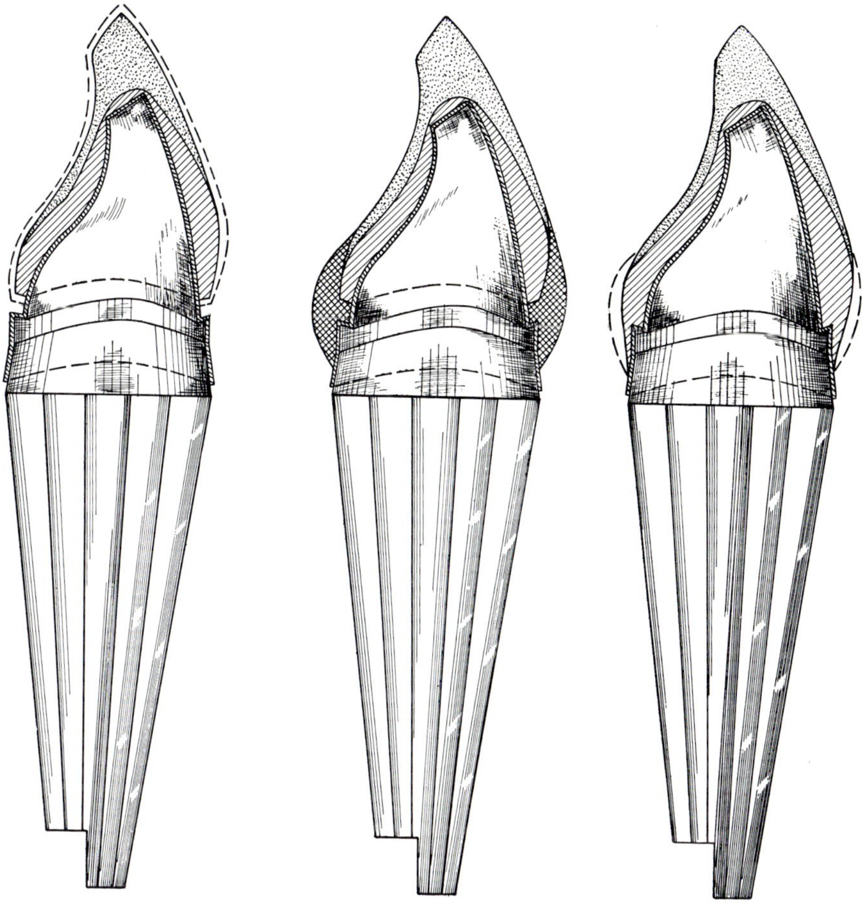

Fig. 26-23. A, Space in gingival area caused by volatilization of wax and shrinkage of porcelain during firing. **B,** Gingival space at shoulder filled with body-colored porcelain and extended incisally and over platinum gingivally. **C,** Shrinkage of fired porcelain applied in **B.**

gingival area is also the gingival color.

If any other additions or alterations are necessary, these are made at this time before the second bisque bake. Additions to the incisal part of the crown are made with the enamel-colored porcelain.

The crown with its freshly added porcelain is now removed from the amalgam die and placed on the tray. The same procedure is followed in the second bisque firing as for the first. In this instance the temperature is also carried to 100° F. below the glazing point of the porcelain.

When the crown is again removed from the muffle and has cooled to room temperature, it is replaced on the amalgam die and the contour and occlusion are verified. It will be recalled that, prior to the second firing, porcelain not only was packed into the gingival space, but also was extended to cover the apron. It is now necessary that the porcelain and the platinum apron that lie rootwise beyond the shoulder be removed before the gingival fit of the crown can be verified (Fig. 26-23, *C*).

TRIMMING AND FITTING CROWN

A ⅞ inch coarse carborundum paper disk is used to cut away this excess porcelain and platinum around the gingival area, while the porcelain crown is seated on the amalgam die. In cutting, the disk is held at such an angle to the crown periphery that a slight gingival convexity is developed on the labial and lingual surfaces (Fig. 26-24, *A* and *B*). Compressed air should be applied to the crown while the cutting is in progress; under no circumstance should this excess porcelain be reduced with stones.

If the patient is present, the crown may be placed at this time on the prepared tooth and tested for fit, contour, contact, and occlusion. The gingival fit is carefully examined with a No. 17 explorer, which is gently carried beneath the crest of the gum tissue and which, with slight lateral pressure, is drawn incisally to determine if any overhang of the porcelain exists. If such overhanging is found, it is trimmed on the amalgam die and again returned to the tooth for verification of fit. When all requirements of contour and occlusion have been satisfied, the crown is returned to the muffle for final glazing. Before doing so, however, the surface of the crown should be carefully examined for any particles of dirt, carborundum, or other foreign matter; if present, these may best be removed under running water with a stiff

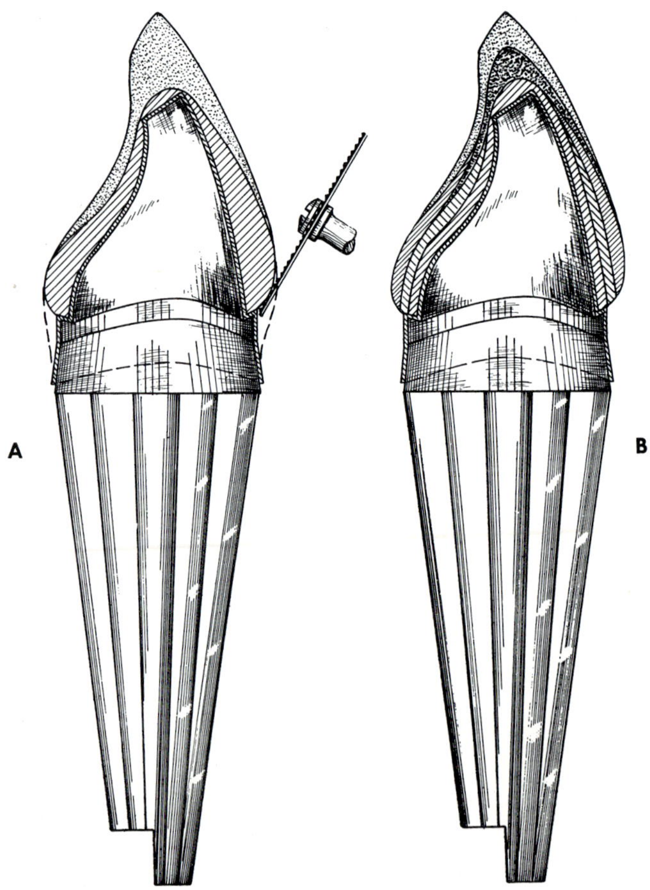

Fig. 26-24. A, Cutting away porcelain which extends beyond shoulder and contouring crown. **B,** Crown given final firing to acquire glaze; note several body colors in this crown.

brush. Sometimes it is advisable to boil the crown in acid or place it in an ultrasonic cleaner to remove the dirt.

FINAL GLAZE

The crown is carried through the final firing process until it has reached a stage of complete vitrification; the temperature and time employed will depend entirely upon the type of porcelain used.

The crown is permitted to cool to room temperature when it is ready for its final fitting on the prepared tooth. It will be noted that the crown in Fig. 26-24, *B* is made with several incisal and gingival colored porcelains. It is well to leave the platinum matrix in the crown during this step, since, if it is found necessary to add porcelain to the contact areas or to some other area, this may be done and the crown again returned to the muffle; this would not be a safe procedure if the matrix had already been removed.

REMOVAL OF MATRIX

Before the crown is cemented to the natural tooth, the platinum matrix is removed. This may be readily done by peeling away the margin of the platinum at the shoulder with a sharp instrument around the entire periphery of the crown, gradually rolling the platinum toward the inside of the crown. The loose edges of the matrix are now brought toward each other, grasped with a pair of tweezers, and gradually peeled away from the inner surfaces of the crown.

Where desirable, the inner porcelain surface, which is smooth, may be roughened with stones or etched with hydrofluoric acid; this procedure, however, is rarely necessary with the complete veneer porcelain crown.

CEMENTING CROWN

After the platinum is removed, the crown should again be placed on the natural tooth and tested for final fit. It is suggested that before final cementation a small amount of the cement powder be mixed with water and glycerin, placed in the crown, and the effect noted on the color of the porcelain veneer crown. If satisfactory, the cement powder is washed out and the crown thoroughly dried.

After the correct shade of cement has been determined, the natural tooth is thoroughly cleaned and dried; rarely, a very thin coat of cavity lining is applied to the coronal portion of the preparation, care being taken not to get any of the lining on the shoulder.

REMOVAL OF EXCESS CEMENT

To assist in the removal of the cement from the outer surfaces of the porcelain crown after its cementation, beforehand, it is well to moisten a pellet of cotton with very thin oil and lubricate the outer surfaces of the gingival portion of the crown; here again, extreme care should be exercised not to get any of the lubricant on the shoulder of the porcelain crown. After the crown has been cemented, the thin film of oil will facilitate the removal of all cement from the gingival crevice area, leaving the crown free of all cement. When cementing a complete veneer porcelain crown, extreme care must be exercised so that no air is trapped within the crown when filling it with cement. After the cement has set and the excess around the gingival area has been removed, the functional relationship is again verified. Just before dismissing the patient, a mild astringent is applied to the soft tissues which are gently massaged while several syringefuls of lukewarm water are gently sprayed upon them.

USE OF PREFIRED VENEER

Because of the difficulty sometimes experienced in matching the color and in obtaining the correct labial anatomy in a porcelain crown by the method just described, Dr. George Thompson in 1920 suggested the use of a high-fusing denture tooth, ground out on the lingual side in such a manner that the remaining labial section could be used as a veneer. This veneer was then placed against the labial surface of the platinum matrix and the balance of the crown was built up with medium- or low-firing porcelain. One of the difficulties encountered in this technic was the displacement of the facing from its correct alignment due to the shrinkage of the lower firing porcelains.

Recently a technic has been presented by Sacchi and Paffenbarger[3] which reduces the shrinkage to a minimum by incorporating the ground porcelain powder made from a high-fusing porcelain tooth (2350° F.), with low-firing porcelain (1875° F.)

THE DIRECT FABRICATION OF RESTORATIONS WITHOUT FOIL ON A REFRACTORY DIE

A materials system and use technic have now been developed by Vickery, Badinelli, and Waltke[4] at the Ceramco, Inc., Research Department that permit the construction of porcelain jacket crowns, porcelain or gold inlays, and porcelain-gold butt shoulder restorations without the use of platinum foil upon a permanent refractory ceramic die prepared directly from the original tooth impression. Through elimination of intermediary steps in preparing secondary impressions and matrices, fabrication is speedier, improved fit and adaptation are obtained, and, in addition, the original die is recovered intact. The neutral tone of the die system and absence of matrix further permit the technician to be aware, at all times, of the true color of a porcelain restoration.

Die properties

The die material, a refractory powder of controlled composition, particle size, and physical properties, is prepared as a castable slurry by admixture with a solution of a refractory binder. Variation of the powder of liquid ratio drastically alters some properties of the die and a ratio of 5:1 is used for optimum results (Table 26-1). The die slurry is poured into the impression and, after an incubation period of approximately 25 minutes, sets through a mildly exothermic reaction. The set model, removed from the impression, is fired to 1860° F. at 75°/minute to stabilize the system. Deviation from this firing schedule of more than 20°/minute, or heating above

Table 26-1. Effect of powder : liquid ratio on Ceramco-die properties

P/L ratio	4:1	4.3:1	4.6:1	5:1	5.3:1	5.6:1	6:1
Mixing	Very thick	Thick	Thick	Optimum	Thin	Thin	Very thin
Working time (minutes)	1	1	3	7	7	8	10
Set time (minutes)	10	10	15	20 to 25	30	40	60
Accuracy percent	-1.5	-1.0	-0.2	- 0 + 0.2	-0.6	-1.0	-2.0
Hardness (BHN)	20	20	30	59	40	30	30
Transverse strength (p.s.i.)	Nil	Very slight	1,000	10,000	1,000	1,000	1,000

1875° F., is inadvisable as the die does not then replicate the original preparation.

Toreskog, Phillips, and Schnell[5] examined various conventional die materials for dimensional accuracy, abrasion resistance, and detail production. Employing the test methods applied by these workers, we obtain for the present material the data given in Table 26-2. Comparable values for other die materials (nonfireable) are also presented. The die composition compensates for shrinkage in impression materials and, correctly handled, dimensional accuracy of −0.0 to +0.2 percent is obtained.

For a die to be used as a substrate in the firing of porcelain, however, properties additional to those described by Toreskog and associates are required. Coefficients of thermal expansion and thermal conductivity of the die and superimposed porcelain must be so matched that compression bonding of the two does not occur on

Table 26-2. Ceramco-die physical characteristics

	Ceramco-die	*Comparison*
Dimensional accuracy (percent)	−0.0 to +0.2	±0.4
Hardness (Brinell)	59	15 to 90
Abrasion resistance (Volume loss/mm.)	.0024 sharp .0012 blunt	.002 to .25 sharp .001 to .123 blunt
Detail duplication	7	4.6 to 7
Modulus of rupture (p.s.i.)	500 green 10,000 fired	— —
Density	2.46	—
Thermal conductivity	0.025 cal./sec./cm.	—

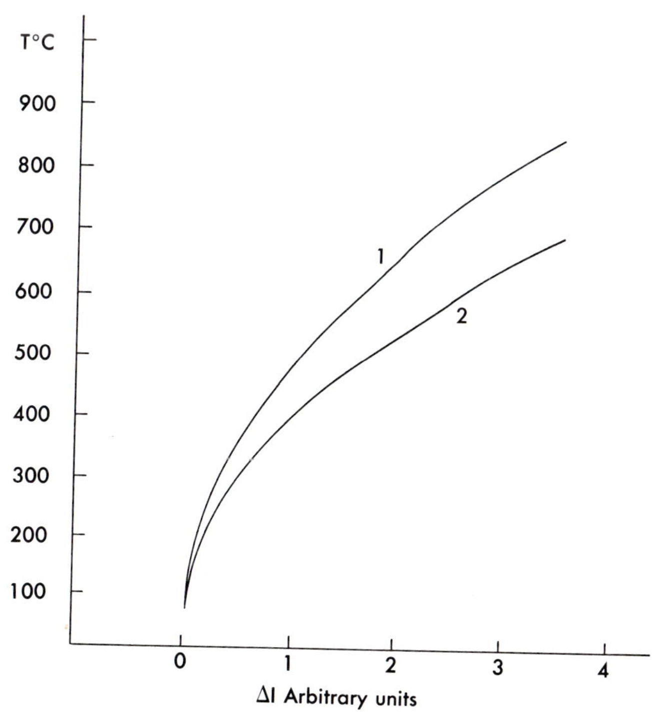

Fig. 26-25. Relative thermal expansivities of the present dies and porcelains. (Courtesy Ceramco, Inc.)

firing and that the porcelain does not craze. Fig. 26-25 shows the relative thermal expansivities of the present die and porcelain.* The die material must be thermally stable, showing no residual dimensional change or loss of physical integrity over several thermal cycles. The die composition does undergo a phase transition during initial firing to 1860° F., but subsequent thermal treatment to this temperature has no other effect.

As indicated, compression bonding of porcelain and die is avoided through control of thermal expansion coefficients. Attachment of porcelain by "wetting" is prevented by establishing an interphase high-surface energy boundary. This is obtained by applying, to the surface of the die, a suspension of appropriate refractory in a film-forming medium. This suspension dries rapidly to a hydrophobic film, which initially prevents porcelain slurry from being drawn into the die structure by capillarity and, on firing, the high-surface energy refractory content prevents wetting of the die by the semiviscid porcelain. The procedural application of this separating medium is simple. Ceramic or high-temperature metal dowels have been used successfully with this new die system.

Die and model preparation

The following technic is used in preparing one-impression models and dies from impressions taken in silicone or polysulphide rubber, compound, or wax. Interaction occurs between the die slurry and hydrocolloid and this negates use of impressions in such aqueous media. Even where rubber is used, the impression should be quite dry in order to maintain accuracy of reproduction and the *cast die should not remain in the impression for longer than 2 hours before removal for firing.*

The die powder and liquid binder are thoroughly mixed in the correct proportions and teased, under vibration, into the individual prepared tooth impressions, making sure that saddle areas are covered. Use of a fine probe and a "painting" manipulation help the slurry to penetrate into all crevices of the indentation. After the impression is filled to the proper level (3 to 4 mm. above the gingival margin), high temperature dowels are inserted into the refractory slurry and accurately positioned, vertically and laterally, by the aid of pins. The cast is allowed to set for approximately 25 minutes. The working-time of the slurry, about 7 minutes, provides adequate time to prepare a segment of an arch of single units in this manner.

After the preliminary set, wax beads or extensions are luted onto the projecting ends of the dowels, the exposed base of the die is painted with separating medium and the exposed dowels are lightly lubricated (Fig. 26-26). The medium dries rapidly and the body of the model is then poured in model base composition up to the margin of the impression. Twenty-five minutes are again allowed for the model to set, and the whole cast may then be lifted from the impression. The dies are examined for surface defects such as bubbles, undercuts, or exigent material; these are eradicated either by local addition of die slurry or by carving. Where small amounts of die are added on, these are allowed to set and contours are trimmed before firing the model. To permit subsequent removal of the individual dies, interproximal saw cuts are made, where appropriate, down to the layer of separator.

After drying out at low temperature, the model is fired to 1860° F. at 75°/minute. Half-jaw models should be "soaked" at this temperature for 1 to 2 minutes; full arch models will require 2 to 3 minutes heat soak to ensure complete thermal penetration of the die. After removal from the furnace, the fired model is allowed to

*Ceramco Porcelain: Ceramco, Inc., Long Island City, N. Y.

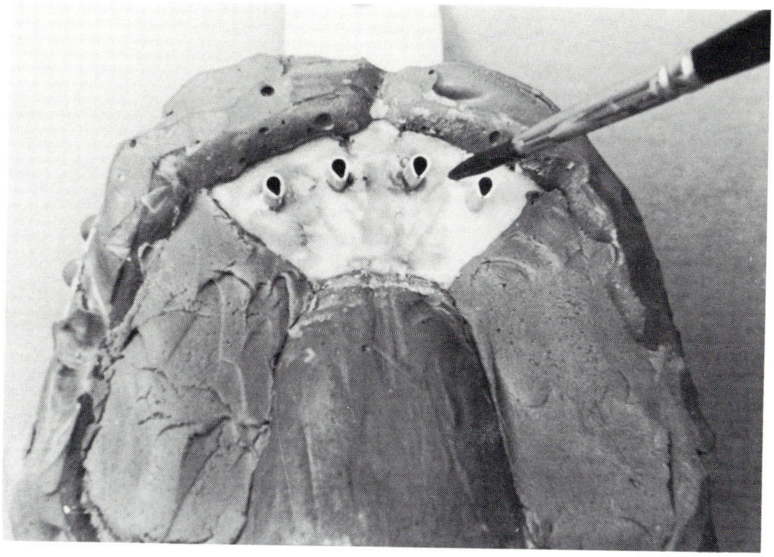

Fig. 26-26. Application of separator to die base. (Courtesy Ceramco, Inc.)

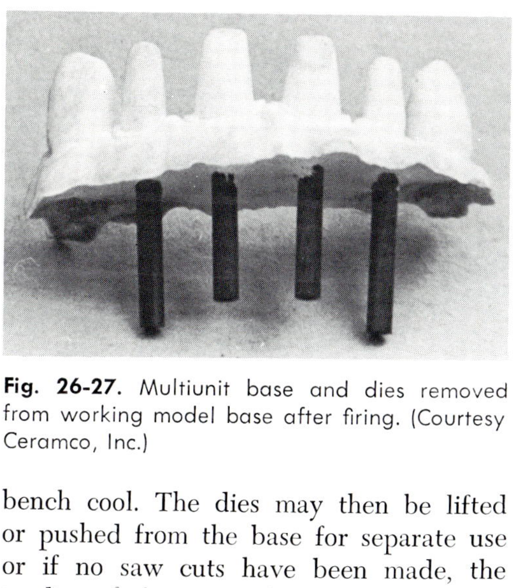

Fig. 26-27. Multiunit base and dies removed from working model base after firing. (Courtesy Ceramco, Inc.)

bench cool. The dies may then be lifted or pushed from the base for separate use or if no saw cuts have been made, the totality of the cast refractory die may be extracted (Fig. 26-27).

When the impression is in compound in a copper band, an extension to the band is made with gummed paper and the die slurry is teased and vibrated into the impression and extension as before. Dowels may be inserted or die slurry may be added to fill the paper tube extension. The slurry is allowed to set for 25 minutes, the paper is peeled off, the copper band and compound are warmed slightly to soften the impression, and the die is pulled out. The elongated stem thus obtained is trimmed and tapered in the usual manner, and the die is fired to maturity (Fig. 26-28, *A*).

Alternatively, for single or multiple units in compound where dowels have been used, the fired dies may be accurately reinserted in one piece into the master impression, the dowel stems and die bases lubricated, and conventional stone poured to provide the model base.

Jacket crown fabrication

Before applying porcelain to the fired die, two generous coats of separating medium are applied to the preparation surface. The first coat covers all but the shoulder (Fig. 26-28, *B*). The second coat covers the crown and shoulder, and extends 2 mm. below the margin (Fig. 26-28, *C*). Care must be taken to ensure that the first coat is thoroughly dry (5 minutes) before applying the second. The separating medium used at this stage is blue, thus enabling the technician to see clearly that

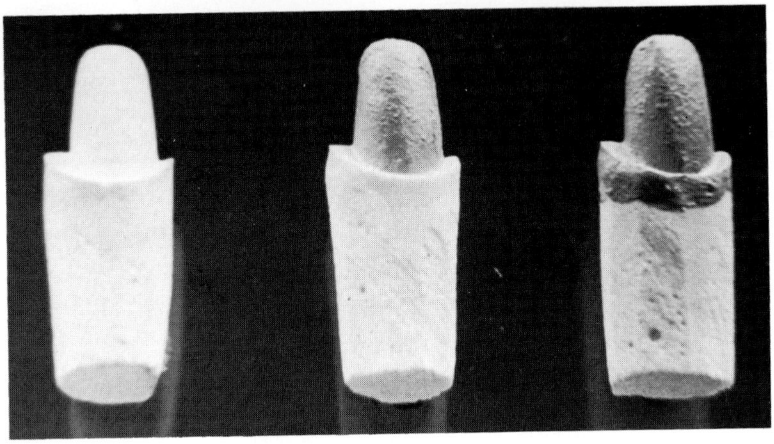

Fig. 26-28. Separator coverage. **Left to right:** no application; first coat; second coat. (Courtesy Ceramco, Inc.)

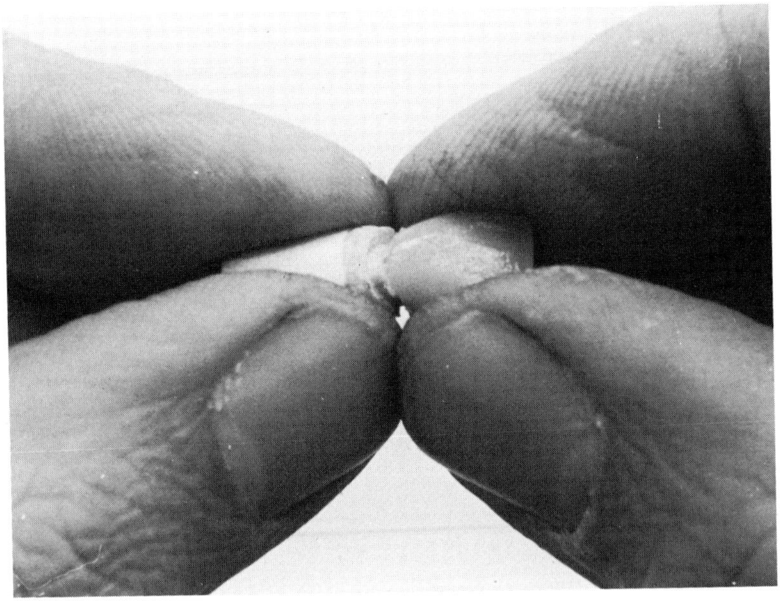

Fig. 26-29. Removal of porcelain jacket from die. (Courtesy Ceramco, Inc.)

the whole preparation surface is covered and to more clearly define margins. It is urged that, *wherever wet porcelain is to be applied to a subjacent die surface, that die surface must be precoated with separating medium.*

The medium dries to a relatively hard smooth, glossy film and porcelain may now be constructed on this surface by normal technic, except that no "ditching" is necessary and porcelain is not extended past the margin. The firing cycle used is that prescribed for Ceramco porcelain, i.e., a few minutes preheat at 1200° F., firing to 1700° F. under vacuum at 80 to 100°/minute, release of vacuum, and finalization of bake to 1800° F.

After firing and bench cooling, the jacket is removed from the die by a gentle pull. To avoid nonparallel pulling forces,

A

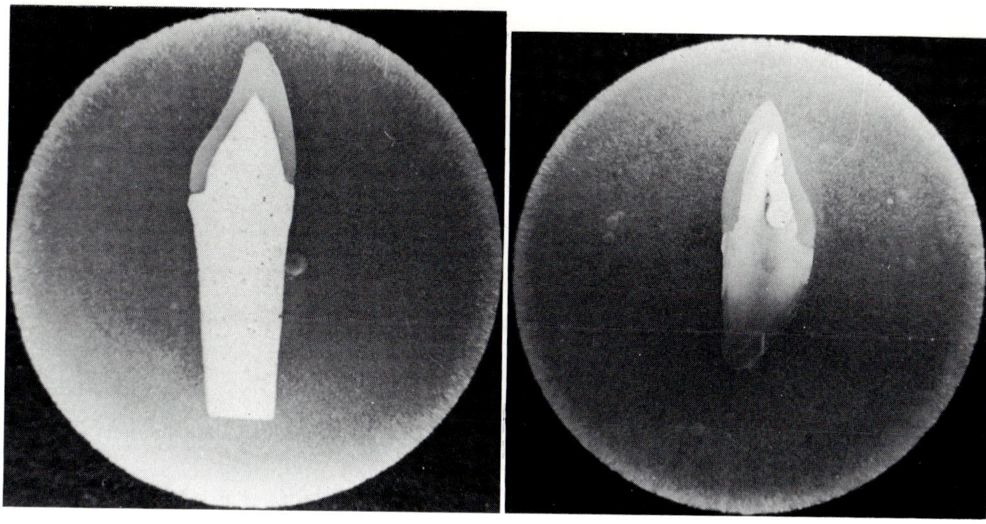

B

Fig. 26-30. Fit of porcelain jacket. **A,** Gingival shrinkage after first bake. **B,** Marginal shoulder fit after final glaze. (Courtesy Ceramco, Inc.)

detach the jacket from the die as shown in Fig. 26-29, with the thumb and forefinger of one hand pressing against the same digits of the other. A fine golden residue remains on the inside of the jacket and on the surface of the die; this is readily removed from both with a stiff bristle brush. The crown is now reseated and ground as necessary, making sure that the jacket is washed and completely dried before proceeding.

One layer of dentin- colored separator is then applied to the entire die surface, extending 2 mm. below the margin; it is allowed to dry.

The two separating media referred to are essentially the same. That used initially is colored; the lighter colored separator referred to here permits the technician to observe the true color of the restoration.

The jacket crown is replaced on the die with firm pressure and is most usually well seated marginally. Sometimes, through localization of dimensional bulk a slight hairline withdrawal may occur at labial or lingual margins. Whether such minimal spaces are seen or not, moist porcelain is brushed into the margin and condensed by vigorous dry brushing from cervical toward incisal areas. The corrected jacket is then taken through normal staining and glazing cycles and, after cooling, cleaned internally.

Fig. 26-30, *A* shows the marginal and internal fit obtained in a jacket crown prepared by one bake and a glaze firing (Fig. 26-30, *B*). The sections are of a die prepared against an impression of the tooth shown. The improvement of adaptation over preparations using platinum matrices is quite clear, the closeness of apposition being accentuated by elimination of the tinner's joint in the foil.

A further benefit inherent in this technic is that the interior surface of the fired jacket is not glassy smooth, but matte, and thus provides for better cementation retention on the prepared tooth.

BUTT-SHOULDER RESTORATIONS (FIG. 26-31)

The die is prepared and fired to maturity as previously described, care being taken to ensure the absence of undercuts. Two coats of separating medium are applied and the wax build-up is carried out directly on the thus prepared surface. The wax pattern is sprued and vented con-

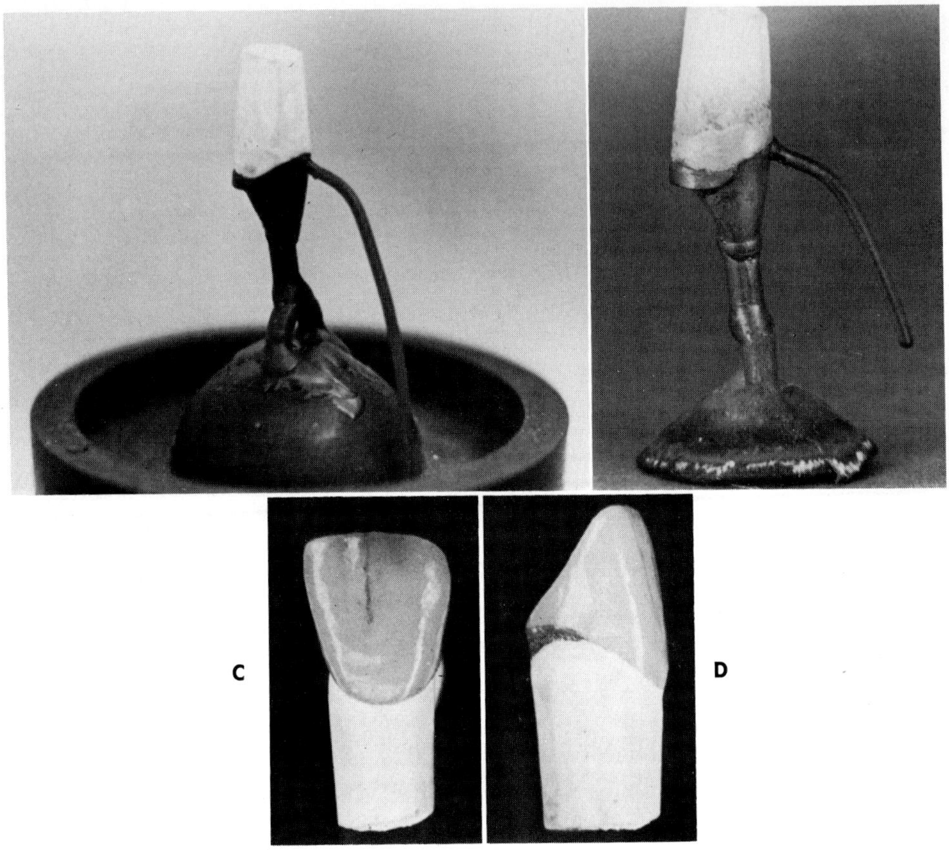

Fig. 26-31. Butt shoulder restoration. **A,** Die waxed up, sprued, vented, and ready for investment. **B,** Die and coping removed from investment after casting. **C,** Labial appearance of restoration after added porcelain construction. **D,** Proximal appearance of total restoration. (Courtesy Ceramco, Inc.)

ventionally and the whole unit, without detaching the wax from the die, is invested, dewaxed, and cast conventionally.

After cooling, the investment is broken from the casting ring. The gold coping will be found to be correctly seated on the die, from which it may be removed by gentle, parallel pulling. The coping is separated from the sprue and vent, and traces of separator are removed from the inner surface of the coping and the surface of the die. The coping may then be reseated and ground and polished where necessary. If metal conditioning agents are to be used, they are fired onto the coping and placed on a sagger tray. The die should not be fired to the temperatures required by these materials.

Opaque porcelain is applied to the coping conventionally and fired. The cool preparation is then replaced on the die, which has been prepared with one generous coat of dentin-colored separating medium around the shoulder and margin where porcelain will make contact. Porcelain is constructed on the metal and exposed in the usual way and is fired, stained, and glazed. Fig. 26-31, *C* and *D,* shows the final adaptation obtained.

TECHNIC RESUME

Ceramco complete porcelain veneer crown: steps

Step 1: Root preparation.

Step 2: Select and fit dowel if pulpless tooth.

Step 3: Take impression in polysulfide rubber, silicone, or compound material.

Step 4: Die and cast preparation. Mix high temperature refractory die material powder and liquid in 5:1 proportions.

Step 5: Pour die material into impression of the tooth preparation and the approximating teeth or edentulous areas 3 to 4 mm. above the gingival margins.

Step 6: Place a high-temperature—resistant dowel into the soft refractory material in the impression. Stabilize the end of the dowel in a vertical position with pins or plastic locks attached to the sides of the impression borders. Allow the material to set within 7 minutes.

Step 7: Set aside and permit a final set for 25 minutes.

Step 8: Paint the base of the poured die with a separating medium and lubricate the exposed ends of the dowels with petrolatum.

Step 9: Pour the model base in Ceramco model refractory material to fill the rest of the impression and allow it to set for 25 minutes.

Step 10: Separate the case from the impression and, if satisfactory, make interproximal cuts on either side of the refractory die base.

Step 11: The cast and die are now slowly dried and inserted into the muffle at 1000° F. very slowly. The temperature is raised 50 to 75°/minute to a temperature of 1800° F. and held for 2 or 3 minutes.

Step 12: The cast is removed from the furnace and bench-cooled to room temperature.

Step 13: Cast is mounted in articulator against the opposing occluding cast.

Step 14: The cuts may now be extended, if necessary, and the individual die may be raised by pushing up on the end of the die, which is exposed through the tunnels formed in the cast by the wax or plastic pin extension that was volatilized in the firing process.

Step 15: The die is next prepared for fabrication of the crown.

Fabrication of ceramco complete porcelain veneer crown

Step 1: Apply one coat of the yellow separating medium to the fired die, covering only the coronal axial surfaces but not the shoulder of the die. Let it dry for 5 minutes. Apply a second coat; this time the blue separating medium is used and applied not only to the entire coronal portion but also to the shoulder and 2 mm. below the outer margin of the shoulder. When the blue coat of separator has dried in 5 minutes it enables the ceramist better to see the shoulder margin when applying the porcelain later. Precoating the die is essential before applying any wet porcelain.

Step 2: The crown is now built up in the customary manner except that no provision is required for cervical shinkage of the porcelain in firing such as ditching or wax or film at the shoulder.

Step 3: The crown is slowly dried, preheated, and inserted at 100 to 1200° F. into the muffle. The temperature is increased 80°/minute to 1700° F. under vacuum. At this temperature the vacuum is released and temperature continued to 1800° F. If the crown is to be fired under atmospheric condition then it is not raised above 1700° F. at this time.

Step 4: Remove and allow to cool to room temperature under Pyrex cover. When cool remove the crown from the die with the opposing finger method.

Step 5: With a stiff bristle brush remove the fine yellow residue from the die surface and from inside the crown.

Step 6: Wash and dry and reseat the crown on the die. Shrinkage may be observed at the cervical edge of the crown. Apply a coat of dentin-colored separator and let it dry for 5 minutes. Reseat the crown and brush a drop of slurry on the gingival porcelain, which will act as a vehicle for conveying the particles of porcelain into the deep areas of the crevice. Trying to pack a drier mass of porcelain into the crevice may leave air pockets beneath the surface, subsequently leaving a thin layer of glazed porcelain at the shoulder edge. This may fracture away easily in subsequent manipulation. Vibrating the dowel during the application of the porcelain into the crevice will facilitate its going to the bottom of the space. Excess moisture is absorbed with a cloth or tissue paper during the process of condensation. Any porcelain extending beyond the outer angle of the shoulder should be carefully brushed away from the die.

Step 7: The die with the built-up crown is now dried, preheated, and carried to a glaze temperature at atmospheric conditions to 1800° F.

Step 8: When glazed it is removed and allowed to cool under a pyrex dish until room temperature is obtained. It is then removed from the die with the opposing finger method.

Labial butt shoulder restoration: steps

Step 1: Die prepared as usual for the complete porcelain veneer crown. Where a metal casting is to cover the coronal portion of the preparation leaving, however, the labial shoulder exposed, it will be necessary to prepare the die in a special manner prior to waxing the design of the coping. The entire die is covered with a tin foil substitute.

Step 2: Forming the wax pattern on the die to the desired design.

Step 3: The pattern is left on the fired die, sprued, vented, and invested in the usual manner.

Step 4: The wax is eliminated and cast in metal in the usual manner.

Step 5: The sprue is removed, cleaned and polished, and reseated on the die. If conditioning agents are needed, these are applied on the die separately.

Step 6: Apply opaque porcelain to the cast coping and fire. Remove from the furnace and let cool.

Step 7: Paint die with two coats of dentin separator on shoulder and outer margin of shoulder; let dry 5 to 10 minutes.

Step 8: Apply tooth-colored porcelain on opaqued metal and the labial shoulder die surfaces. Dry and fire according to firing schedule.

Step 9: Remove from furnace and let cool under Pyrex cover to room temperature.

Step 10: Remove crown from die with the opposing finger push method.

SELECTED REFERENCES

1. Peyton, F. A., and others: Restorative dental materials, ed. 2, St. Louis, 1964, The C. V. Mosby Co.
2. Skinner, E. W., and Phillips, R. W.: The science of dental materials, Philadelphia, 1967, W. B. Saunders Co.
3. Sacchi, H., and Paffenbarger, G. C.: Simple technic for making dental porcelain jacket crowns, J.A.D.A. **54**:366, 1957.
4. Vickery, R. C., Badinelli, L. A., and Waltke, R. W.: The direct fabrication of restorations without foil on a refractory die, J. Prosth. Dent. **21**:227, 1969.
5. Toreskog, D., Phillips, R. W., and Schnell, R. G.: Properties of die materials, J. Prosth. Dent. **16**:119, 1966.

GENERAL REFERENCES

Argue, J. B.: Esthetic value of porcelain in fixed bridge restorations, J.A.D.A. **21**:90, 1934.

Argue, J. E.: Aesthetic castings for bridge abutments on anterior teeth, Oral Health **20**:571, 1930.

Argue, J. E.: The porcelain jacket crown, J.A.D.A. **26**:1472, 1939.

Avary, H.: Porcelain jacket crowns, J.A.D.A. **15**: 601, 1928.

Bartels, J. C.: Dental ceramics, J. Prosth. Dent. **11**:537, 1961.

Bartels, J. C.: Preparation of the anterior teeth for porcelain jacket crowns, J. South. California D. A. **30**:199, 1962.

Both, H. S.: Less operative trauma in preparing vital teeth for jacket crowns, New York J. Dent. **9**:154, 1939.

Bronstein, B. R.: Problems in porcelain rehabilitations, J. Prosth. Dent. **17**(1):79-87, 1967.

Clark, B. E.: Manipulation of dental porcelain, J.A.D.A. **22**:33, 1935.

Conod, H.: Étude sur la statique de la couronne jaquette, Rev. mensuelle Suisse d'Odontol. **47**: 485, 1937.

Cowger, G. T.: Class V porcelain inlays utilizing a cast matrix, J. Prosth. Dent. **11**:146, 1961.

Cowger, G. T., and Dunkin, R. S.: A nonmetal die for porcelain jacket crown fabrication, J. Prosth. Dent. **17**:577, 1967.

Ewing, J. E.: Atypical porcelain jacket crown preparations, J. Prosth. Dent. **2**:815, 1952.

Feinchneider, I. L.: Ceramique en art dentaire, J. Canad. D. A. **27**:829, 1961.

Gill, J. R.: Simplifying the construction of the porcelain veneer crown, D. J. Australia **24**:62, 1952.

Gill, J. R.: Pyrochemical reactions in the firing of porcelain, J.A.D.A. **18**:280, 1931.

Hama, M.: Studies on physical properties of low fusing porcelain and its clinical techniques, Nippon Dent. Col. An. Pub. **4**:1, 1967.

Hodson, J. T.: Phase composition of crown and inlay porcelains, J. Dent. Res. **38**:483-490, 1959.

Hodson, J. T.: Preliminary study of dental porcelains, J. South. California D. A. **26**:334, 1958.

Hodson, J. T.: Phase composition of crown and bridge porcelains, J. Dent. Res. **38**:483, 1959.

Hodson, J. T.: Some physical properties of three dental porcelains, J. Prosth. Dent. **9**:325, 1959.

Holland, M. W.: Improved method for securing the impression and die for porcelain jacket crown construction, Dent. Clin. N. Amer., p. 125, March, 1959.

Klaffenbach, A. O.: Factors in fusing of dental porcelain, J.A.D.A. **26**:1786, 1939.

Klaffenbach, A. O.: Science, art and fundamentals involved in porcelain jacket crown prosthesis, Australian J. Dent. **55**:88, 1951.

Kramer, A. G.: and Kelner, S.: New concept in jacket crown construction, D. Digest **68**:264, 1962.

Kulp, P. R., and others: Impact test for dental porcelain, J. Dent. Res. **40**:1136, 1961.

Le Gro, A. L.: Ceramics in dentistry, Brooklyn, N. Y., 1925, Dent. Items Int. Publishing Co.

Lehman, M. L.: X-ray analysis of dental porcelains; the polariscope, Brit. D. J. **111**:291, 1961.

Lehman, M. L., and Hampson, E. L.: Study of strain patterns in jacket crowns on anterior teeth resulting from different tooth preparations, Brit. D. J. **113**:337, 1962.

Malson, T. S.: Protection for jacket crown preparations, Ohio D. J. **33**:139, 1959.

Michanowicz, A. E., and Michanowicz, J. P.: Endodontic access to the pulp chamber via porcelain jacket crowns: procedure and type of instrumentation, Oral Surg. **15**:1483, 1962.

Mitchell, R. G.: Methods used to obtain optimum esthetics in the porcelain gold crown, Texas Dent. J. **85**(5):7-11, 1967.

Morris, M. L.: Artificial crown contours and gingival health, J. Prosth. Dent. **12**:1146, 1962.

Moulton, G. H.: Porcelain veneer crown, North-West Dent. **38**:363, 1959.

Nuttall, E. B.: Factors influencing success of porcelain jacket restorations, J. Prosth. Dent. **11**:743, 1961.

Pettrow, J. N.: Practical factors in building and firing characteristics of dental porcelain, J. Prosth. Dent. **11**:334, 1961.

Pruden, W. H., II: Porcelain veneer crown, J. Prosth. Dent. **10**:955, 1960.

Richard, E. L., and Brodtmann, N. V.: Cast copings for jacket crowns, J. Prosth. Dent. **12**: 129, 1962.

Sacchi, H., and Paffenbarger, G. C.: Simple technic for making dental porcelain jacket crowns, J.A.D.A. **54**:366, 1957.

Saklad, M. H.: Disclosure of cleavage and fracture lines in porcelain restorations, J. Prosth. Dent. **8**:115, 1958.

Sandler, A. C.: Acrylic trial copings for balanced fixed bridgework, J.A.D.A. **63**:484, 1961.

Sayre, L. D.: Physics and mechanics involved in serviceable porcelain jacket crown restorations, J.A.D.A. **31**: 3, 1942.

Schneider, A. E.: The preparation of a tooth for a porcelain veneer crown, Chicago, 1916.

Sharp, T. B.: Preparation for and construction of baked porcelain crowns and inlays, J. Prosth. Dent. **9**:113, 1959.

Skinner, E. W., and Fitzgerald, P. A.: Physical properties of dental porcelains, J.A.D.A. **25**: 861-865, 1938.

Swann, A. J. N.: Fabrication of atmosphere-fired porcelain jacket crowns utilizing vacuum-fired facings, Dent. Pract. (Bristol) **19**(4):131, 1968.

Vehe, W. D.: Some basic principles underlying porcelain veneer crown technic, J.A.D.A. **17**: 2167, 1930.

Vehe, W. D.: A consideration of the porcelain veneer crown from the standpoint of the general practitioner, Illinois D. J. **1**:453, 1931-1932.

Vehe, W. D.: Tooth preparation for porcelain veneer crown, Minneapolis Dist. D. J. **23**:23, 1939.

Vines, R. F., Semmelman, J. D., Ise, P. W., and Vines, R. P., Jr.: Mechanisms involved in securing dense, vitrified ceramics from preshaped partly crystalline bodies, J. Am. Ceramics Soc. **41**:304, 1958.

Vines, R. F., and Semmelman, J. O.: Densification of dental porcelain, J. Dent. Res. **36**:950, 1967.

Walton, C. B., and Leven, M. M.: Preliminary report of photoelastic tests of strain patterns within jacket crowns, J.A.D.A. **50**:44, 1955.

Watanabe, K., and others: Experiment on the physical strength of porcelain shell faced jacket crown, Odontology (Tokyo) **53**:72, 1966.

Wheeler, R. C.: A comparison of periodontal attachment levels: anteroposteriorly, D. Digest **41**:261, 1935.

Wheeler, R. C.: Important considerations in porcelain veneer restorations, Illinois D. J. **16**: 131, 1947.

Wilson, H. J., and Whitehead, F. I. H.: Comparison of some physical properties of dental porcelains, Dent. Pract. (Bristol) **17**(10):350, 1967.

Yock, D. H.: Porcelain jacket veneer crown preparation, Iowa D. J. **43**:267, 1957.

Chapter 27

Tooth preparation: construction of dowel crowns—anterior and posterior teeth

EARLY TYPES OF DOWEL CROWNS

Crowns with dowels are generally used when it is impossible to restore the tooth by means of fillings or other crowns that do not involve the removal of the pulp. Every other restorative method should be considered before using a crown that requires the removal of the pulp. If used, every precaution must be taken in such instances that the pulp canal is properly filled and that the periapical tissues are not infected.

A root to be acceptable for this type of crown must be sound biologically; also it must have sufficient strength and enough tooth tissue left to withstand the forces to which it will be subjected. It must also have a periodontal membrane attachment of sufficient amount and an alveolar bone that is adequate both in amount and distribution.

Dowel crowns are usually employed on anterior teeth, although they may be successfully used on the posterior ones.

The coronal portion of the restoration may be of gold, of porcelain, of acrylic resin, or may be a combination of gold and porcelain. The dowel is generally an integral part of the restoration.

Dowel crowns depend for their retention and resistance to displacement primarily upon the dowel that extends into the root canal. There are some modifications of these crowns that employ a cap; these may be either swaged, cast, or of fired ceramic and are made to encircle the periphery of the preparation, thus adding considerable retention.

Manufactured dowels may be used or they may be made to fit the individual case. The manufactured dowels usually consisted of a pin with a shoulder near the cervical end; from this point the pin tapered apically. The dowel extended for several millimeters incisally from the shoulder. Because of the forces to which the dowel was subjected, it was usually made of an alloy of the gold and platinum group of metals.

TYPES OF CROWNS

There are several types of crowns that may be used with dowels; the first of these is the all-metal cast gold crown, similar to the one described in Chapter 23.

All-metal gold cast type

These may be either of the shoulder or the shoulderless type. Where the crown portion of the tooth remains, the preparation is identical with that previously described except that, after the pulp has been removed and the canals properly filled, one or more of the canals are reamed out and a dowel of cheap metal wire of suitable length and gauge is fitted.

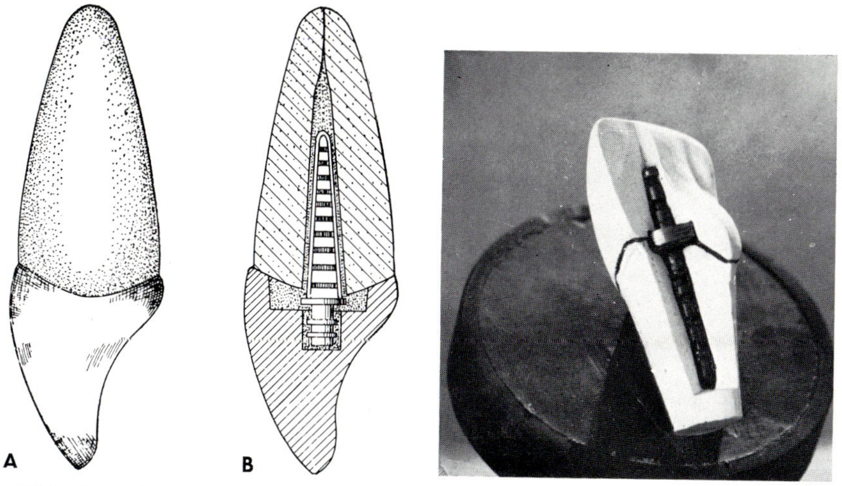

Fig. 27-1. Use of detached type of dowel with all-porcelain crown. Cross sections show relative position of dowel in root and in base of crown. Cement unites tooth, dowel, and crown into one rigid unit (not manufactured today).

When the crown is cast, the dowel is locked in the casting and is made an integral part of the restoration. This type of crown may have a labial veneer of fused porcelain or acrylic resin.

Where the coronal portion of posterior tooth has been largely destroyed either by caries or accident; the root face is prepared, if possible, with a shoulder and a plateau similar to the preparation made in Fig. 23-2. Where, however, it is impossible to prepare a shoulder, two or more planes are prepared in the root face; these planes should be so placed that they will help resist the forces developed during masticatory movements.

Detached dowel type

The second type of crown employing a dowel was one in which the dowel was detached, while the coronal part of the crown consisted entirely or almost entirely of porcelain (Fig. 27-1). This crown was known as the plain Davis crown.

Cast metal base type

When the coronal portion of the natural tooth had been decayed or destroyed to a point below the gingival line so that the crown and root planes could not be perfectly adapted to each other or their peripheries made to coincide, a cast metal base was interposed between the base of the crown and the root face (Fig. 27-2).

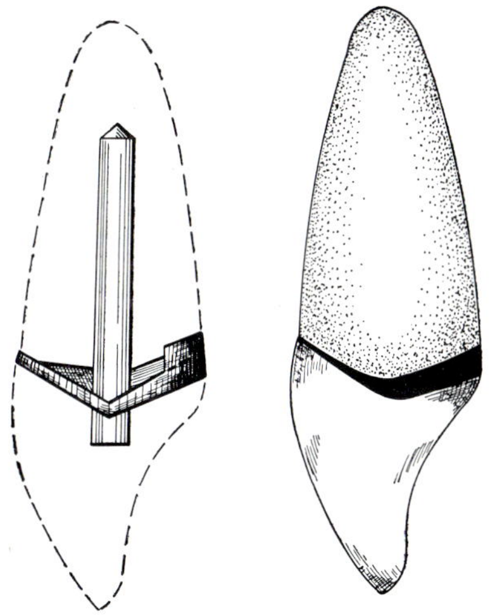

Fig. 27-2. Cast base and dowel and finished crown used when decay of tooth extended below gingival plane.

Fused porcelain base type

Still another method was employed in adapting a complete porcelain crown to a root face; this consisted of interposing

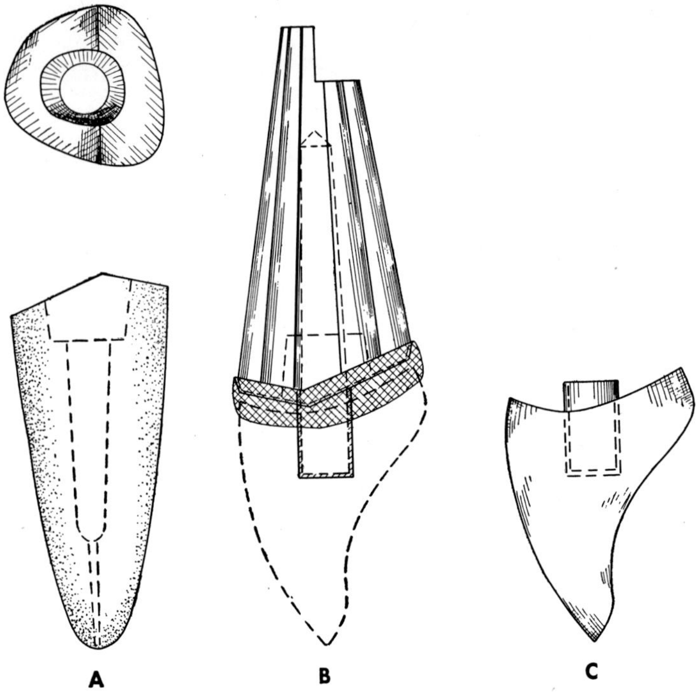

Fig. 27-3. A, Root prepared for fired porcelain base crown. **B,** Platinum ferrule adapted to dowel extension. **C,** Ferrule fitted to opening in base of porcelain crown. This is then replaced on die over which platinum cap has been swaged. Crown, ferrule, and platinum cap are waxed as shown in **B.**

and fusing porcelain between the base of the crown and the root face. The interposed porcelain is fused to and made an integral part of the porcelain crown. Fig. 27-3 shows the steps of the root preparation, swaging the 0.001-gauge platinum ferrule, and the interfaces between the root base and the crown surface.

Swaged iridioplatinum base

A modification of the latter type of crown employed a 40-gauge, swaged iridoplatinum cap soldered to an iridioplatinum post. The coping was made a permanent part of the crown by fusing porcelain between the coping and the crown (Figs. 27-4 to 27-7). This type of crown had a permanent matrix 40-gauge iridioplatinum interposed between the base of the crown and the root face. This shouldered coping encircled the root and reduced to a great degree, the danger of root fracture. This type of crown was especially valuable where the restoration was likely to be subjected to excessive forces; it had been used with complete satisfaction for over 35 years.

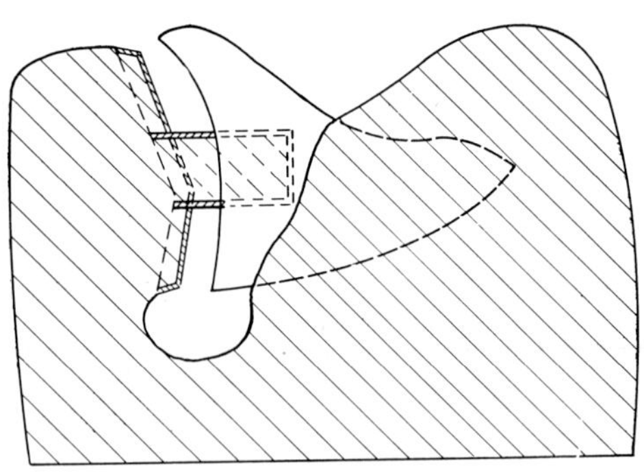

Fig. 27-4. Crown, ferrule, and 0.001-inch platinum cap invested and wax eliminated; porcelain baked between crown and platinum cap.

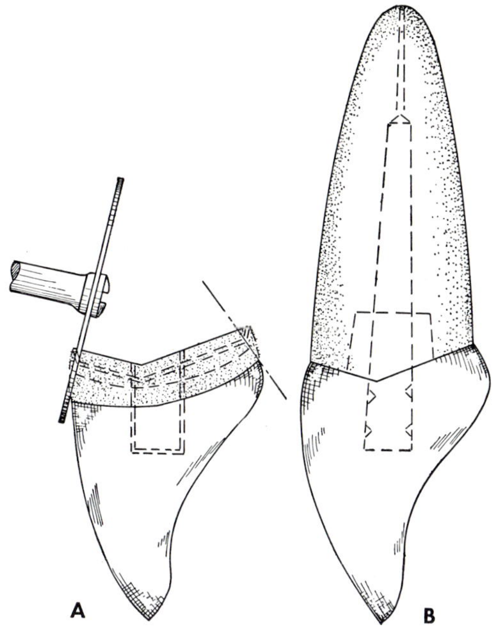

Fig. 27-5. A, Grinding excess porcelain around gingival periphery. **B,** Finished crown with detached dowel in position.

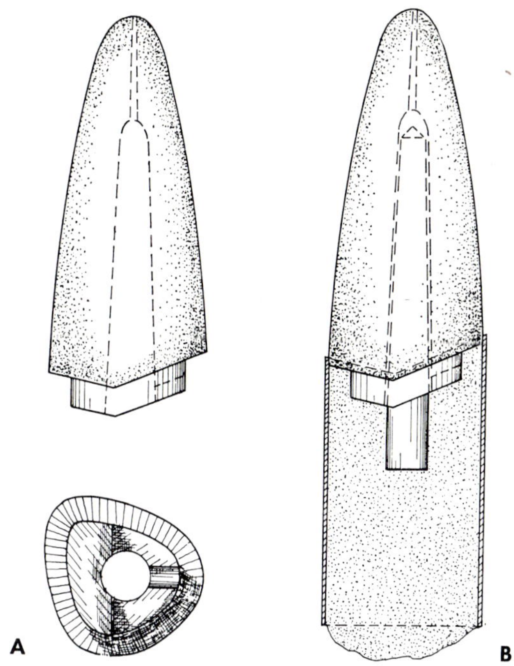

Fig. 27-6. A, Root prepared with shoulder and plateau for swaged platinum plate coping, having iridioplatinum dowel. **B,** Modeling compound impression of root with dowel in place.

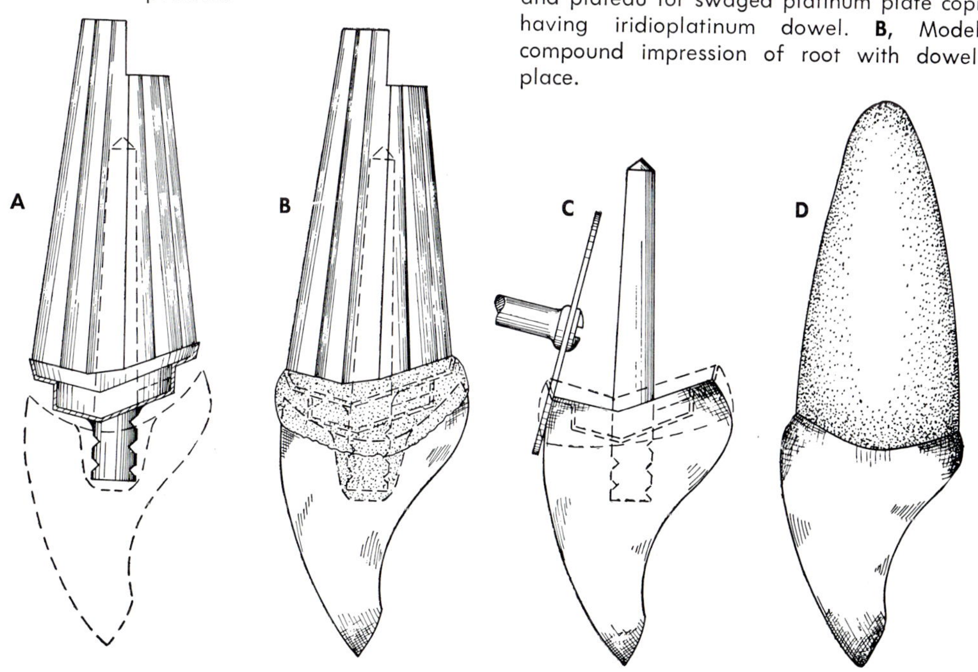

Fig. 27-7. A, Die with 40-gauge iridioplatinum swaged cap soldered to dowel. Crown aligned and centered over dowel extension. **B,** Porcelain baked between and over coping and porcelain crown. **C,** Removing excess porcelain from gingival region. Note that platinum coping remains integral part of finished crown, which is finished flush against outer angle of shoulder preparation. **D,** Completed crown.

RICHMOND CROWN

One of the oldest types of crowns utilizing a dowel is the cast or soldered gold crown, which employes a porcelain veneer facing; this is better known as the Richmond crown (Fig. 27-8, A). Although it may be used as an individual restoration, it is indicated primarily as a bridge retainer on pulpless, anterior teeth whose coronal portion has been destroyed so that it is impossible to use a partial veneer retainer. While it is not used as extensively as formerly due to the difficulty and meticulous skill required for its fabrication, there are conditions which arise that are met very satisfactorily with this type of restoration.

Types and component phases of construction

The component parts of a Richmond crown are a porcelain facing, usually the pin type, and a coping, which are united and held together either by means of solder or by an intermediary casting.

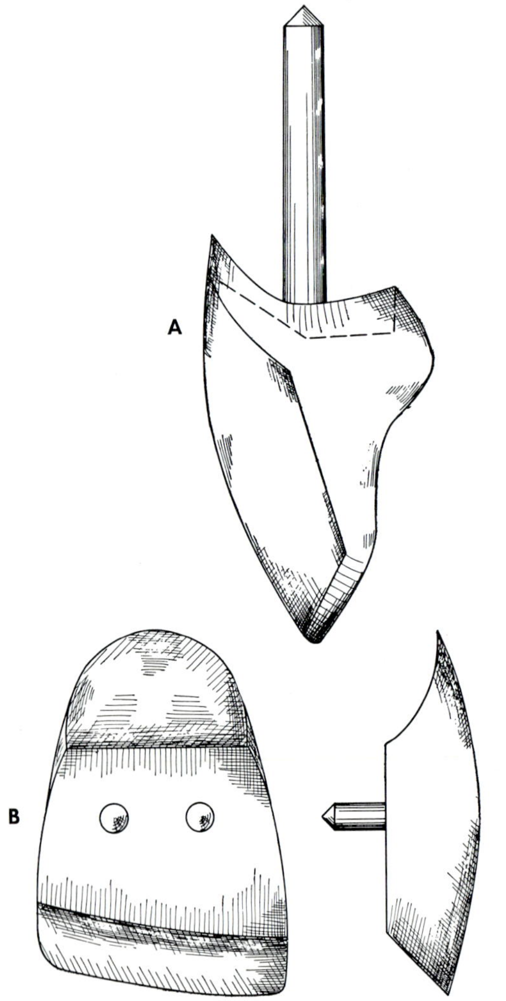

Fig. 27-8. A, Finished Richmond crown. Note incisal protection of gold and position of gingival margin of facing in its relationship to coping. **B,** Gingival portion of facing ground to fit coping; incisal area beveled for protection with gold. Note round pin facing.

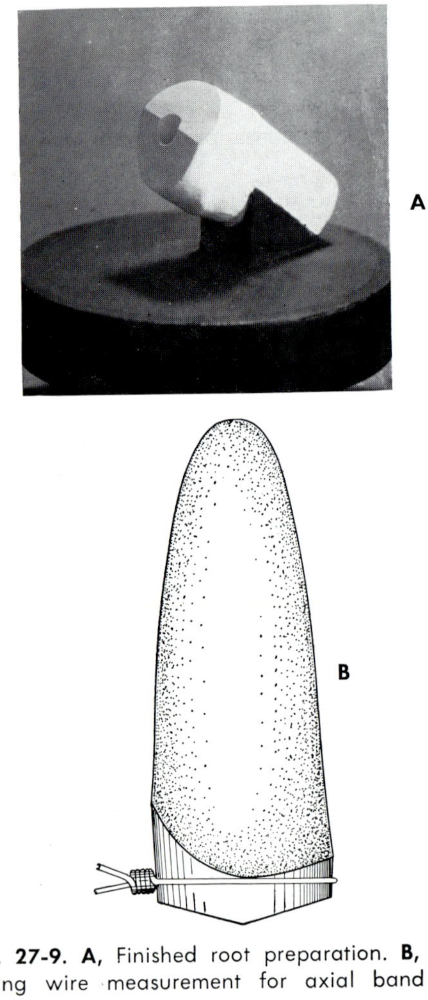

Fig. 27-9. A, Finished root preparation. **B,** Securing wire measurement for axial band of coping.

The facing. The facing used may be the short or long thin type or any of the removable or interchangeable varieties. (Fig. 27-8, *B*).

The coping. The coping consists of (1) a metal cap fitted to the root face and (2) a dowel extending into the root canal (Figs. 27-17, *A*, and 27-22). The general shape of the root preparation is that of a frustum of a cone with its base line slightly beneath the crest of the gum tissue; its narrower end consists of a labial and a lingual plane. The labial plane is slightly beneath the crest of the labial gingiva, while the lingual plane is left 2 mm. above the gingiva (Fig. 27-9, *A*).

There are two available methods for constructing the root cap for the coping: (1) the adapted axial band with soldered cap, and (2) the one-piece swaged cap with axial band. The adapted axial band type is discussed first.

Figs. 27-9, *B*, to 27-14 show a 22-carat, 29-gauge gold plate band constructed and fitted cervically and contoured to parallel the curvature of the gingiva. The labial half of the band together with the labial surface of the root preparation are now reduced slightly below the crest of the gum tissue (Fig. 27-14). The band is then removed from the root and a piece of 36-gauge, 24-carat gold plate is soldered to the incisal end of the band (Figs. 27-15 and 27-17, *A*). When desired, this cap may also be constructed by swaging the 36-gauge, 24-carat gold plate over an amalgam die made from an individual impression taken of the prepared root (Figs. 27-17 to 27-22).

Cast type Richmond crown

Still another method of constructing the Richmond crown eliminates the use of the swaged backing entirely. The ground facing is waxed directly to the coping and

Text continued on p. 590

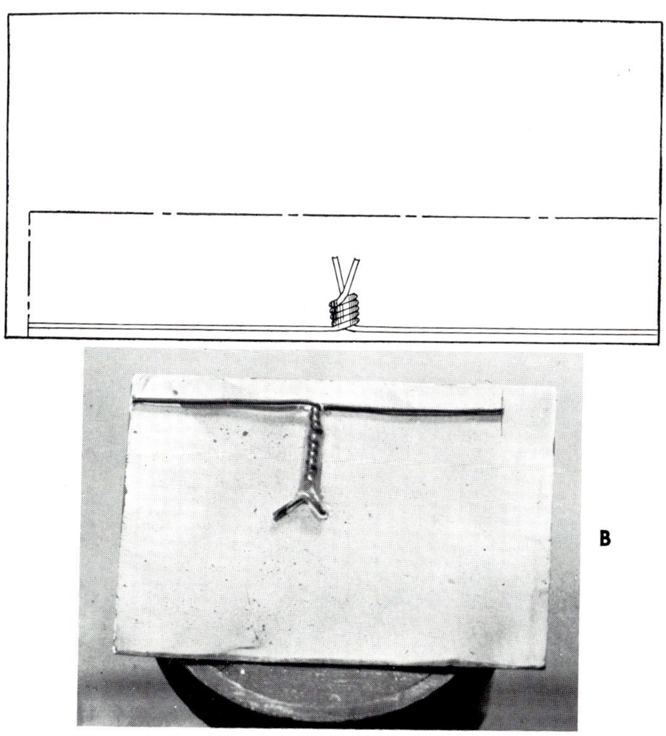

A

B

Fig. 27-10. Transferring measurement to gold plate.

A

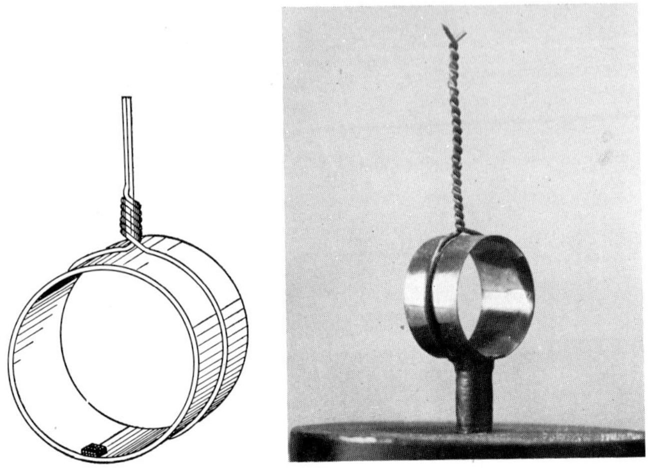

B

Fig. 27-11. Soldering axial band.

A

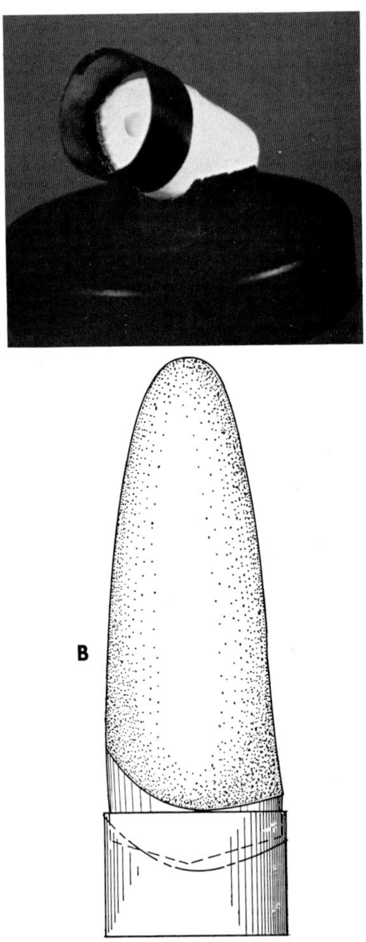

B

Fig. 27-12. Initial step in fitting axial band to root preparation.

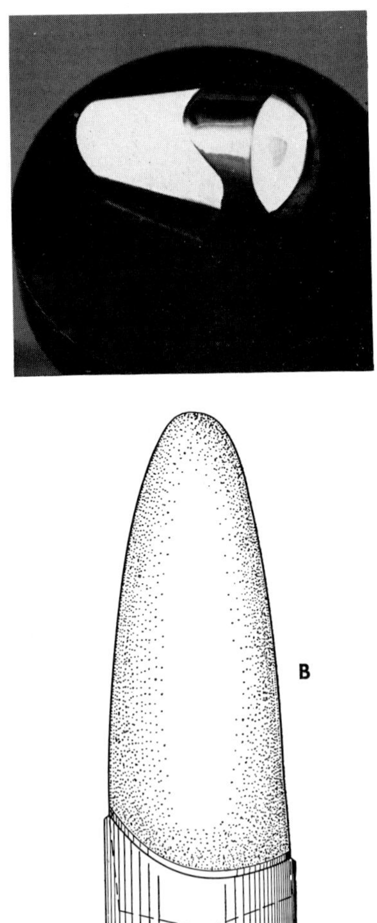

A

B

Fig. 27-13. Band fitted to root preparation and contour of gingiva.

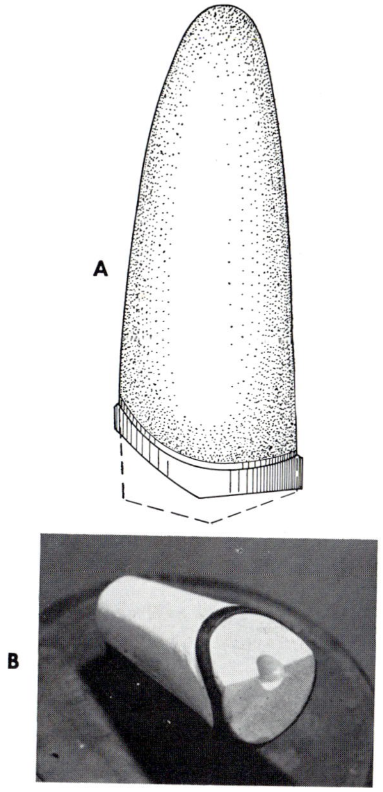

Fig. 27-14. Band trimmed to correct labial, **A,** and lingual, **B,** heights.

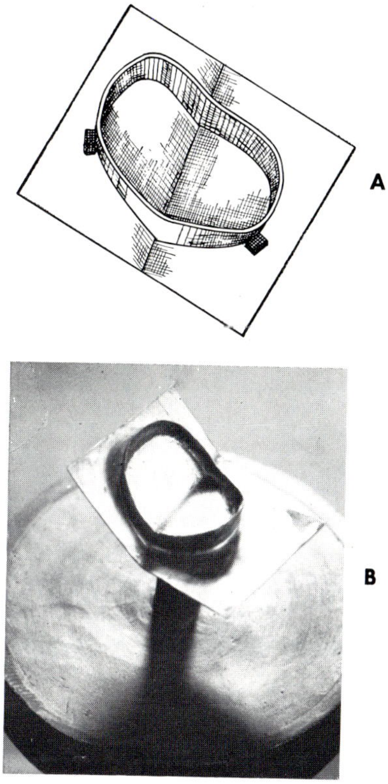

Fig. 27-15. Gold plate soldered to axial band.

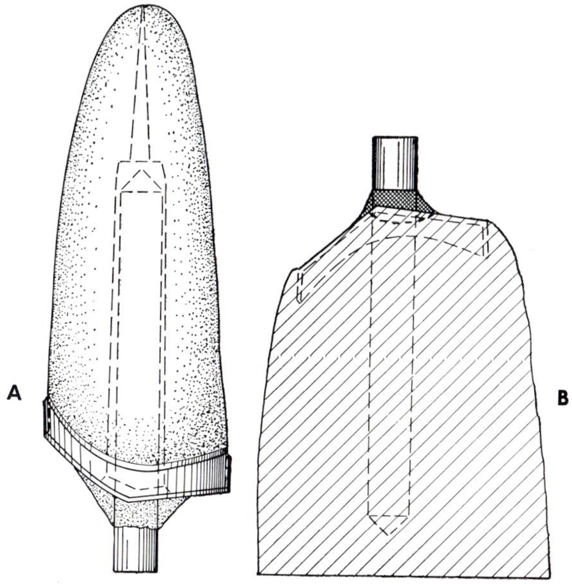

Fig. 27-16. A, Finished cap united with dowel by means of sticky wax, ready for investing. **B,** Cap and dowel invested and united by means of solder, forming coping; note dotted line, showing countersunk depression in root canal opening.

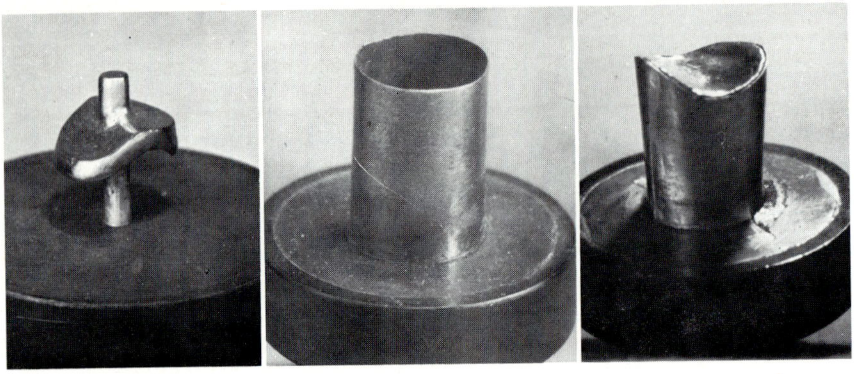

A B C

Fig. 27-17. A, Finished soldered coping. **B,** Copper band to be prepared for swaged type coping impression. **C,** Compound impression material placed in contoured copper band.

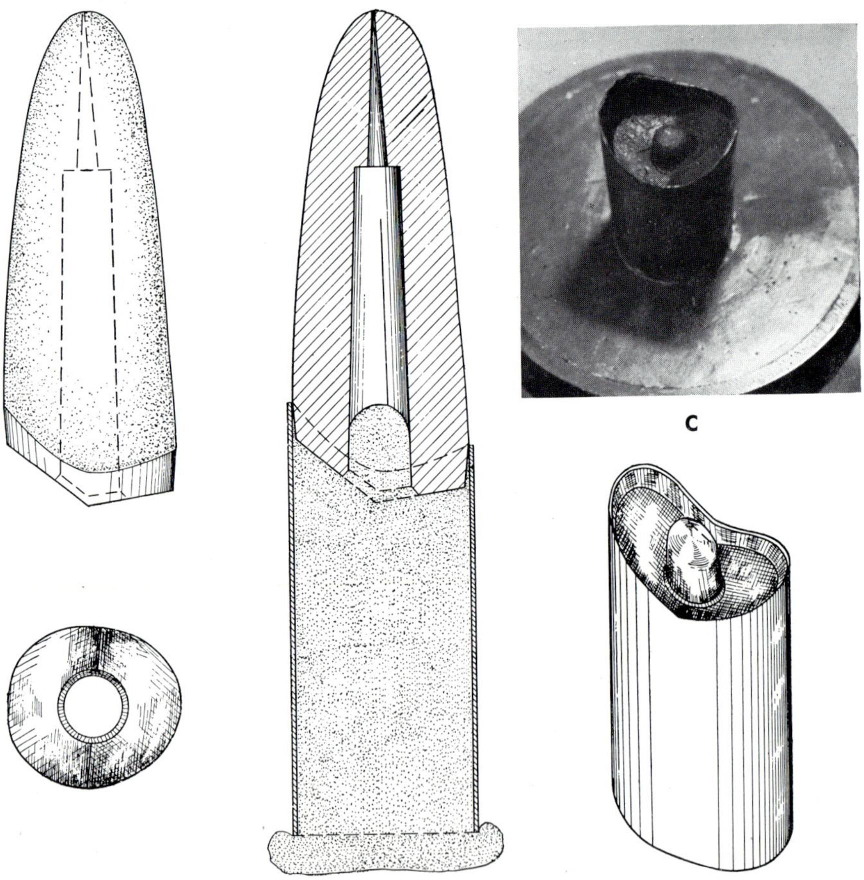

A B C D

Fig. 27-18. A, Where cap is swaged from one piece of metal, root is prepared as shown. **B** to **D,** Modeling compound impression taken in copper band.

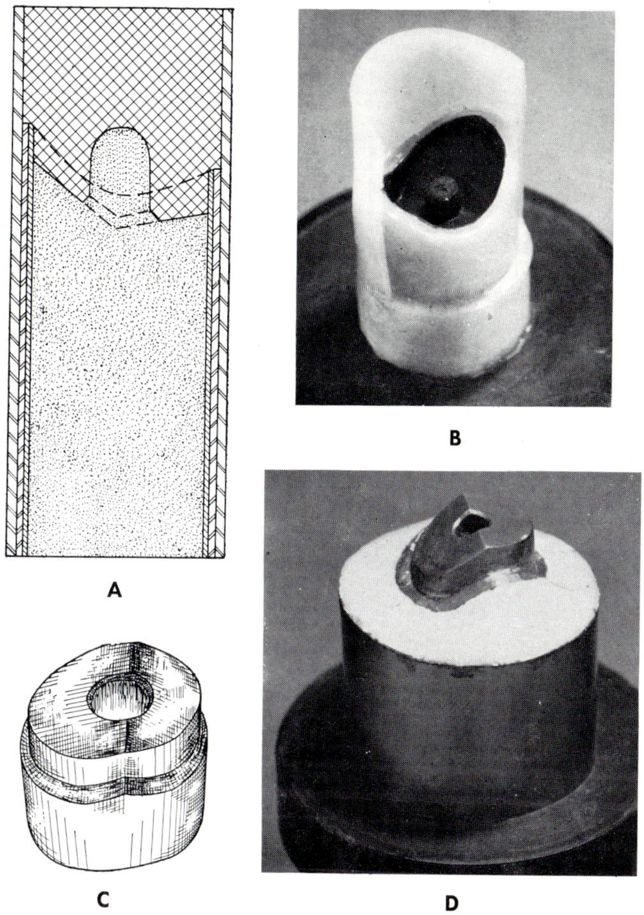

Fig. 27-19. A and **B,** Copper band and impression encircled with sheets of wax and packed with amalgam. **C** and **D,** Amalgam dies.

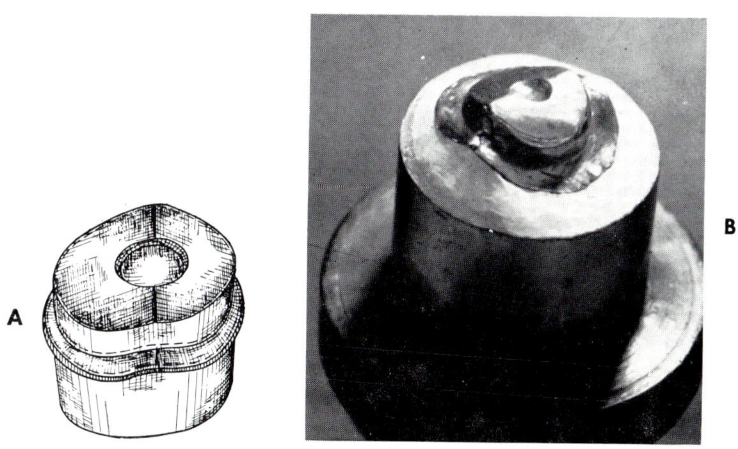

Fig. 27-20. Cap partially swaged and having excess at gingival margin.

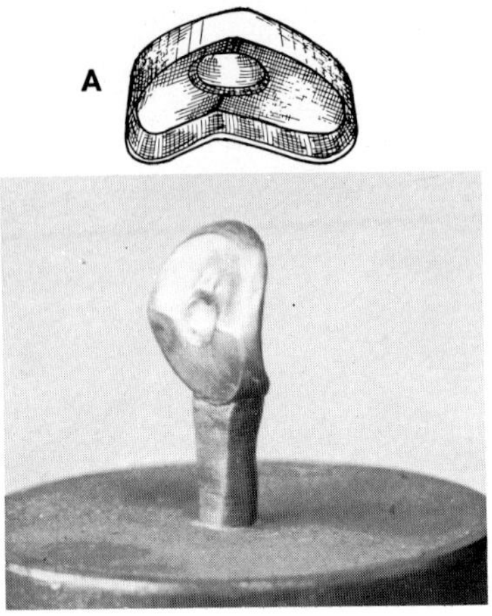

Fig. 27-21. Finished swaged caps.

is withdrawn from the waxed crown before it is invested and cast.

Root preparation

The enamel in the gingival region is removed with enamel cleavers, using the same technic as described in Chapter 24, where the subgingival collar of enamel is removed for a complete veneer porcelain crown.

After the enamel has been removed with cleavers, the axial surfaces of the prepared root are smoothed with thin-bladed files which are kept away from the bottom of the gingival crevice.

The preparation then appears as shown in Fig. 27-9, *A;* its general shape is that of the frustum of a cone with its base lying slightly beneath the crest of the gum tissue and its narrower end consisting of a labial and a lingual plane.

Wire measurement. The next step is securing the wire measurement of the root for the construction of the cap (Fig. 27-9, *B*). This may be constructed (1) directly on the prepared tooth by fitting an axial band to which an incisal cover is soldered, or (2) by the indirect method, when the entire cap is swaged from one piece of metal.

A 36-gauge wire loop measurement is taken of the preparation, at a point even

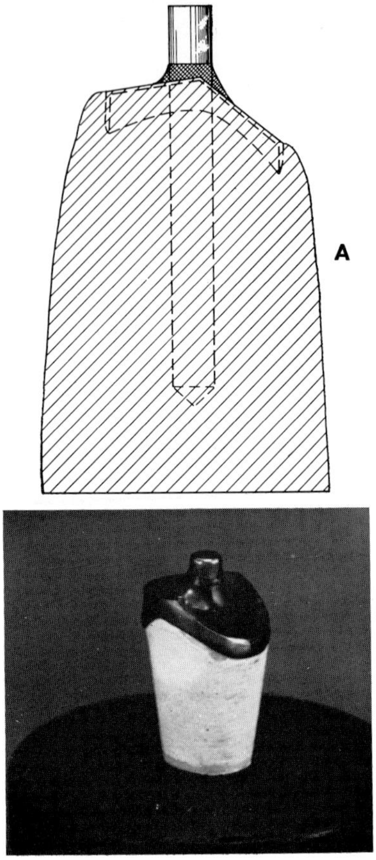

Fig. 27-22. Cap waxed, invested, and soldered to dowel, forming coping.

with the crest of the proximal gum tissues (Fig. 27-9, *B*).

Construction of the cap. After the wire loop has been cut opposite the twist, it is straightened and its length marked on a piece of 22-carat, 29-gauge gold plate, as shown in Fig. 27-10, *A* and *B*. The height of the band is slightly greater than the distance from the lowest point in the curvature of the gingivae to the highest incisal point on the root preparation.

The band is then shaped to form a ring, care being taken that the edges of both ends of the band are in absolute contact. A small piece of 22-carat solder is placed on the inside of the band in such a way that it bridges across the joint of the two ends. It is well to apply some flux to the joint before the application of the solder (Fig. 27-11, *A* and *B*).

The band and solder are carried into a Bunsen flame; as the solder melts, it flows into the joint, uniting the two ends of the band. If the difficulty is experienced of having the edges of the band open, these may be held together by applying a loop of untinned iron wire around the outside of the band, as shown in Fig. 27-11, *B*. This will keep the edges of the band in contact during the soldering operation.

The gold ferrule is now carried over the root preparation, as shown in Fig. 27-12, *A*, and placed cervically until the margin of the ferrule comes in contact with the crest of the proximal gum tissue (Fig. 27-12, *B*). By repeatedly scribing, trimming, and retrying the band on the prepared tooth, the margin of the band is finally made to parallel the curvature of the gum tissue (Fig. 27-13, *A* and *B*). It will be noticed at this point that the gingival periphery of the band is now at a lower level than the plane at which the wire root measurement was originally taken and according to which the size of the band was determined. This is a desirable condition, since the 22-carat gold plate band will readily stretch when slight pressure is applied at its incisal end.

The gingival margin of the band is next lowered beneath the crest of the gum tissue and into the gingival crevice. Before doing so, however, it should be determined how far the margin of the band is to be lowered. If the base of the prepared frustum lies 1 mm. beneath the crest of the gum tissue, the margin must necessarily stop short of that distance. It is probable that 0.75 or 0.5 mm. will be the correct distance, in which event a scratch is made on the labial and lingual surfaces of the gold band about 0.5 mm. from the gingival margin, following which the band is replaced on the tooth and gently pressed rootwise until the labial and lingual scratches on the band are level with the crest of the gum tissue on these surfaces. This technic places the gingival margin of the band a uniform distance beneath the crest of the gum tissues around its entire periphery (Fig. 27-13, *B*).

The height of the band is then reduced on the labial surface to a level where it would not be visible (Fig. 27-14, *A*). That on the lingual surface, however, is left high, approximately 2 mm. above the crest of the gum tissue, in order to afford greater resistance to displacement from the lingual side (Fig. 27-14, *B*).

The band is again returned to the tooth, when it will be found that the labial part of the band is now even with or slightly below the crest of the gum tissue in that area. If the labial part of the root preparation extends incisally beyond the margin of the band, it is reduced with a Densco 5J stone until its plane corresponds with the labial margin of the band.

As shown later, it is necessary that the labial plane of the root preparation be a flat surface so that the correct alignment of the facing may be more easily accomplished.

The band is then removed from the root and a piece of 36-gauge, 24-carat gold plate soldered to the incisal end as shown in Fig. 27-15, *A* and *B*. The excess plate is removed with shears and disks, care being taken to leave a square edge between the soldered plate and the axial band.

The cap is now ready to be soldered to the dowel.

After a clasp metal dowel of suitable gauge and length has been fitted in the root canal, it is removed, and the pulp canal opening is countersunk 0.5 mm. with a No. 10 round bur (Fig. 27-16, *B*). This depression allows a greater amount of solder to unite the cap to the dowel.

Construction of the coping by direct method. The cap is returned to the root and that part overlying the pulp canal is burnished with an egg-shaped burnisher into the countersunk area. The dowel previously fitted is now forced through the cap and into the root canal, which has been previously enlarged to the proper diameter. The dowel extends incisally 2 to 3 mm. beyond the root cap.

A small amount of sticky wax is melted around the dowel and the cap, filling the countersunk space (Fig. 27-16, *A*). When the wax hardens, the dowel and cap are carefully removed from the root and invested for soldering (Fig. 27-16, *B*).

If the cap fails to come away with the dowel, it may be necessary to put a small amount of plaster of Paris over the cap and the dowel, which, when set, will ensure their removal in their correct relationship to each other.

A small amount of soldering investment is then mixed and applied to the inner surface of the cap and around the dowel, as shown in Fig. 27-16, *B*. After the investment has hardened, the sticky wax or the plaster impression is removed, and the surfaces of the cap and the dowel are thoroughly cleaned and fluxed.

The investment is slowly dried over a Bunsen flame, increasing the heat gradually until it is brought to a high temperature; this may be hastened by means of a blowpipe flame.

A small amount of 20-carat solder is now melted to unite the dowel and cap, completely filling the countersunk space. The cap united to the dowel is known as the "coping" (Fig. 27-17, *A*).

After the coping is recovered from the investment, it is cleaned and boiled in acid to make certain that all traces of investment have been removed. When washed and dried, it is tried on the tooth to make certain that the correct relationship exists between the cap, the dowel, and the soft tissues.

Construction of the swaged coping by indirect method. In order to construct a swaged coping by the indirect method, the steps of construction differ somewhat. It will be recalled in the previous technic that after all the enamel was removed from the gingival region of the tooth, the next step was taking a wire measurement and fitting the gold band. In the indirect method a wire measurement is also taken, but a copper band matrix is fitted instead of the gold band (Fig. 27-17, *B*).

After the gingival margin of the copper band has been trimmed to parallel the gingival crest of the gum tissue, it is filled with modeling compound and laid aside for subsequent use (Fig. 27-17, *C*).

With root-facing diamond stones or with the steel root facers, a labial plane is sloped gingivally to terminate even with or slightly below the crest of the gingival tissue. The lingual plane, although it is sloped slightly cervically, is left approximately 2 to 3 mm. in height, as shown in Fig. 27-18, *A*. The root canal opening is then countersunk with a No. 10 round bur.

The next procedure is taking an impression of the preparation in modeling compound in the copper band previously fitted to the root, as shown in Fig. 27-18, *B*. When the impression is taken, it is examined to make certain that all the surfaces and margins are accurately reproduced. It is also essential that the impression show the outline of the base of the frustum of the cone preparation, as shown in Fig. 27-18, *B* to *D*.

The impression is then wrapped with two thicknesses of wax, as shown in Fig. 27-19, *A* and *B*, and an amalgam die (Fig. 27-19, *C* and *D*) is constructed.

A piece of 36-gauge, 24-carat gold plate is cut sufficiently large to cover the face of the die as well as the axial surfaces of the preparation to the finishing gingival line.

The die is oiled and the piece of gold plate centered over it; with finger pressure the gold plate is initially adapted to the root face.

The plate is then removed and boiled

in acid if it is contaminated by mercury or amalgam; then it is brought to a cherry red color in a Bunsen flame and quenched in water, thus restoring its soft working qualities. It is returned to the die and by successive steps is adapted to the root face and the axial surfaces (Fig. 27-20).

It is possible to obtain perfect adaptation by manual swaging only, using finger pressure, pieces of hard wood, and gold files. Round or smooth surface burnishers should not be used, as they have a tendency to work-harden gold plate, causing folds to develop. Repeated heating and quenching during the swaging of the cap will facilitate the quick and accurate adaptation of the metal to the amalgam die.

After the cap has been swaged and trimmed to its correct gingival peripheral outline, some operators give it one or two sharp blows in a swager. In doing so, however, care must be exercised not to tear the cap.

The finished cap (Fig. 27-21) is similar to the two-piece cap except that the inner surface of the swaged cap comes in complete surface contact with the axial surfaces of the root preparation, while the two-piece cap has only a peripheral line contact on the axial surfaces.

When swaged, the cap is returned to the prepared tooth where it is waxed and then permanently united to the dowel by means of solder (Fig. 27-22, *A* and *B*).

The steps in the completion of the Richmond crown are identical with the one-piece swaged or the two-piece banded copings.

Selecting, grinding, and backing facing. The next procedure is the selection, grinding, and backing of the porcelain facing and the establishing of its correct relationship with the coping and the adjoining teeth. These steps are performed on working models containing the cast of the arch involved in the restoration and the cast of the opposing arch; both are mounted on an articulator, which maintains them in their correct relationship to each other and which reproduces their related movements in the mouth.

Taking the bite and impressions. A bite and two impressions are taken and, where necessary, a face bow is used to transfer the centric arch relationships to the articulator.

Where an individual crown is under construction, a sufficient number of natural teeth are usually present to establish the correct occlusal relationship between the two arches. Where a wax bite is necessary, it is suggested that 60-gauge tin foil be placed between two pieces of pink base-plate wax and trimmed to conform roughly to the outline of the arch; this double wafer of wax with interposed tin foil is then softened by thorough heating and the patient is instructed to close upon it. In taking the bite, no effort is made to carry it beyond the tips of the cusps. Where the cusps and inclined planes of the opposing teeth have been worn into close contact with each other, the tin foil will stretch without tearing and afford an accurate seat for both casts. After the wax has cooled, it is carefully removed from the mouth and laid aside.

Constructing working models. An impression is then taken of the entire opposing arch in hydrocolloidal or a rubber type impression material; this is later poured in artificial stone or electroformed.

An impression of the other arch containing the coping is then obtained with plaster of Paris. This impression should also include the entire arch, especially where the restoration involves a bicuspid or molar. Whichever material is used, care must be taken that the model reproduces the natural teeth accurately, particularly those teeth that are immediately adjacent to the crown under construction. Of equal importance is the correct alignment and position of the coping in the impression before the model is poured and the maintenance of the correct relationship while the model is poured.

Before pouring the model, the axial

walls on the inside of the coping and the sides of the dowel are painted with a very thin film of wax. That portion of the cap which rests on the root face and the gingival margin of the cap, however, should not be covered with wax, since they furnish the definite seat for the coping during its removal and replacement on the model during the construction of the crown. After the models are constructed and mounted on the articulator, a small flame is carefully applied to the incisal surface of the coping; this melts the film of wax and allows the withdrawal of the coping from the working model. After all the wax has been removed from the dowel and inner surfaces of the coping, it is oiled slightly and replaced in its position on the model.

It is advisable at this time to cut a small hole at right angles to the labial aspect of the stone model opposite the apical end of the dowel, exposing it slightly. Later, the waxed crown may be removed from the model by inserting a blunt instrument into the opening and prying up on the end of the dowel.

Selecting the facing. The next step is the selection of the facing. A facing of the correct shade, mesiodistal width, and a slightly longer gingivoincisal length is selected. The additional length allows sufficient porcelain for grinding-in the facing accurately at the gingival. For the soldered type of Richmond crown, the short, pointed platinum pin facing is usually used, although the flat pin type may also be employed (Fig. 27-23).

Grinding the facing. As the first step, it is well to fit the gingival or ridge lap of the facing to the coping. Not only should the porcelain be ground to conform to the mesiodistal curvature of the labial gum tissue and coping, but also the lingual surface of the ridge lap should be hollowed out, so that the facing has a line and not a surface contact with the cap. Such a line contact makes it pos-

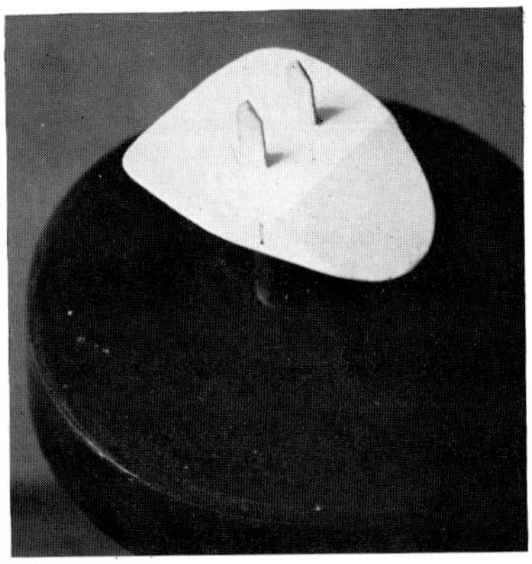

Fig. 27-23. Flat pin facing is sometimes used.

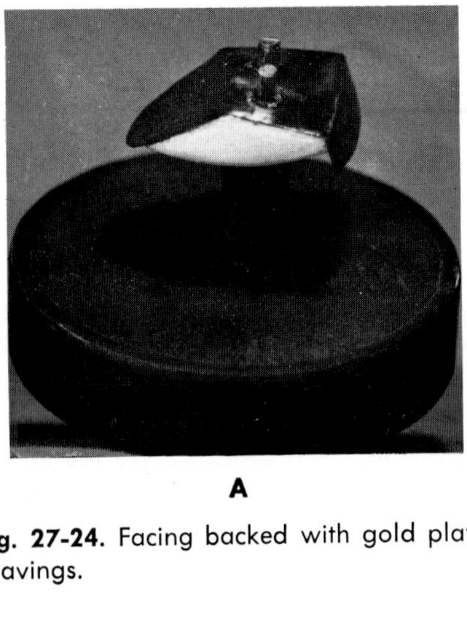

A

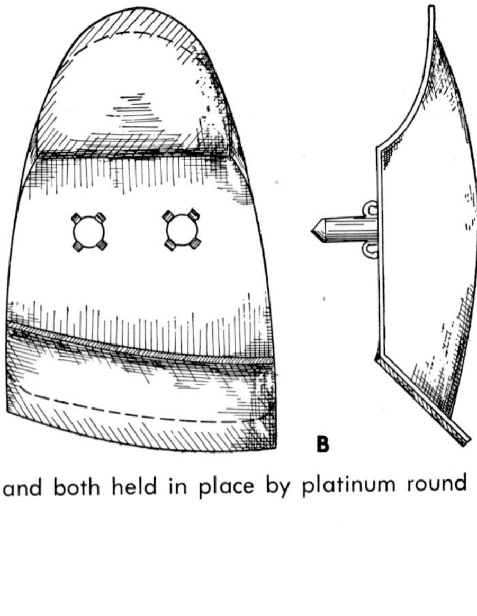

B

Fig. 27-24. Facing backed with gold plate and both held in place by platinum round pin shavings.

sible later to move the incisal edge of the facing labially or lingually, without creating an opening along the gingival margin (Figs. 27-24 and 27-25).

When grinding porcelain facings, the stone should revolve from the labial toward the lingual to preclude the possibility of chipping the labial surface.

Beveling the incisal edge. After the facing has been ground to its proper length, the incisal edge is beveled toward the lingual surface at an angle of 45° with the plane of the lingual surface. This is done to allow for a sufficient thickness of gold to cover the incisal edge in the finished crown. Occasionally, in close bite cases the lingual surface of the facing is hollow-ground from the incisal edge to a point 0.5 mm. above the platinum pins,

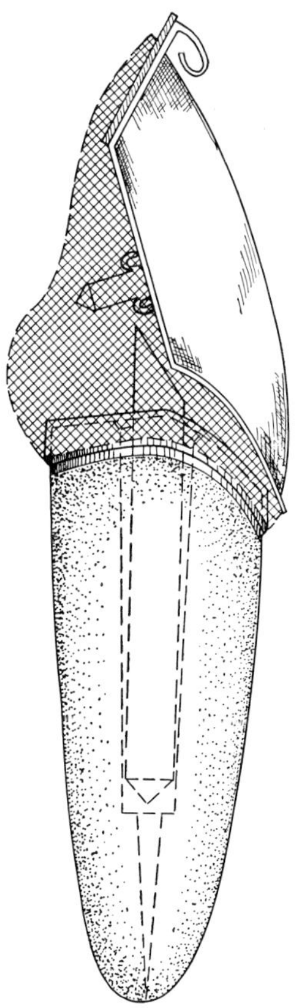

Fig. 27-25. Facing and coping waxed in their proper relationship to each other.

with but a very narrow, supplementary incisal bevel placed along the incisal edge. Such treatment of the facing gives room for a greater bulk of gold in this region; however, it is more difficult to control the shade of the facing when so ground (Figs. 27-24 and 27-25).

Backing the facing. In the soldered Richmond crown it is necessary to back the facing with gold plate (Fig. 27-24). Thirty-six gauge, 24-carat gold plate is used because of the ease with which it may be swaged to the facing. A piece of gold plate, the width of the facing but slightly longer than the length of the lingual surface from the incisal edge to the cervicogingival margin, is cut and made smooth. This is laid flat on a hard rubber cork, and the facing, with the pins pointed down, is centered over it in such a position that the gold extends slightly beyond the gingival and incisal edges. By applying slight pressure to the facing, the pointed platinum pins perforate the plate, and the rubber cork roughly conforms the backing to the lingual surface of the facing.

By the use of finger pressure, the rubber cork, and the convex side of a gold file applied with a rolling motion, it is possible to conform the gold plate closely to the facing. During the process, however, it may be necessary several times to remove the backing, heat and quench it in water; this renders the gold plate again workable after it has been work-hardened during the swaging process.

That part of the gold backing which extends beyond the facing is sheared flush with all the margins, except on the incisal and cervical borders, where it is permitted to extend from 0.25 to 0.5 mm. beyond the porcelain. The backing is removed for the last time, heated and quenched, after which the incisal and gingival planes are slightly bent toward each other. When replaced on the facing, these bent planes of the backing are held in close contact with the porcelain.

To be certain that the backing is kept in close contact with the facing, two or more shavings are planed from the platinum pins with a No. 20 straight chisel; these shavings, still attached to the platinum pins, are then bent against the backing, locking it firmly against the porcelain. This is a much better procedure than bending the entire platinum pins against the backing, because the stresses developed by bending the pins may result in a checked facing in the completed crown.

Incisal reinforcement. To ensure adequate protection of the incisal edge, some operators solder 27-gauge clasp metal plate along the incisal plane before the final adaptation of the backing (Fig. 27-24, *B*).

Alignment of backed facing. The facing with its backing is now ready to be fitted to the coping. After placing some soft carding wax on the coping, the facing is correctly aligned with the adjacent teeth. If the dowel extends too far beyond the coping so that it prevents the proper alignment of the lingual surface of the facing, a part or all of this extension may be removed with stones. It should also be observed whether a sufficient space exists between the lingual surface of the facing and the incisal edges of the opposing teeth to allow for an adequate amount of solder in this region.

In order that the necessary convexity in the cervicolabial region as well as a continuity of surface be established from the margin of the coping to the incisal, and in order to have the least amount of gold showing at the gingival margin, the backed facing is lowered cervically just enough so that its gingival margin drops below the labial plane of the coping; the backing must, however, be in contact with the coping. This procedure also brings the labial surface of the facing into the position formerly occupied by the enamel of this region (Fig. 27-25).

Assembling and finishing the crown. Having established these relations, the remaining space between the backing and the coping is filled with sticky wax. The entire coping and backing of the facing are covered with wax, except a small area along the incisal edge. Here the wax stops on a line lying opposite to the incisal edge of the labial surface of the facing (Fig. 27-24, *A* and *B*). This leaves a narrow strip of gold backing along the incisal edge exposed and not covered by wax. Sometimes a small shaving of gold is cut along the incisal edge and bent labially, as indicated in Fig. 27-25, to assist in holding the backing in contact with the facing during the soldering operation.

When the crown is completely waxed, it may be removed from the cast by inserting a blunt instrument in the hole beneath the apical end of the dowel and applying upward pressure. To simplify the investing and soldering of the crown, a

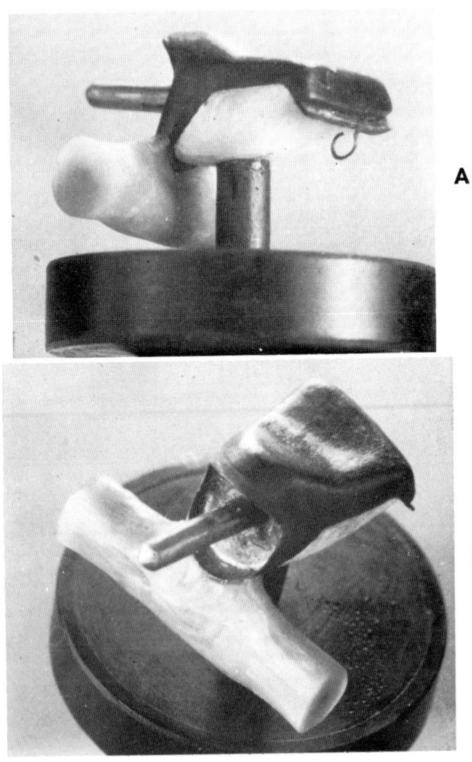

A

B

Fig. 27-26. Roll of wax 0.062 inch in diameter attached to labial portion of coping.

small roll of base-plate wax, ¾ inch in length and ¹⁄₁₆ inch in diameter, is attached on the labial surface between the margin of the coping and the margin of the backing (Fig. 27-26, *A* and *B*).

Investing the crown. A mix of crown and bridge investment is made and a small amount placed on a glass slab. After the inner surfaces of the coping have been filled with investment, the waxed crown is gently forced into the investment on the slab, the labial surface of the crown facing downward (Fig. 27-27). There should be at least ½ inch of investment material between the labial surface of the crown and the base of the investment, in order to avoid fracture of the investment during the soldering operation. When investing the crown, it should be placed in such a position that the incisal bevel is

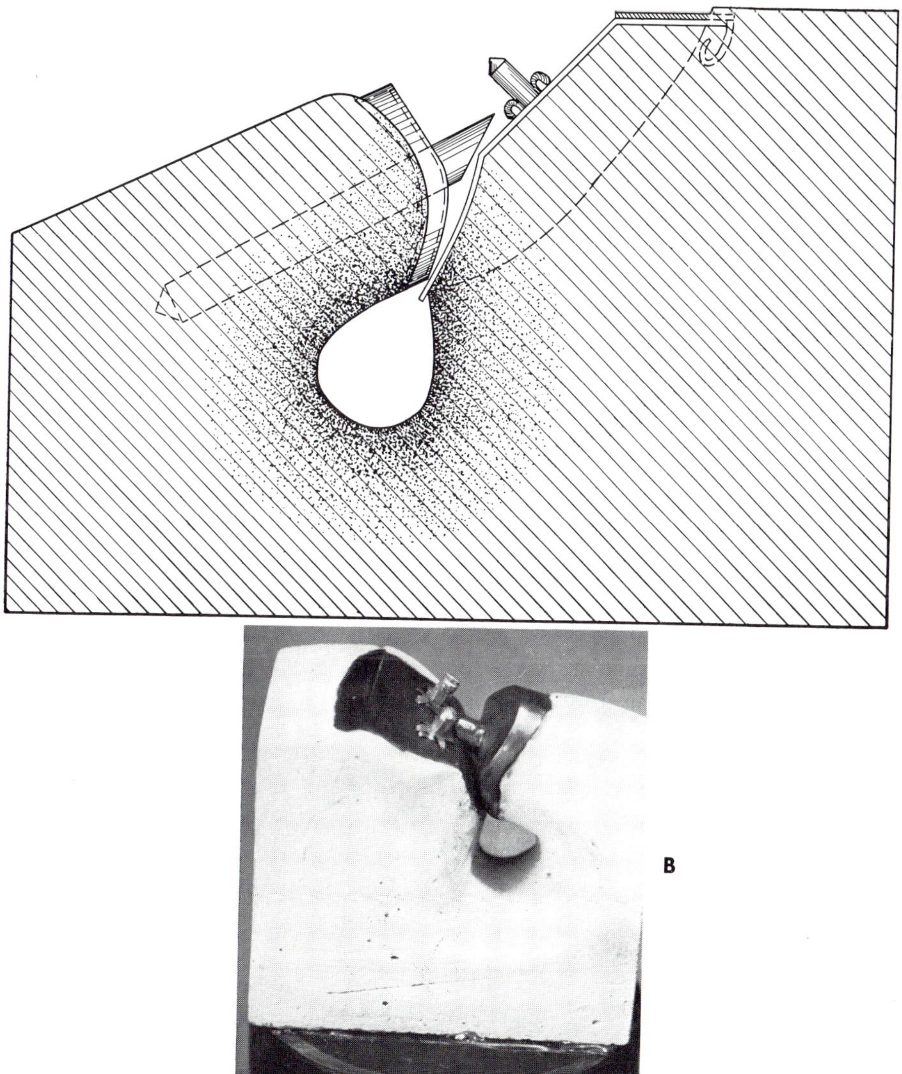

A

B

Fig. 27-27. Crown invested, **A,** and wax eliminated with boiling water, **B.** Note position of facing, which facilitates soldering of crown. Only those metal surfaces are exposed which are to be soldered.

higher than the coping. This facilitates the flow of the molten solder into the deepest portions; likewise, it simplifies contouring the lingual surface. In investing, it is absolutely essential that all porcelain be covered with investment material; if left exposed, there is danger of checking or fracturing the facing.

One of the most frequent errors committed in investing Richmond crowns is the use of an unnecessarily large amount of investment material. Only a sufficient amount is necessary to protect the facing and maintain its alignment and to prevent the fracture of the investment through its base. Fig. 27-27, *B*, shows the respective parts of the crown in position after the wax has been boiled off. It is observed that the entire facing is protected with investment material, while the entire coping and backing are exposed, with the exception of the incisal edge of the backing, which is covered and held in position by the investment. The illustration also indicates the manner in which the small shaving of gold along the incisal edge keeps the gold backing in close contact with the facing.

Removal of wax. A simple yet efficient method of removing the wax from the invested crown consists in directing a small stream of boiling water against the wax. A tin ladle with a hole drilled in its bottom is an excellent instrument for this purpose. The small stream of water can be directed accurately, and any melted wax in the pan of boiling water floats on the surface of the water in the ladle, while the clean water empties through the hole in the bottom. Wax should not be removed by placing the investment and crown in a pan of boiling water, since, in removing if from the water, a thin film of the wax will be spread over the entire surface.

Fluxing the crown. When all the wax has been removed, a small amount of petrolatum flux is applied to the exposed metal surfaces. This flux should be applied with a toothpick or some other small object, in a quantity sufficient only to cover all the exposed gold surfaces. More than this is unnecessary and is very likely to result in its reaching the porcelain, causing it to check. This is one of the most frequent causes of checked porcelain facings.

Heating the investment. Another cause of checking a facing is the too rapid heating or cooling of the investment. Therefore, after the flux has been applied, the invested crown is placed above a small Bunsen flame or in a low temperature furnace and is heated slowly until thoroughly dried. The heat may be gradually increased to a point where, when the blowpipe flame is applied to the investment, it immediately glows red. When this degree of temperature has been reached, it is safe to proceed with the soldering of the crown.

If an attempt is made to solder a Rich-crown before the investment is heated sufficiently, gold solder will fail to flow freely; if the blowpipe flame is applied persistently to such a crown, there is great danger of burning both the backing and the coping. If the investment is properly heated, the crown can be readily soldered even with 22-carat solder without danger of burning the backing.

Soldering the crown. A strip of 20-carat gold solder, held in soldering pliers, is dipped in soldering flux, and the end of the strip is then carried into the deepest portion of the V-shaped opening between the coping and the gingival margin of the backing.

The reducing flame of the blowpipe is applied and the solder is permitted to fill this opening. Care must be exercised that this initial flow of solder also fills the small, triangular space lying between the gingival margin of the band and the cervical margin of the backing. The flame of the blowpipe should be so adjusted that it is a quiet, reducing flame, from 5 to 6 inches long. The reducing portion of the flame should be used; otherwise, the solder will oxidize, and difficulty will be experienced in making it flow properly.

Additional application of the solder is made, covering the coping, the incisal edge, and the lingual surface of the backing. By carefully controlling the blowpipe and the solder, it is possible to develop the lingual contour, leaving but little to be removed by grinding.

Having completed the soldering operation, the invested crown is removed from the soldering block or spider, covered with a Pyrex dish, and allowed to cool to room temperature before the investment is removed.

When cooled, the investment is carefully removed and the crown is brushed clean, boiled in acid, and washed in water.

Grinding and finishing the crown. The surplus gold at the gingival and incisal margins is then removed. Since it is dangerous to use revolving engine stones, the excess gold is taken down by means of gold files, the cutting being done from the gold toward the porcelain. In reducing the excess at the gingival, the correct curvature of this surface must be kept in mind constantly in order that the finished crown shall be correctly contoured in this region.

Incisal bevel. The incisal gold is beveled in such a way that the plane of the gold edge is continuous with that of the labial surface of the porcelain facing. By beveling the protecting gold tip in the manner shown in Fig. 27-28, *A*, any light striking it is deflected and becomes invisible from the labial aspect, since it blends into the shadows of the oral cavity.

ALUMINOUS PORCELAIN CROWN WITH CERAMIC BASE FUSED TO DOWEL*

With the advent of new high-heat refractory investment and the recently developed aluminous porcelains, an all-porcelain crown can be fabricated in which the metal dowel is ceramically fused within the crown as an integrated unit.[1-7]

The plateau type of root preparation (Fig. 27-28) is practical and strong. The root canal is suitably enlarged to accommodate a 16-, 14-, or 12-gauge dowel wire, depending upon whether it is to be used in a lateral, central, or cuspid tooth. That portion of the dowel within the root canal is slightly tapered, while the other end is extended 3 to 6 mm. beyond the root face. An oval tube (Fig. 27-29, *A*) No. T1, T2, or T3, depending upon the size of the dowel selected, is tried for fit over the dowel wire (Fig. 27-29, *B*).

If the dowel extends 4 mm. beyond the root face, the tube to be later cut will be 3 mm. in length. However, prior to cutting off the predetermined length of alumina tube from the piece as it comes from the manufacturer, two slots are first cut through the mesial and distal walls

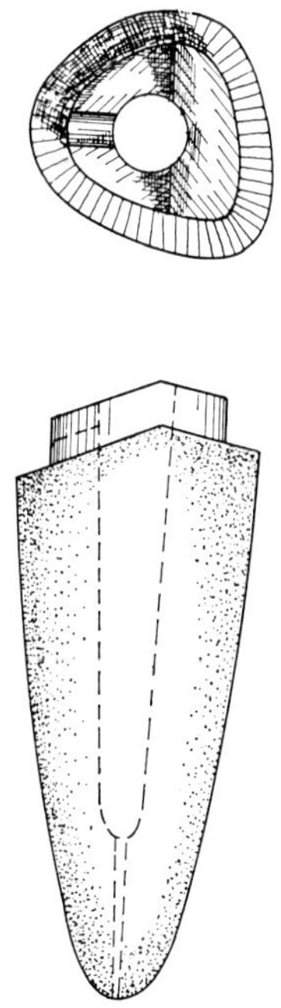

Fig. 27-28. Root prepared with shoulder and plateau for swaged platinum foil coping, having iridioplatinum dowel.

*The modified method of applying and firing of the aluminous types of porcelain is based on the research of Dr. J. McLean, described in Chapter 36.

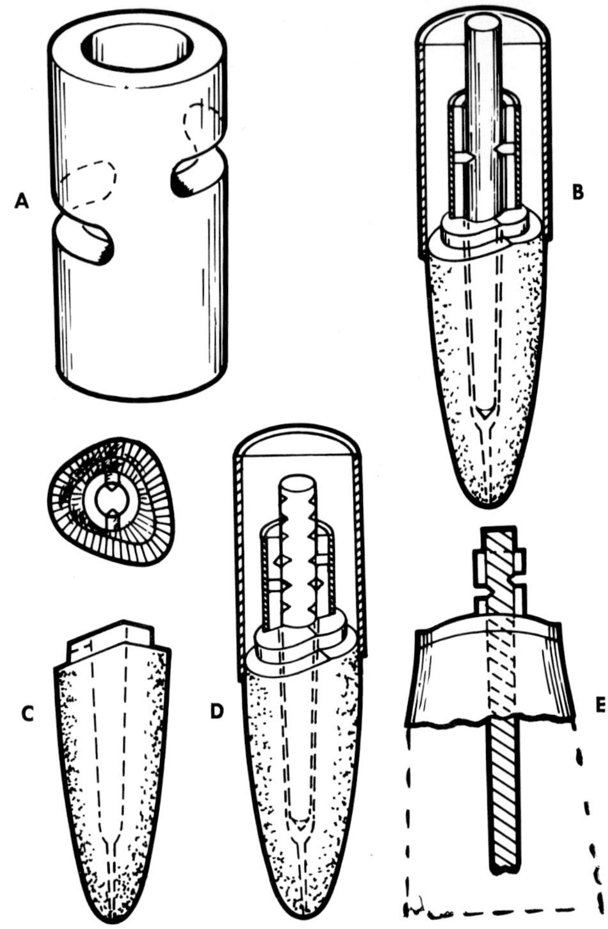

Fig. 27-29. Preformed high-alumina ceramic reinforcement tubes. **A,** Alumina-reinforced ceramic tube with two opposite slots cut. **B,** Tube slipped over dowel; slight cuts made into dowel through two slots, luted with sticky wax. **C,** Cross section of tube seen in **B,** at level of slots in tube; slight cuts into side of dowel. **D,** Vertical section of wax-luted dowel and tube in polysulphide rubber in copper tube impression. **E,** Dowel-tube impression poured in Steele's high-temperature refractory model material, for uniting both parts with high-fusing ceramic core material. (Courtesy Columbus Dental Mfg. Co.)

of the tube with a very thin knife-edged diamond disk at opposite and different levels, about 1.5 mm. from the end of the tube (Fig. 27-29, *A*). The selected dowel wire of the proper gauge is inserted into the tube, and slight cuts are made into the dowel wire through the two openings previously cut in the oval tube (Fig. 27-29, *B* and *C*). At a later time, high-fusing core material will be placed in these cuts establishing a ceramic key and locking the dowel to the tube and crown into an integral unit.

The predetermined length of dowel is cut. No specific measurement is given for a dowel length; however, a safe rule to follow at the beginning is to have the dowel length equal to half the cervico-incisal length of the anterior tooth to be restored.

When the dowel length is determined, it is tapered slightly and placed into the prepared root canal. The slotted T1 tube is slipped over the protruding end of the canal of the dowel so that the bottom of the tube rests firmly on the root surface. A small bead of sticky wax is melted into the two slots in the tube and into the dowel cuts. The ends of the tube and the dowel are also lightly packed with sticky wax.

The next step is taking the customary type of polysulfide rubber impression in a copper band (Fig. 27-29, *D*) and then utilizing the syringe and perforated impression tray technic. When the material has set, the impression is removed, carrying with it the dowel with the alumina tube waxed to it. If it does not come away with the impression, the dowel with the tube is removed from the tooth and replaced accurately in the impression. The root portion of the dowel is still exposed, while the other end containing the alumina tube is within the rubber impression material. The exposed dowel portion is lubricated with a lubricant, usually petroleum jelly or Steele's Die Film.

Steele's high-temperature refractory model material (Die-Mod) is placed into the area containing the root face impression, bringing the refractory material to 4 mm. above the end of the dowel (Fig. 27-29, *E*). This is allowed to harden for 25 minutes. It is removed from the impression and fired to a temperature of 2065° F., which is 50° above the fusing temperature of the high-fusing core material. After removal from the muffle, it is allowed to cool to room temperature. The refractory die holds the dowel and the piece of slotted alumina tube over the end of the dowel. The refractory tube is tapered and replaced into the polysulfide rubber tray and copper tube impression. A small ball of wax is placed over the end of the dowel and Steele's Die Film is applied to the exposed base of the die material while the dowel is lubricated with petroleum jelly. The working model is poured in hard stone and mounted in an articulator in centric relation with the opposing cast. When the casts are separated from the bite registration, care must be taken that no particles of investment or debris lie between the dowel and the slotted alumina tube.

The removable die may now be used for the construction of the aluminous porcelain crown by one of two available technics. The first method employs a swaged 0.001-gauge platinum coping; the second utilizes a separating medium only, which is applied to the fired refractory die, eliminating the necessity of using a platinum foil between the porcelain and the die. The type of crown employing the platinum coping will be considered first.

ALUMINOUS PORCELAIN DOWEL CROWN USING PLATINUM COPING

A small hole is made through a piece of 0.001-gauge platinum foil sufficiently large to be adapted to root face and to the shoulder of the preparation, and to extend 1 mm. actually beyond the edge of the shoulder. The platinum is carefully burnished over the root face and the shoulder of the die, then extended at least 1 mm. apically beyond the outer cavosurface angle of the shoulder (Fig. 27-30). Repeated annealing of the platinum foil during the swaging process may be necessary to avoid tearing the foil. When perfectly adapted to the die the coping should be tested for easy removal without distortion. The slotted piece of alumina tubing, ceramically welded to the dowel, is placed over the preparation so that it rests firmly against the swaged platinum; the slot in the tube and the cut in the wire are synchronized and rigidly locked with fused porcelain (Fig. 27-30).

With a minimum amount of sticky wax the alumina tube is attached lightly at its base to the platinum coping. If no undercuts exist in the tooth preparation or the die it should be possible to lift

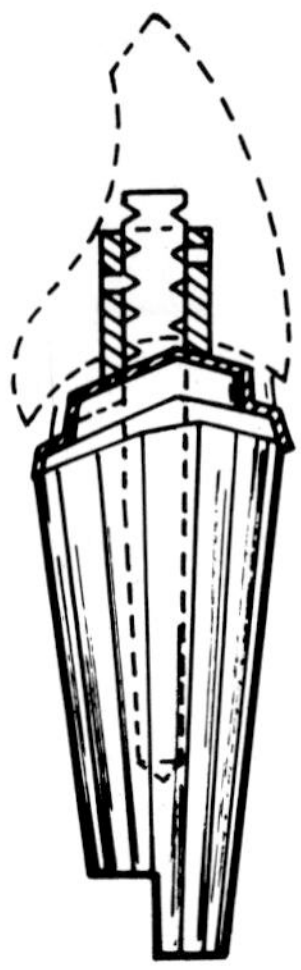

Fig. 27-30. High-temperature alumina reinforcement tube and dowel interlocked by fused porcelain, seated on platinum matrix prior to porcelain application.

the alumina tube with the platinum matrix gently by the exposed end of the dowel. Tacking the alumina tube to the platinum foil coping stabilizes the platinum on the die during subsequent application of core porcelain material.

A very thin film of wax or clear shellac is painted with a small brush over the platinum that covers the shoulder and over 1 mm. of the platinum apron extending on the side of the die. The film, wax, or shellac will burn away clean during the firing procedure; this allows the porcelain core material to shrink away from the platinum, leaving it in its original swaged position on the die. To eliminate any air space that exists between the inner surface of the alumina tube and the dowel, also between the slots in the tube and the dowel, water is applied with a brush. The water displaces the air and acts as a vehicle to carry the initial particles of core material through the slots into the space between the inner walls of the tube and the dowel. When the core porcelain is vibrated into the two slots of the tube it will form a ceramically fused key, locking the alumina tube to the previously made cuts in the dowel. This gives a ceramically fused unit of the alumina tube, dowel and the platinum, and core material over which the crown will be constructed.

The next step is the application of Steele's high-fusing core porcelain to the platinum coping and to the alumina tube-dowel. High-fusing core porcelain (2012° F.) is mixed to a thick, creamy consistency. With a small brush it is applied to the platinum coping on the die and over the alumina tube encircling the dowel.

Continuing with the brush technic, high-fusing core porcelain is applied additionally in small increments to the shoulder and over the root face surface area until the contour of the core is developed (Fig. 27-33). *No core material is applied to the coping beyond the outer angle of the shoulder.* If any should accidentally lodge on the platinum apron it should be removed to the edge of the shoulder preparation.

After the contouring of the core has been completed it is advisable to brush-whip the material in order to further condense and smoothen it. The fire cycle is carried through as outlined in Chapter 35.

When the temperature in the muffle has reached 1922° F., the core is removed and allowed to cool to room temperature under a Pyrex cover. It will be noted that a space exists at the shoulder where the core material has pulled away from the platinum during the firing process. (Fig. 27-31). If there is any doubt that the matrix is not in complete adaptation to the die, it should be reburnished.

Next, the space between the fused core and the platinum matrix is filled with additional core porcelain. Attempting to fill the space directly by spatulating wet porcelain into it is likely to leave air pockets covered over by a thin layer of core material. It is necessary first to displace the air in this space with water; as pre-

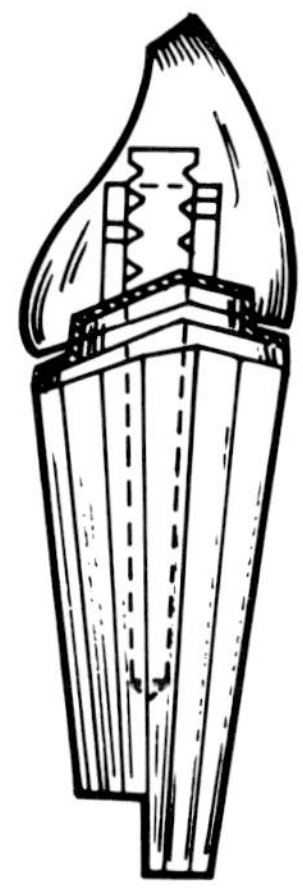

Fig. 27-31. Shrinkage of core porcelain at cervical shoulder after first firing.

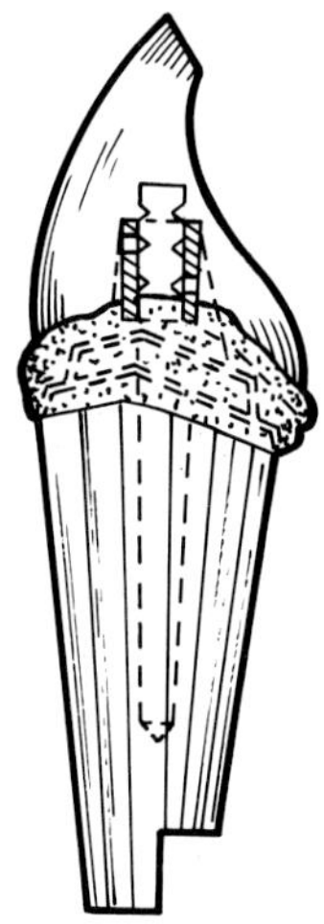

Fig. 27-32. Core porcelain placed into shrinkage crevice and contoured over exposed platinum apron.

viously stated, the water serves as a vehicle in carrying the added core material into the deepest area of the gingival crevice. With light vibration of the die with the serrated side of the spatula, the particles are carried into the deepest portion of the crevice, bringing excess moisture to the surface, where it is absorbed by tissue or by a cloth (Fig. 27-32).

After the space has been completely filled, more procelain is added over the platinum apron gingivally; it is again fired at high-fusing core or low-fusing core porcelain temperature. When cooled to room temperature, any slight excess convexity of core is disked to the margin of the platinum shoulder (Fig. 27-33).

The crown morphology is next developed with successive applications of body dentin and enamel porcelains. Stains, translucents, and neck dentin may be incorporated as desired and as explained in Chapters 25 and 26. The built-up crown is slowly dried, placed in a furnace, and brought to an eggshell sheen stage. If no changes are necessary, the crown may be fired to a final glaze.

After withdrawal from the furnace it is allowed to cool to room temperature under a Pyrex glass. When completely cooled it may be immersed in distilled water and the crown removed from the refractory die. Care must be exercised not to fracture the cervical core collar within the crown that encircles the plateau of the tooth preparation (Fig. 27-33). The platinum foil coping is now carefully removed and the crown is ready for placement on the tooth.

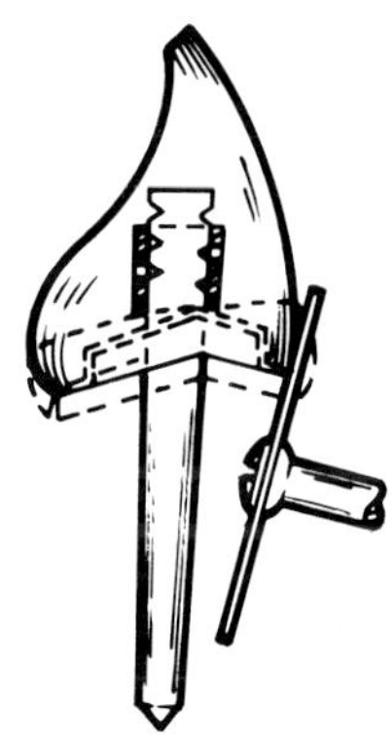

Fig. 27-33. Disking away excess cervical porcelain and platinum matrix apron to gingival margin of crown prior to its glaze firing.

The advantages of this type of crown are several. First, the problem of masking the color of a cast gold core is eliminated because of the reflectivity and compatibility of the color of the core material with the dentin and enamel porcelains. The retention of the crown to the dowel does

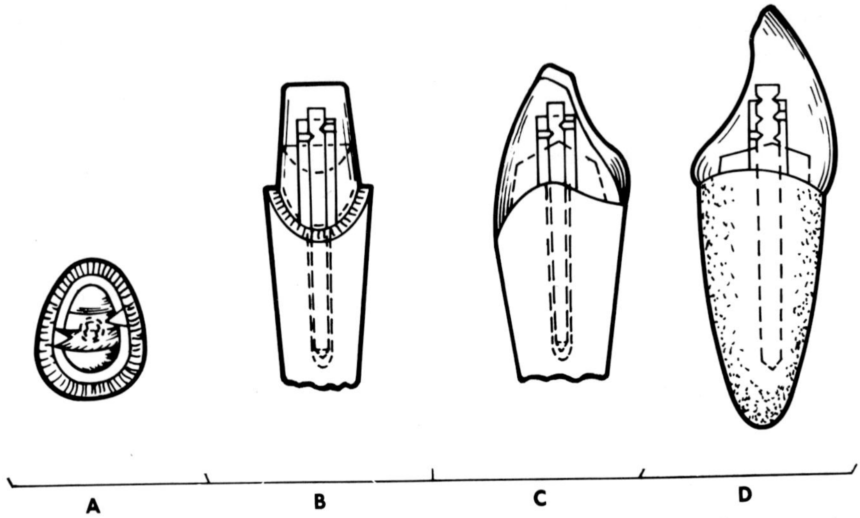

Fig. 27-34. Steps in construction of aluminous porcelain dowel crown without use of metal coping.

not depend upon cement, since there is a physical and chemical bond between the core material and the alumina tube and between the inner surface of the tube and the surface of the metal dowel inside the tube. This type of crown does not require two separate cementations of the crown and the dowel or of a porcelain jacket crown to a cast gold core with a dowel.

ALUMINOUS PORCELAIN DOWEL CROWN WITHOUT A METAL COPING (FIG. 27-34)

The root preparation, the construction of the tooth dowel, and the high-temperature refractory die are the same as in the previous type of crown. The following steps are likewise similar to the stage where the upper and the lower working casts are mounted in an articulator. The removable refractory die with its tube-dowel is removed from the working cast and henceforth the steps of fabricating the crown differ. No platinum matrix is utilized (Fig. 27-34, *A*). Instead, two coats of separating material are applied to the root face shoulder and to 1 mm. of the side of the root die and allowed to dry for 5 minutes each. Care must be exercised not to apply the separator to the slotted tube or any part of the dowel. The separating material is applied in a manner similar to that used on the previous type

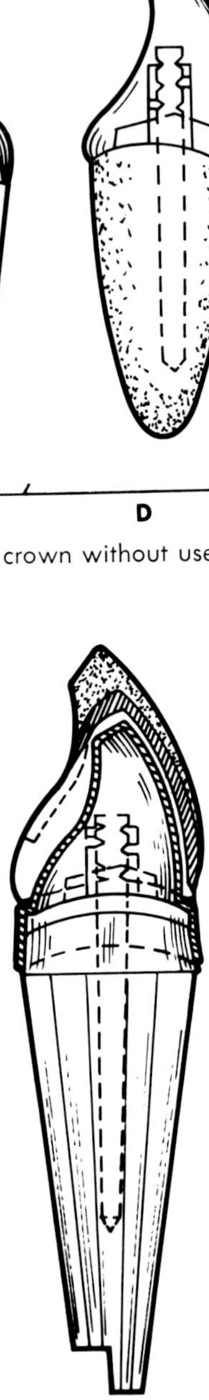

Fig. 27-35. High-fusing porcelain core used in place of customary crest gold core for porcelain veneer crown.

of crown. By means of the brush technic high-fusing core material is applied in small increments to the slotted tube and into the two slots made on each side of the tube. Additional high-fusing core porcelain is added until the entire tube is covered as is the end of the dowel (Fig. 27-34, *B*). By additional increments the root face of the die is next covered with the core material, likewise the shoulder to the outer edge (Fig. 27-34, *C*). The core is now built up in the customary way as previously explained, except that no provision is made for the ceramic shrinkage of the porcelain in firing by ditching or wax fill, since a separating medium has been used over the shoulder.

The built up high-fusing core is slowly dried and preheated before the open door and then inserted into the muffle. As previously, the temperature is increased 50° F./minute to 1700° F. if under vacuum. At this temperature the vacuum is released and the temperature is raised to 2012° F. under atmospheric conditions and held for 7 minutes. However, if the crown is to be made entirely under atmospheric conditions then the temperature of the high-fusing core is immediately carried to 2012° F. temperature. Low-fusing core material is carried to 1900° F. in 6 to 8 minutes. The die and the fired core are removed from the muffle and allowed to cool to room temperature, preferably under a Pyrex cover. It will be observed that a slight shrinkage may also have occurred at the cervical margin, the core material having pulled away from the refractory die.

If a fine yellow residue is visible on the shoulder, it should be carefully brushed away with a fine camels' hair brush. Another layer of separating material should be applied to the shoulder and onto the sides of the *die*. When this has thoroughly dried, a creamy slur of the core material is made and carefully painted into the space between the core porcelain and the shoulder of the die. The same procedure is followed as previously of drying the moist porcelain, adding high-fusing core porcelain, and inserting it at 1700° F. temperature and gradually raising the temperature at 50°/minute until 2012° F. has been attained. When cooled, the crown core on the die is removed and allowed to cool to room temperature. The gingival portion of the crown should be in apposition with the shoulder of the die.

The subsequent firings of dentin and enamel porcelains can be safely carried out without any danger of further shrinkage of the core material, inasmuch as the dentin and enamel porcelains are fired at a lower temperature than core porcelain.

The final buildup of the crown in dentin and enamel aluminous-porcelain together with any color and stain modifications are completed in the manner previously described (Fig. 27-34, *D*).

After the final glaze of the crown it is removed from the muffle and placed under a Pyrex dish and allowed to cool to room temperature. When thoroughly cooled the crown may be grasped and removed from the refractory die by the opposed finger-pressure technic.

SELECTED REFERENCES

1. McLean, J. W., and Hughes, T. H.: The reinforcement of dental porcelain with ceramic oxides, Brit. Dent. J. **119**:251, 1965.
2. McLean, J. W.: The alumina tube post crown, Brit. Dent. J. **123**:87, 1967.
3. Vines, R. F., and others: Mechanisms involved in securing dense vitrified ceramics from preshaped partly crystalline bodies. J. Amer. Ceram. Soc. **41**:304, 1958.
4. McLean, J. W.: The alumina reinforced porcelain jacket crowns, J.A.D.A. **75**:621, 1967.
5. Skinner, E. W., and Phillips, R. W.: The science of dental materials, Philadelphia, 1967, W. B. Saunders Co.
6. Warsaw, S. I., and Seider, R.: Comparison of strength of triaxial porcelains containing alumina and silica, J. Amer. Ceram. Soc. **50**(70): 337, 1967.
7. Columbus Manufacturing Company: The complete Steele's technic, Columbus, Ohio, 1969, Columbus Mfg. Co.

GENERAL REFERENCES

Baker, C. R.: Dowel crowns, J.A.D.A. **61**:479, 1960.

Colley, I. T., Hampson, E. L., and Lehman, M. L.: Retention of post crowns, Brit. Dent. J. **124**:63-69, 1968.

Frank, A. L.: Protective coronal coverage of the pulpless tooth, J.A.D.A. **59**:895, 1959.

Gerstein, H., and Burnell, S. C.: Prefabricated precision dowels, J.A.D.A. **68**:787, 1964.

Goodman, J. B.: Immediate transfer coping for full coverage of teeth, New York J. Dent. **26**: 156, 1956.

Hamilton, A. I.: Porcelain dowel crowns, J. Prosth. Dent. **9**:639, 1959.

Holt, J. K.: Anterior post crowns, Brit. D. J. **113**:299, 1962.

Larato, D. C.: Single unit cast post crown for pulpless anterior tooth roots, J. Prosth. Dent. **16**:145, 1966.

Reed, G. M.: New conception in precision dowels, J.A.D.A. **74**:321-324, 1968.

Richard, E. L., and Brodtmann, N. V.: Cast copings for jacket crowns, J. Prosth. Dent. **12**: 129, 1962.

Sickelmore, F. A.: Post crowns—some weaknesses, Brit. Dent. J. **107**:306, 1959.

Wallace, F. H.: Resin transfer copings, J. Prosth. Dent. **8**:289, 1958.

Chapter 28

Construction of working models

TRANSFER TO ARTICULATOR: FUNCTIONALLY GENERATED PATH METHOD

The working model consists of the maxillary and the mandibular casts mounted on an articulator in such a relationship to each other and to the instrument that they reproduce as nearly as possible the same orientation that exists in the mouth when the jaws are in centric relation to each other. In addition to the correct anteroposterior relationship it is necessary that the correct vertical position of the occlusal plane be established.

Crowns and fixed partial dentures are usually constructed on the models involved in the restoration. These may be made of plaster, soldering investment, artificial stone, low-fusing alloy, or a combination of metal and artificial stone, or they may be electroformed with copper or silver.

TREATMENT OF THE RIDGE MUCOSA

Before an impression is taken of the arch involved in the restoration, it is advisable to consider possible treatment of the edentulous ridge area.

In the discussion of the maxilla and the mandible in Chapter 6, it was seen that the tissue which covers the ridge of the edentulous space differs in its physical and anatomic characteristics and in the extent of its distribution, i.e., it may be thin or firm or it may be thick, spongy, and pendulous in character. It is also important to examine the pontic regions on the labial or the buccal surfaces where the relatively immovable mucosa blends into the very mobile border tissues. This is important, as will be shown in the discussion of the position occupied by the gingival area of the pontic in its relationship to the mucosa (Chapter 30).

When the mucosa is thin, immovable, and firm, it is not generally necessary to treat the ridge before the impression is taken; where it is flabby, thick, and pendulous, it may be advisable to shrink the ridge by means of an astringent applied before taking the impression—sometimes the dentist may have to resort to surgical removal of ridge tissues. The necessary establishment of the correct amount of interface contact between the pontic and the ridge may be accomplished in two ways: first, the edentulous ridge on the working cast may be relieved by scraping, which causes the pontic to exert the necessary degree of contact with the mucosa; or second, this relief may be embodied in the model by shrinking the ridge tissues before the impression is taken. The latter method of shrinkage is controlled physiologically by the relative thickness of the mucosa that covers the bony ridge. Because it is desirable to have a slight contact of the pontic against the ridge in proportion to the increased thickness of the mucosa, the physiologic shrinkage of the tissue will automatically establish the correct amount of contact relationship, and hence an impression taken in this condition of the gum will produce a model whose ridge is of reduced dimensions of the normal size of the ridge.

Such a pontic constructed to contact the shrunken ridge on the working model, when later transferred to the mouth, will establish a relationship with the mucosa, now returned to its normal size, which is physiologically compatible with the tissues since the interface contact between the ridge mucosa and the glazed surface of the pontic is not of sufficient magnitude or area to cause either a resorption of the bone or a hypertrophy of the mucosa.

TYPES OF IMPRESSIONS AND WORK MODELS

The type of impression taken and the material used for the model will determine the kind of impression tray used. The most frequent is an impression taken in one of the elastic impression materials. These are fully discussed in Chapter 21.

If rapid-setting plaster is used, the impression when set is removed in sections, which are reassembled accurately in the impression tray. The bridge retainer previously cast and fitted is removed from the abutment teeth and seated exactly in its respective positions in the impression. It is important that it occupies the same relative positions in the impression that it did in the mouth.

Soldering-investment model

If the pontic is to be soldered to the retainers directly on the working model, the model is made of soldering investment. In this event the inner or the exposed surfaces of the retainers, now seated in the impression, are coated with a thin film of antiflux; the plaster impression is treated with shellac and a separating medium. When the separating medium has dried, the impression is submerged in water for 3 to 5 minutes, after which a mixture of soldering investment is poured into the impression, care being taken not to dislodge or move the seated retainers while the investment is poured. It is essential that no air bubbles be trapped, as these result in a weakened model.

When the investment has set, the plaster impression is carefully removed, leaving a model made of soldering investment containing the bridge retainers held firmly in their correct position. The model is now ready to be placed in the wax bite or bite-frame registration and mounted on the articulator.

This type of model has the advantage that, after the pontics are constructed, they may be aligned, waxed, and soldered to the retainers without removing the retainers from the model. The disadvantage, however, lies in the possibility of the retainers being dislodged from the relatively weak soldering investment model, thus losing their correct relationship. Furthermore, unless extreme care is exercised, the occlusal contour and relationship of such a model is quickly destroyed because of the relative softness of the soldering investment material.

Low-fusing alloy model

Another method of constructing working models from plaster impressions utilizes low-fusing alloy for part or all of the model (Fig. 28-1). The exposed cavity surfaces of the retainers seated in the plaster impression are coated with a thin film of antiflux. If the inner surfaces of crowns or large extracoronal retainers are not convergent, these should be slightly corrected with some molding clay. The posterior border of the impression, as well as the buccal and labial areas, are built up with a small roll of molding clay in order to confine the molten alloy when it is poured into the impression. Before pouring the alloy into the impression, it is essential that all free moisture be removed. The desired condition of the plaster surface develops after it has been permitted to stand at room temperature for one-half hour after its removal from the mouth.

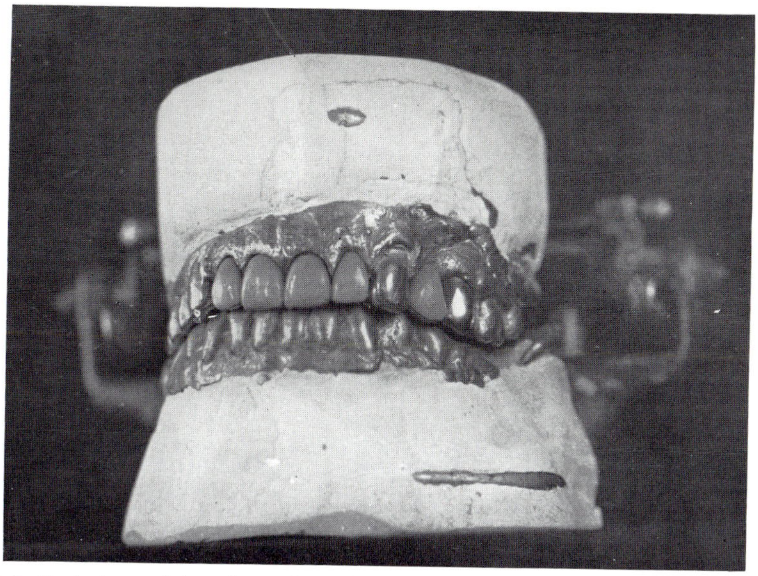

Fig. 28-1. Technic model with teeth and ridges in low-fusing metal; base is stone.

The low-fusing alloy should not be overheated but should be poured at a temperature slightly above its fusing or melting stage. Several of the low-fusing alloys made by reputable manufacturers are suitable for this purpose.

If the model is to be made entirely of alloy, it is advisable, first, to pour that part of the impression which contains the retainers. After this has solidified, the other sections are poured; finally all sections are united. The threaded ends of small screws or friction washers are embedded in the alloy before it solidifies, leaving heads and a part of the washer exposed. The heads are later engaged in the stone when the rest of the cast is completed in stone. Because the molten alloy which comes in contact with the solidified portions remelts the solidified surfaces slightly, the result is a fused union of the several metal sections. The method tends to reduce the total amount of possible shrinkage of the metal model.

When completely solidified, the metal model with its bridge retainers is recovered from the plaster impression. If properly fluxed on their inner surfaces and if no undercuts exist, the retainers can be removed from the metal model repeatedly and replaced without losing their correct position on the abutment teeth.

The metal model with its retainers is now ready to be placed in the registration bite and mounted on the articulator by means of the facebow.

The advantages of such a model are many, since the material of which it is constructed allows for considerable wear without the danger of breaking off the abutment teeth or losing their correct anatomic form or occlusal relationships. It also presents a ridge of the edentulous area to which pontics may be accurately ground and fitted. Where a broken-stress type of bridge is constructed, the removal of the retainer for cutting the keyway is allowed, after which it is replaced with the assurance that it occupies its original position in the metal model. Furthermore, extensive bridges restoring two or more missing teeth permit the construction of the bridge in two parts. One pontic may be soldered to each of the retainers, after which the two parts are reassembled on the metal model and the correctness of their relationship verified; the two sections of the bridge may then be placed in the mouth for the final impression. The impression for the final soldering operation may be taken with a quick-setting stone, occlusal index in the mouth, or on the metal model.

One possible objection to the alloy model is the possibility of dislodging the retainers from the impression while pouring the metal. This danger may be overcome by holding the retainers in position with a wire while the metal is poured; the wire is then left embedded in the metal. As many wires are used as there are retainers, and each abutment is poured and allowed to solidify before the balance of the model is poured.

Combination model of alloy and stone

A combination model of low-fusing alloy and artificial stone may also be constructed from a complete plaster impression. In this method a small ring of molding clay is built around each retainer in the impression. After the antiflux has been applied to the retainers, low-fusing metal is poured into the retainers inside the individual rings of clay, and small screws or washers are inserted into the molten metal as previously described. After the metal has solidified, the molding clay is removed, leaving the metal screw or washer rim extensions exposed. The rest of the plaster impression is treated with shellac and a separating medium, after which the impression is poured in artificial stone. When separated, the model consists of artificial stone, with the exception of the abutment teeth carrying the retainers; these are made of the low-fusing alloy. It is claimed that this technic reduces to a minimum the amount of distortion resulting from the shrinkage present in an all-metal model.

The most important requirement in the construction of any type of working model is the necessity for the bridge retainers to occupy the same relative positions in the working model that they occupied on the abutment teeth. The slightest dislocation in any direction will result in a misfit of the finished restoration, necessitating a dissembling and a resoldering of the component parts of the bridge.

Working models for indirect technic

When the indirect technic is employed, the cast retainers are constructed on dies made of stone, amalgam, or electroformed copper or silver. These may be removable or be an integral part of a solid model. The technic employed when stone dies are used is fully discussed in Chapter 21; those utilizing the rubber type impression materials to form silver or copper electroformed models are discussed in Chapter 21.

Transfer copings. Bailey[1] offered the following technic, which is also usable with the electroformed or stone dies, for individual dies are made of amalgam.

Since this technic employs the indirect method, the first step requires that impressions of the prepared abutments be obtained and that amalgam dies be constructed. After this has been done, the correct transfer of the relationship of the dies from the mouth to the model is obtained; for this, Bailey uses "transfer inlays" and copings. These may be constructed of low-fusing metal or casting gold made directly on the dies. The transfer inlays and copings are then placed on the abutment teeth in the mouth and a combination impression of modeling compound and hydrocolloidal material is taken, with the transfer copings in position. The transfer inlays and copings come away with the impression and are used to seat the original metal dies in their correct relationship in the impression; from this the bridge retainers are constructed on the amalgam dies by the usual indirect method.

Transfer copings may also be made by wrapping a piece of paper around the antifluxed die and by pouring low-fusing metal against the cavity side of the die. The bases of the dies are made of a uniform height.

Taking the impression. In taking the impression of the arch with the transfer copings in place, a water-cooled tray is used with the reversible agar-agar type of hydrocolloid impression material. The bottom of the tray is first lined with tin foil, on top of which is placed a melted layer of black modeling compound; the balance of the tray is then filled with 115° F. hydrocolloidal material (Fig. 28-2). The compound is applied only to that part of the tray which lies opposite to the teeth carrying the transfer copings.

While taking the impression, the tray is carried occlusally until the bases of the transfer copings are embedded in the compound. The compound and colloidal material are then chilled; when removed, the impression carries with it the transfer copings. The metal dies are now seated in their respective transfer copings and are attached to them with sticky wax so that they remain in their correct positions during the pouring of the model.

To permit removal of the metal dies from the working model, Bailey suggested the use of prepared copper bands that surround the root portion of the dies and that facilitate their removal and replacement in the model. The same result may be obtained by forming a 60-gauge tin foil or a 40-gauge copper matrix around the base of the metal die that has been previously tapered. When the model is poured, the tin foil or copper matrix is held by the artificial stone, permitting the withdrawal of the amalgam dies. (See Chapter 21 for additional methods.)

FUNCTIONALLY GENERATED PATH METHODS: HANAU, JELENKO

Working models and opposing anatomic casts may be mounted in their correct relation to each other in an instrument of simple design and using minimum ancillary equipment.[3-5] A similar result can be attained by utilizing more advanced designs of instruments in conjunction with a hinge axis facebow and using the check bite method. It is then possible to record and transfer the dental arch relationships, not only to each other in centric occlusal closure but also in their eccentric relationships to the temporomandibular articula-

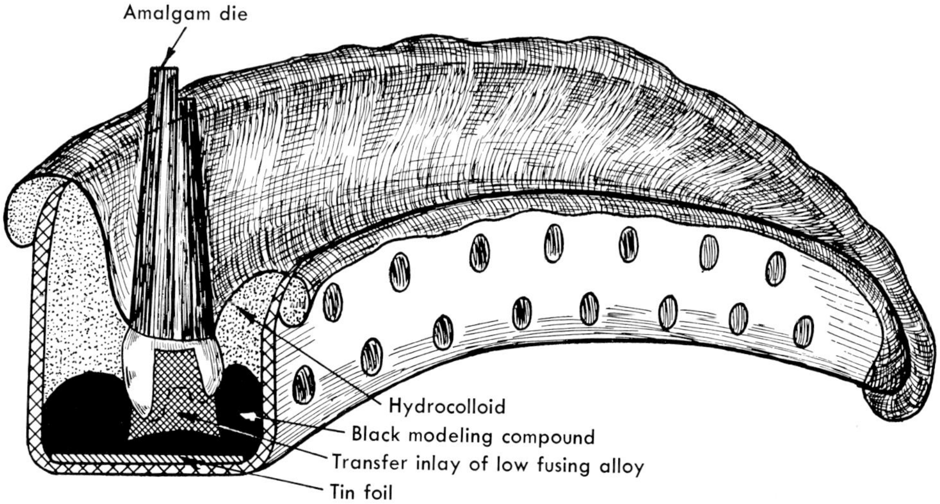

Fig. 28-2. Cross section showing transfer inlay or coping, amalgam die, and combination modeling compound and hydrocolloid impression taken in water-cooled tray. (After Bailey.)

tion. This method and instrumentation is fully discussed in Chapter 29.

A third method of recording and measuring functional relationships of the mandible to the glenoid fossae likewise utilizes a hinge axis facebow, registration tray (or clutches), and a more complicated method of recording the movements and positions of the mandible by graphically identifying the actual paths traveled by the mandible and adjusting the articulator to these recordings so that the same position and movements can be simulated with the least distortion. This method is fully discussed in Chapter 37. The latter method is designated as the gnathologic-pantographic method and is mostly employed in the extensive dental rehabilitation of the patient and in research.

An original concept of obtaining and mounting casts in constructing a simple unilateral fixed partial prosthesis was developed and described many decades ago.[5] With the development of newer materials and instruments the technic has been refined so that restorations may now be made which fulfill many functional and biologic requirements. The method is known as the "Functionally generated path" technic.

Hanau twinstage occluder method

The mounting instrument for the casts is a relatively simple articulator (Fig. 28-3) and the materials used are those customarily found in the dental office. No facebow or extraoral registrations are utilized. A wax record is obtained of the position and movements of the mandible in its centric and in its functionally eccentric positions. The wax record contains the functionally generated paths established by the cusps and ridges of the teeth as the mandible glides from its centric relation, over the opposing teeth, into protrusive and lateral functional paths. The morphology of the cusps and their relationship to the opposing fossae and sulci are likewise registered in the wax.

When quick-setting stone is poured into the wax record and allowed to harden, it gives a positive counterpart of the paths and is designated as the "positive functional core." It is a static record of dynamic or functional movements. Later, when incorporated into one of the casts

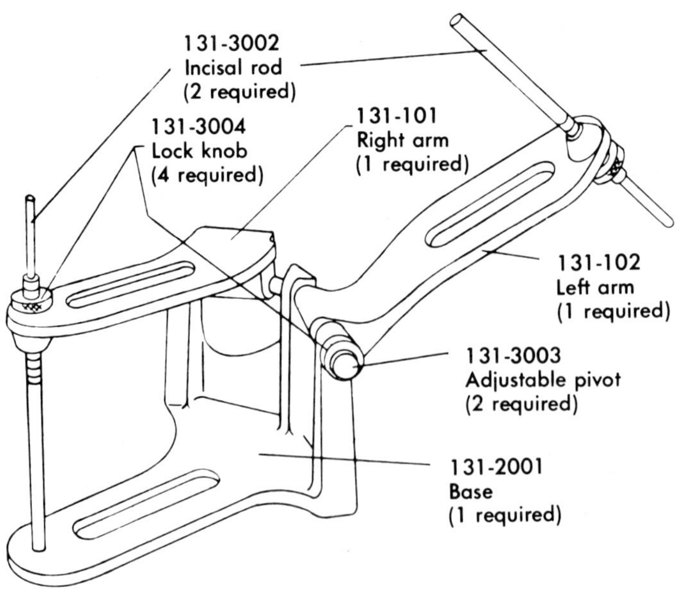

Fig. 28-3. Hanau twinstage occluder. (Courtesy Hanau Co.)

mounted in the articulator, it opposes the working cast of the bridge, and serves as a guide in establishing the occlusal anatomy of the opposing pontics and bridge retainers.

For a unilateral prosthesis, three casts are required: (1) a working cast of the prepared abutments with their removable dies (Fig. 28-4, *B*, lower); (2) an opposing anatomic cast (Fig. 28-4, *A*, upper); and (3) an opposing positive-functional-core cast (Fig. 28-5, *C*). The articulator (Fig. 28-5) must be capable of accurately relating the working cast *(B)*, interchangeably with the anatomic cast *(A)*, and with the positive-functional-core cast *(C)*.

The instrument must be sturdy and rigid enough to prevent any change in the vertical dimension or centric relation between the working cast (*B*), the anatomic *(A)*, or the positive-functional-core cast *(C)*.

A positive rotational axis is maintained by releasing the lock knob 131-3004 at an adjustable pivot, 131-3003. When the fixed brass pivot of right arm 131-101 or left arm 131-102 is in its tapered seat of base 131-2001, the adjustable pivot is brought

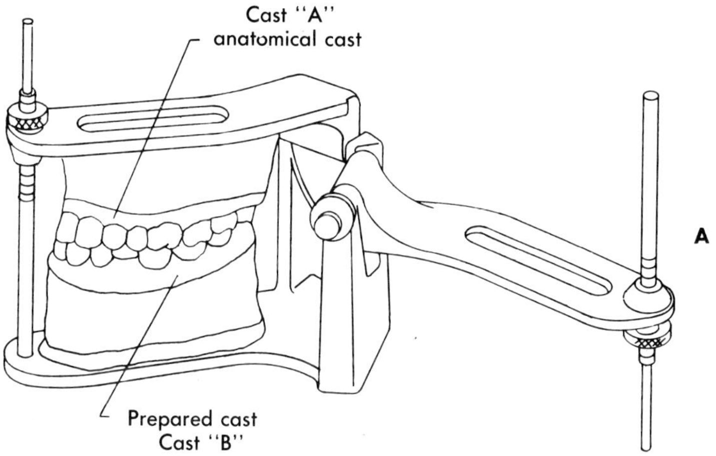

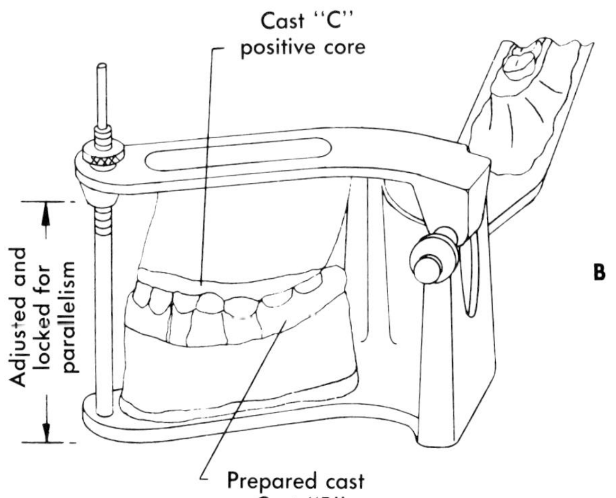

Fig. 28-4. A, Articulator with anatomic cast (A) and prepared working cast (B) in centric relation occlusion. **B,** Articulator with prepared cast (B) and positive-core cast (C) in centric relation occlusion. (Courtesy Hanau Co.)

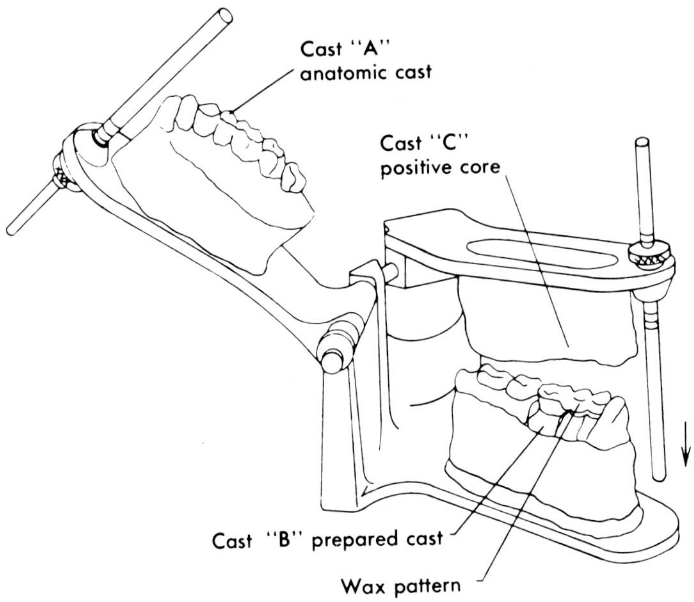

Fig. 28-5. Articulator with prepared cast (B) mounted and related to positive-core cast (C) in centric relation. Anatomic cast (A) mounted on additional upper bow of open instrument, also in centric relation to working cast. (Courtesy Hanau Co.)

into direct contact with the tapered seat of arm and is locked.

A vertical adjustment of incisal rod 131-3002 is accomplished by releasing lock knob 131-3004 and rotating the rod to its position. Tighten lock knob to retain its position.

1. Before undertaking any multitooth restorations, a complete radiographic and oral examination, study casts, diagnosis, and plan of treatment should be established. A determination should also be made whether any prerestorative treatment is indicated such as orthopedic or periodontic, likewise the equilibration of occlusion. If deemed necessary, these must be performed prior to the preparation of the abutment teeth.

2. An alginate impression is taken of the unprepared lower quadrant in which the fixed prosthesis $\overline{/4-6}$ is to be placed. It should include at least one tooth anterior and one posterior to the abutment teeth. The impression, upon removal from the mouth, is placed immediately into a moisture-saturated, covered container for later use (Step 7) in constructing an acrylic splint or platform (Fig. 28-6). The platform will support the wax layer in which functional paths are generated.

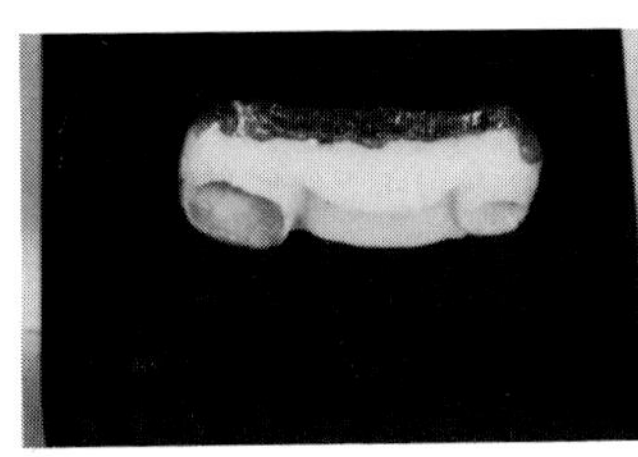

Fig. 28-6. Acrylic splint or platform used to support occlusal recording material.

3. The abutment teeth are prepared and an impression of the upper and lower quadrants is taken simultaneously, at centric relation, using a check bite tray (Fig. 28-7).

4. The prepared teeth in the lower section of the impression are poured in die stone (cast B); tapered dowel pins are inserted parallel into the stone, which is allowed to harden completely.

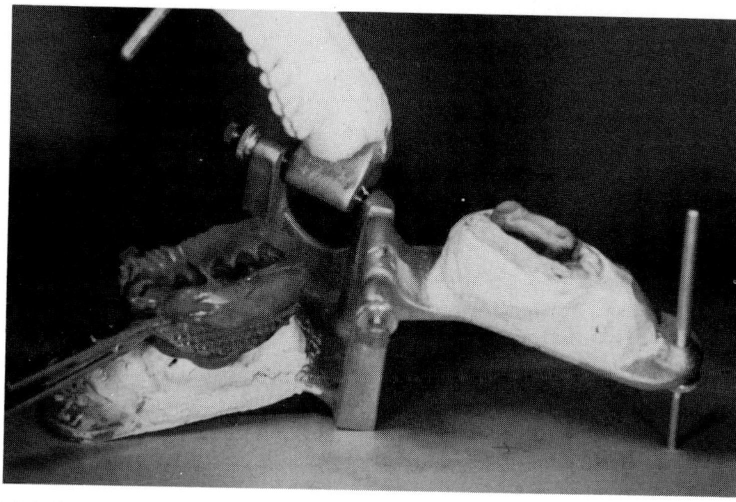

Fig. 28-7. Working cast with removable dies of preparations made and attached to lower arm of articulator. Open arm of articulator has anatomic cast poured in and separated from upper part of check bite tray impression.

5. Upon complete hardening of the stone dies, the exposed base of dies and tapered dowel pins are lubricated, and the lower section is poured in colored stone. This forms the prepared working cast seen in Fig. 28-7. When this is completely set, stone is poured into the upper portion of the impression; this produces the anatomic cast.

6. Without removing the casts from the check bite tray impression (Step 3), the upper and lower casts are attached to the upper arm (131-101) and lower base (131-2001) with stone (Fig. 28-4). This method preserves the centric relation of the casts. (Separate, individual impressions of the upper and lower may be taken in lieu of a dual check bite impression; however, this necessitates a separate centric relation record for final mounting of all casts.)

7. The alginate impression in the humidor taken in Step 2 is removed and all moisture is eliminated. The alginate material between the abutment teeth is reduced to the width of the widest abutment tooth.

8. Lubricate prepared abutments, adjoining teeth, and surrounding tissue with lubricant and flow a medium-thin mix of self-curing acrylic resin into the impression taken in Step 2. Let it set slightly.

9. Reposition it in the mouth and hold for 3 to 5 minutes or until it sets to a firm doughy consistency. Remove tray from the mouth and, if the acrylic mass remains on the teeth, remove it carefully so as not to distort it.

10. Quickly trim excess resin and undercuts and replace splint in the mouth. Let it polymerize until hard.

11. Remove and reduce occlusal portion of the acrylic splint until there is 3 to 4 mm. clearance and *no contact with any opposing teeth in centric or lateral positions of the mandible.* (When desired, a cast-metal tray may be made previously in the laboratory on the study models.)

12. Remove, dry, and place a 3 to 4 mm. layer of a recording material or a tacky wax on the occlusal area of the reduced splint, an amount slightly higher than the cusps of the adjoining teeth. (Fig. 28-6).

13. The splint must fit rigidly on the prepared teeth without displacement. It may be necessary to cement it with temporary cement, keeping the surface of the wax clean. (Avoid cementing, if possible.)

14. Have patient close in centric, then open. Repeat, to verify correct closure; then open.

15. Have patient close in centric and glide into protrusive and open.

16. Have patient close in centric and glide into right lateral, and open.

17. Have patient close in centric, then glide into left lateral and open. If desirable, all three steps may be repeated.

18. A small mix of fast-setting stone is carefully painted with a brush or finger over and into the functionally generated paths; extend the stone over the occlusal one or two teeth adjoining the unprepared teeth, to a thickness of ¼ to ½ inch. A strip of perforated tray metal is laid across the top of the soft stone to reinforce it. This forms what is called the "positive-functional-core" (Fig. 28-13). It is the dynamic record of centric relationship and all functional paths of occlusion. It discloses the physiologic effects of muscular guidance, condylar inclination, incisal tooth relationships, and established proprioceptive patterns. It contains the centric position and the functional paths of the teeth which later determine the occluding morphology of the teeth to be restored in the bridge pontics and retainers.

19. The splint with its stone functional-core is removed from the mouth and is placed in warm water; the two parts are separated. Any remaining wax in the core is removed with hot water and the core is laid aside to be built up later with stone.

20. It is next necessary to construct a third cast, *C*, incorporating the functional-core and relate this cast to the working cast already mounted to the base of the articulator. The first step is to raise the anatomic cast mounted on the upper arm (131-101) out of the way, and then to lower the other upper arm (131-102). Adjust the lock incisal rod (131-3002) for parallelism with previous position of upper arm and base of articulator. The functional-core prepared in Step 19 is now checked for accuracy of fit on prepared working cast *B*. The core is built up on the metal strip side with stone to a height coming within ⅛ to ¼ inch of the upper arm (131-102). When the stone has set, the built-up core is again checked accurately to the lower working cast and luted to it with sticky wax. A new mix of stone is made and a layer of ½ inch is applied to the stone core to attach it to the upper arm, which is gently lowered until the incisal rod comes in contact with the base of the articulator. When the stone sets thoroughly, the luting wax is removed with hot water (Fig. 28-8). It has been found that the building up of the stone core, while an additional step, minimizes the possibility of loosening or displacing the core when luted alone directly to the working cast. Any movement or shifting of the core would defeat the entire purpose of the technic.

21. The next step is waxing, carving, and finishing the wax patterns of the pontics and retainers. The anatomic and the functional-core casts are now related to the functions and requirements of the working cast. To serve their purpose, each upper cast must be mounted in the articulator in identical centric relation to the lower working cast.

The anatomic cast determines, in the waxing process, the final size of the teeth, their contour, and the position of cusps and sulci (Fig. 28-9). The functional-core-cast gives the physiologic occlusion in centric and in functional relations (Fig. 28-8). The pontics and retainers are waxed according to one's concept of correct morphology and occlusion but are overbuilt slightly higher occlusally. The occlusal wax is melted lightly with a wax spatula and allowed to lose its glaze. The lubricated functional-core-cast is brought down gently in centric closure until the incisal rod touches the metal base of the articulator. An identical pattern is now formed in the inlay wax as was previously made in the functionally generated wax in the mouth in centric relation. Other tooth patterns will also be observed—fossae and furrows made by cusps and marginal ridges, and sharp-edged ridges indicating sulci and spillways.

The contour and peripheral outline of the occlusal table will indicate where the buccal and lingual excess wax should be trimmed away.

Following the preliminary trimming and carving, talcum powder or white shoe polish is applied to the occlusal portion of the functional-core-cast, which is lightly tapped against the wax surfaces in the working model. High points and areas that prevent contact of the incisal rod with the base of the articulator will be disclosed. These should be reduced judiciously and the dusting and closing repeated. When there is no wax disclosure upon incisal pin contact with metal base, over-reduction of wax has taken place. If all cup-fossae occlusal morphology has been established and proper axial surface contour attained,

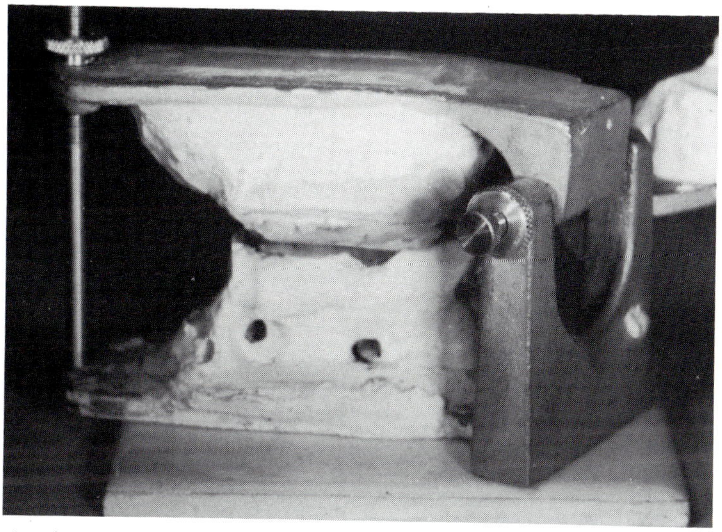

Fig. 28-8. Acrylic splint covered with registering material and its functional-stone core are positioned on working cast.

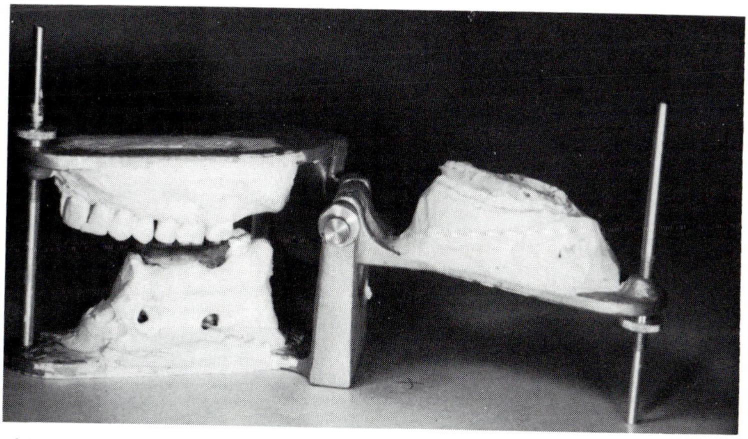

Fig. 28-9. Positive functional-core cast raised and replaced by anatomic cast.

then we can expect biologically and functionally acceptable occlusion.

During the process of adjusting the wax carvings for occlusion and tooth form and buccolingual position in the arch, it is well to check intermittently the progress of our work with the anatomic cast, which is also mounted in the same centric relation with the working cast as is the functional-core cast. The functional-core cast, however, is the final appraiser of occlusal compatibility.

Wax patterns are finished on the removable dies and may be semifinished and tried on the working model against the functional-core-cast, before investing the restoration for soldering. After soldering, the restoration is again tried in the working cast against the functional-core cast. If satisfactory, it is given its final polish and cemented on the prepared teeth.

22. This technic with slight modifications may be used on single tooth or multiple tooth restorations, both unilaterally and bilaterally.

Jelenko Verticulator method (Fig. 28-10)

An instrument of a different design, the Jelenko Verticulator has also proved satisfactory and is ideally suited to crown and unilateral fixed partial denture prostheses, especially where the occlusion is normal. It is so constructed that no movement takes place between the two casts during the mounting procedures and it maintains the same relationship between the upper and lower casts as exists at the time of registration and mounting.

The steps of procedure and their purposes are similar to those considered in the previously described method but are adapted to the verticulator instrument.

Master model is shown in Fig. 28-11 with cavities prepared in the two upper bicuspids and a crown for the first molar.

The functional bite material has been applied as previously to the platform of the acrylic splint, which is placed in position over the prepared teeth (Fig. 28-12). The bite material registers the centric position as well as the protrusive and both lateral paths created by the opposing teeth.

Rapid-setting stone has been painted into the paths registered in the bite material (Fig. 28-13). A narrow strip of thin perforated metal plate is placed on top of the stone to serve as a strengthener to the stone functional core. The core is next attached to the working model, which in

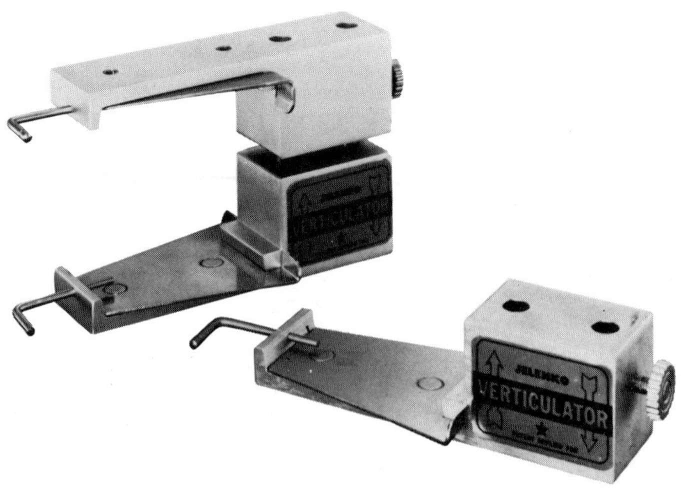

Fig. 28-10. Jelenko verticulator. (Courtesy J. F. Jelenko & Co.)

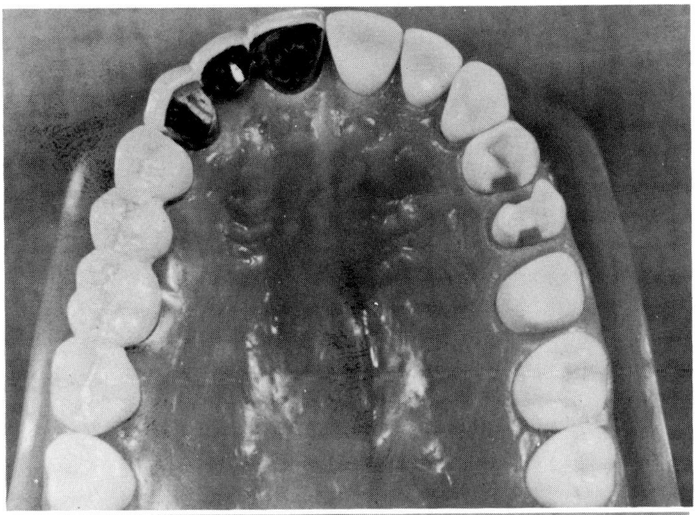

Fig. 28-11

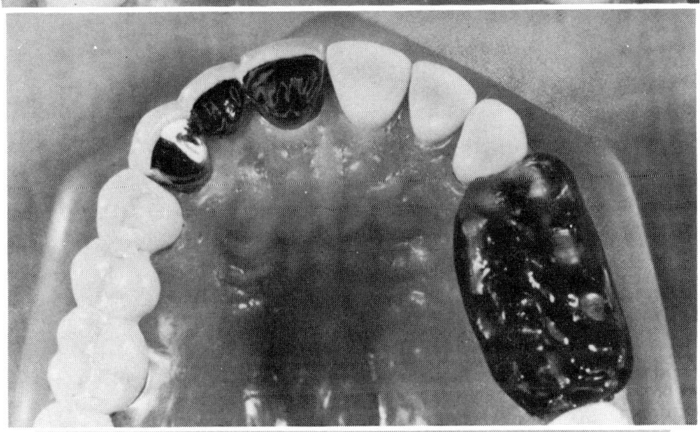

Fig. 28-12

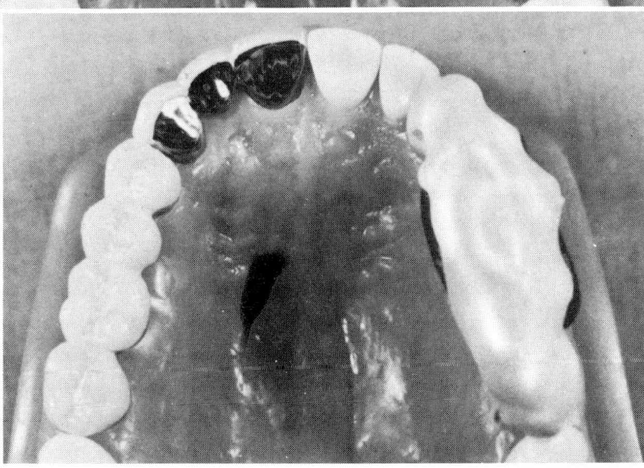

Fig. 28-13

Fig. 28-11. Master model with teeth prepared in upper molar and bicuspids. (Courtesy J. F. Jelenko & Co.)

Fig. 28-12. Functional bite material applied to platform of acrylic splint with functionally generated paths registered. (Courtesy J. F. Jelenko & Co.)

Fig. 28-13. Rapid-setting stone painted into paths registered in bite material. (Courtesy J. F. Jelenko & Co.)

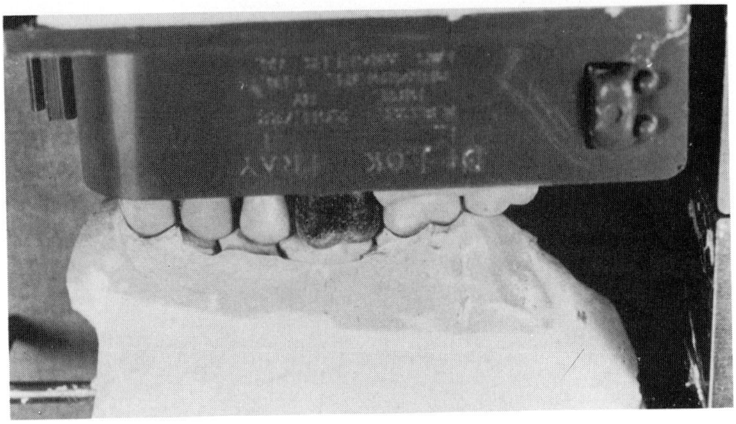

Fig. 28-14. Working model attached to one segment of verticulator. (Courtesy J. F. Jelenko & Co.)

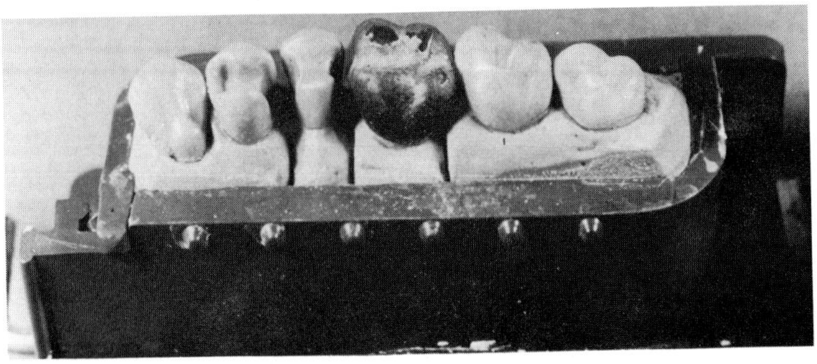

Fig. 28-15. High spots registered on wax crown to be reduced with wax carver. (Courtesy J. F. Jelenko & Co.)

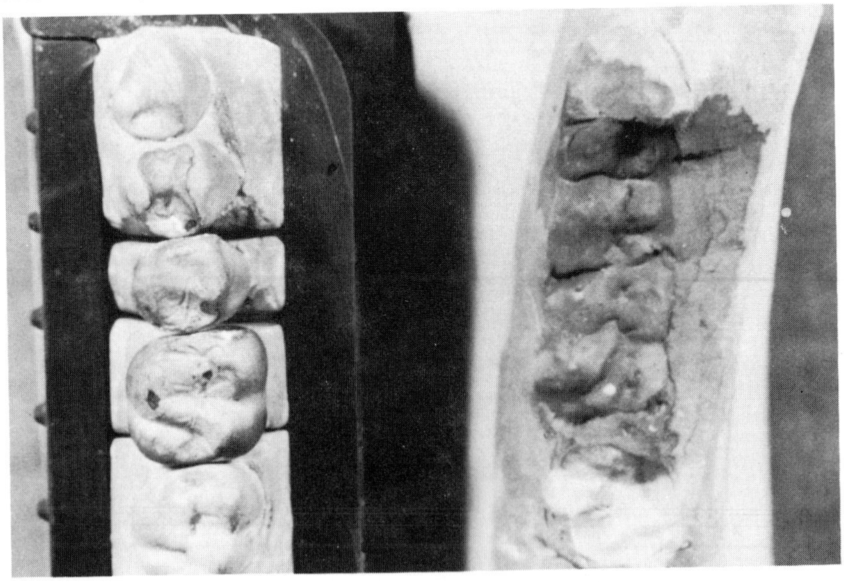

Fig. 28-16. Opposing functional-core arm of instrument in contact with patterns. (Courtesy J. F. Jelenko & Co.)

turn is attached to one segment of the verticulator (Fig. 28-14).

The molar crown is waxed on the die in the working model, the occlusal surface of the pattern is painted with powder, and contact is made with the functional core. This records the high spots on the occlusal surface of the wax crown pattern (Fig. 28-15). It is advisable to wax each of the prepared teeth separately. After this is done the three completed wax patterns are replaced on the dies in the model to establish and verify the position and contour of the contacting areas. The patterns are then invested and cast.

Closure of the instrument discloses any high spots on the wax occlusal surface, which are carefully reduced with the wax carver (Fig. 28-15).

After the three patterns have been completed separately and their contact areas verified, the opposing arm of the instrument is again brought in contact simultaneously with the patterns (Fig. 28-16).

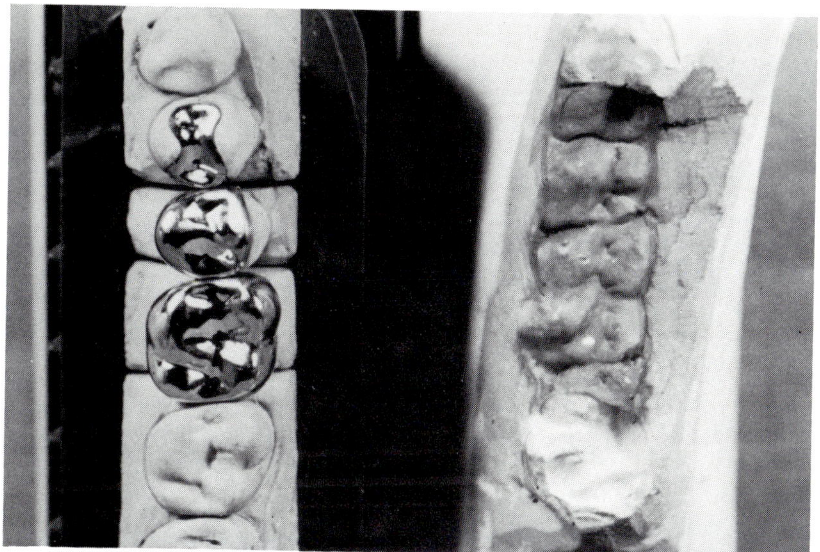

Fig. 28-17

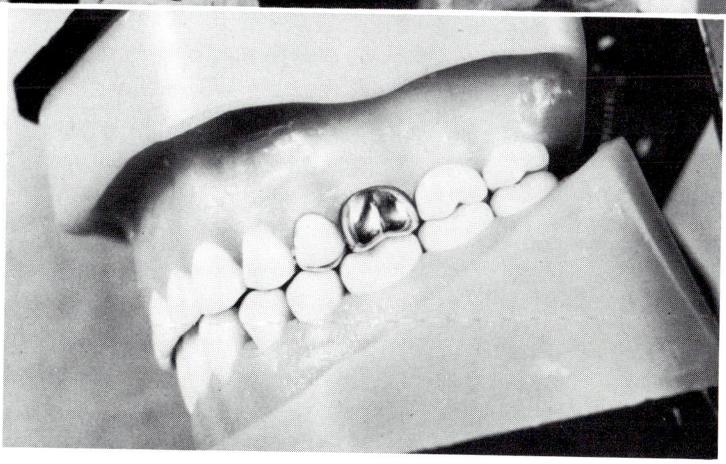

Fig. 28-18

Fig. 28-17. Castings cleaned and placed in work models on dies. (Courtesy J. F. Jelenko & Co.)

Fig. 28-18. Cast restorations in centric and functionally generated occlusion. (Courtesy J. F. Jelenko & Co.)

If any high spots show, the wax is trimmed and the castings are then made.

The castings are cleaned and placed in the work models on the dies and checked against the opposing functional core; if any high spots are present they are corrected (Fig. 28-17).

The three cast restorations are in centric and functionally generated occlusions (Fig. 28-18).

SELECTED REFERENCES

1. Bailey, E. E.: A master model technique for the construction of inlays, crowns, and bridgework, D. Digest **42**:118, 1936.
2. Rubinstein, J.: Simplified impression technic for bridge and precision cases, D. Digest **65**: 457, 1959.
3. Meyer, F. S.: Can the plane line articulator meet all the demands of balanced and functional occlusion in all restorative work? Colorado S.D.A.J. **17**:6-16, 1938.
4. Meyer, F. S.: The generated path technique in reconstruction dentistry, J. Prosth. Dent. **9**:354-366, 1959.
5. Meyer, F. S.: A new, simple and accurate technic for obtaining balanced and functional occlusion, J.A.D.A. **21**:195-203, 1934.

GENERAL REFERENCES

Benfield, J. W.: Di-Lok system with functionally generated paths, work simplification in dental practice, Philadelphia, 1964, W. B. Saunders Co.

Beck, H. O.: Choosing the articulator, J.A.D.A. **64**:468-475, 1962.

Chouraqui, M.: Critical study of various impression technics for fixed dentures: attempt at simplification, Rev. Franc. Odontostomat. **15** (7):931, 1968.

Cowell, T. A., and Moore, J.: New technic for sectional model production for inlay and bridgework, J.A.D.A. **71**:1388, 1965.

Granger, E. R.: The principles of obtaining occlusion in occlusal rehabilitation, J. Prosth. Dent. **13**:714, 1963.

Henschel, C. J.: Impressions for bridge assemblage, Oral Hyg. **52**:57, 1962.

Jankelson, B.: Technique for obtaining optimum functional relationship for the natural dentition, Dent. Clin. N. Amer. pp. 131-141, March, 1960.

Moses, C. H.: Theory and practice of impression making, J. Ontario D. A. **38**:6, 1961.

Nevin, J. J.: How to get the best results in crown and bridge work: the impression procedure, Cal. **23**:3, 1961.

Potter, H. R., and Smith, D. E.: Fitting of abutment castings; impression; stone casts; articulators, Pacific D. Gaz. **39**:779, 835, 1931.

Pruden, W. H.: Development of occlusion where total reconstruction is contraindicated, J. Prosth. Dent. **16**:549, 1966.

Pruden, W. H.: Occlusion related to fixed partial denture prosthesis, Dent. Clin. N. Amer., p. 121-136, March, 1962.

Sendax, V. I.: Master impression technique foı fixed and precision removable bridge restorations, D. Digest **68**:554, 1962.

Skurnik, H.: Functional interarch relationships recorded in wax, J. Prosth. Dent. **21**:283, 1969.

Thomas, C. B.: Fixed bridge assembled in the mouth, D. Digest **65**:409, 447, 496, 542, 1959.

Wormley, J. H., and others: A simplified procedure for remounting dentures, J. Prosth. Dent. **16**:675, 1966.

Zimmermann, E. M.: Modifications of functionally generated path procedures, J. Prosth. Dent. **16**:1119, 1966.

Zola, A.: Acrylic resin transfer pattern, J. Prosth. Dent. **9**:278, 1959.

Chapter 29

Procedure for transfer to articulator using adjustable hinge axis face bow and interocclusal records*

The modern practitioner must be a diagnostician and must apply his knowledge and judgment to the plan of treatment. The study of casts that have been anatomically related to one another in the articulator is essential to diagnosis based on scientific knowledge. The dental profession's major objective is to prevent dental disease and disorders. Such diagnostic procedure makes possible early recognition of disorders to which we may apply preventive measures.

When prevention is impossible, early diagnosis should reduce treatment needs to the minimum, thus avoiding more complex conditions requiring major and costly treatment at a later date.

The practicing dentist's decision can be based on scientific knowledge; he is, however, confronted with the fact that there are differences of opinion regarding application of current knowledge. Controversy over advantages of certain equipment makes selection of instruments, facebows, and articulators difficult for him. Unfortunately, the result may be to focus too much attention on a particular design or mechanical aspect, rather than on the underlying anatomic and physiologic principles that apply. Success of treatment depends primarily on a thorough understanding of principles and diligence in carrying out exacting procedures, rather than on mechanical devices per se.

The anatomic and physiologic principles related to the physiology of occlusion have been discussed in detail in other chapters. It is my intent here to offer a procedure based on those principles, applicable to both diagnostic and treatment needs.

The instruments selected are by no means the only ones that might be employed successfully. The articulator (Fig. 29-1) has been selected because it adapts to the direct use of intraocclusal records, thus permitting a procedure involving a minimum number of required steps. Extensive and careful evaluation of clinical results fails to indicate any inadequacy when compared to other instruments and/or procedures. Mindful that we must make certain decisions based on current knowledge, it is essential that we now accept the fact that we can record and demonstrate an opening and closing axis of the mandible. This is the most important rationale for the use of a facebow in the transfer of the maxillary cast in correct anatomic relationship within the articulator.

McCollum[1] stated: "There is one and

*Text by George H. Moulton, D.D.S., F.A.C.D.; Professor, Department of Crown and Bridge Dentistry; Dean, Emory University School of Dentistry, Atlanta, Georgia.

only one position in which the hinge axis is constant to both the mandible and maxilla." This position is the terminal hinge position of the mandible, or, more specifically, of the condyles in their fossae. It is also described as the most posterior-superior position of the condyles. It must be emphasized that this should be a physiologically acceptable position and should not be obtained by force or by introducing drugs or anesthetics. This is the same condylar-fossae relationship that will again be emphasized in obtaining an interocclusal record of centric occlusion, thus relating maxilla and the mandible to the same axis. Granger[2] stated: "The fact that the hinge axis is constant to the mandible and therefore determines the arc of closure on which teeth meet in every contacting position is of fundamental importance. If it were merely a question of centric closure it would be relatively unimportant." Granger goes on to summarize very well the concept of the hinge axis and the rationale for the use of a hinge axis face bow when he says: "The object of any articulator mounting is to reproduce on a mechanical instrument the same relation of the teeth to the axis of the articulator as the teeth in the mouth occupy to the axis of the condyles." The component parts of the articulator condyles are, therefore, also in their terminal hinge positions during the transfer procedure.

Proponents of the rigid (Snow) face bow discount the importance of the hinge axis, and some question its existence. Instead of locating an axis by trial and error, an arbitrary landmark is fixed by measuring a point 13.0 mm. on a line from the tragus of the ear to the ala of the nose. The styluses of the face bow are then

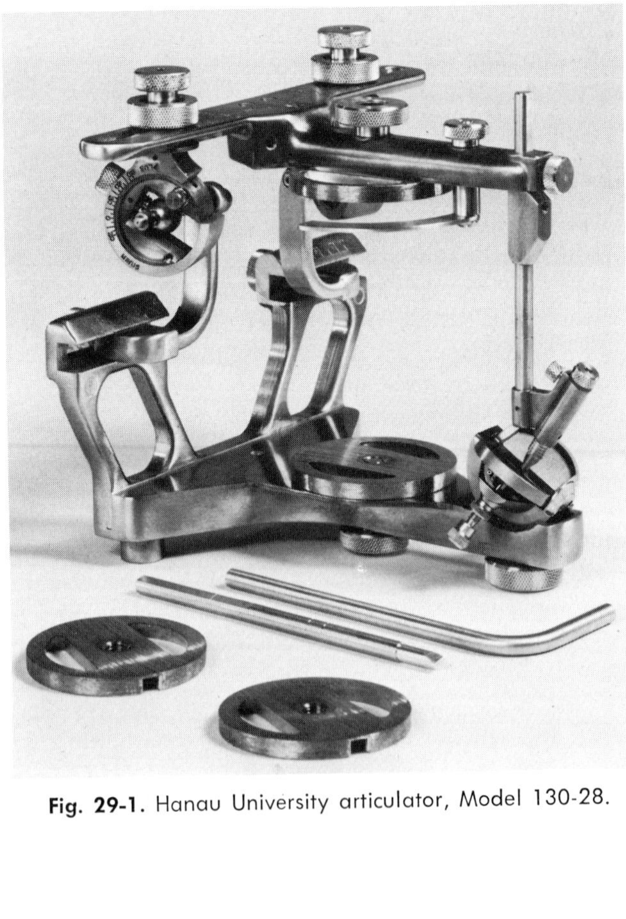

Fig. 29-1. Hanau University articulator, Model 130-28.

placed over these landmarks. Schuyler[3] stated: "We have been told that the face bow as advocated by Snow is valueless. Careful use of it would seem to accomplish at least 90% of the requirements. An effort to reproduce most accurately the axis is commendable."

Faced with these two schools of thought, the operator not planning to use the hinge axis face bow to determine the opening and closing axis should find it helpful to at least palpate the condyles while in their terminal position and mark the approximate center of the condyle. This has been found to be in closer approximation to the recorded axis than the arbitrary landmarks. The adjustable bow also makes it possible to accommodate to the frequent lack of symmetry noted between the two condylar areas.

Because most of the scientific data available at this time seems to support the use of an adjustable hinge axis face bow, this instrument has been chosen to describe this initial procedure in the transfer of the maxillary cast to the articulator.

LOCATION OF THE HINGE AXIS

The plain clutch* tray 135-108 (Fig. 29-2) is adaptable to most lower arches and is available only in this size and contour. This tray may be altered as required, or a special individualized tray may be cast.

*Frequently designated "registration tray" (S.D.T.).

Optionally available is a clutch tray of similar size and contour except that it contains a built-in central bearing screw and has a companion central bearing plate (Fig. 29-3). This central bearing clutch tray is obtainable through your dental dealer and is specified as No. 135-109.

Step 1. The clutch tray consists of a labial and lingual section assembled by screws X-1. The clutch plate 135-3112 is securely attached with two screws X-27 to the flat on the labial of the tray section 135-2004 with the identification mark on the clutch plate at top right. The clutch stem 135-209 is then attached with screw X-27, noting that the identification marks of matched assembly coincide (Fig. 29-2).

Step 2. The assembled clutch tray is securely cemented to the mandibular arch, with the stem extending approximately parallel to the occlusal and saggital planes. It is essential that the tray be anchored firmly to the dentition to prevent even the slightest movement.

Step 3. The face bow (Fig. 29-4) is prepared for maximum adjustability as follows: remove the condylar pointers 135-208 and slide condylar sleeves 135-3606 flush with locknuts 135-3421 and tighten. Position the square section of sliding

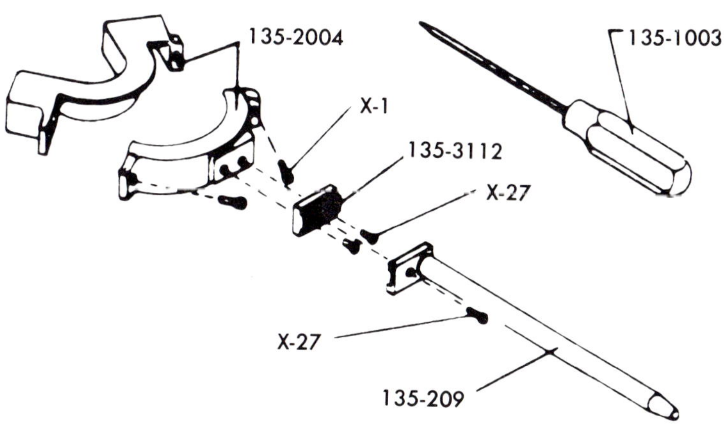

Fig. 29-2. Plain clutch tray 135-108.

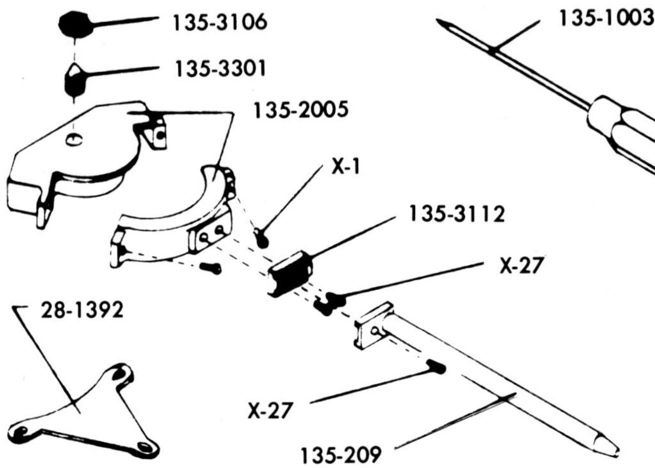

Fig. 29-3. Central bearing clutch tray 135-109.

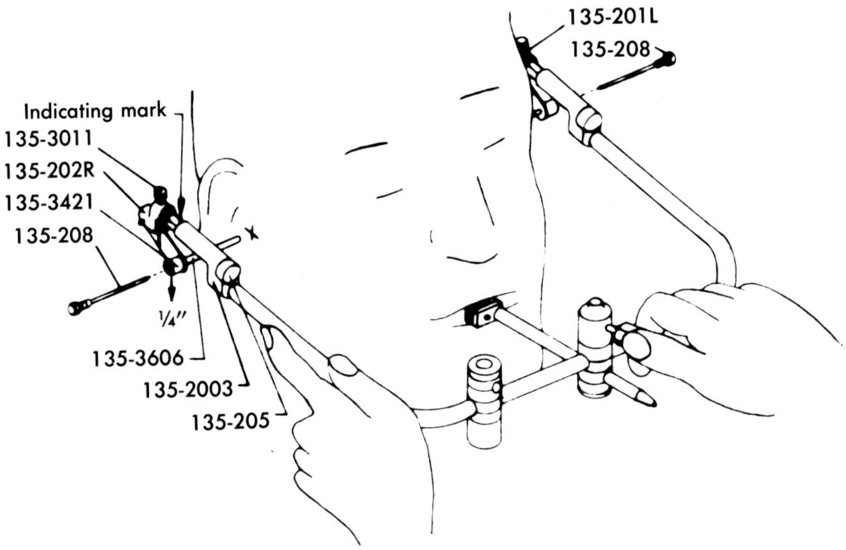

Fig. 29-4. Kinematic transfer bow 135-4 adjusted for application to patient.

frames 135-201L and 135-202R by rotating thumbscrew 135-205 to align the indicating marks with the edge of fixed frame 135-2003. Adjust the thumbscrew 135-3011 to lower the condylar sleeves about ¼ inch from their closed positions.

Step 4. The condyle areas are digitally located and temporarily marked on the patient. The face bow is brought gently over the face with the stem of the clutch tray entering the loose clamp on left side of the bow. With the ends of the condylar sleeves pointing toward, and equidistant from, the temporary condyle markings, the bow is held while the clamp is tightened securely with the wrench.

Step 5. Release locknuts 135-3421 and withdraw condylar sleeves 135-3606 with a rotating motion to permit insertion and threading of the condylar pointers 135-208 to their stops at condylar sleeves. Slide the condylar sleeves with a rotating motion to bring the pointer into close proximity, without touching, to the patient's skin.

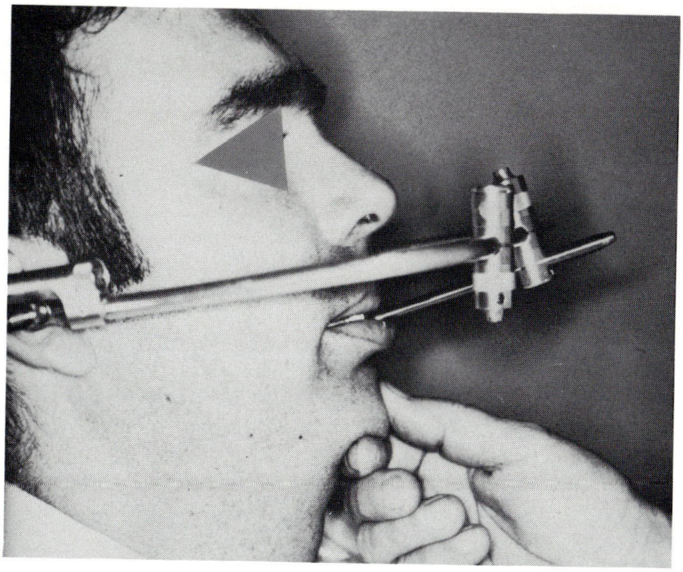

Fig. 29-5. Guiding closure to maintain condyles in terminal hinge position.

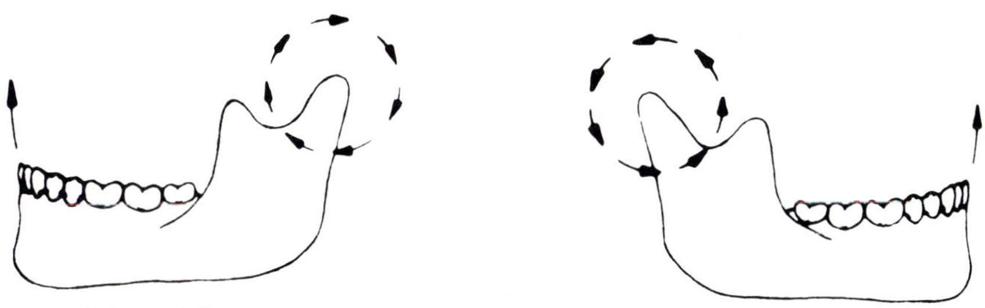

Fig. 29-6. Condyle pointer movement in relationship to hinge axis.

Inward and outward movement of the condylar pointers must be accomplished only by movement of the condylar sleeves, not the condylar pointers, which must remain undisturbed during the axis location procedure.

Step 6. The patient is instructed to open and close within a limited range, not more than 2 cm. The condylar pointers will be observed to move in arcs when not in line with the exact hinge axis. Particular precautions must be taken to prevent incorporation of a protrusive component in the opening and closing movements of the mandible. The operator may have to guide this opening and closing movement to maintain the terminal hinge position (Fig. 29-5). This guidance is usually done by placing the thumb and the forefinger on the chin, and guiding the movement. Force of any kind is contraindicated. Having the patient occasionally protrude and then retrude will help the dentist in developing the clinical "feel" of determining condylar position. It is also advisable to have the patient sit in an upright position with his mandible parallel to the floor. Observe the direction of movement of the condylar pointers only on the closing stroke of the mandible. Fig. 29-6 will aid in making adjustments of the condylar pointers in the correct direction. Anteroposterior adjustments of the condylar pointers are made by turning thumbscrews

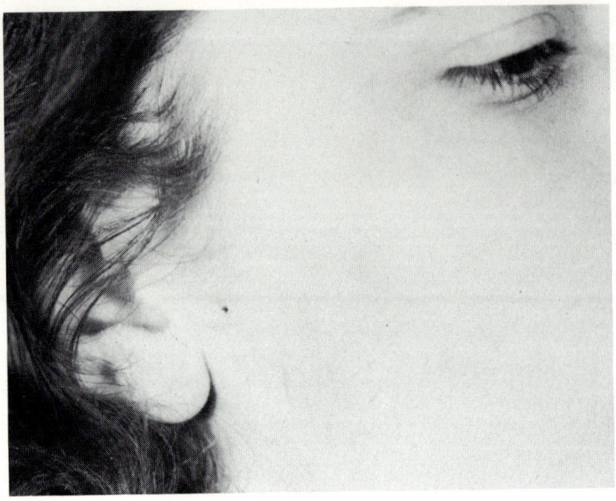

Fig. 29-7. Axis reference marking.

135-205, and adjustments of the pointers above and below the hinge axis are made by the thumbscrews 135-3011.

The farther away the pointers are from the hinge axis, the longer will be the pointer stroke. The pointer stroke will shorten with the approach to the hinge axis. When the pointers are opposite the hinge axis, all movement of the pointers will have been transposed into a strictly rotational axis .

Step 7. When the condylar pointers have ceased to move and are observed to only "hinge" or rotate at fixed points on the face, without a protrusive influence, these points are considered as the Kinematical axis.

The condylar pointers are now disengaged and withdrawn slightly to permit application of a marking medium to the points and they are again engaged to mark the skin (Fig. 29-7). Permanent marks may be obtained by tattooing.

Step 8. To permit safe and convenient removal of the face bow from the patient, the condylar pointers are removed from the condylar sleeves. With the wrench, loosen the clamp supporting the bow and withdraw the entire face bow from the clutch stem. The clutch stem, clutch plate, and two-tray assembly screws are removed in that order to permit the labial and lingual sections of the tray to be removed from the teeth.

Relating the maxillary cast to the terminal hinge position of the mandible

Step 9. The face bow is preadjusted as in Step No. 3.

Step 10. The prongs of the bitefork are covered on both sides with softened wax or any material of the operator's choice. The softened material is seated against the occlusal surface of the maxillary dentition to create a positive index, with the stem of the bitefork extending approximately parallel to the occlusal and saggital plane and chilled while the bitefork is firmly held by the lower teeth. This index of the upper occlusal surface will be used to transfer the maxillary cast to the articulator.

Step 11. The preadjusted face bow is brought gently over the face with the stem of the bitefork entering the clamp of the bow. With the ends of the condylar sleeves pointing toward and equidistant from the hinge axis markings, the bow is held in this position while the clamp is securely tightened with the wrench.

Step 12. Loosen locknuts and withdraw the condylar sleeves to permit inserting

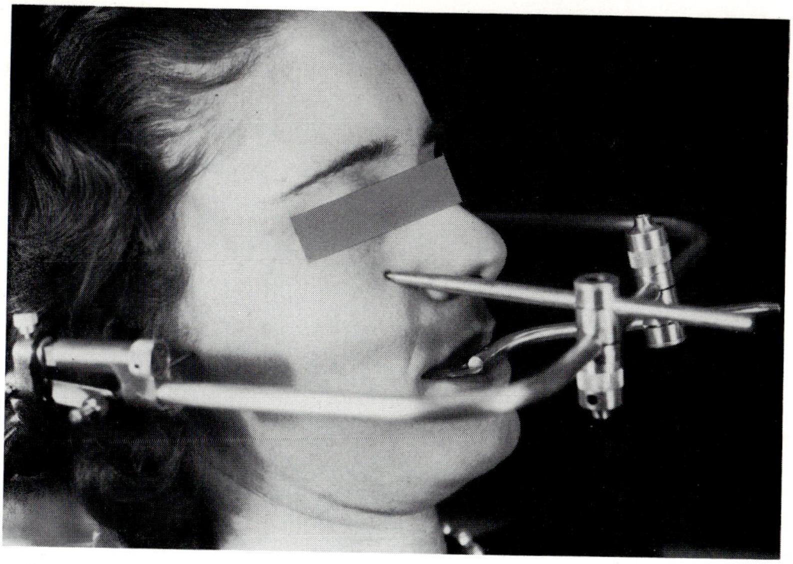

Fig. 29-8. Face bow in position with bitefork and infraorbital marker.

the condylar pointers and screwing them to their stops at the condylar sleeve ends. Slide the condylar sleeves to bring the pointers to the skin while adjusting the thumbscrews for a precise coincidence of the pointers to the hinge axis markings on the skin. When the condylar pointers contact the skin in this exact location, the condylar sleeve locknuts are securely tightened, observing that the bitefork remains firmly seated against the maxillary teeth.

Step 13. The orbital pointer is inserted in the second clamp, and with the pointer lightly touching the face at the infraorbital notch, simultaneously hold the bow and tighten the clamp securely (Fig. 29-8). Observe that the condylar pointer locations have remained consistent with the hinge axis markings.

Step 14. The condylar pointers are unscrewed from their condylar sleeves and removed. The assembled face bow with the bitefork and orbital pointer attached is carefully withdrawn from the patient without disturbing any of the adjustments. The condylar pointers are then replaced in the sleeves in their exact original positions.

Transfer of the maxillary cast to the articulator

Step 15. The articulator is prepared as follows, using no undue force or mechanical aids (Fig. 29-9).

1. Release centric locks 130-3109, rotate condylar guidances 130-137 to a minus protrusive of approximately 25, and remove the upper member of instrument.
2. The right and left condylar shaft supports 130-2018 and 2019 on the lower member are adjusted symmetrically to 55 mm.
3. Incisal guide 130-108 is set at 10 degrees.
4. Petroleum jelly, oil, silicone, or Teflon is applied to all surfaces exposed to the mounting medium.
5. Mounting plate 130-2012 is attached to the upper member.
6. Median of the scribed lines on the straight incisal pin 130-3007 is adjusted flush with the lower surface of the upper member.

Step 16. Remove the calibrated shafts and firmly attach the axial cribs 135-110 with thumbscrews 135-210 (Fig. 29-10).

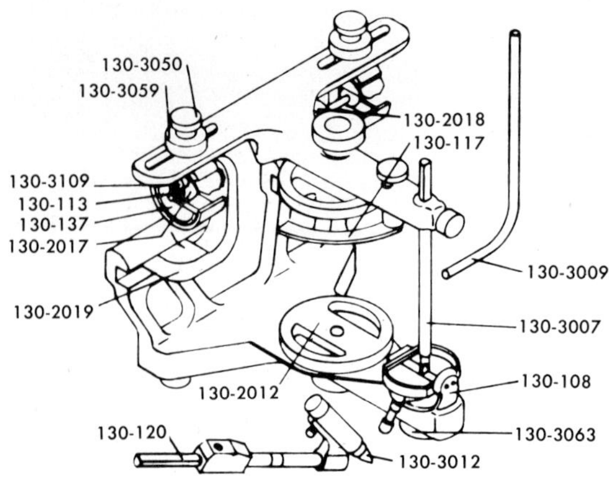

Fig. 29-9. Hanau University articulator, Model 130-28: identification of parts.

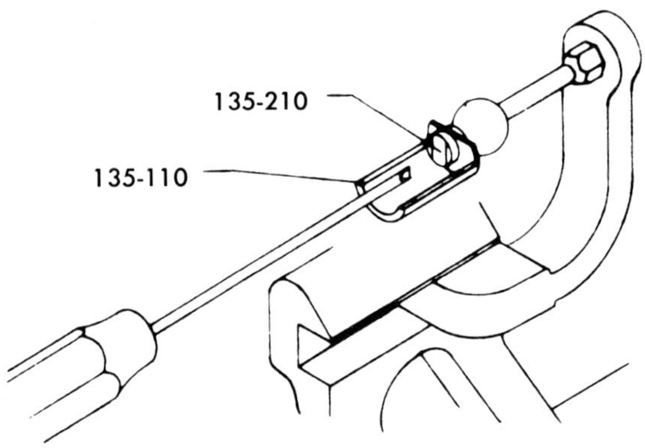

Fig. 29-10. Attachment of axial cribs.

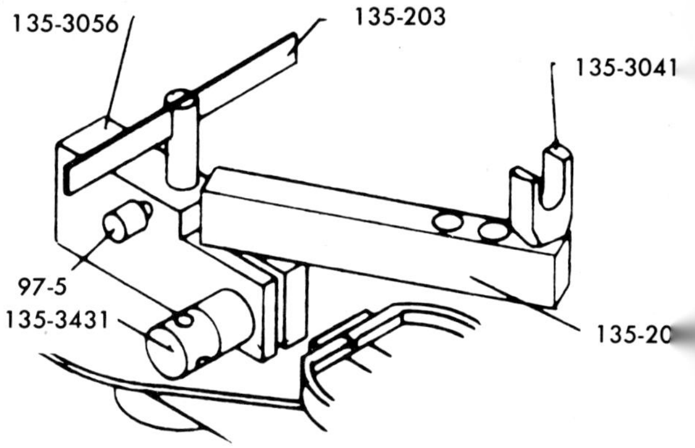

Fig. 29-11. Mounting support.

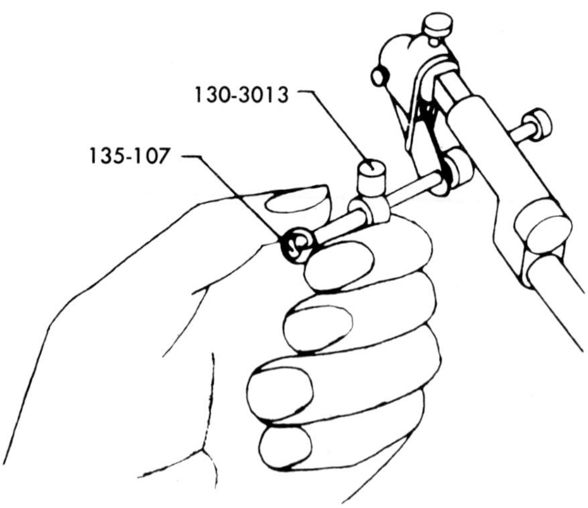

Fig. 29-12. Axial aligners placed on condylar pointers.

Step 17. Tightly attach mounting block 135-3056 to the lower member of articulator (Fig. 29-11). Lockscrew 135-3431 is loosened by wrench (previously used on face bow clamps) to permit the lateral adjustment bar 135-204 to rotate freely. Thumbscrew 97-5 is loosened to lower pivot 135-203. This cast support has an extension that is removed and used only in the event of a steep mounting of the cast, which may require vertical adjustment in excess of that otherwise afforded.

Step 18. Axial aligners 135-107 are placed over condylar pointers of face bow and are locked by thumbscrews 130-3013 when they abut the condylar sleeves (Fig. 29-12). The face bow is positioned so that

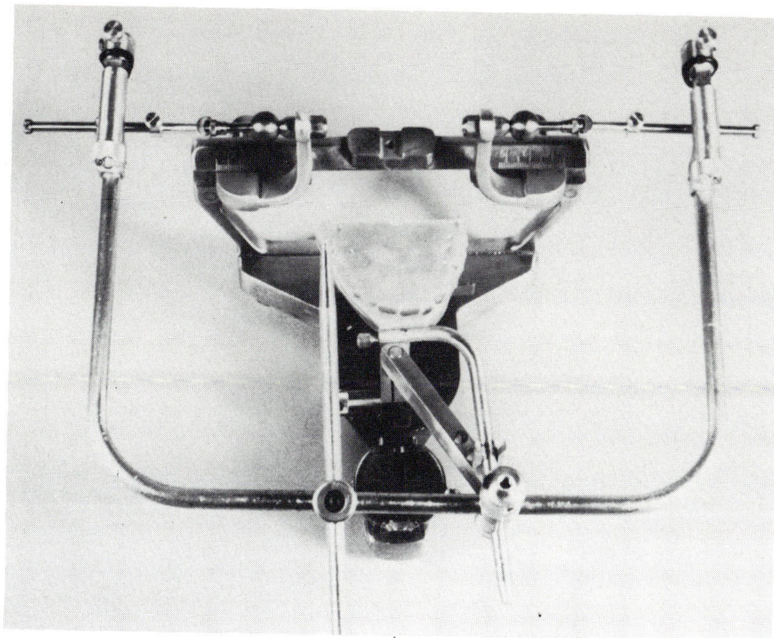

Fig. 29-13. Adjustment of the extendible condylar shafts to correct intercondylar distance.

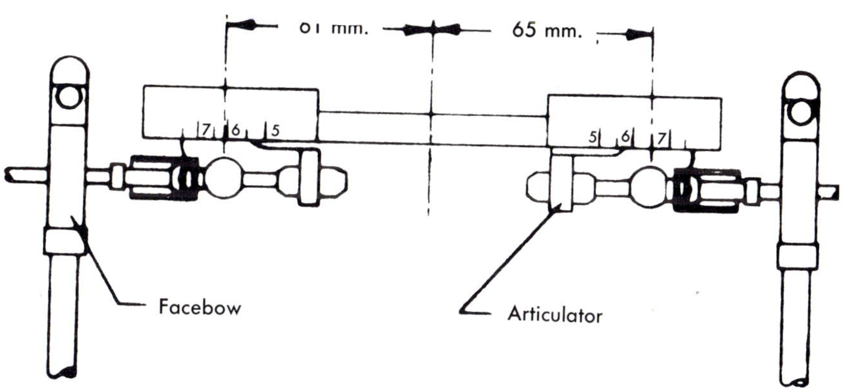

Fig. 29-14. Gauging by contacting of condylar pointers with thumbscrews on condylar shafts.

the axial aligners are resting firmly in the axial cribs while the third point of suspension, the bitefork stem, rests in the bitefork swivel 135-3041 (Fig. 29-13). The bitefork swivel is placed in the appropriate hole of the lateral adjustment bar.

To permit suspension of the axial aligners in the cribs, it may be necessary to increase, or decrease, the original 55 mm. setting of the condylar shaft supports.

Step 19. Carefully increase the intercondylar distance to contact the condylar pointers with the detent in thumbscrews on end of condylar shaft (Fig. 29-14). The sum total of the scale reading on the frame of lower member are added and then divided by two and noted. (Example [Fig. 29-15]: the left scale registering 65 is reduced to 63. The right scale registering 61 is increased to 63.)

Step 21. When the detents in center of thumbscrew on end of both condylar shafts equally touch without strain the condylar pointers of the facebow, the lock-

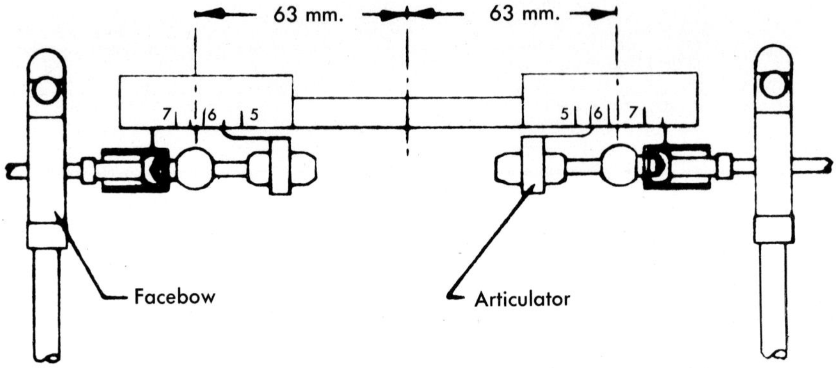

Fig. 29-15. Symmetric adjustment of intercondylar distance.

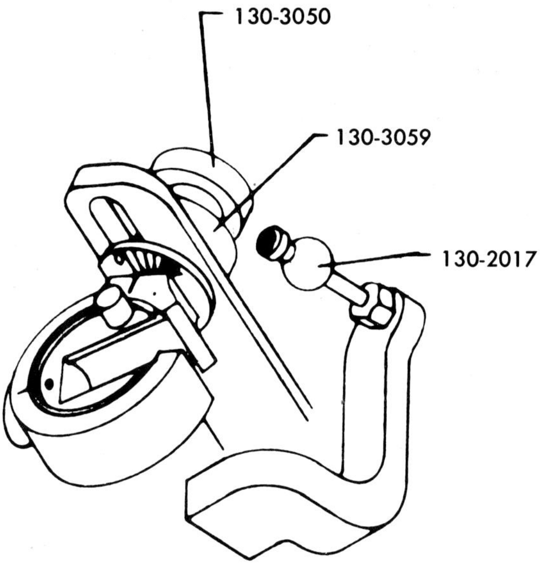

Fig. 29-16. Condylar guidance set at zero degree lateral and placed over condylar element.

screw 135-3431 is securely tightened by wrench (Fig. 29-11).

Upon tightening, verify the symmetry of an unstrained adjustment by lightly lifting the bitefork stem in and out of the bitefork swivel 135-3041. No drag or lateral displacement must be observed, and any evidence of improper alignment requires repeating the two preceding steps.

Step 22. The cast support is now raised until the pivot contacts both sides of the bitefork and is locked by the thumbscrew to prevent any vertical displacement caused by the additional weight of a maxillary cast and the mounting medium (Fig. 29-13). An extension has been provided if the steepness of the cast requires additional vertical adjustment for this support.

Step 23. The condylar guidances on upper member are set at "zero" degree lateral of the calibration at underside of upper member by releasing and then tightening thumbnut 130-3050 (Fig. 29-16).

Replace the upper member of articulator by increasing or decreasing the intercondylar distance of the right and left condylar guidances by thumbnut 130-3059

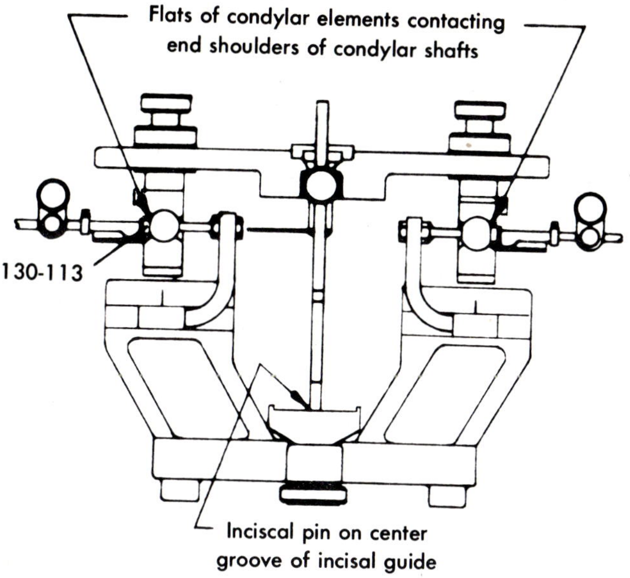

Fig. 29-17. Intercondylar distance adjustments corrected with incisal pin on center groove of incisal guide.

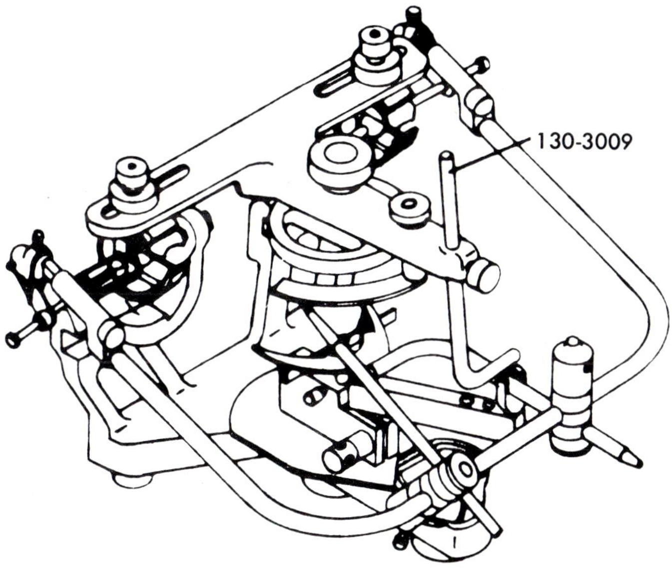

Fig. 29-18. Mounting pin adjusted in contact with stem of bitefork to align orbital pointer with orbital indicator.

to permit entry of the condylar elements 130-2017 into their respective condylar guidance slots. Orbital indicator on upper member may be rotated to prevent any mechanical interference. Tighten the centric locks to restrict the instrument to opening and closing movements only. The protrusive of condylar guidances is set at 30 degrees.

Step 24. Increase the intercondylar distance of the right and left condylar guidances to contact the flats of the condylar elements with the end shoulders of the condylar shafts 130-133 (Fig. 29-17). The

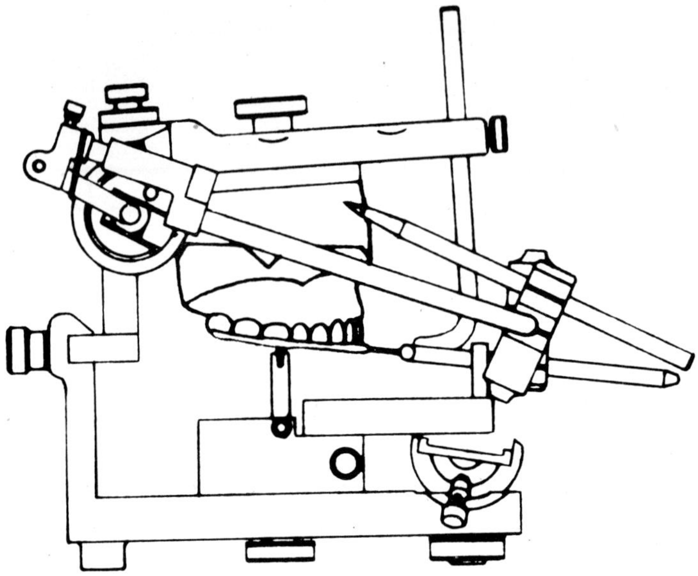

Fig. 29-19. Maxillary cast mounting to upper member of articulator, using "split cast" method.

flattened end of the incisal pin must be exactly coincident with the center groove of the incisal guide when the condylar guidances are tightened. Note that no perceptible sideshift of the condylar shafts in their elements exists.

Step 25. The mounting pin 130-3009 is inserted in place of the incisal pin and the bent end of this mounting pin is seated on a stable contact of the bitefork stem (Fig. 29-18). The upper member is simultaneously adjusted vertically until the orbital pointer is level with the horizontally adjustable orbital indicator on the articulator.

The orbital indicator is removed from the articulator and the maxillary cast is now mounted by the usual technique, using the mounting pin as the vertical static stop instead of an incisal pin.

Step 26. The maxillary cast, ground flat on its mounting side and properly V notched on its peripheral mounting border for the "split-cast" method, is lubricated with a thin coating of petroleum jelly or other separating medium. Boxing wax may be wrapped around it to provide a form into which the countersection is poured.

The cast is then securely seated and luted to the index on the bitefork to maintain the accurate relationship to the hinge axis.

Step. 27. The upper member of the articulator is swung back, and a mounting medium of suitable consistency is placed on the cast. The upper member is swung forward to embed the mounting plate and bring the mounting pin to the static stop on the bitefork stem.

Complete the mounting with a spatula and remove excess material to expose top surface of the mounting plate for convenient removal and accurate reattachment of the cast to the instrument (Fig. 29-19).

Step 28. Upon complete set of the mounting medium, remove the face bow, axial cribs, face bow mounting block, and mounting pin.

Step 29. Trimming of the maxillary mount is completed to present a sharply defined line at the junction to the cast and to eliminate any possible interference with the function of the instrument.

Step 30. The adjustable incisal pin 130-

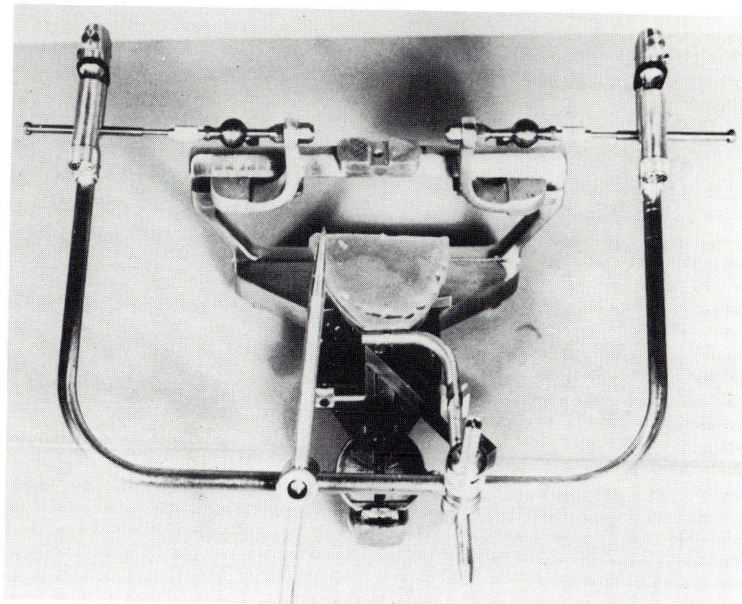

Fig. 29-20. Experimental model (XP) of modified hinge axis face bow.

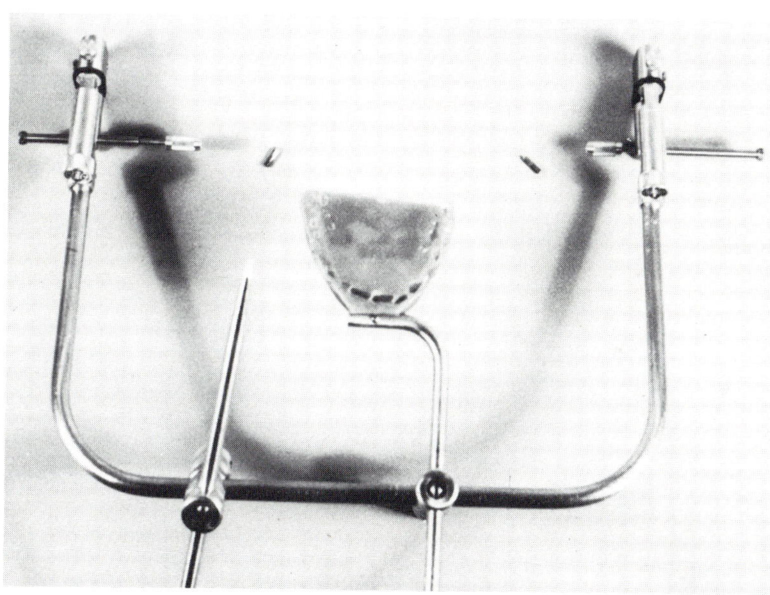

Fig. 29-21. Condylar pointers removed.

120 is now attached with the indicating line on the vertical portion aligned flush with the lower surface of upper member (Fig. 29-23).

The calibrated angle pin 130-3012 is adjusted to the median line and locked. Release the locknut of the incisal guide slightly and, while tilting the guide anteroposteriorly, observe that there is no vertical displacement of the upper member. Should there be, it is eliminated by raising or lowering the vertical portion of the pin and tightening the thumbscrew to maintain its position. When so adjusted, the relocating collar is brought into contact with the underside of the upper member and securely locked. Subsequent removal and replacement of the incisal pin is facilitated by this preset collar, assuring exact repositioning. Reset the incisal guide to "zero" degree and lock. Attach a mounting plate to the lower member.

MODIFICATION OF FACE BOW (XP)

The hinge axis face bow has been modified and the experimental (XP) model is shown in Fig. 29-20. The modifications result in certain advantages. First, it elimi-

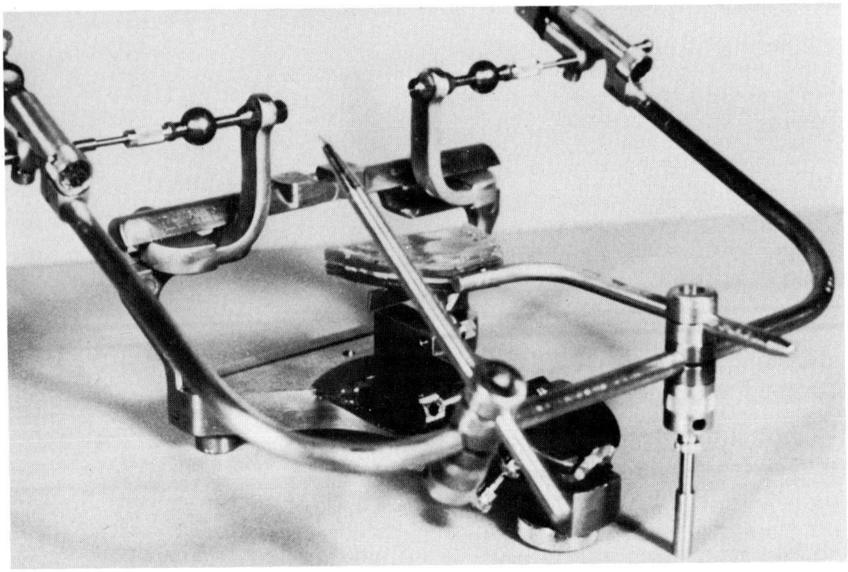

Fig. 29-22. XP Model, using bench top support for bow.

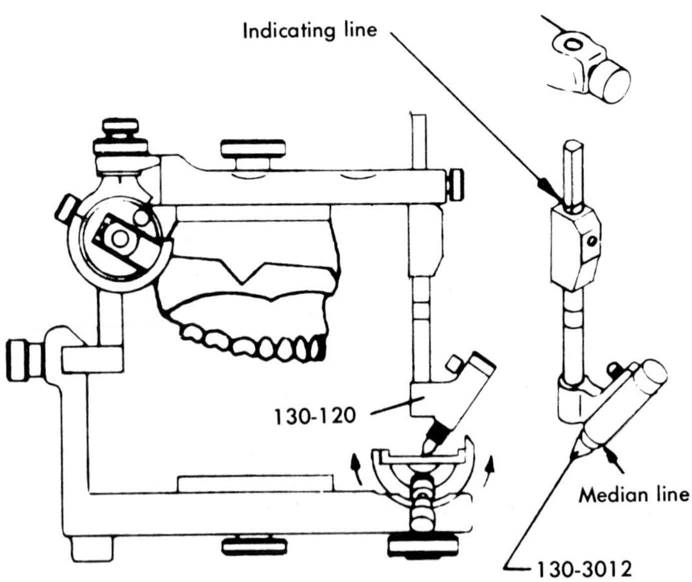

Fig. 29-23. Adjustable incisal pin attached to upper member.

nates the need for axial aligners and cribs. Secondly, upon removal of the condylar pointers (Fig. 29-21) the mechanism for attachment to the condylar shaft of the articulator provides for greater stability (Fig. 29-20). It also provides for more universal usage in that it can be used to relate to an arbitrary landmark, or to determine the opening and closing axis by scientific trial and error. It may be used with a mounting jig or the position of the bitefork support may be reversed, which then provides for the same table support as for the Snow face bow (Fig. 29-22). This modification is adaptable to all uses.

CENTRIC OCCLUSION OR CENTRIC RELATION

The next step in our transfer procedure is to relate the mandibular cast to the already transferred maxillary cast. For emphasis, the quote from Granger[2] is repeated. "The object of any articulator mounting is to reproduce on a mechanical instrument the same relation of the teeth to the axis of the articulator as the teeth in the mouth occupy to the axis of the condyles." In this concept, the condyles must again be positioned in their terminal hinge position when the interocclusal record for transfer of the mandibular cast is made. This is the same condylar position described for recording the opening and closing axis of the mandible, and the axis position to which we related the maxillary cast. This interocclusal record is called a "centric relation record" or a "centric occlusion record." I prefer the term "centric occlusion," in that crown and bridge prosthodontics is concerned with the dentulous patient. After completion of the mounting procedure and removal of the interocclusal record, the occlusion of the teeth resultant of mandibular closure with the condyles remaining in their terminal hinge position is my preferred definition of centric occlusion.[4] It is from this relationship that a study of occlusion must begin, as the resultant closure may bring all teeth into harmonious relationship (Fig. 29-24) to one another, or it may identify a deflective occlusal contact (Fig. 29-25). If a deflective occlusal contact exists, one can observe a slide to maximum intercuspation (Fig. 29-26). This resultant relationship is eccentric occlusion. It has also been termed acquired centric or dual occlusion, and has been described by others as a failure of centric occlusion to coincide with centric relation.

The requirement that this interocclusal record represents a mandible-to-maxilla relationship with the condyles in their

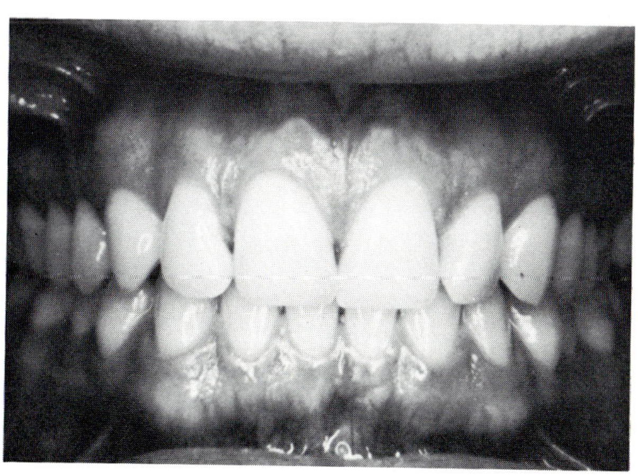

Fig. 29-24. "Ideal" occlusion. Condyles in their terminal hinge position.

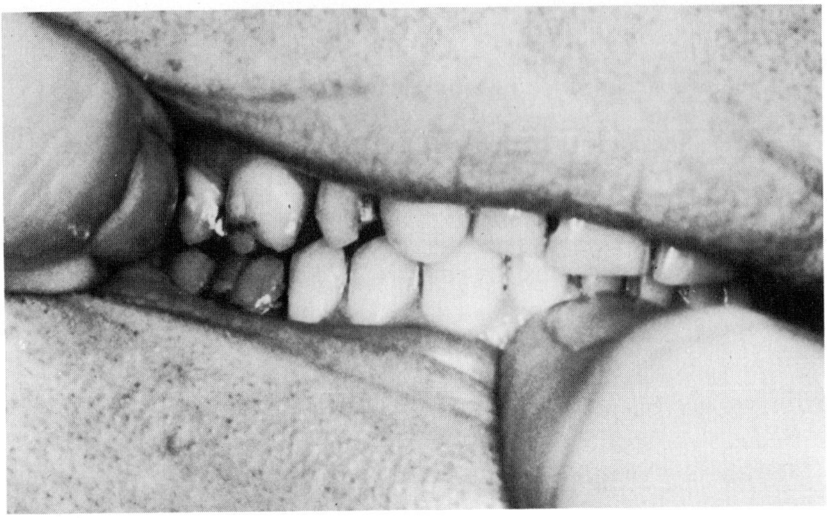

Fig. 29-25. Closure to deflective occlusal contact. Condyles in their terminal hinge position.

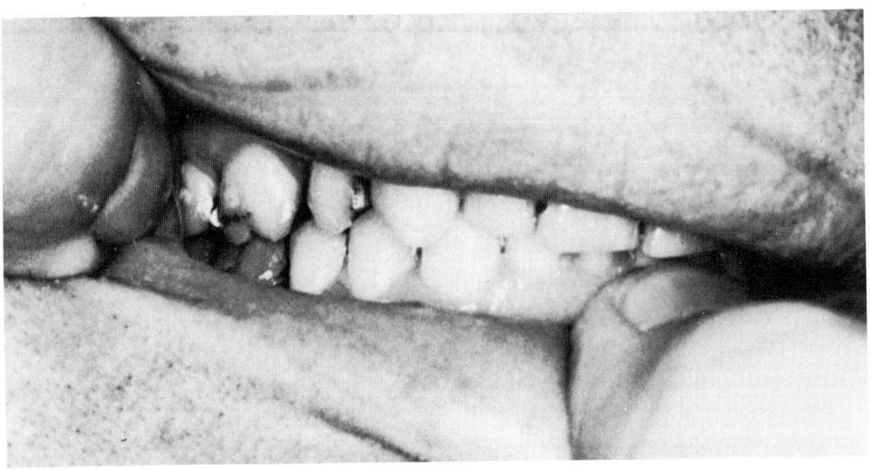

Fig. 29-26. Mandible deflected; condyles translated; maximum intercuspation; eccentric occlusion.

terminal hinge position has often been the cause of confusion and controversy. This record should not be thought of in terms of whether or not it represents a functional relationship. Whether or not a patient occludes in this terminal position during function is not germane to the procedure. This record, and those used to set an instrument, must result in a duplication, in an articulator, of all tooth relationships (within functional range) that occur in the mouth. The tooth contact made in the terminal position is one of these relationships. Whether or not to restore in this position is a diagnostic decision based on at least several factors. Above all, this decision should not be confused with the required record, to transfer and to set an articulator.

PREPARATION OF INTEROCCLUSAL RECORD

Regular pink base-plate wax is used to obtain the recordings. Some advocate the use of other materials. The importance of the materials per se is not paramount, but rather the concept of correct relationships that are to be registered. In preparing for

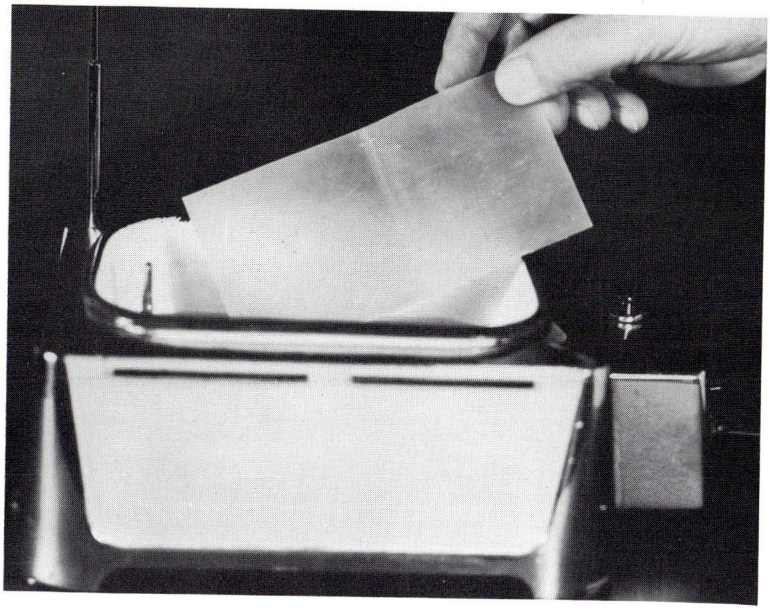

Fig. 29-27. Wax uniformly softened in water bath.

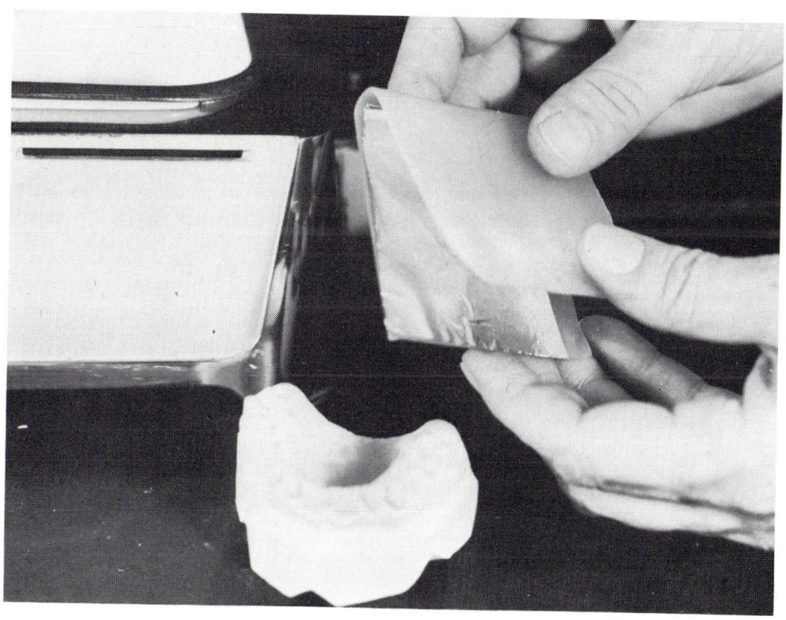

Fig. 29-28. 0.002 inch tin foil interlayed between doubled-over sheet of wax.

a wax record it is essential that "the wax" is uniformly softened, preferably in a water bath (Fig. 29-27). One or more thicknesses of 0.002 inch tin foil should then be interlayed between the doubled over sheet of wax (Fig. 29-28). For the protrusive, also right and left lateral records, two thicknesses of the foil are recommended because of the greater bulk. The purpose of the tin foil is to give reinforcement to the softened wax so that its form can be maintained throughout the various procedures. Collapsing or bending of the prepared checkbite during registration would

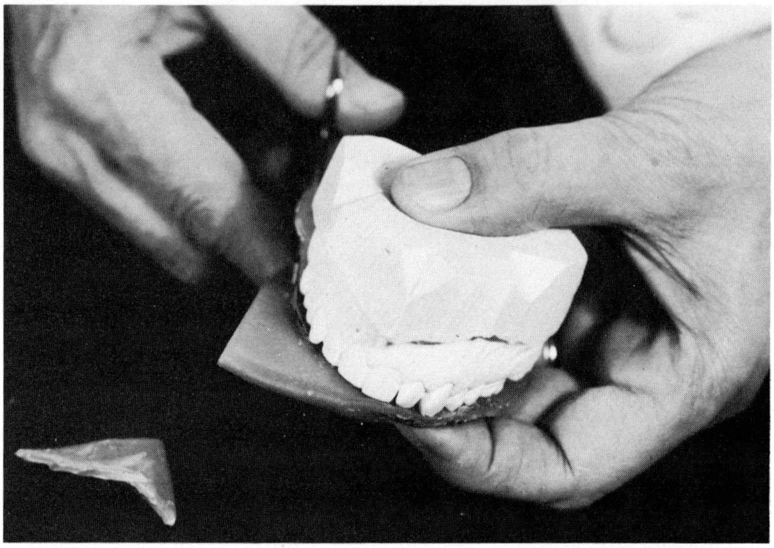

Fig. 29-29. Preliminary fitting and trimming wax record to correct dimension.

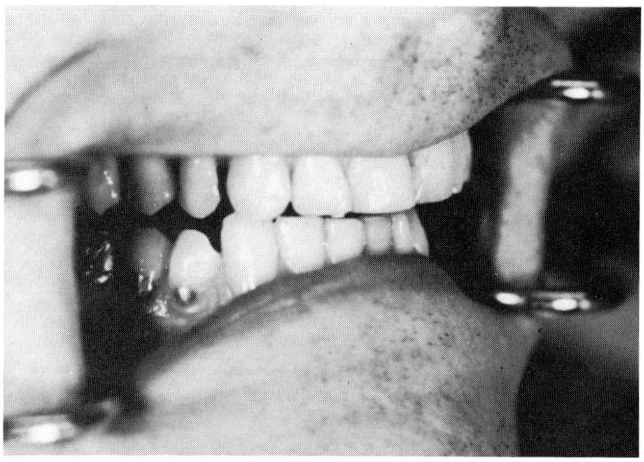

Fig. 29-30. Predetermination of required thickness of wax record.

result in its contacting other thant the occlusal surfaces of the cast. The object is to use the least amount of indexing (Fig. 29-29). The index should involve the minimum of tooth surface, thus avoiding wax contact with soft tissue. To do so would inhibit accurate seating of the record into a stone cast. The tin foil will also discourage actual tooth contact, which is not desirable, especially if deflective occlusal contacts exist.

Although one doubled sheet of baseplate wax is usually adequate in thickness for centric relation registration, this must be determined by observing the interocclusal distance between the teeth in each relationship to be recorded (Fig. 29-30). The instructions are the same for the preparation of all wax records.

Recording centric occlusion

The prepared record is then carried to the mouth. The record is placed on the occlusal surfaces of the maxillary teeth (Fig. 29-31). The patient is "talked" into allowing guided closure, and is told

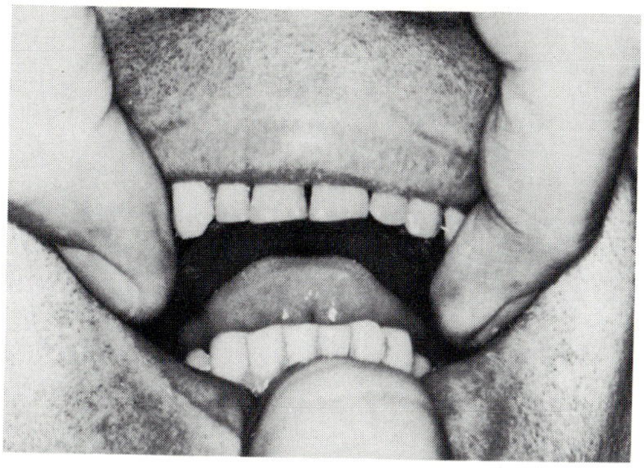

Fig. 29-31. Relating wax record to maxillary arch.

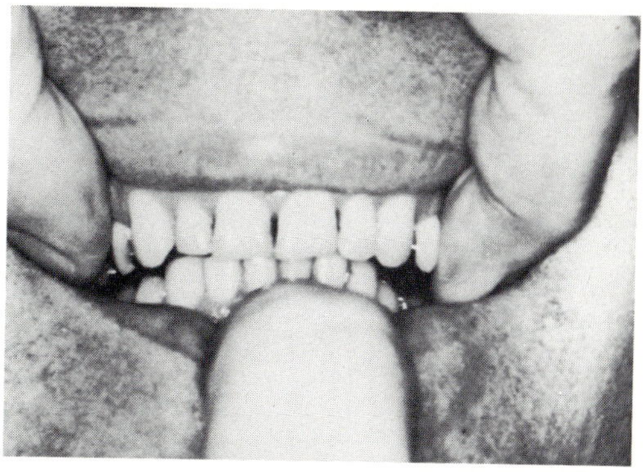

Fig. 29-32. Making centric occlusion record. Index produced; condyles in terminal hinge position.

to tap his teeth on the wax (Fig. 29-32). This is not a relaxed state that would result in an inferior position of the condyle. The patient is doing the opening and closing movement; therefore the muscles are bringing the condyles in a superior as well as a posterior fossa relationship. This exercise should have been carried out several times before introducing the wax record into the mouth so that the patient is familiar with these instructions. He is told *not* to bite into the wax but to gently tap his teeth on the wax. Detailed though it is, this will avoid a common error, particularly if a deflective occlusal contact exists. This procedure will result in obtaining an index of both maxillary and mandibular teeth in the uniformly softened wax. If in doubt as to the terminal position of the condyle, it is well to have the patient fully protrude, and then retrude. With the thumb and forefinger on the patient's chin, the operator can "sense" the condylar position. The record can then be air-chilled, removed, and placed in room-temperature water. All excess should be trimmed (Fig. 29-33). The record is replaced on the teeth as dictated by the index, and is rechecked for accuracy.

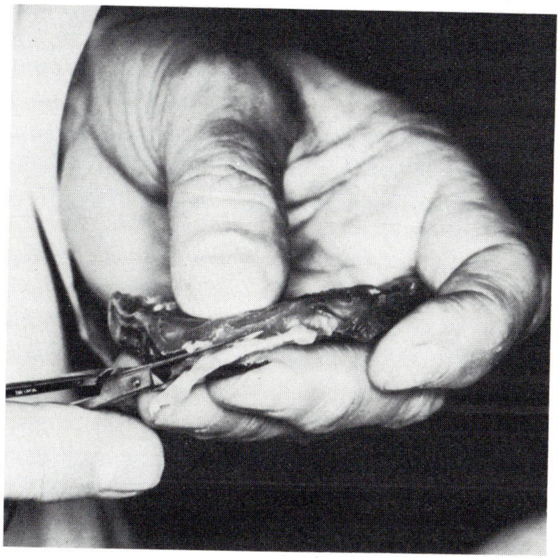

Fig. 29-33. Trimming excess from record prior to rechecking for accuracy.

TRANSFER OF MANDIBULAR CAST IN CENTRIC OCCLUSION

Step 31. The articulator is inverted and the mandibular cast is placed on the maxillary cast without the aid of the centric relation record (Fig. 29-34). Measure and note the "X" dimension.

Step 32. Accurately seat and lute the centric occlusion record between the maxillary and the mandibular casts. Adjust the calibrated angle pin so that the distance "X" is the same as previously determined when the centric relation record was not in place. This procedure compensates for the thickness of the centric record when it is later removed (Fig. 29-35).

Step 33. The lower member of the articulator is swung back slightly and a

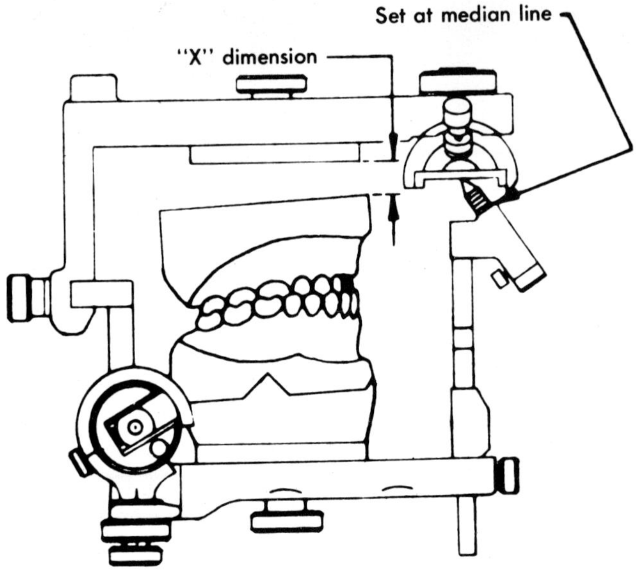

Fig. 29-34. Mandibular cast related to maxillary cast. Condyle element locked in terminal position. Articulator inverted to facilitate mounting and "X" measurement.

mounting medium of suitable consistency is placed on the cast. The lower member is then swung over to embed the mounting plate as well as to bring the incisal pin into contact with the incisal guide, making absolutely certain that the condylar elements are locked against their stops in a centric position (Fig. 29-36).

Step 34. Upon completion of the mounting, the interocclusal record is removed and the calibrated angle pin is raised out of contact with the incisal guide.

RECORDS FOR SETTING THE ARTICULATOR

The transfer procedure at this point has accomplished the positioning of the casts in the correct anatomic relationship to the opening and closing axis of the articulator. The relationship to the axis of the condyles of the patient has been reproduced within the articulator. Both the mandibular and maxillary casts are related to the terminal hinge position, the only position in which the hinge axis is constant to both the maxilla and mandible. The interocclusal record of centric occlusion can be removed, and opening and closing movements and the initial occlusion can be studied. The next step is to make additional records of eccentric records that will be used to set the instrument to reproduce protrusive and lateral movements of the mandible. Granger[2] stated: "The object of an articulator setting is to reproduce the paths of motion of this axis."

Interocclusal record of protrusive relationship

The first interocclusal record used to set the articulator is the record of the protrusive relationship, an end-to-end relationship of the incisors. This record will normally represent the maximum translatory movement of the condyles within normal limits of function. If this record should be one of tooth relationships beyond the normal functional range, it is unlikely that it would be accepted by the articulator. The protrusive record must also be one of wholly protrusive movement, and not one in which a degree of lateral movement is incorporated. Observation of the midline relationship will as-

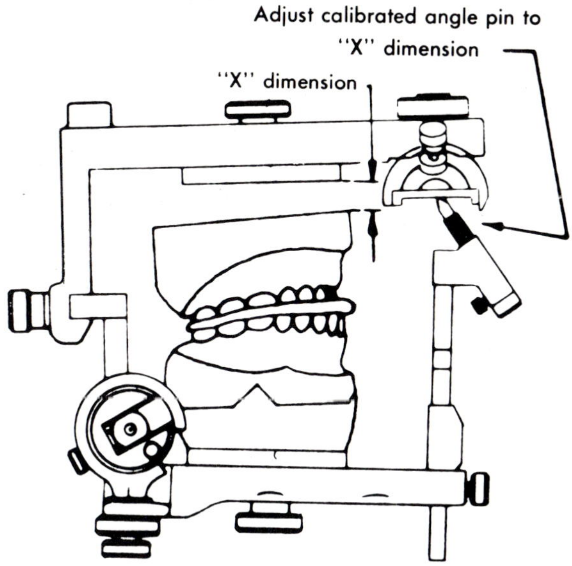

Fig. 29-35. Mandibular and maxillary casts related to interocclusal record of centric occlusion and calibrated angle pin adjusted to previous "X" measurement.

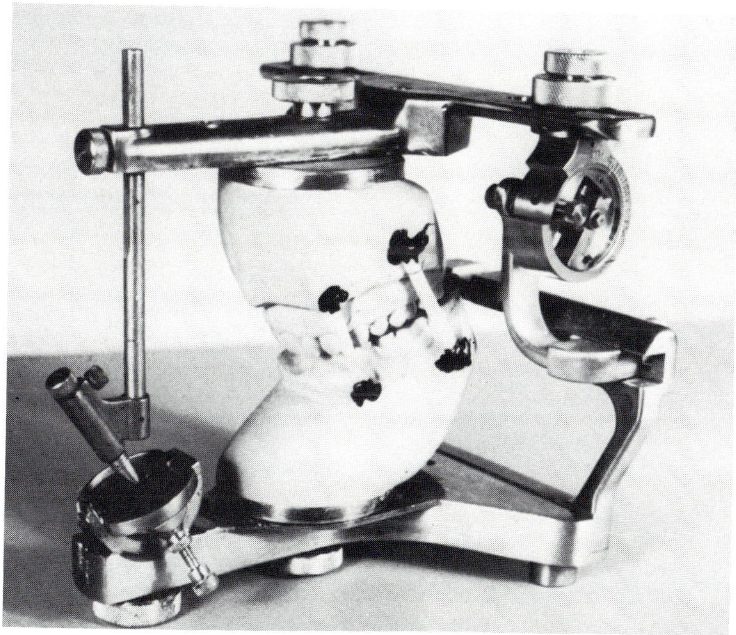

Fig. 29-36. Mandibular and maxillary casts luted together for mounting.

sure accuracy. This record is then used to set the condylar slant.

Setting articulator to protrusive record

Step 35. Centric and protrusive locks of the condylar guidances are released and the lateral of condylar guidances is set at 10 degrees.

Step 36. The maxillary and mandibular casts, with the protrusive record accurately interposed, are related. Some operators prefer to lute them together.

Step 37. The upper member is engaged into the split cast (Fig. 29-37), and the right, then left, protrusive condylar guidances are adjusted until an absolute readaption to the cast occurs (Fig. 29-38). Without deforming the recording surface of the protrusive record, one hand may rest lightly upon the upper member of the instrument, directly over the maxillary cast, in producing a sense of feel during the adjustment.

Step 38. Protrusive adjustments are locked to retain this position. The protrusive record is then removed.

Right and left lateral interocclusal records

An interocclusal record is prepared for recording the lateral relationship. The approximate thickness of wax required to produce an index is estimated by observing the interocclusal distance in the lateral relationship.

The right and left lateral relationships

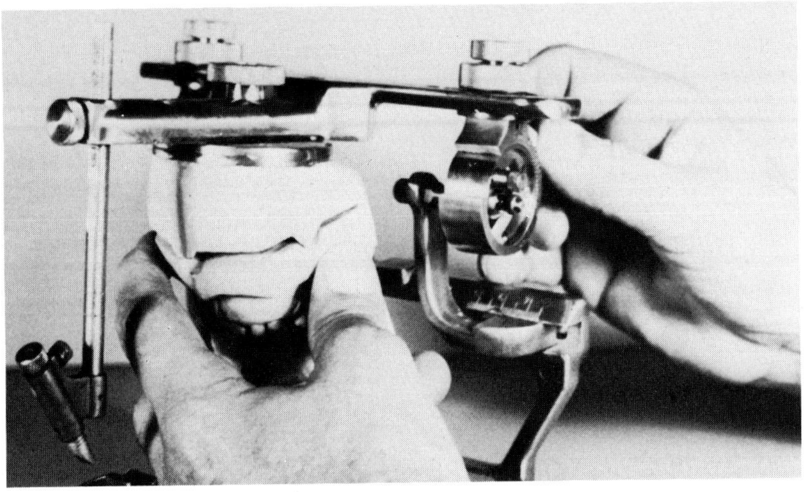

Fig. 29-37. Setting of condylar slant to protrusive record, split-cast procedure.

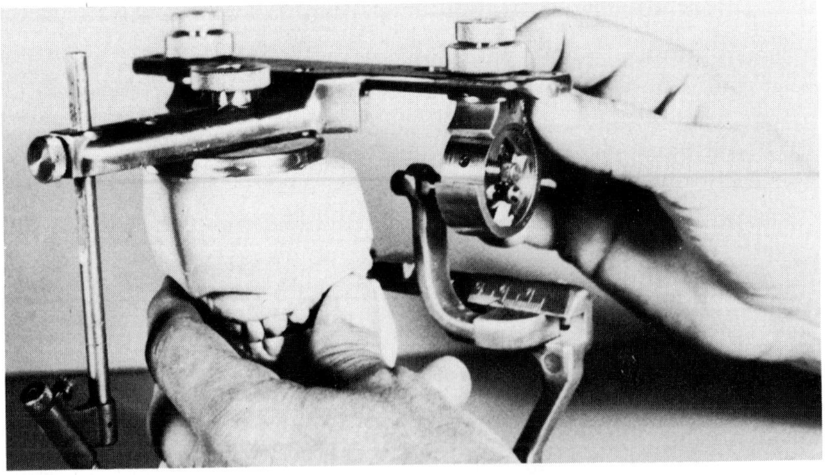

Fig. 29-38. Completion of setting to protrusive record; absolute readaptation assures accuracy.

that must be recorded should represent the maximum amount of condylar movement within the functional range. This position is the end-to-end relationship of the opposing cuspids or a comparable position if the cuspids are missing or malpositioned. This relationship should also be one of lateral movement only and should not contain any protrusive or translatory movement of the working condyle. If a protrusive movement of the working condyle is incorporated into the lateral record, the working condyle will not remain in its terminal position when setting the instrument. If this occurs, a new lateral record should be made. It is recommended that the patient practice, with the operator's guidance, placing the teeth in this lateral position prior to introducing the wax record. Even then the operator will note that he must carefully guide the patient to this position. To determine the accuracy, a perpendicular line drawn on the labial surface of the maxillary and mandibular cuspid may help (Fig. 29-39). One can then determine, with the record in position, whether or not this line is still continuous and therefore not incorporating a protrusive movement. Determination is also made that the recorded relationship is not beyond the functional range. This is emphasized because of the fact that the condyles are capable of assuming positions that a mechanical instrument cannot reproduce. The uniformly softened record is then carried to the mouth in the same manner as described for the protrusive record and the two lateral records (right and left) are made.

This record will have recorded the movement of the axis of the condyle. After setting of the instrument we are therefore able to reproduce the path of motion of this axis. One may speak of this move-

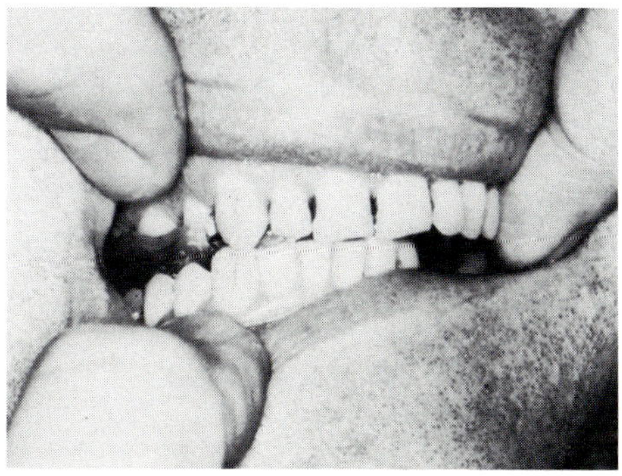

Fig. 29-39. Making interocclusal record of right lateral relationship.

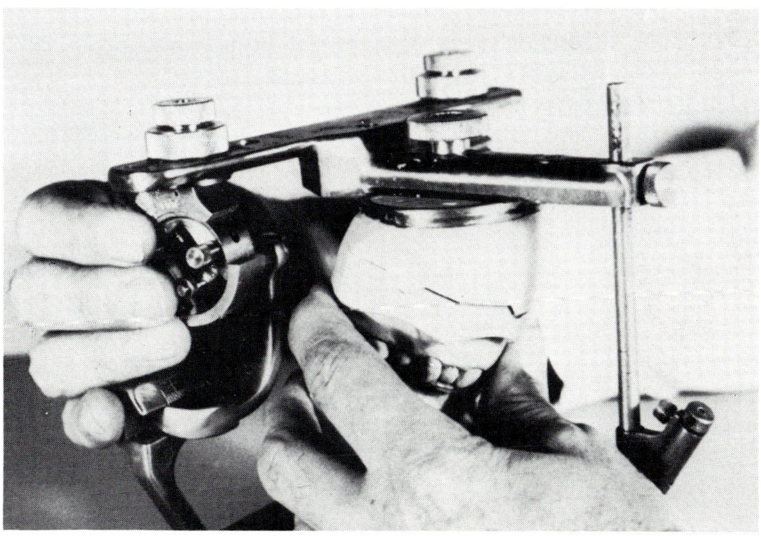

Fig. 29-40. Setting condylar element to lateral record.

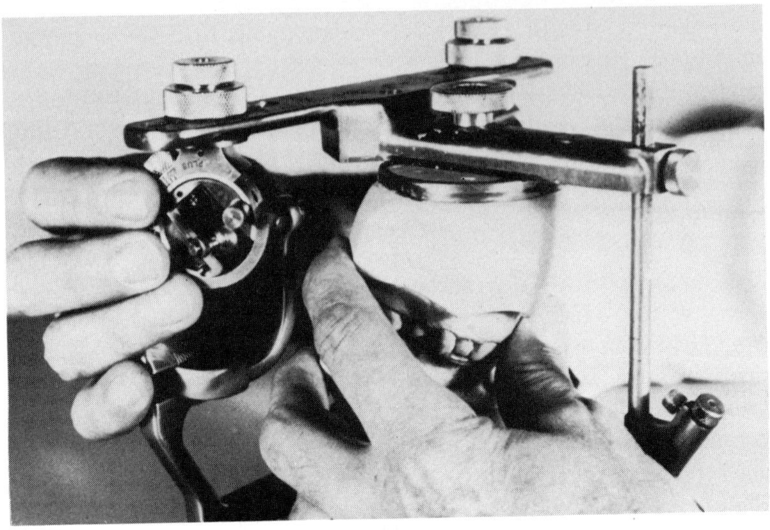

Fig. 29-41. Setting to lateral record complete; absolute readaptation required to assure accuracy.

ment as a "lateral movement" or a "Bennett movement." As Granger[2] has stated: "The term condyle path refers to the protrusive paths of the menisci on the fossae. Bennett movement refers to the lateral paths of the menisci in lateral excursions of the mandible." McCollum[1] stated: "The influence of the Bennett path on cusps of teeth is an intricate and most interesting study. Primarily the Bennett movement influences the position of the cusps in their mesial-distal relationship, due to the fact that a jaw without Bennett movement moves laterally on a shorter radius than one with some or considerable side-shift."

Each lateral record is then used to set the appropriate condylar element. The following instructions must be rigidly adhered to.

Right lateral relation record

Step 39. The right lateral record is accurately seated between the maxillary and mandibular casts.

Step 40. Loosen the thumbnut for lateral adjustment on the balancing side, left of articulator.

Step 41. The components of the mount are brought into light contact (Fig. 29-40) and the left guidance is slowly rotated, increasing the angle of lateral, until the split cast falls into place (Fig. 29-41). In setting to the right and left lateral record a slight change in the protrusive setting may be required to accurately relate the two split-cast components of the mounting. When this is observed, slightly counter-rotate the guidance to contact the condylar element with the end shoulder of condylar shaft and tighten the thumbnut, retaining this lateral adjustment (Fig. 29-42). Remove the lateral record.

Left lateral relation record

Step 42. The left lateral record is accurately seated between the maxillary and mandibular casts.

Step 43. Loosen the thumbnut for lateral adjustment on the balancing side, right of articulator.

Step 44. The split casts are brought into light contact and the right guidance is slowly rotated, increasing the angle of lateral, until the split cast falls into place. When this is observed, slightly counter-rotate the guidance to contact the condylar element with the end shoulder of condylar

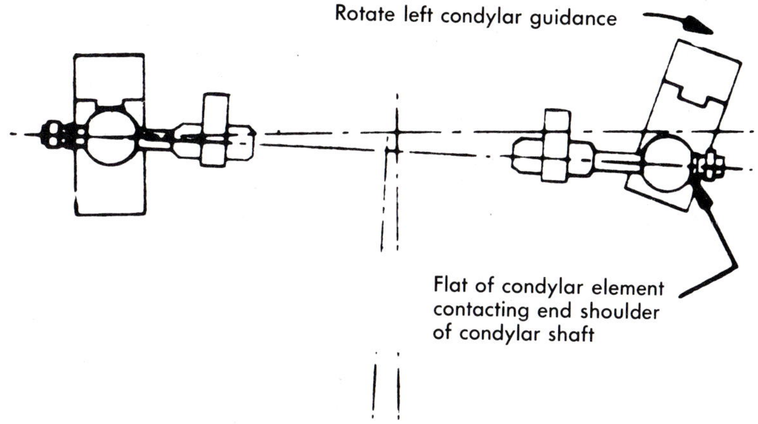

Fig. 29-42. Right lateral relation with flats of condylar element contacting end shoulder of condylar shaft on balancing side.

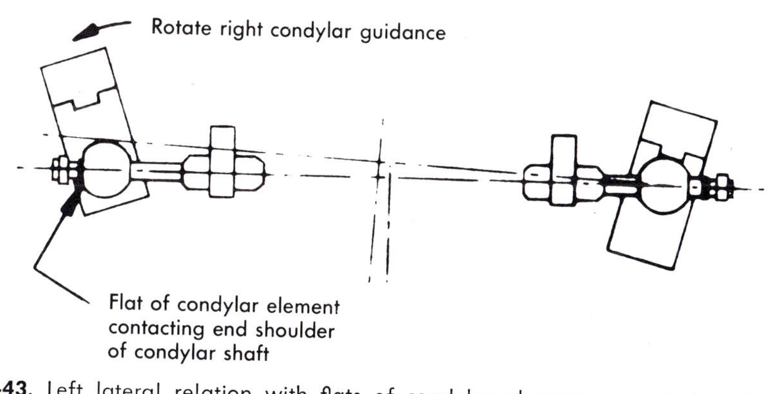

Fig. 29-43. Left lateral relation with flats of condylar element contacting end shoulder of condylar shaft on balancing side.

shaft and tighten the thumbnut (Fig. 29-43). Remove the lateral record.

ADJUSTMENT OF INCISAL GUIDE

Step 45. The components of the split cast mounting are now permanently luted together.

Step 46. With the casts in occlusion, the calibrated angle pin is lowered into contact with the incisal guide and the lockscrew is tightened. If insufficient teeth are present to maintain a previously determined vertical dimension, the angle pin is turned back to the median scribed line at which it had originally been set.

Step 47. The locknut of the incisal guide is loosened, and the incisors are brought into edge-to-edge contact. The incisal

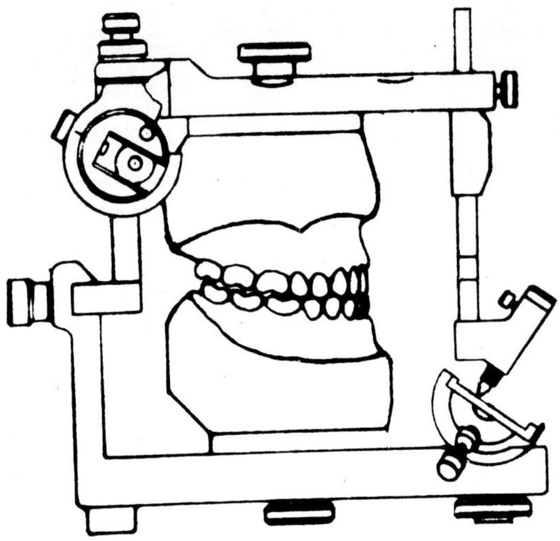

Fig. 29-44. Teeth in protrusive relationship. Incisal guide pin (on left) tilted to make contact with incisal pin.

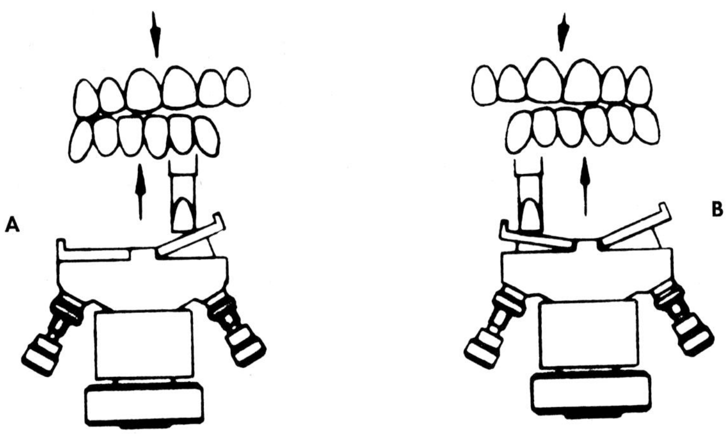

Fig. 29-45. A, Mandible in right lateral relationship; wing of guide is raised to contact pin. **B,** Mandible in left lateral relationship; wing of guide is raised to contact pin.

guide is then tilted anteroposteriorly to make contact with the end of the incisal pin and the locknut is tightened to maintain this position (Fig. 29-44).

Step 48. The casts are now brought into a right lateral excursion and the lateral wing of the incisal guide is raised to contact the edge of the incisal pin and locked (Fig. 29-45, *A*).

Step 49. The casts are then brought into a left lateral excursion and the lateral wing is raised to contact the edge of the incisal pin and also locked (Fig. 29-45, *B*).

Step 50. Record all of the settings for future reference—intercondylar, protrusive, lateral, and incisal guidance.

CHECKING THE ACCURACY OF THE TRANSFER

Previous instructions have described the notching of the maxillary cast and the lubrication of this cast prior to mounting as a part of the "split cast" procedure. Several factors must be emphasized to assure accuracy in the setting of the instrument. After separating the maxillary cast from the upper member of the articulator, the maxillary cast is then related to the mandibular cast as dictated by each of the interocclusal records. This relationship must be carefully maintained while setting the instrument to each record. Do not allow the maxillary cast to be displaced from the index of the interocclusal record. The component of the maxillary mounting attached to the upper member of the articulator is then closed into approximation with the maxillary cast. The appropriate settings, or articulator adjustments, should result in complete readaptation of the split cast components. The resulting relationship should be as precise as before separation. If, in the attempt to set the instrument, the two component parts do not readapt, there is an error in the transfer procedure. Too many have assumed that a small discrepancy is of little importance. This, of course, is not true. The success of this procedure is dependent upon adherence to rigid requirements. Failure to readapt as described suggests an error in the record of centric occlusion (or centric relationship). The experienced operator is less likely to have an error in the face bow transfer of the maxillary cast or in the protrusive or lateral records.

Anatomic and physiologic principles have been applied to the clinical procedure of transfer of casts to an articulator. This procedure satisfies both diagnostic and treatment needs. The instruments selected meet all the requirements to produce the successful clinical result.

SELECTED REFERENCES

1. McCollum, B. B.: Considering the mouth as a functioning unit as a basis of a dental diagnosis; a research report, South Pasadena, California, 1955, Scientific Press.
2. Granger, E. R.: Functional relations of the stomatognathic system, J.A.D.A. **48**(6): 638, 1954.
3. Schuyler, C. H.: Factors of occlusion applicable to restorative dentistry, J. Prosth. Dent. **3**:772, 1953.
4. Moulton, G. H.: The importance of centric occlusion in diagnosis and treatment planning, J. Prosth. Dent. **10**:921, 1960.

GENERAL REFERENCES

Douglas, J. R., and others: "Open rest," a new concept in the selection of the vertical dimension of occlusion, J. Prosth. Dent. **15**:850, 1965.

Gonzalez, J. B., and Kingery, R. H.: Evaluation of planes of reference for orienting maxillary casts on articulators, J.A.D.A. **76**(2):329, 1968.

Graf, H., and Zander, H. A.: Occlusal tooth contacts and electromyography during mastication and swallowing, I.A.D.R. Preprinted Abstracts, No. 167, 1963.

Hickey, J. C., Lundeen, H. C., and Bohannan, H. M.: A new articulator for use in teaching and general dentistry, J. Prosth. Dent. **18**: 425, 1967.

Kawamura, Y., Kato, I., and Takata, M.: Jaw-closing muscle activities with the mandible in rest position, J. Dent. Res. **46**:1356, 1967.

Knap, F. J., and Ziebert, G. J.: Checkbite technique in major oral reconstruction, J. Prosth. Dent. **21**:458-465, 1969.

Mazur, B.: Construction of plastic registration trays, J. Prosth. Dent. **16**(5):904, 1966.

Osborne, J.: Mandibular-maxillary relationships in oral rehabilitation, Int. Dent. J. **16**:398-405, 1966.

Saizan, P.: Muscle mechanisms in centric relation, Rev. Asoc. Odont. Argent. **55**(7):274, 1967.

Shanahan, T. E., and others: Mandibular and articulator movements; physiologic and mechanical concepts of occlusion, J. Prosth. Dent. **16**: 62-72, 1966.

Teteruck, W. R., and Lundeen, H. C.: The accuracy of an ear face-bow, J. Prosth. Dent. **16**:1039-1046, 1966.

Vierheller, P. G.: A functional method for establishing vertical and tentative centric maxillomandibular relations, J. Prosth. Dent. **19**: 587, 1968.

Weiner, M. H.: The physiologic bite in oral reconstruction, Dent. Dig. **71**:540, 1965.

Wormley, J. H., and Brudvik, J. S.: A simplified procedure for remounting dentures, J. Prosth. Dent. **16**:4, 1966.

Chapter 30

Construction of pontics for fixed partial dentures: indications, types, and materials

A pontic is defined as the suspended member of a fixed partial denture or bridge, replacing the lost natural tooth, restoring its function, and usually occupying the space of the missing natural tooth. The pontic is connected to the bridge retainers, which are attached to the remaining natural teeth. This union of the pontic and the retainer may be accomplished by means of a rigid connection, such as a soldered joint, or by means of a nonrigid, flexible union, such as the key and keyway used in the broken-stress type of bridge construction.

REQUIREMENTS OF A PONTIC

In order to fulfill its requirements satisfactorily, a pontic must (1) restore the function of the tooth it replaces, (2) ensure its sanitation, (3) meet the demands of esthetics and comfort, and, finally, (4) be biologically acceptable to the tissues.[1]

TYPES OF PONTICS

Older types

The type of pontic used frequently in the older types of fixed bridge prosthesis caused much harm to the tissues and was largely responsible for bringing about the condemnation of the fixed type of partial denture prosthesis. The older type of bridge construction used a short pin facing whose ridge lap was ground to the labial or buccal contour of the ridge, leaving a pronounced shelf in the linguogingival region; this served as a trap for the accumulation of food and other debris, which was difficult to remove even with a toothbrush (Fig. 30-1). The fermentation of this material resulted in the inflammation of the gum tissues and often in the loss of the entire bridge. These facings, after being ground, were left unglazed, with sharp edges and rough surfaces that were porous and irritating to the tissues. This type of facing was usually backed with 24-carat gold plate and soldered without any or with only partial regard to the proper anatomy of the tooth.

The renaissance of fixed partial dentures had its beginning when the new type of pontic came into existence. In the new type the gingival shelf on the lingual surface is eliminated; the contour is restored in highly glazed porcelain, which usually contacts the mucosa of the ridge and eliminates all food pockets.

Modern types

While it is possible to construct pontics entirely of metal or entirely of porcelain, as in complete porcelain bridges, the type of pontic most generally used today is the combination type. This has the labial, buccal, and gingival portions constructed of porcelain, while the lingual or the occlusal section is made of gold. The combination type of pontic also employs acrylic resins with gold, but it is less desirable than porcelain.

Combination type. The combination type of pontic may have one of three shapes: the conical, the spheroidal, or the ridge lap. These will be discussed separately when the indications and technical steps in their construction are considered.

Among the requisites for a satisfactory pontic, none is more important than the biologic one.

A major contributing cause to the failure of the older types of fixed bridges is found in the fact that, whenever the lingual or the occlusal surface was restored entirely with solder, it was difficult to develop its anatomy in such form as to cause the food during mastication to sweep over the palatal and lingual surfaces without impinging directly upon the gum tissue; lack of such contour caused inflammatory reactions. In the modern types of bridge construction where the correct contours are developed, the food contacts the mucosa in areas where it acts as a massaging and stimulating agent to the tissues.

TISSUE RESPONSE

Where a correct relationship of the contour of the pontic to the gingival ridge exists, the tissues respond so favorably that in many instances it has been observed that the mucosa in contact with the gingival portion of the pontic appears to be a normal free gingiva around the periphery of the pontic. This is one of the most striking evidences of the response of tissues to functional stimulation. Such a favorable reaction does not occur, however, if the pontic is not properly glazed, if it lacks the correct physiologic contact with the mucosa, or if it is improperly contoured.

On the other hand, if the porcelain in contact with the mucosa of the ridge is rough, unglazed, and improperly adapted,

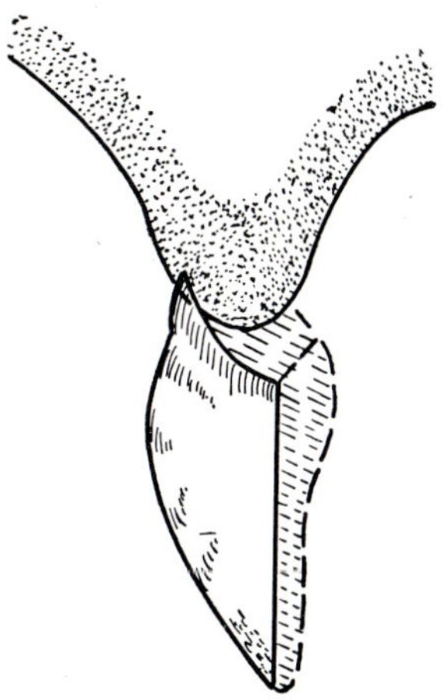

Fig. 30-1. Shelf created at gingival area when facing of pontic is ground as shown above; dotted line represents outline of correct lingual contour.

an unfavorable tissue reaction occurs that very frequently necessitates the removal of the bridge.

So favorably does the mucosa respond to glazed porcelain that it is possible to insert a pontic into an alveolar socket immediately after the extraction of the tooth and obtain a perfect healing of the tissues that touch the glazed porcelain. The mechanical details of constructing this type of pontic are considered later in the chapter, but it is well at this time to consider the biologic reaction of the tissues to the conical, root extension type of pontic.

Biologic reactions to porcelain root extension pontics

Dewey and Zugsmith,[2] in reporting their experimental study of tissue reactions about porcelain roots for fixed bridgework, made some interesting observations.

They pointed out that properly glazed porcelain is practically nonirritating to the soft tissues and that it is, therefore, tissuephile. Because the porcelain tip, which extends partway into the socket, restores to a certain degree the natural environment of the region, their study was directed to learn what tissue reactions actually occurred about the porcelain root extension implanted into the socket; they were particularly interested in verifying the presence or absence of an epithelial covering of the fundus in the ridge next to the porcelain root extension. Their study indicated that, while the inherent tendency of epithelium is to cover free surfaces, it will also extend from the margins of wounds and empty sockets into which porcelain roots have been placed and cover the entire surfaces with epithelium. It was shown that, following extraction, wounds are completely covered with a thin layer of epithelial cells in about 1 week and that after 2 weeks the granulation tissue filling the socket is completely covered with epithelium. This epithelization, they reported, starts as early as 3 days following extraction, and at the end of 3 weeks the epithelial covering resembles a normal epithelial lining.

The report of Dewey and Zugsmith showed further that highly glazed porcelain is apparently nonirritating since the extension of a glazed porcelain pontic does not inhibit the formation of an epithelial lining. They pointed out that such a socket around a porcelain tip pontic is to all intents and purposes a depression on the surface of the mucosa having an epithelial covering continuous with that of the gingiva and developing a local bacterial immunity comparable to that in other parts of the mouth. A porcelain root, since it does not enter into the reactions of the surrounding tissues, is an isolated, nonirritating body that is tolerated by the mucosa.

In using this type of pontic, however, care must be taken not to extend the length of the tip more than one-fourth to one-fifth the depth of the alveolar fundus; also, it must not contact the surrounding alveolar bone.

Changes occurring in ridge

One other observation of biologic significance involves the changes that occur in the normal ridge after the extraction of a tooth. When a tooth is extracted, there is always an accompanying loss of ridge dimensions in that area. This reduction in dimensions usually occurs labiolingually or buccolingually, in addition to a vertical lowering of the ridge. As explained in Chapter 6, the labial and buccal bony processes of the upper arches resorb to a greater extent than the lingual alveolar processes; whereas, in the lower arch there is a more uniform resorption of both the labial and the lingual alveolar plates of bone. This biologic phenomenon has a very practical application in the design of the pontic and establishment of its correct relationship to the ridge; this relationship will be shown later.

Types of mucosa

One other item of clinical significance is the fact that the mucosa covering the ridge is of two types: the one which covers the ridge proper is usually a firm, dense, and immobile type, whereas the other covers the base of the ridge and is a softer and more movable type of tissue. When constructing pontics, this fact should be kept in mind, since that part of the pontic coming in permanent contact with the mucosa is never extended into the region of the movable tissue.

FINISH AND CONTOUR OF PONTICS

If a porcelain pontic is contoured and glazed so that its surface is smooth and impervious to fluids or bacterial infiltration, it will usually be kept clean automatically by the excursion of food; this may be assisted by the use of the toothbrush and ligatures. If the pontic is properly contoured and correctly related to the ridge, there should be no food locks present in the gingival region, either on its buccal or lingual surfaces, to cause food or debris to collect and to produce an unhygienic condition.

To facilitate the hygienic maintenance of the pontics, proper construction requires that the lingual embrasures be widened by narrowing the pontic mesiodistally in its lingual half. This gives the scouring action of the food and the cleaning of the toothbrush an opportunity to keep the surfaces of the pontic in a hygienic condition and the contiguous mucosa in a state of health.

WIDTH OF PORCELAIN FACING

Since the widest part of the pontic mesiodistally is through the gold contact areas and since the pontic is attached to the retainer by means of connectors at these points, the porcelain facing, of necessity, is slightly narrower than the maximum mesiodistal width of the edentulous space. Therefore, should it become necessary to narrow the facing mesiodistally, this is done as described by Clark[3] (Fig. 30-2). This is accomplished by grinding the facing from the buccal surface toward the

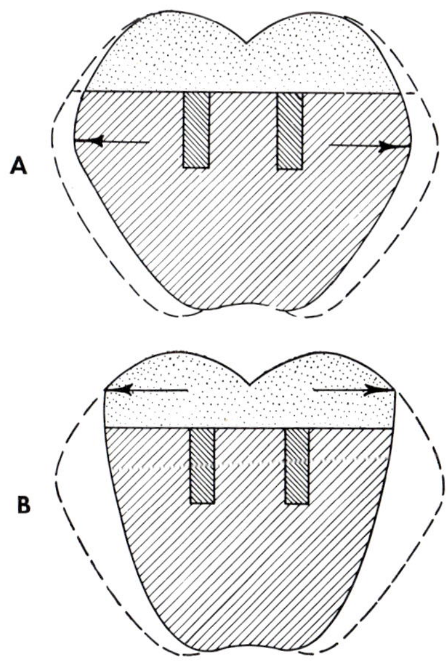

Fig. 30-2. Method used to narrow facing. **A,** Correct. **B,** Incorrect. (From Clark, E. B.: D. Cosmos **64:**809, 1922.)

mesial or distal proximal margins. If the porcelain facing is narrowed by cutting flat surfaces on the mesial and distal areas, the widest part of the pontic will be in porcelain, making it impossible to obtain a correctly soldered union between the pontic and the retainer.

LENGTH OF FACING

Where, for example, a facing for a lower pontic has been ground to the proper occlusal relationship, but it is necessary to shorten it occlusogingivally, this is done also by grinding the buccal surface from the occlusal end of the facing. In this manner the occlusal edge of the facing is kept in the same vertical plane, but is dropped to a lower level (Fig. 30-3). If, on the other hand, the tooth is shortened occlusogingivally by cutting a longer bevel, as shown in Fig. 30-4, the occlusal edge of the facing is carried buccally, resulting in malocclusion and a traumatization of the opposing teeth. (Also see Figs. 30-5 and 30-6.)

BUCCOLINGUAL WIDTH

Because an upper ridge shrinks buccolingually or labiolingually during the healing process following extraction, it is necessary that the pontic also be made narrower in this dimension in order to avoid creating food pockets at the point where the pontic and ridge meet. Failure to do so will create an unhygienic condition in this region.

ABNORMAL CONDITIONS

Where the edentulous space is wider or narrower than the normal, or where the vertical distance exceeds the normal height, the ideas discussed by Blancheri in Chapter 25 can be employed to good advantage.

EMBRASURES

In addition to the wide lingual embrasures so necessary for the hygiene of a fixed partial denture, it is also recom-

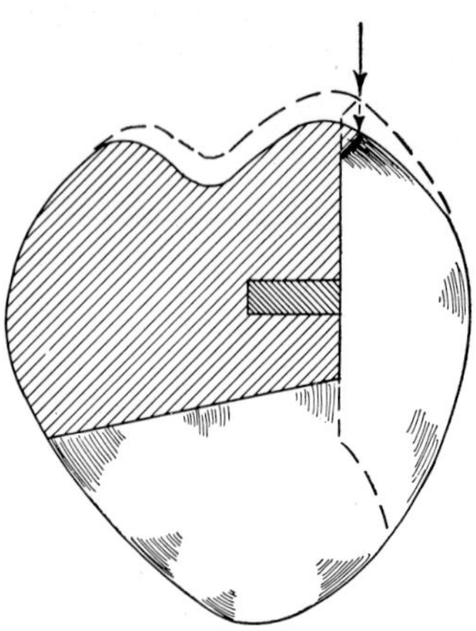

Fig. 30-3

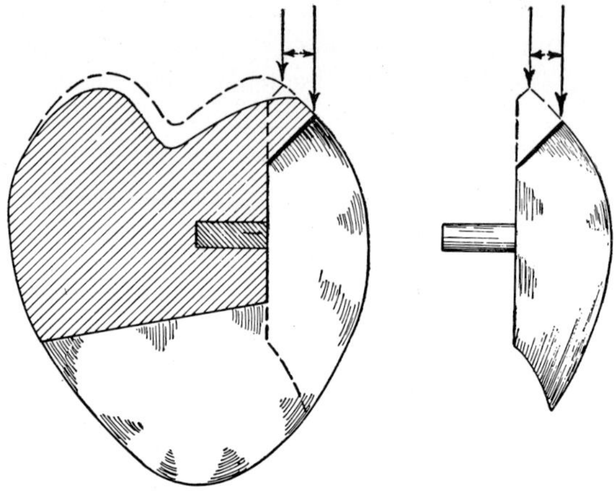

Fig. 30-4

Fig. 30-3. Correct method used to shorten facing occlusogingivally. (From Clark, E. B.: D. Cosmos **64:**809, 1922.)
Fig. 30-4. Incorrect method used to shorten facing occlusogingivally. (From Clark, E. B.: D. Cosmos **64:**809, 1922.)

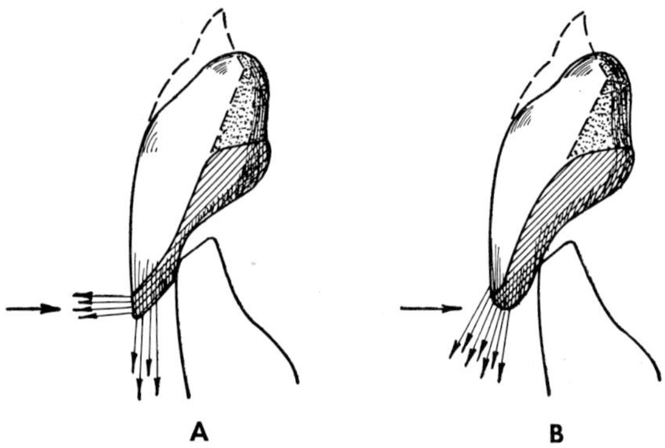

Fig. 30-5

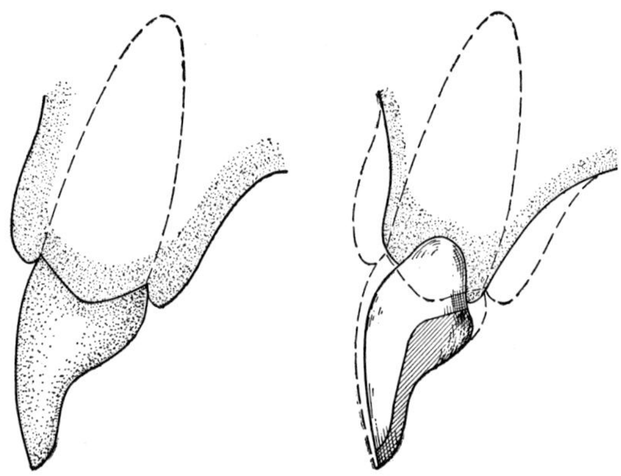

Fig. 30-6

Fig. 30-5. Methods of beveling incisal edge. **A,** Incorrect. **B,** Correct. (After D. Smith.)
Fig. 30-6. Root extension type of pontic used in immediate replacement type of bridge. (After D. Smith.)

mended that, where it does not interfere with the esthetic qualities, there the interproximal or the interdental spaces in the gingival region should be widened to facilitate the dislodgment of food particles. The closer one approaches the conical shape in this portion of the pontic, the more nearly is the ideal developed from the hygienic standpoint. Conical-shaped tips are especially indicated in the lower pontics, since the gingival portion is not usually visible. In the upper, and particularly in the anterior, region, due to esthetic demands, the opening of the interdental spaces to any great extent is limited.

The older types of fixed bridges could not be kept in a hygienic condition, because the porcelain surfaces in contact with or contiguous to the mucosa were ground and left unglazed. It should be a cardinal rule that, whenever ground porcelain comes in permanent contact with the mucosa, it should always be glazed before the restoration is permanently cemented.

SHAPE OF GINGIVAL AREA

One other factor of importance from the hygienic standpoint is the shape of the pontic surface that comes in contact with the ridge. As a rule this surface should always be convex, rather than concave or saddle shaped (Figs. 30-7 and 30-8). This is particularly important in the upper posterior regions where the ridges are relatively wide buccolingually. As will be shown in the discussion relating to the construction of a ridge lap or a spheroidal type of pontic for posterior teeth, all porcelain surfaces permanently contacting the mucosa are made spheroidal or convex.

ADVANTAGES OF PORCELAIN

Although the biologic and hygienic requirements of a pontic are important, the esthetic factors frequently assume major proportions, particularly in the anterior region of the mouth. Because of esthetic considerations, pontics are never constructed entirely of metal in the anterior part of the mouth and rarely are they so made in the posterior. Porcelain, alone or combined with gold on the lingual or the occlusal surfaces, is the material primarily used in visible pontics. It is the material of choice not only because it enables one to restore the proper contour and color of the missing teeth, but also because it reproduces the texture of the remaining teeth. Although it is important to reproduce the correct color, it is equally important to have the correct typal form and outline in order that the restoration may harmonize with the remaining natural teeth.

LENGTH OF PONTIC

Every precaution should be taken during the extraction of those teeth which are to be replaced with bridges in order that the alveolar process and the investing soft tissues are not unduly traumatized or injured, since this causes an abnormal shrinkage and resorption of the residual ridge. Because the ridge does shrink, both

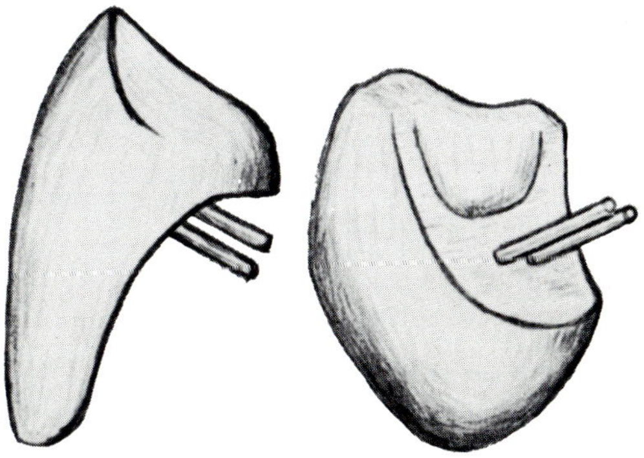

Fig. 30-7. Typical saddle and avoid types of long-pin Harmony facings. (Courtesy D. Smith.)

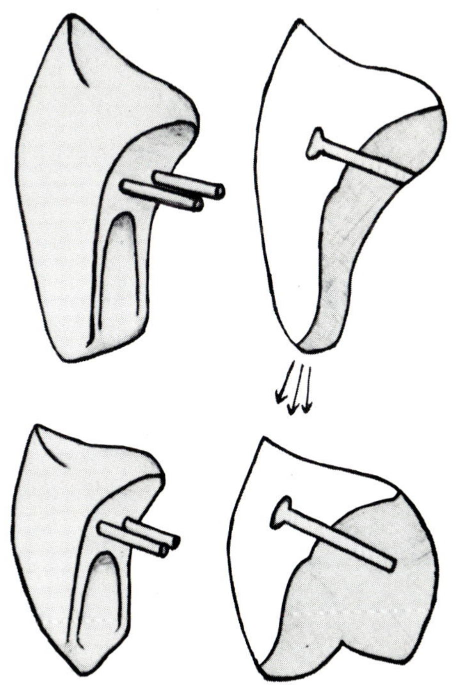

Fig. 30-8. Typical Harmony long-pin facing pontics for anterior and bicuspid restorations. Note compound arch form of backings made possible by integral hollow grinding of facings, which provides adequate metal protection for porcelain. (Courtesy D. Smith.)

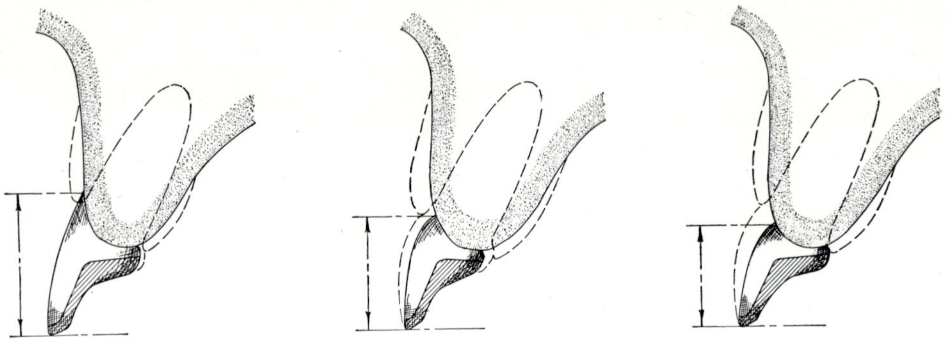

Fig. 30-9. Correct and incorrect lengths of facing as determined by amount of gingival depression. (From Smith, D. E., and Potter, H. R.: D. Digest **43:**16, 1937.)

in a horizontal and a vertical plane, it is essential that the correct length of the pontic be established so that its gingival outline will correspond to a harmonious relationship with the adjacent teeth. This is usually accomplished by depressing the neck of the pontic and changing the greatest convexity of the tooth from the gingival third region to the middle third of the labial surface (Fig. 30-9, *B*).

HIGH LIP LINE AND PONTICS

In those instances where for esthetic reasons a high lip line requires the full mesiodistal width of the pontic, it is so shaped that lingually, to the contact area, it is narrowed very definitely, creating wide lingual embrasures; this harmonizes the esthetic with the hygienic requirements of the pontic. Occasionally, the ridge is resorbed to such an extend that it is impossible to relate the gingival outline of the pontic to it in a way that harmonizes with the neighboring teeth; in such circumstances it is suggested that the correct position of the gingival line be established on the labial surface of the facing and that portion of the pontic which extends rootwise beyond this gingival line be restored in pink porcelain. This procedure usually results in partial success only; it is much better to blend the pink porcelain into the upper part of the pontic without creating a definite, sharp gingival line. The other recourse is the method suggested by Blancheri. (See Fig. 25-12.)

STAINING AND MODIFYING PONTICS

The esthetic factors are sometimes improved by the use of stains or by placing irregular markings on the facing. Very frequently, and this is especially true in the lower anterior teeth, the incisal edge of a pontic is also built up with fused porcelain, which may be modified further by the application of stained porcelain along the incisal edge (Fig. 30-37, *B*). Similarly, wide teeth may be made to appear narrower by convexing their labial surfaces mesiodistally and by rounding the distal or sometimes the mesial angles of the incisal edge. On the other hand, a narrow tooth may be made to appear wider by flattening the labial surface, and extending the incisal edge in a straight line to its full mesiodistal width.

TREATMENT OF INCISAL EDGE

The unnecessary display of gold along the incisal or the occlusal edge of a pontic is one of the most frequent offenders against esthetic appearance. Although it is desirable to have the incisal or the occlusal edges protected by gold to prevent the fracture of the facing, this incisal extension of gold may be made effective, yet invisible, if it is so beveled that it does not reflect the light back in a labial direction (Fig. 30-5: *A*, incorrect; *B*, correct).

As a general rule, it is found that a pontic of a shade slightly darker than the natural teeth is less noticeable than one of a lighter color. Similarly, a tooth that is slightly wider than the natural teeth is less noticeable than one that appears narrower. Much of the artificiality that so frequently proclaims a fixed restoration may be eliminated if the facings are aligned to simulate the natural irregularities which are found in the patient's dentition. All these considerations are especially important from the esthetic standpoint in the anterior region of the mouth.

RESTORING OCCLUSION

Another requirement of an acceptable pontic is one of mechanics of occlusion and of construction. Any pontic to be satisfactory should restore the occlusion characteristic of the natural dentition. It is true that in some instances because of the shifting and rearrangement of the opposing teeth, it may be impossible to build the restoration according to the ideal plan, yet an effort should be made to restore the relationships as near the ideal as the existing conditions permit. A pontic should function properly not only in centric occlusion, but also in the protrusive and the right and left lateral relationships of the mandible. In adjusting these relationships to the opposing teeth, it is essential that the cusps and their inclined surfaces be formed to harmonize with the characteristic shape of the tooth and arch involved in the restoration. Many bridges have failed because they lacked this fundamental requirement. In order to reduce the amount of force transmitted to the abutment teeth, it is advisable generally to narrow the occlusal surface of the pontic mesiodistally in its lingual one-half. In addition to this, supplementary grooves are placed which open lingually through the marginal ridges; natural buccal and lingual grooves are deepened in order to permit the escape of food during the process of mastication. These spillways not only prevent the packing of food in the occlusal fossae, but also facilitate the passage of food into the embrasures to stimulate and massage the tissues.

In spite of any modifications made in the occlusal anatomy or contour of a pontic in order to meet an existing unusual condition, every effort should be made to approach as nearly as possible normal occlusion and tooth anatomy.

METAL PORTION OF PONTIC

In order that the pontic of a bridge may be of service for a long time, it must be made strong enough to withstand the forces to which it will be subjected. That portion of the pontic exposed to these forces is usually made of cast metal or supported by it. This must be sufficient in bulk and distribution and it must be an alloy of the proper chemical formula; finally, it should be properly heat treated if its physical properties are to be developed to their highest degree.

Since few porcelain facings fracture as the result of a direct blow, but rather from a lack of sufficient metallic support against the forces of mastication, one of the first considerations should be a pontic so constructed that all the forces are borne and dissipated by the metal portion of the pontic. Type C casting gold, whose specifications have been formulated by the Research Commission of the American Dental Association at the Bureau of Standards in Washington, D. C., is a suitable type of alloy for this purpose. However, even the use of Type C gold does not eliminate the dangers of fracture or failure, if it is not properly heat treated before the facing is cemented permanently. The suggested heat treatment is discussed later in the chapter. In unusual conditions of excessive forces of mastication, it may be advisable to use the stronger Type D partial denture golds instead of the Type C.

HOLLOW GRINDING THE FACING

It is frequently necessary to hollow grind the incisal portion of the facing on the lingual surface in order to give a greater bulk of metal in this region. This is illustrated in Figs. 30-33 and 30-34. When long pin facings are used in the construction of the pontic, the facing should be ground and related to the cast in such a way that the pins are closer to the cingulum than to the incisal edge of the pontic.

Finally, the pontic should have a sufficient bulk of porcelain at its gingival portion so that it will not fracture easily during the steps of construction or later when placed in the mouth.

No doubt, many other requisites might be mentioned and discussed, but those indicated above, if put into effect, will assure pontics that will be satisfactory biologically, hygienically, esthetically, as well as structurally. Where the short pin facing with a swaged backing and soldered lingual or occlusal contour was formerly used, the majority of bridges today use pontics in which the porcelain facing is removable or replaceable. The one in most general use at the present time is the blunt long pin facing to which is fired a gingival porcelain extension. This is then shaped and fitted to the ridge according to the conditions present. The fired, long pin facing may be placed either in the anterior or the posterior regions and in the upper or lower arches.

REPLACEABLE TYPE OF FACING

Although the long pin facing can be replaced in the event of fracture, this is not accomplished as easily as it can be with a Steele replaceable Trupontic type of facing (Figs. 30-38 and 30-39). This type may be used very satisfactorily and economically where a sufficient vertical distance of the edentulous space exists. More is said regarding this type of pontic later in the chapter where its construction and adaptation are discussed.

A third type of pontic may be constructed, employing porcelain tube teeth or detached post crowns. Although this type of pontic is limited in its application, it is particularly valuable in the posterior region of the lower arch (Figs. 30-42 and 30-43).

SHAPES OF PONTICS AND RIDGES

The selection of the facing for color, size, and form is contingent largely upon the type of ridge present. The ridge may be completely healed, smooth, and well rounded, in which event the pontic will be of the ridge-lap type, sometimes referred to mistakenly as the "saddle" type of pontic.

Where the ridge is partially healed, the type of pontic used is determined by the location of the bridge. If it is located in the posterior part of the mouth, the irregularities of the ridge may be rounded off on the cast and the pontics fitted so that they come in contact with this rounded surface (Fig. 30-13, *B*). Occasionally a depression in the ridge exists in the posterior region, in which event the surface is likewise smoothed, but the concavity or depression is retained, and a spheroidal type of pontic is then fitted into this depression (Fig. 30-13, *C*). Where the irregularities on the cast are marked by unresorbed spicules of bone, it is advisable to remove these by surgical means, since it is difficult, if not impossible to construct a well-adapted porcelain tip to such a ridge.

Another type of ridge to which pontics are fitted is found immediately after extraction and where the so-called immediate replacement type of fixed bridge is placed (Fig. 30-6). The cone-tip, also called the "root-extension," type of pontic is constructed for such conditions where the edentulous space is in the anterior region of the mouth. To employ this type of pontic, it is necessary that, in addition to its being correctly shaped, placed, and glazed, there must also be a sufficient amount of residual alveolar process left after the extraction of the tooth. This type should not be used, however, in those cases in which there is danger of secondary infection occurring. When used in the anterior region, it is usually limited to bridges restoring one and occasionally two missing teeth.

SELECTION OF FACING

Bridge facings may be selected on the cast or the mold of the tooth may be carried directly to the mouth and the proper selection made in that manner. Likewise, after the proper size and form of the facing have been selected, it may be ground to its proper shape directly at the mouth or *on the study cast* before any cutting on the abutment teeth is done. This procedure is especially advantageous in anterior restorations that involve two or more missing teeth. By grinding the facings beforehand in this manner, not only can the esthetic qualities be determined more accurately, but the location of the buccal or labial cavity margins may be placed more accurately when the facing is ground, aligned, and viewed while held temporarily in position with wax. In those bridges soldered with rigid connectors at both ends, the pontic may even be completed beforehand, i.e., the gold portion may be finished even before the retainers are cast.

When grinding a facing to position, not only should every effort be made to establish the correct buccal or labial alignment, but also any characteristics peculiar to the individual's teeth should be reproduced if possible. In the anterior region the slope and the length of the incisal edge should faithfully simulate the neighboring or corresponding tooth.

ALIGNMENT OF PONTIC

Since there is a variation in the amount of resorption that occurs in a ridge following the extraction of teeth, this should be carefully noted because the alignment of the facing is largely contingent upon this factor; in other words, the greater the resorption of the labial or buccal plate of bone, the more will the gingival portion of the facing be depressed lingually. Failure to make the proper amount of such depression at the gingival margin will result in a pontic that has the effect of being either too long or too short. Fig. 30-9, based on the work of Smith and Potter,[4] shows the position of the labial surface of the natural tooth in its relationship to the gingival tissues before extraction; this is represented by the broken line in Fig. 30-9, *A*; the solid line represents the ridge outline following the extraction of the tooth. If the labial surface of the pontic is placed in the same labial plane with that formerly occupied by the natural tooth, the pontic will extend too far gingivally on the labial plane, making the tooth look much longer than the natural tooth which it replaces (Figs. 30-9, *A*, and 30-10, *A*).

By depressing the gingival area of the pontic as shown in Fig. 30-9, *B*, the appearance of proper length is given to the facing at its neck, and the general effect is that shown in Fig. 30-10, *B*.

Where the neck of the facing is depressed too much in its gingival area, as shown in Fig. 30-9, *C*, the general effect is that of a foreshortened tooth and there is the added disadvantage of having food catch in the gingival region.

Figs. 30-11 and 30-12 show the application of the same principle to the bicuspid teeth; Fig. 30-13 shows the molars. In the latter instance, since the esthetic factor is not of such great importance, the pontic may be depressed more at the gingival if this is necessary for hygienic purposes.

In order to facilitate the self-cleansing

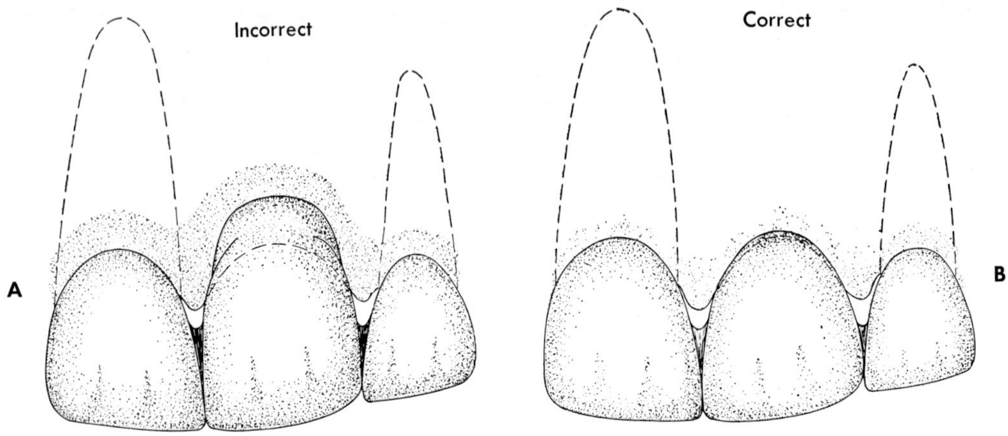

Fig. 30-10. Incorrect and correct gingival lengths of pontic. (After D. Smith.)

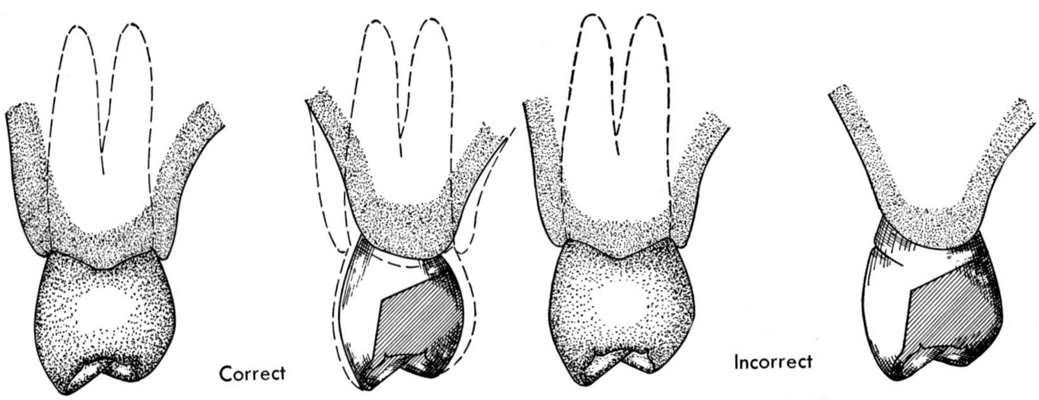

Fig. 30-11 **Fig. 30-12**

Fig. 30-11. Correct length of bicuspid facings. (After D. Smith.)
Fig. 30-12. Incorrect length of bicuspid facings. (After D. Smith.)

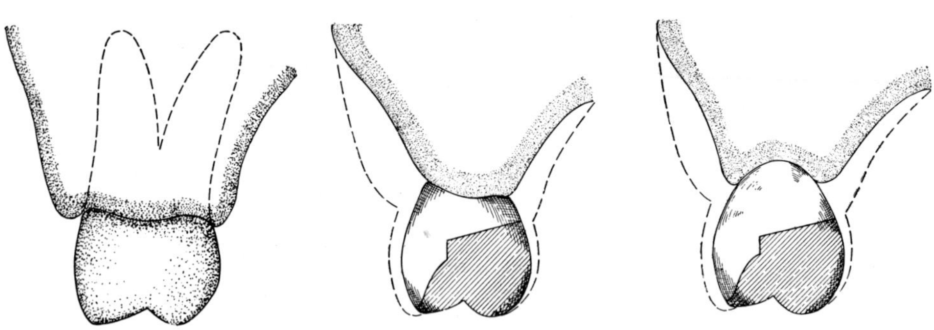

A **B** **C**

Fig. 30-13. A, Natural tooth and investing tissue contours. **B,** Molar pontic in contact with healed, rounded ridge. **C,** Molar pontic fitted to depression in ridge. (After D. Smith.)

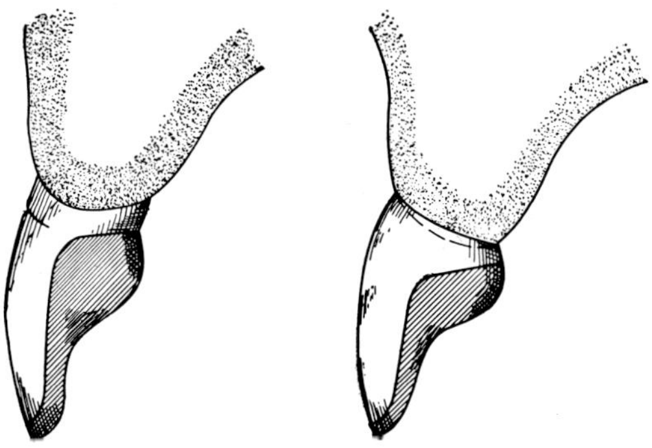

Fig. 30-14. A, True "saddle" pontic; it is concave in all directions. **B,** This pontic, sometimes also referred to erroneously as "saddle type," is convex mesiodistally and spheroidal in lingual half of buccolingual diameter. First type is difficult to keep clean, second is not. (From Smith, D. E., and Potter, H. R.: D. Digest **43:**16, 1937.)

action of the pontic, it is usually narrowed mesiodistally in its gingival third in order to create wide interdental spaces. This may be done freely in the posterior region, but in the anterior teeth it is limited to a large extent by esthetic considerations. Where the lip line is low and covers the gingival portion of the facing, the gingival interdental space may be proportionately increased. In those instances, however, in which the entire labial surface is exposed, the correct mesiodistal width is given to the facing, but the pontic is narrowed greatly in that part which lies immediately lingual to the contact areas. This forms wide lingual embrasures that facilitate the self-cleansing action of the pontic.

RIDGE-LAP AND "SADDLE" TYPES

After the gingival porcelain has been fired to the facing, the correct surface contact relationship must be established between the porcelain and the ridge. Where the ridge is healed, smooth, and well rounded, the ridge-lap type of pontic is usually constructed.

The term "saddle" gives a wrong conception of the exact shape implied by the term. Fig. 30-14, *A*, shows the incorrect shape; Fig. 30-14, *B*, the correct. For esthetic reasons, the pontic must contact the ridge along its labial or buccal margin, both in the anterior and posterior regions of the mouth. From this line of contact the surface of the pontic follows the ridge downward until it reaches the highest point of the ridge; from here it continues lingually, assuming a definitely spheroidal form, and its lingual half emerges lingually as a convex surface.

Considered in its mesiodistal dimension, the contact area between the porcelain and the ridge surfaces is not a complete or continuous one; there is a small, narrow contact isthmus area extending from the buccal or labial margin toward the lingual, but from this narrow band of contact the porcelain slopes away from the ridge tissues into the mesial and distal interdental embrasures, giving the porcelain tip a definite mesiodistal convexity. This shape, shown in Fig. 30-15, creates a self-cleansing arrangement between the porcelain and the mucosa of the ridge, since any food particles carried into this region are easily dislodged mesially or distally into the approximal embrasures.

CONICAL ROOT TYPE

In the immediate replacement type of pontic employing the conical porcelain tip, the same principles of labial alignment mentioned previously are observed. However, instead of fitting the porcelain pontic to a surface contact with a healed ridge, it is extended into the alveolar socket of the extracted tooth to a depth equal to one-fourth to one-fifth the depth of the socket. Nothing is gained by extending these porcelain tips far into the socket, since the bone in the healed socket terminates about 2 mm. from the apex of the porcelain cone. In shaping the porcelain tip, the apex of the pontic should lie in the long axis of the socket; in other words, it should not be brought out labially. Fig.

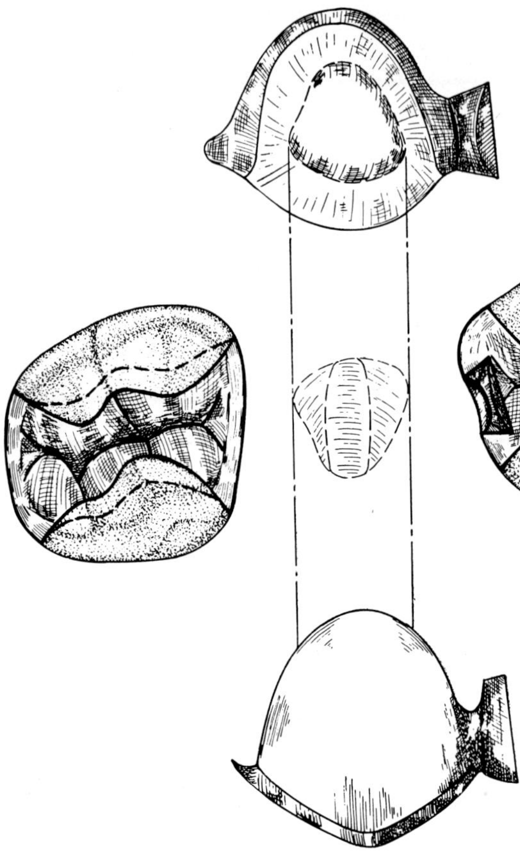

Fig. 30-15. Only narrow oval part of pontic, buccolingually, touches mucosa of ridge; remainder is convex mesiodistally. (From Smith, D. E., and Potter, H. R.: D. Digest **43:**16, 1937.)

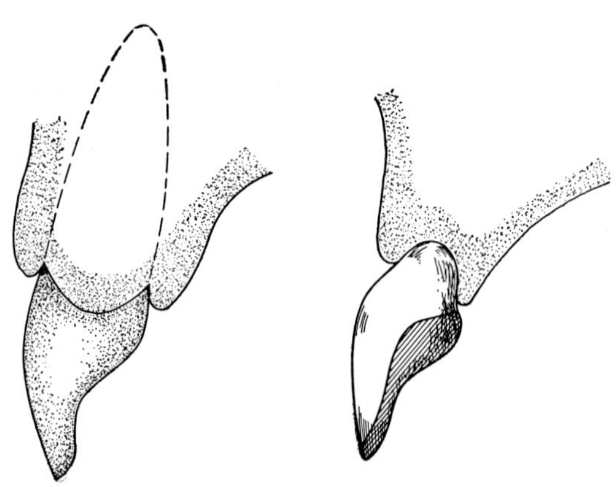

Fig. 30-16. Type of pontic used anteriorly for immediate replacement type of bridge. (After D. Smith.)

30-16 illustrates the relative position of the normal natural tooth and the pontic. In fitting the cone-tip pontic immediately after the extraction of the tooth, under no circumstances is it allowed to come in contact with the alveolar process. The only point of contact between the porcelain and the tissues exists between the porcelain and the free labial gingiva. Even here the peripheral outline of the pontic is made smaller than the circumference of the gingival tissues before the natural tooth was extracted; for, while the porcelain is in contact on the labial side, it is so shaped on the palatal side that a space approximately 1 mm. in width is left between the gingiva and the porcelain. This slack is later taken up when the socket heals and the tissues contract against the cone tip. This method prevents the gingiva on the labial side from slipping up apically during the healing process.

"SANITARY BRIDGES"

The immediate replacement, root extension type of pontic is not used in the lower arch, because it adds nothing to the esthetic values. Pontics constructed for the lower arch are usually conical or spheroidal in shape and are brought in contact with the crest of the ridge, as shown in Figs. 30-17 and 30-18. There are times when

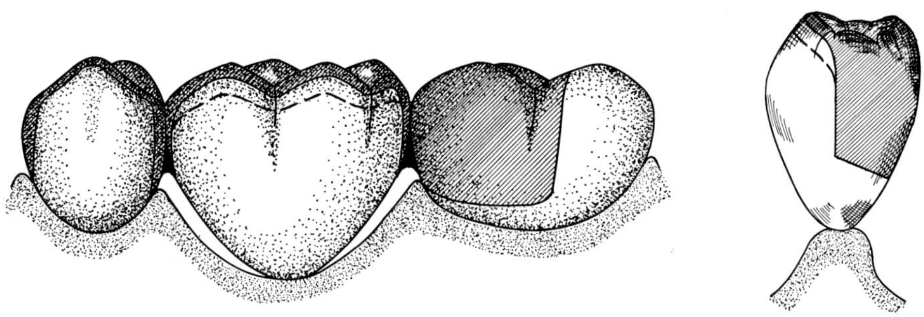

Fig. 30-17. Position and relationship of pontic to mucosa and adjacent teeth. (After D. Smith.)

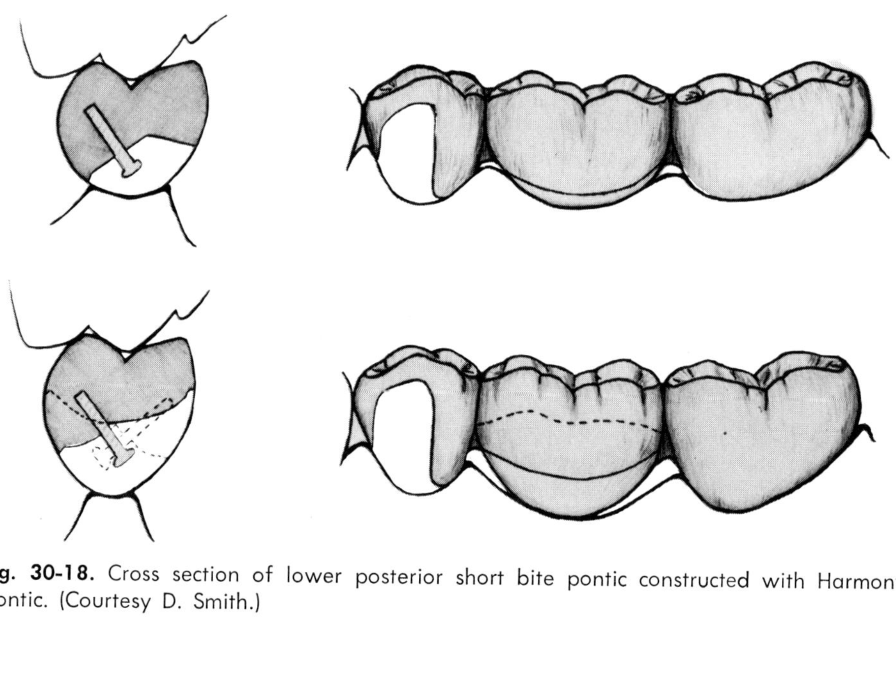

Fig. 30-18. Cross section of lower posterior short bite pontic constructed with Harmony pontic. (Courtesy D. Smith.)

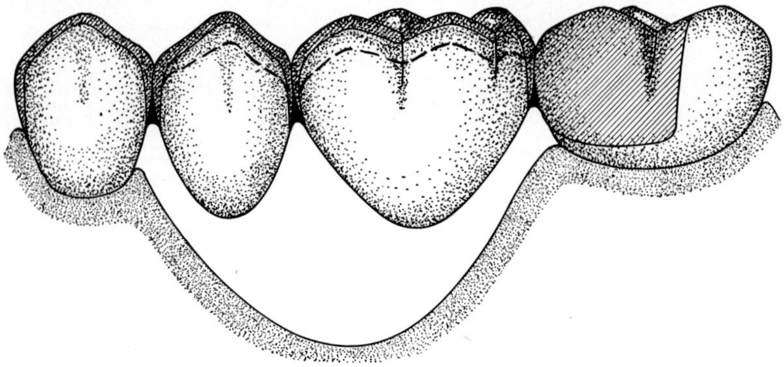

Fig. 30-19. Position of lower pontics where ridge is excessively resorbed. (After D. Smith.)

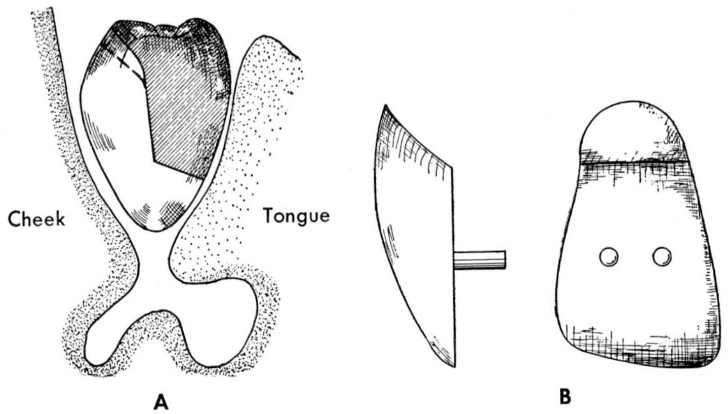

Fig. 30-20. A, Cross section of pontic shown in Fig. 30-19. (After D. Smith.) **B,** First step in construction of pontic is narrowing it mesiodistally in gingival region. This is not done in anterior region where lip is high.

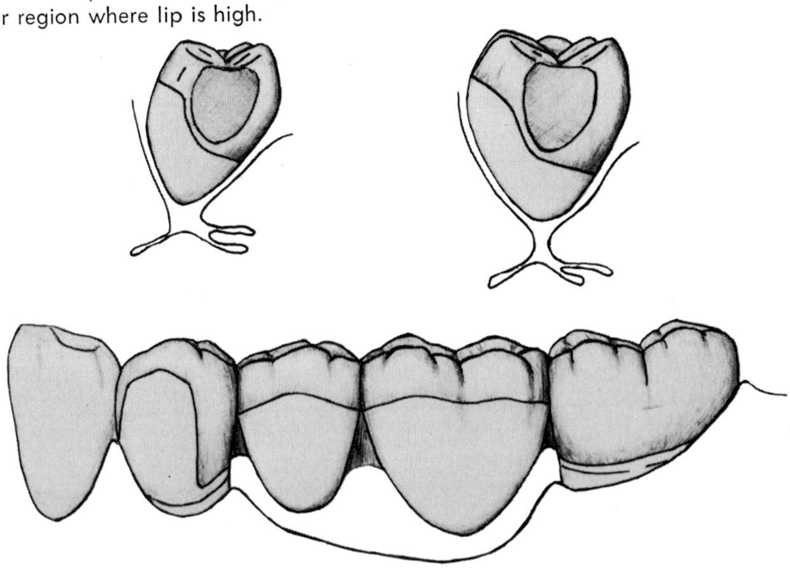

Fig. 30-21. Typical condition of excessive ridge resorption with Harmony pontic form permits contact of cheek and tongue beneath tips to facilitate hygiene. (Courtesy D. Smith.)

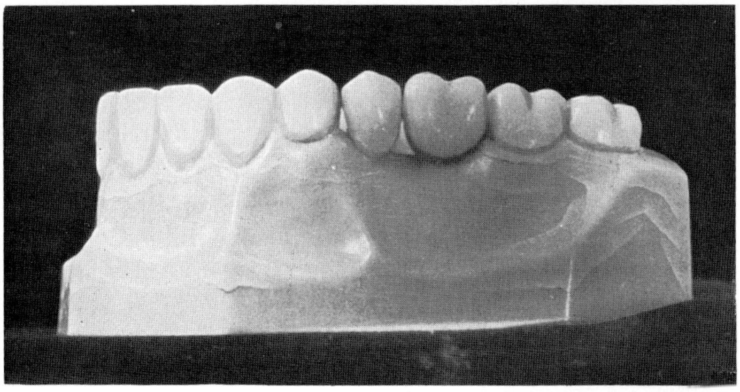

Fig. 30-22. Bicuspid and molar facings narrowed mesiodistally in gingival third. Note gingival embrasures.

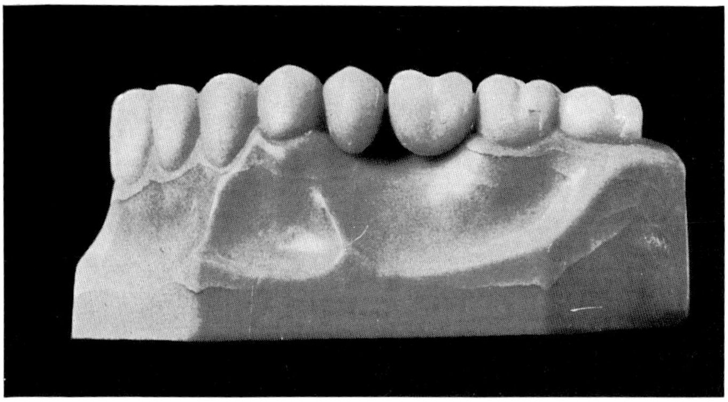

Fig. 30-23. Same region as shown in Fig. 30-22, with facings held in position with wax, ready for pouring of plaster core.

the lower ridge is excessively resorbed; in such instances the pontics may be shortened gingivally so that they do not contact the ridge. Enough space, however, must be left between the pontic and the ridge to permit the tongue and the cheek to keep the underlying porcelain clean (Figs. 30-19 to 30-21). This modification is similar to the so-called sanitary bridges, which were constructed entirely of gold and which were used largely because it was thought they could be kept clean more easily on account of the space existing between the bridge and the crest of the ridge. Clinical evidence has shown, however, that, where the pontics are made entirely of metal, those surfaces facing the ridge are invaribly covered with gelatinous, grayish deposits, in spite of the care a patient may give them. Hence, when a space is left beneath the pontics, the gingival portion of the pontic should be of glazed porcelain.

POSITION OF PLATINUM PINS

When grinding a facing, an effort should be made to position the platinum pins so that they are located in the gingival third of the pontic rather than in the middle or incisal regions. Placed gingivally, the platinum pins are located in that portion of the pontic which restores the cingulum of the tooth; this gives a maximum amount of retention, since the full length of the pins is embedded in the casting. If the pins are located incisally, the pontic of necessity will be thicker, causing an interference with speech or oc-

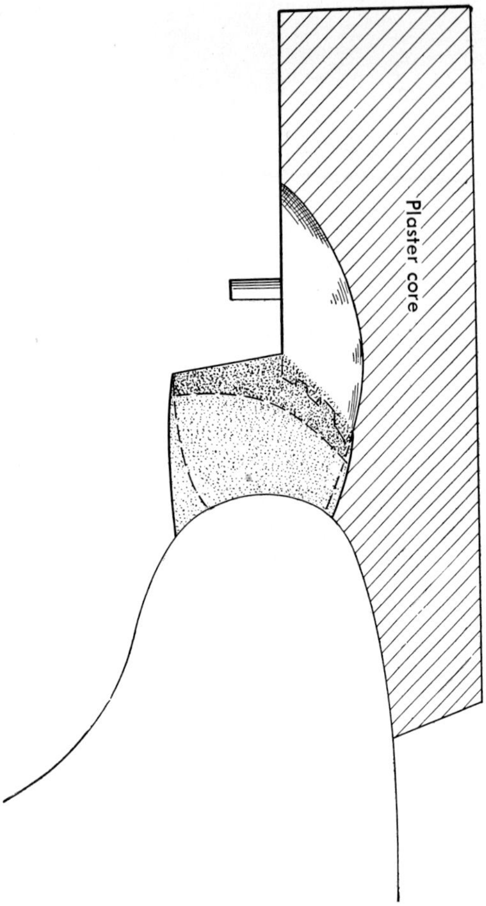

Fig. 30-24. Cross section of plaster core, ridge of working model, and shaded portions of pontic indicating first and second applications of gingival porcelain to facing.

clusion; if the pins are shortened, they lose much of their retention.

When the facing has been properly related to the adjacent teeth and to the ridge, it is narrowed mesiodistally in the gingival one-third (Fig. 30-22). The next procedure is to construct a plaster core to maintain the established relationship of the facing to the cast during the various steps of construction.

CONSTRUCTION OF PLASTER CORE OR INDEX

The facing is held temporarily in position with soft wax applied to its lingual surface (Fig. 30-23). The labial or buccal surface of the facing and the adjacent teeth on the cast are lubricated; a small amount of plaster is mixed and carefully applied to cover the labial or buccal surface of the lubricated model and the porcelain facing extending 0.5 mm. beyond the occlusal edge of the facing (Figs. 30-24 and 30-25). When set, the core is trimmed so that it does not interfere with the closure of the opposing cast mounted on the articulator.

It is essential that the core covers the facing gingivally and interproximally so that when the facing is removed it may be again replaced in its correct position in the core. Some operators make the cores of modeling compound, but experience has shown that the plaster core is preferable.

After the plaster core has set, it is carefully removed from the model; if the facing comes away in the plaster core, it is carefully cleaned of all wax and replaced in the core; the core and facing are then returned to the model (Fig. 30-26). At this time, it is advisable to check the parallelism of the platinum pins in the facing; if out of line, they should be carefully straightened so that they are parallel.

FIRING PORCELAIN TO THE FACING

The next step is firing on the porcelain tip, either the ridge-lap, spheroidal, or the conical types. While there are many instruments manufactured for use in building up the porcelain tip, a very simple contrivance serves the purpose very well and may be made from a K-plier illustrated in Fig. 30-27. A small platform of silver alloy plate is soldered to one blade of the plier, which has been shortened ½ inch. This piece of plate is inclined at a slight angle as shown to give the pontic the necessary slopes for the withdrawal of the wax pattern. The inner surface of the other blade of the plier is hollowed out so that the facing may lie in it and

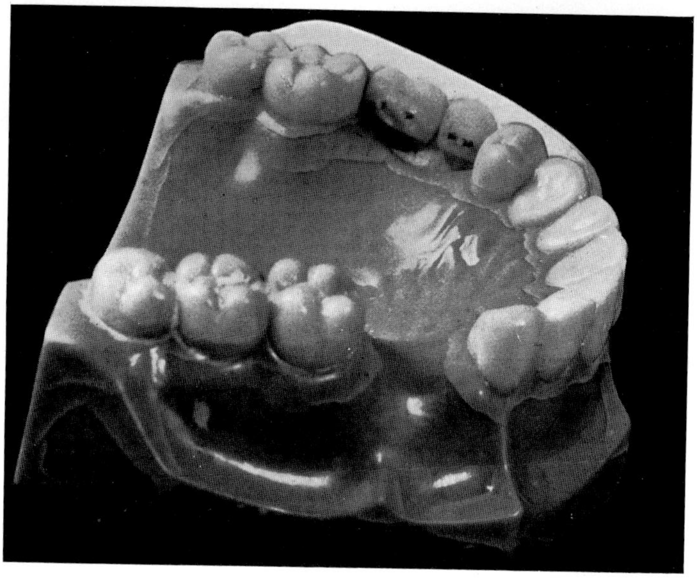

Fig. 30-25. Plaster core with facings held in position after removal of wax on lingual surface.

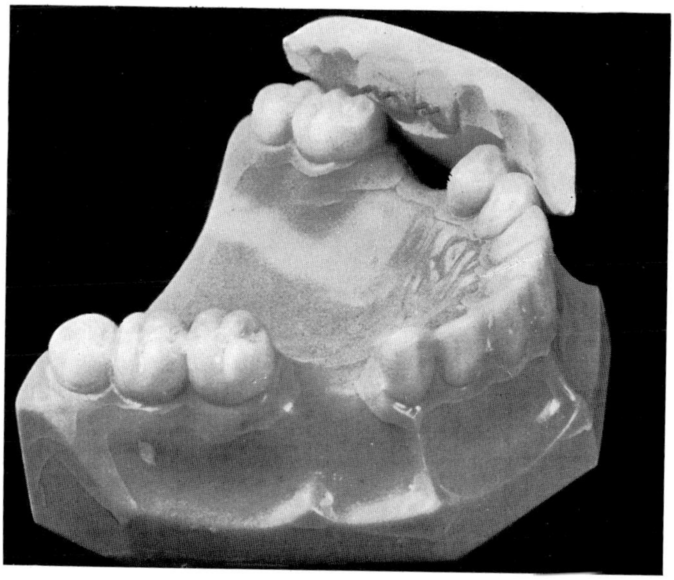

Fig. 30-26. Plaster core and facings, separated from working model.

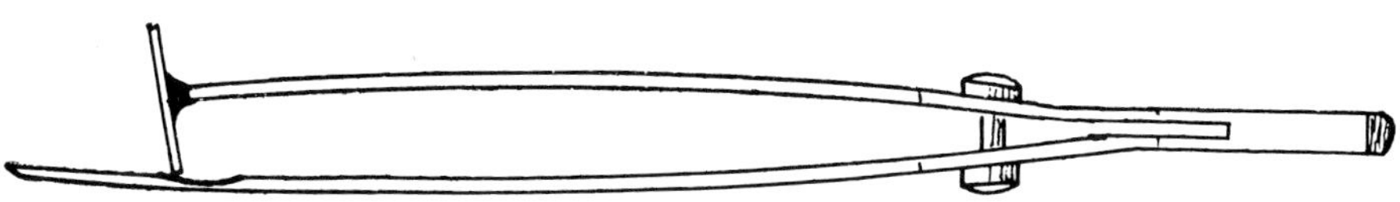

Fig. 30-27. Pontic plier easily made from K-plier; in use for over 40 years.

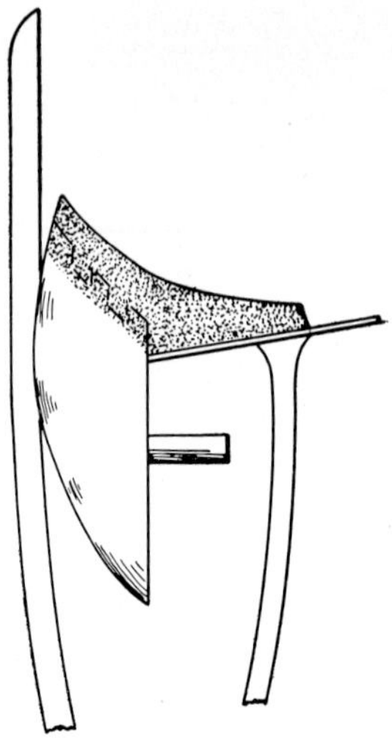

Fig. 30-28. Facing grooved and first application of porcelain made, using pontic plier.

be held firmly during the application of the porcelain.

Usually medium fusing porcelain of 2100 to 2300° F. is employed for firing the porcelain tip, since most facings are manufactured of 2400 to 2500° F. porcelain.

Prior to the application of the medium fusing porcelain, two transverse grooves are cut in the ridge lap of the facing to afford a better mechanical lock for the newly applied porcelain (Fig. 30-28).

The platform of the pontic plier is now lightly lubricated with a thin lubricating oil, not petrolatum, after which the facing is placed in the pliers and securely locked by raising the K-lock. Normally, the sloping platform of the pontic plier is placed as close to the pins as possible, in order to bring the pins in the gingival portion of the pontic. With the facing held firmly in the pliers, a small amount of medium fusing porcelain is applied to the facing ridge lap and vibrated slightly by drawing the porcelain instrument across the sides of the pontic plier. This settles the porcelain against the facing and the platform (Fig. 30-28).

FIRING THE PONTIC "SHELF"

For the first firing of porcelain it is advisable to apply a sufficient quantity to form a definite shelf to which more porcelain may be applied after it is fired. No attempt is made at this time to conform the porcelain to the ridge.

When the first application of porcelain has been properly contoured and condensed, the lock on the pontic plier is released and the facing with its freshly added porcelain is carefully slid off the lubricated platform with a slight lateral pressure of the porcelain instrument.

The facing is then carefully placed on a muffle tray containing coarse silex granules. The facing is placed with the pins pointing downward, care being exercised that none of the newly added porcelain touches the silex. Klaffenbach[5] recommended that two platinum wires be embedded in a fire clay slab and their ends made into two small loops into which the platinum pins of the facing fit; in this way the facing is held suspended above the floor of the tray.

The tray and facing are now placed before the open door of the muffle or in a drying chamber until all moisture has been eliminated. After this, the tray is carefully inserted into the muffle and the porcelain is brought to a low bisque firing.

After the proper degree of vitrification is reached, the current is shut off and the tray with the facing is removed from the muffle and placed under a Pyrex dish to cool slowly. Too rapid cooling of the facing or touching it while hot with a cold pair of pliers is liable to check the porcelain. When cooled so that it can be handled with the bare fingers, the facing is removed from the tray, replaced in the plaster core, and both are returned to the working model. Fig. 30-29 shows the facings and plaster core in this relationship on the model.

The darker area in Fig. 30-25 illustrates that portion of the pontic built during the

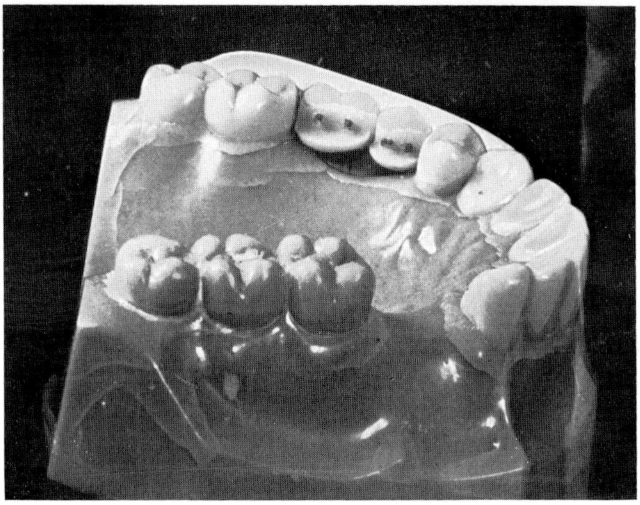

Fig. 30-29. After first firing of porcelain, facings replaced in plaster core to determine amount needed for second addition.

first firing. It is seen that a considerable space exists between the ridge and the gingival surface of the fired porcelain tip. While it is possible to fire on a large bulk of porcelain for the first firing and subsequently grind it to fit the ridge accurately, the technic given here and taught for many years is much simpler and quicker and gives results equal to, if not better than, those obtained by the spot-grinding technic.

In Chapter 17 it is suggested that the tissues of the edentulous ridge be treated with an astringent before the impression is taken; this gives a working model with the ridge in a state of physiological shrinkage or reduction. If the dentist fits the pontic so that it contacts the surface of such a model, he is assured of having the correct degree of interface contact in the finished bridge between the pontic and the mucosa of the ridge.

SECOND APPLICATION AND FIRING PORCELAIN

If the working model is made of metal or if that portion of the model reproducing the edentulous ridge is made of metal, the ridge portion is thoroughly cleaned and burnished with a rounded instrument so that its surface is highly polished and smooth. This, as well as the surfaces of the adjacent teeth, is now lubricated with a thin oil. The facing is removed from the plaster core and that part of the core adjacent to the pontic is thoroughly saturated with lubricating oil. The excess oil is then carefully removed, and the facing with its initial firing of porcelain is now replaced in the plaster core (Fig. 30-29). With the facing held in the plaster core, an additional amount of medium-fusing porcelain is mixed to a wet consistency and applied to the gingival surface of the shelf made in the first firing. Since the plaster core is thoroughly lubricated, none of the moisture is absorbed from the porcelain.

The facing core and the newly added excess porcelain are now carefully placed in their correct positions on the lubricated working model. With a slight tapping or vibration of the working model, the core and the facing with its freshly added porcelain settle into their correct positions on the model, the excess porcelain flowing over and conforming itself to the lingual surface of the ridge and the interproximal

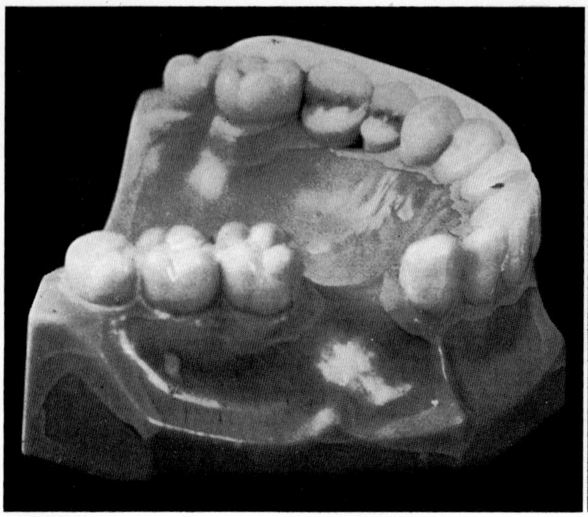

Fig. 30-30

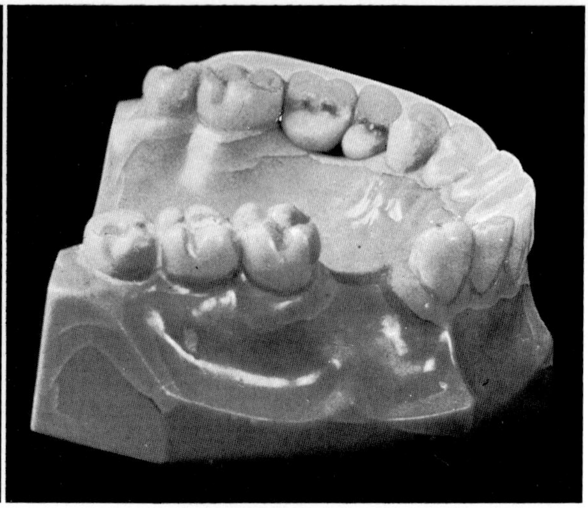

Fig. 30-31

Fig. 30-30. Second application of porcelain. No effort at final contour is made at this time.
Fig. 30-31. Glazed porcelain pontics held in correct position in plaster core.

spaces (Fig. 30-30). Care must be taken that the core and the facing are properly related to the model. After the excess moisture has been absorbed from the second application of porcelain, it is condensed and carved on the model to the approximate contour of the finished pontic; however, a slight excess is allowed (Fig. 30-30). Since the ridge is lubricated, the plaster core and facing with its newly added porcelain can now be raised from the working model in a buccoclusal direction. The gingival part of the pontic will have its gingival surface accurately shaped to fit the surface of the ridge with which it came in contact. No attempt is made at this time to reshape or complete the contour of the pontic. Holding the plaster core firmly in one hand, the pins of the facing are grasped in a pair of pliers and the facings are rolled out of the core in a gingival direction. Any loose particles of porcelain are very carefully removed with a large camel's hair brush, and the facing with its added porcelain is given a second bisque firing.

SHAPING THE PONTIC

When removed from the muffle and cooled to room temperature, the facing with its bisque porcelain tip is replaced in the plaster core and both are returned to position on the working model. It is usually found that the surface adaptation between the ridge and porcelain tip is accurate, but the peripheral outline of the porcelain pontic must now be shaped, with respect to both its buccolingual and mesiodistal aspects. The excess porcelain is ground away with stones, usually narrowing the porcelain mesiodistally in its lingual half and enlarging the interdental spaces. The dotted line in Fig. 30-24 represents approximately the correct amount of reduction made in the pontic after the second firing of porcelain. If for some reason there is too much space between the ridge and the pontic, this condition may be corrected by a third addition of porcelain, which also is brought to a bisque firing; this, however, is rarely necessary. When completely shaped, the ground porcelain surfaces are polished with disks and are

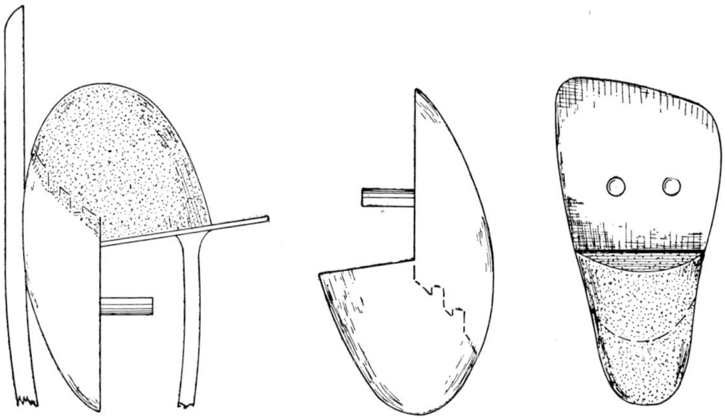

A B

Fig. 30-32. **A,** First application of porcelain for root extension type of pontic. **B,** Finished pontic.

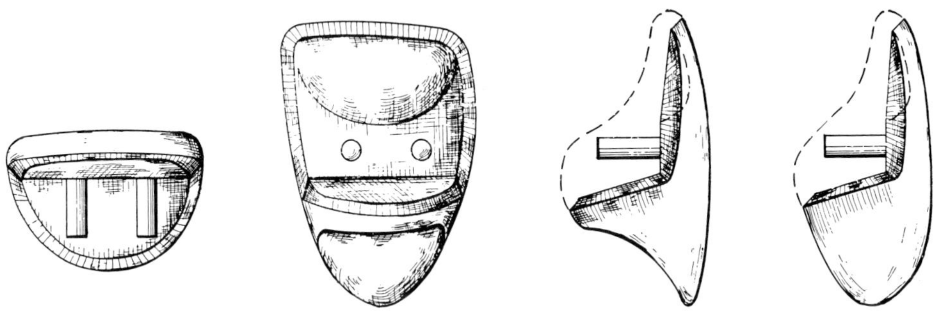

Fig. 30-33. Views of ridge-lap and cone-tip types of pontics. Note marginal bevels and hollow grinding of incisal portion of facing.

cleaned thoroughly, and the pontic is returned to the muffle for its final firing glaze.

After the porcelain pontic has been removed from the muffle and allowed to cool to room temperature, it is replaced in the plaster core and carried to position on the working model; if the gingival fit and contour are satisfactory, the glazed pontic is ready for its final occlusal and marginal grinding (Fig. 30-31).

Where the immediate replacement cone-tip pontic is being constructed, the initial application of porcelain is built cone-shaped as shown in Fig. 30-32, *A*, and a sufficient surplus is allowed for grinding and fitting the porcelain tip to the alveolar fundus in the working model; after this has been done, it is glazed. Fig. 30-32, *B*, shows views of a pontic prepared for the immediate replacement type of prosthesis.

BEVELING AND HOLLOW GRINDING

Since it is necessary to protect the porcelain facing at the incisal or occlusal edge against fracture, the lingual surface is hollow ground from the incisal or occlusal edge gingivally to a point just above the platinum pins. This not only provides an additional bulk of gold for incisal protection, but also makes the facing thinner labiolingually (Fig. 30-33). After this has been done, a narrow bevel is placed around the margins of the facing and the porcelain tip. Beveling the facing this way affords a box-like seat for the porcelain

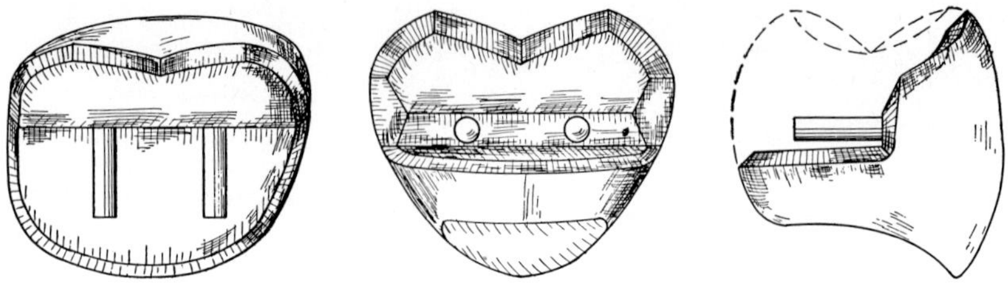

Fig. 30-34. Molar pontic.

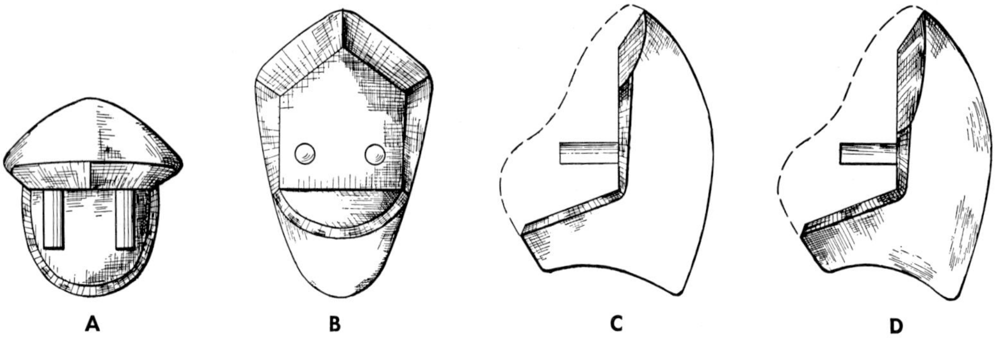

Fig. 30-35. Bicuspid pontic; right pontic hollow ground.

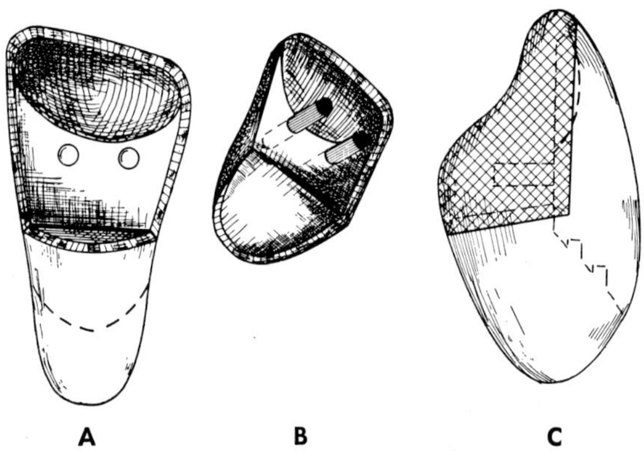

Fig. 30-36. A, Completed porcelain facing. **B,** Lingual portion contoured in inlay wax. Wax pattern has two graphite points inserted in pinholes. **C,** Cross section shows casting fitted to porcelain portion of pontic.

as well as giving it additional protection. Fig. 30-34 illustrates the same principle applied to the molar pontic.

When the 45° incisal or occlusal bevel is employed, only a thin layer of gold protects the lingual surface, as shown in Fig. 30-35, *A* to *C*. The forces exerted along the incisal edge spring the gold over the angle of the porcelain incisal bevel, causing the facing to fracture—hence, the desirability of the hollow-ground principle (Fig. 30-35, *D*).

WAXING THE LINGUAL AND OCCLUSAL CONTOURS

The next procedure is to develop the occlusal or lingual contour in inlay wax. Before applying the wax, however, those surfaces that were ground after the final glazing of the facing are polished smooth with fine sandpaper disks, and all particles of porcelain and other debris are removed; the parallelism of the platinum pins should again be verified (Fig. 30-36, *A*).

The lingual surface of the facing is slightly lubricated with a thin coat of lubricant and inlay wax softened to the proper consistency is pressed against the lingual surface and around the platinum pins. The wax is held under pressure until it has cooled to room temperature.

The plaster core is now removed and the facings are held in their correct relationship in inlay wax. At this time it should be noted whether the wax covers all the porcelain margins. If so, the plaster core is replaced and the excess inlay wax is cut away; the occlusal portion of the wax is then carefully heated to a depth of 1 to 3 mm.

The occlusal surfaces of the opposing cast are then thoroughly lubricated and brought into centric occlusion, leaving their imprints in the softened wax. The excess wax is trimmed away and the surface is again slightly warmed, but not to the point where the previous occlusal markings will be obliterated. The opposing cast is again brought into occlusion and carried through the various lateral and protrusive movements, establishing clearance paths in the wax. Following this, the occlusal anatomy and the axial contour are completed and the wax is smoothed (Fig. 30-36, *B*). Special attention is given to the occlusal carving of the pontics; all natural grooves are accentuated and supplementary ones opening into the lingual embrasures are created through the marginal ridges. The pontic in its lingual half is narrowed mesiodistally, leaving wider lingual embrasures.

Ante[1] stated that in carving the occlusal surface of a bridge pontic "the occlusal surface of a bridge should never be greater than 90 per cent of the combined occlusal surfaces of one tooth, 80 per cent for two teeth, and 70 per cent for three teeth, which it is replacing." Today, over 50 years later, this statement is still a safe guide.

In bridges restoring one missing tooth the dimensions of the pontic approach the normal size. Where two or more missing teeth are replaced, the occlusal surface and the contour of the pontic are drastically modified in order to reduce the surface area that is exposed to the forces of mastication. Where a fixed restoration is opposed by a removable, mucosa-borne partial or complete denture, these precautionary measures are not as essential as when the prosthesis is opposed by natural teeth.

TREATMENT OF PLATINUM PINS

When carving the lingual surfaces of anterior teeth, it is occasionally found that the platinum pins extend lingually through the wax. If this occurs, the pins should not be cut short, but should be left their full length until after the casting is made (Fig. 30-36, *B*). When the bridge is finished, the pins are riveted to the casting at the time the facings are cemented to the bridge.

After the waxed pontic has been properly finished, a sprue former is attached to the lingual surface and the wax portion is carefully removed from the facing. If any difficulty is encountered in separating the inlay wax from the porcelain facing, a piece of sticky wax, attached to the labial surface of the facing, serves as a handle by which the facing is separated from the wax portion. The occlusal or lingual surface of the wax carving is now carefully examined to make certain that all margins are accurately reproduced and that the inner surfaces are smooth and perfectly adapted.

USE OF GRAPHITE POINTS OR METAL PINS

The lubricated surfaces of the wax pattern are brushed clean first with equal parts of hydrogen peroxide and green soap. This is followed by brushing with a wetting agent. Two graphite points or Harmony core metal pins of the same diameter as the platinum pins are now placed in the two pinholes in the labial or buccal surface of the wax pattern. These should be sufficiently long to ensure their being held firmly in the investment while the casting is made (Fig. 30-36, *B*).

The pattern is then invested and cast. After the castings have been cleaned thoroughly, the graphite points, now embedded in the casting, are removed with small, round burs of the same diameter as the graphite points. This is followed by milling the pinholes with a fine cut, tapered No. 600 finishing bur. Care must be exercised not to enlarge the holes beyond the diameter of the platinum pins.

Harmony core pins are available that are made of special metal treated to make it possible to pull them out of the casting with pliers rather than drill out the graphite points. The metal pins may also be replaced in the pinholes of the casting to hold it firmly in the soldering investment and to prevent any solder from accidently filling the pinholes.

The porcelain facing is then replaced on the casting and, if the technical steps have been carefully performed, an accurate fit between the two should result (Fig. 30-36, *C*).

FITTING CASTING TO FACING

Where the facing does not seat entirely, it is possible that all of the graphite has not been removed. The facing should not be seated by cutting off the platinum pins. Sometimes the carbon points are not inserted into the wax pinholes sufficiently deep, in which case it may be necessary to drill the pinhole in the casting a little deeper in order to accommodate the platinum pins; however, care should be taken not to choke the bur in the pinhole and break off its head. Should this occur, the broken bur may be removed by boiling the casting in acid.

At no time should force be used to seat the porcelain facing on the casting, as fracture of the porcelain is likely to result. When fitted, the gold portion of the pontic is polished and finished, after which the facing and gold casting are placed in the core and both are returned to the working model.

The pontics are now ready to be incorporated with the retainers into the complete restoration by means of connectors.

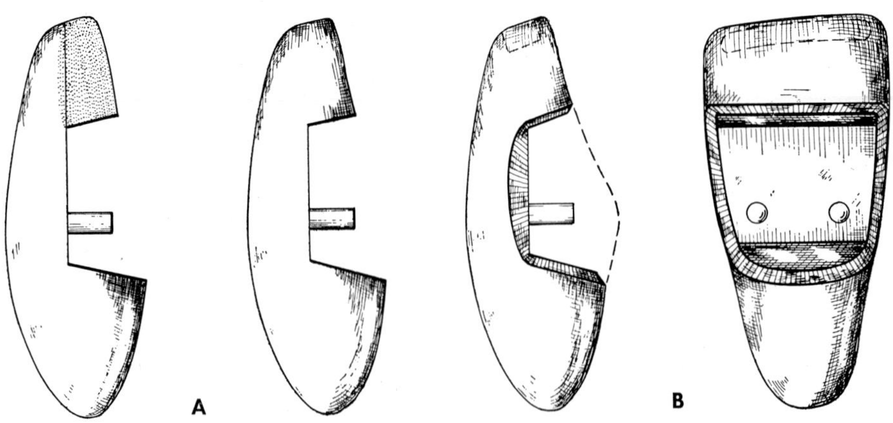

Fig. 30-37. A, Porcelain is sometimes added to incisal edge of lower anterior pontics. **B,** Method of preparing incisal portion for application of stained porcelain.

The procedures are described in Chapter 32.

TREATMENT OF THE INCISAL EDGE

Since the incisal or the occlusal edge of the porcelain facing is protected by a gold casting extending beyond the incisal edge of the facing, it is essential that this extension of metal be beveled in such a manner that light reflected by the incisal gold tip will be directed away from the line of vision (Fig. 30-5). In a lower restoration this is sometimes difficult to do; therefore, porcelain is added along the incisal edge on the lingual surface, as shown in Fig. 30-37, *A*. This incisal addition may

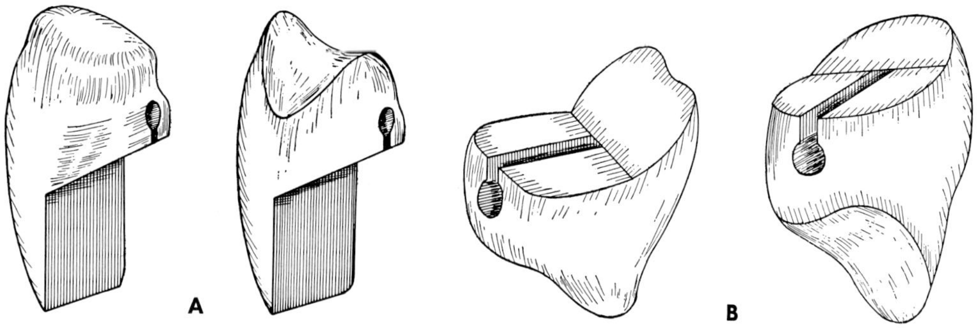

Fig. 30-38. Types of ready-made Steele Trupontic facings for anterior teeth. **B,** Steele Trupontic posterior facings.

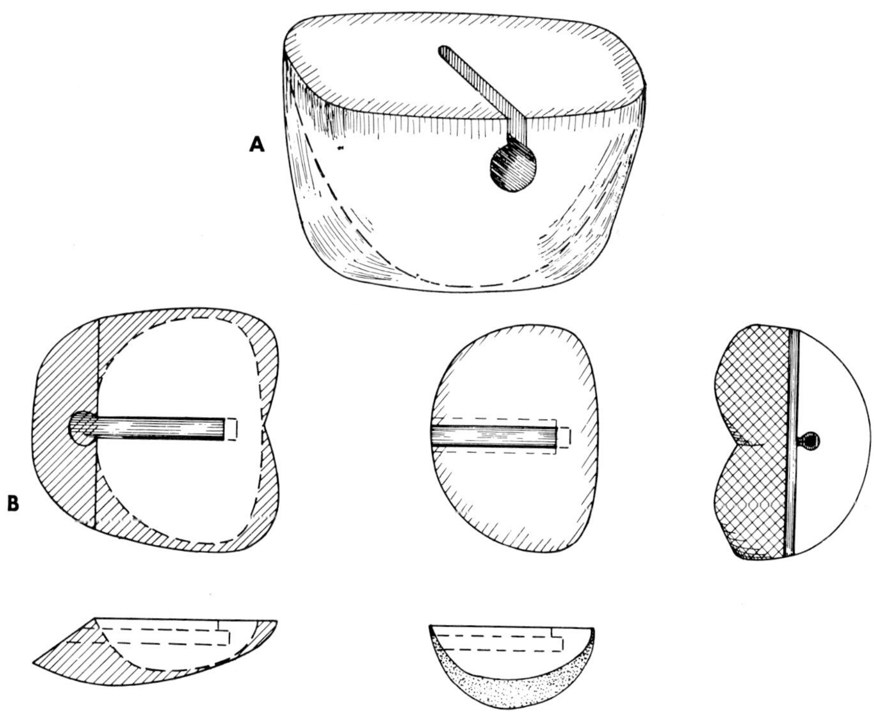

Fig. 30-39. A, Steele type of replaceable facing used in lower posterior pontics. **B,** Steps in construction of pontic shown in **A.**

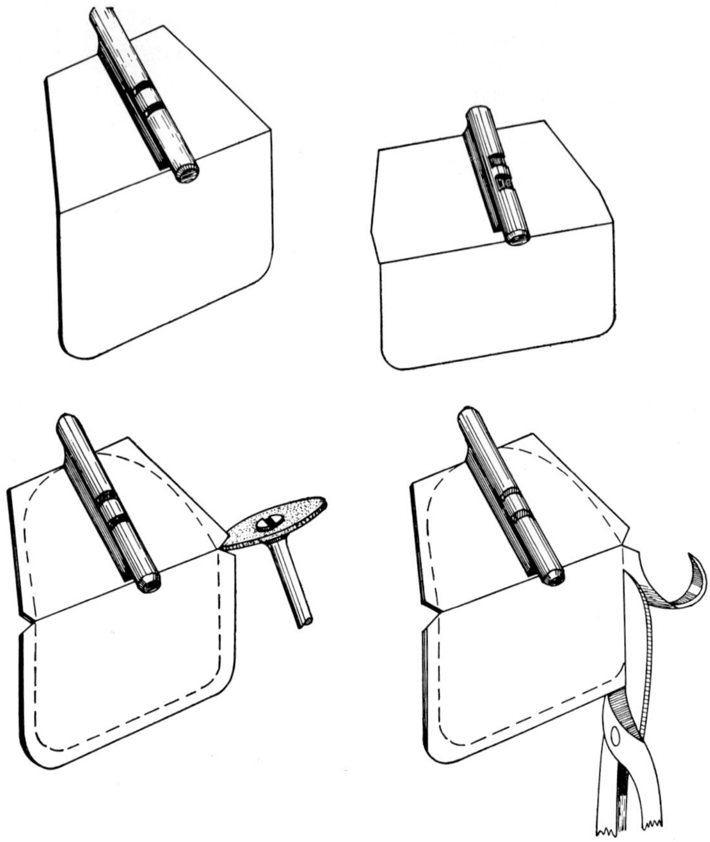

Fig. 30-40. Types of backings used with Steele Trupontic facings. (Courtesy Columbus Manufacturing Co.)

be further modified by cutting a shallow groove mesiodistally along the incisal edge and filling it with stained porcelain; this is then glazed and made an integral part of the porcelain facing (Fig. 30-37, *B*).

After the two additions, one at the gingival and one at the incisal edge, the margins of the facing on the lingual surface are beveled; the gold casting occupies the space between the incisal and gingival porcelain planes.

Ready-made facings also come in replaceable types, such as the Steele Trupontic teeth and others of similar character. Fig. 30-38, *A*, shows two types for anterior replacements; Fig. 30-38, *B*, two types for a posterior replacement in the upper arch; and Fig. 30-39, *A*, a type of pontic usually employed in the lower posterior teeth. Fig. 30-39, *B*, shows the method for constructing the pontic seen in *A*. Fig. 30-40 illustrates backings that are used with the replaceable facings.

Fig. 30-41, *A*, shows a manufactured posterior, replaceable Steele facing pontic.

All these removable and replaceable facings, with the exception of that in Fig. 30-39, *A* and *B*, restore the entire labial or buccal in porcelain; the latter facing restores the gingival two-thirds in porcelain, but the occlusal third of the crown is made of cast gold.

Fig. 30-41, *B*, shows the possibility of combining a regular replaceable Steele

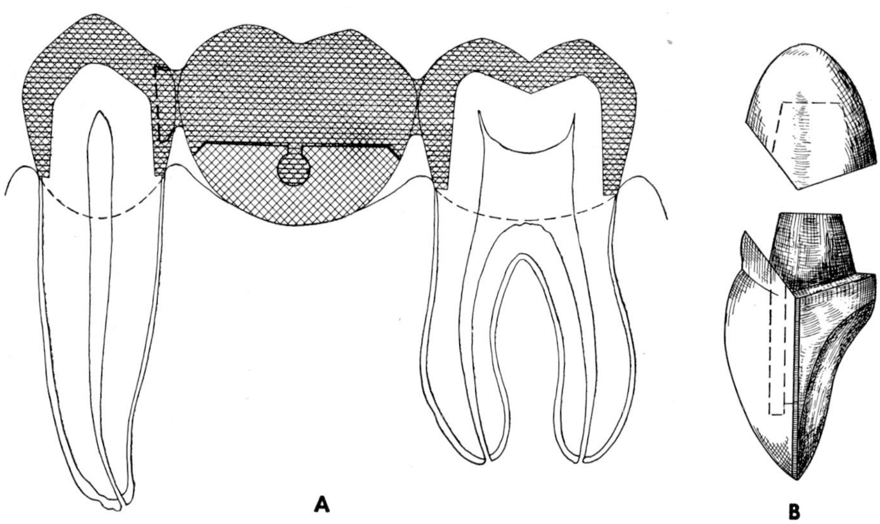

Fig. 30-41. A, Cross section of the bridge having pontic of type shown in Fig. 30-39, A. **B,** Anterior Steele facing; cast gingival part of pontic has gingival core with baked porcelain cap.

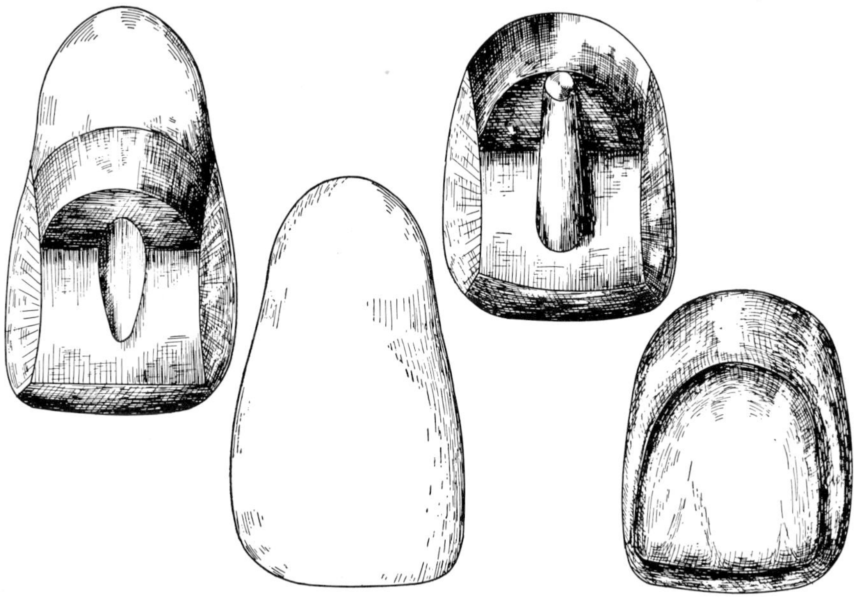

Fig. 30-42. Use of porcelain tube tooth as porcelain facing for anterior pontic. (From Odell, A. W.: D. Cosmos **66**:958, 1924.)

facing with a lingual casting that also has a gingival core extension over which a porcelain cap is fired.

USE OF PORCELAIN TEETH FOR PONTICS

In an effort to obtain the ultimate in esthetics, various other types of pontics have been suggested in which porcelain tube teeth are used in their construction. Odell[6] (Figs. 30-42 and 30-43) showed the use of detached post crowns for anterior as well as posterior teeth. Here, the incisal as well as the entire occlusal surface is covered with cast gold.

More recently Shooshan[7] has developed

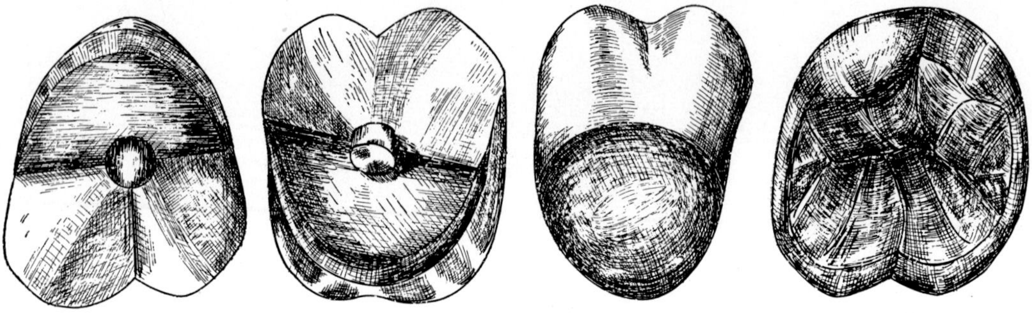

Fig. 30-43. Porcelain tube tooth used in posterior pontic. (From Odell, A. W.: D. Cosmos **66**:958, 1924.)

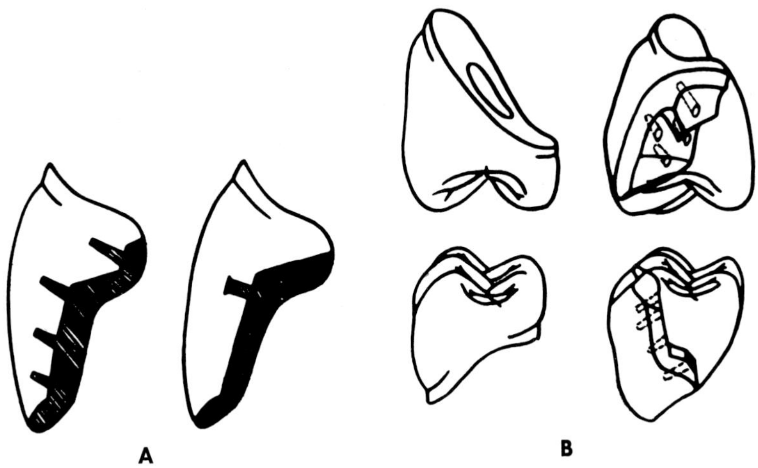

Fig. 30-44. Converting denture teeth into pontic facings by employing reverse-pin principle of retention. **A,** Holes drilled into porcelain; pins cast as part of gold back give retention to facing. **B,** Same principle applied to posterior teeth. (From Shooshan, E. D.: J. Prosth. Dent. **9**:284, 1959.)

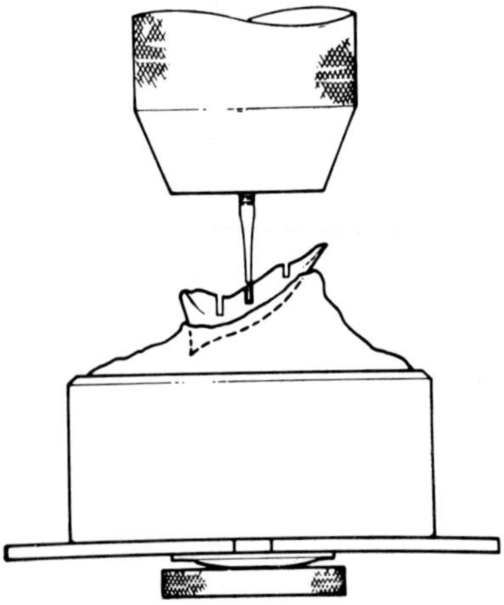

Fig. 30-45. Drilling holes in porcelain facing, using precision drill. (From Shooshan, E. D.: J. Prosth. Dent. **9**:284, 1959.)

the "reverse pin porcelain facing technic" to be used for both anterior and posterior pontics. Instead of retaining the porcelain facings by means of the two platinum pins being cemented into the gold portion of the pontic as is customary (Fig. 30-44, *A*), Shooshan depends upon drilling from three to eight parallel holes into the lingual aspect of the porcelain facing or tooth (Fig. 30-44, *B*). The holes are cut with a Tungsten carbide drill using a precision drill press (Fig. 30-45). The various steps in the conversion of a porcelain denture tooth into a "reverse pin porcelain facing" are shown in Fig. 30-46. The advent of aluminous porcelains has made new types of pontics available.[8, 9]

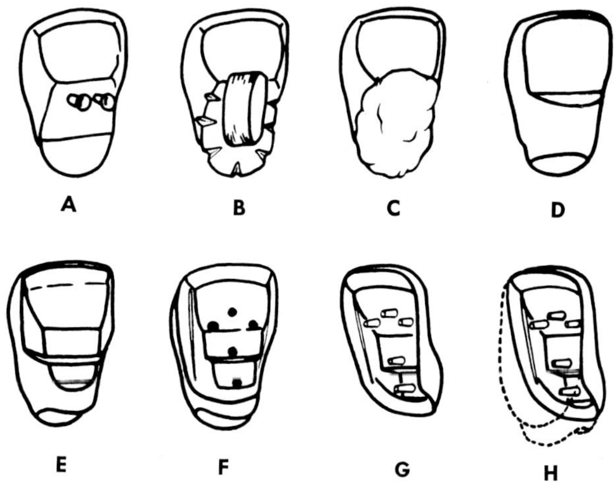

Fig. 30-46. Steps in fabricating reverse pin porcelain facing for central incisor. **A,** Denture tooth of appropriate size, shape, and color is selected. **B,** Pins are ground off, and lingual surface is ground to fit edentulous area. **C,** Porcelain is added to cervical end. **D,** Lingual surface is shaped to fit available space. **E,** Lingual surface is ground to provide space for adequate bulk of gold in backing. **F,** Retention holes are drilled into porcelain. **G,** Backing is waxed. **H,** Backing is cast and placed on facing. (From Shooshan, E. D.: J. Prosth. Dent. **9:**284, 1959.)

SELECTED REFERENCES

1. Ante, I. H.: The fundamental principles, design and construction of crown and bridge prosthesis, D. Items Int. **1:**215, 1928.
2. Dewey, K. W., and Zugsmith, R.: An experimental study of tissue reactions about porcelain roots for fixed bridgework, J. D. Res. **13:**459, 1933.
3. Clark, E. B.: The fixed bridge, D. Cosmos **64:**809, 1922.
4. Smith, D. E., and Potter, H. R.: The pontic in fixed bridgework, D. Digest **43:**16, 1937.
5. Klaffenbach, A. O.: The role of crown and bridge prosthesis in the field of restorative dentistry, J.A.D.A. **25:**536, 1938.
6. Odell, A. W.: The use of detached post crowns for anterior pontics, D. Cosmos **66:**958, 1924.
7. Shooshan, E. D.: Reverse pin-porcelain facing, J. Prosth. Dent. **9:**284, 301, 1959.
8. Columbus Manufacturing Company: The complete Steele's technic, Columbus, Ohio, 1969, Columbus Mfg. Co.
9. McLean, J. W.: A higher strength porcelain for crown and bridgework, Brit. Dent. J. **119:** 268, 1965.

GENERAL REFERENCES

Allison, J. R., and Bhatia, H. L.: Tissue changes under acrylic and porcelain pontics, J. Dent. Res. **37:**66-67, 1958.

Ante, I. H.: Construction of pontics, J. Canadian D. A. **2:**482, 1936.

Boucher, C. O.: Occlusion in prosthodontics, J. Prosth. Dent. **3:**635, 1953.

Boyd, H. R., Jr.: Pontics in fixed partial dentures, J. Prosth. Dent. **5:**55, 1955.

Brecker, S. C.: Clinical approach to occlusion, Dent. Clin. N. Amer. pp. 163-182, March, 1962.

Brice, S. E.: Construction of lower anterior pontics without display of gold, J.A.D.A. **27:**575, 1940.

Brill, N.: Influence of occlusal patterns on movements of the mandible, J. Prosth. Dent. **12:** 255, 1962.

Brill, N., Schubeler, S., and Tryde, G.: Aspects of occlusal sense in natural and artificial teeth, J. Prosth. Dent. **12:**123, 1962.

Brodie, A. G.: Occlusion, New York J. Dent. **29:**60, 1959.

Brotman, D. N.: Contemporary concepts of articulation, J. Prosth. Dent. **10:**221, 1960.

Bruce, R. W.: Clinical applications of multiple unit castings for fixed prostheses, J. Prosth. Dent. **18**(4):359, 1967.

Bruce, R. W.: Evaluation of multiple unit castings for fixed partial dentures, J. Prosth. Dent. **14:**939-943, 1964.

Cavazos, E., Jr.: Tissue response to fixed partial denture pontics, J. Prosth. Dent. **20**(2): 143-153, 1968.

Chasens, A. I.: Effect of traumatic occlusion on the periodontium and associated structures, and treatment by selective grinding of the natural dentition, Dent. Clin. N. Amer. pp. 63-77, March, 1962.

D'Amico, A.: Origin and development of the balanced occlusion theory, J. South. California D. A. **28**:317, 1960.

D'Amico, A.: Functional occlusion of the natural teeth of man, J. Prosth. Dent. **11**:899, 1961.

D'Amico, A.: New concept of functional occlusion of natural teeth in restorative dentistry, Texas D. J. **80**:4, 1962.

Draper, D. H.: Forward trends in occlusion, J. Prosth. Dent. **13**:724, 1963.

Engelberger, A., and others: Diagnosis and treatment of functional disturbances of the masticatory system, D. Abst. **6**:150, 1961.

Ewing, J. E.: Reevaluation of the cantilever principle, J. Prosth. Dent. **7**:78, 1957.

Fedi, P. F., Jr.: Cardinal differences in occlusion of natural teeth and that of artificial teeth, J.A.D.A. **64**:482, 1962; Inform. Dent. **44**:3601, 1962.

Gibson, T. D.: Theory of centric correction in natural teeth, J. Prosth. Dent. **8**:468, 1958.

Goransson, P., and Parmlid, A.: The pontostructor method and a new impression technique, J. Prosth. Dent. **15**:900-907, 1965.

Graf, H.: Occlusal contact patterns in centric relation and centric occlusion, I.A.D.R. **40**: 81, 1962 (abst.).

Granger, E. R.: Occlusion in temporomandibular joint pain, J.A.D.A. **56**:659, 1958.

Granger, E. R.: Establishment of occlusion, the articulator and the patient, Dent. Clin. N. Amer. pp. 527-529, Nov., 1960.

Harbard, W. C.: A simple accurate technic for immediate bridges, D. Digest **50**:500, 1944.

Harmon, C. B.: Pontic design, J. Prosth. Dent. **8**:496, 1958.

Hedges, P. G.: Occlusion as it relates to fixed restorations, J. Prosth. Dent. **13**:499, 1963.

Jackson, G. E.: Functional consideration of the problems of occlusion, Dent. Clin. N. Amer. pp. 355-368, July, 1959.

Jankelson, B.: Dental occlusion and the temporomandibular joint, Dent. Clin. N. Amer. pp. 51-62, March, 1962.

Jankelson, B.: Considerations of occlusion in fixed partial dentures, Dent. Clin. N. Amer. pp. 187-203, March, 1959.

Karlstrom, S.: Pontostruktormetodiken sedd i kasuistikens belysning (A follow-up examination of fixed bridges produced by the pontostructor method), Svensk. tandl. tidskr. **45**: 439-465, 1952.

Klaffenbach, A. O.: Bridge pontics with porcelain tips or saddles, D. Digest **38**:238, 1932.

Klaffenbach, A. O.: The role of crown and bridge prosthesis in the field of restorative dentistry, J.A.D.A. **25**:536, 1938.

Koivumaa, K. K.: Cinefluorographic analysis of the masticatory movements of the mandible, Suom. Hammaslääk. Toim. **57**:306, 1961.

Kurth, L. E.: Monoplane concept of occlusion, Dent. Clin. N. Amer., pp. 199-209, March, 1962.

Legett, L. J.: Bridge pontics, Internat. D. J. **8**:45, 1958.

Lindblom, G.: A new "pontic" construction for fixed bridges, D. Cosmos **75**:230, 1933.

Linkow, L. I.: Contact areas in natural dentitions and fixed prosthodontics, J. Prosth. Dent. **12**: 132, 1962.

Lucia, V. O.: Gnathological concept of articulation, Dent. Clin. N. Amer., pp. 183-197, March, 1962.

Ludwick, W. E.: Construction of immediate temporary bridge, J.A.D.A. **33**:486, 1946.

Meyer, F. S.: Generated path technique in reconstruction dentistry, part II: fixed partial dentures, J. Prosth. Dent. **9**:432, 1959.

Miska, M. G.: Simplified maxillary posterior pontic construction, New York D. J. **28**:276, 1958.

Moulton, G. H.: Importance of centric occlusion in diagnosis and treatment planning, J. Prosth. Dent. **10**:921, 1960.

Pine, B.: Pontics for gold-acrylic resin fixed partial dentures, J. Prosth. Dent. **12**:347-348, 1962.

Podshadley, A. G.: Gingival response to pontics, J. Prosth. Dent. **19**(1):51-57, 1968.

Podshadley, A. G., and Harrison, J. D.: Rat connective tissue response to pontic materials, J. Prosth. Dent. **16**:110-118, 1966.

Posselt, U.: Physiology of mastication; report of a seminar, J. West. Soc. Periodont. **9**:40, 1961.

Posselt, U.: Recent trends in the concept of occlusal relationship, Internat. D. J. **11**:331, 1961.

Posselt, U., and Posselt, A.: Some correlations between the occlusal pattern, function and pathology of the masticatory system, Parodont. **13**:3, 1959.

Posselt, U.: Occlusal relationship in deglutition and mastication, European Orthodont. Soc. Tr. **34**:301 (disc. pp. 311-315), 1958.

Posselt, U.: Occlusal rehabilitation, D. Pract. & D. Rec. **9**:255, 1959.

Poulton, D. R., and Aaronson, S. A.: Relationship between occlusion and periodontal status, Am. J. Orthodontics **47**:690, 1961.

Pruden, W. H., II: Occlusion related to fixed partial denture prosthesis, Dent. Clin. N. Amer. pp. 121-136, March, 1962.

Pruzansky, S.: Applicability of electromyographic procedures as a clinical aid in the detection of occlusal disharmony, Dent. Clin. N. Amer. pp. 117-130, March, 1960.

Ramsey, W. O.: Disorders of the mandibular articulation, J. Maryland D. A. **2**:9, 1959.

Ruhlman, D. C., and Richter, W. A.: A method for pontic stabilization in fixed partial denture construction, J. Prosth. Dent. **17**(4):401-405, 1967.

Schield, H. W.: The influence of bridge pontics on oral health, J. Mich. Dent. Assn. **50**(4): 143, 1968.

Schuyler, C. H.: Factors of occlusion to be observed in everyday practice, J.A.D.A. **57**: 221, 1958.

Schuyler, C. H.: Considerations of occlusion in fixed partial dentures, Dent. Clin. N. Amer., pp. 175-185, March, 1959.

Schuyler, C. H.: Evaluation of incisal guidance and its influence in restorative dentistry, J. Prosth. Dent. **9**:374, 1959.

Schuyler, C. H.: Factors contributing to traumatic occlusion, J. Prosth. Dent. **11**:708, 1961.

Schweitzer, J. M., Schweitzer, R. D., and Schweitzer, J.: Free-end pontics used on fixed partial dentures, J. Prosth. Dent. **20**(2):120-238, 1968.

Schweitzer, J. M.: Masticatory function in man; mandibular repositioning, J. Prosth. Dent. **12**: 262, 1962.

Selberg, A.: An exposition of pontics and their construction for fixed bridges, Illinois D. J. **9**:440, 1940.

Silverglate, L.: A simplified reverse-pin porcelain facing technique, J. Prosth. Dent. **18**:54, 1967.

Silverman, S. I.: Physiology of occlusion, Dent. Clin. N. Amer., pp. 3-17, March, 1962.

Smith, D. E.: Improved porcelain facing design for fixed prosthesis, J. South. California D. A. **23**:34, 1955.

Staffanou, R. S., and Thayer, K. E.: Reverse pin-porcelain veneer and pontic technique, J. Prosth. Dent. **12**:1138, 1962.

Stallard, H.: Physiology of chewing, J. Dist. Columbia D. Soc. **34**:9, 1959.

Stein, S. R.: Pontic-residual ridge relationship: a research report, J. Prosth. Dent. **16**:251-285, 1966.

Stern, R. H.: Dental occlusion; an evaluation of the canine function theory, J. South. California D. A. **30**:348, 1962.

Stuart, C. E.: Why dental restoration should have cusps, J. South. California D. A. **27**: 198, 1959.

Stuart, C. E., and Stallard, H.: Principles involved in restoring occlusion to natural teeth, J. Prosth. Dent. **10**:304, 1960.

Tinker, E. T.: Sanitary dummies, D. Rev. **32**: 401, 1918.

Tylman, S. D.: Anatomic form and function as registered and related to restorative dentistry, Illinois D. J. **25**:221, 1956.

Vaughan, H. C.: Occlusion and the mandibular articulation, Dent. Clin. N. Amer., pp. 37-50, March, 1962.

Weinberg, L. A.: Prevalence of tooth contact in eccentric movements of the jaw: its clinical implications, J.A.D.A. **62**:402, 1961.

Whiteside,, W. D.: Practical mandibular anterior pontic, J. Prosth. Dent. **9**:119, 1959.

Wing, G.: Pontic design and construction in fixed bridgework, D. Pract. & D. Rec. **12**: 390, 1962.

Zander, H. A.: Principles of occlusal adjustment, J. Tennessee D. A. **41**:303, portrait, 1961.

Chapter 31

Gold alloys and soldering operations related to crown and fixed partial prosthodontics

PRINCIPLES OF METALLOGRAPHY AS APPLIED TO DENTISTRY

The ability to interpret the physical phenomena of dental golds is contingent to a degree on a knowledge of the structure of pure metals and their alloys. In order to understand the aggregates, it is necessary to be familiar with the structure and properties of the constituents.

Space lattices

It may be stated that a crystal of metal is that microscopic or submicroscopic volume of metal within which all atoms or molecules have assumed a definite geometric arrangement throughout the grain and that has been allowed to develop without interference so the boundaries of the crystal may have formed into a normal geometric pattern.

A crystalline grain is similar to a crystal in that the internal arrangement of atoms and molecules is the same in both. The difference between the two is that in the case of the crystalline grain, surface boundaries of the grain have been distorted from the regular geometric surface pattern of the crystal, through competition of surrounding grains for material during the formation of the grain.

Material at the boundary of a crystalline grain is usually considered to be stronger and more resistant to the effects of stress than that within the interior of the grain. Slip planes appear within the interior of the grain considerably before they extend to the grain boundaries. This explains perhaps, why small grains are desirable—they interpose more grain boundaries to the path of rupture. (See Fig. 31-4.)

The pattern showing the geometric relation of one atom to another in a crystal is known as the space lattice; the simplest arrangement is the cube (Fig. 31-1). The most common cubic type is the face-centered, which has one atom in each corner and one in the center of each face (Fig. 31-2, *A*). The other type is the body-centered, with one atom at each corner and one in the center of the cube (Fig. 31-2, *B*). In addition to these, there is the hexagonal close packed type (Fig. 31-3). The first two are of special interest to the dentist, since most of the noble metals belong to the first or face-center type. These metals whose crystal have their space lattices arranged on the face centered cubic type of atomic relationship are known to be very ductile and good conductors of heat and electricity. The many phenomena of the physical metallography of the so-called solid metals may be more readily comprehended if we

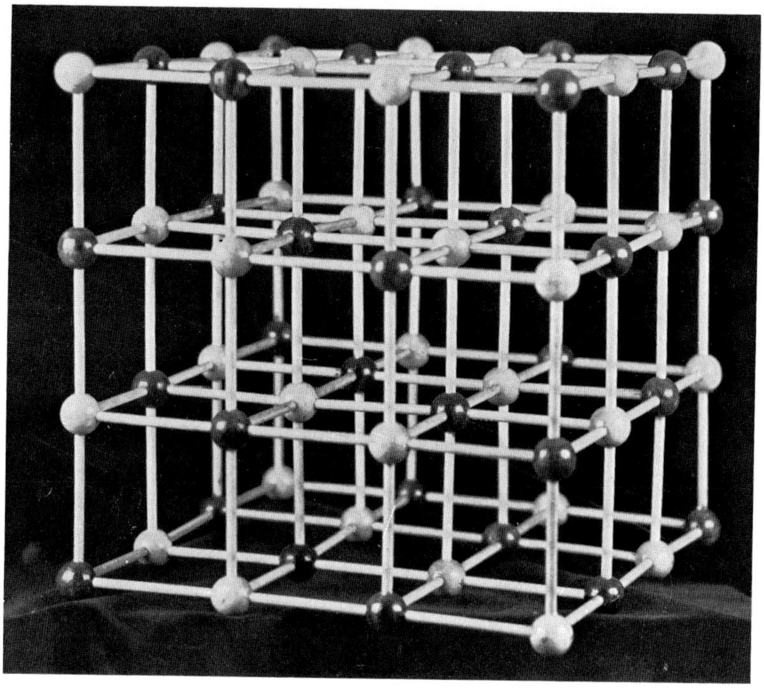

Fig. 31-1. Author's model of cube type of space lattice.

A

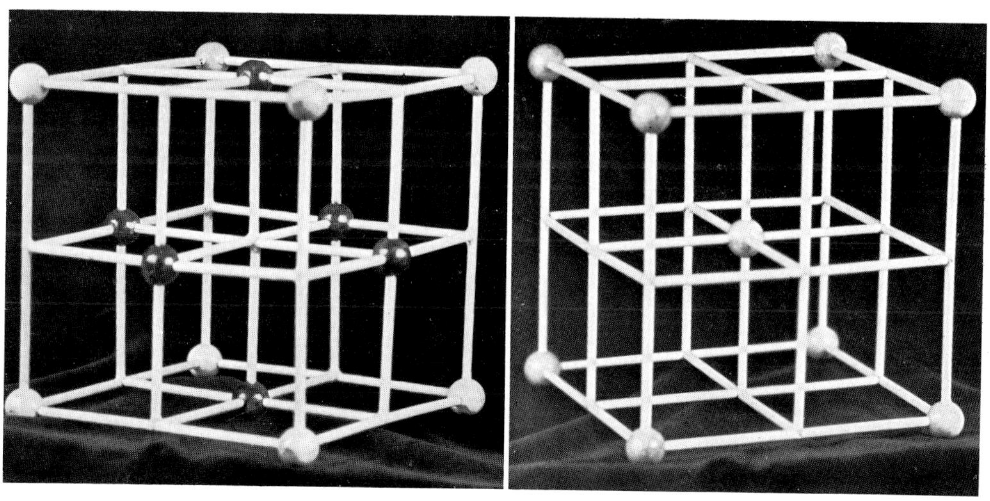

B

Fig. 31-2. **A,** Author's model of face-centered space lattice. **B,** Author's model of body-centered space lattice.

visualize these atoms under proper accompanying heat conditions.

Slip planes

The grain size may be changed by cold working the metal. When this is done, one series of atoms moves along another series of atoms in the crystal along certain planes of weakness called "slip planes" (Fig. 31-4). Face-centered crystals have many slip planes; hence their metals have a high elongation. Face-centered grains appear to have more potential planes of weakness (along which slip planes may develop under stress) than do body centered grains. Hence metals with this type of crystalline structure are usually more ductile than others. It is believed that when slippage occurs within the crystalline planes of a grain, stray atoms or molecules are trapped within the interstices of the normal lattice, thus causing a hardening and strengthening of the material, with a corresponding loss of ductility.

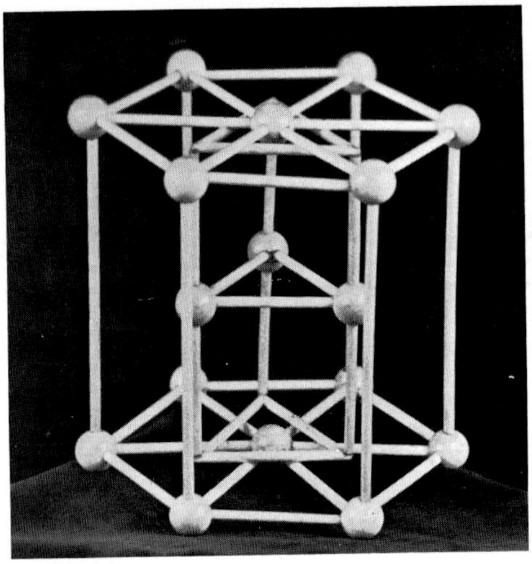

Fig. 31-3. Author's model of hexagonal close-packed type of space lattice.

Pure metals

A pure metal, such as gold, having only one phase in the solid state varies only in the size and shape of its grains, the controlling factors having been mentioned previously. The use of pure gold in dentistry is very limited, owing to certain of its characteristics. Its extreme malleability and lack of response to heat treatment preclude its general use in cast or wrought appliances. Being a pure metal, it solidifies at a single, constant temperature, which makes it a rather difficult material to use when definite and sharp castings are required. It has been found that such castings are more susceptible to "shrink spot" porosity because there is no freezing range during which additional molten metal may be fed into the mold during solidification, which is possible when certain alloys are used. The low proportional limit and ultimate tensile strength, together with a Brinell hard-

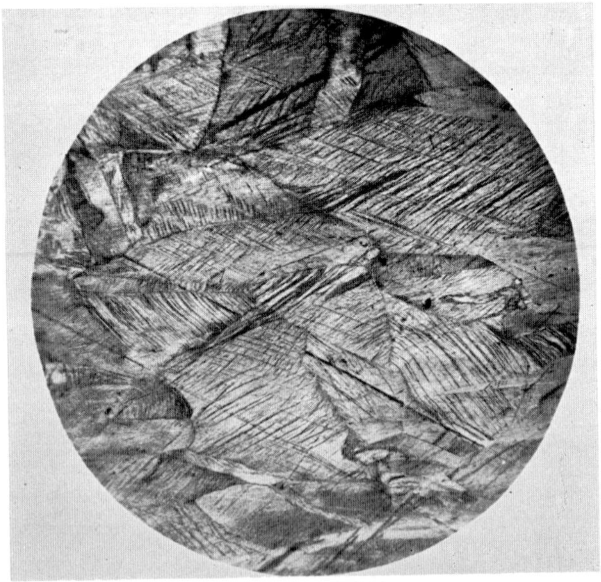

Fig. 31-4. Worked metal showing slip planes.

ness number below 50, make pure gold very limited in its application.

There has been a tendency on the part of some dentists to appraise dental golds only on the basis of carat or fineness. The Bureau of Standards took into consideration the intrinsic value of dental golds when it drew up its specifications, but it did not overlook the fact that, important as the precious metal content of an alloy might be, the ability of such an alloy to resist corrosion in the oral fluids and its suitability, physically and mechanically, for a particular use were more important.

GOLD ALLOYS

To meet the specific and exact requirements of present-day dentistry, it was found necessary to develop alloys of gold that would meet these specifications. It has been determined by Harder[1] that, by using a 10 percent variation of the forty metals, it is possible to obtain 8,039,460 different alloys. Dental gold alloys contain at least two metals, and sometimes as high as seven or eight, among which are included, in addition to gold, the following: copper, silver, platinum, palladium, and nickel. The diversity and complexity of many golds of the past lead one to believe that the bases of their formulas were largely empiric and that their value was largely determined by the market price of the precious metals used. Today, dental gold manufacturers include in their organizations highly trained and well-qualified research staffs whose duty it is to develop alloys to meet the specific requirements of the profession. Reliable manufacturers are cooperating with the Bureau of Standards for the protection of the dentist. The dentist should also cooperate, for his own protection as well as that of his patient.

Types of metal alloys

When two or more metals are fused together, three possible conditions may result, depending on the degree of atomic attraction between the elements.

Distinct separation of each metal. If the degree of attraction between like atoms is greater than that between the unlike, there will not be a close union of the two metals. Each element retains its identity and there will be present two physically distinct phases. Lead and aluminum form such an alloy, if it may be called that.

Metallic compounds. On the other hand, the attraction between the atoms of unlike metals may be so great that they react in definite atomic proportions to form definite metallic compounds. Copper and aluminum form the compound $CuAl_2$; copper and gold, CuAu and Cu_3Au. They are characterized by the fact that they form one phase, possess a distinct crystalline form, usually quite complex, and in many of their properties are different from the constituent metals. Compounds, just as pure metals, have a definite melting temperature, which is usually quite high and sometimes above that of the individual constituents. They are extremely hard and brittle, but they play an important part in the hardening of dental golds when subjected to heat treatment. Two intermetallic compounds are formed in the copper-gold alloys, CuAu and CU_3Au (Fig. 31-5).[2] The first compound contains approximately 75 percent of gold by weight, while the second contains only 50 percent; consequently, the first is of chief interest to us. Copper-gold alloys are solutions in the liquid state as well as in the solid state; but, as the temperature begins to drop slightly below 400° C. (752° F.), if sufficient time is allowed, the compound CuAu begins to form in those alloys whose gold content is from 65 to 90 percent by weight. If the alloy is heated and quenched above this temperature, no compound is formed and the alloy remains soft and workable. For many years, the dental profession took advantage of the changes in the physical properties of copper-gold alloys when

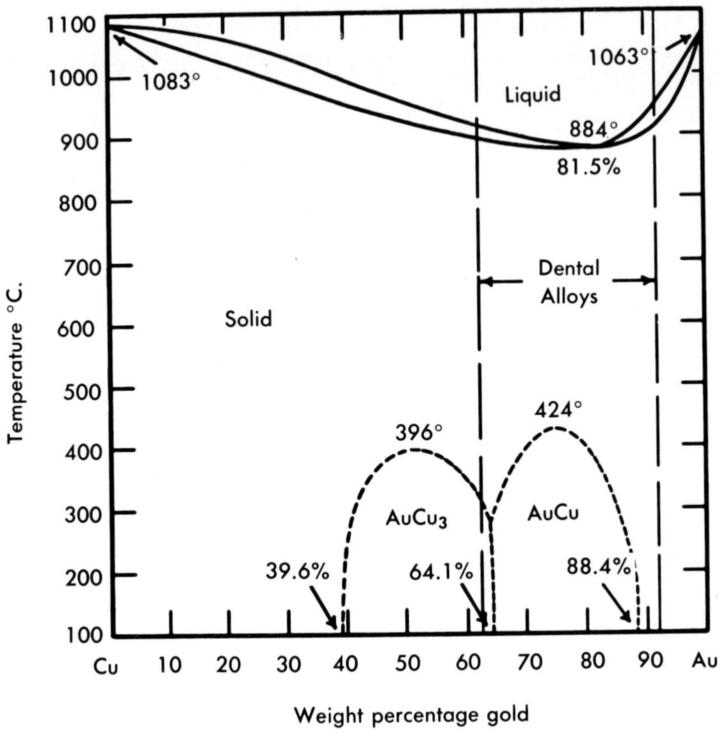

Fig. 31-5. Phase diagram for gold-copper alloys. (Courtesy F. A. Peyton.)

treated in this manner, but the scientific explanation was developed by Kurnakos in 1916.[3] More recently, Wise[7] has shown that the compounds PdCu and PtCu are important in the precipitation hardening of the quaternary dental alloys of the systems Pt-Au-Ag-Cu and Pd-Au-Ag-Cu.

Solid solutions. The third possibility that exists as a result of bringing two or more metals together is the formation of solid solutions. In this event the unlike atoms have a greater affinity than the like atoms, but not of a sufficient degree to form compounds. The constituents of such an alloy are true solutions in both the liquid and the solid states, and the atoms of the constituents are interchangeable in the crystalline structure. The element whose space lattice persists is the solvent; the other, the solute. Solid solutions do not follow any valence laws but merge in any proportions. They likewise merge their individual properties so that there is a gradual variance from 100 percent properties of one to 100 percent of the other. The gold-copper and the gold-platinum alloys are solid solutions with the added compounds formed in the lower temperatures. The structure of the solid solution crystal appears homogeneous. The addition up to a certain point of a solute to the solvent of a solid solution generally hardens and strengthens the alloy. The maximum hardness usually occurs where one space lattice changes over to another. It has been suggested that possibly there is an atomic dispersion of the components in solid solutions. When the addition of one metal to another continues to form a solid solution, it has been found that the maximum hardness of the solid solution is attained when 50 atomic percent of each metal has been included.

Difference between solid solutions and pure metals. There is one distinct difference between solid solutions and pure metals, compounds, and eutectics. The latter freeze at a constant temperature; whereas, a solid solution freezes or melts through a range of temperature. When the percentage of solute is very small, the solid solution may freeze very much like a pure metal; but, as the percentage of the solute is increased, a freezing temperature range is established within which solidification takes place. It is this characteristic that makes solid solutions so acceptable for the casting of dental appliances. There is an interval of time during which some of the metal entering the mold starts crystallizing, while additional molten alloy is still available.

This, with other means at the dentist's disposal, enables him to eliminate shrinkage porosity to a great degree. The first crystals to freeze out are richer in the metal whose addition raises the freezing temperature, leaving a melt richer in the metal that lowers its freezing temperature. After the solution cools slightly, other crystals are formed, but they are of a slightly different composition from the first. Consequently, when the entire mass is solidified, there is a difference in the composition; it is not homogeneous—hence the necessity for proper heat treatment of the alloy to obtain uniform diffusion.

Gold-copper alloy

The copper-gold system is one of the important dental alloys. The two metals form a continuous series of solid solutions above 400° C. (752° F.). Below this temperature, the compounds CuAu and Cu_3Au also form. The solid solutions crystallize with the face-centered cubic arrangement of atoms. At approximately 75 percent by weight of gold and a temperature of 885° C. (1625° F.), the solution passes through a point where the liquid and solid lines meet. Otherwise, the usual temperature range prevails. To become workable, an alloy should be heated and quenched above 450° C. (842° F.). If a hard alloy is desired, heat treating at slightly above 300° C. (572° F.) is necessary, resulting in the formation of compounds. Alloys containing less than 68 to 75 percent by weight of gold are not indicated for use in the mouth.

Specifications of alloys

Every dentist should be qualified to select the proper gold for his restorations. To do this, he must be able to decide what demands will be made on the prosthesis under service conditions, and second, to determine what materials possess the necessary properties to fulfill the requirements. Today, it is not necessary to compromise the type or design of a dental structure because of inferior materials or uncertainty as to their physical properties. Manufacturers now specify the minimum precious metal content and the quantitative behavior of the metal under load. In fact, were a dentist to ascertain the exact time, amount, and location of the various forces to which an appliance would be subjected, he could select materials and so design the structure as to meet these requirements to a nicety. Physical properties of the materials could be selected to give a maximum of service with a minimum of bulk. The art of restorative dentistry could more nearly be made an exact science. (See Chapters 39 and 40).

Although the dental profession does not yet utilize sufficient detailed biophysical data to make such an analysis of oral conditions, most practitioners are able to judge in a general way whether the appliance will be subjected to great loads. If, therefore, the dentist understands the properties of available alloys and certain laws of structural engineering, he is in a position to select intelligently the materials and design that will meet the demands made on them during construction and subsequent service in the mouth. Possessing a fundamental knowledge of their physical properties also enables the dentist to make a comparative selection of alloys of different manufacture.

Classification of inlay casting golds

To assist the dentist in his selection, the Bureau of Standards, in cooperation with the manufacturers, has classified inlay casting golds into four general types: Type I, A for the soft, Type II, B for the medium, Type III, C for the hard, and Type IV, D for the very hard.

In the Type I, A group are included those alloys having a minimum precious metal content of 83 percent and a Brinell hardness number of 40 to 75 percent, but with a very low yield point and a high elongation. Type II, B has a precious metal content of at least 78 percent, a Brinell hardness number of 70 to 100, a yield point minimum of 22,000 pounds per square inch, and an elongation of 18 percent. Type III, C contains metals of 78 percent precious metal content, a Brinell hardness number of 90 to 140, a yield point of 27,000 pounds per square inch, and an elongation of 12 percent. Type IV, D contains metals of 75 percent precious metal content, Brinell hardness of 130 to 200, tensile strength of 90,000 PSI, and an elongation of 2 to 10 percent. Each group is characterized by certain properties. Type I, A is very soft and ductile, permitting a great deal of burnishing, but it has the disadvantage of being difficult to cast and has a tendency to flow and to deform under stress.

Type II, B is harder, but with a reduced elongation, which makes this type suitable for small castings where the loads will be moderate and the bulk of material sufficient for strength.

Type III, C has a high Brinell hardness number, indicating extreme hardness, and a high tensile strength and proportional limit. These golds are indicated for average bridge retainers that will be subjected to normal loads.

Type IV, D has a very high Brinell hardness number and a high tensile strength with lowered ductility and toughness. These alloys are indicated for thin castings and bridge retainers, subject to extremely high loads of all kinds.

Physical properties of alloys

Some manufacturers have developed wrought alloys with a Brinell hardness number of 300 to 400 and a tensile strength in excess of 150,000 pounds per square inch. The tensile properties of a dental gold usually determined are ultimate tensile strength, proportional limit, and percentage of elongation. Ultimate strength indicates the load at which the alloy breaks and is usually expressed in pounds per square inch. This indicates the amount of resistance that a metal will offer before it ruptures. When the percentage of elongation is taken into account with ultimate strength, an index of the possible amount of cold work that can be tolerated by a structure is given. It is sometimes said that dental appliances are not subjected to direct tension in the mouth. It cannot be denied that every time a piece of metal is adjusted by bending, a part of the structure is subjected to a stretching force or tension. Similarly, we find that when forces are exerted on a bridge, one surface may be under compression, but the other may be under tension.

The determination of only the ultimate tensile strength, without a knowledge of the proportional limit and the percentage of elongation of a metal, would give us only a limited insight into its properties. Proportional limit is the point in the stretch of a metal where the increase in length ceases to be proportional to the increase in load. Percentage of elongation measures the increase in length, between its unstressed length and rupture, of a gauge length, marked on the test bar before load was applied. The proportional limit of a metal indicates that unit stress at which the initial permanent deformation takes place. It also indicates the resistance of a metal to any permanent deformation, such as occurs when clasps or wires are bent. High proportional limits should be found in metals used for clasps, thin bridge retainers, bars, or connectors, and other parts that will be subjected to extreme forces. Fortunately, most metals having a high proportional limit also have a high ultimate strength. A low proportional limit metal is sometimes indicated in a casting that is to be burnished, but even then an effort should be made to obtain the highest ultimate tensile strength possible.

Elongation is an index of the amount that a metal can be bent, swaged, burnished, or otherwise permanently deformed before breaking. Alloys with an elongation of less than 1 percent are extremely brittle and of little dental use. The normal range of percentages of elongation, for casting golds, extends from about 22 percent or more for soft alloys or for high-strength alloys in the softened condition, to about 4 percent in the heat-hardened condition. Alloys having high elongation are usually soft. In selecting a material for clasps that will call for adjustments, it is well to select one having considerable elongation.

The product of percentage of elongation plus ultimate tensile strength indicates the toughness of a material, i.e., high elongation with high ultimate strength gives a tough metal. A high ultimate strength with low elongation gives a brittle metal, while high elongation with low ultimate strength are characteristic of a very soft metal. It can be seen that materials covering a wide range of hardness and other properties for required services are at the disposal of the dentist.

Gold alloys and their specifications

The following formulas for gold alloys, together with their specifications of physical properties (Tables 31-1 to 31-4), are

Table 31-1. Specifications for dental golds, Types IA, IIB, and IIIC

Casting golds	*Composition*	*Physical properties*	*Values*		*Fusion temperature*
Type IA inlay gold					
Gold	84⅓	M.P.*			1786° F.
Pt	1	B.H.N.	65		
Ag	11	Y.P.	11,000		
Cu	3⅔	U.T.S.	34,000		
		Elong.	22%		
Type IIB inlay gold					
Gold	80	M.P.			1722° F.
Pt	2	B.H.N.	92		
Ag	12	Y.P.	22,500		
Cu	6	U.T.S.	45,000		
		Elong.	18%		
Type IIIC inlay gold					
Gold	74	M.P.			1758° F.
Pt	3				
Pd	2		*Quenched*	*Oven-cooled*	
Ag	10	B.H.N.	118	188	
Cu	10	Y.P.	31,000	57,000	
Zn	1	U.T.S.	50,500	80,000	
		Elong.	16%	4%	

**M.P.*, melting point; *B.H.N.*, Brinell hardness number; *Y.P.*, yield point; *U.T.S.*, ultimate tensile strength; *Elong.*, elongation.

Table 31-2. Type IV, D bar, clasp, saddle, and bridge retainers

Casting golds	*Composition*	*Physical properties*	*Values*		*Fusion temperature*
Gold	67.25	M.P.*	*Quenched*	*Oven-cooled*	1706° F.
Platinum	4.25	B.H.N.	140	225	
Silver	12.00	Y.P.	39,500	72,000	
Copper	11.00	U.T.S.	73,500	111,000	
Zinc	2.00	Elong.	10-14%	2-4%	
Palladium	3.50				

**M.P.*, melting point; *B.H.N.*, Brinell hardness number; *Y.P.*, yield point; *U.T.S.*, ultimate tensile strength; *Elong.*, elongation.

Table 31-3. Specifications for dental gold solders

	No. 1 18 carat .650	*No. 2 20 carat .739*	*No. 3 22 carat .802*
Gold	65	74	80.2
Silver	15	11	8.3
Copper	12½	10½	8.5
Base metal alloy	7½	4½	3
Total	100	100	100

Table 31-4. Group I—regular high-grade solders

Solder	*Approximate range (° F.)*	*Solder*	*Approximate range (° F.)*
14 (416 Fine)	1295 to 1400	18 (615 Fine)	1365 to 1480
14 (437 Fine)	1260 to 1410	18 (625 Fine)	1360 to 1480
16 (500 Fine)	1300 to 1425	18 (650 Fine)	1380 to 1480
16 (530 Fine)	1315 to 1425	20 (667 Fine)	1406 to 1480
16 (560 Fine)	1330 to 1420	20 (708 Fine)	1415 to 1495
18 (585 Fine)	1370 to 1460	22 (750 Fine)	1440 to 1530
18 (600 Fine)	1340 to 1465	22 (802 Fine)	1485 to 1585

typical of the type of materials used today in practice.

HEAT TREATMENT

In the case of many gold alloys, predetermined heat handling of the alloy designed to produce desired physical properties is known as heat treatment. Some alloys may have their elastic strengths almost double from that of the soft ductile condition to the hard condition by proper heat treatment and may still retain enough toughness for necessary impact resistance.

These desirable ends are accomplished in gold alloys by carefully regulating, in the case of softening, the going into solid solution of certain chemical combinations in the alloy or, in the case of hardening, of regulating the falling out of solution of the same solutes or chemical compounds. These purposes may only be accomplished by careful attention to the heat conditions that will accomplish the desired ends. The quenching of gold alloys to soften them and quenching of some steels to harden them only reflects differences in the characteristics of the two metals.

Grain structure may be refined, in the case of many steels, through proper heat regulation. This is because steel is allotropic, i.e., exists in different space lattice forms at high and low temperatures. Gold alloys are not allotropic and do not have this possibility.

The base metal alloy as used only in these formulas consists of two parts zinc and one part tin or 66⅔ percent zinc and 33⅓ percent tin.

In order to soften a gold alloy that has been hardened either as a result of working or previous heat treatment, it is generally agreed that the structure be heated to 700° C. or 1292° F. and quenched. When an alloy is so treated, a relatively high degree of elongation, a low tensile strength, a low degree of hardness, and a low elastic limit are secured. As a result, a soft and weak metal is obtained. When an appliance is in this condition, it may be adapted, swaged, bent, and worked to a maximum degree without danger of fracture. It is not advisable to exceed a temperature of 800° C. or 1470° F. or to go below 400° C. or 752° F. before quenching.

Through the employment of a suitable tempering process, the appliance may be given a high tensile strength, medium elongation, a high elastic limit, and a high Brinell hardness number; this gives an alloy that is hard and tough. There are several methods of heat-treating alloys. By improper heat treatment there is often obtained a very brittle and useless structure. Improper heat handling may result in a relatively high ultimate tensile strength, a high hardness, and an elongation of less than 1 percent. This condition may result when a large casting is permitted to cool slowly in the investment. Such large appliances should, after a lapse of 10 minutes, be plunged in water.

Two methods of heat treatment

According to the hardening treatment developed at the Bureau of Standards and generally recommended, the structure after quenching is heated to a temperature of 450° C. or 842° F. and gradually cooled within 30 minutes to 250° C. or 482° F. This is usually done in an oven whose temperature and time may be controlled. It has been found that if an alloy subjected to this method of hardening develops the desired properties, similar effects may be obtained by the so-called age hardening, in which case the appliance is submitted to a specific temperature for a definite number of minutes for specific alloys, after which it is removed and immediately allowed to cool to room temperature. Most of the reliable gold manufacturers have determined age-hardening data for their specific alloys. This treatment can be given either in an air oven or in a liquid held at constant temperatures. Many investigators prefer and recommend the method of aging at fixed temperatures.

Shell made the following distinction between annealing, tempering, age hardening, and low temperature hardening:

"(1) Annealing is a heat treatment which softens the metal and is usually accompanied by a decrease in tensile strength or proportional limit, but an increase in elongation. (2) Tempering is a heat treatment which results in a reduction of the hardness, and 'tempering' is not a good term to use when referring to the type of heat treatment which takes place in gold alloys between 482° C. (900° F.) and 141° C. (300° F.). (3) Aging or age hardening is a heat treatment which occurs over a period of time, usually at room temperature. Aging is not a good term to use for this type of heat treatment, although it is preferable to 'tempering.' (4) Low temperature hardening is recommended for use in referring to the heat treatment of gold alloys. Although the temperature may be as high as 421° C. (800° F.), this is still a low temperature treatment as compared with annealing at 700° C. (1300° F.), or melting and soldering at temperatures exceeding 871° C. (1600° F.)."[4]

Results of heat treatment

The advantage of heat treatment is that, by developing the desirable qualities to a maximum, it is possible to construct appliances of minimum bulk and greater comfort and service at less cost.

In addition to the chemical changes taking place within solid metals, resulting in formation of compounds, by proper heat treatment the homogeneity of metals also can be modified. Solid solutions are seldom homogeneous when cast, but they are made so through diffusion when properly heat treated.

Many failures are the result of improper heat treatment, whether intentional or accidental. To avoid difficulties, it is advisable to adopt a standard method, preferably the one recommended by the manufacturer of the gold alloy.

SOLDERING

Two pieces of metal or alloy may be united by means of welding or by soldering. Since welding is rarely employed in dental operations, attention is directed to the soldering process. The operation of soldering may be performed either by the use of an intermediary metal or alloy or by the direct fusion of the two parts of the metal; the latter process is known as autogenous soldering. This method is employed primarily in fusing the ends of gold bands for crowns. The other method of soldering, which employs an intermediary metal or solder, is the one most generally used and consists of uniting two pieces of metal by means of a melted alloy, which fuses and adheres to the surfaces of the metals being united.

The composition of solders previously given is typical of the types used in dental practice.

Requisites of a solder

Skinner lists the following requisites for a satisfactory dental solder: "(1) It must not be corroded or tarnished by the mouth fluids. (2) Its melting point must be lower than that of the metal upon which it is employed, in order that the latter may not be fused during the soldering operation. (3) Its color should match that of the metal employed. (4) It should flow properly and smoothly over the surfaces of the parts being joined. (5) Its physical properties should be at least as good as those of the metal, in order that the joint may not be a source of weakness."[5]

Factors involved in successful soldering

In addition to the use of the proper solders, there are other factors that enter into the successful soldering operation. One of the first and most important considerations is the matter of cleanliness. The surfaces to be united by means of solder must be absolutely clean and free from metallic oxides, particles of soldering investment, and any contamination by the base metals, such as lead or tin from a metal working model. To assure the cleanliness and freedom of the gold retainers from base metal contamination, these should be thoroughly cleaned by boiling in one part acid to two parts water before they are assembled in the impression prior to running up the investment cast. It has also been found that solder flows more freely on a surface that is polished smooth than on one that is rough.

Another factor is the proper exposure of the area to be soldered by trimming away the investment in this area so that the soldering flame can be properly applied without overheating the investment, thus avoiding contamination from sulfur gases.

Use of flux and antiflux

Those surfaces that have been covered by sticky wax prior to their investment should have the wax removed by a stream of boiling water directed upon the surfaces to be soldered. While the gold parts and the investment are still warm, a small amount of petrolatum flux is applied to the surfaces to be soldered. Only a small amount of flux is needed to cover these surfaces. Fluxes are used primarily to cleanse and protect the surfaces against oxides. Among the more commonly used fluxes are borax or sodium tetraborate, potassium nitrate, or potassium carbonate and pulverized charcoal, also one suggested by Ryge[6]: dehydrated borax 56 percent, boric acid 36 percent, silica 8 percent. These are fused and ground into a fine powder, then mixed with petrolatum or alcohol.

Position of parts to be soldered

Another important factor to consider in soldering is the proximity of units to be soldered. The prime purpose of investing the two parts of a bridge in soldering investment is to maintain their relative positions while they are being united with solder. Because gold alloys expand when they are subjected to soldering temperatures, it is not advisable to have the proximal surfaces of the pontic and retainer in contact because, when heated, they expand and cause the investment to crack or the expansion warps the bridge out of line. For this reason it is suggested that a space be left between the two invested parts, of 0.005 to 0.001 inch increasing as the length of the component sections of the bridge are increased.

To assist the solder in bridging the space between the two parts, an occlusal spur is extended from the pontic over onto the marginal ridge of the retainer.

Perdigon and van Eepoel[7] suggested a technic for soldering a bridge whereby the step of investing is eliminated. After the retainers are waxed, a plastic or wax button is attached to the side of the pattern proximating the pontic area. After the crowns are cast, the pontic is carved in wax which is well secured to the buttons extending from the sides of the crowns. Next, round plastic sprues, 14-gauge, are attached to the occlusal surface of the cast crowns, and a 12-gauge sprue is attached to the wax pontic. All three sprues are connected together. The entire assembly is removed from the cast, invested, and cast. The cast assembly is replaced on the working model to verify fit; if satisfactory, flux and a small piece of solder are applied between the pontic and each crown. The assembly is removed and held over a Bunsen flame until the solder flows. The author claims a minimum of distortion and shrinkage by this method.

The soldering flame

The correct flame and its correct use are equally important in the soldering oper-

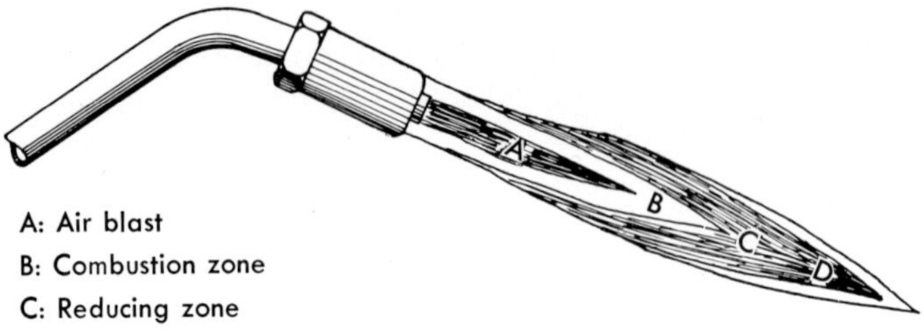

Fig. 31-6. Blowpipe flame and zones.

ation. In examining Fig. 31-6 of a flame, it will be noticed that there are several zones. The first, *A*, indicates the air blast coming from the center of the nozzle; *B* indicates the area of partial combustion where the air and the gas are mixed; zone *C* is the reducing zone or the deoxidizing flame and is usually represented as a pale blue color. This region may be readily located if a piece of oxidized copper or a penny is placed in the blowpipe flame, when it will be noted that the metal immediately brightens in the area covered by the flame in this zone. This zone contains highly heated but unburned hydrogen, which, when it contacts an oxidized surface or an oxide, combines with the oxygen and leaves the surface free of oxide. The tip or the end of the flame, *D*, represents the oxidizing flame or zone and is the area of complete combustion. The application of this part of the flame to the metal surfaces to be soldered results in their oxidation and the necessity of applying additional flux in order to clean the surface. The proper use or misuse of the soldering flame very often determines the success or failure of a soldering operation. In addition to the use of the proper flame, the parts soldered should not be exposed to unnecessary heat or maintained at a high temperature for a long time. The objective in soldering is to make the solder flow where it is required as quickly as possible and at as low a temperature as is consistent with the soldering operation. If the invested bridge or crown is heated correctly, i.e., a temperature of 1200 to 1300° F., before the blowpipe is brought to play upon the parts to be soldered, and if the parts are clean and properly fluxed, there will be little trouble in making the solder flow easily. Solder should be selected for each particular appliance so that its maximum melting range will be approximately 120 to 140° F. below the initial melting point of the parts soldered. The fusing range of solder from the solid to the liquid state should not exceed 100° F.

Results of excessive heat

If an excessively high melting range solder is used, requiring excessive heat, the surfaces of the two parts being soldered may also fuse to the point where the parts are excessively weakened. Fig. 31-7 shows solder flowed on wire, the flame having been removed as soon as the solder flowed. There was no overheating of the solder, and it will be noted that there is also no solution of the wire in the solder.

In Fig. 31-8 the same materials were used, but in this instance the solder was kept molten for 45 seconds after it had flowed on the wire. The marked solution of the wire can readily be seen, resulting in a very definite weakness in this area.

Solder usually comes from manufacturers in strip form. It may be used in this form when the lingual surface of a crown is being soldered or when it is possible to feed the strips continuously into the invested work. Where, however, small joints

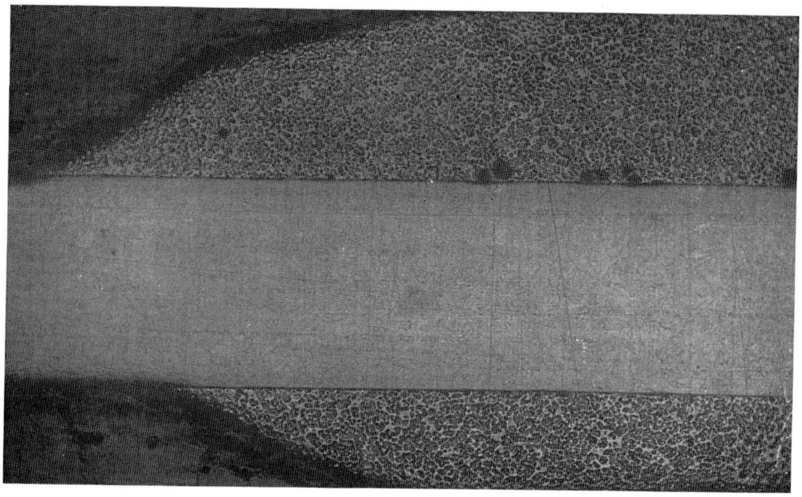

Fig. 31-7. Solder correctly applied to gold alloy wire; no overheating. (Courtesy J. M. Ney Co.)

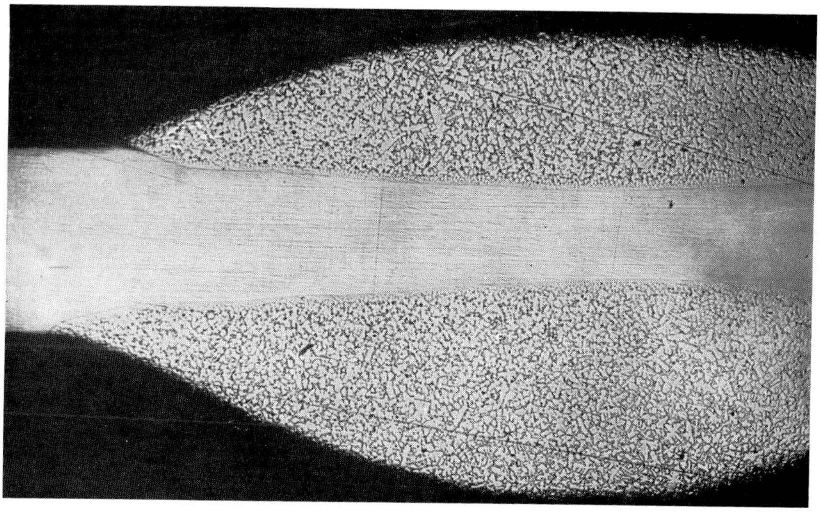

Fig. 31-8. Improperly soldered wire. Note solution of wire in solder. (Courtesy J. M. Ney Co.)

are to be made or narrow margins are to be soldered, the strips may be cut into small pieces, ⅛ or $\frac{1}{16}$ inch in length. These pieces are then taken up with soldering tweezers and carried to the exact location where the solder is to flow.

Position of invested crown or bridge

To assist the proper flow and placement of the solder, the crown or the bridge should be so invested that the molten metal will be carried to place by gravity. Furthermore, the bridge should be so invested that, after the wax is boiled out, the parts to be soldered can be easily exposed so that the flame has ready access to the surfaces to be soldered. It is extremely difficult to apply the reducing zone of the soldering flame into a deep pocket.

Temperature of investment

To solder successfully, the investment must be heated to a temperature not to exceed 1200 to 1300° F. Investment begins to give off harmful quantities of sulfur gases after a temperature of 1300° F. Higher temperatures could lead to contamination of the gold alloy contained in it. If long continued it may result in serious embrittlement. Until this temperature is reached, the blowpipe should not be applied to the exposed metal parts. Once the proper degree of temperature has been obtained, it will be found that the solder flows readily.

Because solder flows by capillary attraction, every effort should be made to have the contiguous parts within 0.005 to 0.01 inch of each other and still not in actual contact. On the other hand, it must be remembered that the weakness of a soldered joint increases in proportion to its increased width. Therefore, an excessive amount of solder should never be used.

Excessive use of flux

The excessive use of flux will result in a pitted soldered joint and a weak union. If the solder is exposed to an oxidizing flame, the base metal ingredients of the solder are oxidized, causing the solder to ball and not flow freely. The addition of flux and the use of the reducing flame will rectify this condition to a degree, but there is always danger of burning and overfusing the parts being soldered.

Location and amount of solder

In soldering a pontic to a retainer, the solder should be limited to the occlusal one-half region and should be circular in shape. Every effort should be made to confine the solder to the smallest possible area consistent with strength and to prevent its coming in contact with the margins of the retainers.

Occasionally, the surfaces to be soldered are not clean and, as a result, the solder surrounds this area, leaving an empty space between the two surfaces. Subsequently, during use, the bridge breaks at this point because of the lack of complete fusion of solder between the two contiguous surfaces.

PROCEDURES FOLLOWING THE SOLDERING OPERATION

After the bridge or the crown has been soldered, it should be set aside and allowed to cool for 15 minutes. The invested bridge may then be placed in tepid water, the investment removed, and the crown or the bridge examined to see if the solder has flowed where wanted and in a sufficient amount. If satisfactory, any excess is removed with stones and the joint polished with disks.

Pickling and contamination

Pickling is very important from the standpoint of discoloration. Many dentists use dirty acid in their pickling baths. The acid is used over and over without changing; consequently, it becomes discolored from the load of oxides removed from other castings. Pure acid is inexpensive, and the insurance against damage to the finish of the casting is amply worth changing the acid bath quite often.

When dirty acid is used for pickling, especially when the castings are allowed to lie in it for some time, the contaminated acid gets into small defects or pockets that lie near the surface having minute openings to the surface. These sometimes are not removed when the casting is cleaned and polished. Later, this embedded contaminated acid mixes with saliva, exudes, and spreads in a ring over the surface. These rings from numerous microscopic defects spread and finally meet to produce surface discoloration, causing concern to the patient and the dentist. A little attention to the cleanliness of the pickling solution will solve this problem.

Special tweezers should also be used that are not soluble in the pickling acids.

The prosthesis is then placed in an acid

dish and heated to the boiling point. It is then washed in water, after which it is tried in the mouth and the necessary adjustments made. If satisfactory, the bridge is given its final finish and polish, after which it is hardened by heat treatment in order to restore its desirable physical properties. After heat treatment, it is cleaned, dried, and ready to be permanently cemented.

SELECTED REFERENCES

1. Harder, O. E.: Modern dental metallography, Minneapolis, 1930, Burgess Roseberry Publishing Co., p. 28.
2. Peyton, F. A., editor: Restorative dental materials, ed. 3, St. Louis, 1968, The C. V. Mosby Co.
3. Kurnakos, N., Zemczuzny, S., and Zasedatelev, M.: Transformations in alloys of gold with copper, J. Inst. Metallurgy **15**:305, 1916.
4. Shell, J. S.: Advantages in the use of safe heat treating technics for gold alloys, D. Craftsman, **12**:6, 1938.
5. Skinner, E. W., and Phillips, R. W.: The science of dental materials, ed. 6, Philadelphia, 1936, W. B. Saunders Co.
6. Ryge, G.: Dental soldering procedures, Dent. Clin. N. Amer., p. 747, Nov. 1958.
7. Perdigon, G. J., and van Eepoel, E. F.: Minimizing solder joint warpage in fixed partial denture construction, J. Prosth. Dent. **7**:244, 1957.

GENERAL REFERENCES

Ady, A. B.: Effect of solidification time of the microstructure and physical properties of dental gold casting alloys, J. D. Res., **45**:921, 1966.

Asgar, K., and Peyton, F. A.: Flow and fracture of dental alloys determined by a microbend tester, J. D. Res. **41**:142, 1962.

Asher, H. H., and Comstock, J. A.: Some causes of variation in hardness of gold-copper castings, J. D. Res. **13**:407, 1933.

Bien, S. M., and Ayers, H. D., Jr.: Autoradiographs of solder joints with Fluorine, J. D. Res. **38**:428, 1959.

Bjorn, E.: Are fined-grained castings homogeneous?, Evensk Tandlak. T. **55**:73, 1962. (Sw.)

Bjorn, E., and Wennstrom, A.: Dental gold alloys and their properties under varying heat treatment, Svensk Tandlak. T. **55**:633, 1962. (Sw.)

Buckley, H. E.: Crystal growth, New York, 1951, J. Wiley and Sons.

Chatelain, J. L.: Removable bridges and removable fixed bridges (fixed detachable), Internat. D. J. **7**:563, 1958.

Coleman, R. L.: Physical properties of dental materials (III), D. Cosmos **68**:743, 1926.

Coleman, R. L.: Some effects of soldering and other heat treatments on orthodontic alloys, Internat. J. Orthodontia **19**:1238, 1933.

Council on Dental Research: American Dental Association adopts revision of American Dental Association Specification No. 5 for Dental Casting Gold Alloy, J.A.D.A. **62**:755, 1961.

Council on Dental Research: American Dental Association adopts revision of American Dental Association Specification No. 2 for Casting Investment for Dental Gold Alloy, J.A.D.A. **63**:317, 1961.

Dell, C. L.: Dental solders and soldering technic, Chron. Omaha D. Soc. **18**:302, 1955.

Dykema, R. W.: Study of the effects of certain variables on the comparative strengths of soldered and cast bridge joints, Alum. Bull. Indiana Univ. School Dent., March, 1962, p. 16 (abst.).

Eick, J. D., and Hegdahl, T.: Segregation in dental gold casting alloys, J. Dent. Res. **47**:1118, 1968.

Eick, J. D., and others: Chemical composition of dental gold casting alloy and dental wrought gold alloy, J. Dent. Res. **48**:1284, 1969.

Engel, F.: Soldering of fixed bridge-work without distortion, Internat. D. J. **7**:566, 1957. (abst.).

Fairhurst, C. W., and Ryge, G.: Effect of certain variables on the strength of soldered joints, I.A.D.R. **35**:109, 1957 (abst.).

Fusayama, T., and Ogata, K.: Casting shrinkages of inlay golds of known composition, J. Prosth. Dent. **16**:1136, 1966.

Going, R. E., and others: Marginal penetration of dental restorations by different radioactive isotopes, J. D. Res. **39**:273, 1960.

Hedegard, B.: Homogenization: a clinical study of its significance in crown and bridge prosthesis, Trans. Roy. Sch. Dent. (Sweden) **1**:3-26, 1958.

Hedegard, B.: Studies in crown and bridge prosthesis (homogenization of dental alloy castings; a clinical study), Tr. Roy. Schools Stockholm & Umea, no. 1, 1958, pp. 3-21.

Hollenback, G. M., and Skinner, E. W.: Shrinkage during castings of gold and gold alloys, J.A.D.A. **33**:1391-1399, 1946.

Jeffries, Z., and Archer, R. S.: Science of metals, New York, 1924, McGraw-Hill Book Co., p. 250.

Jeffries, Z., and Archer, R. S.: The slip interference theory of the hardening of metals, Chem. & Metall. Eng. **24**:1057, 1921.

Jelenko, J. F. and Co.: Crown and bridge construction: a handbook of dental laboratory procedures, ed. 5, New York, 1963, The Company.

Kaires, A. K., and Thompson, J. C.: Effect of heat treatment variables on the microstructure and hardness of a cast dental gold alloy, J. D. Res. **38**:888, 1959.

Kozak, S. F., and Ryge, G.: Porosities in dental gold castings, I.A.D.R. **34**:89, 1956 (abst.).

Kurnakos, N., Zemczuzny, S., and Zasedatelev, M.: Transformations in alloys of gold with copper, J. Inst. Metallurgy **15**:305, 1916.

Lain, E. S., and Caughron, G. S.: Electrogalvanic phenomena of the oral cavity caused by dissimilar metallic restorations, J.A.D.A. **23**:1641, 1936.

LeClaire, A. D.: Diffusion of metals in metals, Progr. Metal Phys. **1**:306-379, 1949.

Meyer, F. S.: Elimination of shrinkage and distortion at solder joints, North-West Dent. **37**: 113, 1958.

Meyer, S. S.: Elimination of distortion during soldering, J. Prosth. Dent. **9**:441, 1959.

Meyers, R. E., and Pfeiffer, K. R.: Effect of varying conditions on time required to cast gold under air pressure, J.A.D.A. **27**:530, 1940.

The Ney Gold Handbook, Hartford, Conn., The J. M. Ney Co., 1956.

Nielsen, J. P., and Tuccillo, J. J.: Grain size in cast gold alloys, J. D. Res. **45**:964, 1966.

O'Brien, W. J., and others: Wetting characteristics of dental gold solders, I.A.D.R. **40**:93, 1962. (abst.).

Perdigon, G. J., and Van Eepoel, E. F.: Minimizing solder joint warpage in fixed partial denture construction, J. Prosth. Dent. **7**:244, 1957.

Peyton, F. A.: Flexure fatigue studies of cast dental gold alloys, J.A.D.A. **21**:394, 1934.

Pokorny, D. K.: Fixed bridge failures, J. Michigan D. A. **43**:203, 207, 1961.

Reinfelder, K. F., Gervoir, W. J., and O'Brien, W. J.: Mechanical properties of high-fusing gold alloys, J. Prosth. Dent. **21**:523, 1969.

Ritze, T. E., and Thayer, K. E.: Bridge soldering procedure, Iowa D. J. **47**:11, 1961.

Ryge, G.: Dental soldering procedures, Dent. Clin. N. Amer., p. 747, Nov., 1958.

Ryge, G., Kozak, S. F., and Fairhurst, C. W.: Porosities in dental gold castings, J.A.D.A. **54**: 746, 1957.

Samuels, L. E.: A study of the deformed layer produced on metal surfaces of mechanical machining, abrasion and polishing operators, Electroplat. and Metal Finishing, **10**:279-285, 1957.

Schoolden, E. A.: Some notes on the joining of metals—soldering, D. Technician **14**:88, 1961.

Shell, J. S.: Advantages in the use of safe heat treating technics for gold alloys, D. Craftsman **12**:6, 1938.

Shell, J. S.: Some factors influencing specific gravity determination of cast gold alloys, J. D. Res. **45**:337, 1966.

Shell, J. S., and Hollenback, G. M.: Abrasion rate on gold castings, J. Calif. Dent. Assn. **42**:5, 1966.

Shell, J. S., and McCormack, D.: Roentgenographic examination of dental gold alloys, J.A.D.A. **18**:2193, 1931.

Skinner, E. W.: Effect of nucleation of gold alloys, I.A.D.R. Abst. No. 188, 1966, p. 85.

Skinner, E. W., and Lasater, R. L.: Abrasion of dental gold alloys, J. Dent. Res. **21**:103, 1942.

Soremark, R., Freedman, G., Goldin, J., and Gettleman, L.: Structure and microdistribution of components of gold alloys, J. Dent. Res. **45**:1723, 1966.

Souder, W. H., and Paffenbarger, G. C.: Physical properties of dental materials, Washington, D. C., 1942, U. S. Govt., National Bureau of Standards Circular C 433, pp. 69, 80.

Steinman, R. R.: Warpage produced by soldering with dental solders and gold alloys, J. Prosth. Dent. **4**:394, 1954.

Swartz, M. L., Phillips, R. W., and El Tannir, M. D.: Tarnish of certain dental alloys, J. D. Res. **37**:837, 1958.

Tammann, G.: Metallography, New York, 1925, Chemical Catalog Co., p. 264.

Tylman, S. D.: Gold alloys: an evaluation of research data in relation to clinical requirements, J.A.D.A. **21**:1426, 1934.

Vines, R. F.: Heat treatment of dental gold alloys, J.A.D.A. **25**:1817, 1938.

Winslow, M. B.: Fixed splint and bridge assembly, J.A.D.A. **51**:47, 1955.

Wise, E. M., Crowell, W. S., and Eash, J. T.: Role of platinum metals in dental alloys, Am. Inst. Min. & Met. Engineers **99**:363, 1932.

Chapter 32

Assembling retainers and pontics utilizing connectors (nonrigid and rigid)

CONSTRUCTING CONNECTORS

With the plaster core holding the finished pontic in position as described in Chapter 30, the pontic is fastened with sticky wax on its lingual surface to the adjacent retainers in order to verify the correctness of its alignment, adaptation to the ridge, and esthetic features. With posterior bridges this may be done satisfactorily on the model, but it is much better done directly in the mouth in anterior bridges. Occasionally a slight shifting or discrepancies occur during construction of the core and fitting of the backings to the porcelain facings, which necessitates a realignment of the pontics; this may best be verified by trial in the mouth.

If everything is satisfactory, the next step is the construction of the connectors. As stated previously, there are two methods by which pontics may be united with retainers: (1) directly on a model made of soldering investment, or (2) by the use of registration cores or indexes that enable the dentist to remove the pontic and retainers from the model and solder them together, after which they are replaced on the model.

When only one tooth is restored in a fixed restoration, the pontic may be soldered to one retainer only, after which the soldered portion and the remaining retainer are placed back on the abutments, another occlusal plaster index is taken, and the final soldering operation is performed. The reason given for not soldering both terminals at one time is that occasionally a drifting of the teeth occurs in the mouth between the time that the impression for the bridge is taken and the time when the bridge is ready to be soldered on the investment model; hence the advisability of two or more soldering operations.

The soldered connector

The soldered joint should not fill the entire vertical interproximal space occlusogingivally; it should be rounded in form and occupy the region of the contact area, i.e., it is limited to the occlusal half of the interproximal space. The soldered joint should not extend too far buccally or lingually, since it is necessary to have a correct lingual embrasure between the pontic and the retainer.

When a bridge has two pontics, these preferably should be carved and cast as one unit, thus eliminating one soldered joint.[1] The soldered connector should be smooth, highly polished, and without sharp fissures so that the patient can easily keep this area clean.

Special care should be taken in constructing the soldered connector not to flow the solder buccally or lingually too near the margins of the retainers, since the solder might flow inside of the retainer; flowing the solder too near the margins would also prevent the accurate finishing of the margins of the retainer after the bridge is cemented. However, the precaution must be taken to have a sufficient amount of metal through the soldered area vertically to be able to withstand the forces of mastication.

Use of core or index

With the facing and the cast pontic fitted and held in position in the labial plaster core (Fig. 30-31), the pontic is waxed to the adjacent retainers; a lingual core, either of modeling compound or of dissolving plaster, is made; in posterior teeth the lingual core is made to include the occlusal surfaces also (see Chapters 30 and 39).

When the lingual core has hardened, the labial plaster core is removed, after which the lingual core with the pontic is withdrawn from the working model. Should the pontic remain on the model, it is removed and replaced in the lingual core in its correct position. The retainers are likewise removed from the working model and placed in their respective positions in the core.

The porcelain facing is then removed from the cast pontic, after which the gold pontic casting and the two retainers are carefully waxed to place in the core; some sticky wax is then carefully flowed between the retainers and the pontic in the area to be soldered. If a crevice or opening exists on the labial aspect between the pontic casting and the retainer, this should be carefully filled with soft carding wax, care being exercised not to flow the wax on the labial surface of the cast pontic; here again the wax should be kept sufficiently away from the margins of the retainer to prevent any solder from flowing too closely. It must be kept in mind that solder fills in all space previously filled with wax. Next, the labial surface of the cast pontic is painted with antiflux to prevent solder from flowing onto this surface; it is well also to paint the outer surface of the bridge retainer along its margin, a strip about 0.5 mm. in width, to prevent solder from approaching the margin too closely.

If the metal pins were used instead of graphite pins when casting the pontics, these should be reinserted into the pinholes as a precautionary measure against solder flowing into the holes and to help to stabilize the position of the pontics in the investment during the soldering operation.

INVESTING THE BRIDGE

A small amount of soldering investment is then mixed and applied to the labial or buccal surfaces of the retainers and the pontic. Some investment is also placed on a glass slab, and the core, with its retainers and pontic covered with the soldering investment, is inverted and settled into the investment on a glass slab. In investing, care must be exercised that the soldering investment is worked into all angles and against all surfaces, in order later to control the flow of the solder during the soldering operation.

After the investment has set, which usually takes from 20 to 30 minutes, the lingual core is removed. If modeling compound is used, the compound is softened by placing the invested case and core in a pan of warm water until the compound is softened to a point where it may be removed without disturbing the cast pontic or the retainers. If dissolving plaster has been used for the lingual core, it is placed in a pan of cold water that is gradually heated until it reaches the boiling point, whereupon the plaster disintegrates, leaving the pontic and the retainers clean in the investment.

If any sticky or soft carding wax remains in the interproximal space between the cast pontic and the retainer, this should be removed by pouring a small stream of boiling water on it. This will leave the lingual interproximal space between the pontic and the anterior retainer exposed from the incisal edge to the gingival ledge; on the posterior teeth, the interproximal space will also be exposed occlusally between the adjoining proximal ridges.

PREPARING THE BRIDGE FOR SOLDERING

The invested bridge, still warm from the boiling water, is now prepared for the initial soldering. (See Chapter 31 for a discussion of soldering and its metallurgical aspects.) A small amount of petrolatum flux is placed between the retainer and the cast pontic. Only enough flux should be applied to those surfaces to be soldered. It is not necessary to have more flux than is needed, because this causes pits to develop in the finished soldered joint. The invested bridge is then slowly dried over a small flame, after which the heat is raised until the investment and bridge are brought to a dull red heat. Meanwhile, the solder has been selected and cut into suitable pieces or strips, fluxed, and laid aside, ready for use. Usually 22-carat solder is used for this initial soldering operation.

If the investment and bridge are heated uniformly and to a sufficiently high temperature, little difficulty is experienced in flowing the solder evenly and quickly. If they are insufficiently heated, however, the solder fails to flow and is likely to spheroid and oxidize.

Another method of soldering is to place the fluxed bridge in a furnace; it is heated gradually to the melting temperature of the solder used. The invested bridge is then removed from the furnace to a soldering block, fluxed, and solder quickly applied to the joint. Using a reducing flame, the solder will flow instantly and cleanly.

Some advocate that the individual units of a bridge be assembled in proximal contact with each other to prevent the contraction that accompanies a soldered joint. It must be remembered that gold and its alloys expand when they are heated to soldering temperature, and, if these parts contact each other, it is likely that the expansion may cause the dislodgment of the units or the cracking of the investment. Hence, it is advisable to leave approximately a 0.005-inch space between the two proximal metal surfaces to be soldered together. Because it is difficult to bridge a gap with solder, it is recommended that an occlusal slot be cut in the marginal ridge of the retainer and a spur of wax extended from the pontic into this groove, which is then reproduced in the gold casting. The spur then bridges the 0.005-inch gap into which the solder follows, uniting the two parts (Fig. 32-4).

UNITING THE PARTS OF THE BRIDGE

In those bridges having two pontics, it is advisable to solder one pontic to each of the retainers, leaving the space between the two pontics to be soldered later. Better still, the two pontics may be cast as one unit, thus eliminating one solder joint.

When the soldering operation has been completed, it should be observed whether the solder has filled the space completely and whether it extends labially and occlusally into the desired areas. If satisfactory, the bridge is allowed to cool, after which it is cleaned, boiled in acid, and washed; it is then ready for a trial in the mouth.

TRIAL IN MOUTH

If the restoration is extensive and complex, the two sections are examined to see whether the articulation and the occlusion are satisfactory; any major adjustments and corrections can also be made at this time. Likewise, the porcelain facing is inserted into the cast pontic to verify its adaptation to the ridge. Any adjustments of contour or outline should be made at this time. If found necessary to grind the porcelain pontic on surfaces that come in permanent contact with the mucosa, these surfaces should be reglazed. At this time, also, the soldered joint and the bridge retainers are shaped and polished to a fine sandpaper finish.

TAKING FINAL IMPRESSION

If the bridge fulfills the requirements of occlusion, contour, and esthetics, the two parts are united with wax or with self-curing resin in the mouth and a small plaster impression is taken of the assembled parts, applying the plaster to the lingual surfaces in an anterior bridge, while the lingual and occlusal surfaces are included in a posterior bridge. This impression may be taken in a small teaspoon tray or with a flat piece of perforated tray material.

In taking this impression, the correct relationship of the assembled parts must not be disturbed. When the plaster has set, the impression is removed and the units of the bridge are removed from the abutments and reassembled in the impression in their correct position. The porcelain facing is again removed and the two parts of the bridge are waxed to the impression; a small amount of sticky wax is flowed into the space to be filled with solder. The labial surface of the cast pontic, as well as the margins of the retainer, is again covered with antiflux, and the plaster impression is given a coat of separating medium. After it has dried, a small amount of soldering investment is mixed and poured against the labial surface and around the entire exposed portions of the two parts of the bridge.

A simpler method is the use of a self-curing resin instead of the plaster index. After the two segments fit satisfactorily, the resin is applied with the brush-add-on technic to the open joint and extended over the two bridge sections in sufficient amount to lock them rigidly in a splint. When the resin has hardened completely in the mouth, it is removed with the bridge parts securely locked to each other. This is invested in soldering investment. When the investment has set completely it is placed in the burn-out muffle, where the resin will be eliminated. The exposed metal portions are fluxed and soldered in the usual manner.

FINAL SOLDERING OF BRIDGE

If a plaster core was used, this is permitted to set, after which the plaster index is carefully removed, leaving the lingual and occlusal surfaces in posterior teeth exposed, ready for the application of flux and solder. When the invested case has been heated to the proper temperature, solder is flowed between the cast pontic and the bridge retainer, the same precautions being exercised as previously. When cool, the finished bridge is removed from the soldering investment, cleaned, boiled in acid, washed and carried to the mouth for final fitting and verification of occlusal relationships in centric, lateral, and protrusive movements of the mandible. If the contact areas are satisfactory, the bridge is then ready for the final finish, polish, and heat treatment, which will be discussed later.

CEMENTING THE BRIDGE

After proper heat treatment, the bridge is cleaned and dried and the porcelain tip facings are next cemented on. The bridge and the porcelain facings are thoroughly cleaned and dried, and cement of the proper color is mixed to a thick, creamy consistency. With a small, sharp instrument, the pinholes in the cast pontics are filled with the cement; at the same time the lingual surface of the porcelain pontic and the buccal surface of the cast pontic are covered with a thin layer of the cement. The porcelain pontic is now carried to position, centered, and firmly pressed to place. Pressure is maintained on the facing for several minutes until complete crystallization of the cement has occurred. The excess cement is removed, and the gold margins surrounding the porcelain are finished with fine polishing disks.

In thin anterior teeth where the platinum pins of the facing extend lingually through the cast pontic, the pins should not be cut off before the facing is cemented to place. These are left long so that they may be riveted after cementation.

Before the facing is cemented, the opening of each pinhole on the lingual surface is slightly countersunk with a No. 600 bur in such a way that the cuts incline toward the center of the lingual surface. After the facing is set, the protruding ends of the pins are bent toward each other on the lingual, and the excess is ground off with stones and smoothed flush with the lingual surface, thus riveting the facing to the casting.

THE BROKEN-STRESS PRINCIPLE

Clinical evidence of over 40 years indicates that when all factors are equal, the bridge having a rigid or soldered connector is more successful percentagewise, both biologically and mechanically, than one employing a so-called broken-stress.

There are times when the so-called broken-stress principle is employed in fixed partial denture prosthesis, in which case one of the connectors between the pontic and the retainer is made nonrigid.

Nonrigid connector

The nonrigid connector consists of two parts: (1) The keyway, sometimes referred to as the "dovetail," is a depression cut in one of the retainers, usually the anterior one—the keyway is widest at its occlusal opening, from which point it gradually tapers gingivally, terminating in a flat gingival seat (Fig. 32-1); (2) the key, sometimes called the "lug," is a tapering piece of metal, usually cast, which fits the keyway exactly and which is attached to and

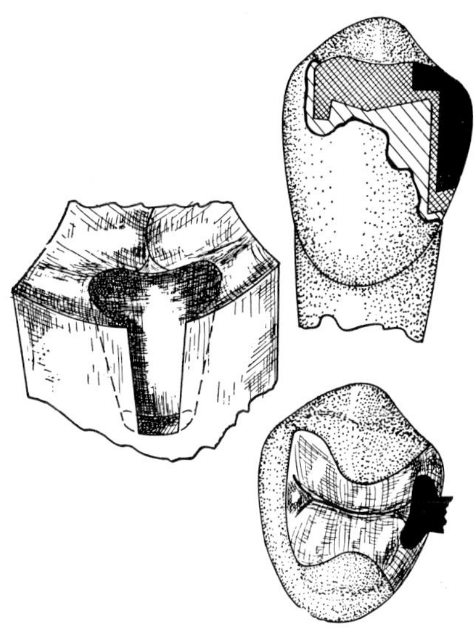

Fig. 32-1. Oval-shaped keyway.

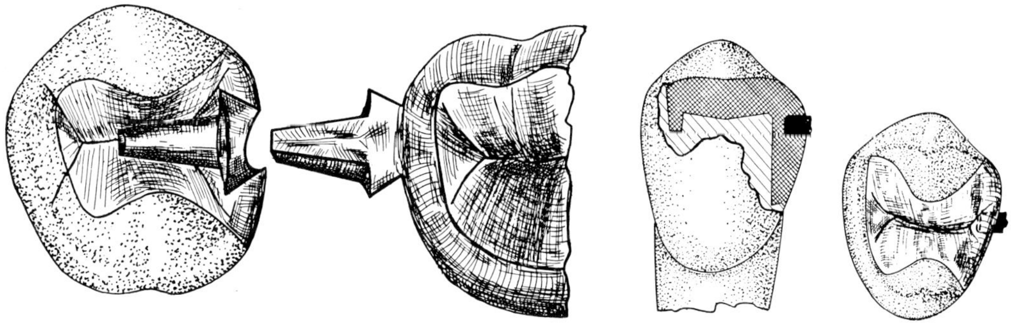

A B

Fig. 32-2. A, Occlusal extension type of keyway broken-stress connector with occlusal extension. (After D. Smith.) **B,** Subocclusal type of key and keyway broken-stress connector.

made a part of the pontic. An occlusal extension is often added to the key in order to give more stability to the connector and to place the stress in the center or in the long axis of the tooth (Fig. 32-2, *A*).

Advantages of its use. It is claimed by some that whenever two abutment teeth, one at each end of a bridge, are soldered rigidly together, there is a slight interference with the physiologic, individual movement of both teeth. In addition, any forces imposed upon one of the abutments are said to be transferred directly to the other through the medium of the intervening soldered pontic. A review of Chapters 10 and 11 is suggested at this point.

An advantage claimed for its use is one of mechanics and esthetics. Its use allows the employment of the simpler types of retainers, which require less cutting of tooth structure and which usually result in a more esthetic type of restoration. The simpler types of inlay retainers are usable because they are not called upon to withstand the displacing forces present when the pontic is soldered directly to the retainer. The use of this type of connector also permits the dentist to finish and cement one retainer before the balance of the bridge is cemented. It is used mainly when two terminal abutment teeth incline toward each other, preventing the vertical insertion of a rigidly soldered restoration.

Because torque is one of the most harmful forces to which an abutment may be subjected, the nonrigid, sometimes also called the "semifixed," connector has been advocated because it does not transmit the torsional forces from the bridge proper to the anterior retainer.

Notwithstanding some advantages, the broken-stress principle is not universally applicable in fixed partial denture prosthesis. It should not be used in connection with bridges having long spans; it is primarily indicated in short-span bridges, especially those restoring one tooth.

Its use is indicated more in the posterior region than in the anterior part of the mouth. Even under those conditions favorable to its use, it is contraindicated if one of the abutment teeth is unduly loose in its socket. Using the broken-stress principle in loose teeth will only hasten the time when the abutment will loosen completely and the bridge will be lost.

When used, the nonrigid connector should not have an unlimited movement of the posterior abutment; neither should there be more movement than the tooth normally has. The use of the nonrigid connector is contraindicated in the anterior four-, five-, and six-tooth bridges, particularly if the preparations of such bridges can be paralleled so that a fixed bridge can be constructed. Where only one tooth is replaced, the key and keyway principle functions satisfactorily provided it uses the precision type key.

When the opposing natural teeth strike the abutment in which the keyway lies and the distal extension of the bridge and its distal abutment have no opposing occlusion or an occlusion with a mucosa-borne partial denture, the broken-stress connector should not be employed; the bridge should be soldered rigidly at both ends. If this is not done, the bridge and its key will egress occlusally out of the keyway.

When employed, the nonrigid connector is usually placed in the distal surface of the anterior retainer; this is usually the weaker of the two retainers involved in the bridge.

When used in anterior teeth, the broken-stress may be placed on the lingual or in the proximal surfaces; when used in posterior teeth, it not only involves the proximal, but occasionally also extends well into the occlusal surface.

Nonprecision types of broken-stresses

There are several types of nonprecision broken-stress connectors, the simplest of which consists of a semicircular or triangular groove cut in the retainer with the key resting in this groove. Although this may be used on either the anterior or the posterior teeth, it is rarely employed because its shape does not afford much resistance to the displacement of the key from its keyway. Formerly it was used extensively on the posterior teeth, but, because of its inherent retentive weakness, it has been supplanted by the type that employs a proximal, tapering key and keyway (Fig. 32-1).

The keyway. The keyway or dovetail type of nonprecision broken-stress may be of several different shapes. It may be round, T-shaped, or oval; the ones most generally used are the T-shaped and the oval varieties. The keyway is usually prepared in the anterior retainer and is made with walls that diverge very slightly from the gingival to the occlusal, while the buccal, lingual, and gingival walls are dovetailed (Fig. 32-1).

In cutting the keyway, an effort should be made to have it twice as long occlusogingivally as it is wide buccolingually, and it should be at least 1 mm. wide at the gingival wall.

In those bridges which restore a molar or two pontics, an occlusal extension is made mesially from the key and terminates in the center or the long axis plane of the tooth (Fig. 32-2, *A*).

In order to limit the amount of occlusal movement of the key in its keyway, it is slightly modified, as will be explained later, in such a way that it can be clinched in position after the bridge has been cemented (Fig. 32-5).

There is another type of nonrigid connector sometimes employed known as the proximal, subocclusal rest (Fig. 32-2, *B*). In this type a slightly tapered opening is made in the proximal surface of the anterior retainer slightly below the marginal ridge in the region of the contact area. Into this is placed a tapering pin or key, which is an integral part of the cast pontic. The amount of movement is controlled largely by the degree of taper given to the wall of the keyway. Although this type of connector prevents any occlusal displacement, it is not generally used because the key is easily dislodged distally in the event of a slight posterior drift of the bridge and because it necessitates the cementing of both retainers at one time when the bridge is set.

This latter type of broken-stress is sometimes modified by forming a sphere or disk which is engaged in the keyway in such a way that it cannot be pulled out distally (Fig. 32-6).

While the technic of constructing the broken-stress type of connector is not difficult, it is accurate and exacting in its requirements.

Steps in constructing nonprecision keyway. The first step is the preparation of the keyway in the anterior retainer. While this may be done in the casting, a great deal of time, material, and effort can be saved by shaping the keyway in the wax pattern before it is cast, and by performing the final finishing in the casting.

The distal surface of the wax pattern of the retainer to receive the keyway should be slightly overcontoured and the surface slightly flattened to allow a greater bulk for the cutting of the keyway. Provision is also made for the keyway by modifying the tooth preparation in its distal surface with a so-called box type preparation.

While it is desirable and customary in simple operative restorations to contour the marginal ridge of an inlay to simulate the natural contour, where the casting is used for a broken-stress keyway, the marginal ridge is built to a higher occlusal plane and its margin is left straight and is not rounded. This is done so that a sufficient amount of gold is left in the cast retainer after the keyway has been cut to permit the clinching of the key in the keyway after the bridge is cemented (Fig. 32-5).

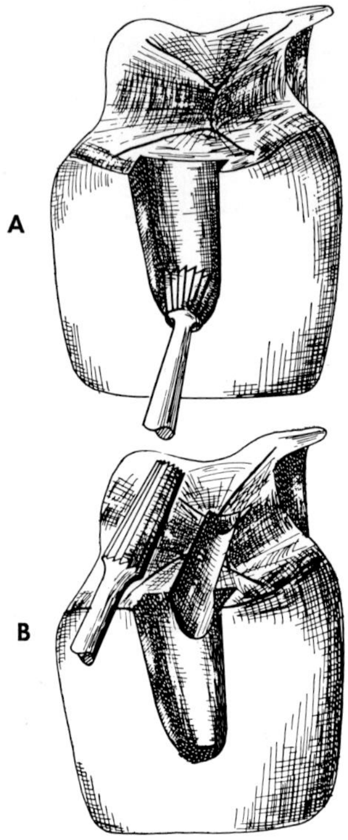

Fig. 32-3. Instrumentation used in preparing occlusal extension type of stress-breaker. (After D. Smith.)

The cutting of the dovetail or keyway in the wax may be done while the wax pattern is in the tooth or the removable die. In either event a line should be scratched on the proximal surface of the wax pattern indicating the direction in which the posterior retainer withdraws from its abutment. Where the access is good, it is possible but difficult to cut the keyway in the pattern while it is in the mouth. Therefore, it is recommended that a sprue former be attached to the complete wax pattern in its occlusoproximal portion and withdrawn from the tooth.

A groove extending occlusogingivally is now cut in the axial surface, using a No. 700 or 701 cross-cut fissure bur until the bur has been carried into the wax to the depth of its diameter. It is then laid aside, and with an inverted cone bur, No. 37, 38, or 39, depending upon the size of the bridge and the retainer, the groove made by the No. 700 bur is extended laterally in a buccal and lingual direction so that these walls are undercut. An inverted cone bur is then carried gingivally so that the gingival wall is also undercut as shown in Fig. 32-3, *A*.

During the cutting of the keyway in the wax pattern, every effort should be made not to distort the wax pattern or to injure its margins. When any doubt exists, it is better to return the wax pattern to the tooth and again verify its fit and marginal relationship.

Metal or carlion keys are available that can be waxed into the wax pattern (Fig. 35-7); after the casting is made, the key is removed by boiling in acid or with a bur, leaving the desired shape of keyway.

As previously stated, the keyway should be approximately twice as deep as it is wide buccolingually, and it should be 1 mm. wide at the gingival wall. The divergence of the keyway occlusally from the gingival wall should be very slight, inasmuch as an excessive flare will make it difficult to clinch the key into position after the bridge is finished.

After the proximal portion of the keyway has been prepared, the retainer is then invested, cast, and tried in the tooth and its fit is verified.

The keyway in the casting is now smoothed by milling it out with a finishing bur or with a dull inverted cone bur. The walls of the keyway must be highly polished, smooth, and free from all undercuts or nodules.

Where desirable, the next step is the preparation of the occlusal extension with a No. 700 or 701 cross-cut, tapering fissure bur. The groove is placed in the center of the sulcus and is carried mesially until it terminates at or slightly beyond the center of the tooth. As shown in Fig. 32-3, *B*, the bottom of the groove is rounded and is wider toward the keyway than it is at its mesial extremity.

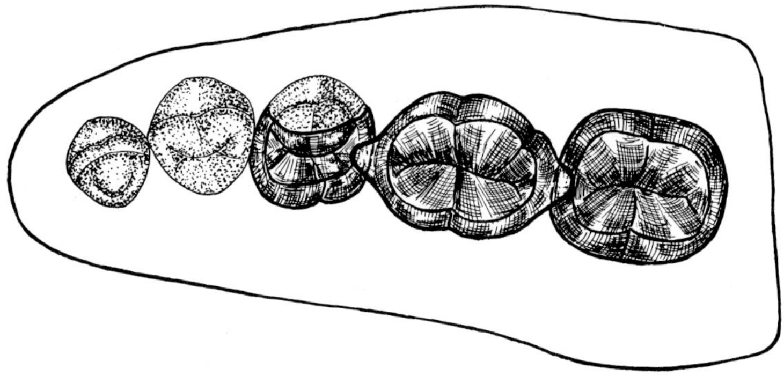

Fig. 32-4. Cast pontic with two occlusal extensions resting in depressions cut in two retainers.

Later, when the key is cast as a part of the pontic, it will have the shape shown in Fig. 32-2, *A*.

Construction of nonprecision key (broken-stress). To construct the cast key that fits into the prepared keyway, the prepared retainer is placed in the anterior tooth and the other retainer is seated in the posterior abutment; the bite, impression, and shade are taken and the working model is constructed.

After the pontic facing has been glazed and the occlusal and lingual portions have been completed in inlay wax, it is temporarily laid aside. The keyway in the anterior retainer is now slightly lubricated and a small amount of softened inlay wax is pressed into it, care being taken not only that the wax fills the keyway, but also that all its margins are completely covered. The wax is then chilled and the excess removed, and the remaining part is carved to complete contour with the exception of the marginal ridge, which is left high and straight up. With a small explorer, the waxed key is now gently removed and replaced to make certain that there are no undercuts present and that the wax has been forced into all the sharp angles of the keyway.

The waxed pontic is replaced on the working model and the wax key is replaced in the keyway and then attached to the wax pontic by passing a heated small, round instrument between the two pieces of wax.

After cooling, the excess wax is removed and any additional contour developed that may be necessary.

The sprue is carefully attached and both wax pontic and key are now removed in one piece from the working model. If the union between the two parts is satisfactory, the facing is removed, graphite points are inserted into the pinholes, and the wax pontic with its key is invested and cast.

After the casting has been cleaned, the graphite or metal points removed, and the facing tried for fit, the pontic is returned to the working model, whereupon the key should slide into the keyway without any difficulty. If it does not seat easily, it should not be forced, but should be reexamined to see if there are any globules or rough areas in the casting. If any exist, these should be carefully removed and the casting replaced. Usually it will go to place with finger pressure or with a slight tap of the mallet. It should also be tested for any lateral movement.

Completing the bridge. If the fit is satisfactory, the pontic is ready to be attached to the posterior retainer. As previously suggested in the construction of rigid, soldered connectors, a slight occlusal depression is cut through the marginal ridge into which extends an occlusal spur from the pontic (Fig. 32-4). With the key on the mesial margin and the small gold spur extending on the distal margin of the pontic, it is easily seated into its correct relationship with the model and the two retainers.

Although it is possible to solder the distal connector directly on the model, it is suggested that the two retainers be removed from the model and seated in the natural teeth in the mouth, and that the cast pontic be examined directly in the mouth for correct occlusal relationship and fit of the porcelain pontic against the ridge. If the key and keyway fit accurately, it will be found that the pontic maintains its correct position without any difficulty. If the pontic does not hold tightly, it may be held lightly with some sticky wax while a plaster impression is taken with a tongue blade. The technic of using self-curing resin may also be employed instead of plaster. The two retainers and the pontic are then removed and seated in the plaster impression, and a model of soldering investment is poured; the distal joint is then made with a soldered connector.

Cementing the bridge. When soldered and cleaned, the two parts of the bridge are returned to the mouth and verified for fit. If satisfactory, the bridge is finished, polished, and heat treated prior to cementation of the facings. In cementing a broken-stress type of bridge, the anterior retainer is first cemented in the tooth, finished, and polished, after which the distal portion of the bridge is cemented.

Clinching the key. Before doing so, however, Smith[2] suggests that the key be so prepared that it can be clinched in position after the bridge has been cemented. This is accomplished as follows: with a small gold file or with a small knife-edged disk, a small, triangular portion of the metal is cut away on each side of the key from the occlusal surface gingivally to one-third the occlusogingival height of the key. This will leave a small, triangular space between the key and the margins of the keyway; arrows point to relieved areas (Fig. 32-5). After the posterior portion of the bridge has been cemented to place, this small, triangular space is eliminated by turning in the margins or edges of the keyway with a mallet and gold plugger points in such a way that the key is now grasped or clinched in the keyway

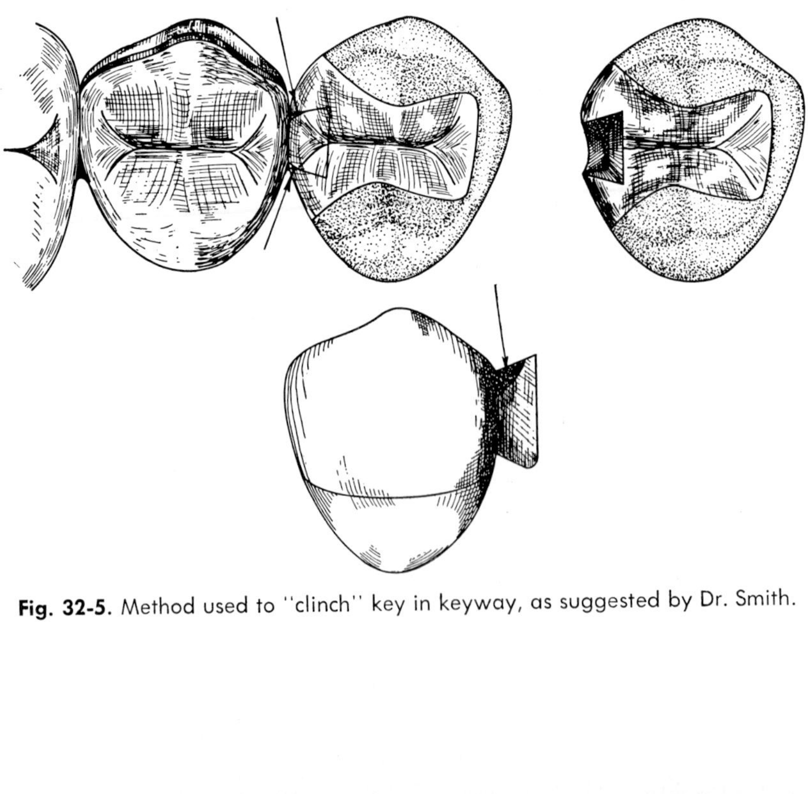

Fig. 32-5. Method used to "clinch" key in keyway, as suggested by Dr. Smith.

so that its occlusal movement is prevented. This explains why the marginal ridge of the retainer is left high and straight so that there may be an excess of gold to lock in the key.

In posterior teeth both the buccal and lingual margins may be clinched. However, in the anterior teeth, due to the shape of the lingual surface, only the lingual wall of the keyway is clinched over the key. This, however, is sufficient.

Modified types. Several modifications of the stress-breaker type of connection have been suggested.

Subocclusal spherical keyway. Starr[3] recommended a subocclusal spherical keyway in which the peripheral outline of the keyway is undercut, using a round bur, not smaller than a No. 6; this is then antifluxed with a small pellet of cotton saturated with aromatic spirits of ammonia, then filled with wax subsequently cast as an integral part of an extension of the pontic. The key is cast directly into the round keyway which is cut in the distal surface of the anterior casting. After the pontic is cast, the key is locked in position in the anterior retainer, permitting only a rotary motion

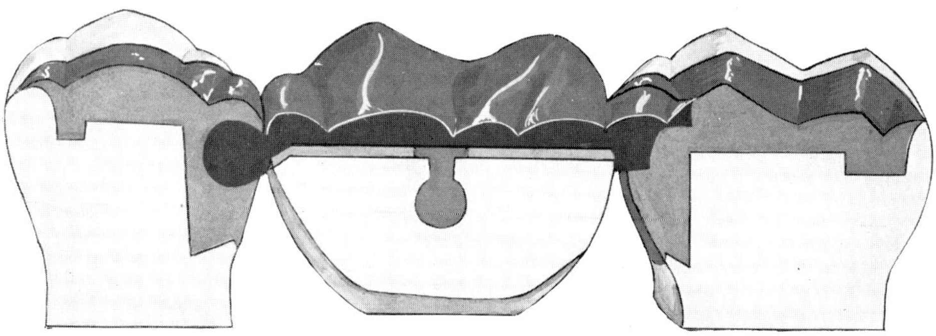

Fig. 32-6. Subocclusal type of nonprecision key and keyway stress-breaker. (Courtesy Dr. F. Starr.)

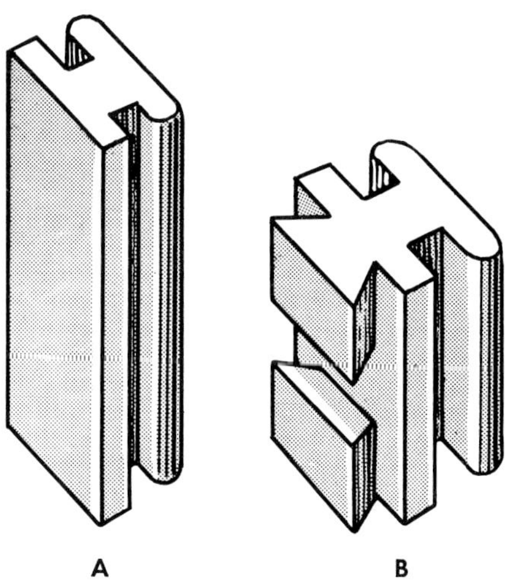

Fig. 32-7. Stern precision rest used as precision type of key in cast keyway. (Courtesy Stern Dental Co., Inc.)

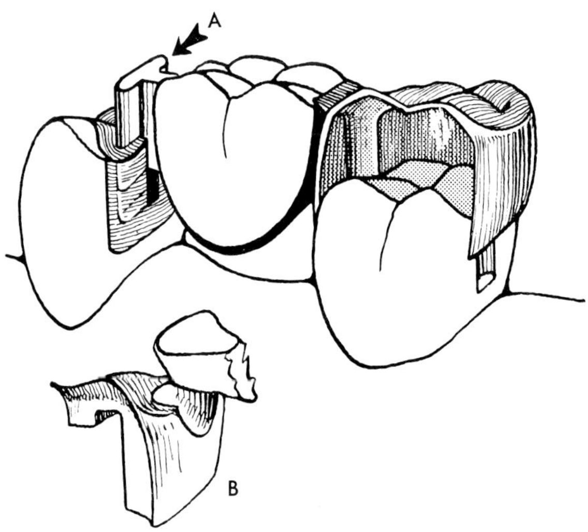

Fig. 32-8. A, Precision fit of Stern's manufactured key into keyway cast in inlay retainer. **B,** Incorrect type of nonprecision key. (Courtesy Stern Dental Co., Inc.)

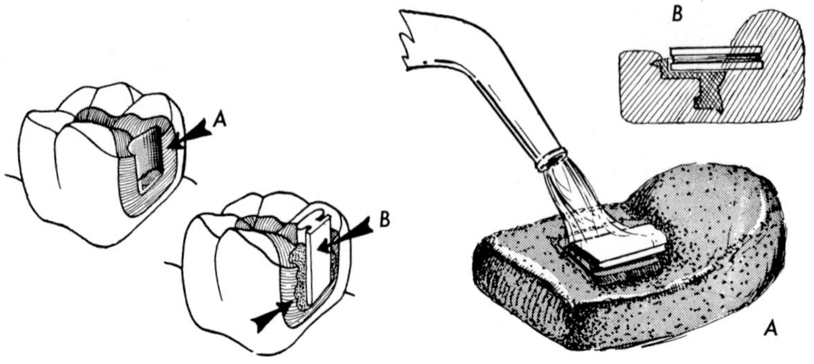

A B

Fig. 32-9. A, Stern's precision key broken-stress connector. (**A,** Recess cut out of wax pattern to accommodate key. **B,** Special alloy former waxed into wax pattern. After casting is made, former is removed by boiling in acid, leaving keyway into which key fits precisely) (Fig. 32-10, B). **B,** Keyway may also be formed in retainer by soldering former into inlay after it is cast. Later, former is dissolved in acid. (Courtesy Stern Dental Co., Inc.)

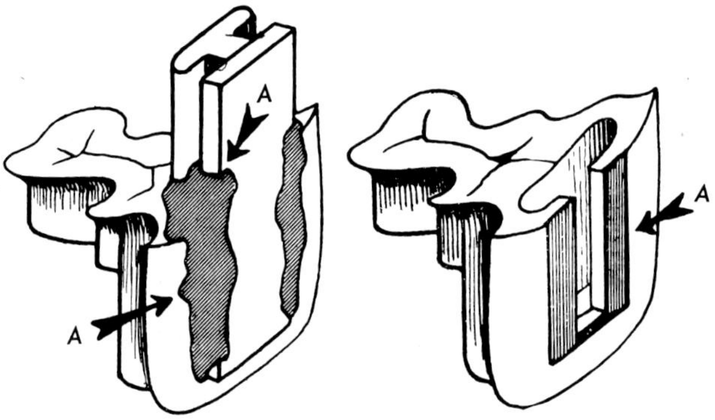

A B

Fig. 32-10. A, Enlarged view of Fig. 32-9, A. **B,** Retainer after keyway-former has been dissolved in acid, leaving precisely fitting keyway for precision key. (Courtesy Stern Dental Co., Inc.)

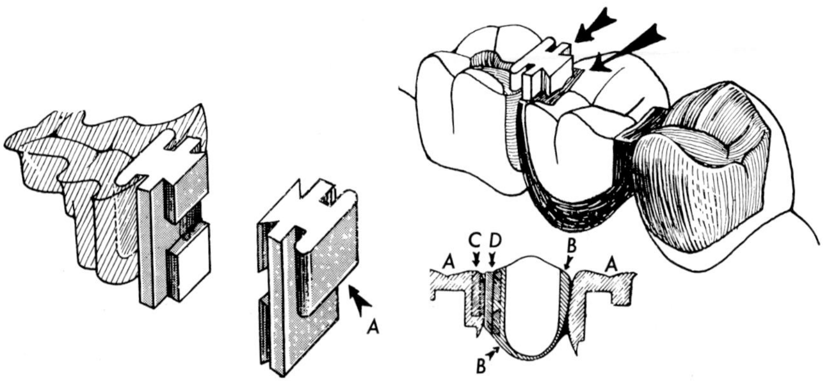

A B

Fig. 32-11. A, Key is fitted into keyway with precision fit. **B,** Key inserted into keyway and shank of key is waxed to pontic boxing. (Courtesy Stern Dental Co., Inc.)

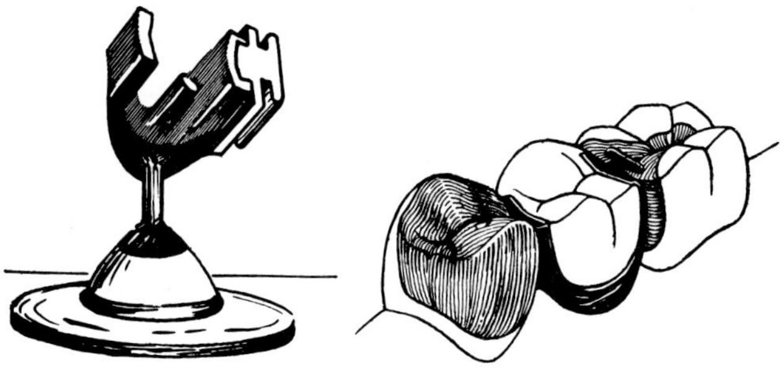

A B

Fig. 32-12. A, Stern's key waxed to wax housing of pontic ready to be cast. **B,** Finished bridge; soldered connector at one end and Stern's precision broken-stress connector at other. (Courtesy Stern Dental Co., Inc.)

between the posterior part of the bridge and the anterior retainer (Fig. 32-6).

Precision types of broken-stress connectors

In addition to the nonprecision type of broken-stress connectors just described, it is recommended to use any of the standard manufactured precision types, such as the Chayes and Stern.[4] When used, the box or keyway portion of the precision attachment is soldered or cast into the anterior retainer, after which the frictional precision rest or key is united to the pontic portion, either by casting or by soldering. There are many sizes and shapes available, and, when properly used, they are preferred to the nonprecision types.

The technic for the use of the Stern precision rest or connector is illustrated in Figs. 32-7 to 32-12.

SELECTED REFERENCES

1. Klaffenbach, A. O.: The role of crown and bridge prosthesis in the field of restorative dentistry, J.A.D.A. **25:**536, 1938.
2. Smith, D. E.: Twenty-five years of fixed bridgework, J. South. California D. A. **3:** 794, 1939.
3. Starr, F. C.: The Starr attachment. Personal communication.
4. Precision rests, their function and technic for use, Mt. Vernon, N. Y., 1939, Stern Dental Co., Inc.

GENERAL REFERENCES

El-Ebrashi, K., Asgar, K., and Bigelow, W. C.: Electron microscopy of gold soldered joints, J. Dent. Res. **47**(1):5-11, 1968.

Fairhurst, C. W., and Ryge, G.: Effect of certain variables on the strength of soldered joints, I.A.D.R., 35th meeting, Atlantic City, N. J., 1957, Preprinted Abstracts.

Gilson, T. D., Asgar, K., and Peyton, F. A.: The quality of union formed in casting gold to embedded attachment metals, J. Prosth. Dent. **15:** 464-473, 1965.

Lasky, M. C.: Semifixed bridgework, J.A.D.A. **70**(3):648-651, 1965.

Litvak, A. L.: A study of the microstructure and physical properties of electro-soldered joints, Northwest. Univ. Bull. **65:**4-12, 1965.

Markley, M. R.: Broken stress principle and design in fixed bridge prosthesis, J. Prosth. Dent. **1:**416, 1951.

Mason, H.: One piece castings of gold bridges, North-West Dent. **38:**289, 1959.

Meyer, F. S.: The elimination of distortion during soldering, J. Prosth. Dent. **9:**441-447, 1959.

Ryge, G.: Dental soldering procedures, Dent. Clin. N. Amer. 1958, pp. 747-757.

Stackhouse, J. A., Jr.: Assembly of dental units by soldering, J. Prosth. Dent. **18**(2):131, 1967.

Wetterstrom, E. T.: Use of Jelenko vacuum porcelain furnace for soldering, Thermotrol Technician **22:**1-4, 1968.

White, M. L., and Drobek, J.: Effect of residual abrasives on wettability of polished gold surfaces, J. Phys. Chem. **70:**3432-3436, 1966.

Winslow, M. B.: Fixed splint and bridge assembly, J.A.D.A. **51:**47, 1955.

Chapter 33

Installation, maintenance, and repair of crowns and fixed partial prostheses

After the fixed bridge has been heat treated and cleaned, it should be given a final trial in the mouth to determine that the bridge goes to place without requiring excessive force and without causing the displacement of the abutment teeth. Dentists may set bridges temporarily to allow the abutment teeth "to adjust" themselves so the bridge may be cemented at a subsequent sitting. When this is necessary, usually some malrelation has occurred during the assembling of the bridge; if the malrelation is evident it is advisable to unsolder the bridge, take a new bite and impression, and resolder the appliance.

TESTING THE BRIDGE BEFORE CEMENTATION

A final test of the fit of the bridge before cementation is valuable in that the margins and their adaptation at the gingival border may be verified, and any necessary modifications may be made.

The contact areas should be tested with a ligature and, if found misplaced or insufficiently tight, the bridge should be reinvested and the contact areas corrected, even though the procedure requires an additional sitting for the patient.

It is well to verify the occlusion of the restoration with its opposing teeth in centric, lateral, and protrusive positions of the mandible. If any interference exists, this may be verified and located; the bridge is removed and the high points corrected. This is more comfortable for the patient than if the grinding is done after the bridge has been permanently cemented.

A final examination of the relationship of the pontic to the ridge is also made at this time. This is especially important in those restorations which are of the immediate replacement type and which employ the cone root extension type of pontic. If it is found necessary to grind the gingival surface of the pontic, it should be reglazed before the bridge is cemented.

In the final examination of any bridge it is advisable to remove the facing so that the metal structure alone is tried in the mouth without any interference from the porcelain members of the restoration. These may be placed later and their fit also verified separately.

SETTING THE BRIDGE TEMPORARILY

In the case of the immediate replacement type of restoration it is advisable to place the bridge initially with temporary cement to make certain that the porcelain pontic extension placed into the alveolar socket will not hinder proper healing of the tissues. The patient is dismissed for 3 days to 1 month, after which time the bridge is removed and the alveolar fundus is examined. If there is no sign of infection and if the healing is satisfactory, the entire bridge is cleaned thoroughly, washed in alcohol, dried, and prepared for final cementation.

PREPARING THE ABUTMENT TEETH

If a rubber dam was used during the preparation of the abutments and if properly made temporary coverings kept the prepared surfaces free of saliva, debris, and oral bacteria, very little more needs to be done to the abutments except to remove the temporary cement and to dry the cavity walls thoroughly. If, on the other hand, the prepared teeth were exposed to saliva, it is necessary that they be thoroughly cleaned and dried. Selberg[1] recommended that, immediately after the cavity has been prepared, it be painted with a cavity varnish to seal the tubules against the ingress of saliva and bacteria and then a protecting band or celluloid cap be placed on the tooth.

He also recommended that just before cementing the bridge to place a disclosing solution be used to determine whether the preparation is clean. He claimed that washing the tooth with an aqueous 70 to 80 percent solution of alcohol is not sufficient to clean the tooth surfaces. He suggested that a solution of glycerin and iodine or Mercurochrome be used and that any areas that absorb this solution be thoroughly scoured with pumice or alumina powder to assure a thoroughly cleaned surface.

Other operators suggest wiping the surfaces of the preparation with cotton pellets wet with body temperature water to remove all surface debris. After complete drying of the moisture with cotton pellets, the cavity is then wetted thoroughly with a 3 percent hydrogen peroxide solution, which is permitted to remain for 5 minutes. The cavity is again dried with pellets, following which, a thin coat of cavity varnish is applied, care being taken to avoid covering the cavity margins. When the varnish has completely dried, the restoration is cemented.

SELECTION AND MIXING OF CEMENT

The selection and mixing of cement are important operations in the success of a fixed partial denture, individual crown, or facing.[2] The color of the cement may influence to a marked degree the final color of a complete veneer porcelain crown or the facing of a fixed bridge; hence, great care must be exercised in selecting cement of the proper color. The selection may be facilitated by mixing a small amount of the cement powder with water and placing this mix in the crown and then on the prepared tooth. By repeating this trial process, the exact shade may be selected, after which the cement powder is mixed with the cement liquid. The same method of trial for color selection may be used for bridge facings.

Where complete metal crowns or three-quarter veneer retainers are employed, the selection of the color of cement used is less critical; still it is advisable to select a color which approximates that of the tooth. This is particularly true in the anterior part of the mouth, where the use of a dark cement might darken the normal shade of the natural tooth.

The zinc phosphate cements are generally used in dentistry[3] and consist of a zinc phosphate powder mixed with phosphoric acid. Many crowns and bridges, perfect from a mechanical standpoint, fail biologically because they are improperly cemented.

Essentials of correct cementation

There are certain rules and procedures that must be followed and executed accurately to cement a restoration successfully.[4-6] First, the abutment teeth and the bridge must be absolutely clean and dry, for as yet there is no cement which is hydraulic or which will harden perfectly in the presence of moisture. Second, the cement mix must be kept dry until the initial set has occurred. Third, the correct proportions of the powder to the liquid should be used in order to develop the optimum qualities of the cement. Fourth, both the powder and the liquid should be kept absolutely clean of any foreign particles or debris. Fifth, the liquid should be kept in a well-stoppered bottle so that it may maintain its proper water content. If the bottle is left open and the liquid is allowed to evaporate, the setting time of the cement will be retarded; on the other hand, if the liquid is diluted with water, the setting time of the cement is hastened. The setting time is further influenced by the speed with which the powder is incorporated into the liquid; the faster this is done, the quicker the cement sets, but prolonging the mixing time retards the speed of setting. By increasing the ratio of powder to liquid, the cement will set faster than when the correct powder-liquid ratio is used.

Because the presence of cement crystals from a previous mix accelerates the setting time of cement, it is essential that a clean glass slab and a stiff, stainless steel spatula be used for each mix. A slab that is deeply scratched or a spatula that has particles of cement adhering to it should not be used.

LUBRICATING THE BRIDGE

In order to ensure the complete and easy removal of the cement from the prosthesis after the cement has hardened, it is suggested that all surfaces, except those coming in contact with the prepared tooth, be lubricated very lightly and the excess lubricant wiped off. Care must be exercised not to allow any of the lubricant to come in contact with the inner surfaces of the retainers. The lubricant will facilitate the removal of the excess cement from the gingival crevice and from the interdental spaces after the final cementation.

The prepared teeth should be thoroughly cleaned, dried, and, where possible, place the rubber dam prior to cementation of of the bridge before the prosthesis is cemented.

After the correct amounts of powder and cement liquid have been placed on the glass slab, the powder is divided into six portions, and one small part is incorporated into the liquid and thoroughly spatulated into a smooth, homogeneous mixture. After this, the second, third, and the other parts are successively added until the desired consistency is obtained.

Difficulties in cementing crowns

A perplexing situation occasionally arises during the cementation of a prosthesis. Although a crown or a bridge fits accurately before it is cemented onto the tooth, after the cement has set, occlusion sometimes feels high and the margins of the retainers rise above the enamel margins.[7] In the case of a complete crown this happens when, as the crown is pressed to place, some of the cement is trapped between the occlusal surface of the tooth preparation and the inside of the crown, thus preventing its escape around the periphery and resulting in the incomplete seating of the crown. To avoid this difficulty, some dentists suggest drilling a small hole through the occlusal or the buccal surfaces of the crown near the occlusal third to permit the escape of the cement while the crown is being forced to place. This small opening is later filled either with gold foil or with a gold wire of the same diameter as the opening. The gold foil or the wire is then finished flush with the surface of the crown.

This difficulty may also be overcome by cutting four grooves on the inside of the crown to within 0.5 mm. of its peripheral margin. The cement trapped in the occlusal region then has an avenue of escape toward the peripheral margin. This method avoids the necessity of cutting through the occlusal or the buccal surfaces of the finished crown. A similar displacement arises with the three-quarter partial veneer or the intracoronal MOD type of retainers; here, however, the difficulty is due to the fact that sustained pressure on the restoration is not maintained while the cement is setting. Occasionally, some air is trapped between the preparation and the casting; when the pressure on the retainer is released before the cement has fully set, the compressed air expands[8] and raises the inlay from the prepared tooth. Aqua regia may be applied to the inside of the crown some time prior to cementation to create space for cement.

CEMENTING THE CROWN OR BRIDGE

With suitable instruments, a small amount of the cement is applied to the inner surfaces of the retainers or the crown; the balance of the cement is applied to the prepared surfaces of the abutment teeth, following which the prosthesis is carried to place with firm pressure; the excess cement meanwhile escapes gingivally and around the margins of the restoration.

When the crown or bridge is firmly seated on the tooth, it should be tapped gently with a mallet and an orangewood stick; sometimes, it is well to have the patient bite on a small stick of wood placed between the restoration and the opposing teeth. Additional pressure may be had by applying pressure to the lower border of the mandible. If the restoration is a porcelain veneer crown or a porcelain bridge, the tapping with the mallet and orangewood stick is omitted; likewise, caution should be exercised if the patient is permitted to bite on a piece of wood; instead, a small piece of rubber dam may be interposed between the restoration and the opposing natural teeth so that the pressure is safely cushioned. The pressure should be continued for at least 10 minutes, after which time the excess cement may be removed. During the time that the cement is setting, it should be kept absolutely free of moisture.

Although some dentists advocate the use of a rubber dam while cementing crowns and bridges, the field of operation may be kept dry by the judicious use of cotton rolls, cotton roll holders, and the saliva ejector.

Where a dowel type of crown is to be cemented, provision must be made for completely filling the root canal with cement, so that it securely holds the dowel of the crown. The cement may be carried into the canal by means of root canal plugger points or by manufactured celluloid tubes made especially for this purpose. These tubes, which have long, thin extensions, are filled with cement; the point is then inserted into the canal and gradually withdrawn while the cement is squeezed through the opening of the tube; thus the canal is completely filled, after which the dowel crown is inserted.

After all the excess cement has been removed, it is advisable to paint the margins of the cavity and restoration with cavity lining before dismissing the patient.

PROCEDURES FOLLOWING CEMENTATION

After the crown or bridge has been cemented and the excess cement has been removed, the occlusion should again be verified by testing it with carbon paper and a sheet of warmed wax. If any slight interferences exist, these should be adjusted before the patient is dismissed; if this is not done, the resulting trauma may produce a periodontitis or an inflamed pulp.

The surrounding soft tissues should now be bathed with lukewarm water and the interproximal spaces tested with a ligature to make certain that no particles of cement remain.

Before dismissing the patient, a roentgenograph should be taken of each abutment or crowned tooth to make certain of the accuracy of the gingival or peripheral fit and to be sure that no particles of cement remain undetected. A complete record of the existing conditions should be taken, and these data recorded on crown and bridge record sheets for future reference and study.

SCOPE OF MAINTENANCE

In order to render a complete maintenance service, it is essential that complete records be kept of every prosthesis placed. These records should include radiographic,[9, 10] clinical, and dynamic data. This phase of dental practice is one of the most neglected, and yet it is one of the most important from the standpoint not only of rendering the patient a complete service, but also of enabling the dentist to study the results of his restoration.

When a crown or a bridge has been cemented and the patient dismissed, it is presumed that it has been installed and finished in such a way that it meets all the requirements, both biological and mechanical.

Under such circumstances, it appears that little is left to be desired either from the patient's point of view or that of the dentist. Yet, many dentists know that sometimes patients with apparently ideal and perfect prostheses return in a course of a few years with the restorations in such a condition that not only are the function and the anatomic form destroyed to a large extent, but frequently other additional damage has been sustained by the teeth and tissues that were normal and healthy at the time the prosthesis was installed. If patients with restorations that fail do not return, the dentist loses a rare opportunity to study the reason for the failures.

There are times when some minute yet important irregularity escapes his attention when the appliance is placed. Unless the patient returns for a periodic examination, the condition may grow progressively worse until the damage sustained is so extensive that, by the time the patient returns, it is irreparable.

A complete maintenance service commences before the work is started by the dentist and includes (1) roentgenographs of all the teeth taken prior to the construction of the prosthesis and (2) an accurate set of study casts. These records should also include (3) a record of the profile of the patient as well as (4) the color of the natural teeth. These data are then filed for future reference and comparative study.

As previously stated, (5) every crown or fixed partial denture should also be roentgenographed immediately after its installation, since this will enable the dentist to locate immediately any discrepancies of fit or unobserved remnants of cement.

In extensive oral rehabilitation it is also recommended that another set of study casts be made after final cementation. These may prove very valuable at some later date to determine if any significant changes have taken place in the occlusion that may require attention. The casts may also prove valuable in the event that they are needed as legal evidence if the patient became involved in an accident that damaged his teeth.

PURPOSE OF MAINTENANCE SERVICE

The patient should be fully informed of the purpose of such a procedure; namely, that these steps are taken as precautionary measures, and for purposes of future comparative study of the supporting bone and tissues. Intelligent patients will realize that the dentist is taking every possible measure to ensure the continued satisfactory condition of the restoration.

By following this procedure, every tooth carrying a crown or a bridge retainer is fortified with two roentgenographic records, one prior to and one following its reconstruction. It is well at this time, also, to inform the patient that, although the prosthesis is a mechanical appliance, it is also a part of his biologic entity and that changes may occur in the existing biologic status. The patient should also be impressed with the need and importance of subsequent roentgenographs taken at periodical intervals following the installation of the appliance. This is especially important if an abutment tooth is pulpless.

OCCURRENCE OF CHANGES

It should be explained to a patient that changes can and do occur, not only in the individual tooth, but also in groups of teeth. These changes may be due to normal processes accompanying normal function, in which event there usually is no harmful result. On the other hand, slight changes may cause an unfavorable tissue reaction and, unless recognized and corrected in its early stages, may result in serious damage.

Those patients who have been under the constant care and observation of their dentist may occasionally require the extraction of a tooth because of a suspected or questionable periapical condition. If complete previous periodical clinical and roentgenographic records are available, a comparative study of the questionable tooth may disclose that the existing condition is not one in the initial stages of degeneration and destruction, but, on the contrary, that it may be in the process of regeneration and repair; therefore, the tooth is not sacrificed needlessly.

RECORDING THE ORAL AND GENERAL HEALTH

In addition to complete roentgenographic and dynamic examinations, it is advisable at the time to determine and record the general health of the patient as well as the existing oral health. It should be routine practice to classify the patient with reference to susceptibility to caries. During the subsequent periodic clinical examination, it is advisable to make a detailed study of the condition of each crown and bridge retainer from the standpoint of caries and a study of the condition of the pulp.

This may be done with electrical and thermal tests. These findings should be accurately recorded showing the degree of response obtained to the tests and the date that they were done. These findings should be accurately recorded to show the date and the degree of response to the tests.

During these visits of the patient, the condition of the investing soft tissues, the ridges underlying the pontics, and the condition of the enamel should be carefully examined. If there is evidence of inflammatory processes existing around the soft tissues, the causes should be determined and corrected. If a recession of the ridges has occurred, a decision must be made whether or not additional porcelain is to be added to the pontics, and, if so, whether it should be done immediately or at a subsequent time. Occasionally, a hypertrophy of the tissues permits an unsanitary condition to develop, in which case it may be necessary to remove the porcelain member of the bridge and modify it or even to remake the entire bridge.

ROENTGENOGRAPHIC DATA

Roentgenographic interpretation is sometimes questionable and usually subjective, yet by means of it one can establish a norm for osseous and periodontal tissues. Through roentgenographic study it is possible to make comparisons of the bone as to its structural form, resorption, or increased calcification. These observations may be recorded on charts as shown in Figs. 33-1 and 33-2. It will be seen that any changes noted may be designated either in the gingival, the middle, or the periapical thirds of the root. Similar observations and recordings may be made with reference to the periodontal membrane.

Because the age of the patient is known and the degree of function of any particular tooth may be determined, the dentist is enabled to judge whether the periodontal membrane is normal or excessively thickened and whether any pathologic process exists. A series of roentgenographic and clinical records extending over a period of years simplifies the task of detecting any changes that occur.

RECORDING METHOD OF TOOTH PREPARATION

The crown and bridge history records the method by which the tooth was prepared to receive the crown or the bridge retainer. As stated in a previous chapter, warm water of approximately 110° F. should be sprayed on the stone and the tooth during the cutting process. Where this method is employed, it should also be recorded. If an anesthetic is used in the preparation of the teeth, the record should indicate whether it is infiltrative or block anesthesia. Finally, if neither anesthetics, hot water, nor cocoa butter is used, this also should be recorded.

While the use of an anesthetic is usually advisable in certain cases for cavity preparation, in a large majority of patients, if the instrumentation and the operative technic are carefully and exactly performed, it is possible to prepare every type of preparation with a minimum amount of pain. The danger in the use of an anesthetic during cavity preparation is that it removes the danger signals and very frequently results in the exposure of pulpal horns or in injury to the pulp by overheating the tooth by cutting too rapidly. Clinical records show that the lowest percentage of injury or mortality of teeth occurs when the water and cocoa butter technic is employed.

Records have been kept for over 40 years on the relative cleanliness and susceptibility of patients in relation to their crown and fixed partial denture require-

CROWN - BRIDGE HISTORY

Name   Patient No.   File No.

Address   Age   Date Completed

Tooth / Crown / Bridge			Examined / Date	Pulp		Condition of Paradontal Tissues										Bite		Abrasion			Re-grind		Prepared						Occlusion			Health			Therapeu.
						Gingival			Osseous			P. M.				LLBS					M. M.														
						1. Buccal 2. Lingual 3. Proximal			1. Gingival 2. Middle 3. Periapical			1. Gingival 2. Middle 3. Periapical																							
Fixed	Semi-Fixed	Removable		Vital	Non-Vital	Normal	Recession	Inflamed	Normal	Absor't'n	Calcif'c'n	Normal	Thickened	Pathologic	Improving	Restored Side	Opposite Side	Uniform	Lab. Occl.	Ling. Occl.	Attachments	Pontic	Hot Water	Infiltration	Block	Dry	Cleanliness	Susceptibility	Normal	Distal	Mesial	Poor	Fair	Good	

(17286)

Fig. 33-1. Filing envelope used for crown and bridge records and roentgenographs.

ments. The results of these earlier tabulations are recorded in Chapter 9.

It is also advisable to record the condition of the patient's general health, whether it is poor, fair, or good.

In addition to the study casts which are filed, the crown and bridge record indicates whether the occlusion is normal or in mesial or distal relationship. In the last column of the history sheet the file number and record are given of any crown or abutment tooth that has previously had its pulp removed and the root canal filled.

All such ground surfaces should be highly polished and refinished to their original state. In the case of porcelain, if the ground surface is in permanent contact

CROWN - BRIDGE HISTORY

Name JONES, Mrs MARY **Patient No.** 6945 **File No.** BSF51

Address 8750 LOLA AVE. **Age** 33 **Date Completed** 4-4-24

Tooth / Crown / Bridge			Examined Date			Pulp		Condition of Paradontal Tissues: Gingival (1. Buccal 2. Lingual 3. Proximal)			Osseous (1. Gingival 2. Middle 3. Periapical)			P. M. (1. Gingival 2. Middle 3. Periapical)				Bite LLBS		Abrasion			Re-grind M. M.		Prepared						Occlusion			Health			Therapeu.		
Fixed	Semi-Fixed	Removable				Vital	Non-Vital	Normal	Recession	Inflamed	Normal	Absor'tl'n	Calcif'c'n	Normal	Thickened	Pathologic	Improving	Restored Side	Opposite Side	Uniform	Lab. Occl.	Ling. Occl.	Attachments	Pontic	Hot Water	Infiltration	Block	Dry	Cleanliness	Susceptibility	Normal	Distal	Mesial	Poor	Fair	Good	LOC. THERAP. #677	L5	
	1		4	4	24	✓		✓			✓			✓				25	35						✓				+	+			✓			✓			
	3					✓		✓			✓			✓				60	80						✓														
	5						✓		✓			✓		✓				40	60									✓											
	1		11	13	24	✓		✓			✓			✓				28	35																	✓			
	3					✓		✓			✓			✓				65	80																				
	5						✓		✓			✓		✓				50	60																				
	1		10	23	25	✓		✓			✓			✓				30	35										+	−						✓			
	3					✓		✓			✓			✓				65	80																				
	5						✓		✓			✓		✓				40	60																				
	1		12	16	26	✓		✓			✓			✓				30	35																				
	3					✓		✓			✓	✓		✓				70	80																	✓			
	5						✓		✓					✓				50	60																				
	1		11	17	28	✓		✓			✓			✓				30	35										+							✓			
	3					✓		✓			✓			✓				70	80																				
	5						✓		✓			✓		✓				50	60																				

(17286)

8 7 6 5 4 3 2 1	1) ~~2~~ 3) ~~4~~ (5) 6 7 8	Ed. Collins
H G F E D C B A	A B C D E F G H	

CROWNS—ATTACHMENTS

Tooth	Vital	Pulpless	Type
L1	✓		DL inlay
L3	✓		3/4 crown
L5		✓	Gold Crown

PONTICS

Tooth	Type
L2	Ridge LAP
L4	Ridge LAP

2000—8-39—17286-S

Fig. 33-2. Record pertaining to semifixed bridge extending from central incisor to second bicuspid with intervening cuspid support.

with the soft tissues, it should be reglazed. Likewise, if it is found necessary to grind the natural teeth, these should also be highly polished not only to avoid any discomfort to the patient, but also to preclude the possibility of decay.

RECORDING STRENGTH OF BITE

Also at the final sitting, a record is determined of the strength of the bite. For the purpose of studying dynamic tabulations, a gnathodynamometer, an instrument that records the bite pressure in pounds, is used, if advisable. The record is first taken on the teeth carrying the bridge and then on the corresponding teeth in the other segment of the arch. If it is a two-abutment fixed partial denture, the force determinations are made on each of the abutment teeth, as well as on their mates in the opposite segment of the arch. It will be found that in obtaining this record it is not only the musculature, but also the sensitiveness and the tolerance of the periodontal membrane that are the determining factors in the force registered.

It has been observed in those patients who return regularly at 6-month intervals that after the first year there was usually a definite increase in the pressure tolerance of the periodontal membrane; likewise, a comparison of the roentgenographs showed a reorientation of the bony trabeculae that sustained the new forces on the restored teeth.

As previously stated, it has been observed clinically that a tooth out of function or with greatly reduced function may be quite immobile as compared to a normally functioning tooth; yet a comparison of their respective dynamic tabulations shows the less mobile tooth is not capable of sustaining the same degree of pressure as the corresponding tooth having greater mobility. This important clinical factor should be established and then supplemented with roentgenographs.

VALUE OF ACCURATE RECORDS

To construct an appliance mechanically satisfactory and biologically acceptable to the tissues is indeed an accomplishment; to maintain it in a healthy and serviceable state for a long period of time is a real service.

The dental profession is missing one of its rare opportunities if it fails to maintain a complete and accurate follow-up record of its crown and bridge restorations.[10, 11] Each year there are thousands of bridges inserted, each of which, if carefully recorded, would afford unlimited possibilities for clinical study. Likewise, many well-constructed and well-planned bridges are lost annually because of the oversight or the possible slight mishap which may have occurred to a restoration and which was permitted to continue uncorrected, resulting finally in the loss of the tooth and the restoration.

The crown and bridge history, as shown in Fig. 33-1, is printed on envelopes in which the originals or duplicates of patient roentgenographs may be filed. They are convenient for comparative study each time the patient returns. Fig. 33-2 shows a record taken from the file, indicating the conditions found and recorded during subsequent visits of the patient.

TIME OF SUBSEQUENT EXAMINATIONS

The interval between periods for roentgenographic and clinical examinations of the patient is determined to a large extent by the condition and type of supporting teeth, the type and extent of the restoration, the habits and health of the patient, and possibly the type of occlusion present. In each instance, however, a definite time should be designated for the subsequent examination. If the patient is convinced that this service is more than mere routine procedure, accompanying regular semiannual prophylaxis, he will regard it as part of a preventive and maintenance service closely related to his continued health.

CONSTRUCTING ADDITIONAL STUDY CASTS

During the periodical examinations of the patient, it may be advisable to take impressions and make study casts for comparison of the occlusal relations of the two sets of models. Not infrequently a shifting or dislocation of a tooth due to a misplaced or a miscontoured contact area is found, disclosing an occlusal disharmony that developed since the prosthesis was made or since the last set of casts was obtained. The presence and the degree of abrasion or attrition may also be determined and recorded in the sixth column of the crown and bridge history. If it is found that certain points of occlusal interference exist that need adjustment, the amount may be determined and the correction made before extensive periodontal destruction has taken place. When such corrections are made, they should be recorded on the chart, and the reason for performing this service should be explained to the patient at the time. Most patients will appreciate a corrective and a preventive maintenance service of this character.

INSTRUCTION IN THE CARE OF THE PROSTHESIS

Finally, before the dismissal of the patient, it is advisable to instruct him regarding the use and care of the prosthesis. One should advise the patient in a broad general way as to what service he may expect, the limitations of the use of an artificial appliance, and the care expected of him in the maintenance of that appliance in a usable and sanitary state.

The patient should be informed that vital tissues are not static and, as a result of changes in the supporting tissues, adjustments may be necessary from time to time. To do so satisfactorily, the patient should be made to realize that the dentist must have the cooperation of the patient in order to help maintain the usefulness of the crown or fixed partial denture. Many patients spend considerable sums of money in keeping their teeth in repair and in replacing those lost, and yet they are not informed as to their duties in keeping the appliances in a clean and healthy condition. This the dentist can do nicely by demonstration and careful subsequent examinations of the patient's mouth.

A conscientious program of maintenance and follow-up service on the part of the dentist will prove to be one of his most valuable assets, in that it sustains an interest in dental care on the part of the patient and at the same time helps to maintain the patient contact which is extremely important to a successful practice.

REPAIR

The repair of crowns and fixed partial dentures presents problems that frequently test the ingenuity of the dentist. While in some cases it is possible to remove crowns and bridges and subsequently recement them, in the large marjority of cases that require repair a complete remake of the appliance, in whole or in part, is usually much more satisfactory.

When repair is possible, it is frequently a makeshift arrangement to tide the patient over a period of economic stress or lack of time until a new restoration can be made.

CAUSES FOR REMOVAL OF PROSTHESES

While some crowns can be removed and repaired sufficiently well to use them again, in bridge repairs, other than fractured facings, it will be found that once the bridge is removed it is usually remade in whole or in part. Crowns and bridges are removed because of decay occurring around the periphery of the crown or the margins of a retainer. Where the decay cannot be removed and suitably replaced with a filling without destroying the usefulness or the esthetic effects of the restoration, the prosthesis is usually removed.

Another cause for removing crowns is the fact that opposing teeth may wear through the occlusal surface and expose the underlying tooth preparation. This condition will not develop if the dentist originally takes the necessary precautions to have a sufficient amount of metal in the occlusal portion of the crown to withstand the abrasive action of the opposing teeth. Where an opening develops in the occlusal surface, resulting in an extensive decay of the underlying coronal portion of the tooth, it sometimes becomes necessary to cut away the entire occlusal portion of the crown in order to remove all the decay. It is then usually advisable to remove and remake the entire crown. Where the decay has exposed the pulp, the axial surfaces of the crown are left in position until after the tooth has been treated and the root canals filled.

Where the opening through the occlusal surface of the crown is small and where no extensive decay has developed, it is often possible to repair such a condition by cutting a typical occlusal cavity and making a cast inlay, which, when set, repairs the crown and restores it to full usefulness.

Occasionally, an opening is made through the occlusal surface of a crown or retainer in order to treat the pulp as the result of trauma or a severe blow. In this event, an opening is made of such shape that it later may be filled with a gold casting.

REMOVAL AND REPAIR OF GOLD CROWNS

Complete gold crowns may be removed in three ways. If the gold crown has a contoured axial band and swaged occlusal surface of gold plate, it may be slit on the buccal surface gingivoclusally with a crown slitter. In using this instrument, care must be exercised, in placing the blade of the slitter, not to lacerate or injure the buccal gingival tissues. After the slit has been made, the two cut ends of the axial band are pried away from the axial surface of the tooth, thus breaking the cement seal and axial continuity of the band. With a prying motion directed occlusally, the crown is then easily dislodged.

Such a crown may be repaired by boiling the crown in acid to remove the cement and debris and by then bringing the two cut ends of the band together with contouring pliers. A small piece of 0.001-inch platinum matrix is placed on the inside of the band opposite the slit. A small amount of sticky wax is melted between the cut ends of the band, filling the opening and attaching the platinum against the inner surface of the crown.

The crown is filled with investment and the wax boiled off, fluxed, and soldered. The excess solder and platinum from the inner surface are now removed and the crown is finished; and if it is satisfactory, it is recemented.

Where a crown slitter is not available, the cut extending occlusogingivally on the buccal surface may be made with a No. 700 crosscut fissure bur. This, however, cuts away a little more of the gold plate than does the slitter. The two ends of the band are aligned as previously described, and the repair is made by the same method.

Where a complete veneer gold crown consists of an axial band plus the cast gold contour or where the crown is entirely cast, it is not possible to use the crown slitter due to the thickness of the metal on the axial surfaces; neither is it advisable to cut through with a fissure bur, since it is rather difficult, if not impossible, to peel back or pry open the two cut ends. For such crowns, a small hole is drilled through the buccal surface just below the plane of the occlusal surface of the prepared tooth. This is carried in a lingual direction between the occlusal surface of the crown and above the occlusal plane of the preparation. This opening is made of a sufficient size to permit the insertion of a round, long instrument with which the crown is then gently raised in an occlusal direction. The leverage force exerted against the prepared tooth beneath the crown is usually sufficient to dislodge the crown from its preparation.

The crown is then boiled in acid to clean it of its cement and other debris, after which a small piece of gold foil is placed in the opening and then filled in with 22-carat solder. If desirable, a small piece of 0.001-inch platinum matrix material may be placed on the inner surface of the opening, wax may be placed in the hole, and the crown invested. After the wax has been boiled out, solder is flowed into the cut, after which the platinum on the inside of the crown is removed with stones. The crown is then finished, polished, and recemented.

Another method is to insert a specially designed screw, which, when turned, engages the metal with its threads and mechanically dislodges the crown by breaking the cement union.

REPAIR OF PORCELAIN CROWNS

Occasionally, the entire crown or a portion of it is fractured as a result of a blow, necessitating removal of the crown. At other times it is necessary to remove crowns because of gingival irritation resulting from an improper fit or a lack of correct gingival fit. Where a complete veneer porcelain crown is fractured or shows a gingival irritation, the removal of the crown and its complete remaking are usually required. This latter type of crown may best be removed by first cutting, in the labial surface from the incisal edge gingivally, a groove of sufficient depth to expose the cement lying between the tooth preparation and the inside of the crown. By inserting a No. 20 chisel into the groove, half the crown may be easily broken off, after which the other or remaining portion is easily dislodged. A new porcelain crown is then made and cemented to replace the one removed. For this reason it is good practice to identify and retain all amalgam dies used for the construction of complete veneer porcelain crowns, so that they are quickly available in the event of subsequent fracture.

REMOVAL OF CROWN WITH DOWEL

Sometimes it is necessary to remove a dowel-type crown; since this type of crown has an attached dowel, its removal presents a more difficult problem. It is a dangerous procedure to try to remove an attached dowel crown by pulling and prying or by leverage action, because of the possibility of fracturing the root.

Due to the multilation accompanying the removal of a dowel crown, it can rarely be repaired and used again. Since the access to the dowel is usually covered by solder on the lingual surface and since porcelain is present on the labial surface, it is first necessary to sever the crown from the dowel. This is done by drilling a hole through the lingual surface, directing the bur or the bibeveled drill in the direction of the dowel. An effort is made to cut through the dowel slightly below the plane of its attachment to the root coping. Once the dowel has been cut, the crown portion drops off, leaving the remainder of the dowel within the root canal. The dowel is now removed by the following technic.

Removal of dowel

First, it is determined whether there is a greater amount of tooth structure on the labial or the lingual aspect of the remaining portion of the root. If there is more root substance on the labial, then most, if not all, of the cutting to follow is done on the labial surface.

The smallest round bur, S. S. White No.

½, is placed against the labial surface of the remaining dowel and a semicircular cut is carried mesiodistally back and forth until a groove approximately 1 mm. in depth is made in the root dentin and cement adjacent to the metal dowel. During the entire operation, while cutting into the dentin and cement, an effort should be made *to keep the bur constantly touching the metal dowel.* In this way the danger of cutting through the side of the root and perforating it is minimized.

After this initial narrow groove has been cut in a mesial to distal curve next to the dowel, the No. ½ bur is replaced by a No. 1 or No. 2 bur and the groove is enlarged by the size of the second bur. It should now be possible to look into this groove and see where the cement is in contact with the dowel; if not, a larger-sized bur may be used to increase still further the width of the semi-circular groove extending in a mesial to distal direction. If the cement is visible, then the smallest bur is again placed in the handpiece and the operation repeated, sinking the groove apically another millimeter and again enlarging it as previously.

This operation is repeated until the labial surface of the dowel is exposed from mesial to distal to a depth equal to at least one-half the length of the dowel remaining in the canal. The roentgenograph will usually disclose the length of the broken-off dowel remaining in the root canal. It is now only necessary, with gentle force, to pry the metal dowel from a lingual direction, gradually loosening the cement bond on the apical one-half length of the dowel, which has not been freed with burs. If care is exercised and if the proper amount of controlled leverage is applied, the dowel will be moved into the space created by the grooving, whereupon it is carefully raised out of the canal with an instrument.

Occasionally a dowel will break off so deep down in the root canal that this technic cannot be employed. The alternative method is one which may be successfully used, but it is rather risky.

In this alternative method the root canal immediately above the remaining portion of the dowel is enlarged with a No. 6 round bur. When proper vision has been established within the canal, the smallest round bur, No. ½, is centered and gradually sunk into the end of the dowel itself to a depth of ½ or 1 mm. This is then followed by the next larger round bur and the process repeated until the dowel is milled out to its full circumference. The process is then repeated step by step until all or most of the metal is removed. The danger, however, lies in the difficulty of cutting directly into metal of a very limited surface area, for the bur is likely to slip off and go through the side of the root, perforating it. The first method is preferable.

In every instance in which a dowel must be removed it is advisable to caution the patient that one cannot assure him of ultimate success. This is one of the most difficult and delicate operations that a dentist is called upon to perform in his practice.

Extreme caution should be observed when using the so-called dowel puller or other forms of mechanical traction, because of the possibility of root fracture.

REMOVAL OF BRIDGES

Bridges are usually removed because of the failure of one or more of the bridge retainers, or because of a break occurring through the body of the bridge, usually at the soldered joints. If one or more of the retainers are complete cast gold crowns, they are opened along the buccal surface by the method described previously, whereupon the bridge may be readily removed by wrapping several strands of ligature over the pontic section of the bridge and then pulling occlusally. In those bridges using intracoronal inlays or three-quarter partial veneer retainers, it is frequently necessary to cut through the occlusal or lingual portion of the castings in order to release the bridge from the abutment teeth. Where the occlusal portion of the cast retainer is sufficiently thick, it is possible to dislodge it by first cutting a small, round hole through the occlusal surface, after which the opening is threaded to accommodate a small screw. When the turning screw reaches the occlusal surface of the prepared tooth, an additional turn or two will cause it to lift the inlay from the prepared tooth. This procedure is then repeated with the other retainer, whereupon the bridge is readily dislodged. These small openings are repaired by the process previously described. After the repairs have been made to the individual retainers, the two parts of the bridge are reassembled in the mouth, and, if the margins and the peripheral fit have not been disturbed, a tongue blade, plaster impression is taken, and the cast is invested in soldering investment, soldered, finished, and recemented to place.

In place of using the occlusal plaster or stone index method, the two segments of the fixed partial denture may be repositioned on the abutments and locked with an application of self curing acrylic resin to form a splint. When the resin has set, it is placed in a burn-out oven at low temperature, where the resin volitalizes leaving the joint clean for repairing in the usual manner.

REMOVING AN ALL-PORCELAIN BRIDGE

Occasionally, it is necessary to remove an all-porcelain bridge for root canal treatment; otherwise the bridge is quite satisfactory and could be recemented if its removal were effected without fracture. A simple and effective technic for removing an all-porcelain bridge or an individual complete veneer porcelain crown is the following. For removing a porcelain bridge, four lengths of waxed dental floss are twisted into a single strand and passed in the gingival interdental spaces between the pontic and the porcelain retainers. The strand is then brought over the occlusal surface and across the intervening pontic into the anterior interdental space, through which it is also passed. This forms a loop, which grips the bridge near its two rigid connectors. The two ends of the twisted strands are permitted to hang occlusally.

A piece of softened modeling compound is next applied to the lingual surface of the bridge, care being exercised that the compound is forced into the interdental spaces and brought in contact with the lingual surfaces of the bridge. The compound is then adapted occlusally so that it covers the lingual half of the occlusal surface. After it has hardened, the compound core is removed and the occlusal part is trimmed to a flat buccal plane, mesiodistally. The core is lubricated and replaced against the lingual surfaces of the teeth. Another piece of soft modeling compound is then placed against the buccal surface of the bridge and the buccal half of its occlusal surface; it stops against the flat surface of the lingual core. The two cores are now seared together in the mouth with a small spatula.

The bridge is now embedded between the two modeling compound cores, while the two strands of floss hang occlusally several inches in length.

The two modeling compound cores are gripped firmly with the fingers of one hand, while the strands of ligature are wrapped around the fingers of the other. With a firm grip and occlusal pull, the bridge is usually dislodged without fracturing. This is possible because the traction is equalized by the modeling compound cores placed against the buccal and lingual surfaces.

The bridge is then cleaned, and, after the necessary root canal treatment of the abutment is completed, it may be recemented.

REMOVAL OF COMPLETE PORCELAIN VENEER CROWN

A complete porcelain veneer crown may also be removed by searing modeling compound to the entire exposed surfaces of the crown; after the compound has hardened, the crown can often be removed by exerting traction on the compound in a line parallel with the long axis of the preparation.

In removing bridges having inlays or three-quarter partial veneer crowns as retainers, it is usually necessary to remake the retainers either because of warpage of the casting or fracture of the cavosurface margins of the tooth.

The repair of a complete porcelain veneer crown is sometimes made on a tooth whose pulp is treated without removing the crown. This procedure usually involves cutting an opening through the lingual surface of the crown with a diamond stone or bur to allow access to the pulp. After the treatment and the filling of the root canal have been completed, the lingual opening then may be filled with a porcelain filling.

Repair of crown or bridge facing

Fracture or the loss of the porcelain facing of a crown or bridge is not an infrequent occurrence.[12] Where the facing has loosened from the crown or from the gold portion of the pontic without fracturing it may be cleaned and recemented, provided that it is a long pin or a Steele replaceable type of facing (Fig. 33-4). Such a facing, if fractured, can be readily replaced after an impression has been taken of the labial or buccal surface of the crown or pontic, a die constructed, and another facing ground to fit it.

A more serious situation confronts one, however, when a soldered short pin facing fractures and the two platinum pins are left embedded in the gold portion. Such a fracture may be repaired by first cutting off the protruding platinum pins and that part of the gold bevel which protects the incisal edge; this leaves a flat surface from the gingival to the incisal edge.

A Steele removable facing is then selected and ground to fit this surface. A small amount of soft wax is applied to the cast backing incisogingivally, and the fac-

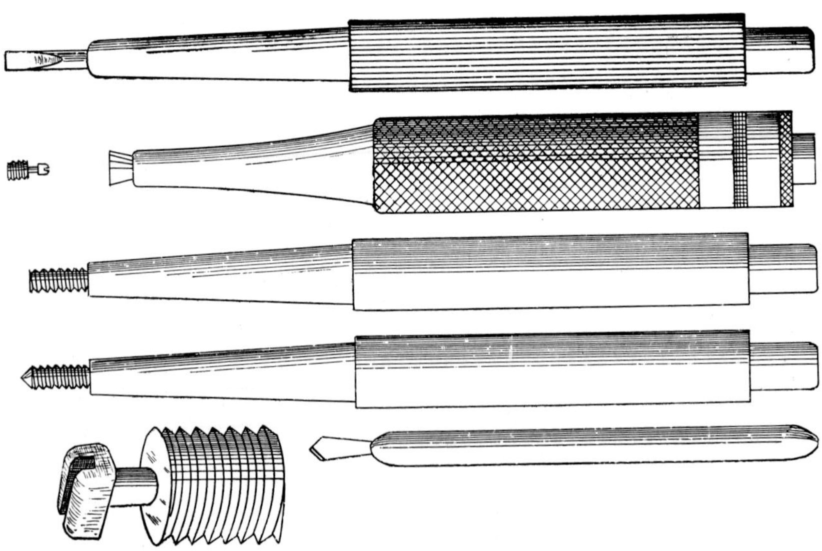

Fig. 33-3. Repair kit for use with Steele facing for Graver method of repair.

ing is pressed against it so that the groove on the back of the facing leaves a slightly elevated rib in the wax.

Two small holes are then drilled in the backing, threaded with a small tap, and two Steele screws inserted. Only the heads are permitted to protrude beyond the backing. Fig. 33-3 shows the drill, tap, screwdriver, and the repair screws. The Steele facing is slipped over these, and, if the fit, contour, and mesiodistal width are satisfactory, it is cemented in place.

In employing this type of repair, it is essential that a sufficient amount of gold extend beyond the incisal edge of the facing to protect it against further fracture.

A Steele facing also may be used to replace a fractured facing on a bridge that does not employ the baked porcelain type of pontic. Fig. 33-4 shows the technic that prepares a cavity in the pontic.[13] The slot on the back of a Steele facing is then filled with wax and united to the wax pattern made in the cavity prepared in the pontic. The facing is removed and the casting is completed, after which the casting is cemented into the gold pontic; the facing is then cemented on the ribbed portion of the casting.

REPAIRING LONG PIN PONTIC; HYDROCOLLOID TECHNIC

Procedure.[14] Remove pins and cement from the backing and with a 699 crosscut taper fissure bur, ream out the pinholes

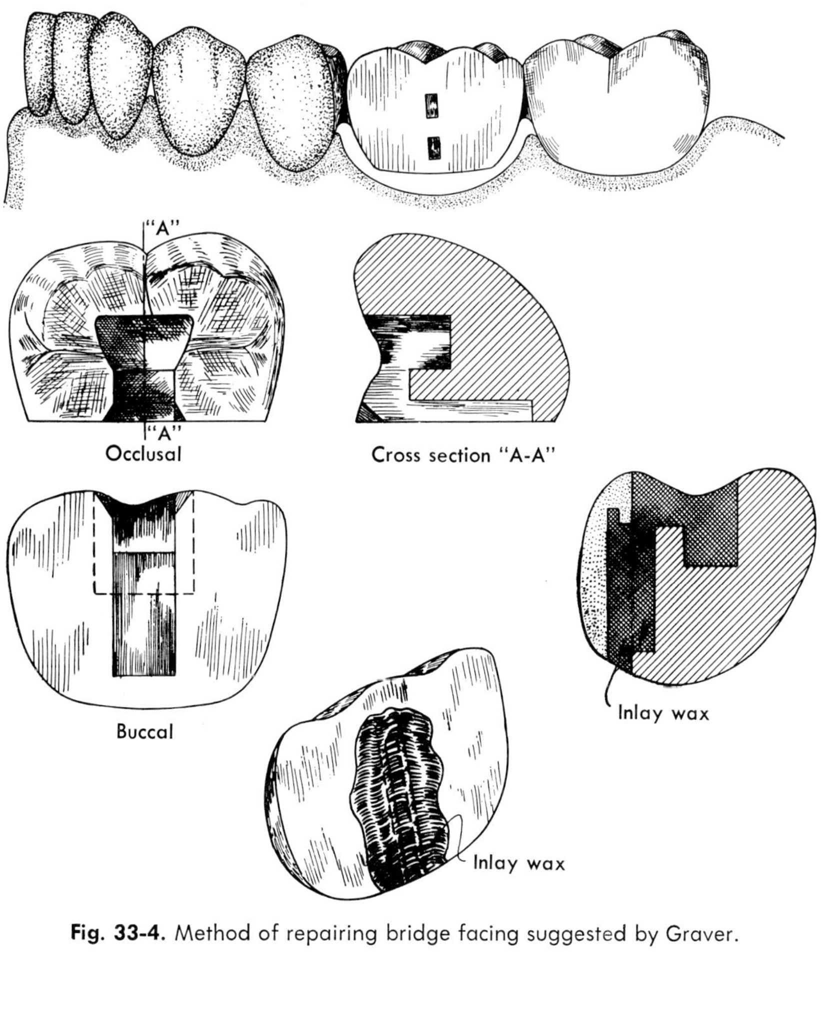

Fig. 33-4. Method of repairing bridge facing suggested by Graver.

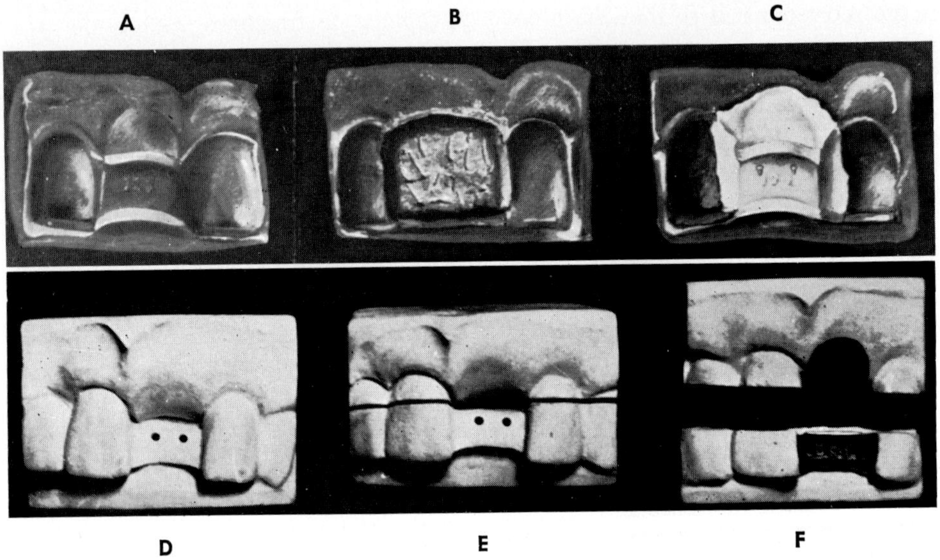

Fig. 33-5. Whittemore technic to repair bridge with fractured pin facing.

in the backing. Do not enlarge the pinholes (Fig. 33-5).

Prepare a small block of modeling compound, about ¾ inch in length and about ½ inch in breadth and thickness. Chill, then warm one surface over a Bunsen burner flame until it is quite soft.

Press the softened surface against the labial or buccal surface of the backing and the adjacent teeth to get a good impression of the required area (Fig. 33-5, *A*).

When completely hardened, remove the compound, chill it, and cut out a shallow recess in the impression side. This recess should relieve the backing area and at least half the buccal or labial areas of the adjacent teeth, leaving enough of the surface imprints of the adjacent teeth so that the compound core can be returned accurately to its original position (Fig. 33-5, *B*).

Wipe the surface of the compound in the cutout area with a pledget of cotton dipped in chloroform.

Place cotton rolls in the mouth, and thoroughly dry the backing with a blast of air. Be particularly careful to blow all moisture out of the pinholes.

The hydrocolloid should have been previously liquefied in an all-metal small syringe with a 21-gauge cannula.

Place the tip of the cannula in the pinhole and inject it full. Do the same with the other pinhole. Inject more material over the backing. Fill the cutout area of the compound core with hydrocolloid, and press the core to its correct position and chill.

Some hydrocolloid will come through to the lingual surface and cause too much of an overhang for correct removal of the impression. Remove any such excess, and withdraw the impression buccally or labially in line with the pin (Fig. 33-5, *C*).

Box and pour the impression with Diolite or a similar stone. Let the stone set until it is hard, and separate the impression. An accurate duplicate of the backing, pinholes, and adjacent teeth should result (Fig. 33-5, *D*).

With a fine jeweler's saw, cut from the labial or buccal side down into the stone die so that the blade passes between the model of the crest of the ridge and the gingival margin of the model of the backing (Fig. 33-5, *E*).

Do not cut entirely through the die. Cut far enough so that the die may be

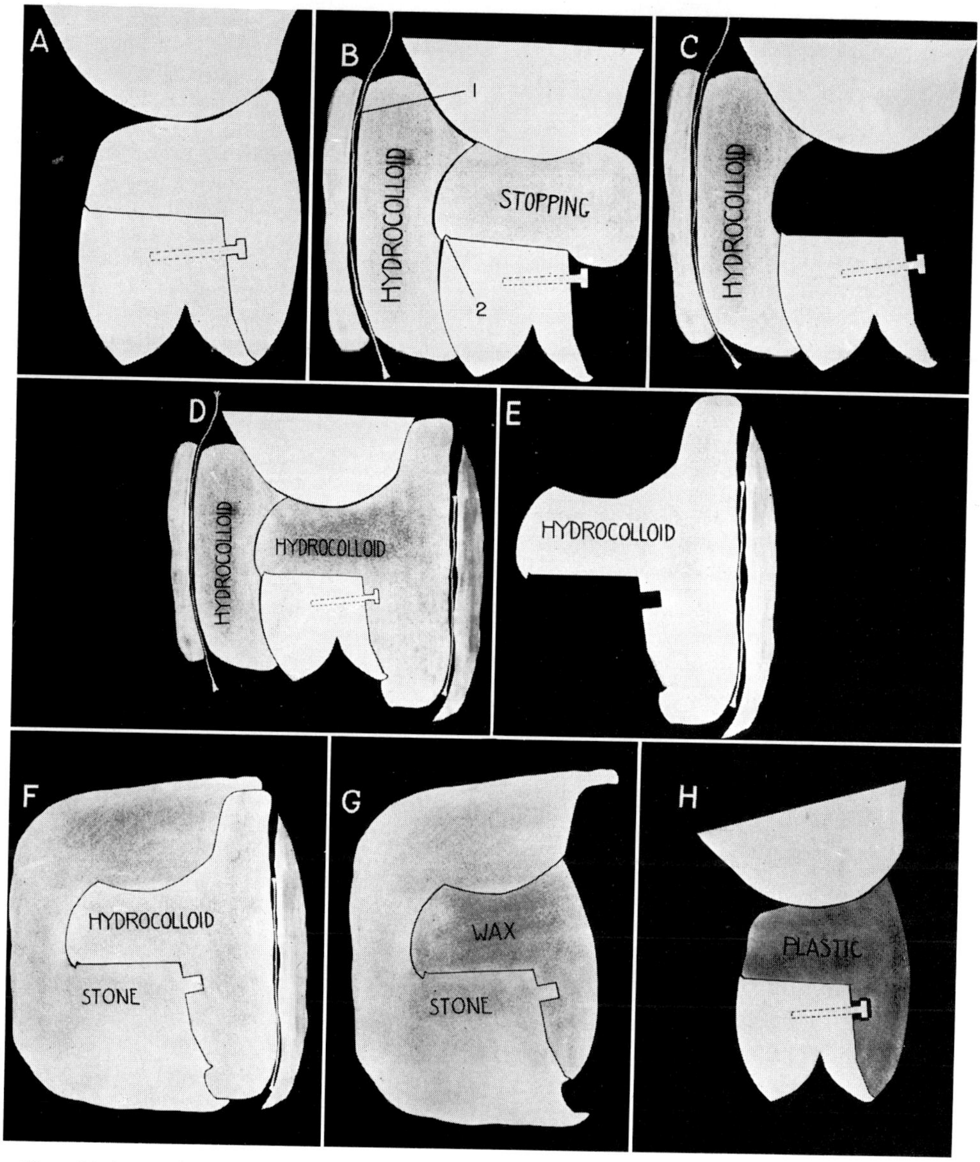

Fig. 33-6. Hydrocolloid technic for replacing long-pin, porcelain-facing, acrylic pontic. (Courtesy Dr. M. J. Thompson.)

broken apart. Leave sufficient die material to fit the halves together after the die is split.

Blacken the surface of the areas representing the backing and the crest of the ridge with a carbon pencil. Proceed to grind in the new facing to fit the backing and ridge accurately (Fig. 33-5, *F*).

The following method utilizes hydrocolloid to take the impression for the fractured pontic.[15] A stone model is then constructed, on which a processed acrylic resin facing is made.

Fig. 33-6, *A*, shows a typical porcelain, long pin facing with cast-gold, occluso-lingual part.

The space (Fig. 33-6, *B*) previously occupied by the porcelain is filled with soft wax or stopping, and a matrix of hydrocolloid is made for the lingual surface, extending mesially and distally. A length of gauze, No. B-1, is used in the construction of the matrix to provide reinforcement and a means of handling. It is necessary to extend the stopping slightly past the gold margin, No. B-2.

The stopping is removed, and hydrocolloid is injected into this most critical space (Fig. 33-6, *C* and *D*) and chilled. During the process a strip of gauze is laid over the surface and a second portion of hydrocolloid is added to reinforce the material when it is chilled.

Next, the hydrocolloid is removed and the area around the platinum pins is cut out to form a rectangular groove (Fig. 33-6, *E*). A heavy mixture of hydrocal is vibrated over the impression (Fig. 33-6, *F*).

The wax pattern for the facing is shaped on the model, and the two are placed in a flask (Fig. 33-6, *G*). The acrylic resin opposite the heads of the platinum pins is grooved for mechanical retention upon cementation (Fig. 33-6, *H*).

Fractures of porcelain facings usually result from an insufficient amount of gold protection along the incisal or occlusal edges. If the precaution is taken to have a sufficient amount of metal in this region, the percentage of fractures and repairs can be reduced to a minimum.

Fractures of crowns are most frequent in the complete veneer porcelain types; these result either from an improperly prepared tooth or from the application of unusual or incorrectly applied stresses. Therefore, before repairing or replacing a crown or a bridge facing, an effort should be made to determine the cause of fracture in order to avoid its recurrence.

When bridges fracture through soldered joints, it is usually due to a disregard of some of the principles of soldering or bridge design.

SELECTED REFERENCES

1. Selberg, A.: Modern fixed partial denture restorations, J.A.D.A. **23**:460, 1936.
2. Volland, R. H., Paffenbarger, G. C., and Sweeney, W. T.: A study of zinc phosphate cement, J.A.D.A. **22**:1281, 1935.
3. Paffenbarger, G. C., and Souder, W.: Physical properties of the zinc-phosphate cement, Tr. Ninth Internat. D. Cong., p. 347, 1936.
4. Bassett, R. W.: Solving the problems of cementing the full veneer cast gold crown, J. Prosth. Dent. **16**(4):741, 1966.
5. Horn, H. R.: The cementation of crowns and fixed partial dentures, Dent. Clin. N. Amer., March, pp. 65-81, 1965.
6. Kaufman, E. G., Colin, L., Schlagel, E., and Coelho, D. H.: Factors influencing the retention of cemented gold castings: the cementing medium, J. Prosth. Dent. **16**:731-739, 1966.
7. Trail, J. S., and Sausen, R. E.: Investigation of cavity-sealing properties of zinc phosphate cement, J. D. Res. **41**:525, 1962.
8. Fusayama, T., Ide, K., Kurosu, A., and Hosoda, H.: Cement thickness between cast restorations and preparation walls, J. Prosth. Dent. **13**:354, 1963.
9. Babbit, B.: Complete records in the dental office, J. Ontario D. A. **37**:22, 1960.
10. Frykholm, K. O., and Lysell, L.: Different systems for the recording of teeth and teeth surfaces, Internat. D. J. **12**:194, 1962.
11. Holder, M.: Maintaining an effective recall system, Dent. Clin. N. Amer., pp. 141-149, March, 1961.
12. Denen, H. E.: Technic for the replacement of broken anterior bridge facings, D. Digest **52**:142, 1946.
13. Graver, C. J.: Bridge repair technic, D. Digest **41**:193, 1935.
14. Whittemore, W. C.: Trulyte new hue pontics, New York, 1946, Dentists' Supply Co.
15. Thompson, M.: A standardized indirect technic for reversible hydrocolloid, J.A.D.A. **46**:1, 1953.

GENERAL REFERENCES

Anderson, J. R., Jr., and others: Physical properties of some zinc oxide–eugenol cements, J. Dent. Res. **45**:379-387, 1966.

Armen, G. K., Jr., and Mahler, D. B.: Addition of silver amalgam alloy to zinc phosphate cement, J. D. Res. **38**:756, 1959 (abst.).

Baraban, D. J.: Cementation of fixed bridge prosthesis with zinc oxide-eugenol cements, J. Prosth. Dent. **8**:988, 1958.

Barber, D. B., and Massler, M.: Penetration of isotopes through liners and bases under silicate cement restorations, J.A.D.A. **65**:786, 1962.

Barry, A. L.: Safe silver nitrate technic, D. Survey **37**:884, 1961.

Bodecker, H. W. C.: The metallic inlay, Berlin, 1911, Hermann Meusser, chap. 11, pp. 131-147.

Boucher, C. O.: Maxillomandibular relations and records, Tr. Am. D. Soc. Europe **68**:8, 1962 (abst.).

Bowen, R. L.: Adhesive bonding of various materials to hard tooth tissues, J. Dent. Res. **44**: 690, 1965.

Brannstrom, M., and Nyborg, H.: Dentinal and pulpal response, IV; pulp reaction to zinc oxyphosphate cement, Odont. Revy. **11**:37-50, 1960.

Brauer, G. M., and others: Improved zinc oxide-eugenol type cements, J. D. Res. **41**:1096, 1962.

Buonocore, M., Azevedo, N., and Dalton, E.: Evaluation of cavity liners for permeability and adhesion to dentin, J. New York Dent. Assoc. **28**:239-244, 1962.

Buonocore, M., Wileman, W., and Brudevold, F. A.: A report on a resin composition capable of bonding to human dentin surfaces, J. Dent. Res. **35**:846-851, 1956.

Burhani, H.: Protection of dentist's health against air turbine dangers, Rev. Dent. Syrie **3**(1):5-14, 1967.

Eichner, K., Lautenschlager, E. P., and Von Radnoth, M.: Investigation concerning the solubility of dental cements, J. Dent. Res. **47**:280, 1968.

Everett, F. G., and others: Treatment of hypersensitive dentin, J. Oral Ther. **2**:300-310, 1966.

Ewing, J. E.: Temporary cementation in fixed prosthesis, J. Prosth. Dent. **5**:388, 1955.

Friffin, J. R., and Ware, Al: Evaluation of dental cements, Australian D. J. **5**:285, 1960.

Galligan, J. D., Schwartz, A. M., and Minor, F. W.: Adhesive polyurethane liners for anterior restorations, J. Dent. Res. **47**:629, 1968.

Gardner, A. F., and Higel, R. W.: Evaluation of agents used in cavity sterilization, Australian D. J. **7**:53, 1962.

Gilmore, H. W.: Clinical study of the marginal leakage of restorative materials as determined by Ca^{45}, Alum. Bull. Indiana Univ. School Dent., March, 1962, p. 14 (abst.).

Going, R. E.: Cavity liners and dentin treatment, J.A.D.A. **69**:415, 1964.

Gordon, S. G., and Halpern, I. L.: Medical aspects of dental patient history, Oral Surg. **15**: 1270, 1962.

Graver, C. J.: Bridge repair technic, D. Digest **41**:193, 1935.

Grieve, A. R.: Finishing cavity margins Brit. Dent. J. **125**:12-17, 1968.

Horn, H. R.: Improved cementation, J.A.D.A. **63**: 812-820, 1961.

Iwamoto, T.: Study on the porosity in thin films of zinc phosphate cement, Acta Odont. Scand. **24**:35-46, 1966.

Jendresen, M. D., and others: A comparative study of four zinc oxide and eugenol formulations as restorative materials, part I, J. Prosth. Dent. **21**(2): 1969.

Johnson, W. W., and Wick, F. H.: Cavity liners versus phosphoric acid, D. Progress **1**:215, 1961.

Jorgensen, K. D.: Factors affecting the film thickness of zinc phosphate cements, Acta Odont. Scandinav. **18**:479, 490, 1960.

Jorgensen, K. D.: Structure of the film of zinc phosphate cements, Acta Odont. Scandinav. **18**: 491, 1960.

Kamienski, M. A.: Something new in dental charts and filing, J. Ontario D. A. **38**:11, 1961.

Kamoi, K., and Yasuda, K.: The evaluation of varnish type cavity lining materials of acrylic direct filling resins, Jap. J. Conservative Dent. **2**:19-36, 1968.

Kanai, S., and Fusayama, T.: Effect of a cavity varnish on the retention of restorations, J. Dent. Res. **47**(3):403, 1968.

Kaufman, E. G., Coelho, D. H., and Colin, L.: Factors influencing the retention of cemented gold castings, J. Prosth. Dent. **11**:487-502, 1961.

Khowassah, M. A., and others: The sealing properties of methyl 2-cyanoacrylate as an adhesive in dentistry, J. Dent. Res. **45**:376, 1966.

Langeland, K., and Langeland, L. K.: Pulp reactions to crown preparations, impression, temporary crown fixation, and permanent cementation, J. Prosth. Dent. **15**:129-143, 1965.

Mahler, D. B., and Armen, G. K., Jr.: Addition of amalgam alloy to zinc phosphate cement, J. Prosth. Dent. **12**:157, 1962.

Morrow, T.: Recall system important part of bookkeeping, D. Survey **36**:233, 1960.

Mosteller, J. H.: The prevention of postoperative thermal sensitivity, Dent. Clin. N. Amer., pp. 881-888, Nov., 1963.

Mullins, H.: Value of periodic recalls, Cal. **25**:8, 1962.

Myers, G. E.: Status report on zinc oxide-eugenol and modified cements, J.A.D.A. **76**(5):1053, 1968.

Nakazawa, S.: Research on superfinishing abrasives of alumina, D. Bull. Osaka Univ. **1**:99, 1960.

National Institute of Dental Research: Adhesive

restorative dental materials, Washington, D. C., 1964, 1966, U. S. Government Printing Office.

Norman, R. D., Swartz, M. L., and Phillips, R. W.: Studies on film thickness, solubility, and marginal leakage of dental cement, J. Dent. Res. **42**:950-958, 1963.

Norman, R. L., Swartz, M. L., and Phillips, R. W.: Studies on the solubility of certain dental materials, J. D. Res. **36**:977, 1957.

Oldham, D. F., Schwartz, M. L., and Phillips, R. W.: Retentive properties of dental cements, J. Prosth. Dent. **14**:760-768, 1964.

Phillips, R. W., and others: Zinc oxide and eugenol cements for permanent cementation, J. Prosth. Dent. **19**:144-150, 1968.

Pinto, J., and Buonocore, M.: Effects of bases and cavity liners on marginal penetration of filling materials, I.A.D.R. **40**:88, 1962.

Ritchie, G. M.: Repair of coronal fractures in upper incisor teeth, Brit. D. J. **112**:459, 1962.

Sheets, C. E.: A split cast procedure for the replacement of pontics, J. Prosth. Dent. **16**:5, 1966.

Swartz, M. L., and others: Strength, hardness and abrasion characteristics of dental cements, I.A.D.R. **40**:86, 1962 (abst.).

Swartz, M. L., Phillips, R. W., Day, R., and Johnston, J. F.: A laboratory and clinical investigation of certain resin restorative and cementing materials; part I, in vitro tests on adhesive characteristics; part II, a twenty-eight month clinical evaluation of a resin cement, J. Prosth. Dent. **5**:698, 705, 1955.

Swartz, M. L., and others: Role of cavity varnishes and bases in the penetration of cement constituents through tooth structure, J. Prosth. Dent. **16**(5):963-972, 1966.

Trail, J. S., and Sausen, R. E.: Investigation of cavity-sealing properties of zinc phosphate cement, J. Dent. Res. **41**:525, 1962.

Troxell, R. R.: Polishing of gold castings, J. Prosth. Dent. **9**:668, 1959.

Chapter 34

History and development of metal-ceramic fixed partial dentures (bridges); early types to present-day restorations

The biologic compatibility and the esthetic qualities of glazed porcelain have directed the attention of the dental profession for many years toward the possibility of constructing serviceable bridges made entirely of porcelain. Efforts along this line were initiated over 60 years ago by endeavoring to replace lost teeth in this manner. Lakermange and Gonon[1] reported that in 1884 Parmely-Brown constructed porcelain bridges which consisted of teeth fired to a porcelain bar; the terminal ends of the bar were embedded in cavities prepared in natural teeth and were held in place by gold fillings or crowns.

In 1906 and 1907 Roussel and Goslee and later Capon suggested the use of porcelain bridges which used platinum Richmond crowns or complete veneer platinum crowns as retainers; these were united together by a platinum bar to which platinum pin facings were soldered; the bridge was completed by firing the occlusal surfaces and lingual contour in porcelain.

Later, when the Land porcelain veneer crown was more generally used, a missing tooth was frequently replaced by firing the pontic entirely of porcelain and uniting it directly to the veneer crown without the use of any platinum bar.

As the principles of correct tooth preparation for the reception of complete porcelain veneer crowns were better understood, porcelain bridges were made, employing two complete porcelain veneer crowns as retainers, between which was suspended the pontic, also made entirely of porcelain. No metal was used in the construction of this type of crown other than the 0.001-inch platinum matrix, which, however, was always removed prior to the cementation of the bridge.

In an effort to extend the usefulness and the application of the all-porcelain bridge, this type of restoration was gradually used to restore two, three, and sometimes even four missing teeth, as in an anterior cuspid-to-cuspid fixed bridge. Due to the lack of sound judgment frequently displayed in the selection and construction of this type of bridge, many failures resulted, and the all-porcelain bridge gradually fell into disrepute and disuse, except in those partially edentulous mouths where only one tooth was restored.

Because the porcelain bridge possesses so many good qualities, the dental profession turned its attention to the development of a technic that would retain all the good and desirable qualities and which would also reinforce the porcelain so that it could withstand the forces to which it might be subjected in the mouth.

INDICATIONS AND CONTRAINDICATIONS FOR PORCELAIN BRIDGES

As stated previously, an all-porcelain bridge may be utilized in a short span, i.e., where only one tooth is missing. It may be safely used in a longer span provided (1) that not more than two missing teeth are replaced, (2) that the average poundage the patient is capable of exerting is not excessive, and (3) that the natural teeth are not worn down to the degree where the bite is very close or (4) where it exists in an end-to-end relationship. When the last two conditions exist, a porcelain bridge is contraindicated.

The porcelain bridge is primarily indicated in the anterior region of the mouth because of its high esthetic qualities.

Since one of the basic requirements of fixed bridge construction is the conservation of the pulp, porcelain bridges are usually placed on teeth that are carious or malformed or that have been damaged accidentally. It is not advisable to cut into a sound healthy tooth in order to place a porcelain bridge so long as there are other means and other methods available for the replacement of the lost teeth without extensive cutting of the tooth. Sometimes the shock to the pulp resulting from an extensive preparation is too great for its survival. Similarly, porcelain bridges, whether reinforced with metal or not, are *contraindicated in younger patients,* but they may be safely used in older patients in whom one may expect the pulp to be protected sufficiently by a deposit of secondary dentin.

Porcelain bridges are not usually placed for patients who do not habitually take good care of their mouths. Likewise, this type of bridge is contraindicated where the position, relationship, or torsional forces will be so great that the structure will not be able to overcome the existing handicaps.

TYPES AND CONSTRUCTION OF PORCELAIN BRIDGES

Porcelain bridges are divided into two general classes: (1) the all-porcelain bridge, in which the restoration is made entirely of porcelain; and (2) the porcelain bridge, which employs a metal reinforcing framework.

The all-porcelain bridge

As previously stated, the customary all-porcelain bridge is extremely limited in its use, being employed primarily in restoring one missing tooth, and then only when its environment is most favorable and the occlusion is normal.

The procedures involved in the construction of the various types of porcelain bridges will be considered, the first being the all-porcelain bridge constructed without any metal reinforcement.

Construction of the all-porcelain bridge. The usual type of all-porcelain bridge that does not employ a reinforcing metal framework is indicated primarily when one tooth is replaced in the anterior region of the mouth; this is usually the upper lateral incisor (Fig. 34-1). In order to use this type of restoration successfully, the occlu-

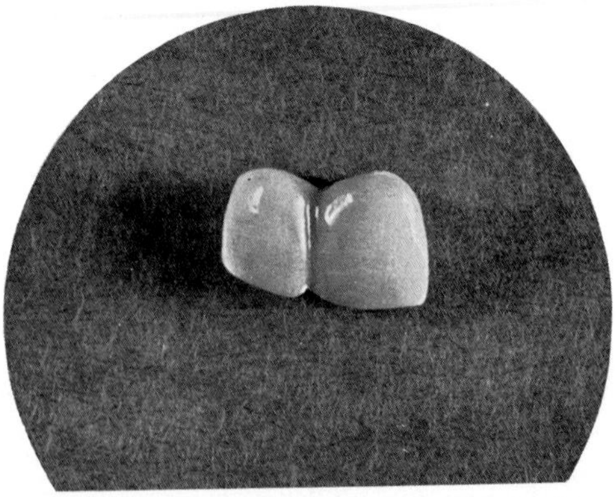

Fig. 34-1. An all-porcelain type of cantilever bridge. (Courtesy Dr. F. Felcher.)

sion must be normal and the edentulous area should not exceed the normal mesiodistal width of the lateral incisor being restored. Where the space is wider or where the occlusion is exceptionally strong, it is advisable to employ an additional abutment and construct a three-tooth bridge, either of the fixed or of the semifixed type. When the cantilever type of all-porcelain bridge is constructed, the abutment is prepared with the same type of shoulder as for a typical complete veneer porcelain crown. After the amalgam die has been constructed and properly oriented in the working model, a 0.001-inch platinum matrix is made as for a regular porcelain crown.

Next, a small piece of platinum matrix material is burnished to the edentulous ridge of the working model, after which the abutment tooth is built in porcelain as for a complete veneer crown. At the same time that the crown is built, the pontic is shaped to its approximate contour by applying porcelain to the piece of platinum covering the ridge; the pontic is made an integral part of the porcelain veneer crown.

After the veneer crown has been relieved at the gingival margin, the bridge is brushed smooth with a camel's hair brush and the entire structure is carefully removed from the amalgam die and model. The piece of matrix covering the ridge remains attached to the porcelain bridge. It is placed on a tray covered with coarse silex powder, so that only the gingival portion of the platinum matrix and the piece of platinum covering the ridge rest on the silex. No porcelain should touch the silex granules.

After the bridge has been thoroughly dried in front of the open muffle or in the drying chamber, it is then given a bisque firing.

When cool, the bridge is removed from the muffle and replaced on the amalgam die. The matrix of the crown is reburnished to the amalgam die at the gingival margin, after which the gingival edge discrepancy is filled in with porcelain; any other modifications of contour are also made at this time. The bridge is then carefully removed and given another bisque bake.

Following this, the bridge is replaced on the die and working model for any further modifications or adjustments. After the crown and the pontic have been contoured to the desired shape and fitted properly to the gingival shoulder, the bridge is fired to a glaze, after which it is removed from the muffle and allowed to cool slowly to room temperature under a pyrex cover. Slow cooling is necessary in order to avoid internal stresses developing within the porcelain.

Where two complete veneer porcelain crowns are used as abutments to support an intervening pontic, the steps of construction are similar, with the exception that one additional crown is made separately. When the bridge and the second abutment crown have been fired the second time and ground to proper contour and relationship, the two parts of the bridge are placed in the mouth, waxed together, removed, and invested in a high heat investment material. A rigid joint is then completed by fusing porcelain between the pontic and the second porcelain crown. It may require one or two firings to complete the operation.

The metal reinforced bridge

The porcelain bridge more generally used today is one in which a cast metal reinforcement is employed.

Early types of reinforcement. The metal reinforcement may be of several types; in the first type the metal structure consists of two platinum alloy copings that are made to fit the vital abutment preparations; these are then united by means of a platinum alloy plate or bar. The bar is united to the abutment copings or "adapt-

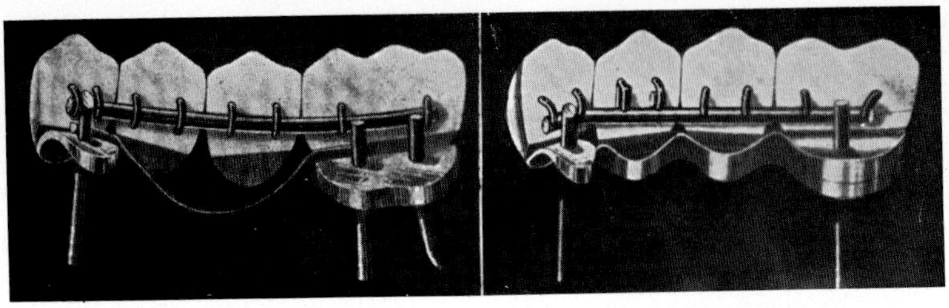

Fig. 34-2. Early types of reinforced porcelain bridges. (After Prothero.)

ers," as they are sometimes called, by means of a soldered union. After the bridge has been completed, the metal reinforcing framework is embedded within the porcelain bridge and remains as a permanent part of the structure.

The second type of metal reinforcement uses various gauges of iridioplatinum wires that extend horizontally through the body of the bridge and are wound around the two abutment teeth; the horizontal strands of wire are then reinforced by a coil-like winding of additional iridioplatinum wires. This entire reinforcing structure also becomes a permanent part of the finished bridge.

The third type of metal reinforcement is also made of the platinum group metals, but the metal framework is cast, instead of being assembled and soldered wrought metal. Each of these three types will be discussed, and the original technics will be presented.

First type of reinforced bridges using wrought metals. The first type, the porcelain bridge employing a metal reinforcement constructed of wrought platinum plate and bar material, assembled by soldering, is one of the oldest types. Fig. 34-2 illustrates this older type of construction. Although certain elements of strength were incorporated in this type of bridge which were lacking in the all-porcelain appliance, it also possessed many inherent weaknesses. Because the union between the facings and the platinum bar was formerly united with pure gold or gold-platinum solder, this frequently loosened and proved a serious weakness. Moreover, the metal used for this framework was pure platinum, which does not possess the strength needed for functional purposes. Later a 25 percent iridioplatinum alloy was used; this possessed the necessary physical properties to withstand masticatory forces and also lent itself to the procedures involved in the construction of the bridge. It was found in the older types of reinforced bridges that cleavage planes were established at the point where the porcelain came in contact with the platinum bars. In addition to this the design of metal framework used prevented the proper contouring of the bridge to make it easily cleansable.

The next step in the development of the reinforced porcelain bridge took place when suitable alloys and platinum solders were developed for this purpose. The alloying of 5 to 25 percent iridium with platinum and the development of a platinum alloy solder furnished the dentist with materials that enabled him to use the alloys in smaller quantities, yet have the necessary strength; it was also possible to distribute it in such a way that the maximum of strength was available without establishing dangerous cleavage planes in the porcelain.

Since this type of bridge could be placed on abutments with vital pulps, it employed bands made of iridioplatinum fitted around the axial surfaces of the preparations and united by means of bars of various shapes. The axial bands, also called adapters, copings, or caps, frequent-

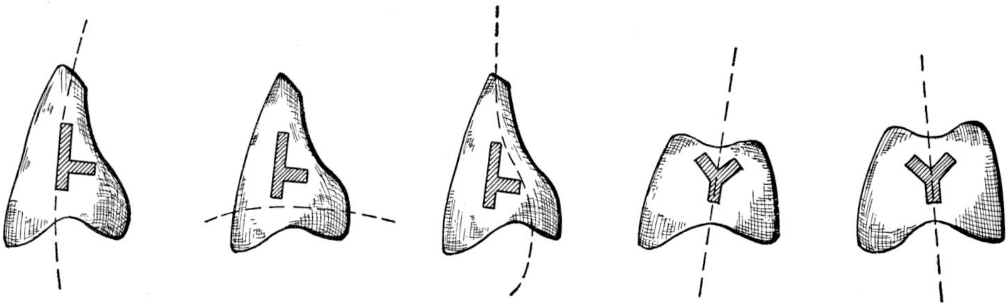

Fig. 34-3. Shapes and positions of stress bars as suggested by Swann.

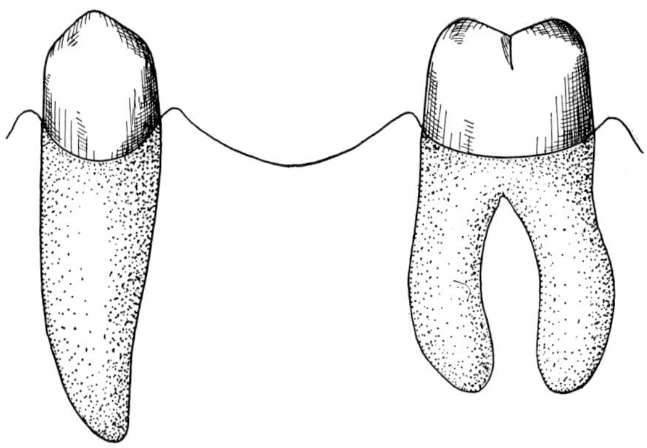

Fig. 34-4. Shoulderless preparations for reinforced porcelain bridge.

ly caused the failure of the entire bridge, because they were not made of sufficiently heavy gauge metal and because they engaged too little surface of the preparation. The band material used was 35-gauge iridioplatinum plate having a 5 percent iridium content. This was found to be too weak and as a result the alloy was changed to a 20 to 25 percent iridium content, giving a much stronger and tougher metal for this purpose.

Swann type. A new technic was suggested by Swann[2] for the construction of the coping or adapter; it was made in two pieces soldered together in such a way that a double thickness of the iridioplatinum plate extended over the axial angles of the preparation. This will be illustrated and explained later in the chapter.

In an effort further to increase the strength of the metallic structure, the connecting bar, which formerly consisted of a round bar or a flat piece of metal, was changed to a Y or T shape; its purpose was to resist the torque imposed upon the bridge (Fig. 34-3). These bands or copings were usually used in conjunction with the shoulder type of preparation, and the gingival margin of the band terminated slightly short of the gingival shoulder.

Hovestad type. Occasionally, it was necessary to prepare the abutment without a gingival shoulder, and for such a preparation (Fig. 34-4) Hovestad[3] designed a cap or axial band which was fitted to the preparation just as is the axial band for a complete gold veneer crown. At the gingival periphery of this band, however, he soldered a reinforcing strip of iridioplatinum wire. The technic for constructing this band is described by him as follows:

First, the cap and band are made of 35 gauge, iridioplatinum plate, 5-20% iridium. The band is adapted to a lap joint, and the joint is sol-

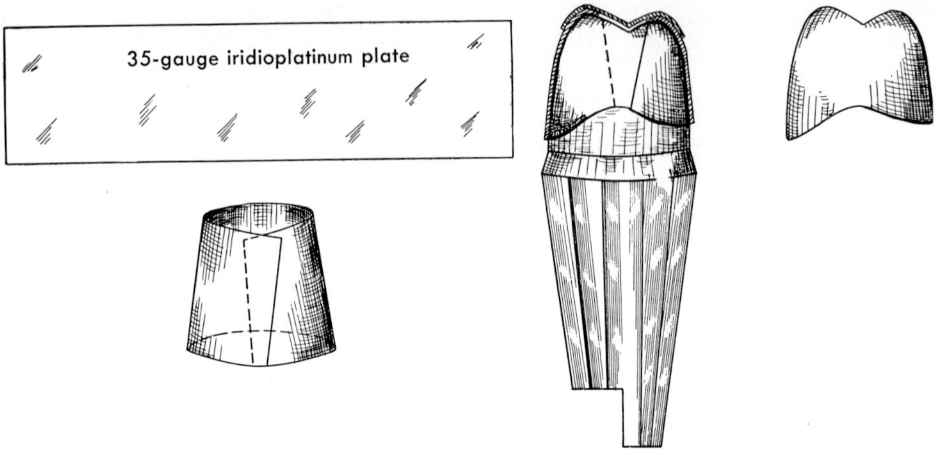

Fig. 34-5. Steps of constructing an iridioplatinum cap as suggested by Hovestad. (From Hovestad, J. F.: D. Items Int. **58:**239, 1936.)

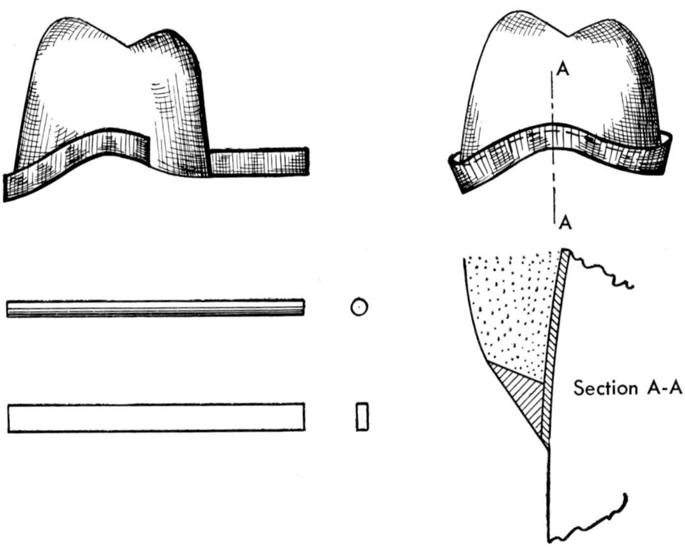

Fig. 34-6. Details of constructing Hovestad cap. (From Hovestad, J. F.: D. Items Int. **58:** 239, 1936.)

dered with platinum solder [Fig. 34-5, *A*]. Second, the band and cap are made in two pieces, and the cap is soldered to the band with a lap joint, using the same platinum solder which united the edges of the band [Fig. 34-5, *B*]. Third, 19-21 gauge iridioplatinum wire, 20% iridium, is made half-round in shape, and is attached to the periphery of the band with platinum solder. The edge of the shoulder is filed thin to give it an appearance of cervical contour to the restoration at this point [Fig. 34-6]. This half-round wire lends great strength and rigidity to the restoration. Fourth, when the abutments are joined together with the bridge frame, the supporting truss is fitted to the respective band with as much of a lap joint as the space available will permit.*

Fig. 34-7 shows the abutment caps united with the Y-torque bar; Fig. 34-8 is the finished bridge.

Felcher type. Felcher,[4] employing a similar principle, constructed his adapter of 0.002-inch platinum matrix in which the lap joint was brazed together. He also

*From Hovestad, J. F.: Porcelain bridges, D. Items Int. **58:**239, 1936.

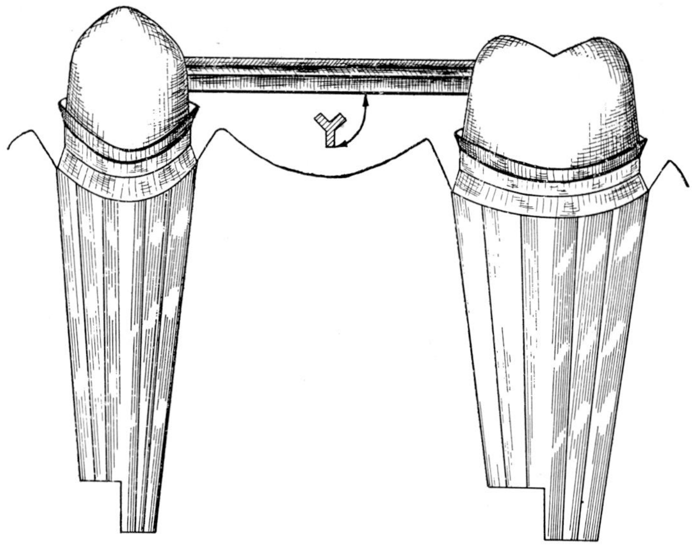

Fig. 34-7. Two completed caps united by means of Y shaped stress bar. (From Hovestad, J. F.: D. Items Int. **58:**239, 1936.)

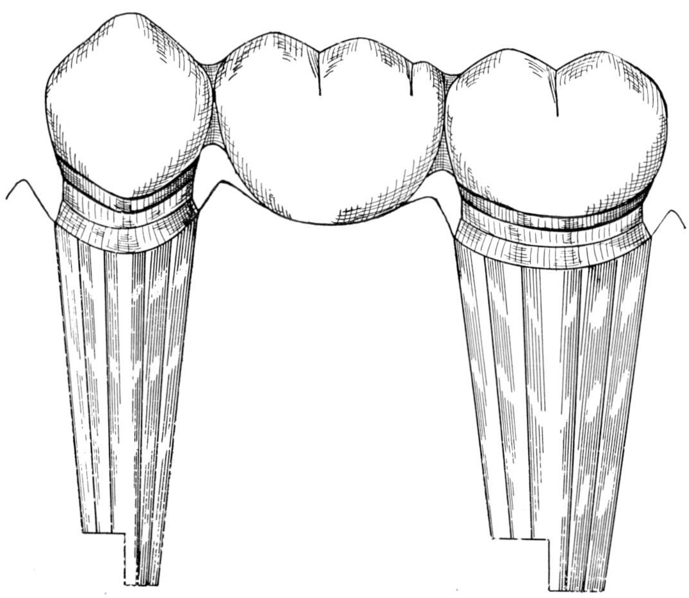

Fig. 34-8. Completed Hovestad reinforced porcelain bridge. Note that narrow margin of metal is exposed around gingival periphery. This is not visible in lower posterior region. (From Hovestad, J. F.: D. Items Int. **58:**239, 1936.)

reinforced the gingival periphery in whole or in part with an iridioplatinum wire to form a finishing shoulder at the gingival periphery. He modified the connecting bar by brazing two pieces of flat plate metal to it in a vertical position in the region to be occupied by the porcelain pontic (Fig. 34-9).

Although a fair degree of success had been obtained with the various types and methods of constructing the metal reinforcing structure in porcelain bridges, be-

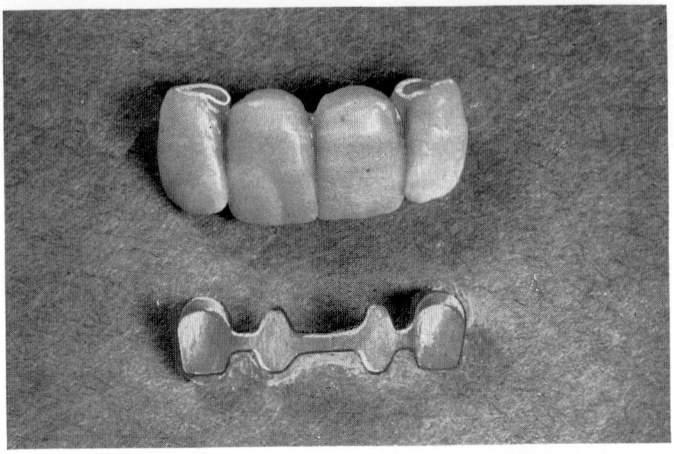

Fig. 34-9. Felcher type reinforced porcelain bridge. (From Felcher, F. R.: D. Digest **43**:24, 1927.)

cause of the difficulty in adapting the iridioplatinum plate and the high heat necessary in the soldering operations, a small percentage of dentist did their own laboratory work for this type of prosthesis. A majority depended to a large degree for this service upon laboratory technicians, who in some instances were not sufficiently trained or who were not conversant with the forces to which the appliance would be subjected in the mouth. Hence, with this type of prosthesis many failures resulted which could have been avoided if a technic had been used in which the metallic structure could be waxed and cast by the dentist himself, if it needed to be, just as he could cast an inlay or a partial denture. When a casting technic was developed that was comparatively simple and that was made available to the dentist, it was quite likely that a new impetus was given to this type of work and its development and use took place on a larger scale than existed at that time.

Second type, using cast iridium or palladium platinum alloys reinforcement framework. Several attempts had been made to cast iridioplatinum for reinforcing porcelain bridges, one of which was described by Hovestad.[3] The difficulty in this technic was due largely to the investment used for casting, since it did not possess the necessary physical properties to withstand high temperatures and still produce an accurately fitting casting. Johnson[5] developed a casting method and the necessary casting investment for constructing reinforcing structures. The design of his structure, however, differed from that suggested by Swann, Felcher, or Hovestad in that it was based on a cross-stayed, truss principle, using round bars in such a manner that the T-bar principle was utilized without having the solid T-shaped mass of metal in the center of the bridge and without forming cleavage planes in the porcelain. Fig. 34-10 illustrates such a truss between two abutment caps. This, Johnson claimed, definitely eliminated the planes of cleavage which were present with the Swann T-bar or with the brazed, vertical plate types of reinforcements.

Granger,[6] also employing the cast principle for the construction of the reinforcement structure, modified the connecting bar so that an axial ferrule or coping of iridioplatinum metal is cast in the region of each pontic of the bridge. This ferrule is then united to the retainers, which may be either a platinum coping, cap, crown, cast platinum inlay, or partial veneer crown. Figs. 34-11 to 34-16 are photographs of such connecting trusses.

More recent developments by Therma-

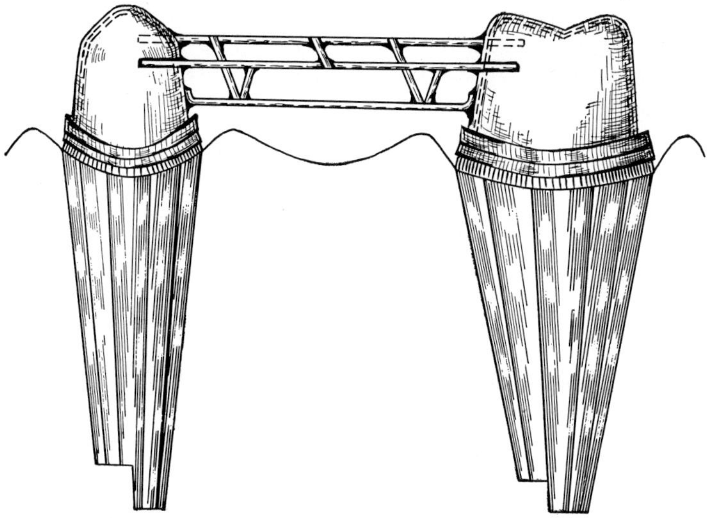

Fig. 34-10. Principle of reinforcement recommended by Dr. C. W. Johnson.

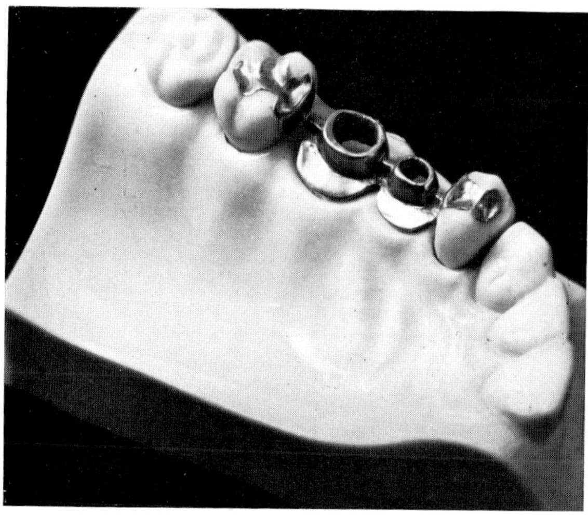

Fig. 34-11. Cast iridioplatinum structure soldered to two retainers; lingual view.

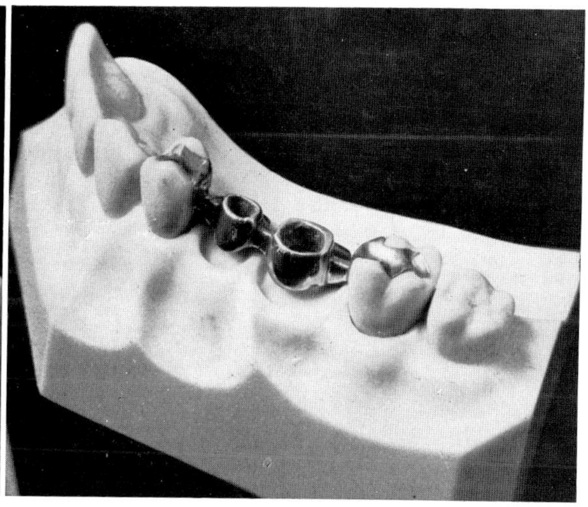

Fig. 34-12. Labial view of model shown in Fig. 34-11.

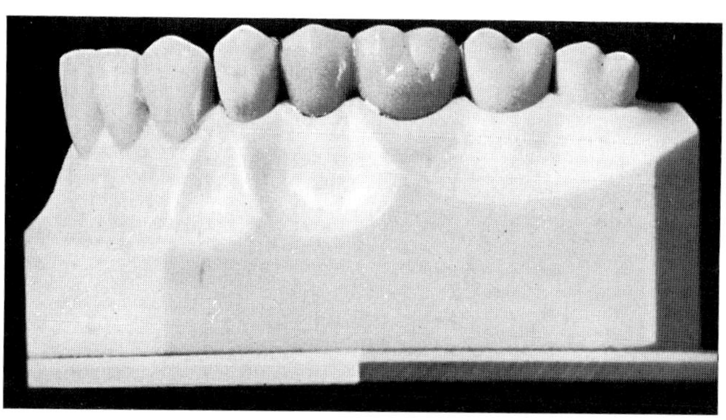

Fig. 34-13. Buccal view of finished bridge.

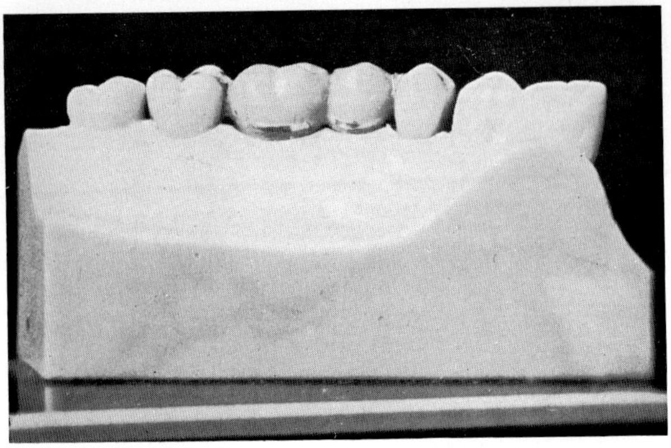

Fig. 34-14. Lingual view of finished bridge.

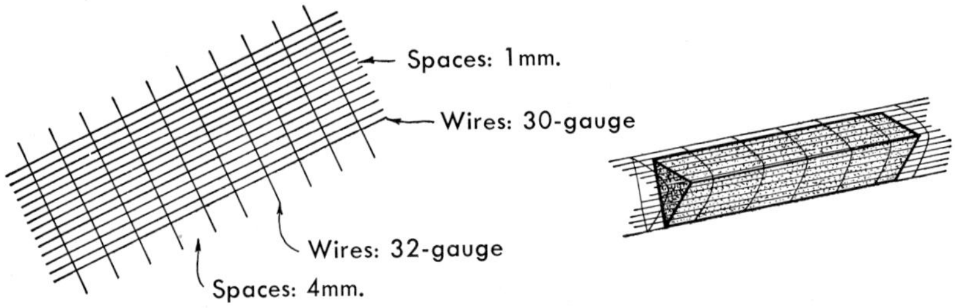

Fig. 34-15. Webbing used to reinforce porcelain bridge. (From Lakermange, R., and Gonon, P.: J. Am. D. Club Paris **2**:1, 1934.)

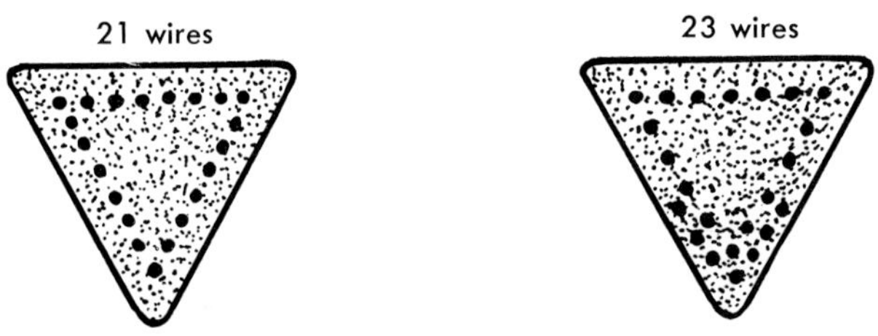

Fig. 34-16. Two methods of distributing reinforcing wires in beam. (From Lakermange, R., and Gonon, P.: J. Am. D. Club Paris **2**:1, 1934.)

lite,[7] Micro-Bond,[8] Ceramco,[9] and Steele's Aluminous Porcelains[10] are those in which (1) the coefficients of expansion and contraction of the porcelain and the alloy have been balanced and (2) a definite bond obtained between the porcelain and the alloys. These types of bridge and technics for their construction are given in Chapters 35 and 36.

The third type: use of reinforcement wires. The third type of metal reinforcement involves the use of iridioplatinum reinforcement wires, the technic for which was evolved and reported by Lakermange and Gonon.[1] It is little used today.

It is known that porcelain has a resistance to compression far in excess of amalgam. The weakness of porcelain, however, lies in its lack of resistance to bending forces. This is borne out clinically by the fact that complete porcelain veneer crowns are capable of withstanding large amounts

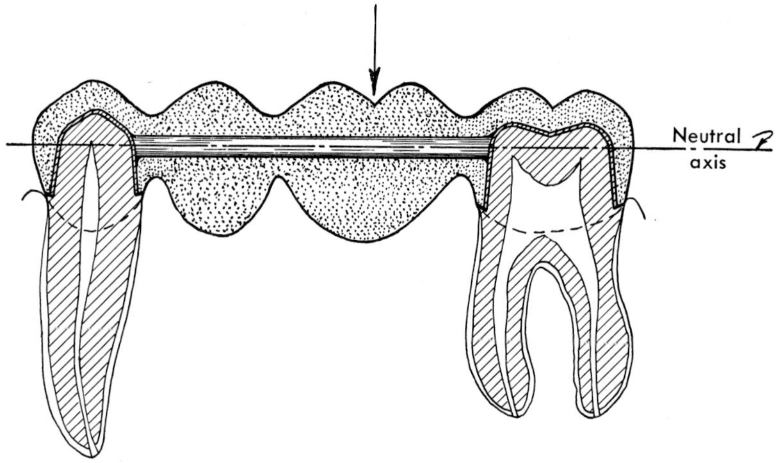

Fig. 34-17. Reinforcing bar placed in line with neutral axis furnishes minimum amount of resistance to fracture. (From Lakermange, R., and Gonon, P.: J. Am. D. Club Paris **2**:1, 1934.)

of compressive force, provided the tooth is so prepared that the preparation absorbs the forces through planes placed at the correct angles. Similarly, it is borne out clinically that unsupported porcelain fractures very easily.

Because a porcelain bridge is comparable to a simple beam in its reactions to applied forces, Lakermange and Gonon conducted a series of experiments to determine the means best suited in a porcelain bridge to counteract bending forces. They also conducted tests to determine the form and type of metal alloys best suited to accomplish this purpose.

Their initial tests involved a study of the forces necessary to break solid beams of porcelain that did not contain any reinforcing structure. These they were able to fracture under loads varying from 19 to 24 kg.

The next series of tests were made on porcelain cylinders of identical dimensions, except that they were reinforced with a 25 percent iridioplatinum wire webbing or netting, as illustrated in Fig. 34-15. These beams, reinforced with an equal distribution of the wires around the three surfaces of the beam, broke under a load of 68 kg.

Position of reinforcement. By redistributing the reinforcing wires so that a greater number were placed in the region lying below the neutral axis, as shown in Fig. 34-16, 80 kg. were required to break the porcelain beam. Tests conducted by the author (S.D.T.) have verified these findings and have shown also that the power of resisting fracture decreases as the reinforcing metal wires approach the level of the neutral axis. If the wires or a metallic bar is placed at the neutral axis line, it fails to serve any purpose, since it lies in a plane that has a zero longitudinal strain (Fig. 34-17). Since porcelain itself is capable of resisting great compressive forces, a reinforcing metallic structure placed above the neutral axis fails to add any resistance to forces. Moreover, placing a heavy metal bar through the neutral axis merely sets up lines of cleavage in the porcelain bridge. The metal reinforcement in the bridge should be lowered beneath the neutral line axis as far as the design of the structure permits it to meet the hygienic requirements.

Even modifying the circular rod into a Y or a T shape does not change the condition very much.

Lakermange and Gonon conducted further experiments to determine the relative

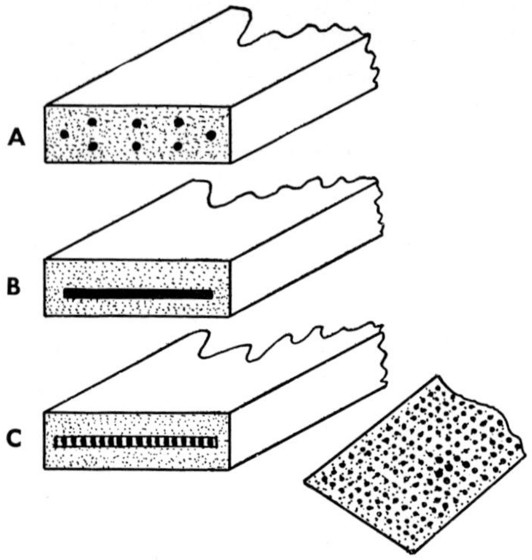

Fig. 34-18. Different methods of distributing reinforcing metal. (From Lakermange, R., and Gonon, P.: J. Am. D. Club Paris **2**:1, 1934.)

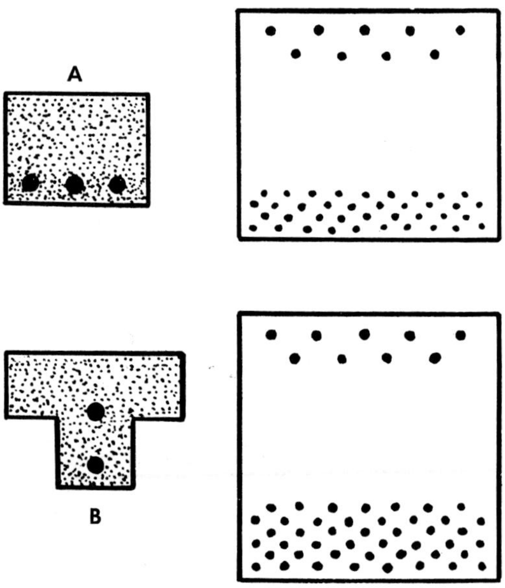

Fig. 34-19. Various methods of distributing reinforcing rods in concrete beams. (From Lakermange, R., and Gonon, P.: J. Am. D. Club Paris **2**:1, 1934.)

values when using the same amount of reinforcing metal but applied in different shapes and distribution. Fig. 34-18 represents three samples of reinforcing metals having the same total cross-sectional area; *A* contains eight wires of 0.8 mm. in

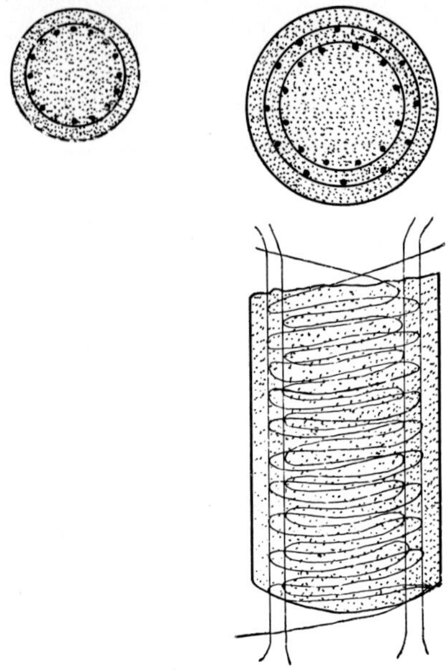

Fig. 34-20. Methods of reinforcing pillars subjected to compressive forces. (From Lakermange, R., and Gonon, P.: J. Am. D. Club Paris **2**:1, 1934.)

diameter, having a total cross section of approximately 4.2 mm. The metal used in *B* and *C* is in the form of a plate 8 mm. wide and 0.5 mm. thick; this also has a cross-sectional area of approximately 4.2 mm. It will be noted that in the latter two, the shape and position of the metal plate are such that it lies in the neutral axis region and sets up definite cleavage planes.

Reinforced concrete beams, when used in construction projects, usually have the reinforcing metal distributed as illustrated in Fig. 34-19, *A;* where greater loads are to be carried, the beams are reinforced as illustrated in Fig. 34-19, *A,* where, it will be observed, the greater proportion of reinforcing metal lies below the neutral axis of the beam. Figs. 34-19, *B,* and 34-20 shows the same principle of distributing reinforcing metal in pillars designed to withstand compressive as well as stretching forces.

In Fig. 34-21 the two diagrams on the left, having the total amount of metal in one piece centrally located, are the least desirable methods to use. The third dia-

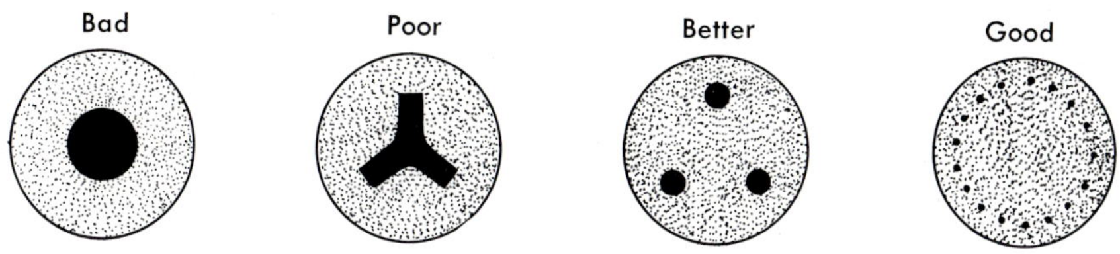

Fig. 34-21. Four methods distributing approximately same amount of reinforcing metal. (From Lakermange, R., and Gonon, P.: J. Am. D. Club Paris **2**:1, 1934.)

gram, wherein the total volume is divided between three reinforcing rods, is better, but the method shown on the extreme right indicates the best arrangement of the reinforcing rods. The maximum resistance, however, may be obtained by winding, in addition, a circular armature around the longitudinal rods, as shown in the fourth illustration.

Lakermange and Gonon found that, in order to prevent surface cracking, it is necessary that a covering of material equal to at least two diameters of the reinforcing rods or wires be applied to the outside surface (Fig. 34-22). In porcelain bridgework, however, this amount is usually greater, because, if the iridioplatinum wires are brought close to the surface, they show through the porcelain. This difficulty, however, is largely overcome by the application of semiopaque porcelain, which covers the reinforcing iridioplatinum wires.

With these facts in mind, Lakermange and Gonon developed a system of reinforced porcelain bridgework that depends upon the use of iridioplatinum wires of relatively small gauge, distributed through the porcelain bridge and around the abutments in such a way that the reinforcing metal furnishes a maximum resistance to tension with a minimum use of metal and an almost complete elimination of cleavage planes (Figs. 34-28 to 34-36).

Construction of wrought-metal reinforced bridges. The construction of reinforced porcelain bridges employing wrought metals for the framework is somewhat different from all-porcelain bridges. The copings or adapters are usually constructed of an iridioplatinum alloy of 5 to

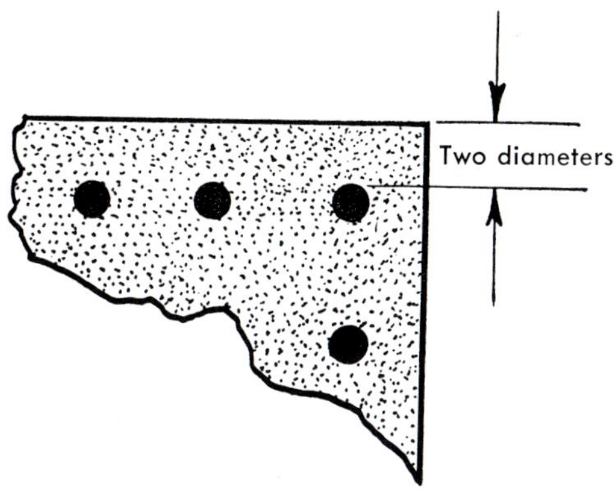

Fig. 34-22. To prevent surface cracking, surface material must be equal in thickness to at least two diameters of reinforcing wire. (From Lakermange, R., and Gonon, P.: J. Am. D. Club Paris **2**:1, 1934.)

25 percent iridium in plate form and 40- to 19-gauge in thickness.

The connecting bar between the two copings or adapters may be either round, L, Y, or T shaped; sometimes it is merely a plate of metal to which additional pieces of alloy are soldered or brazed to reinforce the porcelain. Fig. 34-3 shows a cross section of the T and the Y shaped Swann type of bar used for this purpose. Fig. 34-9 shows the modification of the truss bar as advocated by Felcher. This so-call stress bar, is usually made of iridioplatinum varying from 15 to 25 percent iridium.

The solder used for uniting the copings with the stress bar is a 75 to 25 percent platinum-iridium alloy.

The Swann adapter. There are several types and methods of swaging the iridoplatinum coping or adapter. The one suggested by Swann and Megaw, consisting of two pieces welded together, later was the

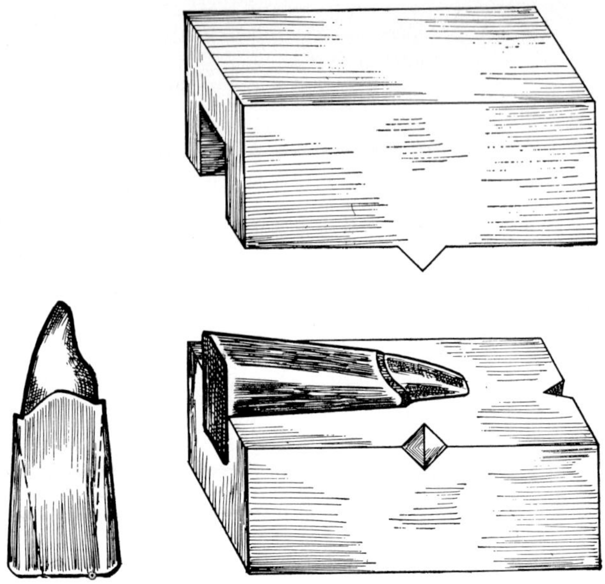

Fig. 34-23. Two-section plaster mold of die and matrix. (From Swann, H.: Torque resisting porcelain bridge, Chicago, 1931.)

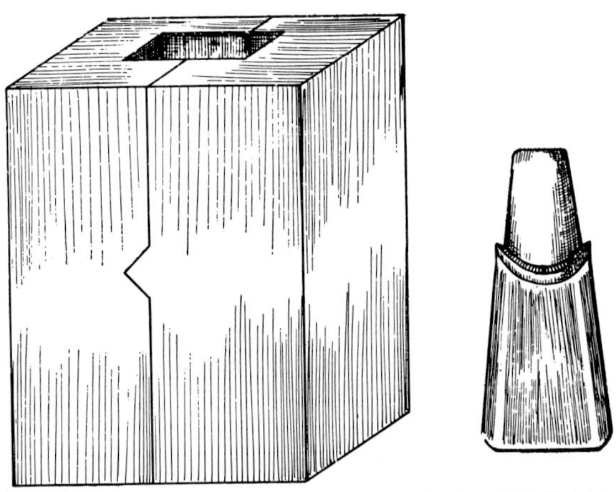

Fig. 34-24. Assembled plaster mold and die. Die may be made of low-fusing metal or preferably of hard technic metal. (From Swann, H.: Torque resisting porcelain bridge, Chicago, 1931.)

one more generally used for bridge restorations. The first step in the construction of the adapter or coping requires amalgam dies of correctly prepared teeth, properly oriented in their working casts.

A platinum matrix, 0.001 inch thick, is adapted to the amalgam die. The iridioplatinum reinforcement coping must be made to fit over the 0.001-inch platinum matrix. Since this material is thin, the burnishing or swaging of the iridioplatinum plate over it would cause it to tear; therefore, a die is made of metal that reproduces the shape of the 0.001-inch platinum matrix on the amalgam die. A two-section plaster mold is made of the amalgam die with its platinum matrix as shown in Figs. 34-23 and 34-24. Low-fusing metal is then poured into the mold, producing a metal die which reproduces the exact di-

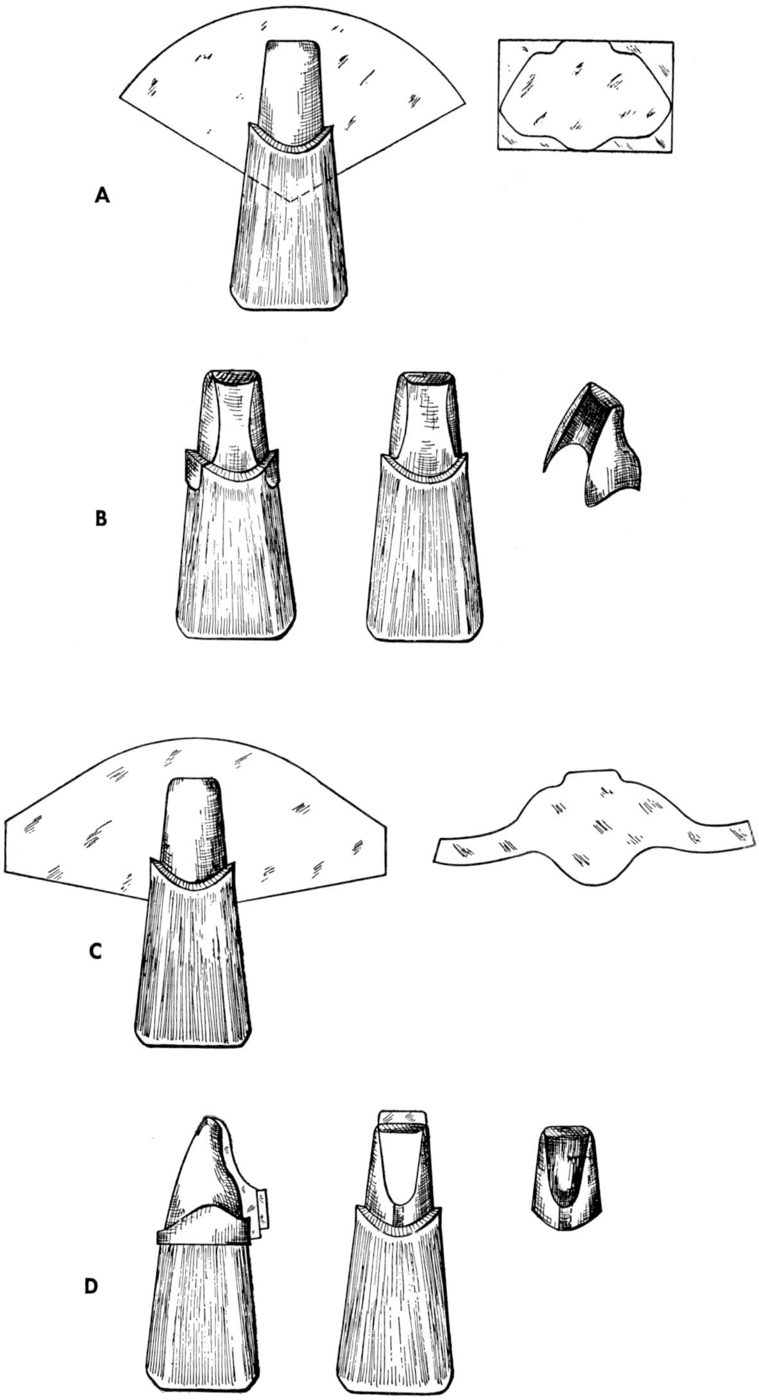

Fig. 34-25. A, First step in construction of Swann cap. **B,** Lingual part of cap. **C,** First step in adapting labial part of cap. **D,** Labial and lingual parts assembled, and completed Swann cap for anterior teeth. (From Swann, H.: Torque resisting porcelain bridge, Chicago, 1931.)

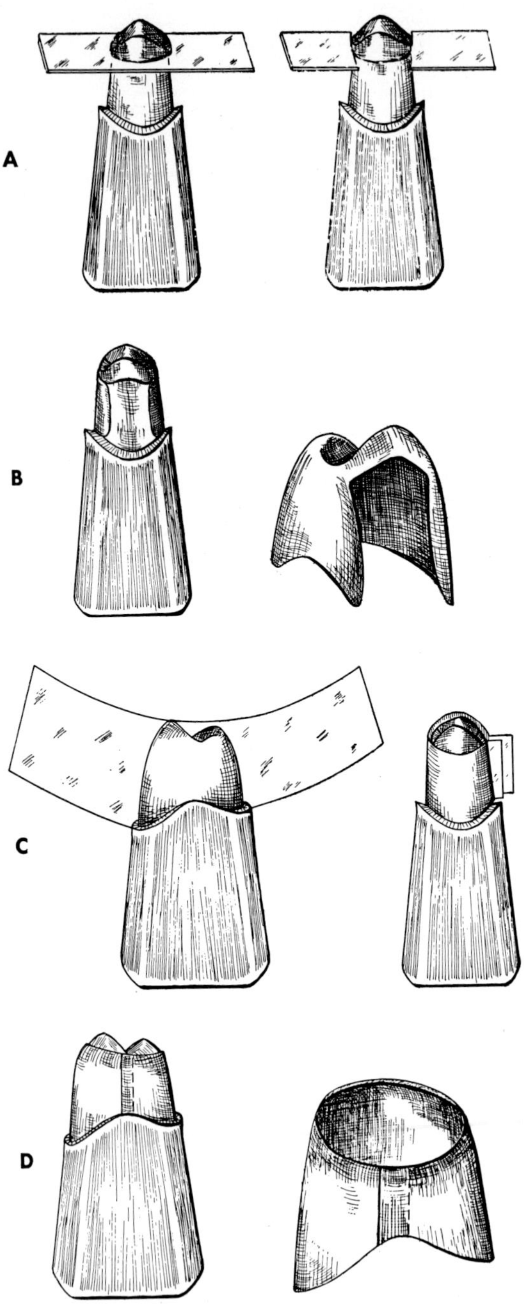

Fig. 34-26. A, First step in adapting cap to occlusal and two proximal surfaces. **B,** First portion of cap completed. Note buccal and lingual surfaces are exposed. **C,** Adapting axial band portion of cap. **D,** Two parts of band assembled and soldered to form posterior Swann cap. (From Swann, H.: Torque resisting porcelain bridge, Chicago, 1931.)

mensions of the tooth preparation covered with its 0.001-inch matrix. If a die of a harder material is desired, softened inlay wax may be forced into the plaster sectional mold, and the wax model is reproduced by casting it either in hard technic metal or in a silver-copper alloy. The coronal portion of such a die is now larger than the natural tooth preparation by the thickness of the 0.001-inch matrix. The platinum reinforcement coping is now constructed and fitted on this enlarged die. Iridioplatinum plate, 38- to 40-gauge and 15 to 25 percent iridium, is used for this purpose. The copings for both the anterior and the posterior teeth are made in two pieces, which are subsequently united by brazing with platinum solder. Fig. 34-25 shows the various steps in the construction of such a reinforcement coping for an anterior incisor. Because of the difficulty of manipulating the iridioplatinum plate, it is advisable first to make a tin foil pattern for the lingual surface, bringing it around to the proximal and onto the labial surface as shown. A piece of iridioplatinum plate is then cut out to conform to the outline of the tin foil pattern. By successive steps of burnishing, swaging, annealing, and trimming, the iridioplatinum plate is adapted to the lingual and the two proximal surfaces and is overlapped on the labial surface around the two line angles. A slight extension is left to cover the incisal plane. The gingival margin is trimmed so that it terminates just short of the inner line angle formed by the axial surface and the shoulder.

The same procedure is followed in adapting the labial portion of the iridioplatinum reinforcement coping. When completed, the iridioplatinum plate covers the labial and the two proximal surfaces and that portion of the lingual surface extending around the cingulum of the tooth. The two parts, labial and lingual, are now waxed on the lingual surface, invested in high heat investment, and united with irid-

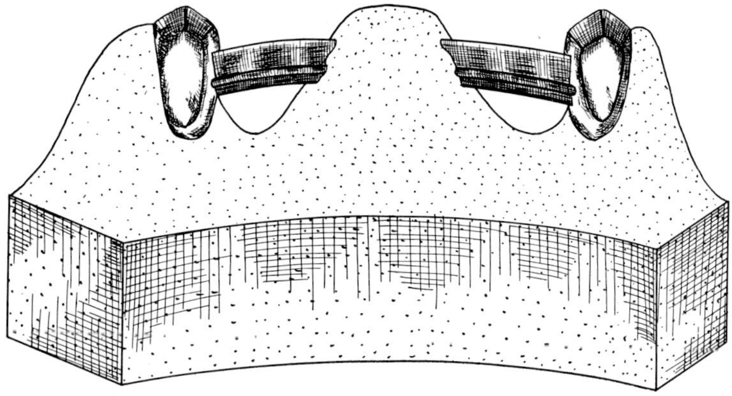

Fig. 34-27. Method of investing stress bar and caps for soldering. (From Swann, H.: Torque resisting porcelain bridge, Chicago, 1931.)

ioplatinum solder. It will be observed that there is only one thickness of metal on the labial and lingual surfaces, but that all other surfaces have two thicknesses of the reinforcing plate.

The coping is placed back on the enlarged, hard metal die and swaged to conform it accurately. After this has been done, the reinforcement coping is placed on the original amalgam die, which is covered with the 0.001-inch platinum matrix. Since the coping was fitted and swaged to the enlarged die, it also fits over the platinum matrix.

For the posterior teeth, Swann suggested that the reinforcement coping be made in two sections, which ultimately are also fused together with platinum solder. Fig. 34-26 shows that portion of the coping which is swaged to cover the occlusal and the two proximal surfaces. It will be noted that the buccal and the lingual surfaces are open, except the part near the cusps.

With this completed and in position, another piece of iridioplatinum metal is cut in strip form and wrapped around the axial surfaces of the enlarged die, encircling the inner section of the coping. The two parts are waxed together, invested, and soldered; this gives a coping having one layer of metal on the occlusal, the buccal, and the lingual surfaces and having two thicknesses on the two axial surfaces. The gingival margin of the posterior coping is also trimmed so that it is just short of the inner angle formed by the axial surface and the shoulder.

Uniting the copings with a stress bar. Where the shoulder type of preparation is made, the Swann type of reinforcement coping just described is preferable. Where, however, the shoulderless type of preparation is employed, the reinforcement coping may be made according to the methods of Hovestad and Felcher. Following the completion of the two reinforcement copings, a stress bar of the proper shape and design is selected and contoured to correspond to the general curvature of the ridge mesiodistally. The two copings and the bar are then waxed, removed from the model, invested in high heat soldering investment, and soldered with iridioplatinum solder. When investing the assembly, care should be taken that the surfaces to be united with solder are fully exposed and accessible to the blowpipe flame; this may be done by placing a small amount of investment over the center of the bar, leaving its two ends exposed as shown in Fig. 34-27.

The soldered iridioplatinum framework is now cleaned by boiling it in hydrofluoric acid to remove all traces of the investment, after which it is replaced on the amalgam dies in the working model, which are covered with the 0.001-inch platinum matrices.

A small amount of sticky wax is melted between the reinforcement copings and the platinum matrices, uniting them. Both are removed from the amalgam dies and the entire assembly is invested in high heat investment placed on a muffle tray. Care must be exercised that none of the investment comes in contact with the iridioplatinum framework or the outer surfaces of the platinum matrices. The tray with the mounted metal structure is then inserted into the muffle and gradually heated until all traces of wax have been eliminated and the investment material is thoroughly hardened. The tray with the metal structure is then removed and allowed to cool.

Application and firing of porcelain. A small amount of opaque porcelain is mixed and a thin layer is applied to cover the entire iridioplatinum framework, including the gingival periphery of the coping but not the 0.001-inch platinum matrix material. The entire structure, still mounted on the tray, is now carried to a temperature about 100° F. below the glazing point.

After the appliance has cooled, a second application and firing of porcelain is made; this time, however, equal parts of opaque and of translucent gingiva-colored porcelain are used; this gives a semiopaque porcelain. This also is applied with a brush in a thin layer, this time covering not only the entire iridioplatinum structure, but also the 0.001-inch platinum matrix, and carrying it close to the outer edge of the matrix shoulder. It is then dried and fired to a temperature approximately 80° F. below the glazing point.

When cool, the structure is given a third application of porcelain. This time, however, the standard gingival and the incisal porcelain colors are used. At this time also the reinforcement copings are covered with gingival porcelain in an amount ordinarily used for the first bake of a complete veneer porcelain crown. At this time a foundation core, using the gingiva-colored porcelain, is also built on the bar in the region of the pontic. The bridge is then dried, inserted in the muffle, and brought to a fusing point approximately 60° below the glazing temperature of the porcelain. For this bake gingival porcelain also covers the remaining portion of the shoulder and the platinum apron extending beyond the shoulder.

After the bridge has been fired and removed from the muffle and allowed to cool, it is removed from the investment on the tray and tried on the working model. If satisfactory, the abutment teeth and the pontics are built to complete contour with the proper gingival and incisal colors. Vertical cuts between the crown and the pontics are then made in the porcelain down to the foundation porcelain on the stress bar. This is done to enable the porcelain to shrink toward separate centers, leaving shrinkage spaces between the pontics and the crowns.

When the bridge is removed from the muffle and allowed to cool, definite spaces will be found where the vertical cuts were made. These spaces are now filled with porcelain and the necessary contour is developed. It is advisable to overcontour slightly at this time, in order to have sufficient porcelain for the final grinding and adjusting of the bridge. While the final glaze may be given at this stage, it is a better practice to bring the firing point of this bake approximately 20° F. below the glazing point of the porcelain. The bridge may then be tried again on the model for final adjustment and verification of fit, after which the final glaze is given. In all the firings, particularly the last three, it is important that the temperature be raised and subsequently lowered very gradually to avoid the possibility of internal stresses developing within the bridge, which ultimately might cause a fracture or failure of the bridge.

Before the bridge is permanently ce-

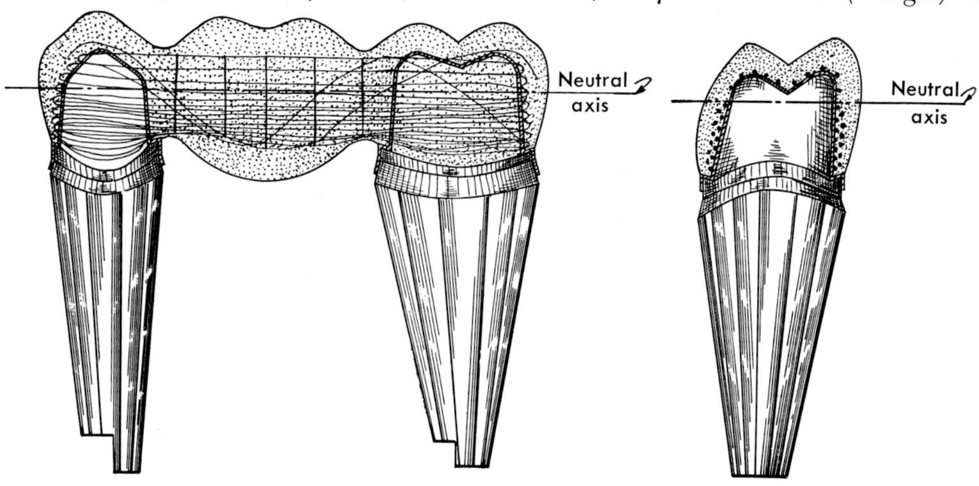

Fig. 34-28. A, Cross section of porcelain bridge showing distribution of reinforcing wires. **B,** Buccolingual cross section through molar retainer, showing distribution of reinforcing wires of webbing. (From Lakermange, R., and Gonon, P.: J. Am. D. Club Paris **2**:1, 1934.)

mented, the 0.001-inch platinum matrices are removed from both of the crowns. The gingival shoulders of the crowns consist entirely of glazed porcelain, the metal reinforcement copings lying within the angle of the shoulder preparation and in contact with the axial surfaces of the tooth.

The same precautions should be observed in the shaping and the glazing of the gingival portions of the pontic as in other types of bridge construction. If the stress bar has been properly placed, it should not be visible; neither should it interfere with the proper contouring and shaping of the interdental and interproximal spaces of the bridge.

In those bridges that employ shoulderless preparations, 0.001-inch platinum matrix is used, since the iridioplatinum reinforcement coping itself constitutes the gingival margin of the porcelain crown.

Wire reinforcement method of Lakermange and Gonon. Reinforced porcelain bridges not using copings of wrought iridioplatinum plate metal, but wire instead, are made by a method which is comparatively simple and which is within the ability of the average dentist to construct. Fig. 34-28, *A* illustrates a cross section of a bridge reinforced by the method recommended by Lakermange and Gonon. It will be noted that the two abutments are prepared with shoulders to receive complete veneer porcelain crowns. Longitudinal reinforcement wires extend from one abutment to the other, with the greater proportion of the wires lying below the neutral axis. It will be observed in Fig. 34-28, *B,* that the crown is reinforced by a circular winding of reinforcing wires in accordance with the principle of reinforcement used in pillars sustaining heavy compressive and bending forces.

No reinforcement adapters or copings are made for the individual abutments other than the 0.001-inch platinum matrix regularly employed in the construction of a complete porcelain veneer crown.

After the two matrices have been constructed on the amalgam dies seated in the working model, they are covered with a thin layer of gingival-colored porcelain, which is brought to a bisque firing (Fig. 34-29). The next step is to grind a prismatic piece of high-fusing porcelain to fit between the two abutments (Fig. 34-30). This piece extends horizontally, mesiodistally, from one abutment to the other

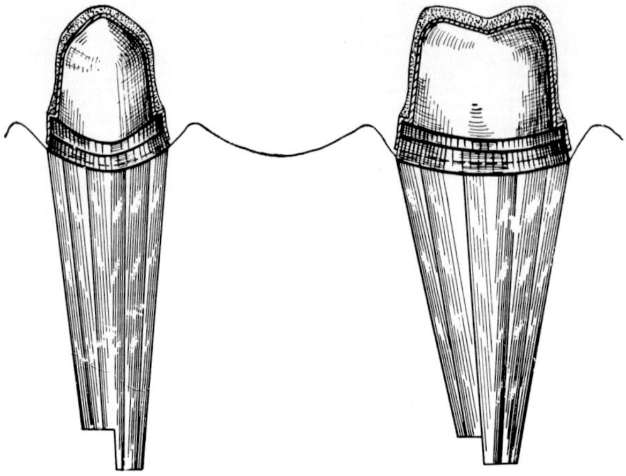

Fig. 34-29. Platinum matrix, 0.001 inch, adapted to amalgam dies. Thin layer of gingival porcelain is baked on. (From Lakermange, R., and Gonon, P.: J. Am. D. Club Paris **2:** 1, 1934.)

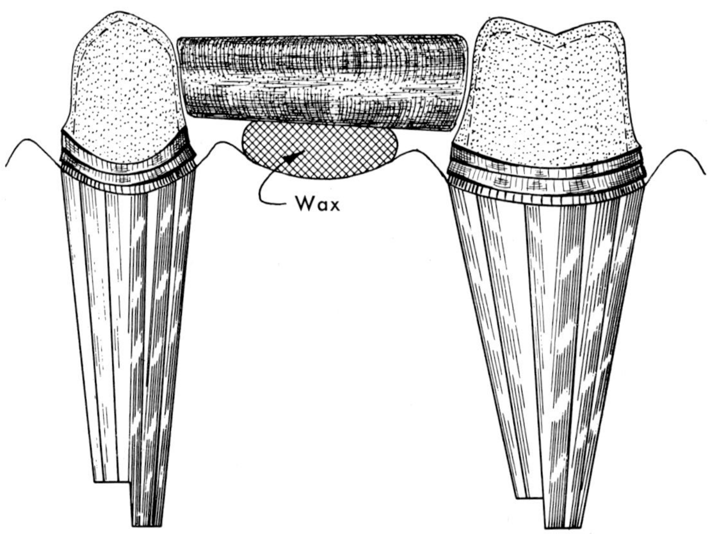

Fig. 34-30. Prism of high-fusing porcelain ground to fit between two retainers and held in position with wax. (From Lakermange, R., and Gonon, P.: J. Am. D. Club Paris **2:** 1, 1934.)

and is given the general shape of a pontic; it is wider at the occlusal area and tapers gingivally, as shown in Fig. 34-31. The porcelain prism is now wrapped with the 25 percent iridioplatinum webbing of the gauges indicated in Fig. 34-15, *A*. The overlapping of the webbing is made at the gingival border, at which point there is the greatest need for resistance to tension. The ends of the longitudinal wires are permitted to extend mesially and distally beyond the porcelain prism and are left sufficiently long that they may be wrapped around the platinum matrices of the abutment teeth. The lateral wires forming the armature may be removed from the netting that extends beyond the length of the prismatic porcelain core.

The porcelain core is supported between the two platinum matrices and ground so that it touches the two proximal surfaces without too much pressure. The wires of

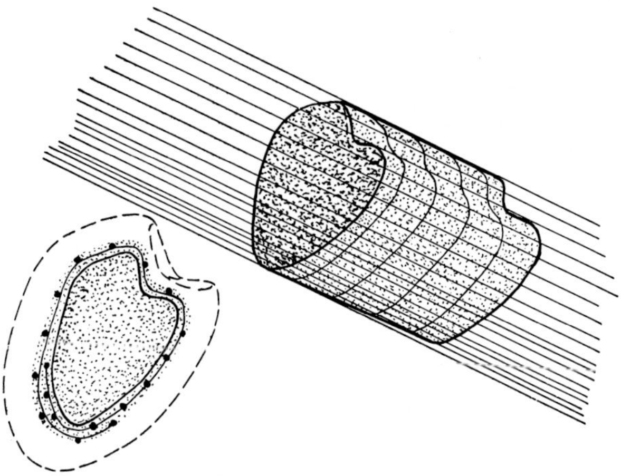

Fig. 34-31. Porcelain prism roughly shaped and wrapped in reinforcing metal webbing. Note that circular reinforcing wires cover only prism. (From Lakermange, R., and Gonon, P.: J. Am. D. Club Paris **2**:1, 1934.)

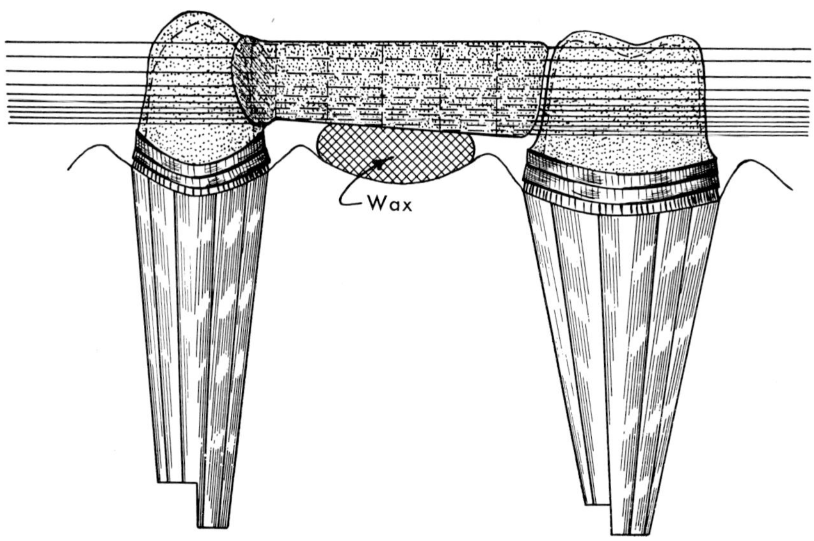

Fig. 34-32. Prism wrapped in webbing, replaced between two retainers; ends of wires straightened and one end of prism united to one retainer with baked porcelain. (From Lakermange, R., and Gonon, P.: J. Am. D. Club Paris **2**:1, 1934.)

the webbing extending beyond the porcelain prism are roughly adapted to the labial and lingual surfaces of the matrices covered with the initial bake of porcelain. The porcelain prism is fused to one of the platinum matrices by applying a small amount of porcelain between the prism and the matrix covered with an initial bake of porcelain (Fig. 34-32).

The porcelain prism or core and the matrix are returned to the amalgam die on the model, and the wire extension of the webbing is wrapped and wound around the labial and the lingual surfaces of the line angles of the tooth. It is not necessary that these wires be wrapped completely around the labial and lingual surfaces; it suffices if both ends of the wires overlap each other by at least 2 mm. Usually such an overlap of wires may be made entirely on the distant or remote proximal surface (Fig. 34-33). Ad-

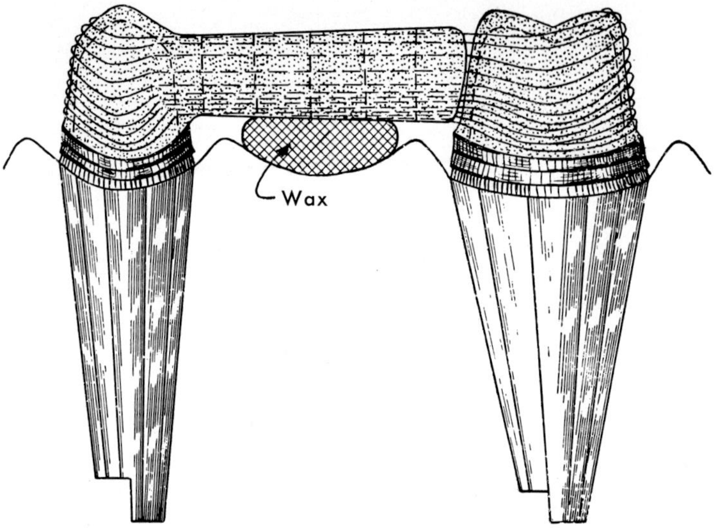

Fig. 34-33. Ends of wire wrapped around two retainers and porcelain applied and baked over bicuspid wire webbing. (From Lakermange, R., and Gonon, P.: J. Am. D. Club Paris **2**:1, 1934.)

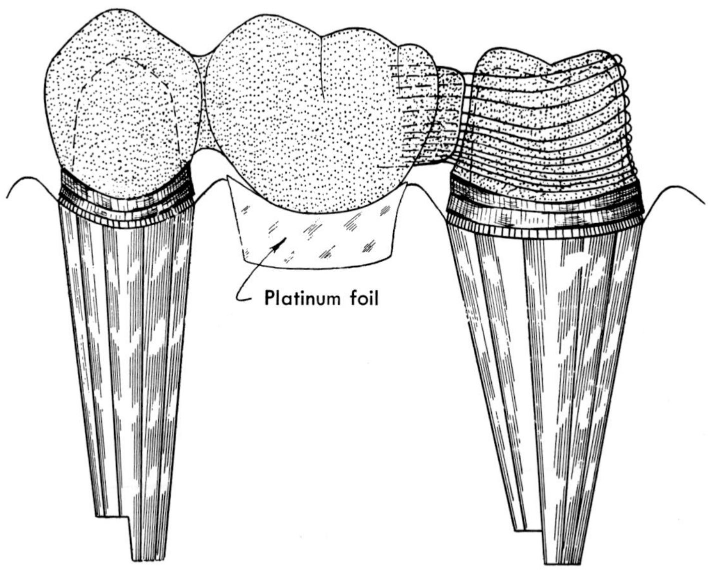

Fig. 34-34. Bicuspid retainer and molar pontic contoured in porcelain and baked. Note platinum foil covering ridge. (From Lakermange, R., and Gonon, P.: J. Am. D. Club Paris **2**:1, 1934.)

ditional gingival-colored porcelain is then added to cover the wires, and the entire structure is given a bisque firing.

It should be noted at this time that the porcelain core has been attached and fired to one retainer only, the other still remaining unattached. When cool, the one retainer and the core are now built in porcelain to their full contour and brought to a high bisque bake. This portion of the bridge is now nearly complete (Fig. 34-34).

The next step involves the construction and completion of the second retainer, but

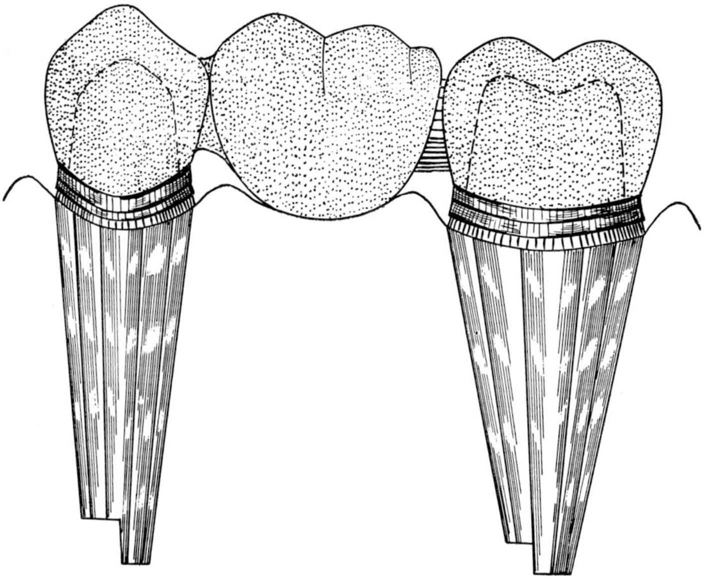

Fig. 34-35. Molar retainer baked; note there is still no rigid union between pontic and molar retainer. (From Lakermange, R., and Gonon, P.: J. Am. D. Club Paris **2**:1, 1934.)

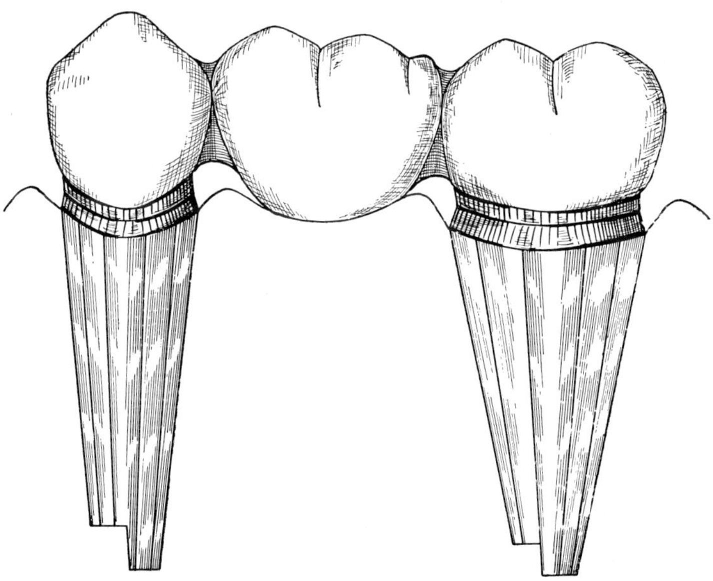

Fig. 34-36. Final union of pontic with molar crown; completed bridge is set after 0.001 inch platinum matrices are removed from retainers. (From Lakermange, R., and Gonon, P.: J. Am. D. Club Paris **2**:1, 1934.)

without uniting it to the entire bridge. This procedure is very important, since it allows a final trial on the model before the completion of the bridge. The wires of the webbing extending distally are, therefore, adapted to the buccal and lingual surfaces of the platinum matrix covered with a thin layer of porcelain. The wires are then covered with the gingival-colored porcelain and brought to a bisque firing, thus uniting the matrix of the second retainer to the iridioplatinum wire webbing extending from the porcelain core (Fig. 34-35). It should be observed, however, that no rigid union has been made between the pontic portion of the bridge and the second retainer; the only connection exists by virtue of the iridioplatinum wires between the two parts. If the relationship is satisfactory, porcelain is added between the second retainer and pontic, rigidly uniting the two parts of the bridge. After the final contour and adjustments have been made, the bridge is glazed and ready for cementation following the removal of the platinum matrices from both retainer crowns (Fig. 34-36). Fig. 34-28, *A*, shows the approximate relationship and position of the reinforcement wires in relationship to the bridge proper.

SELECTED REFERENCES

1. Lakermange, R., and Gonon, P.: Bridges in reinforced porcelain, J. Am. D. Club Paris **2**:1, 1934.
2. Swann, H.: Torque resisting porcelain bridge, Chicago, 1931.
3. Hovestad, J. F.: Porcelain bridges, D. Items Int. **58**:239, 330, 418, 509, 615, 1936.
4. Felcher, F. R.: Platinum reinforced porcelain restorations, D. Digest **43**:24, 1937.
5. Johnson, C. W.: Los Angeles, Calif. Personal communication.
6. Granger, E. R.: Platinum-iridium castings; a new concept of the dental casting process, J.A.D.A. **27**:1718, 1940.
7. Ney-Oro P-16, Thermalite Porcelain Manual, Hartford, Conneticut, 1968, The J. M. Ney Co.
8. Micro-Bond High-Life Porcelain Technic, Chicago, 1967, Austenal Co.
9. Ceramco Basic Porcelain Manual, Woodside, New York, 1963, Ceramco, Inc.
10. Steele's Aluminous Porcelain Technic Book, Columbus, Ohio, 1968, Columbus Dental Mfg. Co.

GENERAL REFERENCES

Argue, J. E.: Esthetic value of porcelain in fixed bridge restorations, J.A.D.A. **21**:90, 1934.

Bassman, A. H.: Baked porcelain fused to gold, Fort. Rev. Chicago D. Soc. **42**:11, 59, 1961.

Bastian, C. C.: The porcelain jacket crown and its application to bridgework, J. Michigan D. Soc. **24**:27, 1942.

Baum, L., Hayden, J., Jr., and Bonlie, D.: Cast restorations with baked porcelain incisal edges for fractured young permanent incisors, J. Dent. Child. **28**:177, 1961.

Bjorn, E., and others: Element distribution in gold-platinum alloys; a pilot study with the electron micro-probe, Acta Odont. Scand. **23**:323-334, 1965.

Brecker, S. C.: Porcelain baked to gold—a new medium in prosthodontics, J. Prosth. Dent. **6**:801, 1956.

Brewster, C.: The alloy of platinum with iridium, D. Cosmos **2**:352-354, 1860.

Brickman, B. M.: The light and color phenomena in teeth and dental porcelains, D. Cosmos **74**:666, 1932.

Cohen, M.: Use of porcelain in development of better dentistry, D. Survey **6**:28, 1930.

Dennison, E. A.: Vita air and vacuum fired porcelain, D. Technician **11**:28, 1958.

Felcher, F. R.: Modern dental porcelains, J.A.D.A. **23**:1009, 1019, 1936.

Felcher, F. R.: Problems involved in reinforcing under porcelain, J.A.D.A. **26**:1284-1288, 1939.

Felcher, F. R.: Platinum reinforced porcelain restorations, D. Digest **43**:24, 1937.

Gonon, P.: Indications and technique of construction of porcelain bridges, Tr. Eighth Internat. D. Cong. **9**:68, 1931.

Gonon, P., and Lakermange, R.: Bridges de porcelaine armee suivant les methods d'amature de beton, Odontologie **72**:540-564, 1934.

Hovestad, J. F.: Practical dental porcelains, St. Louis, 1924, The C. V. Mosby Co.

Hovestad, J. F.: Use of porcelain rods in dental ceramics, D. Items Int. **57**:22, 1935.

Kingery, W. D.: Introduction to ceramics, New York, 1960, John Wiley & Sons.

Land, C. H.: Porcelain dental art, Dent. Cosmos **45**:437-444, 1906.

Le Gro, A. L.: Ceramics in dentistry, Brooklyn, N. Y., 1925, Dental Items of Interest Publishing Co.

Le Gro, A. L.: Renaissance of dental ceramics, D. Cosmos **69**:1129, 1927.

Squires, W. A.: Bridges—present status of porcelain bridgework, J.A.D.A. **25**:570, 1938.

Chapter 35

Current dental restorations utilizing ceramics fired to gold-alloy castings (Thermalite, Micro-Bond, Ceramco porcelains)

A later development by Granger[1] gave accurate iridioplatinum castings of individual crowns and complete reinforced fixed partial structures. Granger modified the stress bar or truss by designing ferrule-shaped copings for the pontic section of the truss (Figs. 34-11 to 34-14).

Complete description of the Granger reinforced porcelain bridges has been given in previous editions of this textbook. Discussion of the Micro-Bond palladium-platinum alloy types of porcelain bridges are also found in the previous editions. While both the Granger and the platinum alloy types of Micro-Bond are satisfactory from the standpoint of utility and esthetics, the comparatively high cost of materials and the time involved in their construction, plus the need for unusually skillful technicians to perform the necessary work, make it necessary to confine the discussion here to the more generally used present-day ceramic-metal types of bridges employing the gold alloy metals.

The science of metallurgy of precious metals has advanced greatly in the last decade, as has the knowledge and application of the high-temperature refractory casting investments. This has enabled the dentist to obtain accurately fitting cast metal structures that support the fused porcelain components of a ceramic-metal fixed partial prosthesis. The coefficients of expansion and contraction of the alloys and porcelains have been balanced and the molecular bond obtainable today between metal and porcelain has eliminated the necessity for basic mechanical retention between the two.

With a properly designed structure of metal, the present special gold alloys bonded molecularly to porcelain are sufficiently strong to meet the requirements to which the structure will be subjected, inasmuch as these alloys are comparable to the Type IIIC and Type IV casting gold alloys generally used in fixed partial denture construction.

USE OF THERMALITE 1750° F. PORCELAIN AND NEY-ORO P-16 CASTING GOLD

Among the list of gold alloys available are those of Ney-Oro P-16, with Thermalite porcelain, 1750° F.[2]; Micro-Bond High Life with Micro-Bond porcelain[3]; and Jelenko and Aderer golds, used with Ceramco porcelains.[4] The physical

Table 35-1. New hue and bioform shade guides

Shade	Porcelain		Opaque	
	Gingival	*Incisal*	*Gingival*	*Incisal*
		Trubyte new hue vitality scale		
60	60N	(2)91 + (1)60N	G	H
61	61N	(1)90 + (1)WP	(1)D + (1)A	(1)H + (1)A
62	62BN	90	G	H
65	65BN	(2)91 + 65BN	(1)F + (1)G	H
66	66BN	(2)90 + (1)66BN	(1)D + (1)G	H
67	67BN	(2)91 + (1)67BN	D	H
68	68N	(2)91 + (1)68N	(1)D + (1)G	H
69	69BN	(2)92 + (1)69BN	(1)D + (1)H	H
77	77BN	(2)92 + (1)77BN	(1)F + (1)H	H
78	78N	(2)92 + (1)78N	F	H
81	81BN	(2)92 + (1)81BN	F	H
87	87BN	92	F	H
		Trubyte bioform (vacuum) shades		
59*	59*	(1)59 + (1)95	(2)G + (1)A	(2)G + (1)A
60	60B	96	F	(1)H + (2)A
62	62BN	(3)90 + (1)62BN	(2)G + (1)H	H
64	64B	(2)91 + (1)Trans.	D	H
65	65BN	(3)91 + (1)65BN	(1)F + (1)G	H
66	66BN	91	(1)G + (1)D	H
67	67BN	(3)91 + (1)67BN	D	H
68	68B	(3)91 + (1)Trans.	(1)D + (1)G	H
69	69BN	(2)92 + (1)69BN	(2)G + (1)H	H
70	70B	(3)91 + (1)70B	F	H
77	77BN	(2)92 + (1)77BN	(1)F + (1)H	H
81	81BN	(3)93 + (1)81BN	F	H
82	44	(1)92 + (1)Ging. Bl.	F	(1)F + (1)H

properties of four casting gold alloys used for ceramic-metal prosthodontics are listed later in this chapter. The numerical values for Brinnel hardness shown later are those obtained after the casting has been subjected to the temperature and time cycles required to fire the porcelain to it.

One manufacturer (Ney Co.) states that the strength of the P-16 gold alloy is ample not only for individual crown castings but also for long-span bridges if correctly designed. Its hardening mechanism is such that the firing procedures make the casting stronger than it was in its original cast condition.

Casting investments designed specifically to be used with the higher fusing gold alloys must be used. The following investments are satisfactory: Ransom and Randolph HFG, Whip-Mix Ceramigold, and Kerr Ceramvest. The manufacturers' instructions for the use should be meticulously followed in investing, burning out, and casting. A detailed consideration of these factors is given later.

After the Ney-Oro P-16 casting is recovered from the investment it is boiled in hydrochloric acid, following which it is stoned and finished with a rubber bonded abrasive wheel. Sharp margins are produced at the veneer areas with straight fissure burs. Pickle the casting again for

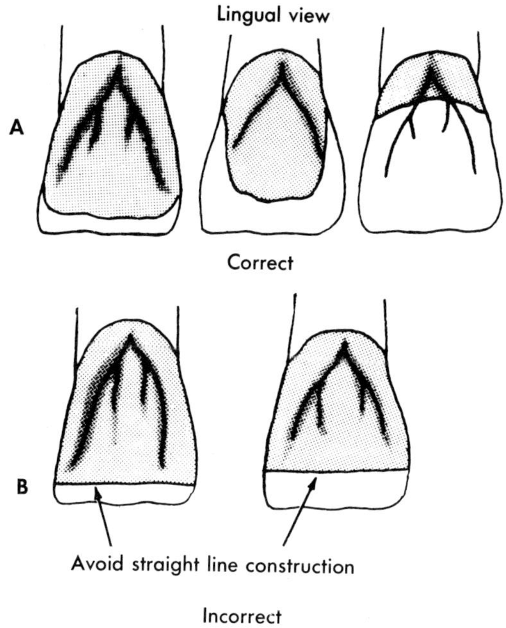

Fig. 35-1. A, Correct lingual design of casting. **B,** Incorrect design. (Courtesy J. M. Ney Co.)

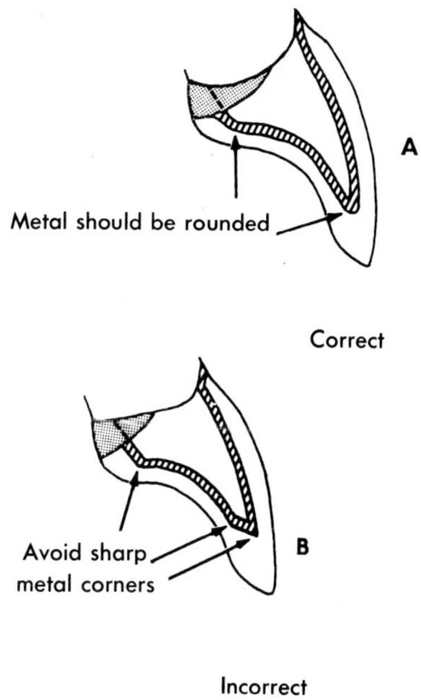

Fig. 35-2- A, Correct proximal, incisal, and gingival design. **B,** Incorrect design. (Courtesy J. M. Ney Co.)

two hours in hydrofluoric acid; rinse thoroughly in clean water.

The following procedures and shade guides are given by the manufacturer for the use of Thermalite porcelain 1750° F. on Ney-Oro P-16 gold alloy (Table 35-1). The technic requires meticulous attention to certain details of preparation and procedures to obtain its maximum benefits.

The tooth preparation is similar to that for a porcelain veneer or a Hollenback crown, namely, a shoulder on the labial aspect, and either a shoulder or a chamfer on the lingual aspect. A removable die of amalgam, stone, or an electroplated one, properly oriented in a working model, is required. As with all veneered cast-gold crown preparations, a sufficient amount of tooth structure must be removed to leave sufficient labial room for the gold and the porcelain veneer.

In waxing and finishing the cast gold crown the labial aspect also is given special shape. Fig. 35-1, *A*, shows the correct lingual designs of the casting; Fig. 35-1, *B*, the incorrect. Fig. 35-2 shows the incorrect and the correct views of the proximal, incisal, and gingival design. More complete discussions of the importance of correct design of the cast structure is given subsequently. Figs. 35-3 and 35-4 show other types of crowns made by the Ney-Oro, P-16, Thermalite technic.

The application of bonding agent

Mix the Bonding Agent thoroughly with a spatula until it has a creamy consistency. With a #1 or #2 Red Sable Brush, apply a uniform coating to the metal surfaces which are to receive the porcelain. Dry the coating slowly and thoroughly in front of the furnace. While advancing the work into the furnace, additional fuming may take place. After this ceases, the metal is heated to 1800-1825°, held for 10 minutes, and removed from the furnace. There should be a uniform grey matte coating. Wrinkled areas resulting from too rapid firing during the fuming period may be scraped with a spatula. A second coat of the Bonding Agent is applied and carefully dried. The metal is then returned to the furnace and taken to 1800-1825° where it is held for 10 minutes.

The Bonding Agent is a precious metal dispersion which alloys with the casting gold. It is completely resistant to hydrofluoric, sulphuric, and hydrochloric acids. If porcelain is stripped with hydrofluoric acid, the bonding film will remain

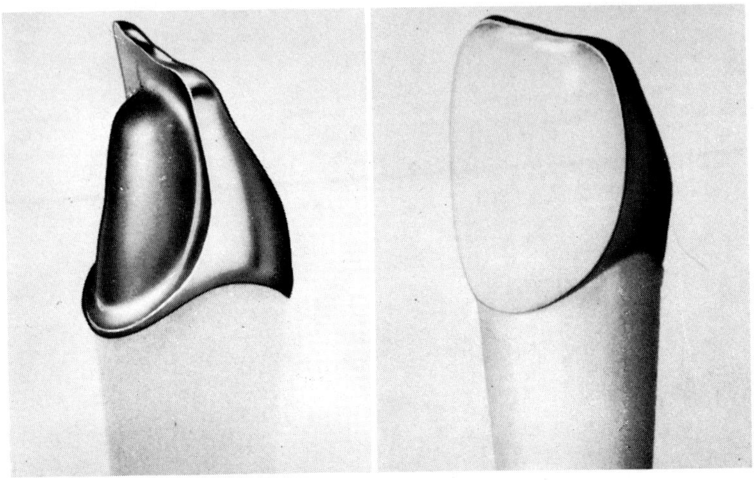

Fig. 35-3. Correctly prepared casting and finished crown with fused Ney-Oro porcelain veneer. Incisal edge protected with gold. (Courtesy J. M. Ney Co.)

intact. However, since the metal has been exposed to acid, a burn-out at 1800° F. for five minutes will be required to clean and de-gas the metal prior to porcelain re-application.

The brush is cleaned with turpentine. Should the Bonding Agent thicken, it may be thinned with oil of turpentine.

Opaque

Application. The selected opaque is mixed with distilled water to a light cream-like consistency and brushed onto the metal casting. Absorb the excess water with an absorbent tissue. One application is generally sufficient, since Thermalite Opaques have excellent hiding power.

Air-firing. Dry the work carefully in front of the muffle and insert into the muffle slowly. Raise temperature 100° a minute to 1750° F. Hold for two minutes, remove work from furnace, and cool slowly under a glass cover.

Vacuum-firing. Vacuum-firing is optional, but if used, follow these suggested steps: After drying the opaque in front of the muffle, insert the work into the furnace slowly and raise the temperature to 1200° F. Hold for 1 or 2 minutes, apply about 19 inches of vacuum, and raise the temperature to 1750° F. at the rate of 100° a minute. Hold at 1750° for two minutes, remove the work from the furnace, and allow it to cool under a Pyrex glass cover.

Any grey areas which appear after cooling are too thinly covered with opaque. Apply additional opaque where it is required and repeat the firing schedule. Areas with shrinkage cracks were dried too rapidly before firing. If metal is exposed, reapply opaque and refire; otherwise, merely smooth with a clean mounted stone.

First bake (biscuit):

Preparation:

1. Place the opaqued castings back on the model and relieve any copings which did not seat properly with diamond points.
2. Soak the stone model in water to prevent it from absorbing water from the porcelain while it is being applied.
3. The porcelain placed over the edentulous areas beneath pontics must have a smooth surface and must separate easily from the model. Place a piece of damp tissue paper over the pontic area after the porcelain has been built up. This tissue can be easily removed.
4. If the model is not mounted on a metal articulator, set a steel burr into the model with plaster. Stroking the shank of the burr with a serrated tool will provide the required vibration for flowing and condensing the porcelain.
5. Spatulate the selected porcelain thoroughly on the slab until every particle is wet and the mix has a creamy consistency.

Porcelain application:

1. Build up the bridge with the gingival porcelain. Vibrate and pack as tightly as possible.
2. Bevel the tips and apply the incisal blend.
3. The anatomy of each tooth is now carved and the teeth separated from each other by slicing through between them to the opaque. This permits the teeth to shrink in firing without shrinkage cracks appearing between adjacent teeth. Next, shape the embrasures. Finally, add sufficient porcelain to the contact areas to compensate for shrinkage during

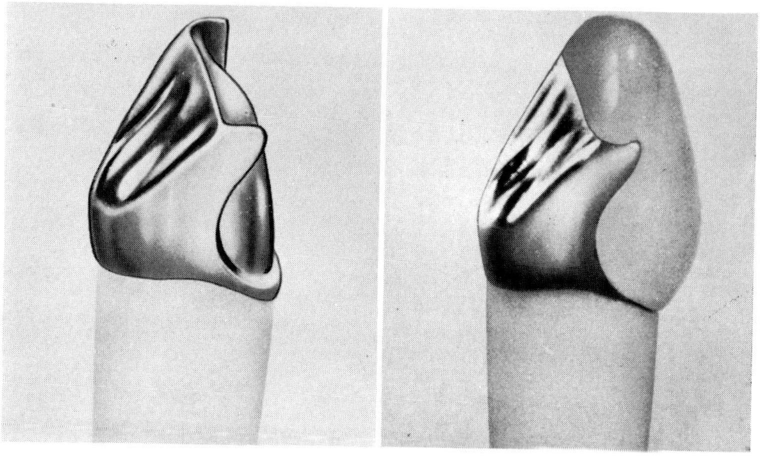

Fig. 35-4. Ney-Oro type of crown having entire incisal portion of porcelain. (Courtesy J. M. Ney Co.)

firing, and the work is ready for the furnace.

1. *Air-firing:*

a. Dry the work carefully in front of the muffle, starting at 1200° F. and allowing the furnace temperature to cool to 1000° F.

b. After drying, insert slowly and wait for a few minutes until the furnace temperature again reaches 1200° F. This will burn out organic matter such as oil, tissue, lint, etc.

c. Raise the temperature 100° a minute until 1650° F. is reached, and hold two minutes for a bake. Remove from the furnace and cool under a Pyrex glass.

d. After recontouring, if additional porcelain is needed, repeat the firing cycle.

e. A surface glaze may be obtained by firing to 1650° F. and holding for two minutes.

2. *Vacuum-firing:*

a. Dry the work carefully in front of the muffle, starting at a furnace temperature of 1200° F. and allowing it to cool to 1000° F.

b. After the drying, insert slowly and wait for a few minutes until furnace temperature reaches 1200° F. again. This will burn out organic matter such as oil, tissue, lint, etc.

c. Apply a minimum of 19 inches of vacuum and raise the temperature 100° a minute until 1650° F. is reached and hold two minutes for a bake. Remove from furnace and cool under a Pyrex glass. Increasing the vacuum intensifies the color.

d. After recontouring, if additional porcelain is needed, repeat the firing cycle.

e. A surface glaze may be obtained by refiring to 1650° F. and holding for two minutes. A vacuum is unnecessary on glaze bake.

Second bake:

Preparation:

1. Fit the copings back on their dies and soak the stone model in water.
2. Check the bite and grind the porcelain into proper occlusion where necessary.
3. Shape the anatomical contours, embrasures, saddle areas, etc.
4. Clean the bridge thoroughly with a brush and follow with immersion in the ultra-sonic cleaner. It is essential that grinding residue be removed before additional porcelain is applied. If diamond wheels have been used, be careful not to leave metal smears on the porcelain. Residues from grinding stones may produce black specks or bubbles. If rubber wheels have been used, any residue not removed will discolor the porcelain with a green stain after firing.

Porcelain application:

1. Add porcelain to complete the anatomical form, and if necessary, add to the occlusal surface, contact points, and saddle areas.
2. Fire as for the first bake.
3. If the work is to be tried in the mouth, it is desirable to fire to a slightly higher temperature to reduce the possibility of absorption of foreign materials.

Clean-up.

1. Reseat the bridge on the model, and check the bite, saddle areas, and contours. Be sure that the dies seat properly. Remove any porcelain from the inside of the copings.
2. If the case is large and fuses unevenly because of unequal proximity to hot muffle walls, it is helpful to wet-pumice the porce-

A

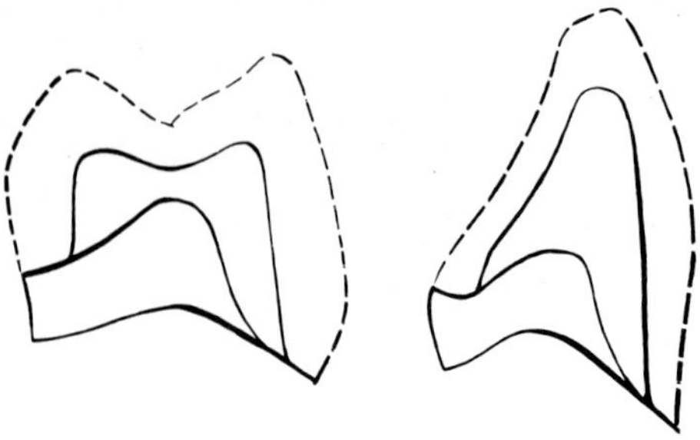

Fig. 35-5.

A, Complete porcelain coverage is strong and esthetic; correct shape of metal core in relation to thickness and contour of porcelain.

B

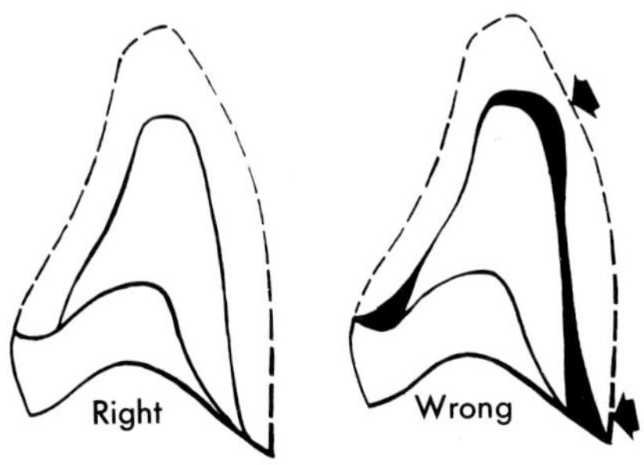

B, Metal should be constructed to provide for uniform thickness of porcelain. Labial surface is weak at incisal and gingival areas.

C

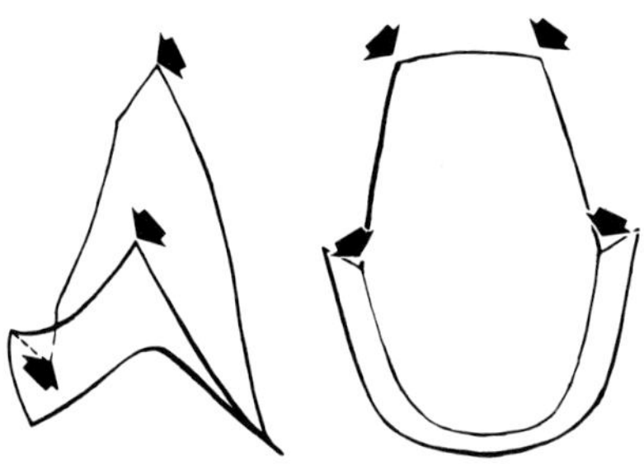

C, To provide maximum fusion of porcelain to metal, avoid sharp corners and undercuts. Eliminate potential cleavage points created by sharp angles.

D

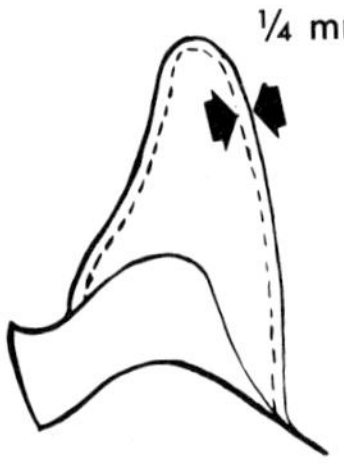

D, On those surfaces where there is insufficient space, minimum thickness of metal is 0.25 mm. where porcelain is to be applied.

E

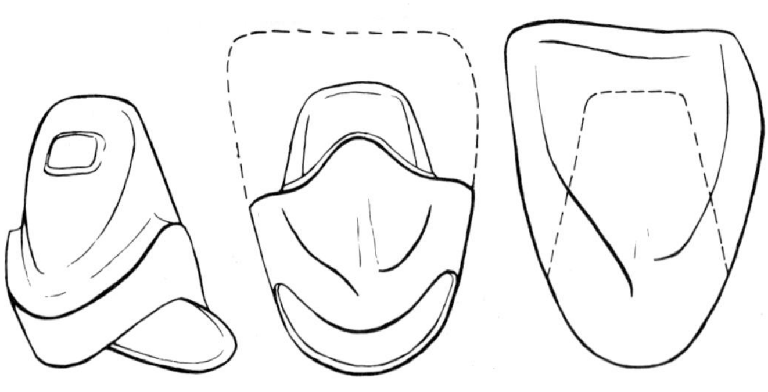

E, Some solutions for those instances when there is not enough room for metal and for porcelain: **left,** island of metal in lingual incisal area of incisal occlusion; **center,** gingival half covered with metal on lingual; **right,** complete porcelain coverage. Note that full porcelain coverage, or as nearly full coverage as possible, makes the strongest restoration.

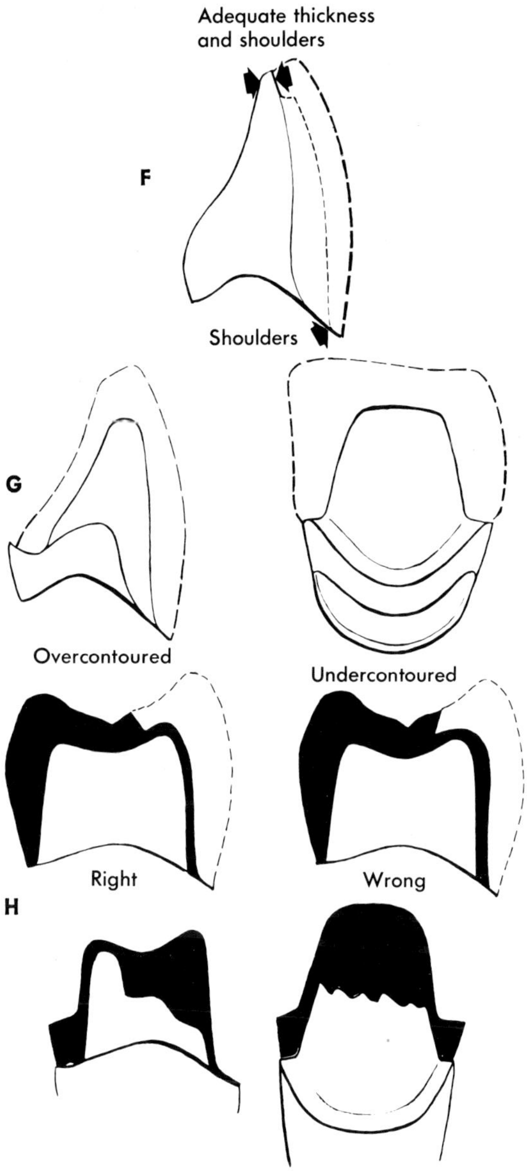

Fig. 35-5, cont'd.
F, Two important considerations in veneer types of crowns are: (1) incisal or occlusal metal edge should be heavy enough to resist burnishing; (2) there should be incisal and gingival shoulder to support porcelain.
G, Metal should always be shaped and contoured to provide harmonious blend with porcelain at finish lines. Right or slightly obtuse angle of metal at porcelain-metal junction is most desirable contour.
H, Broken or badly decayed abutments should be restored to normal contours. (Courtesy Dr. R. Vining and Howmet Co.)

lain to produce a smooth finish on the biscuit bake. The texture is then more uniform, the color is easier to see, and the final glaze can be accomplished with less firing.

3. Clean the work in the ultra-sonic cleaner, and it is ready for the try-in or finishing.

Finishing:

Preparation. If the bridge has been tried-in, wash it thoroughly with a bristle brush, and follow with about 15 minutes cleaning in the ultrasonic cleaner. When major corrections in color or anatomy are required after the try-in, a third bake will be necessary.

Porcelain application. It is desirable to fire the third time at the lowest possible firing temperature. The wet-pumice polishing described above is helpful. Apply stain where required.

Firing. Heat the case to 1650° F. for two minutes without vacuum. It is unnecessary to return vacuum-fired porcelain to the furnace after spot-grinding. Any spot-grinding done after glazing may be wet-pumice polished, further polished with tin oxide, and finished with white rouge. Fit the case back on the model and the work is completed.

Stains: Thermalite stains are color concentrates which are finely ground and designed to mature with the porcelain. These are versatile materials, and may be used in any or all of the porcelain additions. Stains should be mixed with Steele's Liquid Medium. They will serve best when they are always available, pre-mixed with Medium, and spaced neatly on a glass slab which is covered when not in use.

Fused porcelain will always look more natural if some of the many characteristic stains found in the mouth are reproduced in it.

Thermalite's reliability is not confined to the ceramist; this reliability extends to the dentist and, perhaps most important of all, to the patient. The dentist will find the final fitting pleasant and the patient will find restoration beautiful, long lasting, and trouble-free.*

TECHNIC FOR CONSTRUCTING MICRO-BOND HI-LIFE RESTORATIONS

The combination of Hi-Life gold and Hi-Life porcelain (Figs. 35-5 to 35-8) makes possible restorations with both natural appearance and the strength and tissue compatibility needed for maximum service. This information is offered to aid

*From Instruction Manual, Thermalite 1650, Bloomfield, N. J., 1963, American Thermocraft Co.

in obtaining the maximum results with these materials. Careful adherence to this technic will make it possible to construct restorations of exceptional beauty and service (Figs. 35-5 and 35-6).

The discussion has been divided into three parts: (1) Metal phase, (2) Porcelain phase, and (3) Trouble shooting (listing some of the most common errors and describing their cause and solution).

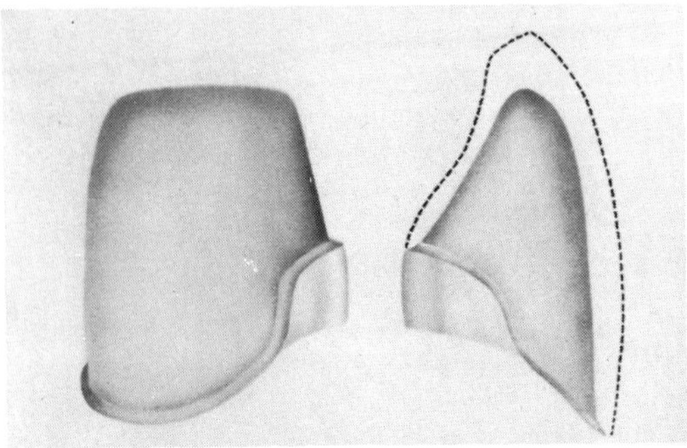

Fig. 35-6. Casting with heavy linguoproximal coping used with complete porcelain coverage of crown. (Courtesy Dr. R. Vining and Howmet Co.)

METAL PHASE

The importance of the design and construction of the metal substructure cannot be overemphasized. It is important not only from the standpoint of strength, but also for its effect on the esthetic result of the final restoration. This is especially true with Hi-Life porcelain, with which a new theory for achieving shades of a vital and natural appearance is employed. The color is concentrated in the undercoat and covered with a layer of more translucent porcelain, thus creating a more faithful duplication of the natural dentition.

Because of the strong influence of final shade by the undercoat, uniformity of thickness of the body porcelain becomes most important. Position and design of the metal substructure greatly determine the

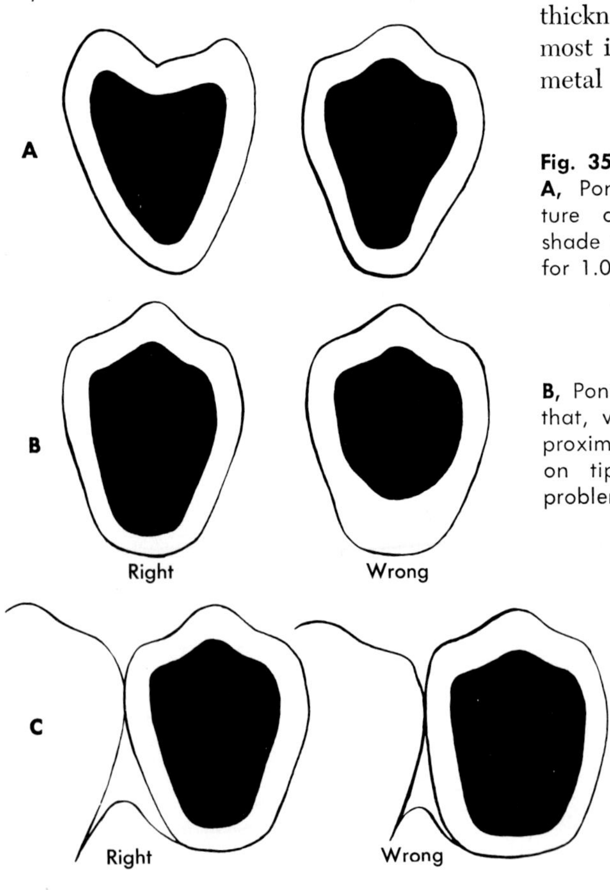

Fig. 35-7.
A, Pontic should be contoured to be miniature of finished unit's size, location, and shade to ensure consistency; they should allow for 1.0 to 1.5 mm. thickness of porcelain.

B, Pontics should be long enough gingivally so that, when undercoat is applied, there is approximately 1.0 mm. space for body porcelain on tip. Shorter pontic will create shading problems for ceramist.

C, Pontic tips should be narrow enough mesiodistally to maintain normal tooth width and to avoid broad, bulky appearance. This will also provide open interdental space, allowing ease of cleaning and affording fewer opportunities for periodontal involvement. (Courtesy Dr. R. Vining and Howmet Co.)

A1

A2

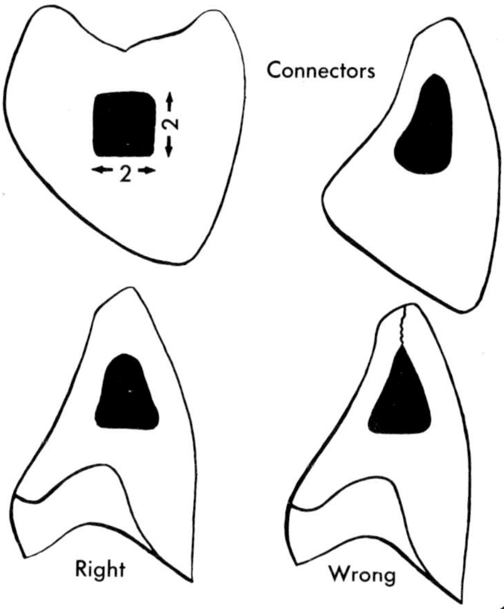

Fig. 35-8.
A1, Metal in connector should be approximately 2.0 sq. mm. in size. Size can be varied to fit different situations (for example, 1.0 mm. × 3.0 mm., or 1.5 mm. × 2.5 mm.). **A2,** Different bridges will dictate their different configurations; most important is that cross section of connector never has area of less than 2.0 mm. (4.0 sq. mm.).

B

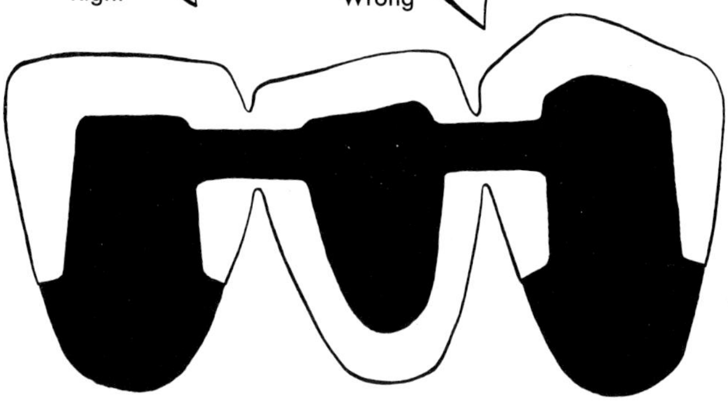

B, Connector should always pass through what would be normal contact area of teeth being replaced. This allows for creation of normal embrasures and interdental spaces. This area will normally be marginal ridge area of die on bicuspids and molars. Connectors will be in incisal third between centrals and laterals, in middle third between laterals and cuspids.

C

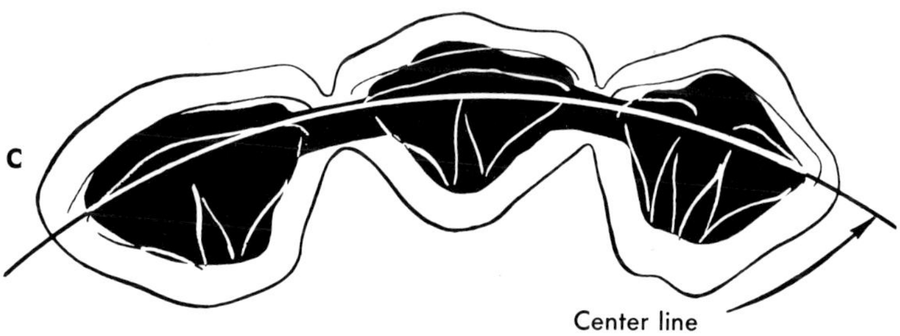

C, All connectors on anterior bridges should be placed slightly lingual of center line from incisal aspect.

D

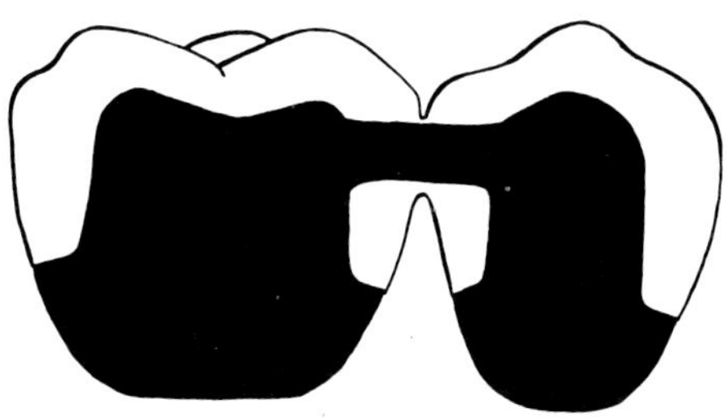

D, Incisal or occlusal surface of connector should never have sharp edge, which presents cleavage point to porcelain.

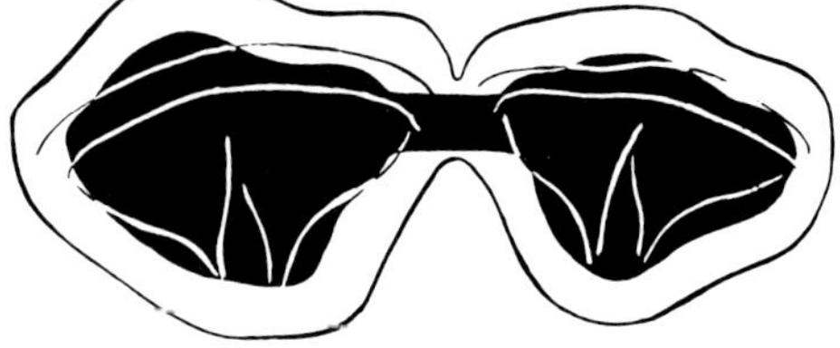

E

E, Connector should be contoured interproximally to allow for equal porcelain coverage on adjoining teeth. In most instances, this connector should be 2.0 mm. from distal of one unit to mesial of adjoining unit. (Courtesy Dr. R. Vining and Howmet Co.)

thickness and contour of the final porcelain restoration.

The following are some general rules to remember when constructing the metal work.

Pontics. Pontics should be designed and constructed according to the principles listed for abutments (Fig. 35-7). In addition, there are several points of specific importance that must be considered.

Connectors. There are a number of important design principles relating to multiple unit connectors that must be adhered to if the maximum in esthetics and strength of a bridge are to be achieved (Fig. 35-8). When an irregular arrangement is desired, it may be necessary to modify the guides given in Fig. 35-8.

Spruing

1. Use large sprues, preferably straight 10-gauge sprues.
2. Sprue bridge on model waxing one sprue to each unit. Join sprues together with additional wax. This serves as added support when removing bridge from model.
3. If a reservoir sprue is used, the reservoir must be not more than 1/16 inch from unit in order to properly "feed" the casting during the cooling and shrinkage period. If a unit has more mass than the reservoir, thicken the reservoir so that its mass will be greater than the unit it feeds. If reservoirs are close together join them with a little wax.
4. The total length of the sprue from button to each unit should be ¼ inch. In spans of considerable length or curvature, the button need not be round but may follow the general curvature of the span being sprued.
5. Sprue units so the abutment openings are facing up to avoid trapping air during investment procedure.
6. Sprue posterior pontics into the heaviest cusp. Sprue anterior veneers at the incisal junction of the thick lingual wax and thin labial wax.
7. The sprued bridge should be waxed on the crucible former to allow ¼ inch of investment over the pattern. This allows for escape of gas from the mold when the metal is cast.
8. "Wax out" potential thin, sharp, fragile investment areas that might fracture and become incorporated into the in-rushing metal.

Investing and burnout (using Ceramigold investment—Whip Mix Corp.)

1. Line casting ring with one layer of asbestos and brush entire surface with melted wax.
2. Mix Ceramigold investment liquid with tap water on liquid ratio—1 part water, 1 part Ceramigold investment liquid.
3. Use 14 ml. of the liquid and 100 gm. of Ceramigold investment. Mix for 20 seconds in a mechanical mixer or hand spatulate for 30 to 45 seconds. Vacuum mixing equipment is recommended.
4. Fill the investment ring around the patterns using technics to avoid trapping air.
5. Allow investment to set for 90 minutes before burnout.
6. Place ring in furnace at room temperature. Bring furnace temperature to 1500° F. and soak for 90 minutes.

NOTE: The following is a hygroscopic procedure for those who prefer that technic.

Hygroscopic technic
1300° Technic for M. B. gold castings

Ceramigold investment	60 grams	120	240	480
Ceramigold liquid	6½ cc.	13	26	52
Water	3½ cc.	7	14	28

Invest and place ring to half its height in water bath at 100° F. Allow to set in bath for 30 minutes. Remove from water bath and allow to stand on bench for 15 minutes and then place into cold oven

Table 35-2. Physical properties of four casting gold alloys for ceramic-metal prosthodontics

Ney-Oro P16 gold alloy	*Micro-Bond gold alloy*	*Jelenko, Ceramco No. 1*	*Aderer, Ceramco No. 1*	*Physical properties*
2020-2170° F.		2150° F.	2160° to 2240° F.	Melting range
57,000	63,000	51,000	51,000	Ultimate tensile strength, psi
155	143 after firing	150	150	Brinell hardness
3%	5%	3%	3%	Elongation
2300° F.	2350° F.	2300° F.	2300° F.	Casting temperature
	18,000,000			Modulus of elasticity
42,000 psi	50,000 (0.2% offset psi)	33,000	150	Yield strength
2150° F.	2200° F.	2150° F.	2160° F.	Fusion temperature

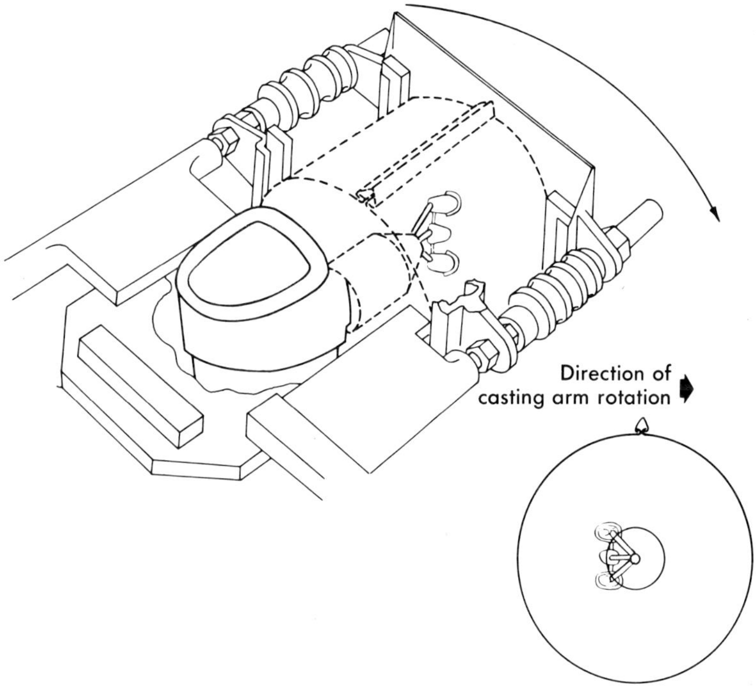

Fig. 35-9. Ring placed in casting machine.

and bring to 1300° F. Soak at 1300° F. for 1 hour and cast.

Table 35-2 is a listing of the comparative physical properties of four generally used gold alloys employing Thermalite, Micro-Bond, and Ceramco porcelains.

Casting (Fig. 35-9)

1. Equipment—Mecco torch (present Micro-Bond torch) using single orifice tip. The recommended torch tip is the Mecco WG-8.
2. Fuel—gas-oxygen.

3. Flame—use a reducing flame with a 1¼ inch inner cone and an 8 to 9 inch entire cone length.

4. Melting—heat alloy *without* flux in a regular unlined Vitallium crucible. Use a new crucible and identify so it will be reserved for Hi-Life Gold only. (Do not use a crucible where flux has been applied and *never* flux the alloy.) As alloy becomes molten, it is first shiny and then a dark film forms over the surface. The alloy should be further heated until the melt becomes clean, bright, and very fluid in appearance.

5. Cast the alloy into the mold and allow it to bench cool until it reaches handling temperature.

6. Knock off gross investment and sandblast to remove remaining material. Set sandblast air pressure at 30 pounds or less. Sand or glass beads may be used.

Electromatic control settings for electromatic casting machine

Range switch	Temperature 2350° F.	Soak time 45 seconds
Micro-Bond gold Centrifuge 380 rpm	Centrifuge acceleration 0 for less than an ounce, 10 for an ounce or more Radiation pyrometer angle—forward	heat low

The ring should be placed in the casting machine so that the units to be cast are trailing the direction the arm is spinning (Fig. 35-9).

Soldering

1. Surfaces to be joined must be clean and free of oxide. Metal-to-metal contact is most desirable for maximum accuracy (flat surface contact is best).

2. Invest units in Howmet all-purpose soldering investment.

3. Boil off wax and heat model to dry.

4. Apply soldering flux to areas to be soldered if necessary. NOTE: Joints will be stronger if soldering can be accomplished without use of flux.

5. Use gas-oxygen soldering torch with reducing flame for the soldering operation.

6. Heat investment until metal becomes cherry red, apply fluxed Micro-Bond gold solder to areas to be joined and apply flame to solder. When solder flows freely, remove flame immediately and allow the cast to bench cool. CAUTION: Use only enough flux to accomplish soldering.

Preparation of metal for porcelain application

A. Grinding and cleaning
   1. Rough grind with hard mounted stone all metal surfaces to which porcelain is to be applied. Clean mounted stones are excellent for this operation.
   2. Clean metal in ultrasonic cleaner or wash thoroughly with detergent and stiff brush (Fig. 35-10).
   3. Rinse metal well in clean water.

B. Bonding agent application and degassing
   1. Dry metal thoroughly. Avoid handling with fingers.
   2. Apply an even coat of Micro-Bond gold bonding agent to metal to receive porcelain. Brush out gross excess to avoid bubbling. NOTE: Stir bonding agent thoroughly and often—ingredients tend to settle very rapidly.
   3. Place in front of furnace muffle until thoroughly dry, usually 5 to 7 minutes. CAUTION: Too rapid a dry-out will cause a darkening and bubbling of bonding agent, leading to gassing problems when porcelain is applied.
   4. Insert into furnace at 1400°

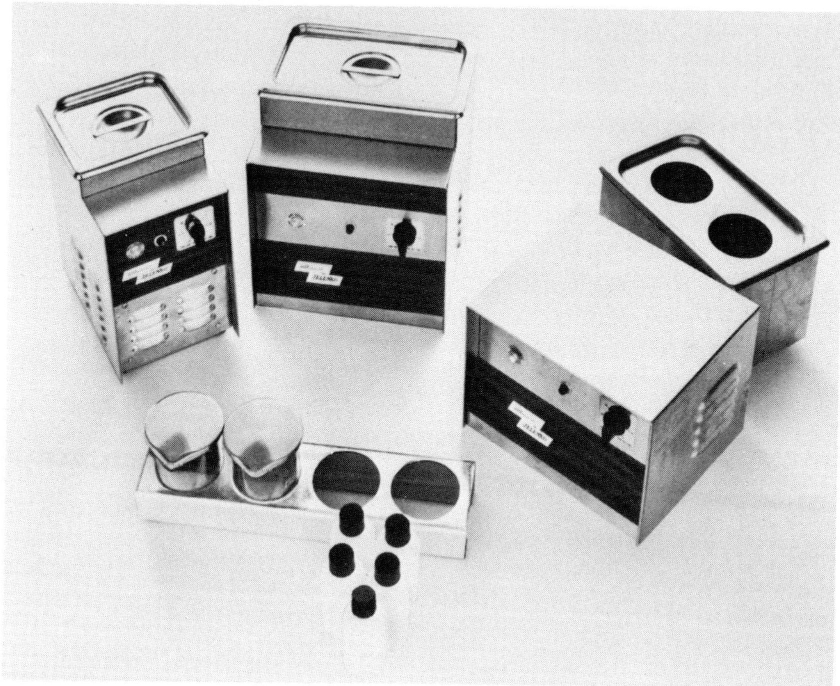

Fig. 35-10. Ultrasonic equipment. (Courtesy J. F. Jelenko Co.)

F., close door, and raise furnace temperature to 1875° F. under full vacuum.

5. Hold at 1875° F. for 5 minutes, remove metal, and cool on bench.
6. Restoration is now ready for porcelain application. NOTE: Some technicians prefer to do this in two steps. Run restoration to 1840° F. for 5 minutes under full vacuum, remove and allow to cool, then apply bonding agent. Run furnace to 1875° F. and take restoration out immediately.

PORCELAIN PHASE

Description of Hi-Life porcelains. Hi-Life porcelains are carefully formulated fine grain powders that glaze at 1800° F. They are supplied premixed in the thirteen shades of the Bioform Shade Guide.

Undercoat porcelain. Hi-Life Undercoats are supplied in thirteen shades of intense opacity and color, plus unstained for alterations. This intensity of color helps create a more life-like appearance by duplicating the effect of nature where the dentin color reflects through a layer of enamel. The extreme opacity makes it possible to block or mask out the metal with a very thin coat.

Body porcelains. The Body porcelains are supplied in thirteen premixed Bioform shades, plus unstained. These porcelains are formulated to be compatible with the equivalent undercoat shade and help create the same effect.

Incisal porcelains. The Incisal porcelain is supplied in two degrees of translucency, Standard Incisal and Translucent Incisal. The Standard Incisal matches Bioform Incisal, while the Translucent Incisal is for those units where a great degree of translucency is desired.

Color modifiers. These porcelains are

for modifying basic shades and are supplied in orange, peach, yellow, gray, pink, brown, white, and blue.

I. Firing information on Hi-Life porcelain
   A. All bakes are entered into muffle at 1400° F.
   B. Heat rise should be between 75° F. and 100° F./minute.
   C. Undercoat and glaze bakes are without the use of vacuum.
   D. All bisque bakes are under a vacuum of 27 inches.

II. Firing chart for average unit

	Enter unit at	*Remove from furnace*	*Vacuum*
Undercoat	1400° F.	1700° F.	No
First Bake	1400° F.	1750° F.	27″
Second Bake	1400° F.	1775° F.	27″
Glaze	1400° F.	1800° F.	No

III. Undercoat application and firing
   1. Mix the desired shade of undercoat porcelain with Hi-Life undercoat liquid. This mix should have the consistency of heavy cream.
   2. Apply a thin uniform coat, using a brush, to one unit at a time. Vibrate lightly to level coating and go on to the next unit.
   3. Dry out in front of open muffle, insert in furnace at 1400° F. and run up to 1700° F., remove, and allow to cool in open. NOTE: If undercoat is applied too heavily a slight checking may be noted. This will cause no problem; proceed with build-up.

IV. First build-up and bake
   1. Mix desired body porcelain with liquid and proceed with build-up using any acceptable technic for condensing. (Liquid is 7 parts distilled water with 1 part Micro-Bond liquid concentrate.)
   2. Mix Standard Incisal porcelain, 3 parts, with body porcelain, 1 part. NOTE: This ratio may be altered to create more or less translucency as desired.
   3. Complete build-up using Incisal mix.
   4. It is recommended on multiple units that interproximal slices be made using a razor blade. This allows each unit to shrink within itself making a denser porcelain.
   5. Dry out and preheat in front of muffle. Insert at 1400° F. and fire to 1750° F. under 27 inches of vacuum.
   6. Grind to desired shape and contours using sandpaper disks and stones.
   7. Clean thoroughly in ultrasonic cleaner and rinse under tap water. The units are now ready for any additions or corrections.

V. Second bake
   1. Add necessary additional porcelain to restoration.
   2. Dry out and preheat in front of muffle. Insert at 1400° F. and fire to 1775° F. under 27 inches of vacuum.
   3. Grind to final contours and clean thoroughly. If additional application is required before glazing, fire to 1775° F. under 27 inches of vacuum.

VI. Glaze bake
   1. Dry out and preheat in front of muffle. Insert at 1400° F. and fire to 1800° F. without vacuum. More glaze may be obtained by soaking unit at 1800° F. for 30 seconds to 1 minute.

VII. Color modifiers

These are intense colors for modifying basic shades and should be used sparingly. The unstained is used to lighten a color intensity. (These modifiers are not to be used to alter undercoat colors; if used they will dilute the opacity of the undercoat.) Undercoat shades can be changed by the addition of small amounts of either a lighter or darker undercoat.

VIII. Incisal porcelains

Standard Incisal, when mixed 3 parts to body 1 part, will produce an incisal likeness that compares to the most commonly used shade guides. Translucent Incisal is an almost clear porcelain and is used when extreme translucency or special effects are desired.

IX. Add-On porcelains

This is a clear porcelain that is used to make small additions, such as contact points, after the glaze bake. It fires to a smooth glaze finish at 1725° F.

X. Characterizing porcelains

Any final characterization can be achieved by using the Micro-Bond Glaze Stain Kit. This kit contains ten stain colors and five gingival tones plus diluter, overglaze, and liquid. The desired effects are achieved by painting on the proper colors, drying out, and air-firing to 1775° F. They will fire to a smooth glazed finish. Complete instructions for staining and over glazing are furnished with the Micro-Bond Glaze Stain Kit.

TROUBLE SHOOTING

Metal phase

I. Incomplete castings
   A. Copings waxed too thin, less than 0.3 mm.
   B. Casting temperature was not hot enough (metal casts at 2350° F.).
   C. More than ¼ inch of investment above highest part of pattern.
   D. Faulty spruing. (See section on Spruing, especially length and gauge.)

II. Porosity
   A. Shrink pot voids—sprues too long and/or too narrow a gauge. Sprues should be ¼ inch long and 10-gauge.
   B. Pinpoint porosity—casting temperature was either too hot or too cold.
   C. Gas porosity—incomplete burnout or too much investment over patterns. Burnout temperature is 1500° F., soak for 90 minutes. Investment covering pattern should be ¼ inch thick.
   D. Button is too small to properly feed casting as it solidifies.
   E. Contamination—remelting spills, using a crucible that had been used for other metals, or in which flux has been used are some of the possible sources of contamination. A new crucible should be labeled Hi-Life and used for that purpose only. Casting flux should never be used.

III. Cracked molds
   A. Placing mold in burnout furnace too soon. (Invested case should set 90 minutes before burnout.)
   B. If invested case is allowed to set in open overnight or longer, it should be soaked in a bowl of water for 20 minutes before placing in furnace.

Porcelain phase

I. Bubbling and darkening of the Bonding Agent.
   A. Too short dryout time or too close to heat. Bonding agent, because of liquid media used, requires a long, slow drying out before entry into muffle.

II. Small check marks in fired undercoat
   A. Undercoat applied too heavy or

puddled. Units can be used, but on future cases care should be exercised to achieve a thin uniform application.

B. Insufficient dry out before insertion into muffle.

III. Metal shows through undercoat

A. Undercoat applied too thin; paint another thin coat and refire.

IV. Voids in porcelain at juncture of incisal and body porcelain

A. Body porcelain is too dry; moisten body porcelain with water so that it will properly accept addition of incisal porcelain.

V. A checking or tearing of porcelain particularly at interproximals

A. No interproximal slices or they are not deep enough.

B. An unusually large mass of porcelain in a given area. Metal framework should be constructed to provide for a uniform coverage of porcelain.

VI. Checking of porcelain especially in final bisque bake

A. Porcelain not dried out thoroughly before introduction into muffle. If check lines do not open up, many times this problem can be corrected by refiring units.

VII. Milky appearance to porcelain on second or later firings

A. Not thoroughly cleaned after grinding; all grinding dust must be removed.

B. All traces of detergent or soap not thoroughly rinsed off.

C. Vacuum not sufficient; 27 inches recommended.

D. Vacuum not turned on at 1400° F.

VIII. Black streaks and smudges, particularly in interproximals and at porcelain-metal juncture

A. Metal contamination of porcelain either from dragging metal grindings up on porcelain or from diamond disk. If case is kept wet with water when grinding with diamond disk, chance of contamination is greatly reduced.

IX. Small voids on surface of glazed units

A. Surface not properly filled with porcelain before glaze firing. Can be corrected by filling with thin mix of half body shade and half add-on, fire to 1750° F. without vacuum.

Design of the structure and the technical steps of investing, burnout, and casting of the metal were presented in previous discussions of gold alloys of other manufacturers. All agree on the same basic principles. It is also generally agreed that another fundamental requirement for successful fusion of porcelain to a cast gold alloy is the bond between the metal and porcelain, which would not separate. The nature of this bond has been the subject of much discussion; was it a chemical or a mechanical bond? Shell and Neilsen stated that "the dental porcelain to dental gold bond, if properly made, was primarily one of interatomic bonding. The total bond had a shear resistance of about 10,000-13,000 pcs.; about one-third of this resistance appeared to be due to the van der Waals forces of wetting, and two-thirds appeared to be due to chemical bonding, perhaps a mixture of ionic, covalent, and metallic bonding. A mechanical bond did not play an important role in the bond strength proper. Roughening per se did not add to the shear resistance at the bond."[5]

However, the technics are similar in that all castings are stone finished prior to the application of porcelain, giving a questionable additional mechanically locked bond. However, since stones are usually porcelain contaminants, it is fundamental that all finished castings must be absolutely cleaned, either by mechanical or ultrasonic means prior to the application of porcelain.

It is suggested that, for further insurance against contamination and gassing insert the casting into the furnace at 1200° F. and raise the temperature to 1925° F. and remove.

CERAMCO TECHNIC

Ceramco[4] suggests the following technic in the use of its porcelains. Make a thin mix of Ceramcote Powder and Ceramcite Liquid. Paint a thin wash over the surface to receive the porcelain. Dry by holding the casting inside the furnace vestibule at the end of long tongs. Place on a tray with support at every abutment and fire to 1925° to 1950° F. until a slight sheen is visible. Remove and bench cool.

Ceramco gold* does not require the use of a bonding agent. However, two types of metal surface sealers are available at the user's option. One type is a ceramic base sealer and is called "Ceramcote." It has virtually no color effect on the metal. The other has a gold base and is called "Britecote." It leaves a gold plated effect. The choice of which type to use should be based on shade considerations. Both are efficient sealers and will reduce the potential hazard of outgassing that may result from the presence of subsurface porosity in the casting. Neither type will affect bond strength adversely when properly used.

Britecote is reconstituted by adding a few drops of the accompanying liquid to the dry cake while stirring with a clean instrument. Add liquid and stir until a homogeneous, paint or syruplike consistency is noted.

Paint a coat of Britecote over the porcelain bearing surface. Place on a firing tray with support at every abutment or use one of the custom molded support materials now available for this purpose and dry and preheat by placing in front of the open muffle of a furnace held at 1200° F. Insert at 1200° and raise temperature at a rate of 100° F. per minute until a shiny gold "flash" is observed at or about 1950° F. Hold at this temperature until the shine is replaced by a slight dullness. This indicates the oxide development necessary for bonding. Remove and bench cool. Do not use any acid or pickling bath.

*Ceramco gold is manufactured by J. F. Jelenko Co. and by Julius Aderer Co.

The opaque bake

A. Ceramco Opaque Porcelain serves a threefold purpose.
  1. The principal function of the opaque is to mask out the color of the underlying Ceramco Gold.
  2. The color of the opaque porcelain complements the gingival shades.
  3. The fusing power of Ceramco Opaque Porcelain joins the porcelain to Ceramco Gold in a powerful bond.

How to apply Ceramco Opaque Porcelain

1. *Consistency*—Try to avoid too wet a mix when adding *distilled* water to the opaque powder. A thick creamy mix, which can be comfortably lifted and painted with a red sable brush, is ideal.
2. *Application*—Vibrate the opaque porcelain onto the metal surface with the red sable brush or an instrument if more convenient. This is done by using a short dabbing motion of the hand. Apply to a small area at a time and prevent the opaque from running by blotting with a a clean absorbent tissue or cloth. Try to make the opaque coverage as dense as possible.
3. *Optimum Thickness*—The opaque porcelain must be applied in a layer thick enough to mask out all traces of the underlying metal color. An application of the wet opacifier 0.5 mm. thick, will shrink to a thickness of 0.33 mm. after firing. In most cases this is sufficient coverage. To insure dense opaque coverage, two thinner applications and firings may be substituted for the above.
4. *Firing the opaque porcelain*—Dry the opaqued work by placing it near the open door of the furnace which is being held at 1200° F. As the porcelain dries, evidenced by a chalky appearance, ease it gently and gradually into the hot zone of the furnace.

If vacuum porcelain is being used, apply full vacuum (26" minimum) immediately upon insertion. The heating rate should be between 90 and 100° per minute. Open the vacuum seals at 1700 to 1750° F. and continue to fire in normal atmosphere at the same heating rate until the opaque is observed to be in a "high biscuit" condition. This state is characterized by a grainy yet somewhat shiny surface. In vacuum opaques it occurs between 1820 and 1850° F. when fired at the proper heating rate. Remove the case and bench cool. *Do not cool in the furnace.*

Air-fired opaque is fired at the same rate and in the same manner except for the omission of the vacuum cycle. The "high biscuit" should occur at or near 1800° F.

5. *Corrections*—Examine the opaqued surface after firing. Thin spots, if any, will appear as grayish areas. Any such thin spots are corrected by applying additional opaque and baking as before. Thick or lumpy spots may be ground off. Wash the ground surfaces with a clean bristle brush or in an ultrasonic cleaner. Rinse under clear running water.

Building up for the first bake

A. Condensing or packing Ceramco Porcelain
1. The four principal methods of condensing or packing porcelain are pressure, vibration, brushing (semi-dry), and capillary flow: Vibration and capillary flow are used with the fluid porcelain mix as it is applied.
   a. *Vibration* may be applied directly with the applying instrument or by running a serrated edge along the mold or die.
   b. *Capillary* packing is done by blotting the surface diametrically opposed to where the fresh application of porcelain is made. By this means, the moisture flows through the porcelain mass, drawing the ultra-fine particles inward.
   c. *Pressure* packing is done by placing clean tissue paper over the fingers and pressing.
   d. *Brushing* the well blotted and semi-dry surface with a ⅜″ flat camel's hair brush serves to fill in surface voids and remove loose particles.
2. These four methods of condensing the porcelain may be used separately or in any combination depending upon the geometry of the restoration, e.g., a single veneer may be packed by vibration and pressure while an extensive case with full porcelain coverage will be packed by means of capillary flow and pressure in those spots where it is possible.

B. The Gingival or Body Porcelain
1. *Consistency*—Add *distilled* water to the gingival powder and spatulate to a thick creamy consistency avoiding excessive wetness. Any surplus water should be blotted up.
2. *Application*
   a. Hand vibrate the gingival porcelain over the surface to be covered using a thin spatulate instrument.
   b. In those bridges where porcelain-to-tissue contact is desired for the pontic units, the following technique is recommended.
      1. Soak the model in water until it becomes nonabsorbent.
      2. Adapt a piece of tissue or rice paper over the ridge, using a wet brush.
      3. Flow or vibrate gingival porcelain over the tissue and under the metal pontic form.
      4. Compress and blot.
3. *Shaping*—After the full tooth or bridge has been built up in gingival porcelain, it may be shaped with a carving instrument or by rubbing with clean fingers.

C. Applying the Incisal Porcelain
1. *Beveling*—The technique used in preparing the build-up to receive the incisal porcelain is the same as that used for acrylic. First the incisal or occlusal tips are cut away. Then tapering beveled cuts are made in the labial or buccal surfaces. Naturally, the depth of the cuts made will depend upon the type of blend that is contemplated.
2. *Mixing the incisal*—For most new hue shades add 10-20% of the body blend to the incisal mix. For Bioform shades add 25% or more white modifier to the incisal. This is to control translucency and to attain the characteristic Bioform high value effect. The consistency should be slightly wetter than that used for the gingival build-up.
3. *Applying the incisal*—Distilled water is added to the incisal blend which is spatulated to the same consistency as was the gingival. Vibrate the incisal mix over the prepared surface using an instrument or brush. Blot excess moisture in the usual manner and condense.
4. *Blending the incisal*—Remove excess incisal porcelain and blend by brushing toward the cervical using light strokes with the ⅜″ camel's hair brush.

5. *Carving*—When carving bridges, cut through the porcelain right down to the opaque at all the interproximal and proximal points. This will create separations and prevent excessive distortion when the porcelain shrinks in firing.
6. *Shrinkage*—Ceramic Porcelain [when applied] will shrink from 15% to 18% depending upon [its] density. Therefore, all work must be overbuilt to compensate. In addition to the longitudinal compensation, contact points must be added laterally on single jackets as well as the end abutments of bridges.

DIRECTIONS FOR AIR-FIRED PORCELAIN

The first firing

A. Insertion
   1. The refractory tray bearing the crown or bridge supported at each abutment is placed near the open furnace for drying. As the porcelain dries and the color lightens, move it into the furnace vestibule and toward the hot zone of the muffle in gentle, gradual stages. The entire drying, preheating and inserting process usually takes no longer than five minutes. The furnace is held at 1200° F. during this entire process.

B. Firing
   1. For vacuum porcelain, begin vacuuming as soon as the case has been inserted at 1200° F. Vacuum pressure may range from 26″ to 29″. Set the amperage control to a setting which yields a temperature rise of 90-100° per minute. At a point between 1700-1750° F, "release" the vacuum and continue firing at the same heating rate until a high biscuit bake is observed. This bake is characterized by its shiny yet grainy surface and should be attained between 1775-1800° in vacuum porcelain. Remove immediately and bench cool.
   2. Air porcelain is fired at the same heating rate and to the same appearance. The only difference is the omission of the vacuum cycle. Air porcelain yields a high biscuit at about 1800° F.

The second firing

A. Single Jacket Crowns
   1. Grind away any excess porcelain that prevents correct seating on the die.
   2. Grind into occlusion.
   3. Carve or accentuate the anatomy with stones or discs. Then using very fine carborundum or sandpaper discs, finish the porcelain surface so that it is smooth and and semi-polished.
   4. If no extensive porcelain additions are required, the jacket is . . . ready for glazing. All debris left by the grinding media must be washed [away] with a clean bristle brush under running water. Ultrasonic cleaners may be used but be sure to remove all traces of detergent, if used, by soaking [case] in fresh, clear water.
   5. If a small add-on of porcelain is required, it should be made at this time.
   6. Follow the same firing technique that was outlined for the first bake.

B. Bridges
   1. Grind off any porcelain on the abutment contact [areas] or elsewhere that prevents correct seating on the dies.
   2. Check the bite and grind where necessary for correct occlusion.
   3. Carefully remove any excess labial, buccal, or lingual bulk of porcelain.
   4. Wash the bridge under running water using a clean bristle brush.
   5. Add to the porcelain-tissue contacts by following the technique outlined in [Building up for the First Bake].
   6. Add gingival and incisal porcelain interproximally and recut the separations.
   7. Add incisal blend occlusally where indicated.
   8. Remove the bridge and place it on sagger points near the furnace door for drying.
   9. Follow the same firing procedure as in the first bake and remove the bridge from the furnace as soon as the newly added porcelain shows evidence of a 'shine.'

C. If, after the second bake, additional adjustments are required, the second bake procedure is repeated.

Preparing for the glaze

A. After the bridge has been built up to correct occlusion and contact, and the teeth are properly contoured and separated, it is ready for the final glaze bake.
   1. Carve or accentuate the anatomy with stones or discs. Then, using very fine carborundum or sandpaper discs, finish the porcelain surface so that it is smooth and semi-polished.
   2. Wash the bridge carefully, and examine the surface to make sure that it is clean.
   3. Follow the same procedure as in the previous bakes in inserting and firing the bridge.

GLAZING

A. Ceramco porcelain glazes naturally and does not require the use of special glazing agents. Vacuum is not required.

B. The purpose of the glaze bake is to form a paper thin film of glass on the porcelain surface which will not absorb fluids or odors and will insure maximum tissue tolerance.

C. The glaze bake should not be used to smooth down roughly finished porcelain. The heavy glass formation that results from this incorrect practice causes a loss of sharpness and definition, a burn out of color and severe stresses in the ceramic material. Follow the finishing instructions in VII, A, 1 and form a thin glass coating that coats the anatomical features but does not dissolve them.

D. Always bear in mind that the shine of a glaze increases when the tooth or bridge is wet, and fire your glaze bake accordingly. Avoid overglazing and the glassy 'false tooth' appearance that accompanies it.

E. Ceramco Porcelain will glaze at or near 1800 degrees F. However, do not rely on pyrometer indications alone when firing. Develop the habit of examining the degree of vitrification visually.

STAINING

A. Ceramco Porcelain may be stained by using any stains which fuse in the 1750-1800 degree F. range.

B. Staining with Ceramco stains.

Staining is part of the routine procedure of preparing for the glaze bake. Complete data on the Ceramco color system and staining technique are included in the Ceramco color system manual which accompanies the stain kit.

Table 35-3. Directions for firing Ceramco vacuum porcelain*

Maturing temperature	
Gingival and incisal	1775 to 1800° F.
Opaque	1825 to 1850° F.
Vacuum range	1200 to 1700° F.
Vacuum pressure	26 to 29" Hg
Heating rate	90 to 100° per minute
Glaze bake	Air fired

*Ceramco vacuum porcelain is handled and condensed exactly like Ceramco air-fired porcelain. Britecote or Ceramcote should also be used routinely. The firing of Ceramco vacuum porcelain is done partly under vacuum and partly in normal atmosphere. The same vacuum cycle is used for first bakes as well as for any additions of porcelain.

Table 35-4. Ceramco vacuum bioform shades

Premixed shades			
Gingivals		*Opaques*	
BF 59	BF 68	BF 59	BF 68
BF 60	BF 69	BF 60	BF 69
BF 62	BF 70	BF 62	BF 70
BF 64	BF 77	BF 64	BF 77
BF 65	BF 81	BF 65	BF 81
BF 66	BF 82	BF 66	BF 82
BF 67		BF 67	

Basic shades		
Modifier porcelains	*Opaques**	*Incisals*
BF White	BF White	Incisal BF Light
BF Orange	BF Yellow	Incisal BF Dark
BF Brown	BF Gray	
BF Gray	BF Pink	
BF Pink	BF Orange	
BF Yellow		
BF Blue		

*These basic opaques are the same colors as the basic opaques in the Ceramco Vacuum New Hue kit.

Post completion corrections [new Ceramco 1800 porcelain]

A. If, after a crown or bridge has been fired to a natural glaze, a small addition of porcelain is required, follow the technique suggested below:
   1. Remove all surface glaze with a sandpaper disc.
   2. Re-accentuate the anatomical carving.
   3. Wash under running water.
   4. Make the small porcelain addition and fire to a glaze.*

VACUUM FIRING

Dry the case in the usual manner by placing it near the open furnace door. The furnace should be held at 1200° F. When the characteristic chalky appearance shows that it is dry begin to insert it in gradual stages by moving it toward the hot zone an inch at a time. The total time for the

*From Ceramco Basic Porcelain Manual, Woodside, N. Y., 1963, Ceramco, Inc.

step by step insertion need not exceed 2 or 3 minutes. Maintain the temperature during the insertion period.

As soon as the case has reached the hot zone of the muffle, close the furnace, seal the vacuum chamber, and start the vacuum pump. The recommended vacuum pressure is 26 to 29″ Hg. This pressure should be maintained throughout the vacuum portion of the firing. Raise the temperature at a rate of 90 to 100° F. per minute.

At 1700° F., stop the vacuum pump and open the valves and seals and complete the firing cycle in normal atmosphere as described below.

COMPLETING THE FIRING CYCLE FOR VACUUM OPAQUE

Continue the firing in air at the rate of 90 to 100° per minute until the opaque attains a shiny yet grainy surface. In the case of vacuum opaques this should occur in the 1825 to 1850° range. Remove at once and bench cool.

It is important to remember that the vacuum opaques are higher fusing than the vacuum gingival and incisal porcelains. Also, different shades of vacuum opaques may have slightly differing maturing points due to the varying percentages of high temperature coloring oxides.

COMPLETING THE FIRING CYCLE FOR VACUUM GINGIVAL AND INCISAL

Firing in normal atmosphere after the vacuum period, the temperature increase of 90 to 100° per minute is continued.

At or about 1800° the porcelain should have the characteristic shiny yet grainy appearance. This is sometimes referred to as a "high biscuit bake." Remove at once and bench cool.

GLAZING

It is not necessary to vacuum the glaze bake. However, if a slight addition of porcelain is being made in conjunction with the final glaze bake, follow the vacuum cycle.

SELECTED REFERENCES

1. Granger, E. R.: Platinum-iridium castings; a new concept of the dental casting process, J.A.D.A. **27**:1718, 1940.
2. Ney-Oro P-16, Thermalite Porcelain Manual, Hartford, Connecticut, 1968, The J. M. Ney Co.
3. Micro-Bond High Life Porcelain Technic, Chicago, 1967, Austenal Co.
4. Ceramco Basic Porcelain Manual, Woodside, New York, 1963, Ceramco, Inc.
5. Shell, J. S., and Nielsen, J. P.: Study of the bond between gold alloys and porcelain, J. Dent. Res. **41**:1424, 1962.

GENERAL REFERENCES

Argue, J. E.: The problem of tooth color, J.A.D.A. **24**:1341, 1937.

Baker, C. R.: A porcelain-faced crown, J. Prosth. Dent. Vol. **18**:1-9, 1967.

Bastian, C. C.: The individual unit porcelain bridge, J.A.D.A. **29**:1369, 1942.

Bazola, F. N., and Malone, W. F.: A customized shade guide for vacuum-fired porcelain-gold combination crowns, J.A.D.A. **74**(1):114, 1967.

Bentman, D.: Avoiding the "metal-sag" with porcelain fused-to-metal bridgework, Cereb. Palsy Rev. **1**:9-12, 1966.

Borom, M. P., and Pask, J. A.: Role of adherence oxides in the development of chemical bonding at glass-metal interfaces, J. Amer. Ceram. Soc. **49**:1-6, 1966.

Brecker, S. C.: Porcelain baked to gold—a new medium in prosthodontics, J. Prosth. Dent. **6**: 801-810, 1956.

Brecker, S. C.: Improved porcelain fused to gold bridge, Dent. Clin. N. Amer., pp. 163-173, March, 1959.

Carlsson, B., and Lindholm, R.: Metal-bonded porcelain—a new alternative in crown and bridge technic, Svensk Tandlak T. **59**(6):343, 1966.

Clark, E. B.: An analysis of tooth color, J.A.D.A. **18**:2093, 1931.

Clark, E. B.: The color problem in dentistry, D. Digest **37**:499, 1931.

Clark, E. B.: Tooth color selection, J.A.D.A. **20**: 1065, 1933.

Clark, E. B.: Manipulation of dental porcelain, J.A.D.A. **22**:33, 1935.

Cohen, R.: Improved esthetics and greater strength using porcelain fused to metal crowns and bridges, New York J. Dent. **30**:168, 1960.

Conod, H.: Etude sur la statique de la couronne

jaquette, Rev. Mensvelle Svisse d'Odontol. **47**: 485-529, 1937.

Cowger, G. T., and Woycheshin, F. F.: Gold plating to enhance the appearance of porcelain-faced crowns, J. Prosth. Dent. **11**:925, 1961.

Custer, F., Asgar, K., and Peyton, F. A.: The effect of certain variables in the bond strength of porcelain fused to gold, Internat. A. D. Res. **40**:94, 1962.

Dunworth, F. D.: Porcelain fused to gold, J. Prosth. Dent. **8**:635, 1958.

Dupont, R.: Ceramo-metallic restorations, Int. Dent. J. **18**:288, 1968.

Dykema, R. W., Johnston, J. F., and Cunningham, D. M.: The veneered gold crown, Dent. Clin. N. Amer. pp. 653-669, Nov., 1958.

Ewing, J. E., and Bentman, D.: Porcelain-veneered full-crown restorations made with cadmium patterns, J. Prosth. Dent. **18**:140, 1967.

Fairhurst, C. W., and Leinfelder, K. F.: Heat treating porcelain enameled restorations, J. Prosth. Dent. **16**:554-556, 1966.

Garofalo, F.: Fundamentals of creep and creep rupture in metals, Macmillan Series in Materials Science, New York, 1965, The Macmillan Co.

Gettleman, L., Freedman, G., Shaw, B., Goldin, J., and Soremark, R.: Studies on a new dental casting gold alloy, J. Dent. Res. **45**(3):595-601, 1967.

Hagen, W. H. B.: Combination gold and porcelain crown, J. Prosth. Dent. **10**:325, 1960.

Haggard, C. B.: Clinical aspects of porcelain bonded to gold, Rev. Dent. Liban. **15**:15-19, 1965.

Hama, M., and others: Studies on the baking of the mixed porcelain affixed to porcelain tooth, Odontology (Tokyo) **53**:256-261, 1965.

Harter, J.: Indication and contraindication for ceramic-metallic combinations in reconstruction unit, Rev. Franc. Odontostomat. **9**:834 (corrections, p. 1151), 1962. (Fr.)

Hoffman, E. J.: How to utilize porcelain fused to gold as a crown and bridge material, Dent. Clin. N. Amer., pp. 57-64, 1965.

Howard, W. W.: Porcelain fused to gold for class IV inlays, J. Prosth. Dent. **13**:761, 1963.

Howell, R. A.: Gold/porcelain anterior crowns, Brit. D. J. **111**:118, 1961.

Howell, R. A.: Gold/porcelain bridge work, Brit. D. J. **116**:80-82, 1964.

Johnston, J. F., Dykema, R. W., Mumford, G., and Phillips, R. W.: Construction and assembly of porcelain veneer gold crowns and pontics, J. Prosth. Dent. **12**:1125-1137, 1962.

Kaaber, S.: Dental metal-ceramics: a survey of the development of the enamelling technique in dentistry, Odont. T. **75**:317-340, 1967.

King, B. W., Tripp, H. P., and Duckworth, W. H.: Nature of adherence of porcelain enamels to metals, J. Amer. Ceram. Soc. **42**:504-525, 1959.

Knap, F. J., and Ryge, G.: Study of bond strength of dental porcelain fused to metal, J. Dent. Res. **45**:1047-1051, 1966.

Lakermange, R., and Gonon, P.: Bridges in reinforced porcelain, J. Am. D. Club Paris **2**:1, 1934.

Lautenschlager, E. P., Greener, E. H., and Elkington, W. E.: Microprobe analyses of gold-porcelain bonding, J. Dent. Res. **48**:1206, 1969.

Lavine, M. H., and Custer, F.: Variables affecting the strength of bond between porcelain and gold, J. Dent. Res. **45**:32-36, 1966.

Leibowitch, R.: Porcelain baked on precious metal alloy, Rev. Franc. Odontostomat. **9**:825, 1962. (Fr.)

Leinfelder, K. F., and others: Heat treatment of alloys to be used for the fused porcelain technique: additional data, J. Dent. Res. **43**: 927, 1964.

Leinfelder, K. F., Fairhurst, C. W., O'Brien, W. J., and Ryge, G.: Evolution of gases from high fusing gold alloys, J. Dent. Res. **45**:1154, 1966.

Leinfelder, K. F., O'Brien, W. J., Ryge, G., and Fairhurst, C. W.: Hardening of high fusing gold alloys, J. Dent. Res. **45**:392, 1966.

Leinfelder, K. F., and others: Mechanical properties of high-fusing gold alloys, J. Prosth. Dent. **21**:523-528, 1969.

Leone, E. F., and Fairhurst, C. W.: Bond strength and mechanical properties of dental porcelain enamels, J. Prosth. Dent. **18**:155, 1967.

Lyons, D. M., Cowger, G. T., Woycheshien, F. F., and Miller, C. B.: Porcelain fused to gold—evaluation and esthetics, J. Prosth. Dent. **10**: 319-324, 1960.

Mattox, D. M.: Influence of oxygen on adherence of gold films to oxide substrates, J. Appl. Phys. **37**:3613-3615, 1966.

Meadows, T. R.: Clinical comparison of cast gold crowns with acrylic and with fused porcelain veneer facings, J.A.D.A. **66**:772, 1963.

Medwedeff, F. M.: Porcelain fused to gold: fixed partial dentures, J. Prosth. Dent. **18**: 6-14, 1967.

Morrison, K. N., and Warnick, M. E.: Investment compounded specifically for ceramic procedures, J. D. Res. **38**:762, 1959 (abst.).

Morse, F. F. E.: Porcelain fused to metal; comparisons of the air-fired and vacuum-fired porcelain jacket crowns and porcelain fused to precious metal, D. Pract. **13**:99, 1962.

Mumford, G.: The porcelain fused to metal restorations, Dent. Clin. N. Amer. pp. 241-249, March, 1965.

Mylin, W. K.: Present status of porcelain fused

to metal restorations, J. Kentucky D. A. **14**:152, 1962.

Nally, J. N.: Chemicophysical analysis and mechanical tests of the ceramometallic complex, Int. Dent. J. **18**(2):309-325, 1968.

Nally, J. N., Meyer, J. M., and Monnier, D.: Topographic distribution of certain elements of alloy and porcelain at the level of the ceramic-metallic bond, Schweiz. Mschr. Zahnheilk. **78**(9):868-878, 1968.

O'Brien, W. J.: Significant developments in dental materials, Connecticut Dent. J. **26**:5, 1968.

O'Brien, W. J., Kring, J. E., and Ryge, G.: Heat treatment of alloys to be used for the fused porcelain technique, J. Prosth. Dent. **14**:955-960, 1964.

O'Brien, W. J., and Ryge, G.: Relation between molecular force calculations and observed strength of enamel-metal interfaces, J. Amer. Ceram. Soc. **47**:5-8, 1964.

Pruden, H. H.: Solder connections with porcelain fused to gold, J. Prosth. Dent. **22**:679, 1969.

Ryge, G.: Current American research on porcelain-fused-to-metal restorations, Int. Dent. J. **15**:385-392, 1965.

Schiffer, R.: Soldering technique for high-fusing gold in the porcelain, J. Prosth. Dent. **22**:4, 1969.

Schnell, R. J., Mumford, G., and Phillips, R. W.: An evaluation of phosphate bonded investments used with a high fusing gold alloy, J. Prosth. Dent. **13**:324, 1963.

Semmelman, J. O.: Fusion of porcelain to metal, Conference for Teachers of Dental Materials, Dec., 1961.

Shelby, D. S.: Practical considerations and design of porcelain fused to metal, J. Prosth. Dent. **12**:542, 1962.

Shell, J. S., and Nielsen, J. P.: Study of the bond between gold alloys and porcelain, J. D. Res. **41**:1424, 1962.

Shell, J. S., and Nielsen, J. P.: The strength and nature of the porcelain-to-gold bone, Paper presented before the Dental Materials Group of the International Association for Dental Research Meeting, St. Louis, March, 1962.

Sherring-Lucas, G. M.: Bonded porcelain to gold; Degudent-Swiss Vita VMK technique, Dent. Techn. **19**(11):98-103, 1966.

Silver, M., and Klein, G.: Precision attachments in conjunction with cast platinum-porcelain restorations, D. Digest **62**:296, 1956.

Silver, M., Klein, G., and Howard, M. C.: Platinum-porcelain restorations, J. Prosth. Dent. **6**: 695, 1956.

Silver, M., Howard, M. C., and Klein, G.: Porcelain bonded to a cast metal understructure, J. Prosth. Dent. **11**:132, 1961.

Silver, M., Klein, G., and Howard, M. C.: An evaluation and comparison of porcelains fused to cast metals, J. Prosth. Dent. **10**:1055-1064, 1960.

Smith, B. B.: Considerations in the current use of porcelain to gold, Int. Dent. J. **18**:280, 1968.

Straussberg, G., Katz, G., and Kuwata, M.: Design of gold supporting structures for fused porcelain restorations, J. Prosth. Dent. **16**(5): 928-936, 1966.

Swartz, M. L., and Phillips, R. W.: A study of adaptation of veneers to cast gold crowns, J. Prosth. Dent. **7**:817, 1957.

Toreskog, S.: Metal-bound porcelain—an addition to crown and bridge prosthetics, Sverige. Tandlakarforb. Tidn. **59**(11):495-499, 1967.

Tuccillo, J. J., and Nielsen, J. P.: Creep and sag properties of a porcelain-gold alloy, J. Dent. Res. **46**(3):579-583, 1967.

Vickery, R. C., and Badinelli, L. A.: Nature of attachment forces in porcelain-gold systems, J. Dent. Res. (In press.)

Vining, R., and Lust, J.: Micro-bond presentation: symposium on trends in dental laboratory activities, Walter Reed Hospital, Washington, D. C., 1963.

Warnick, M. E.: Use of porcelain-fused-to-gold in the restoration of fractured young permanent anterior teeth, J. Dent. Child. **29**:3, 1962.

Weinberg, L. A.: A new design for porcelain-fused-to-metal prostheses, J. Prosth. Dent. **17** (2):178-194, 1967.

Woolson, A. H.: Restorations made of porcelain baked on gold, J. Prosth. Dent. **5**:65, 1955.

Yamada, S.: Metal-cast dental porcelain, J. Jap. Dent. Ass. **19**:111, 1966.

Chapter 36

Alumina-reinforced ceramics*

The advantages of the complete porcelain veneer crown have already been described and it still remains in the foremost rank among dental restorations (Chapter 24).

The main disadvantage of dental porcelain is its fragility. It is well known that sudden fracture may occur in a complete porcelain veneer crown that has insufficient or improper tooth support; meticulous attention to the preparation of the complete veneer crown has also been emphasized (Chapter 26).

Fractures in dental porcelain originate from microcracks in the surface (Fig. 36-1). These cracks may be caused during cooling of the porcelain crown resulting in surface stress. The outside layer or skin of the porcelain will cool more rapidly than the interior. Consequently the skin will be under compression while the interior will contain tensile stresses, since its thermal contraction may be partially prevented by the rigid skin that has solidified. Such a differential change may fracture or rupture the skin to produce minute cracks when the opposing stresses try to neutralize each other in this region. Surface grinding effects produced by too coarse an abrasive or overheating will also contribute to the production of microcracks. Fractures in dental porcelain originate from these microcracks at the surface that act as stress concentrators. According to the Griffith Crack Theory, the deeper the crack, the greater the stress concentration; brittle fracture may occur with almost explosive force.

The bonding of porcelain to metal has largely overcome these problems, but frequently with the sacrifice of esthetic properties. One of the limiting factors in the use of bonded-porcelain crowns is that sufficient tooth tissue must be removed to allow for at least 1.5 mm. space for gold and porcelain. This requirement is not safely met and particular difficulty may be experienced in younger patients where extensive removal of tooth tissue is biologically undesirable. Although a thin gold veneer may be placed on the palatal surface of the tooth, the labial surface will often present a greater problem since it is here that strength is dominated by esthetic consideration. Many adult teeth do not lend themselves to thick labial veneers and it is obvious that the metal reinforcement places a heavy demand on the technician's skill in obtaining good color values.

ALUMINA-REINFORCED PORCELAINS

In order to overcome the objections to using metal reinforcement, research has been directed toward formulating higher strength porcelains using alumina crystals as the reinforcing phase.[1, 2] These aluminous porcelains have recently become available; the esthetics obtainable with them are comparable to a modern vacuum-fired, regular porcelain.

It must be clearly understood that the

*Text by John W. McLean, N. D. S., L. D. S., R. C. S.; London, England.

strength of aluminous porcelain, while being nearly double that of regular porcelain, still does not allow the use of these materials on inadequately prepared teeth or where the occlusion contraindicates the use of an all-porcelain restoration. The operator must be aware that he is still limited by the strength of ceramics in thin section and that aluminous porcelain is offered primarily as a replacement for, and to extend the use of, regular porcelain.

High-fusing regular porcelain is composed of a high potash content feldspar together with a 10 to 15 percent content of quartz, the latter possibly acting as a strengthener.

The low and medium fusion porcelains contain feldspar fluxed by a boro-silicate glass, which reduces the firing temperature but at the same time decreases the resistance of the fired body to pyroplastic flow. The regular porcelains may be referred to as glasses since their free crystalline content is very limited. By contrast, the aluminous porcelains contain up to 50 percent free crystalline material and can therefore be classed more accurately as porcelains.

FORMULATION OF ALUMINOUS PORCELAINS

It has been shown that when crystalline grains of high strength and elasticity were introduced into a glass or porcelain of similar expansion, the strength and elasticity of the mixture, when fired, were found to increase progressively with the proportion of the crystalline phase.[3, 4] The choice of high strength crystals that can be used satisfactorily in dental porcelain is limited and research in this field indicated that aluminum oxide (Al_2O_3) was the most promising material for use in complete porcelain-veneer crown powders.[2]

Alumina is the oxide of aluminum commonly extracted from the mineral bauxite, which is mainly a hydrated aluminum oxide. According to normal practice the ore is crushed and ground to –10 mesh and is digested in a concentrated solution of caustic soda. The alumina-bearing liquor recovered from this process is clarified, and the alumina is precipitated in the form of alumina-trihydrate crystals, which are then washed and dried without the removal of the chemically combined water. The alumina-trihydrate is converted to alumina by calcination, usually in a rotary kiln at a temperature of 1100° F., which drives off the chemically combined water in the hydrate to form y-alumina. Further calcination converts it to alpha-alumina.

For ceramic applications, the calcined alpha-alumina is generally ball-milled and commercially supplied as a fine powder, usually below 10 or 20 μ in size. In order to obtain suitable alumina crystals for reinforcing dental porcelain, calcined alumina is fused in an electric arc furnace at approximately 4000° F., where complete melting of the crystals occurs. On cooling, very large crystals of fused alumina are formed and these are then ground and sized by standard mineralogic technics.

The fused alumina crystals are then mixed with specially formulated glass powders of matched expansion to form aluminous porcelain. During firing the glass will melt and flow around the alumina crystals. A strong ionic bond is formed between the glass and alumina phase, resulting in an alumina/glass composite. Theoretically, the inclusion of fused alumina crystals into a glass of similar thermal expansion may be considered as a constant-strain system and the stress in each phase should be proportional to its elasticity. The overall stress applied to the body should lie in value between the stresses in the two phases. If both phases have similar critical strain, the strength of the body will vary with the effective modulus of elasticity, and fracture has an equal chance of starting in either phase. In the absence of thermal expansion differences the fracture passes indiscriminately through the glass

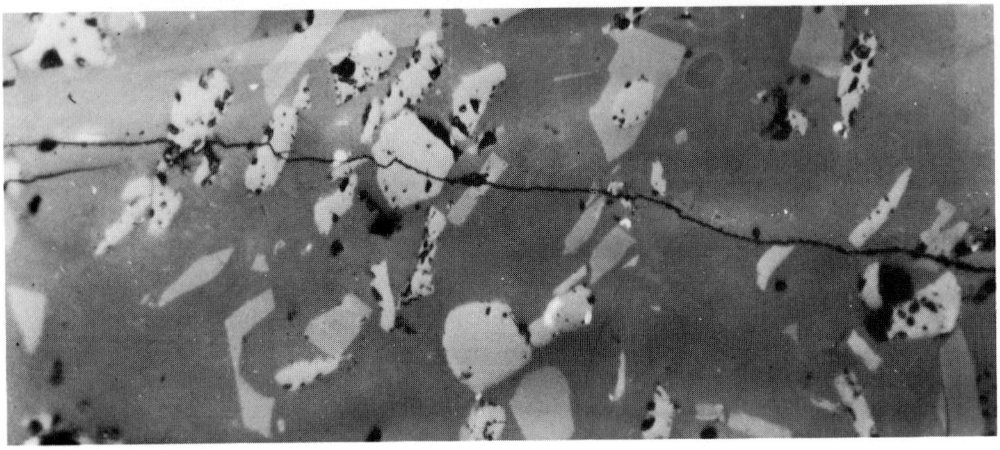

Fig. 36-1. Photomicrograph of fracture path in two-phase system of aluminous dental porcelain reinforced with fused alumina crystals. (Courtesy Eastman Dental Hospital.)

Table 36-1. Modulus of rupture of 50 percent fused alumina content porcelain and a regular medium fusing feldspathic porcelain of the vacuum type

Material	*Modulus of rupture*			*Standard deviation*	*Variance coefficient (%)*
	Average	*Low*	*High*		
Aluminous porcelain 50 percent alumina	22,458	19,335	25,543	2,387	10.63
Regular porcelain medium fusing	11,076	10,079	13,925	1,270	11.47

or the included crystalline grain (Fig. 36-1). Sometimes the crack deviates at the boundary of a grain, presumably to reach a crack already present in the grain, but in *no case does it avoid a fused alumina crystal.*

Ceramics containing more than 75 percent alumina are referred to as *high aluminas;* materials below this level are classed as *aluminous porcelains.*

Dental aluminous porcelain contains 45 to 50 percent by weight of alumina crystals and its strength measured in terms of modulus of rupture (bending strength) can be more than double that of regular porcelain. A typical 50 percent aluminous dental porcelain is compared in Table 36-1 with a regular dental porcelain.

Aluminous porcelain is used in jacket crown work as a core porcelain to strengthen the overlaying enamel and resist the deepening of surface microcracks. By use of an aluminous porcelain core, the higher modulus of elasticity of this material will stiffen the entire ceramic component and improve the resistance of the jacket crown to torque. The esthetic limitations of the anterior metal-reinforced porcelain crown frequently indicate the use of the aluminous porcelain type. Aluminous porcelain has also been successfully used in dowel crowns and many types of bridges. An alumina-reinforced core porcelain, when used as a palatal backing on a jacket crown, will also increase the impact resistance in the biting area.

Indications for use

Aluminous porcelain crowns should not be constructed on conical preparations or

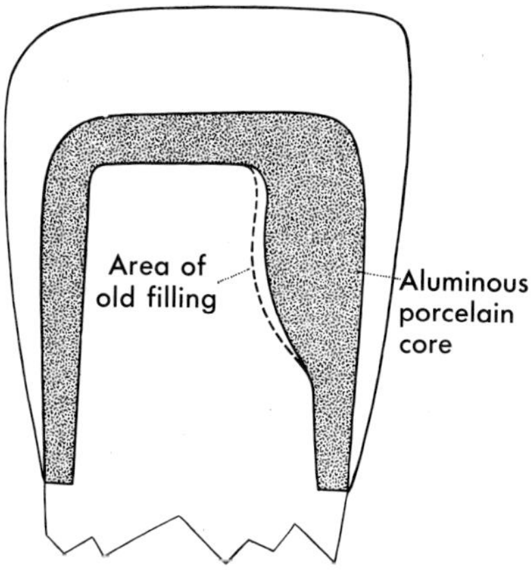

Fig. 36-2. Typical restoration for aluminous porcelain jacket crown, with destruction of tooth dentin; portion restored with core porcelain.

where there is sufficient tooth structure to support the fused porcelain restoration. The preparation must have planes at right angle to the force of mastication (see Chapter 24). The aluminous porcelain veneer crown is not recommended as a general replacement for the porcelain-fused-to-metal restoration and is contraindicated in the closed bite condition where lingual clearance is less than 0.8 mm.

The alumina-reinforced crown is comparable in appearance with a regular vacuum-fired porcelain crown and is more suitable for anterior restorations than metal reinforced crowns when appearance is of paramount importance. Clinical experiments with 1,334 alumina-reinforced porcelain veneer crowns produced a fracture rate of less than 0.5 percent over a 3.5-year trial period.[4] The crowns constructed for these experiments were all reinforced on the palatal surface with aluminous porcelain and the surface was then covered with a sealing glaze. The high strength of the full palatal backed aluminous porcelain core contributed to this low fracture incidence.

The atypical preparation

In many instances the dentist is faced with the problem of restoring a tooth in which destruction of enamel and dentin by caries or placement of fillings has reduced the area of sound tooth structure to a minimal level. It is in this situation that aluminous porcelain has particular value since the additional strength may provide the balance between fracture or a durable restoration. Fig. 36-2 illustrates a typical situation in which the mesial surface of the classical outline form of the preparation has been encroached upon by a filling. It is important when preparing the tooth that *maximum cervical support* is provided for the crown and that the area of the old filling not be restored with cement. The maximum bulk of aluminous core porcelain is used to restore this area, thereby utilizing its mechanical properties to the best advantage. By retaining near parallelism at the cervical third of the rebuilt axial walls, maximum support to the crown is given in this difficult situation.

Principles of esthetics

Ideally, the ceramist should fabricate a custom-built shade guide of complete veneer porcelain crowns and use these in conjunction with shade buttons. Such a procedure is suited to the individual dentist or technician. However, the large laboratory owner is generally presented with a specific shade, selected by the dentist from a modern multiblended vacuum-fired tooth shade guide.

The aluminous porcelains were formulated with this situation in mind and a description of the blending of a vacuum-fired shade guide tooth is most pertinent to the ensuing discussion on aluminous porcelain crown construction.

An examination of a modern multiblended vacuum-fired denture tooth reveals that it comprises four basic colors (Fig. 36-3). These colors consist of a backing porcelain containing the pin anchorage, a darker dentin color that is carried up into the gingival of the tooth to create a dense neck area, and the body or dentin porcelain overlaid by a translucent enamel. This enamel porcelain covers the labial and palatal aspects of the incisal edge and overlays the dentin on the entire labial surface. Various concentrated body and surface stains are applied as "effect" masses. These vacuum-fired teeth simulate a natural tooth extremely well.

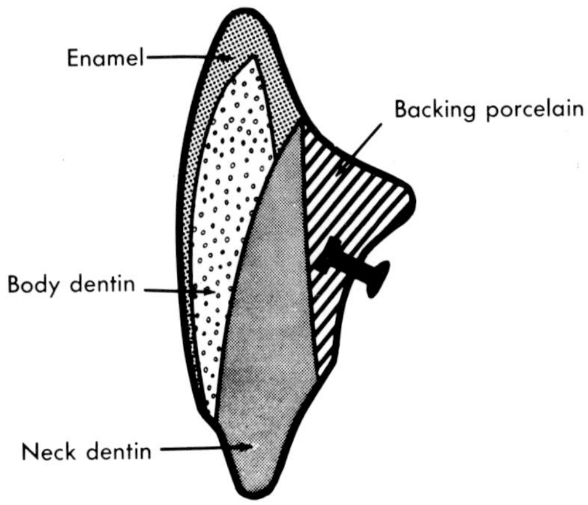

Fig. 36-3. Cross section of multiblended vacuum-fired denture tooth.

In order to duplicate a vacuum-fired shade guide tooth, the aluminous porcelain must be fired in layers corresponding to the thickness of the shade guide tooth enamel and dentins (Figs. 36-4 and 36-5). The aluminous core porcelain will correspond to the dense backing porcelain containing the pin anchorage. *The high strength core must extend to the full contour of the palatal surface and the labial surface is chamfered from the gingival to the incisal so that the core tapers to a thickness of not more than 0.5 mm. at the incisal edge of the preparation. Where the total labial thickness is less than 1 mm., the core may be further thinned in this area, always bearing in mind that at least 0.5 mm. of dentin and enamel porcelain is required to obtain natural blending and depth of translucency.* It is essential to maintain a 0.5 to 0.8 mm. core thickness at the cervical third since this will provide

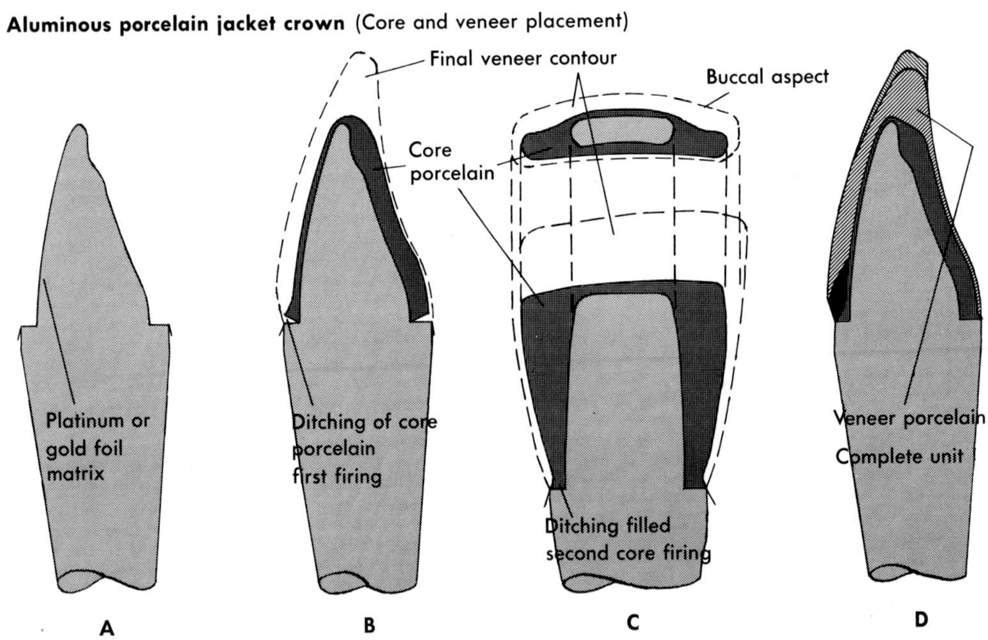

Fig. 36-4. A, Tooth preparation with foil matrix. **B,** First buildup core, "ditched" prior to placement in muffle. **C,** Distribution of core and veneer porcelain for second firing. **D,** Distribution of core porcelain, body veneer porcelain, and enamel veneer porcelain over labial neck dentin.

a strong ring reinforcement. The core can be masked with quite a thin section of gingival or neck dentin in this area and a dense neck area is also beneficial to esthetics.

The gingival or neck dentin porcelain should also be chamfered into the tooth to allow an overlay of body dentin that will establish the main color in the crown. The overlay of enamel porcelain and the incisal translucent will now create a natural enamel effect and provide depth of translucency to the finished crown. It should be noted that the aluminous dentin porcelains are generally more translucent than the porcelains used for fusing to metal and resultantly the overall finish to the crown will provide more lustre and internal light refraction and reflection.

At first sight it may appear that the aluminous core porcelains are very opaque, but a study of Fig. 36-6 will reveal that the current powders that fall within a specific surface area of 1,000 to 1,200 cm.^{2}/g. do provide quite a high degree of light transmission when vacuum-fired. In this case the 1 mm. thick specimens were transmitting over 20 percent light and resultantly these core porcelains will not present such problems as the opaques used in the bonded porcelains where a background of metal is used.

The most common fault observed with the gold-bonded porcelain crown in the anterior region is caused by "metameric color effects" deriving from the use of very opaque backgrounds. Metameric effects are produced by changes in the spec-

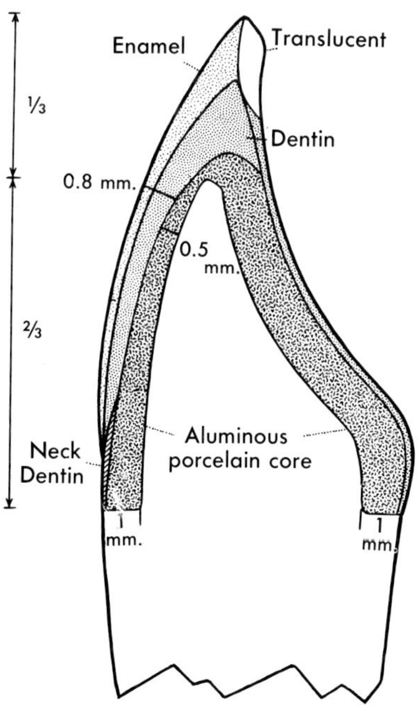

Fig. 36-5. Cross section of aluminous porcelain jacket crown; correct placement of high-strength core porcelain and overlaying veneers of dentin and enamel porcelains.

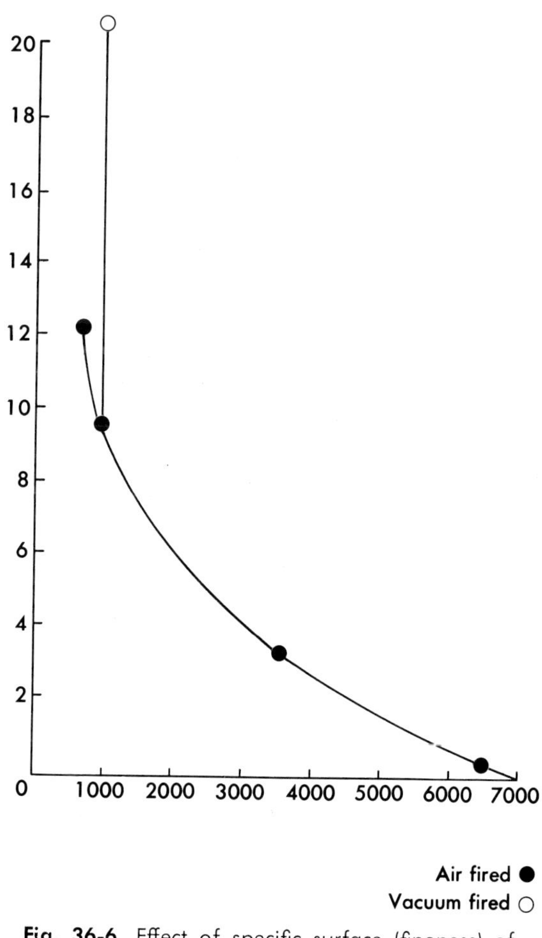

Fig. 36-6. Effect of specific surface (fineness) of alumina on opacity of aluminous core porcelains.

tral distribution of the illuminants, i.e., daylight to artificial light. These changes cause two apparently similar colors to look different and may be explained by the difference in pigments used to obtain the color; porcelain pigments are different from natural enamel and dentin colors.

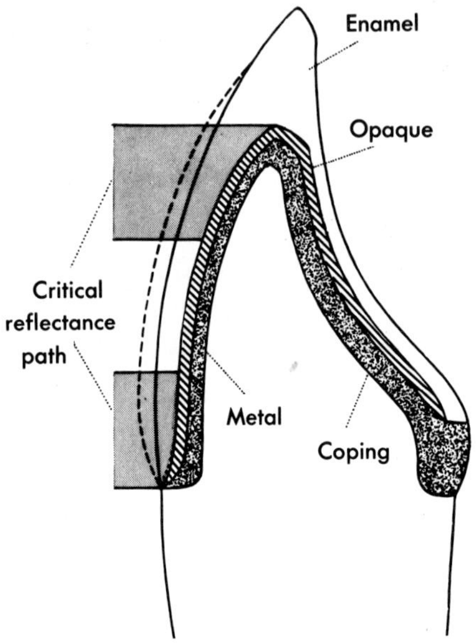

Fig. 36-7. Cross section of fused porcelain to gold crown; critical reflectance paths and area of potential overcontouring.

Fig. 36-7 illustrates the main problem experienced with the anterior porcelain-fused-to-gold crown. Two critical paths of reflectance are generally present and, if there is an inadequate depth of enamel and dentin porcelains the opaques will tend to look chalky and bright yellow in reflected light, particularly of the tungsten type. Because of this deficiency, the technician will borrow space as indicated by the dotted line in Fig. 36-7. The crown is now overcontoured and may create gingival problems due to the creation of a cervical stagnation area (C.S.A.). The gingival contour of a porcelain-fused-to-gold crown will therefore present a greater esthetic problem than the aluminous porcelain crown where no metal background is used. Metameric effects can still be produced with an aluminous porcelain veneer crown and these will generally occur at the incisal third of the preparation when core placement is incorrect and prevents an adequate thickness of overlaying enamel and dentin.

Table 36-2. Aluminous porcelain materials

Materials	*Number of colors*	*Fusing temperature*	*Use*
Low-fusing core	5	1922° F.	Core base for crowns, bridges, etc.
High-fusing core	5	2012° F.	
Dentin	22	1652 to 1742° F.	Main color component
Enamel	4 Air 3 Vacuum	1652 to 1742° F.	Air and vacuum versions of enamel colors
Translucent	(AT #1) 2 (AT #2)	1652° F. 1508° F.	Modifiers and correction materials
Modifiers	13	1652 to 1742° F.	Modifiers for basic color range, mixed with dentin or enamel
Add-On	8	1472 to 1508° F.	Correcting or adding to the fired crown
High alumina reinforcements	1	Stable up to 2732° F.	Strengtheners and substructures for crowns and bridges

Aluminous porcelain materials*

Aluminous porcelain crown powders consist of three main components:

1. A high-strength core porcelain containing as much as 50 percent fused alumina crystals
2. Dentin
3. Enamel veneer powders made from glasses containing a high combined alumina content which overlay the high strength core and give color and translucency to the complete veneer.

Two types of aluminous core porcelains are available.

1. The low-fusing cores, containing 45 percent by weight of alumina crystals and maturing within the temperature range of 1850 to 1922° F.
2. High-fusing cores containing 50 percent alumina crystals that are fired at 2012° F.

The high-fusing core porcelains are stronger but due to their higher alumina content, are more opaque. These materials are better confined to the lingual surfaces. The range of firing temperatures in the core porcelains will depend upon the fusibility of the glass fluxes used as the bonding matrix; these vary from manufacturer to manufacturer. All the materials require similar handling and firing technics but in order to clarify these technics a description will be given of materials maturing in the 1922° F. range for the low-fusing core, 2012° F. for the high-fusing core, and 1652° F. to 1742° F. for the dentins and enamels.

Core material. There are two of these materials, a low-fusing core (LFC) and a high-fusing core (HFC). These core materials are basically the same except for their fusing point. The low-fusing core fuses at 1922° F., while the high-fusing core fuses at 2012° F. Their advantage lies in the fact that they are extremely stable while the lower fusing enamels and dentins are subsequently being fired. After the core has been fired, the platinum matrix can be stripped from it before the lower fusing dentins and enamels are fired, but this is not advised. The foil should be stripped as one of the last steps in construction. The core material is very similar in purpose to a metal reinforcement.

Dentin material. This material forms the esthetic body of the crown and is most important in providing proper shade. It fuses at 1652 to 1742° F.

Air-fired enamel. This is purely what the name suggests and is used as an *enamel or translucent coating* for the crown. It also fuses at 1652 to 1742° F.

Vacuum-fired enamel. This material is substituted for air-fired enamel when vacuum firing is being done. It also fuses at 1652 to 1742° F.

Translucents. There are two translucents, AT 1 and AT 2, both of which are similar and used in a similar way to the enamels. Where vacuum firing is done, these are replaced by the vacuum-fired enamel as in the case of the enamels. AT 1 fires in the normal range (1652 to 1742° F.) of the other overlay materials, while AT 2 fires at 1508° F.

Aluminous porcelains

7 Enamel shades (1652 to 1742° F.)

Air	Vacuum
AE 1—light grey	VE 4
AE 2—blue grey	VE 5
AE 3—grey	VE 6
AE 4—pink yellow	

2 Translucent shades (AT 1—1652° F.; AT 2—1508° F.)

AT 1—light grey tint
AT 2—warm light grey tint; surface glaze and carrier for stain

22 Dentin shades (1652 to 1742° F.)

D 5—light yellow	D 6—white yellow
D 7—grey yellow	D 8—dark yellow
D 9—grey yellow	D 10—brown yellow
D 11—light cream	D 12—grey cream
D 13—cream	D 20—white cream
D 21—grey cream	D 22—grey yellow
D 23—yellow	D 24—yellow grey
D 25—cream yellow	D 26—yellow
D 27—dark yellow	D 31—grey yellow
D 32—brown yellow	D 39—grey cream
D 40—grey	D 41—grey

10 Core shades—low-fusing core (LFC) (1922° F.); high-fusing core (HFC) (2012° F.)

LFC 12—lihgt grey	HFC 8—cream
LFC 13—light yellow	HFC 13—light yellow
LFC 25—dark yellow	HFC 25—dark yellow
LFC 41—grey yellow	HFC 41—grey yellow
LFC 50—white	HFC 50—white

9 Add-On shades (1472 to 1508° F.; shade number corresponds to similar number of dentin porcelain)

AO 5	AO 9
AO 8	AO 20
AO 13	AO 31
AO 23	AO 41
AO 32	

*All references to Aluminous Porcelain are those of Columbus Dental Manufacturing Co., Columbus, Ohio (S.D.T.)

Table 36-3. Formulas to reproduce new hue shades, air-fired

Shade	*Core*	*Dentin*	*Enamel*
59	HFC 13 with wash LFC 12	D 20	1—AE 1 1—D 20
60	HFC 13	3—D 23 ½—D 13	4—AE 1 1½—Dentin mix
61	HFC 13	3—D 20 1—D 5	AE 3
62	HFC 13	3—D 20 1½—D 5 1¼—D 23	4—AE 1 1—Dentin mix
65	HFC 25	2—D 23 2—D 5	4—AE 2 1—Dentin mix
66	HFC 25	3—D 23 ½—D 13	4—AE 1 1—Dentin mix
67	HFC 25	3—D 31 ⅛—D 32	4—AE 2 1—Dentin mix
68	HFC 25	3—D 31 ¼—D 32	4—AE 2 1—Dentin mix
69	HFC 41	3—D 8 1—D 9	4—AE 3 1—Dentin mix
77	HFC 25	4—D 41 ½—D 32	4—AE 3 1—Dentin mix
81	HFC 25	2—D 32 1—D 23	4—AE 2
87	HFC 41	3—D 31 1—D 32	4—AE 2 1—Dentin mix

NOTE: These are basic formulas and are not meant to provide exact shade matches. Variations may be obtained by adding small amounts of other dentins or stains to the basic formulas. Enamels and translucents may be interchanged or mixed together.

CONSTRUCTION OF THE ALUMINOUS COMPLETE PORCELAIN VENEER CROWN

Die preparation and the adaptation of the 0.001 inch platinum foil have been described in Chapter 26; the requirements for constructing an aluminous porcelain crown are identical to the basic methods of constructing a regular vacuum-fired complete porcelain veneer crown.

TECHNIC FOR CONSTRUCTING LOW-FUSING CORE PORCELAIN

The buildup of the core porcelain is best done with the brush technic (Fig. 36-8). A fine sable brush is used. Dip the brush in distilled water and absorb excess moisture on a sponge. The tip of the brush should now have a fine point. The low-fusing aluminous core porcelain is mixed with distilled water on a glass slab to a *thick and creamy* consistency. Never use thin mixes since this can cause separation of the alumina and glass powder. The point of the brush may now be gently pushed into the edge of the porcelain mix so that it picks up a small bead of porcelain. The bead is transferred to the platinum matrix and placed in position on the palatal sur-

Table 36-4. Formulas to reproduce Bioform shades, air-fired*

Shade	*Core*	*Dentin*	*Enamel*
59	HFC 13 with wash LFC 12	D 20	1—AE 1 1—D 20
62	HFC 13	D 5	4—AE 1 2—D 5
65	HFC 25	D 23	4—AE 1 2—D 23
66	HFC 13 with wash M 2	D 25	4—AE 1 2—D 25
67	HFC 25	6—D 25 1/16—M 5	4—AE 1 2—Dentin mix
69	HFC 13	D 10	4—AE 1 2—D 10
77	HFC 13	D 8	4—AE 1 2—D 8
81	HFC 13	3—D 10 1⅛—D 32	4—AE 1 2—Dentin mix

*For vacuum firing, replace the following: AE 1 with VE 4; AE 2 with VE 5; AE 3 with VE 6; AT 1 with VE 4; AT 2 with VE 5.

C—core material; D—dentin material; AE—air-fired enamel material; VE—vacuum-fired enamel material.

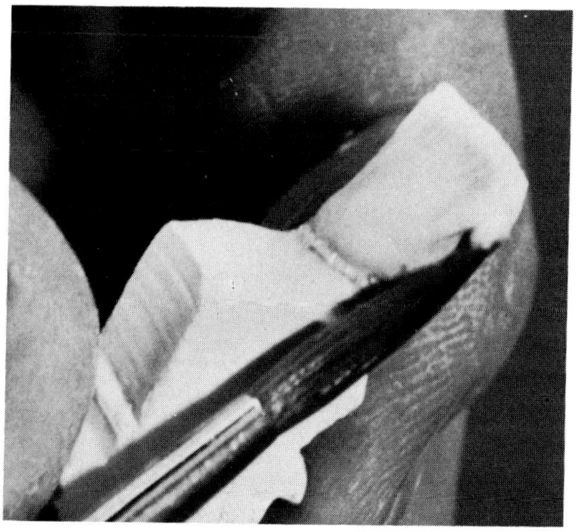

Fig. 36-8. Buildup of porcelain by means of brush technic.

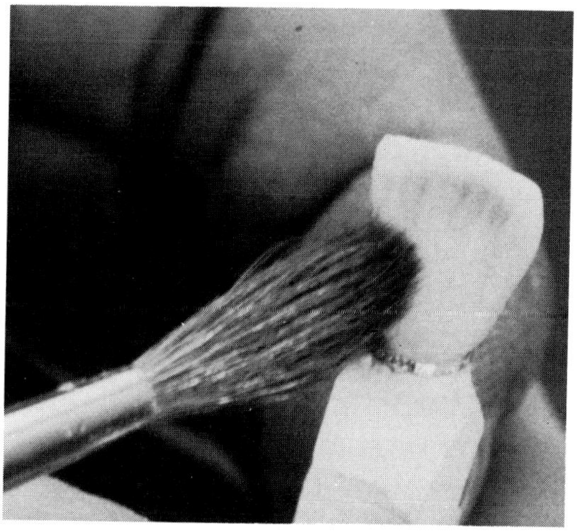

Fig. 36-9. Completed aluminous porcelain core.

face. By repeating these movements the ceramist can quickly build up the core layer to an *even thickness* of approximately 0.6 mm. over the entire crown. Incremental buildup will reduce the trapping of air and rapid placement of the core porcelain in the exact position required will be achieved. There is no excess material, and slumping of the porcelain is avoided by periodically absorbing excess moisture with a paper tissue or cloth. Once the initial buildup of the core is complete, the die is vibrated with a porcelain carver handle and the porcelain core is held on the labial in a folded paper tissue. The tissue may then be folded over the incisal edge to absorb excess water on the palatal surface. Thorough vibration of the aluminous porcelain is essential since this crystalline ceramic will benefit from meticulous condensation. Even vacuum-firing will not eliminate large entrapped air bubbles.

The die is reseated in the model, the surface of the core-porcelain slightly moistened, and further porcelain added on by the brush technic (Fig. 36-8). This additional porcelain should cover the entire lingual surface of the preparation and increase the thickness at the labial cervical collar (Fig. 36-7). The lingual porcelain must be built up to the maximum extent of the occlusion (Fig. 36-9) and finally brush-shaped.

CERVICAL RELIEF

Aluminous porcelain has a 40 percent volume porosity in the powder bed and must shrink on firing like any ceramic material. One of the satisfactory ways of overcoming this shrinkage is to "ditch" the cervical shoulder with a sharp instrument (Fig. 36-10). The clearance of porcelain from this area will allow the main bulk of aluminous porcelain to shrink centrally onto the platinum foil without overdistorting the apron.

It is possible to fire an aluminous porcelain core in one bake but if a precision fit is required, the two-stage cervical relief technic must be employed.

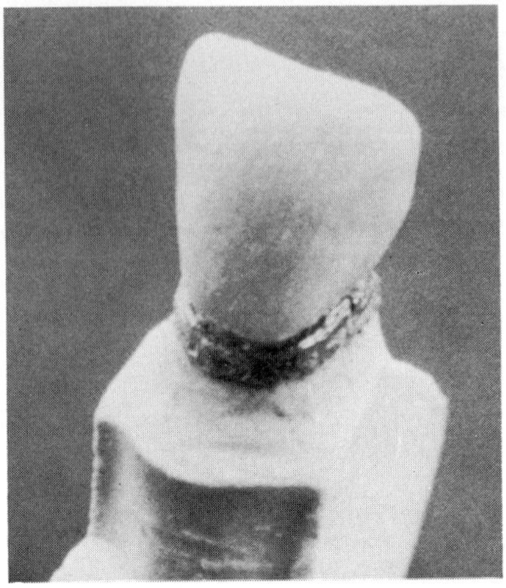

Fig. 36-10. Completed buildup of core porcelain with shoulder "ditched."

The core is now ready for its first firing and it is important for the ceramist to have a good knowledge of processes involved in sintering dental porcelain.

VACUUM-FIRING AND AIR-FIRING TECHNICS

Much controversy surrounds the methods of firing crowns, arising in the main from an incomplete understanding of the sintering or fusion processes that occur during the firing of a porcelain.

There is generally no difference in the chemical composition of the vacuum-fired or air-fired porcelains and often a manufacturer will prepare both materials from the same glass frit. The only difference between the materials is the particle size of the powders and the amount of pigment, opacifiers, or crystalline material used to obtain the dentin or enamel colors. Vacuum-firing porcelain powders generally have a grain size distribution of less than 40 μ with the major distribution in the 5 to 10 μ range. For air-fired porcelains, the largest size may be 70 μ or slightly more, and all sizes less than 7 μ are removed. The air-firing porcelain powders therefore have a natural size distribution between 7 and 70 μ.

All porcelain powders reveal a volume porosity in the dry powder bed of 35 to 45 percent depending on the packing ratio of the powder particles. When these porcelains enter the hot zone of the furnace, each grain will be contacting its neighbor and furnace atmosphere will be present in the void spaces. The grains of porcelain will lense at their contact points and weld together once the softening point of the glass is reached. The entire ceramic body will start to contract, generally *toward its greatest bulk.* The furnace atmosphere or porosity at the grain boundaries will tend to be swept out via these boundaries and, depending on the time/temperature cycle, this porosity can be almost entirely eliminated. The ideal time/temperature cycles are employed by the industrial ceramist where the majority of his work must be air-fired. The "green" ware is placed on trays that enter a tunnel kiln and the ceramic ware is gradually moved along the tunnel until it reaches the hot zone of the furnace. This process can often exceed 24 hours. Gases formed in the ceramic can escape; very high densities are obtainable in the fired body.

The logic of this procedure is self-evident since the sintering or fusion of any porcelain is directed toward eliminating the voids between the powder particles. Furnace atmosphere trapped in these voids can only escape by slow sintering since a rapid rise to the fusion point will merely *seal the surface* and any entrapped air cannot escape. If gas is entrapped in the fired body it may cause the ceramic to "bloat" or swell.

Dental procedures usually demand a quick-firing technic and violate accepted industrial ceramic practice. Vacuum-firing was introduced to mitigate to a certain extent this situation. Vacuum-firing will reduce the size of porosities in a porcelain body, but it will not eliminate them. Quick-firing can still seal the surface and the continued use of vacuum from this point is often useless and can be dangerous, since it increases the risk of bloating. Although vacuum-firing technics were introduced mainly to increase the translucency and homogeneity of dental porcelain, it may also be seen that when properly used, vacuum can also assist in the more rapid escape of gases. An appreciation of the sintering processes of ceramics can therefore give a guide to the successful firing of dental porcelain.

If air-firing methods are employed, a very slow maturation period is required to allow the escape of entrapped gas or air bubbles. Such a procedure can produce an extremely dense ceramic.

In the case of vacuum-firing, the above process should ideally still be the same but the vacuum will assist in the more rapid removal of entrapped gas or furnace atmosphere from the void spaces. Resultantly the firing schedule for a vacuum processed ceramic can be reduced. Vacuum porcelain powders also possess an additional advantage inasmuch as the powder is finer and the void spaces smaller. Any entrapped bubbles will therefore be smaller and remain more discreetly in the fired body. By contrast the coarser air-fired porcelain will reveal larger porosities.

The increasing popularity of the vacuum-fired porcelains is therefore understandable. They can be handled easily, fired more rapidly, and the surface may be ground and repolished more easily. Consistent color and translucency are also obtainable when rapid firing technics are employed, although there is a limit to the speed of this operation.

However, it must be clearly understood that the ceramist can still produce outstanding results with air-fired porcelain, providing he understands the sintering processes involved in firing porcelain crowns. It is possible to produce air-fired crowns that are indistinguishable from vacuum-processed porcelain; air-firing technics are still capable of providing the dentist with a restoration of the highest quality.

Aluminous porcelain when fired is a two-phase crystal-glass solid, and its strength will be influenced by the amount of porosity surrounding the fused alumina crystals. If air-firing technics are used, a *very slow maturation period* is required, thus allowing the gradual escape of entrapped air and gases. The best results will be obtained when a firing schedule of 50° F./minute or less is observed and high densities will be obtained in the fired body. This firing schedule should ideally be used when vacuum-firing on aluminous core porcelain. However, *once the manufacturer's recommended maximum maturing temperature is reached, the vacuum must be broken.* Continued vacuum-firing of aluminous porcelain at high temperature can produce bloating in the ceramic body. Vacuum should only be used to aid the escape of gases and reduce porosity in the porcelain body while the glass phase is softening and starting to flow around the alumina. Once the glass phase has become viscous, prolonged vacuum will cause this phase to bloat and gross weakening of the porcelain will result.

Aluminous porcelain, when completely sintered, should present an egg-shell sheen impervious to the penetration of a water-soluble dye. The cardinal points to bear in mind when firing this new porcelain are the following.

1. Furnace temperature must be at least 400° F. below the maximum recommended maturing temperature when the work is introduced into the hot muffle zone; lower temperatures of 400 to 500° F. can be even more beneficial in producing a dense ceramic.
2. Raise firing temperature slowly at 50° F. per minute.
3. Break vacuum immediately on reaching maximum maturing temperature to prevent bloating.
4. Air-fire work at maximum maturing temperature for a minimum period of 8 minutes. Longer firing will increase the glaze on the surface and can improve the fired density in aluminous core porcelains with a 50 percent alumina content. Periods of up to 30 minutes can be used with absolute safety and there is no risk of spoiling the ceramic. The only precaution required before applying the dentin and enamel porcelain is to *remove any surface glaze on the core with a diamond stone prior to firing the enamel porcelains.*

Aluminous core porcelain—first firing

The core porcelain must be slowly dried in front of the open furnace door for at least 4 minutes. It may then be placed on the firing platform for a further 3 minutes. Modern vacuum furnaces, which employ a push-rod on vertical slide, are ideal for this procedure (Fig. 26-19). The recommended firing schedule for the 1922° F. core porcelain is as follows:

Drying	(Furnace 1750° F.)
Muffle entrance	4 minutes
Firing platform	3 minutes
Apply vacuum	28 inches

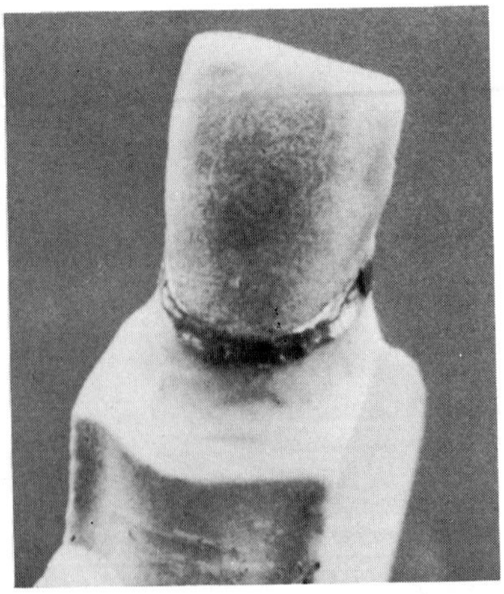

Fig. 36-11. Aluminous core after second firing.

Firing

Enter hot zone of furnace at 1750° F.
Raise temperature to 1922° F. at 50° F. per minute
Switch off vacuum at 1922° F.
Hold at 1922° F. in air for 5 minutes

Cooling

Slow cool to 1500° F.
Remove work and allow to cool at room temperature

Aluminous core porcelain—second firing

The platinum apron is reburnished at the gingival shoulder and more core porcelain applied to fill in the ditched area.

The second firing should now follow the exact procedure adopted for the first firing, except for the final period of maturation in air, which should be extended to 8 minutes (Fig. 36-11).

After cooling the core porcelain, a simple test may be performed to see whether it is fully sintered. A little ink or water-soluble dye is applied to the surface. If the core is not fully sintered, the ink will soak into the pores on the surface and, despite subsequent washing in water, will still be visible. If the core is completely vitrified, the ink may be washed off the surface quite easily and the core porcelain should exhibit an eggshell finish. If there is any doubt over the complete vitrification of the core, it is safer to raise the temperature of the furnace by 20° F. and refire in air for 5 minutes.

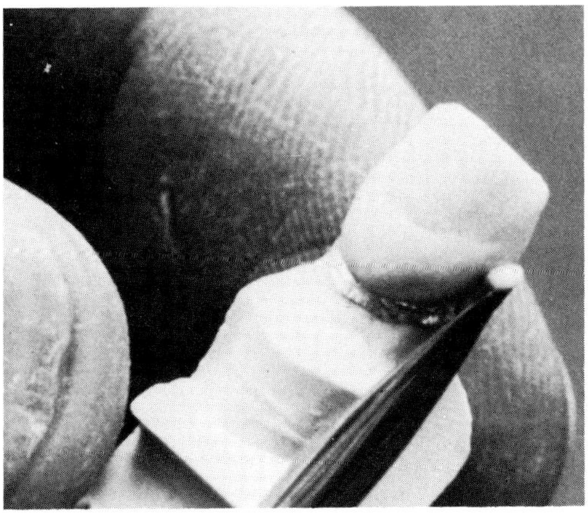

Fig. 36-12. Covering core with body porcelain after second firing.

A thin wash of core porcelain must never be used. Maximum core thickness, particularly on the palatal surface, will provide resistance against torque and improve the thermal shock resistance of the finished crown. If the body of the crown is highly reinforced, the deepening of microcracks on the surface will be resisted by the high-modulus core porcelain.

Application of gingival and body veneer porcelains

An aluminous porcelain veneer powder is selected to match the color of the neck area of the shade guide tooth. A creamy mix of this powder is applied over the core porcelain, also using the brush technic. The porcelain is vibrated and dried with a paper tissue. The main body or dentin color is then applied on all surfaces of the core porcelain and condensed to position (Fig. 36-12). A more intense color may be introduced over this thin layer of dentin to give a central body effect to the tooth in the gingival third (Fig. 36-5). A study of the shade guide tooth will reveal the exact position of these colors. The crown is then positioned on the model, and the palatal and labial areas are corrected with the necessary amount of dentin porcelain to obtain full tooth contour. The incisal edge should also be extended by 1 to 1.5 mm. to allow for firing shrinkage. It is much easier to cut back a fully contoured crown for the enamel application than to attempt to judge the incisal blend at this stage. The crown may be modeled with a brush or porcelain carver to obtain a smooth finish.

Application of enamel veneer porcelain

The dentin is scalloped with a sharp knife to provide the exact depth and blend of enamel porcelain (Fig. 36-13). Blend-

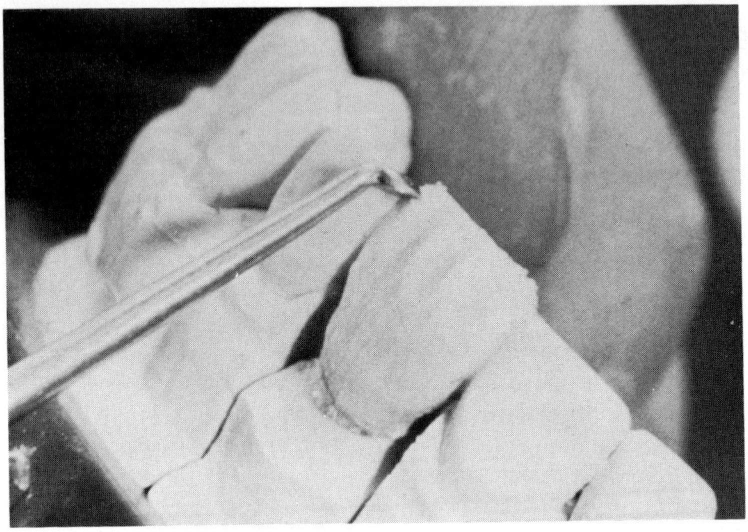

Fig. 36-13. Removal of some dentin porcelain to be covered with enamel porcelain.

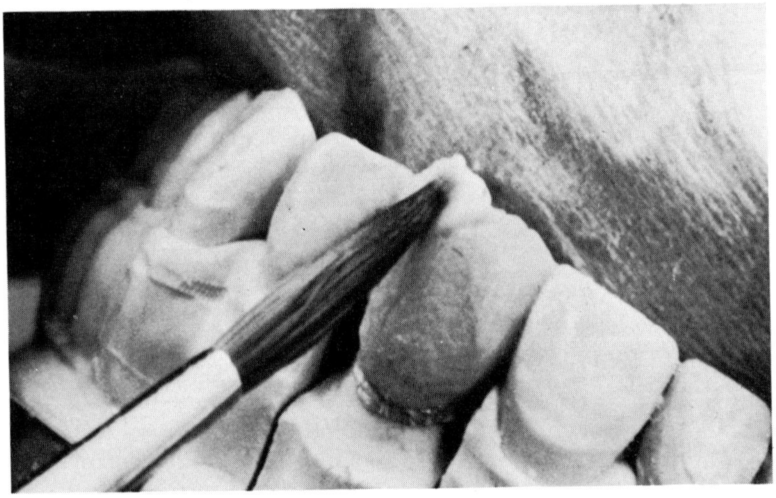

Fig. 36-14. Application of enamel porcelain over incisal dentin body color.

ing of the enamels will be improved if the dentin porcelain is kept moist.

A creamy mix of the enamel porcelain is prepared and applied with a sable brush to the incisal area (Fig. 36-14). The enamel blend may demand complete coverage of the dentin according to the shade and mode of construction of the shade guide tooth. Excess water is absorbed by vibration and brush-shaping but care must be taken not to overvibrate and cause slumping of the porcelain.

Final characterization

The incisal area may be markedly improved in esthetics by the judicious use of translucent porcelain combined with concentrated colors. For example, proximal translucence can be improved by removing a small quantity of enamel porcelain from the mesial and distal surfaces. This porcelain must be removed so that translucent porcelain can be wrapped around the entire proximal surface (Fig. 36-16). White or blue stain may be applied over

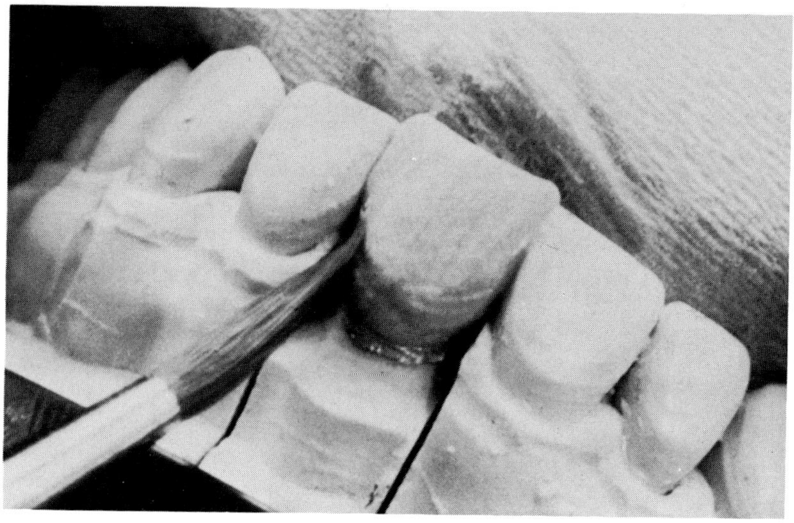

Fig. 36-15. Enamel porcelain applied at incisal and blended gingivally over body porcelain.

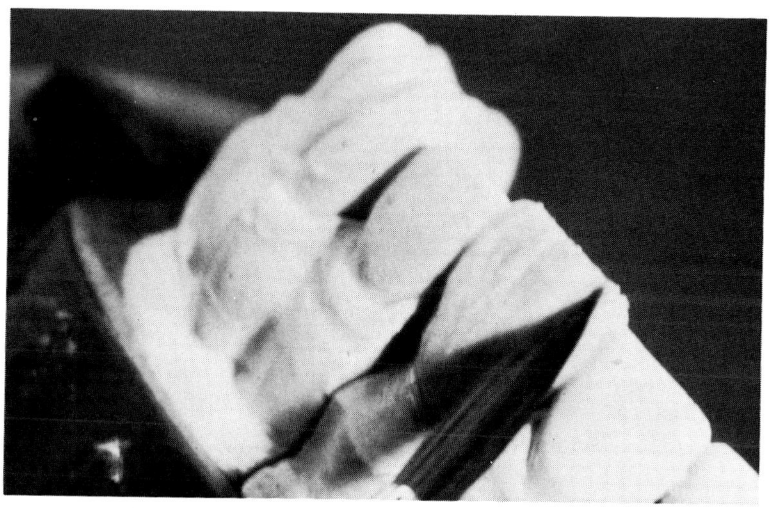

Fig. 36-16. Translucent porcelain applied proximally near incisal third area.

the exposed enamel surface prior to the application of the translucent porcelain, and this will aid the breakup of light and enliven the incisal corners. This stain must be applied in minute quantity and the lightest touch with the brush is necessary to avoid gross effects.

The central areas of the incisal edge may also be scalloped into V shaped grooves and treated similarly (Fig. 36-17). At the bottom of the groove a small quantity of dentin porcelain is laid in, and orange stains blended in at the incisal end of the groove (Fig. 36-18). Enamel porcelain is then blended over the thin dentin layer to create a beveled area exactly similar to the one for the enamel-dentin blend. If the translucent is now applied over the incisal grooved area, it will create a three-dimensional effect (Fig. 36-19). The incisal enamel will appear extremely lifelike and the inlaid concentrated colors

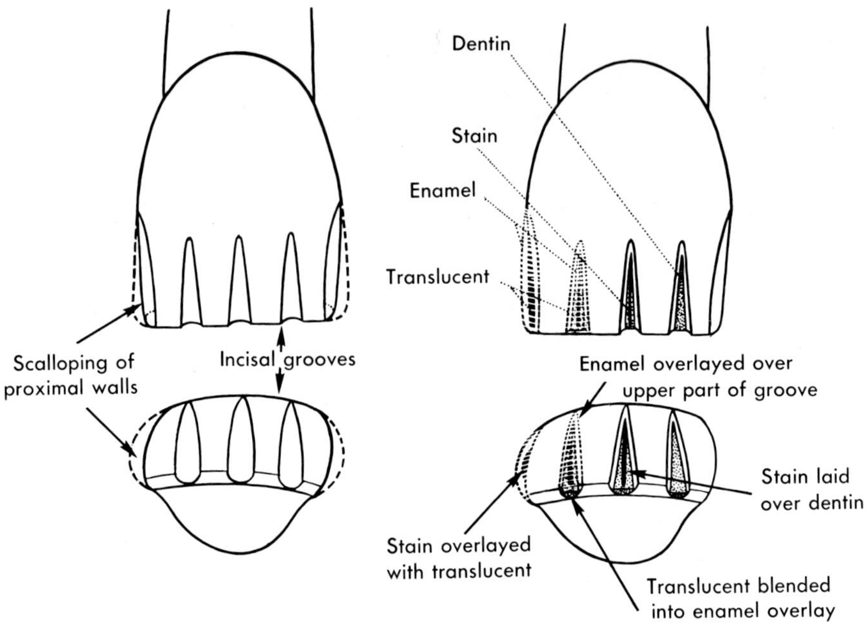

Fig. 36-17. Incisal edge grooved for stains and translucent porcelain.

will reproduce the effect of enamel cracks or striae.

The importance of beveling the enamel porcelain in the groove line should be emphasized since it will prevent a sharp demarcation line from appearing when the translucent porcelain overlays the entire groove. This translucent porcelain must be used in very small quantity since excess material will create a washout effect.

In some cases a sharp incisal blend of translucence is required; this may be simulated by adding additional translucent porcelain behind the incisal edge.

Subtle use of inlaid concentrated colors (modifiers) and translucent porcelains will often transform a porcelain crown that otherwise could look very artificial in the mouth.

ALUMINOUS PORCELAIN INTENSE COLOR MODIFIERS

These modifiers are available in a range of thirteen colors and are used in obtaining shades or variations of shades by adding to or by firing over aluminous porcelain.

M	1—Opalescent	M	7—Dark brown
M	2—White/pink	M	8—Pink
M	3—Ivory/cream	M	9—Grey
M	4—Grey/brown	M	10—Blue
M	5—Light orange	M	11—White
M	6—Orange	M	12—Light cream
		M	13—White/white

These intense colors may be mixed with any of the dentins or enamels in the aluminous porcelain range or used undiluted as they are (fusing temperature—1652° F.).

Contact area adjustment

Once the final buildup of the crown is completed, additional translucent and dentin porcelains (1472 to 1508° F.) may be added to the proximal surfaces to allow for firing shrinkage and the surface gently smoothed with a shipping brush.

Firing the veneer porcelain
(dentin and enamel)
Biscuit firing for 1742° F. porcelain
Air-firing technic
Drying
Muffle entrance for 4 minutes
Firing platform for 3 minutes
(Furnace at 1000 to 1200° F.)

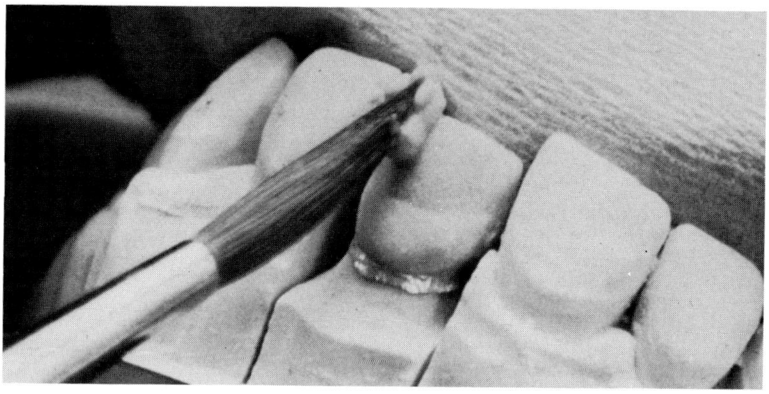

Fig. 36-18. Stain laid in at bottom of groove and covered with enamel porcelain.

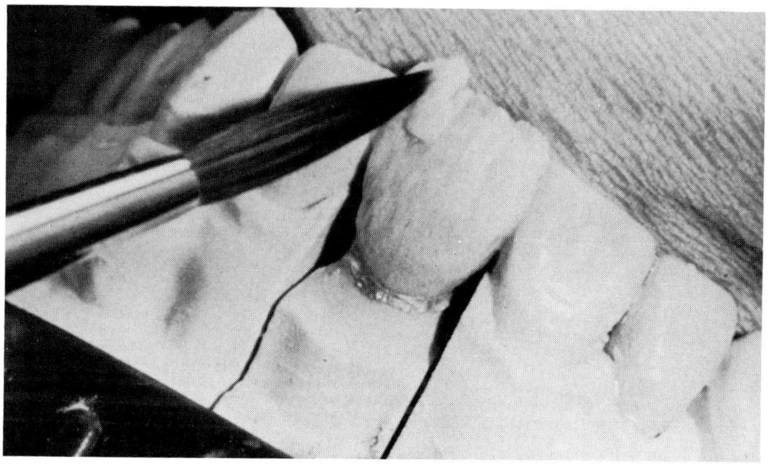

Fig. 36-19. Translucent porcelain applied over grooved area in Fig. 36-18 to complete three-dimensional effect.

Firing

Enter hot zone of furnace at 1000° F.
Raise temperature at 50° F./minute
Hold temperature at 1650° F. for 3 minutes

Vacuum-firing technic

Dry as for air-firing

Firing

Enter hot zone of furnace at 1300° F.
Apply vacuum at 20 inches
Raise temperature at 50° F./minute
Break vacuum at 1650° F.
Hold at 1650° F. for 3 minutes

The surface of the crown should now be at a high biscuit stage. Firing aluminous veneer porcelains to a low biscuit is not recommended since most of these materials are made from isotropic glasses that are improved in color and thermal shock resistance by firing to nearly full maturity. If the crown still presents a low biscuit surface it must be refired for 3 to 4 minutes to increase vitrification.

Grinding and staining

The biscuit-stage aluminous porcelain porcelain crown should preferably be ground with diamond stones used exclusively for this work. After any occlusal or contact area adjustments have been made, the crown may be tried in the mouth. Duplication of the surface anatomy of the adjoining natural teeth may be achieved by grinding the aluminous porcelain surface with very fine diamond wheel stones. Smoother areas may be created by using rubber-bonded carbide wheels, but the surface must be thoroughly cleaned afterward with detergents or an ultrasonic cleaner.

Surface "effect" stains may now be applied and a thin streak of orange stain on a darker dentin color may be applied behind the tip of the incisal edge to produce the slight milkiness present in many natural teeth. Orange or brown stain is also effective when applied on the mesial and distal surfaces since these colors are highlighted through the enamel surface.

Glazing

It should be emphasized that stressing of a complete veneer porcelain crown due to thermal shock is severe when a biscuit fired crown is rapidly introduced into the furnace. Minute thermal cracks can be formed in the glazed surface that are not apparent to the naked eye (Fig. 36-1). Surface weakening via these microcracks is therefore built into the crown. At a later stage the crown may fracture in service due to the deepening of these cracks under occlusal loading, and catastrophic failure may occur when the patient is eating nothing harder than bread and butter.

The ceramist must therefore *take the greatest care in preheating his biscuit-stage crown very slowly in order to ensure that all areas of the crown expand evenly.* The principle of the industrial tunnel kiln is therefore the ideal at which to aim. The crown should be moved stage by stage into the hot zone of the furnace muffle, and simple preheating at the entrance is not sufficient. *A minimum period of 5 minutes should be given to moving the crown into the hot zone and the firing tray should be inserted at 1-minute intervals.*

All glazing must be accomplished in air and where possible a powerful electric lamp will enable the ceramist to view his glazed surface directly. *The recommended glazing period for the 1742° F. aluminous porcelain is 4 to 4.5 minutes.* However, visual inspection of the surface remains the best method of ensuring that the tooth anatomy has been maintained. The aluminous porcelain dentin and enamel porcelains contain a high content of combined alumina and are resultantly very resistant to slump or pyroplastic flow at their recommended maturing temperature. Rounding of angles and loss of detail are invariably produced by glazing at too high a temperature. It is therefore essential to maintain a constant check on the accuracy of the furnace pyrometer and to bear in mind that, if necessary, a little more time spent on glazing at a lower temperature will ensure brighter colors and greater surface detail. Greenish colored porcelain is produced by quick-firing at too high a temperature; the glass is overvitrified. In some cases, it may even devitrify, producing flecked areas in the surface.

THE POSTERIOR ALUMINOUS PORCELAIN CROWN

An alumina-reinforced crown may be constructed on the posterior teeth, but it must only be used where at least 1.0 mm. of core porcelain can be used for occlusal protection. To obtain optimum reinforcement, the core porcelain should contain 50 percent by weight of alumina (high-fusing core) and should cover the entire

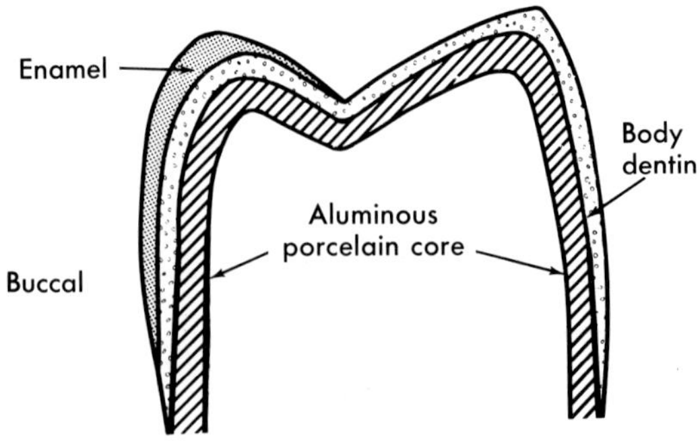

Fig. 36-20. Correct preparation of premolar aluminous porcelain crown.

occlusal and lingual surfaces (Fig. 36-20). Subsequent firing shrinkage will allow sufficient room for a thin layer of dentin and enamel powders. The buccal surface may be completed with the same technic used for the anterior crown.

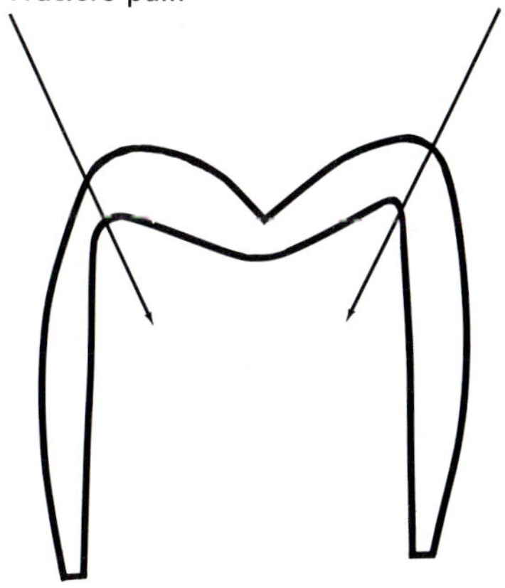

Fig. 36-21. Incorrect preparation of premolar aluminous porcelain crown.

The tooth preparation must simulate the original tooth contour line and present no sharp angles on the occlusal surface (Fig. 36-21). If a thin amount of porcelain is present between the occlusal-axial walls, fracture is almost inevitable.

PREFORMED HIGH-ALUMINA CERAMIC REINFORCEMENTS

High-alumina ceramics used in dentistry generally contain at least 97 percent pure alumina and they differ considerably from aluminous porcelain (Table 36-1).

Aluminous porcelain is a mixture of alumina crystals and a glass flux, and during sintering the glass forms a matrix for the harder and stronger alumina crystals. In the case of high alumina, although small quantities of fluxing agents are used, the main process that occurs during firing is termed "recrystallization."

Many theories exist regarding the ex-

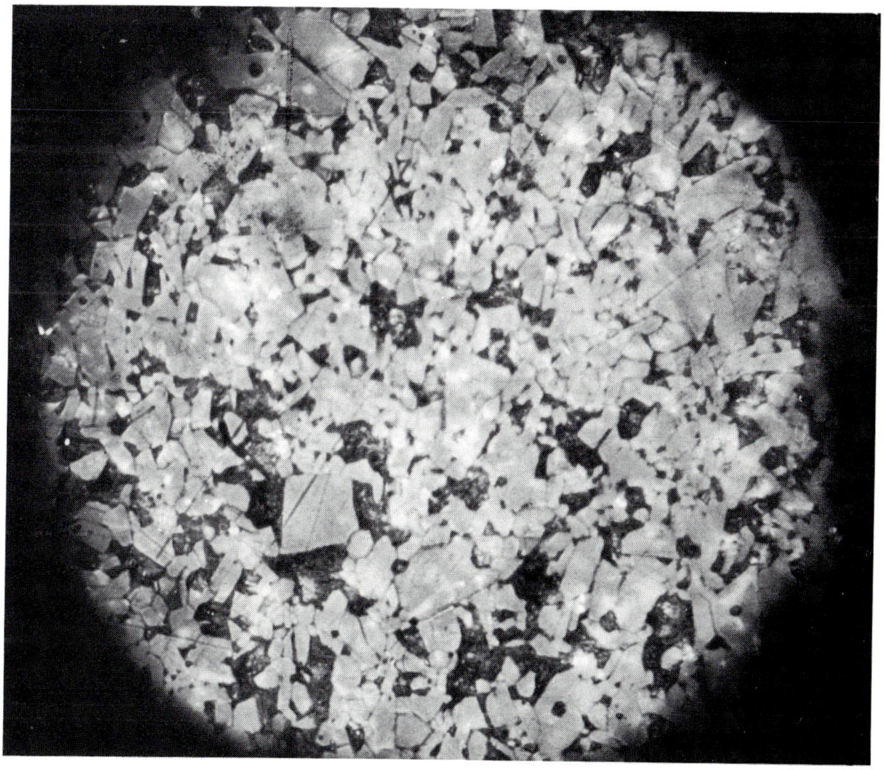

Fig. 36-22. Photomicrograph of recrystallized alumina.

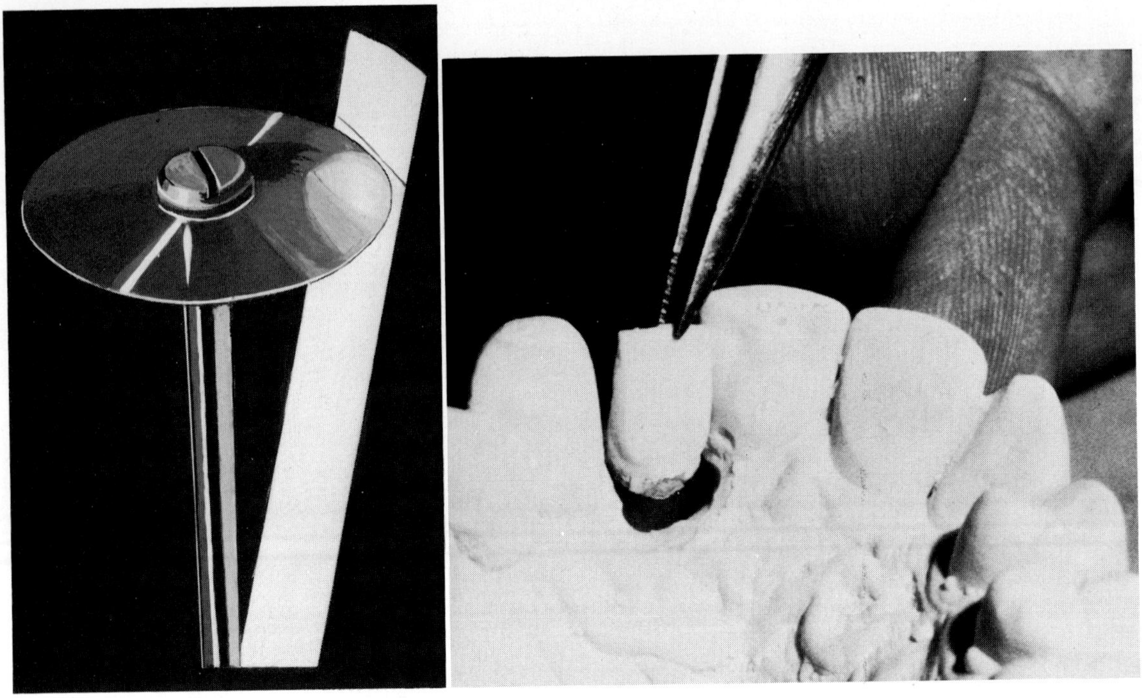

Fig. 36-23. A, High-alumina strip is cut with diamond disk. **B,** High-alumina strip to be placed on lingual surface of tooth in Figs. 36-5 and 36-26, for added strength and translucence.

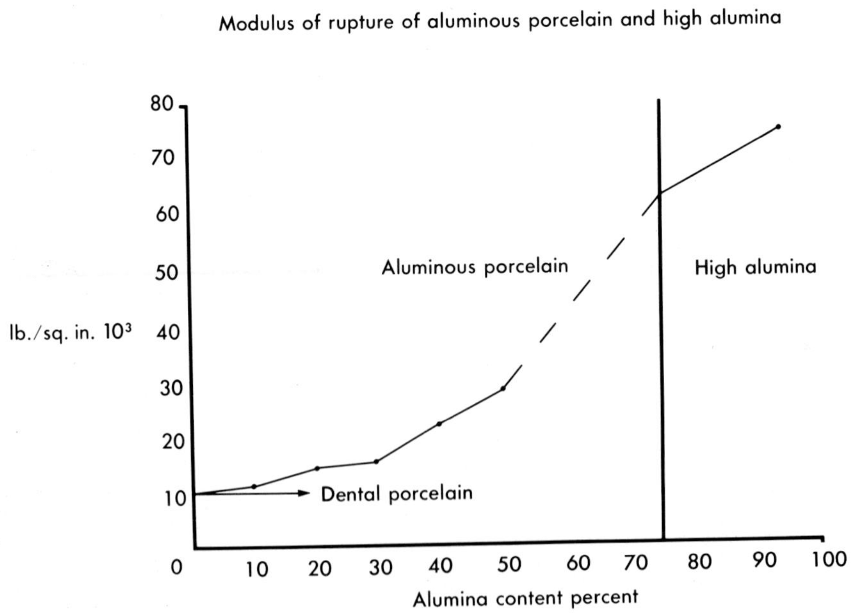

Fig. 36-24

Table 36-5. Preformed high-alumina rods, tubes, and strip*

Type	*No.*	*Length (mm.)*	*Internal diameter (mm.)*	*External diameter (mm.)*	*Uses*
Oval tube	T.1	50	1.5 × 2.0	2.5 × 3.0	Dowel-crowns
Oval tube	T.2	50	1.8 × 2.5	2.8 × 2.5	Dowel-crown tube pontics
Oval tube	T.3	50	2.0 × 3.0	3.0 × 4.0	Dowel-crown tube pontics
Oval tube	T.4	50	2.0 × 2.5	4.0 × 4.5	Tube pontics
Oval rod	R.1	50		2.8 × 3.5	Bridge connectors
Round rod	R.2	50		1.0	Bridge connectors
Round rod	R.3	50		1.5	Bridge connectors
Curved strip	S.1	50		7.1 × 0.7	Reinforced linguals on jacket and dowel-crowns Reinforcement for cantilever bridges
Dovetail—slotted backing	A.1	50		4.0 × 2.27	Facings on metal substructure

*Cutting and shaping of all high-alumina reinforcements are best done using diamond instruments rotating at not less than 20,000 rpm. Areas where the porcelain buildup will contact the model should be treated with a release agent. (Courtesy Columbus Dental Mfg. Co., Columbus, Ohio.)

act processes that occur during the firing cycle of high alumina. However, it appears that during firing, the following steps occur. First, welding occurs at points of contact between adjacent oxide particles, giving rise to a lensing effect as normally occurs in sintering processes, i.e., partial fusion. Migration of atoms then takes place from one particle to another, resulting in a shift in particle boundaries on recrystallization. During recrystallization, the shift in grain boundaries results in the formation of a closely interlocking crystalline structure of considerable strength, the improved packing of the particles resulting in shrinkage of the oxide mass (Fig. 36-22). Fluxes such as CaO_2, SiO_2, TiO_2, and MnO_2 bond the structure together and increase diffusion in the alumina itself.

High-alumina ceramics are made from calcined alumina powders that have been mixed with suitable binders and a release agent. The alumina "dough" can then be automatically dry-pressed or extrusion moulded for use as crown or bridge reinforcements (Figs. 36-23, *A*, and 36-26).

The moulded articles are then slowly oven-dried and fired at a fusion temperature of up to 3012° F., the resulting product being a hard impermeable ceramic of very high strength and chemical resistance (Table 36-6). The fired alumina is considerably stronger than aluminous porcelain and has proved, under clinical tests, to be as strong as current metals (Fig. 36-24).

High-alumina ceramics are colored to a neutral dentin shade using high-temperature resistant pigments such as manganese-alumina pink, vanadium-zircon blue, and praesodymium-zircon yellow. This background of pure color is very receptive to veneering with the more translucent veneer porcelains (Fig. 36-23, *B*). The bonding at the interface between aluminous porcelain and high alumina is of a chemical nature, and an ionic bond between the oxide constituents of both materials is achieved. This can be shown by observation of the fluorescent effect at the interface when examined under ultraviolet light.

High-alumina reinforcements are used to reinforce aluminous complete porcelain crowns and to provide high-strength anchorage systems for bridge pontics, facings, dowel-crowns, and all ceramic bridges. High alumina is supplied in the form of reinforcing rods, tubes, dovetail backings, and sheets (Table 36-5).

PALATAL REINFORCED CROWNS

High-alumina curved strip (S.1)

This method was devised to increase the strength of the complete aluminous porcelain crowns, particularly in the closed bite situation. Clinical experience has indicated that high-alumina strips used as a palatal reinforcement can provide strength in the critical occluding area and prevent midline or half-moon fractures. The technic is particularly useful on the anterior crown where space limits the use of porcelain-fused-to-gold crowns (Fig. 36-25). The high-alumina curved strip becomes an integral part of the core porcelain and will enable aluminous porcelain crowns to be constructed where all-porcelain restorations would definitely be contraindicated.

Technic

As much as possible of the palatal surface is covered with the sheet without interfering with incisal esthetics or lingual contour (Fig. 36-26). The slight curvature of the strip may be orientated in any direction so as to adapt as closely as possible to the palatal form of the preparation. The dentist may wish to bear in mind the curvature of the strip and select a similar diameter cutting wheel with which to prepare the palatal section of the preparation, to ensure a fully fitting insert without leaving an unreinforced area palatocervically. Objections to using such a preformed reinforcement can be raised regarding the universal application of this technic to all preparations since every tooth will differ in palatal curvature. Clinical experience under laboratory conditions has indicated that at least 70 percent of all preparations

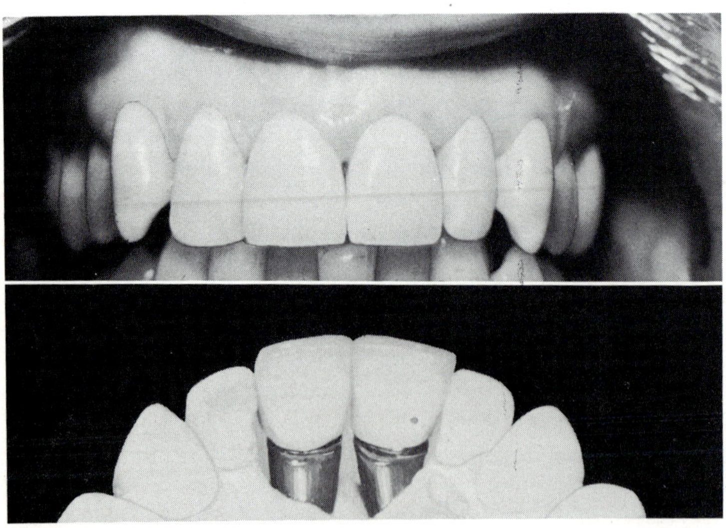

Fig. 36-25. Labial and lingual views of two upper central incisors with aluminous porcelain crowns.

can be fitted with high-alumina sheet reinforcement without interfering with occlusion or esthetics.

The platinum matrix is prepared as for a conventional crown. The alumina strip is applied to the preparation and marked with a pencil to an estimated size and cut off square with a diamond disk. Further shaping is by diamond wheel. Exact contour is not imperative at this stage. A little high-fusing aluminous core porcelain is applied to the palatal area of the preparation and partially condensed by gentle tapping of the model and absorbing with a paper tissue or gauze.

The shaped alumina backing sheet is

Table 36-6. High-alumina reinforcement components

Tensile strength	lb./sq. in.	20,000
Compressive strength	lb./sq. in.	250,000
Bending strength	lb./sq. in.	50,000
Impact strength	Kg.cm.	5.5
Thermal conductivity at 20° C.g.cal./cm.^{2}/sec./ °C./cm.		0.050
Hardness—Moh scale		9
Coefficient of linear expansion—parts/million/C.	20° C. to 400° C. 20° C. to 600° C. 20° C. to 1,000° C.	6.6 7.2 8.2
Porosity	Fuchsine dye penetration Water absorption	Nil Nil
Working temperature, maximum, C.		1,500

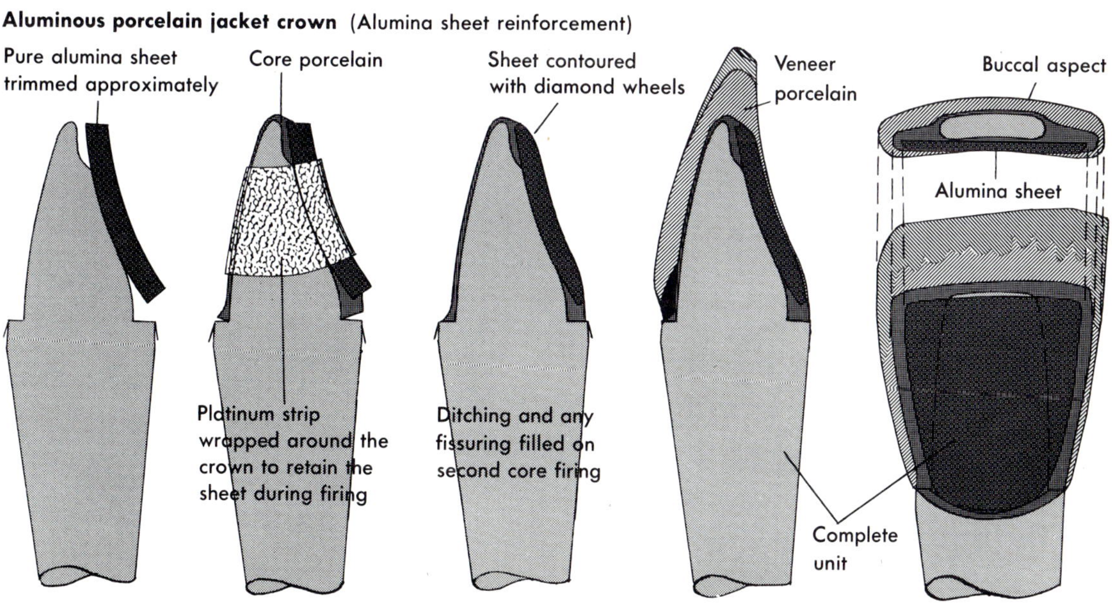

Fig. 36-26. Aluminous porcelain crown built up to full contour with alumina sheet reinforcement on die covered with 0.001 inch platinum matrix.

Table 36-7. Physical properties and characteristics of Hilox alumina*

Tensile strength	lb./sq. in.	20,000
Compressive strength	lb./sq. in.	250,000
Modulus of rupture	lb./sq. in.	50,000
Modulus of elasticity	lb./sq. in.	46×10^6
Coefficient of linear expansion: Parts/million/°C	20° C. to 400° C. 20° C. to 600° C. 20° C. to 1,000° C.	6.6 7.2 8.2
Porosity	Fuchsine dye penetration Water absorption	Nil Nil
Hardness	Rockwell C scale	72

*Courtesy Steatite and Porcelain Products Ltd. (Morgan Crucible Company).

roughened with a diamond wheel stone and any contaminant is removed by heating in a furnace. The backing is then positioned with tweezers and settled into the core porcelain until it is firmly against the platinum matrix. When the opposing teeth are positioned, the insert may tilt slightly if there is contact, pushing it into better adaptation at this point. It is left in this position and more porcelain is added around the proximal and incisal edges, taking care not to trap air under the sheet. The insert is held tightly by finger pressure with a tissue and gently condensed.

At this stage the full core form may be built up, condensed and relieved at the shoulder, taking care not to alter the position of the insert. Alternatively the insert may be fired to the matrix first. Whichever method is used, it is important to retain the insert in close contact with the matrix during firing. This may be done by wrapping a narrow strip of platinum around the complete fabrication, and the ends may be linked by a simple finger-formed tinner's joint. If this is not done, the steam pressure behind the insert during drying may cause the insert to come away from the porcelain or to fall away under its own weight. This stage is fired until complete shrinkage of the added core porcelain has occurred (2012° F.).

The shoulder is reburnished and the cervical space is filled, together with any fissuring around the insert. The core porcelain is then given a final firing of at least 8 minutes at 2012° F.

The edges of the insert are tapered into the core porcelain by contouring with a diamond wheel, and any high points on the occlusion are eased (Fig. 36-26).

The insert should not be thinned to less than half its thickness over a large area, but it has been found reliable to thin a pinpoint area to ¼ mm. If space permits it is desirable (although not critical) to cover the insert with core porcelain. It should, however, be finally covered with at least a thin glaze veneer.

The final buildup is of dentin and enamel as described for the aluminous porcelain crown (Fig. 36-26).

SELECTED REFERENCES

1. Marzahl, H.: Effect of quartz on the strength of porcelain, Ber. Dtsch. Keram. eGs. **32:** 203, 1955.
2. Mattyasovszy-Zsolnay, L.: Mechanical strength of porcelain, J. Amer. Ceram. Soc. **40:**299, 1957.
3. Genin, L. G.: Effect of quartz on the strength of porcelain, Glass and Ceram. (Moscow) **15:**35, 1958.
4. Weyl, von D.: The effect of internal stresses on the structure and mechanical strength of porcelain, Ber. Dtsch. Keram. Ges. **36:**319, 1959.

GENERAL REFERENCES

Adriaasen, J. A. T. Personal communication.

Austin, C. R., Schofield, H. Z., and Haldy, N. L.: Alumina in Whiteware, J. Amer. Ceram. Soc. **29**:341, 1946.

Batchelor, R. W., and Dinsdale, A.: Some physical properties of porcelain bodies containing corundum, Transactions of the 7th International Ceramics Congress, London, England, 1960, p. 31.

Binns, D. B.: Some physical properties of two-phase crystal-glass solids. In Science of Ceramics, vol. 1. London, 1962, Academic Press, Inc.

Blodgett, W. E.: High strength alumina porcelains, Ceram. Bul. **40**:74, 1961.

Brecker, S. C.: Crowns, Philadelphia, 1961, W. B. Saunders Co.

Brecker, S. C.: Clinical procedures in occlusal rehabilitation, Philadelphia, 1966, W. B. Saunders Co.

Charlton, G.: Brit. Dent. J. **119**:452, 1965.

Fonvielle, F. P., and Semmelman, J. O.: Annual Meeting of the I.A.D.R., 1967.

Hasselman, D. P. H., and Fulrath, R. M.: Proposed fracture theory of a dispersion-strengthened glass matrix, J. Amer. Ceram. Soc. **49**: 68, 1966.

Johnston, J. F., Mumford, G., and Dykema, R. W.: Modern practice in dental ceramics, Philadelphia, 1967, W. B. Saunders Co.

McLean, J. W.: A higher strength porcelain for crown and bridge work, Brit. Dent. J. **119**: 268, 1965.

McLean, J. W.: Brit. Dent. J. **119**:268, 1965.

McLean, J. W.: The development of ceramic oxide reinforced dental porcelains with an appraisal of their physical and clinical properties, MDS thesis, University of London, 1966.

McLean, J. W.: The alumina tube post crown, Brit. Dent. J. **123**:87, 1967.

McLean, J. W.: High alumina ceramics for bridge pontic construction, Brit. Dent. J. **123**:571, 1967.

McLean, J. W., and Hughes, T. H.: The reinforcement of dental porcelain with ceramic oxides, Brit. Dent. J. **119**:251, 1965.

Pickard, H. M.: Brit. Dent. J. **117**:517, 1964.

Tylman, S. D.: Theory and practice of crown and bridge prosthodontics, ed. 5, St. Louis, 1965, The C. V. Mosby Co.

Vines, R. F., and others: Mechanisms involved in securing dense, vitrified ceramics from preshaped partly crystalline bodies, J. Amer. Ceram. Soc. **41**:304, 1958.

Chapter 37

Gnathologic procedures utilizing the Denar Model D4-A and pantograph*

The Denar Model D4-A articulator is a precision mandibular movement simulator, a mechanical equivalent of the lower half of the head. The articulator has total capability to reproduce all mandibular movements or jaw positions recorded by any chew-in technic, checkbite, or the more sophisticated method employing a pantograph. The ability of this articulator to accurately reproduce the patient's mandibular movements is limited only by the accuracy of the record to which it is adjusted. The Denar D4-A articulator reduces the diagnostic recordings and resultant movements produced by the articulator to numeric values. This permits the instrument to be reprogrammed for treatment function. The specifications thus established accurately define the parameters within which the restoration is to be constructed in order to eliminate eccentric interferences (Fig. 37-1).

*This chapter is based on the lecture notes, published material, and illustrations of Niles Guichet, D.D.S. (Instructor, University of California Postgraduate School of Dentistry, Anaheim, California), which he used when presenting his philosophy and procedures for occlusal treatment with the Denar Model D4-A articulator and pantograph, and which he prepared in collaboration with Robert J. Pinkerton, B.S., D.D.S., Anaheim, California. Instrumentation and procedures involved in gnathology may at first seem complicated and difficult, but it has been the experience of many teachers that third- and fourth-year dental students have successfully used the hinge axis face bow and the adjustable articulator in dental school clinics, provided that the basic principles of gnathology were taught to them understandably and that these principles were integrated early in their preclinical, technical, and biologic courses. The use of the pantograph with a more refined adjustable articulator brings dental prosthodontics the opportunity to advance another step. (S.D.T.)

ANTERIOR AND POSTERIOR CONTROL AREAS

In the application of an articulator to the fabrication of occlusal restorations, the articulator is programmed to produce a motion that is a determinant of the occlusal anatomy being developed. The motion produced by the instrument is dictated by the settings of its posterior or condylar controls and its anterior or incisal guide control.

Dental articulators are conventionally constructed to be reasonable facsimilies of their anatomic counterparts because this construction provides the most convenient means of producing the desired movements. However, better perspective and understanding can be achieved if the motion produced by the articulator is visualized as a motion that occurs between one movable beam extending anteroposteriorly (one member of the articulator) rela-

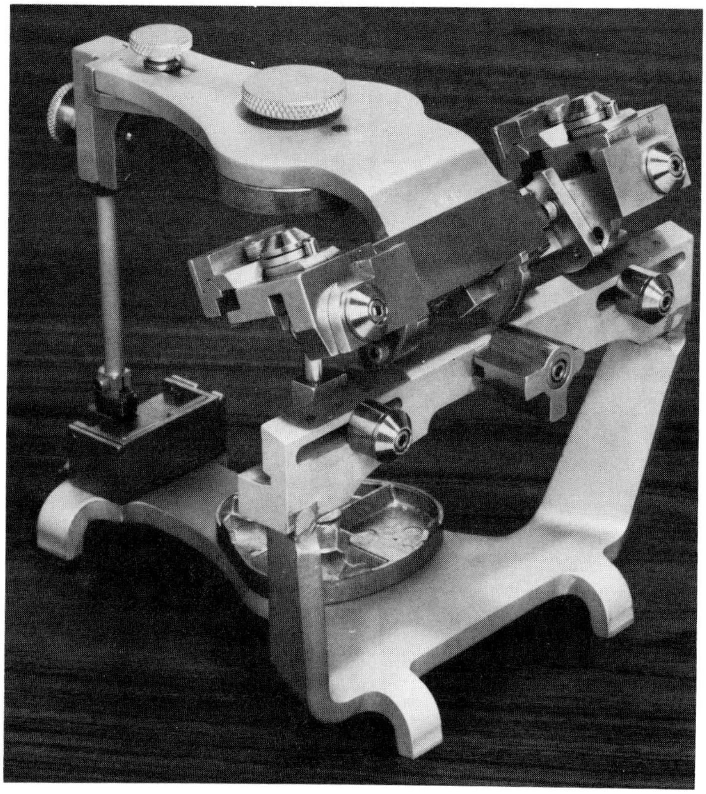

Fig. 37-1. Denar D4-A articulator. (Courtesy Dr. Niles Guichet and Denar Co.)

tive to a second fixed beam running in the same direction (the other member of the articulator). The motion produced by the movable beam is determined by the direction each of its two ends, the anterior and the posterior, is guided. The anterior guide and the posterior guide of the beam have equal influence on the motion produced by the beam regardless of the relative complexity of the guiding controls. The clinical significance of the guide control areas of an articulator is found in the motion produced, not in the manner in which the motion is produced. This is to say that the anterior or incisal-guide-control area is of equal importance to the posterior or condylar-control area.

In practical application, tremendous clinical significance of these control areas is found in their capacity to be precisely readjusted after the diagnosis, so the instrument will produce a motion that facilitates the efficient accomplishment of the prime objective, fabricating the desired occlusion. The ability of the motion programmed in the articulator to be interpreted in calibrated control areas and expressed in numeric values permits the same instrument or another instrument in a remote location to be programmed subsequently without the expenditure of additional time and expense. This is clinically significant in that it encourages the treatment sequence to be accomplished according to the dentist's or patient's desires rather than by instrument limitations.

In the utilization of an articulator to facilitate the fabrication of the desired occlusion, there are three general areas of consideration.

1. *The posterior-control areas (the condylar controls)*. These control areas are

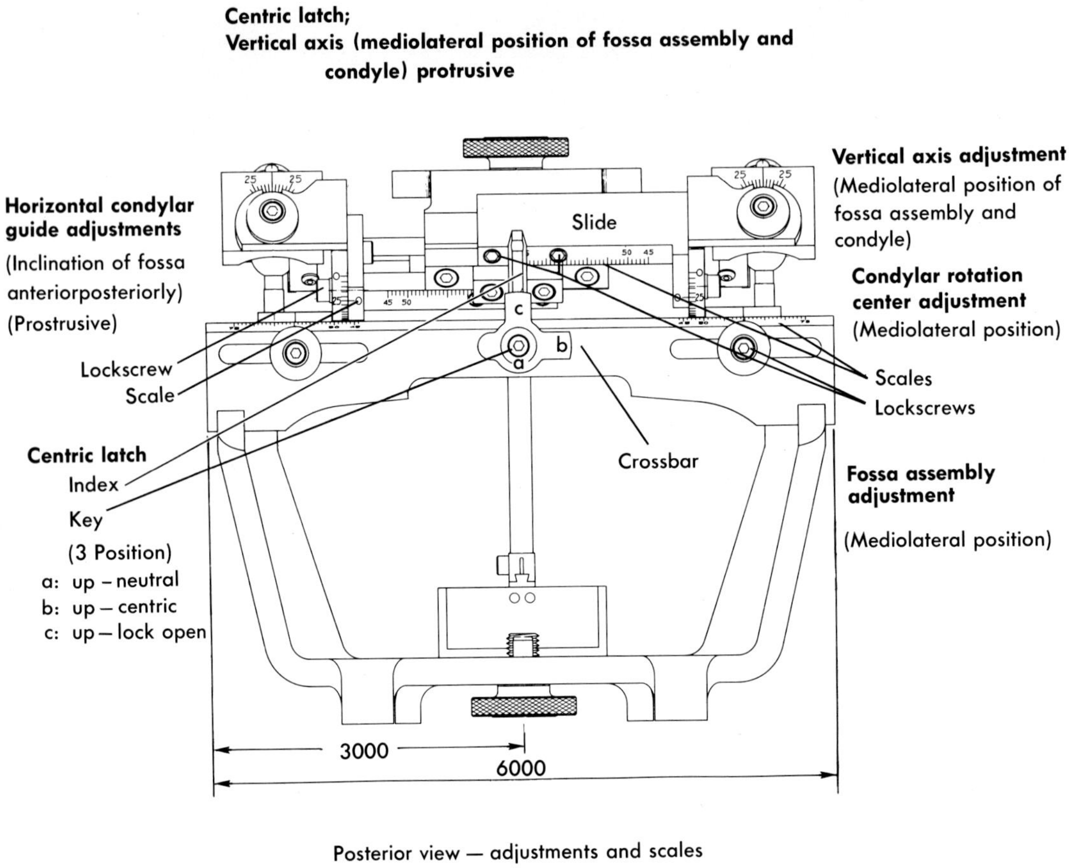

Fig. 37-2. Rear view of Fig. 37-1. (Courtesy Dr. Niles Guichet and Denar Co.)

adjusted in consideration of the patient's temporomandibular joint characteristics, which are identified with the aid of a pantograph or alternate condylar movement recording means such as chew-in techniques (Chapter 20) or checkbite methods (Chapter 29).

2. *The anterior-control area (the incisal guide).* This control area is of equal importance to the posterior-control area. In existing occlusions, it is adjusted in consideration of the vertical overbite and horizontal overjet relation of the anterior teeth. In edentulous mouths the overbite and overjet position of the anterior teeth is established by phonetic and esthetic measurements.

3. *The centric-occlusal position of the mounted casts in proper orientation to the control areas. This is the most important* of the three general areas of consideration. Accurate orientation of the mandibular cast to the maxillary cast at the centric occlusal position is of paramount importance and is often the most difficult and most time-consuming accomplishment of these three areas of consideration in occlusal treatments. Here the dentist must rely on his knowledge of neuromuscular physiology, hinge axis theory, and equilibration, checkbite, and laboratory technic.

ARTICULATOR CALIBRATIONS

In the diagnosis, the articulator is used to measure temporomandibular joint characteristics. *In treatment,* it is used to establish the specifications or measurements to which the restoration is to be con-

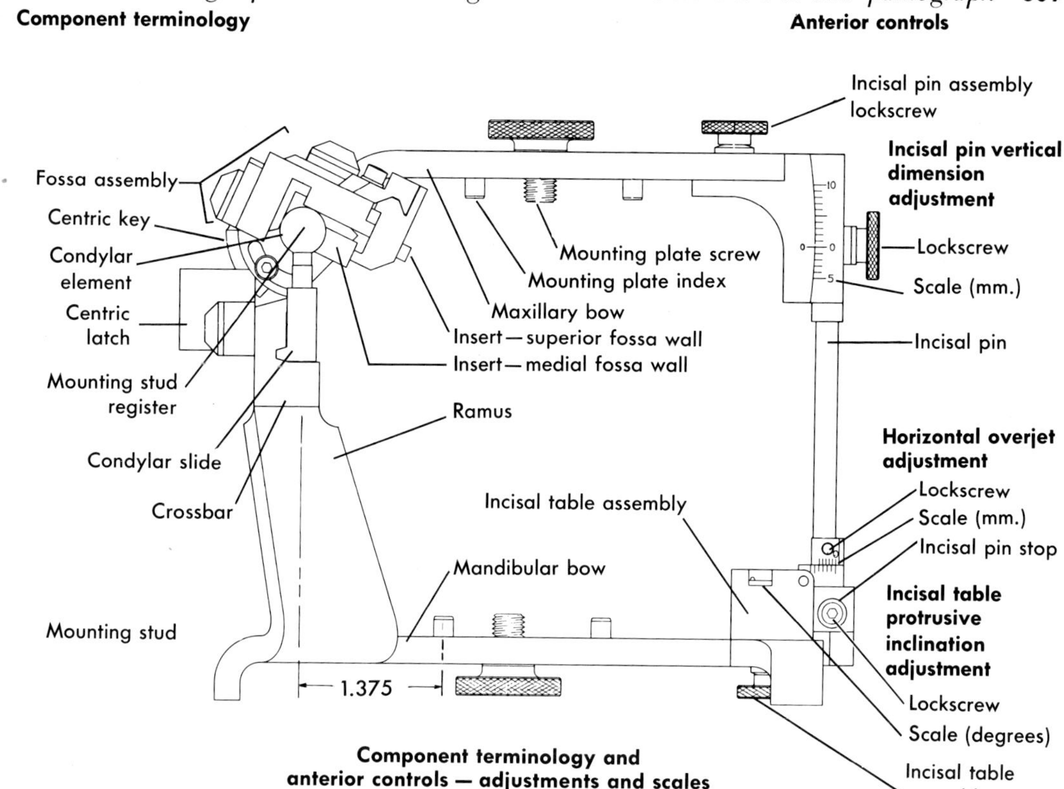

Fig. 37-3. Side view of Fig. 37-1. (Courtesy Dr. Niles Guichet and Denar Co.)

structed. In any measuring procedure, the measurement is made in relation to an initial reference or starting position. In measuring the anatomic determinants of occlusion, the initial references are the *horizontal reference plane* and the *midsagittal reference plane*. These initial reference planes established on the patient are also identified on the articulator, the mechanical equivalent of the lower half of the head.

Horizontal reference plane

The horizontal reference plane of the articulator is the horizontal plane that intersects the centers of rotation in the condylar elements and is parallel to the upper and lower bows of the articulator.

Midsagittal reference plane

The midsagittal reference plane of the articulator is the vertical plane that passes anteroposteriorly through the middle of the articulator.

The diagnostic data registered by the mandibular movement record is interpreted in the calibrated control adjustments of the articulator and expressed in numeric values of millimeters and degrees. These numeric expressions are in relation to specific positions or planes of reference, which can be precisely relocated.

POSTERIOR CONTROL AREAS

Vertical axes of rotation (Fig. 37-2): Expressed in millimeters from the midsagittal plane.

Horizontal condylar path (Fig. 37-3): Expressed in degrees from the horizontal reference plane.

Immediate-side-shift (Fig. 37-4): Expressed in millimeters from the centric position of the mandible.

Progressive-side-shift (Fig. 37-4): Expressed in degrees from the sagittal plane which passes through the point at which the progressive side shift begins.

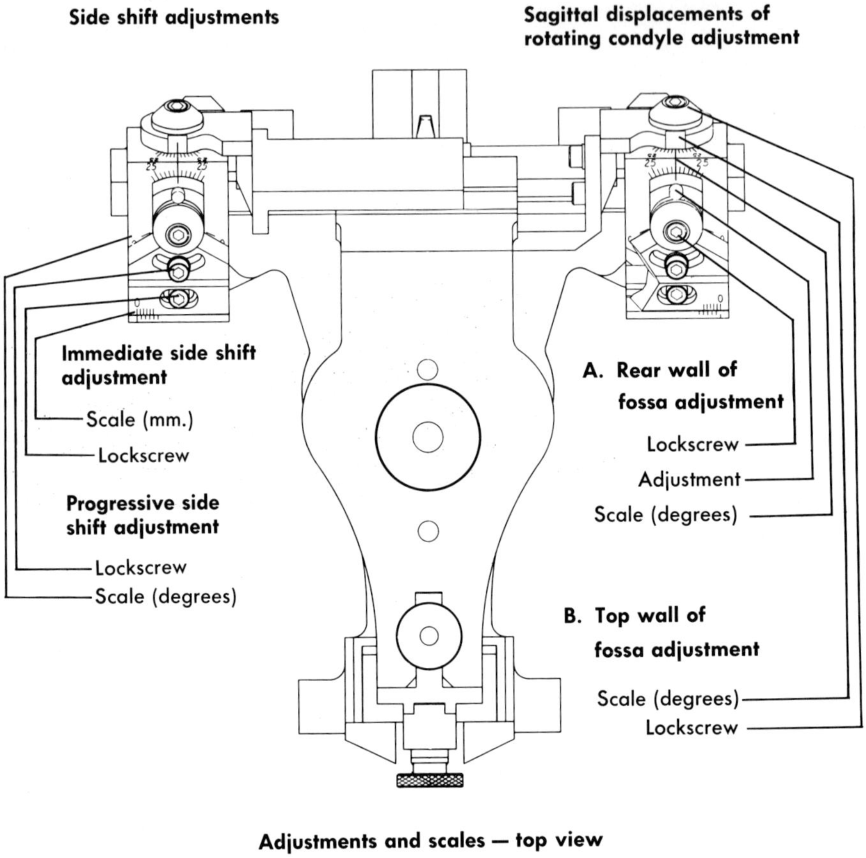

Fig. 37-4. Top view of Fig. 37-1. (Courtesy Dr. Niles Guichet and Denar Co.)

Sagittal displacements of the rotating condyle (Fig. 37-4): Backward or forward; expressed in degrees from the coronal plane; rear wall of fossa adjustment. Up or down; expressed in degrees from the horizontal plane; top wall of fossa adjustment.

ANTERIOR CONTROL AREA

Vertical dimension of the incisal pin (Fig. 37-3): Expressed in millimeters of opening or closing of the articulator in the area of the incisor teeth. In the Denar D4-A articulator, this dimension is read directly on the incisal pin. This calibration was computed on the basis of the average anatomic dimensions of a skull as described by Bonwill being transferred to the articulator so that the plane of occlusion of the anterior teeth would be coincidental to the midhorizontal plane of the articulator. The scale is calibrated in 1 mm. increments.

Horizontal overjet adjustment (Fig. 37-3): Expressed in millimeters from the transverse vertical or coronal plane, which passes through the labioincisal angle of the mandibular anterior teeth. The vernier scale is calibrated in increments of 0.2 mm.

Incisal table, protrusive, and lateral wing adjustments (Fig. 37-3): Expressed in degrees from the horizontal plane. The scales are calibrated in 5° increments.

POSTERIOR CONTROL ADJUSTMENTS

The vertical axes can be adjusted mediolaterally from 45 to 75 mm. mediolaterally as measured from the midsagittal reference plane. The scales for this adjustment are calibrated in 1 mm. increments.

In locating the mediolateral position of the vertical axes, the fossa assemblies must be adjusted first. In order to do this, the fossa assembly slide-lock screws (Fig. 37-2) must be loosened. After the adjustment, the mediolateral position of the fossa can be maintained by gently tightening only one of the lock screws provided on each slide. (Two screws are provided because in some positions one of the screws on the upper slide will be behind the centric-latch index.) The mediolateral position of the condylar elements is subsequently adjusted to a position 1 to 2 mm. lateral to the fossa elements by loosening the condylar rotation centric adjustment lock screw. The upper member of the articulator is then brought to rest on the lower member and the correct mediolateral orientation of the respective members is accomplished by engaging the centric latch in the centric position. The thumb is then used to push the condylar element medially until it engages the medial wall of the fossa; the locknut is secured. It is important that the immediate-side-shift adjustment be set to zero when this adjustment is made.

HORIZONTAL CONDYLAR GUIDE ADJUSTMENT: ANTEROPOSTERIOR ANGLE OF THE EMINENTIA PROTRUSIVE

The anterior position inclination of the superior fossa wall or fossa assembly can be adjusted from 0 to 60° from the horizontal or horizontal reference plane by loosening the horizontal condylar guide lockscrew. The scale for this adjustment is calibrated in 5° increments (Figs. 37-2 and 37-27).

Immediate-side-shift adjustment

Fig. 37-4 illustrates the superior view of the maxillary assembly detailing the immediate-side-shift adjustments. The medial fossa wall can be displaced medially by loosening the immediate-side-shift adjustment lockscrew.

The amount of the displacement and the amount of immediate side shift allowed is indicated on the vernier scale. The adjustment is set to zero when the apex of the reference mark is indexed to

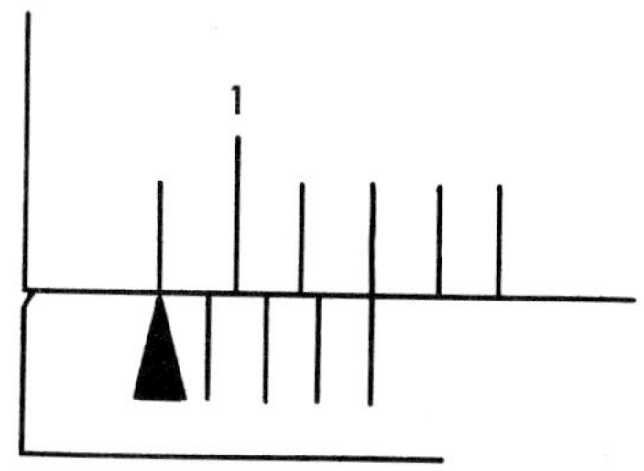

Fig. 37-5. Vernier scale. (Courtesy Dr. Niles Guichet and Denar Co.)

the most lateral mark on the upper scale. The lines on the upper scale marked with the numeral are 1 mm. apart. The lines on the lower scale identified with the reference mark are 0.8 mm. apart. Consequently, when the medial fossa wall is displaced medially 0.2 mm. to allow a 0.2 mm. immediate-side-shift, the second pair of lines will line up indicating the 0.2 mm. displacement. As the medial fossa wall is displaced more medially, each successive pair of lines that registers indicate an additional 0.2 mm. displacement of the medial fossa wall or immediate-side-shift permitted. Fig. 37-5 illustrates this scale with the 0.2 mm. increments on the lower scale marked.

Progressive-side-shift adjustment

Fig. 37-4 illustrates a superior view of a fossa assembly detailing the progressive-side-shift adjustment. The medial fossa wall can be set at any pitch from 0 to 30° to the sagittal plane by loosening the progressive-side-shift lock screw. This permits the mandibular member of the articulator to move progressively laterally as the traveling condyle functions along the medial wall of the fossa (Fig. 37-29).

Sagittal displacement of the rotating condyle; backward and forward rear wall adjustment

Fig. 37-4 illustrates a superior view of a fossa assembly detailing the rear wall adjustment. The posterior fossa wall can be inclined anteriorly or posteriorly 30° from the coronal plane by loosening the rear wall adjustment lockscrew. The degree of anterior inclination of the rear wall is indicated on the lateral portion of the scale. The degree of medial inclination of the rear wall is indicated on the medial portion of the scale. The scale is calibrated in 5° increments (Fig. 37-30).

Lateral condylar path adjustment; lateral adjustment; orbiting path adjustment

As a mandibular lateral excursive movement is made, the traveling condyle moves downward, forward, and inward and orbits around the opposite or rotating condyle (sometimes referred to as the "working condyle" because it is on the working side). The path the orbiting condyle travels along the superior fossa wall will be different from the path it travels when a straight protrusive excursive movement is made. In almost all cases, the anteroposterior inclination of this path to the horizontal plane is equal to or greater than the path traveled in the protrusive excursive movement. The horizontal condylar path adjustment is used to establish this orbiting path on the articulator. Sometimes one horizontal condylar adjustment will establish the correct anteroposterior angle of the eminentia for both the protrusive condylar path and the orbiting path. If it does not, the shallower path is used in routine clinical treatments. (This will be the protrusive path with very rare exceptions.) If the correct angle of the eminentia for both the protrusive path and orbiting path is not established at one horizontal condylar inclination setting and it is desired to accurately reproduce mandibular movement, the anteroposterior angle of the eminentia should be set to the steeper path (generally the orbiting path), and then the correct inclination of the shallower path should be established by custom-grinding the inferior surface of the superior fossa wall.

The superior and medial fossa wall inserts are available in various anatomic curvatures. They are available in nylon for continuous usage and in acrylic. The acrylic inserts are available to facilitate custom modification of these inserts by grinding and the addition of cold-cure acrylic in those cases in which it is necessary to allow the instrument to produce a movement that will enable the pantograph to accurately track the recorded lines. The superior wall inserts are interchangeable, right and left. The medial wall inserts are provided in right- and left-hand sets. A complete stock of other inserts is available.

Custom-grinding inserts

This procedure is generally done only when the articulator is being adjusted to a pantographic recording and it is desired that the styli accurately track the recorded lines in all their detail when this cannot be accomplished simply by selecting the proper fossa inserts and by utilization of the articulator adjustments. Final inserts are selected and the articulator is adjusted to produce the desired movement permitting the styli to track the recorded lines; additional stock must be removed from the inserts in selected areas. These selected areas on the inserts are identified with the aid of carbon paper. Carbon paper is inserted between the condyle and the insert to be modified, and the articulator is moved in a limited excursion where it fails to produce the desired movement. This marks the area of the insert to be modified. The insert is then ground with a Fastcut stone or vulcanite cutter having a ⅜ inch radius. The procedure is repeated until sufficient stock is removed from the fossa-insert so the instrument will produce the desired movement. When the inserts are removed from the articulator, a sharp instrument is used to identify them with the patient's name or number and whether they are right or left so that they can be filed for future reference.

ANTERIOR CONTROL ADJUSTMENTS

Vertical dimension of incisal pin; incisal pin adjustment

The incisal pin assembly can be removed from the articulator without changing the vertical dimension of the incisal pin assembly, by loosening the incisal pin assembly lockscrew (Fig. 37-3). Loosening the incisal pin vertical dimension adjustment lockscrew permits the vertical dimension of the incisal pin to be increased 10 mm. or decreased 5 mm. The scale is calibrated in millimeters in the area of the incisor teeth. Note that the two washers on the incisal pin lockscrew have matching concave convex surfaces that should always face toward each other.

Horizontal overjet adjustment; long centric adjustment

In order to adjust to the horizontal overjet of anterior teeth or to provide for horizontal movement in the articulator to specify an area of centric for complete denture construction, the foot of the incisal pin can be retracted from the inclines of the incisal table by loosening the lockscrew (Fig. 37-3). The foot of the incisal pin rests on the incisal pin stop.

Protrusive inclination of the incisal table; angle of the incisal table anteroposteriorly; anterior vertical overbite adjustment

Loosening the incisal table protrusal inclination permits the incisal table to be inclined upward from 0 to 60° to the horizontal plane anteroposteriorly. This inclination is read on the scale calibrated in 5° increments.

Lateral wings of the incisal table; angle of the incisal table mediolaterally

By loosening the lockscrews on the anterior surface of the incisal table, the lateral wings of the incisal table can be inclined up to an angle of 45° to that member of the incisal table that inclines anteroposteriorly. The adjustable incisal table is replaceable with a custom incisal platform of acrylic, which can be easily modified for special requirements.

INITIAL REFERENCE

In any measuring procedure, the measurement is made in relation to an initial reference or starting position. In measuring the posterior anatomic determinants of occlusion, the initial references are the horizontal reference plane and the midsagittal plane.

Horizontal reference plane

The horizontal reference plane is a plane established on the face of the patient by an anterior reference point and two posterior reference points from which measurements of the posterior anatomic determinants of occlusion are made. The three reference points that locate the horizontal reference plane are arbitrarily established. However, once the measurements are made, the reference points cannot be changed if the measurements are to remain valid.

Anterior reference point

The anterior reference point is a point on the face at some fixed dimension above the incisal edges of the maxillary anterior teeth that will position the plane of occlusion in the middle of the articulator vertically when the maxillary cast is transferred to the articulator in relation to this reference point. The anterior reference point is located in relation to the fixed immovable inner canthus of the eye so it can be permanently recorded and precisely relocated. This reference point is efficiently located with a 43 mm. notch fixed in the Denar Reference Plane Locator.

Posterior reference points

The posterior reference points are two points located one on each side of the face in the area of the terminal hinge axis. These points will be registered by the pantograph and transferred to the horizontal axis of the articulator. The specific influence the location of the terminal hinge or horizontal axis has on mandibular movement is in motion which occurs about that axis, i.e., the opening arc and arc of closure of the mandibular teeth (sagittal plane rotation).*

In fabricating occlusions, the only functional use of an articulator is when it functions in accord with its control areas and is used as a gauge or shearing device in determining the exact shape of the occlusal surfaces. This only occurs when the incisal pin is on the incisal table. In these functional uses, arcs of rotational movement which occur about the horizontal axis are slight and occur only in *eccentric* positions. These arcs are so imperceptibly influenced by the precise location of the horizontal axis that exactness in its location is of no clinical significance.

The only time rotational movement about the horizontal axis can be of sufficient magnitude to be clinically significant is when insufficient consideration given to the precise location of the horizontal axis could cause an error in the occlusion. This could only occur (1) when the mandibular cast is transferred to the articulator by means of a centric record taken at an increased vertical dimension and then by rotational movement about the horizontal axis the correct vertical dimension is restored, or (2) by a significant change in the vertical dimension on the articulator. EXAMPLE: Assume a situation in which the mandibular teeth were disoccluded from the maxillary teeth along an opening arc that occurred by rotational movement about the terminal hinge axis (horizontal) and a centric record taken at an increased vertical dimension. If this centric record were then used to transfer the mandibular cast to an articulator in which the relation of the maxillary cast to the horizontal axis of the instrument did not coincide with the relation of the maxillary teeth to the terminal hinge axis of the patient, when the mandibular teeth are reoccluded to the correct vertical dimension by rotational movement about the horizontal axis of the articulator, they would follow a different arc or path of closure than they traveled in the disoccluding arc. Consequently, they would not return to their original starting position. An error would be introduced in the *centric* occlusal position that could be of clinical importance.

If the mandibular cast is going to be transferred to the articulator by means of a centric record taken at an increased vertical dimension, the posterior reference point must coincide with the terminal hinge axis of the patient and precise hinge axis location is necessary in order to avoid the possibility of this error. In this manner the arc of opening on the patient and the arc of closing on the articulator will coincide and the centric occlusal position will be *theoretically* accurate. Alternately, however, if simultaneous even contacting and indexing of the teeth occur at the correct vertical dimension with the condyles in terminal hinge position, the most accurate way of transferring the mandibular cast to the articulator is by occluding it with the maxillary cast. In this case, rotational movement about the horizontal axis must be of insufficient magnitude for precise hinge axis location to be of any clinical significance. Posterior reference points selected by average anatomic measurements are indicated because precise hinge axis location offers no advantage.

Summary

The manner in which the mandibular cast is transferred to the articulator is the specific determinant of the method employed to locate the posterior reference points.

*A sagittal plane rotation of the mandible is a rotational movement of the mandible in which each point within the mandible stays within its own respective sagittal plane and rotates about an axis (horizontal) perpendicular to that plane.

RULE: If the mandibular cast is to be transferred to the articulator by means of a centric relation record taken at an increased vertical dimension, or if the vertical dimension is going to be changed on the articulator, the posterior reference location (Fig. 37-13).

RULE: If the mandibular cast is to be transferred to the articulator by means of a centric relation record taken at the correct vertical dimension, the posterior reference points may be selected by average anatomic measurement.

NOTE: In extensive reconstruction procedures where the restoration is to be seated in the mouth and subsequently remounted in the articulator by means of a centric relation record taken at an increased vertical dimension for final occlusal correction prior to cementation, precise hinge axis location is always indicated. However, in the diagnostic mounting of study casts or in minor restorative procedures, the mandibular cast is sometimes transferred to the articulator at a minimal vertical opening without precise hinge axis location. In these instances the possible introduction of errors is subsequently eliminated when the restoration is seated in the mouth.

REFERENCE PLANE LOCATION (FIGS. 37-6 to 37-9)

When average anatomic measurements are used in locating the horizontal reference plane, the reference plane location aids can be used to advantage. These consist of:

A. Reference plane locator
B. Reference plane marker
C. 43 mm. notch to locate anterior reference point
D. Hole to locate posterior reference point
E. Millimeter scale
F. Hole to index to reference plane support rod

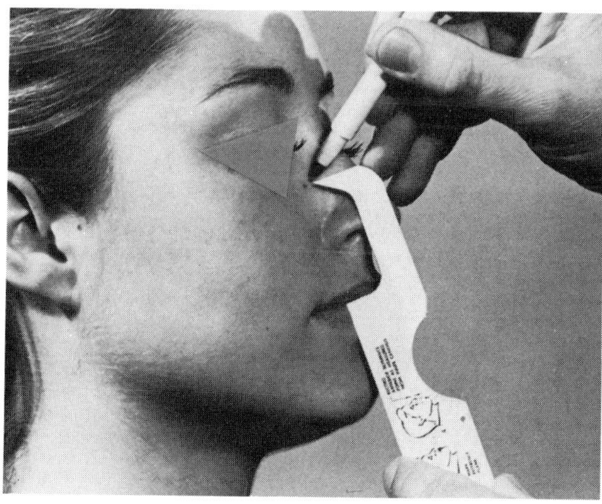

Fig. 37-6

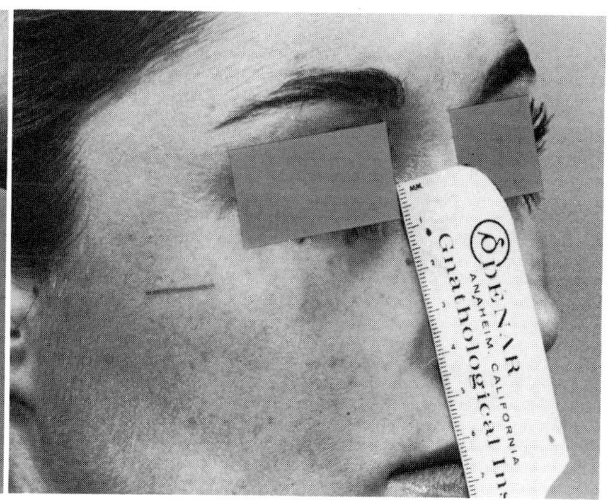

Fig. 37-7

Fig. 37-6. Locate anterior reference point by indexing notch against incisal edge of maxillary anterior tooth or, preferably, lower lip line. (Courtesy Dr. Niles Guichet and Denar Co.)

Fig. 37-7. Record relation of anterior reference to fixed immovable inner canthus of eye so anterior reference point may be precisely relocated if necessary. RULE: If mandibular cast is to be transferred to articulator by means of centric record taken at correct vertical dimension, locate posterior reference points by average anatomic measurement. (Courtesy Dr. Niles Guichet and Denar Co.)

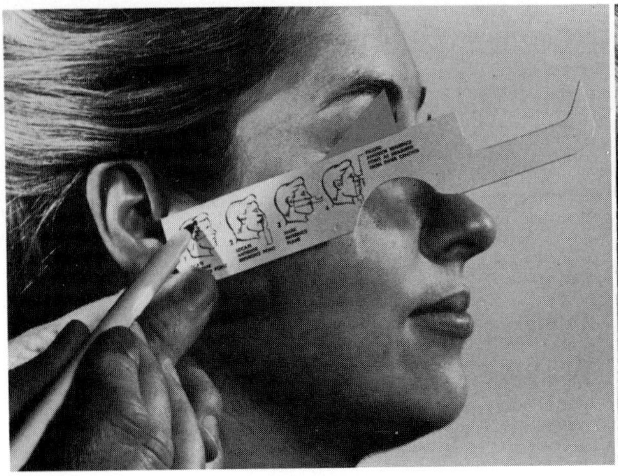

Fig. 37-8

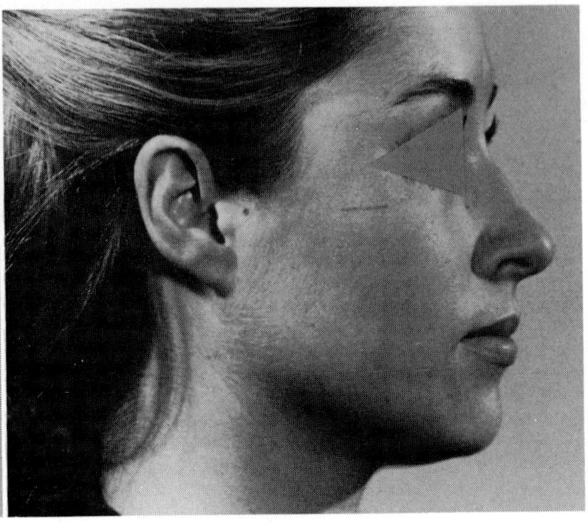

Fig. 37-9

Fig. 37-8. Position reference plane locator forward from middle of upper margin of external auditory meatus to outer canthus of eye and mark posterior reference points through hole provided in reference plane locator. Align reference plane locator between anterior and posterior reference points on right side of patient just out of contact with patient's face so as not to displace skin; scribe reference plane on right side of patient's face. (Courtesy Dr. Niles Guichet and Denar Co.)
Fig. 37-9. Initial references, posterior reference points, and horizontal plane of reference scribed on patient's face. (Courtesy Dr. Niles Guichet and Denar Co.)

CLUTCH CONSTRUCTION (REGISTRATION TRAY)

In order to locate the hinge axis or perform a pantographic survey a pair of clutches* is necessary to index the hinge axis locator or pantograph to the dental arches. Denar provides two clutch formers, a dentulous clutch former and an edentulous clutch former to facilitate the efficient fabrication of clutches. The dentulous clutch former is used for all clutch fabrication except for the totally edentulous patient.

Dentulous patient

An ideal clutch is one that is very thin over the tops of the cusps but thick for rigidity in the central sections without soft tissue impingement. The impressions made by the teeth should be very slight with little or no detail but positive enough to provide accurate indexing to the teeth. With a little experience, this can be accomplished routinely.

The clutch former is a jig mechanism that locates two acrylic clutch frames (Fig. 37-10) in proper position for construction of clutches directly in the mouth. A spacer is used to relocate the lower or upper clutch frame distally to accommodate Class II or Class III arch relations. When the lower clutch frame is repositioned distally with the spacer to accommodate extreme Class II arch relations, the clutch die is pulled to its most distal position and the opening that occurs anteriorly between the clutch frames is occluded with utility wax in order to prevent the bonding together of the upper and lower clutches. Anteriorly the clutch frame has a precision index to which an anterior crossbar assembly can be precisely located. Laterally it has retentive side arms to which cold-

*Such clutches are sometimes called registration trays. (S. D. T.)

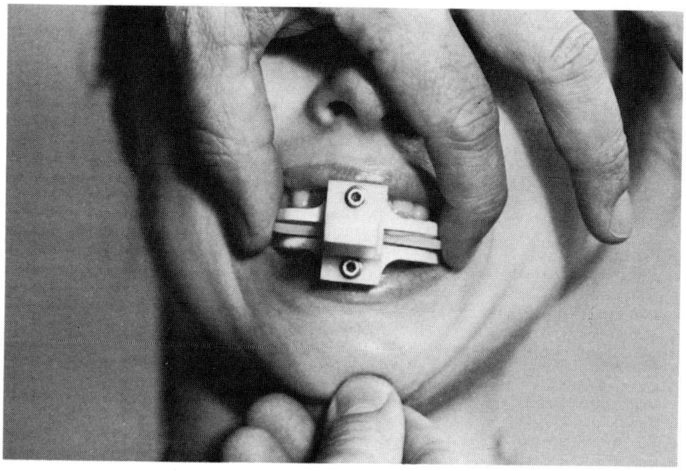

Fig. 37-10. Clutch former in patient's mouth. (Courtesy Dr. Niles Guichet and Denar Co.)

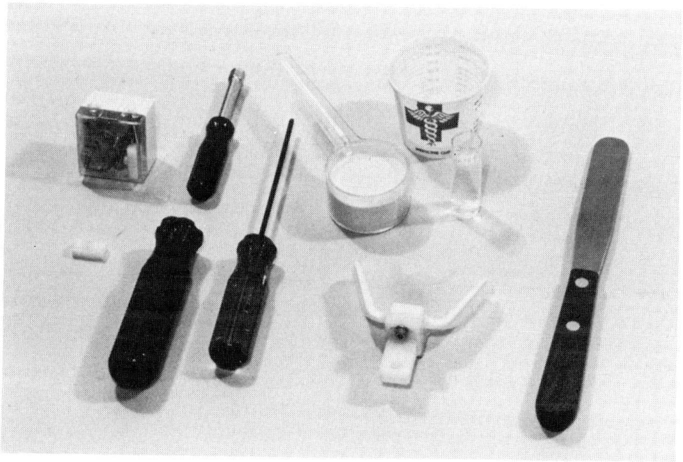

Fig. 37-11. Equipment and material needed for clutch construction. (Courtesy Dr. Niles Guichet and Denar Co.)

cure acrylic will bond. In order to accommodate wide archs, these side arms may be reshaped after warming them over a flame or they may be modified by grinding. Interposed between the clutch frames is the rubber clutch die, which prevents the cold-cure acrylic of the upper and lower clutches from bonding to each other during clutch fabrication. On the inferior surface of the clutch die, a center bearing screw is supported in the correct location for incorporation by the cold-cure acrylic into the mandibular clutch. On its superior surface is a form over which is cast the area in the maxillary clutch, which the center bearing screw will glide when the patient executes mandibular movements. This form, cast in the maxillary clutch, subconsciously encourages (proprioceptively programs) patient cooperation in executing directed excursive movements (Fig. 37-11). Three-quarters of a vial of monomer will produce the correct amount of acrylic to fabricate clutches. Slightly more than half the mix is used to fabricate the upper clutch. Immerse the loaded clutch former in hot water to hasten cure. Allow the acrylic to set beyond the tacky

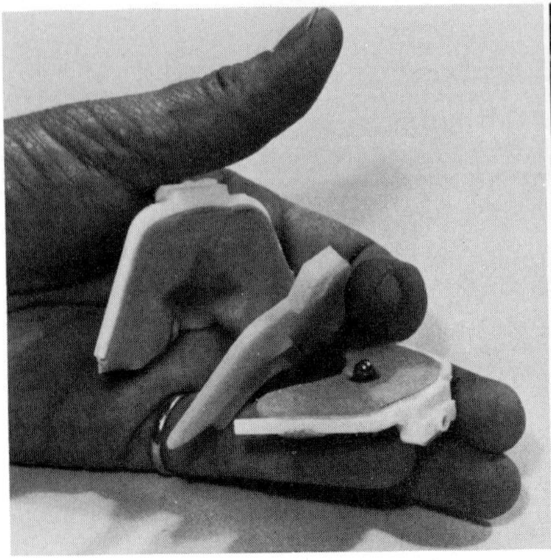

Fig. 37-12

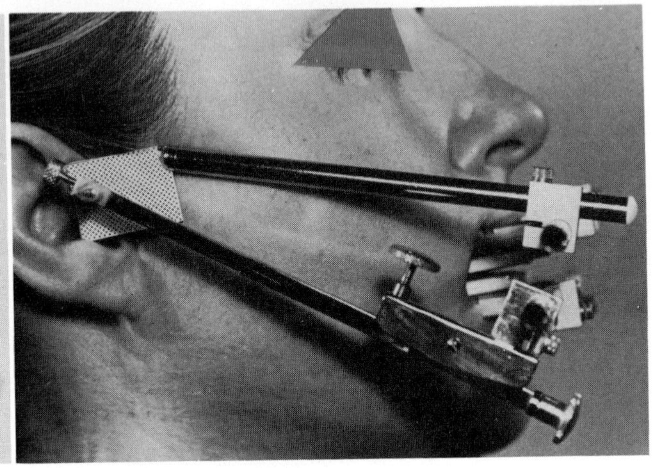

Fig. 37-13

Fig. 37-12. Disassembled clutch former. (Courtesy Dr. Niles Guichet and Denar Co.)
Fig. 37-13. Stylus against micro-dot pattern in hinge axis analyzer. (Courtesy Dr. Niles Guichet and Denar Co.)

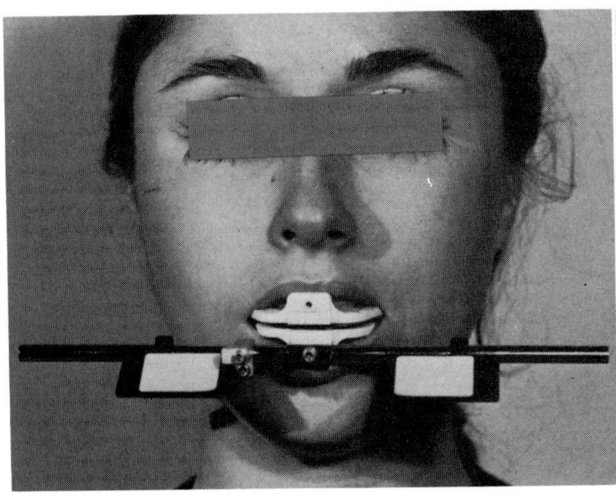

Fig. 37-14

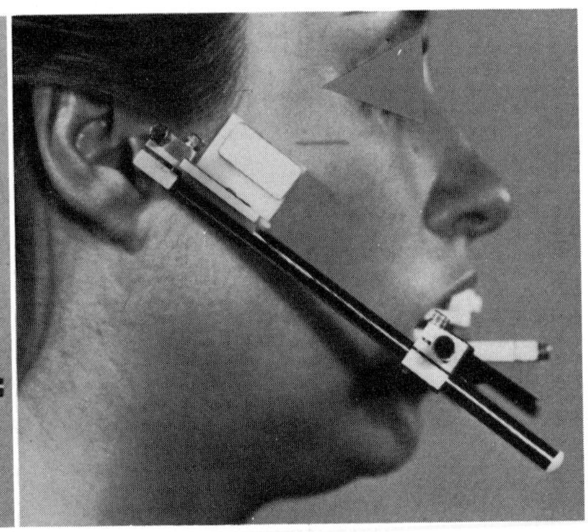

Fig. 37-15

Fig. 37-14. Clutches checked in patient's mouth for stability. (Courtesy Dr. Niles Guichet and Denar Co.)
Fig. 37-15. Reference plane supports rod clamp parallel to reference plane scribed on patient's face. Posterior reference pins are horizontal and lightly touch posterior reference points marked on patient's skin. (Courtesy Dr. Niles Guichet and Denar Co.)

stage to a tough consistency which resists displacement.

While supporting the clutch former in the intermaxillary space with the left hand, guide the patient in terminal hinge closure to obtain desired impressions of teeth. Immediately remove the clutch former from the mouth. When the acrylic has set to a very tough consistency, return the clutch former to the mouth for final cure and maximum accuracy.

Disassemble the clutch former (Fig. 37-

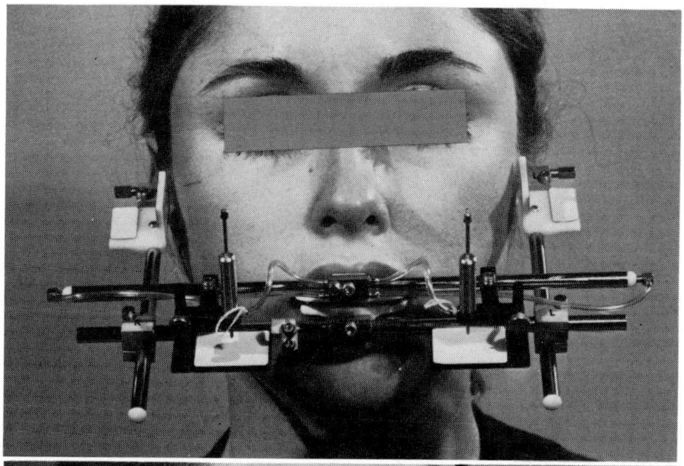

Fig. 37-16

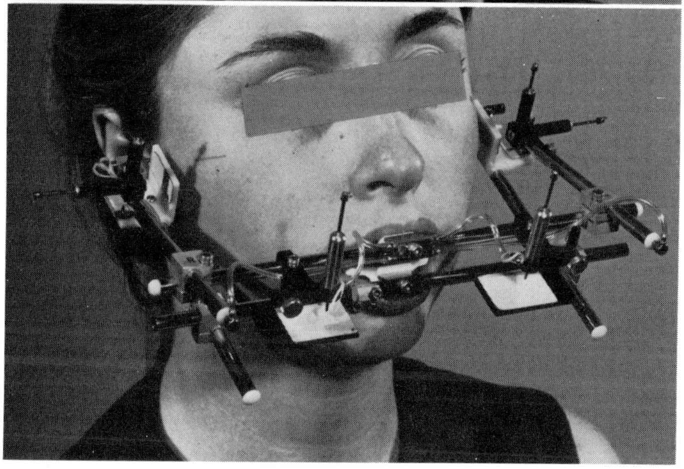

Fig. 37-17

Fig. 37-16. Anterior recorder assembly attached to mandibular clutch. (Courtesy Dr. Niles Guichet and Denar Co.)
Fig. 37-17. Assembled Denar pantograph prior to attachment of control valve to pantograph manifold. (Courtesy Dr. Niles Guichet and Denar Co.)

12). Check the clutches in the mouth for stability (Figs. 37-13 and 37-14). Adjust center bearing screw height so that there is 1 mm. clearance between clutches when the mandible is in the terminal hinge position. IMPORTANT: In attaching anterior crossbar assemblies of the pantograph or face bow to the clutch, always completely index the crossbar assembly and the clutch before inserting the screw. This will support the projecting nozzle on the clutch index and prevent its breakage when the screw is inserted. Always use a screw length that gives full-length thread engagement to the clutch and do not overtighten so as not to strip plastic threads in clutch.

DENAR PANTOGRAPH

The Denar pantograph is a precision mandibular movement recording instrument (Figs. 37-15 to 37-17). It provides the dentist with the most accurate, simplest, and fastest means of recording mandibular movement and jaw positions. Pneumatically powered from the dental air syringe, a push-button controlled device automatically and simultaneously lifts all

Fig. 37-18

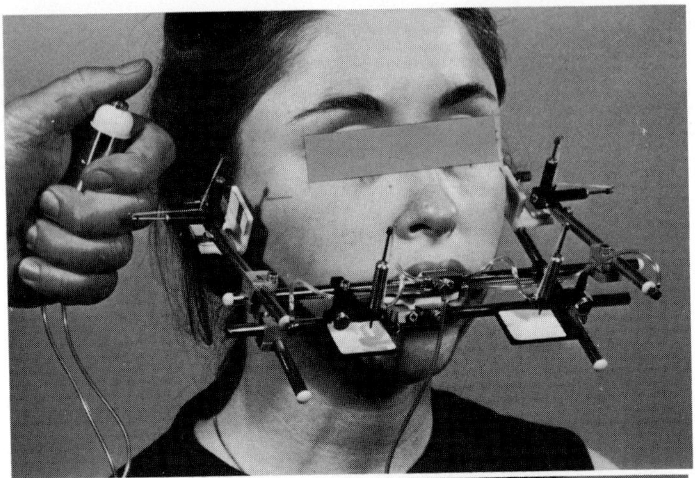

Fig. 37-19

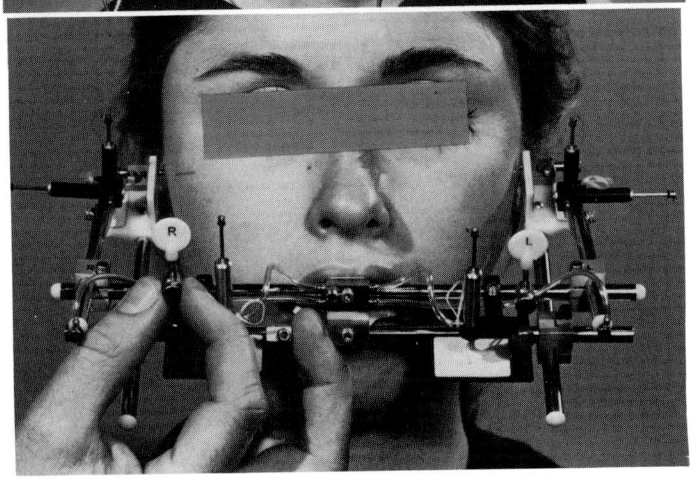

Fig. 37-18. Stylus control valve connected to pantograph manifold; when lever is depressed, styli are held in retracted position. (Courtesy Dr. Niles Guichet and Denar Co.)
Fig. 37-19. Patient in centric relation; heated centric pins are placed into wax wells and are secured. (Courtesy Dr. Niles Guichet and Denar Co.)

styli upon the dentist's command (Fig. 37-18). This enables the dentist to obtain a total recording of the patient's mandibular movements and to discriminate between erratic abnormal jaw movements and pure peripheral movements in a practical efficient manner. Additionally, the pantograph permits each record and procedural step to be double-checked for accuracy before proceeding to the next step. To ensure accuracy, the styli are depressed and their relation to the scribings is confirmed as the patient maintains centric relation (Fig. 37-19). The centric pins are heated and placed into the wax walls and secured.

Although there are many reasons for the dramatic increase in simplicity and ease of operation of the Denar pantograph, one of the most important is the ease of clutch construction.

One-step transfer

The Denar pantograph, unlike original research instruments, can be transferred directly to the articulator, eliminating the necessity of additional procedural steps employing a mounting stand. In addition,

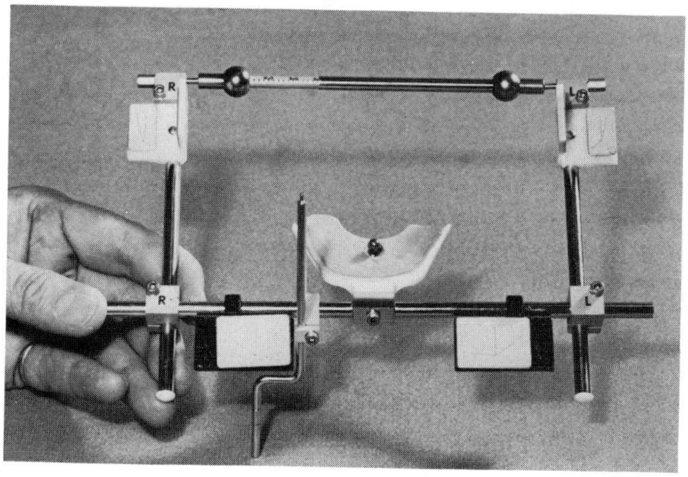

Fig. 37-20. Transfer of pantograph to Denar D4-A articulator. (Courtesy Dr. Niles Guichet and Denar Co.)

due to the rigidity of the pantograph, it can be handled in a rapid manner without fear of loss of tolerance.

Systems approach

The design of the Denar clutch former, pantograph, and D4-A articulator reflects the systems approach to the solution of problems that heretofore prevented the reduction of sophisticated researches to practical application. Engineered into the system's design are features that produce results or conveniences automatically. For example, the center bearing screw of the lower clutch will always be in correct relation to the center bearing screw area of the upper clutch. The crossbars of the pantograph will be properly aligned on the patient's face. The pantograph and articulator design are compatible. The pantograph transfers directly to the articulator. The pantograph is constructed to complement the articulator and the side arms of the pantograph do not crisscross. This allows the upper member of the articulator along with the attached upper members of the pantograph to be lifted easily from their lower counterparts for convenient change or modification of fossa guide inserts. Additionally, since all scribers are constant to the upper assembly, the record tables and recorded lines are constant to the lower assembly and condyles. This allows easy interpretation of the recording. The resultant savings in time and accuracy are of extreme significance to a practicing dentist.

Transferring the pantograph to the Denar D4-A articulator

The posterior reference pins are screwed all the way in and the telescoping mounting axis is expanded to index over the tips of the posterior reference pins (Fig. 37-20). The number on the scale indicates the position to which the vertical axes are adjusted to accept the pantograph. The vertical axes are adjusted to this position.

The articulator is prepared to receive the pantograph by setting the anteroposterior angle of the eminentia to 25 to 30°. The progressive side shift is set to 5°. All other adjustments, including the vertical dimension of the incisal pin and the incisal table adjustments, are set to zero. Mounting studs are positioned in the holes provided in the lateral aspects of the condylar elements.

The recorder is transferred to the ar-

Fig. 37-21

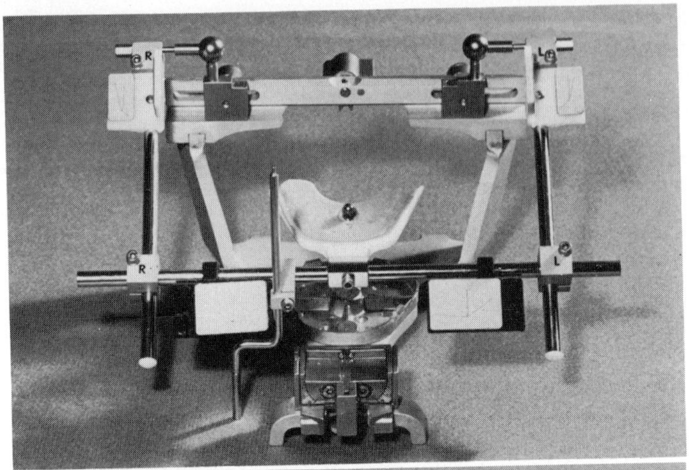

Fig. 37-22

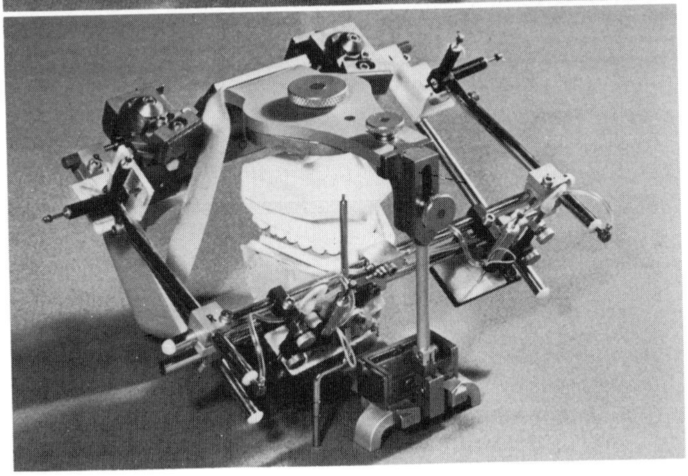

Fig. 37-21. Mounting stand is constructed by attachment of recorder to lower mounting plate with dental stone.
Fig. 37-22. Study cast secured in maxillary clutch for mounting. (Courtesy Dr. Niles Guichet and Denar Co.)

ticulator by indexing the posterior reference pins in the holes provided in the lateral extremeties of the mounting studs (Fig. 37-21). The reference plane support rod is allowed to rest on the surface bearing the articulator. A mounting stand is constructed by attaching the recorder to the lower mounting plate with dental stone.

The upper member of the articulator is positioned on the lower and engaged in the lock open position with the centric latch. An elastic may be used to ensure positive seating of the condyles in their respective fossa. The right and left centric pins are accurately located in their respective guide tubes in exactly the same orientation they had when the wax chilled about them. The scriber is then oriented to the recorder by indexing the centric pins in the impressions they made in the hard inlay wax in the wax wells on the recorder. The maxillary clutch is allowed to rest on the center bearing screw in the lower clutch prior to securing the maxillary clutch to the upper mounting ring.

When the scriber is transferred to the articulator, a cast may or may not be

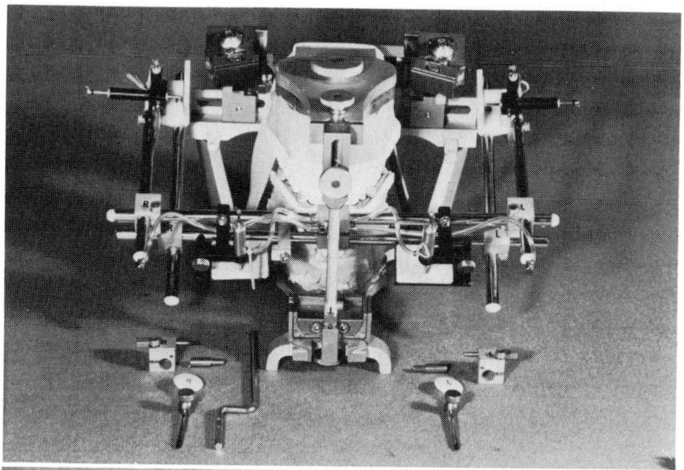

Fig. 37-23

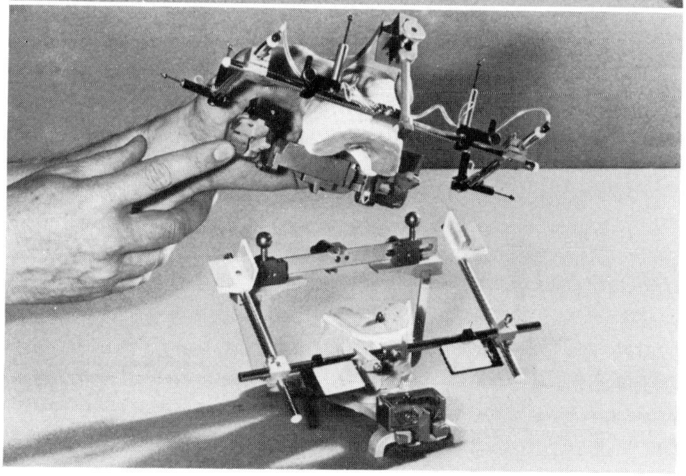

Fig. 37-24

Fig. 37-23. Components removed from articulator-pantograph assembly to facilitate adjustment procedure. (Courtesy Dr. Niles Guichet and Denar Co.)
Fig. 37-24. Maxillary bow with attached scriber assembly removed from mandibular bow for modification of fossa insertion, if desired. (Courtesy Dr. Niles Guichet and Denar Co.)

placed in the maxillary clutch for mounting (Fig. 37-22). In almost all cases, clutches are constructed and the pantographic record is obtained prior to tooth preparation. Generally a study cast—or, if sufficient unprepared teeth remain for accurate orientation of the cast in the clutch, a working cast—is transferred to the articulator simultaneously with the pantograph. If extensive tooth preparation is to be performed, it is recommended that the pantographic record be obtained prior to tooth preparation and subsequently after the teeth are prepared the working cast be transferred to the articulator with a face bow.

If a maxillary cast is to be transferred to the articulator simultaneously with the pantograph, the cast is accurately indexed in the upper clutch and secured with sticky wax. If the cast does not seal accurately in the clutch it may be necessary to remove the maxillary clutch from the scriber and trim away excess acrylic with a vulcanite bur or Fascut stone.

If the dentist elects not to transfer the maxillary cast to the articulator at this time but will transfer only the pantograph to the articulator to diagnose temporomandibular joint characteristics, he will subsequently transfer the maxillary cast to the articulator by means of a face bow. In this case additional retention of the upper clutch should be achieved by adapting additional cold-cure acrylic retentive modules to the superior surface of the clutch.

Fig. 37-23 illustrates a study cast transferred to the articulator simultaneously with the pantograph and secured to the mounting studs, which may interfere with maxillary bow with dental stone. The adjustment of the posterior fossa walls, must be removed. Support the hinge axis reference pin and loosen the hinge axis pin support. Retract the posterior reference pins and remove the hinge axis pin support. The mounting studs can then be removed. Remove the centric pins and the reference plane support rod. Retract the styli. Open the articulator and turn the centric latch to the neutral position.

The maxillary bow with attached scriber assembly can be removed from the mandibular bow for convenient modification of the fossa inserts if desired (Fig. 37-24). Diagnosing temporomandibular joint characteristics by setting the articulator to the pantographic record is described on p. 825.

FACE BOW TRANSFER

A dental face bow is used to transfer a facsimile of the dental structures (maxillary cast) to a mechanical equivalent of the lower half of the head (dental articulator) in the same relation to posterior control areas (fossa-condylar) as the dental structures enjoyed in the patient. The Denar Pantograph also functions as a face bow and can be used to accomplish this procedure (see Fig. 37-20).

Posterior reference points are established and a clutch, edentulous clutch, or bite fork is indexed to the maxillary teeth or arch. The face bow is then attached to one of the aforementioned devices and adjusted so as to register the location of the maxillary arch to the posterior reference points and horizontal reference plane. Subsequently the face bow is used to transfer this relationship to the dental articulator. When a bite fork is used to register to the maxillary teeth, a thin layer of low-fusing impression compound is attached to its superior surface. The compound is flamed to a dead soft consistency and then tempered in a water bath. The bite fork is then carefully and lightly indexed to the maxillary teeth so as not to displace mobile teeth and the compound is allowed to cool. The objective is to achieve slight impressions of cusp tips only without penetration of the compound. The dental cast should then be tried in the bite fork registration to confirm accurate seating.

An anterior crossbar assembly is secured to the bite fork and the assembly is brought to the mouth and indexed to the maxillary teeth. The patient is instructed to maintain the position of this assembly with their thumb.

Orient the face bow side arms so that the posterior reference pins are horizontal and lightly touch the posterior reference points on the patient's face. The posterior reference pins should be completely screwed into their housings when this is done. Secure the side arm clamps as tightly as possible. Adjust the reference plane support rod clamp parallel to the reference plane scribed on the patient's face.

Insert the reference plane support rod in the reference plane support rod clamp, approaching it from its inferior surface. Index the reference plane locator on the reference plane support rod in the hold provided. With the reference plane locator resting on its support rod, adjust the position of the reference plane support rod up or down and, by line of sight, accurately orient the reference plane locator coincidental to the horizontal reference plane on the patient's face by the posterior reference pins and the anterior reference point. Secure the reference plane support rod in its clamp with the offset in the rod to the left. The posterior reference pins are retracted into their housing so as not to scratch the patient's face on removal. The face bow record can now be removed from the mouth and used to accurately relate a maxillary cast in an articulator.

The telescoping mounting axis is extended to index over the tips of the hinge axis pins. The calibrated scale indicates the position to which the vertical axes of rotation of the articulator are adjusted in order to accept the recorder. The vertical axes of the articulator are adjusted to this dimension. Be sure to adjust the mediolateral location of the fossa elements first. Mounting studs are indexed in the lateral aspects of the condylar elements.

The face bow can now be indexed to the articulator by indexing the posterior reference pins in the holes provided in the mounting studs. The maxillary cast is secured to the bite fork with a rubber band or sticky wax. If the maxillary cast is heavy and causes deflection of the face bow, the bite fork should be supported with a maxillary cast support.

The centric latch can be used to hold the articulator in the lock-open position to facilitate laboratory procedures in securing the maxillary cast to the mounting plate. Care should be taken in closing the articulator after the mounting stone has been added to ensure that the condylar elements maintain contact with the superior and rear fossa walls.

Adapt a small piece of wax to the anterior margin of the mounting plate prior to mounting to it. This will provide a key way after mounting into which a plaster knife can be inserted to facilitate easy removal of the mounting stone. The stone is removed from the mounting plate in a manner comparable to opening an oyster.

ADJUSTING THE D4-A ARTICULATOR TO THE PANTOGRAPHIC RECORD

When the pantograph is transferred to the articulator, if the articulator is adjusted to duplicate exactly the temporomandibular joint characteristics of the patient, it will accurately describe the protrusive, orbiting, and rotating condylar paths of the patient and the styli will track the recorded lines. Conversely, if the articulator is adjusted so that the styli accurately track the recorded lines, the temporomandibular joints characteristic of the patient will be simulated in the fossa-condylar control elements of the articulator. Furthermore, these characteristics will have been reduced to a numeric value of millimeters or degrees expressed on the calibrated control adjustment scales of the articulator.

Depending on the dentist's objectives, the articulator may be adjusted so the styli (a) accurately follow the lines, or (b) follow a path relative to the lines. Generally speaking, most accurate reproduction of the patient's mandibular movement can be accomplished most efficiently, by selecting the appropriate fossa inserts and/or by custom modification of these inserts. Fig. 37-25 is a diagrammatic illustration of the pantographic recording tables. The black lines reflect the characteristics of the protrusive condylar path (character and anteroposterior inclination of the eminentia). The shorter light lines reflect the characteristics of the rotating condylar path (sagittal displacements of the rotating condyle—the horizontal table reflects back-forward displacements, the vertical table reflects up-down displacements). The longer light lines reflect the characteristics of the orbiting condylar path (the vertical table reflects the character and anteroposterior inclination of the eminentia; the horizontal table registers timing of the

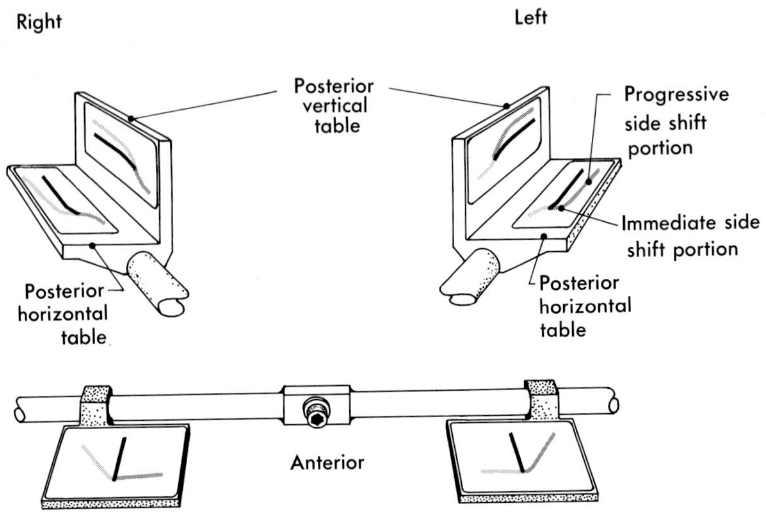

Fig. 37-25. Correlation of pantographic tracings to excursive movements. (Courtesy Dr. Robert J. Pinkerton.)

side shift—immediate and progressive).

When adjusting the D4-A to pantographic writings the operator should be thoroughly familiar with the significance of each line in the tracings and which characteristic of the temporomandibular articulation it most graphically reflects. When studying Fig. 37-25 remember that the styli are fixed to the maxillae and fossae, and that the record tables move with the mandible and condyles. The operator should also be thoroughly familiar with the location of the articulator adjustments that control the mechanical equivalents of these temporomandibular joint characteristics and with the location of the corresponding lock screws and scales of these adjustments.

When setting an articulator to pantographic scribings, the operator should know whether it will be to his advantage or disadvantage to have the articulator accurately reproduce mandibular movement (styli follow the lines) when the articulator is being used in its treatment function to define the occlusal anatomy of a restoration under construction. If it is not to his advantage to have the articulator reproduce mandibular movement, he should know where the stylus should be set relative to the line to have the instrument produce the movements that will dictate the desired occlusal form. This knowledge will permit the operator to set the articulator to the scribings with the minimal expenditure of time and effort so it will produce a movement that will permit the least potential for error.

In adjusting an articulator to pantographic tracings, the operator must manipulate the articulator in a manner to maintain positive contact of the condyles against the appropriate fossa-bearing surfaces. With a little experience the operator will soon develop the best hand grasps of the instrument to accomplish this most conveniently.

The recommended technic to employ in adjusting an articulator to pantographic scribings is to move the articulator in a test excursive movement in the appropriate direction while observing the movement of the styli relative to the line to which it is being adjusted. If a modification of the temporomandibular joint characteristic of the articulator is indicated, this adjustment is made and another test excursion is executed. This procedure is repeated until the desired setting is achieved.

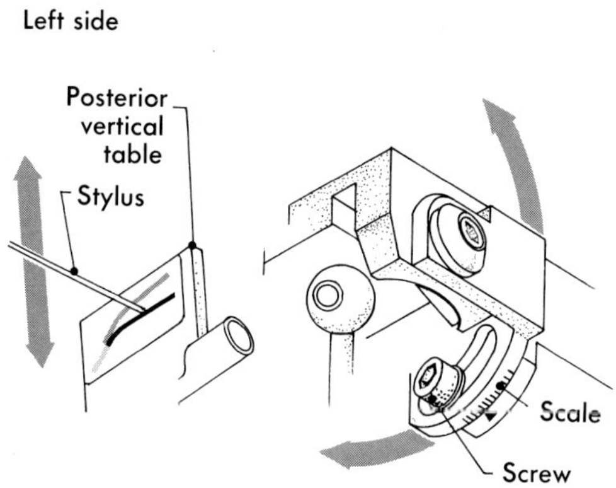

Fig. 37-26. Setting anteroposterior angle of eminentia or protrusive path adjustment (protrusive excursion illustrated). (Courtesy Dr. Robert J. Pinkerton.)

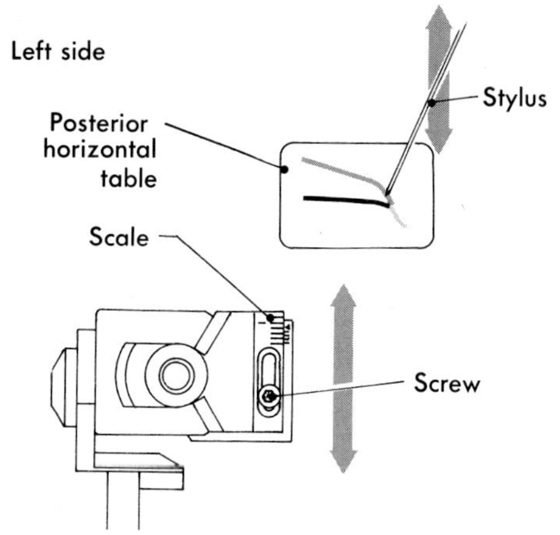

Fig. 37-27. Setting immediate side shift on medial fossa wall adjustment (right lateral excursion illustrated). (Courtesy Dr. Robert J. Pinkerton.)

When the mediolateral location of the condyles is adjusted to accept the pantograph in the transfer procedure, it is located by average anatomic measurement. This location will be confirmed or modified in the following procedure.

SEQUENCE OF ADJUSTMENTS

1. *Protrusive:* The articulator is manipulated so that all vertical styli track the protrusive lines. The protrusive condylar path is adjusted by setting the posterior horizontal styli relative to the black line in Fig. 37-26.

2. *Immediate side shift:* The outer line on the horizontal record table is inspected to determine its character and the appropriate medial fossa wall is selected or the visually determined amount of immediate side shift is introduced into the instrument for trial. The articulator is manipulated in the appropriate lateral excursive movement and the immediate side shift is timed by adjusting the posterior vertical styli relative to the immediate side shift portion of the outer line on the posterior horizontal table, as illustrated in Fig. 37-27.

3. *Progressive side shift:* The articulator is manipulated in the appropriate lateral excursive movement and the progressive side shift is adjusted by setting the posterior vertical styli relative to the outer line on the posterior horizontal table, as illustrated in Fig. 37-28.

4. *Rear wall adjustment (anteroposterior inclination of rotating path):* The articulator is manipulated in the appropriate lateral excursive movement and the rear wall is adjusted by setting

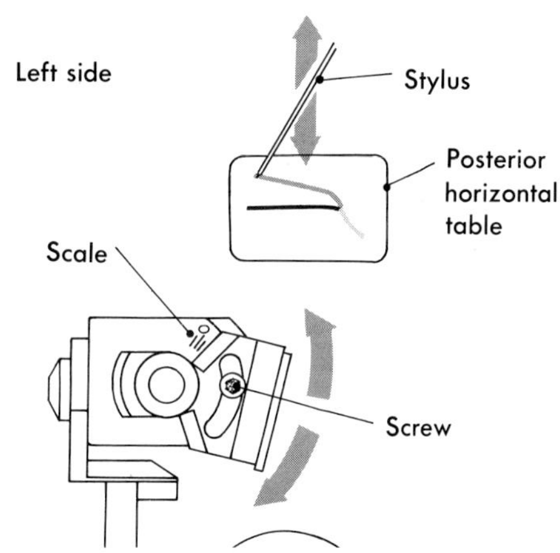

Fig. 37-28. Setting progressive side shift on medial fossa wall adjustment (right lateral excursion illustrated). (Courtesy Dr. Robert J. Pinkerton.)

the posterior vertical styli relative to the short line on the posterior horizontal record table, as illustrated in Fig. 37-29.

5. *Vertical axis adjustment (mediolateral location of fossa condylar elements):* After the rear wall adjustment is made the anterior vertical styli will most often accurately trace the anterior gothic arch tracings. If the styli do not track the medial legs of the tracings accurately, the articulator is manipulated in the appropriate lateral excursive movement and the vertical axes are adjusted until the styli track the medial leg of the anterior tracing. Moving the vertical axes medially relocates the medial leg of the anterior

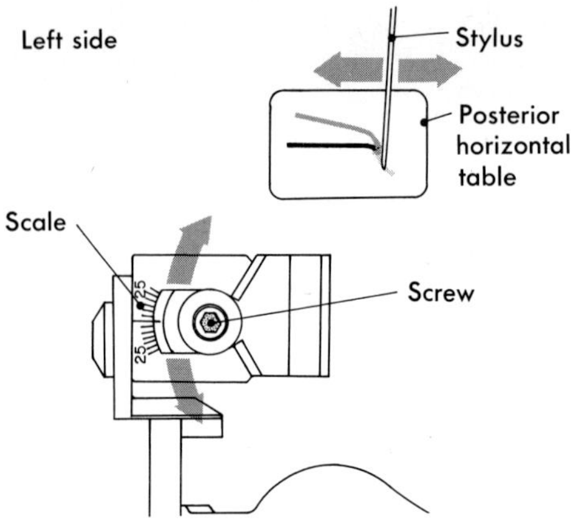

Fig. 37-29. Setting rear wall on forward and backward displacement of rotating condyle adjustment (right lateral excursion illustrated). (Courtesy Dr. Robert J. Pinkerton.)

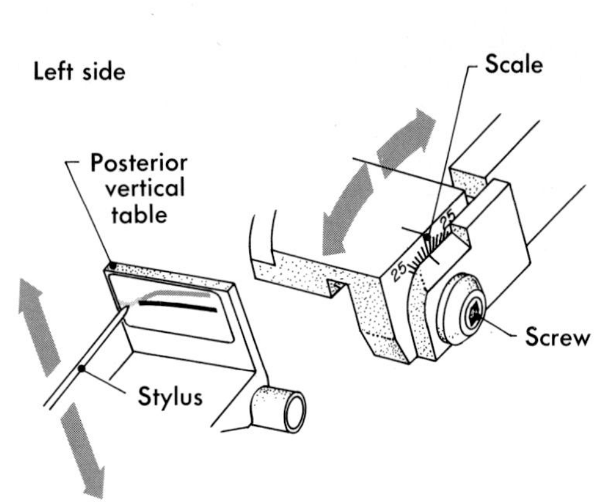

Fig. 37-30. Setting top wall on upward and downward displacement of rotating condyle adjustment (left lateral excursion illustrated). (Courtesy Dr. Robert J. Pinkerton.)

tracing more anteriorly relative to the styli, and vice versa.

6. *Orbiting path:* The articulator is manipulated in the appropriate excursive movement and the anteroposterior angle of the eminentia is adjusted by setting the posterior horizontal styli relative to the long upper (light) line on the posterior vertical record table, as illustrated in Fig. 37-26.

7. *Top wall adjustment (upward-downward inclination of rotating path):* The articulator is manipulated in the appropriate lateral excursive movement and the mediolateral inclination of the superior fossa wall is adjusted by setting the posterior horizontal stylus relative to the short (light) line on the vertical record table, as illustrated in Fig. 37-30.

RECIPROCAL INFLUENCE OF ADJUSTMENT

Reciprocal means "expression of mutual influence or relation." When the pantograph is assembled, although the styli will move in and out of their respective cylinders, they all have certain fixed relations to each other. Therefore when an articulator is adjusted to move one stylus relative to a line, that adjustment may have a mutual or reciprocal influence on other styli relative to their recorded lines. The listed sequence of settings takes into consideration the reciprocal influence of adjustments and sets forth the recommended sequence for most efficient adjustment of an articulator to pantographic scribings. However, an understanding of the reciprocal influence of adjustments is an aid in setting the articulator. These reciprocal influences can be categorized into three classes: (1) protrusive (right and left); (2) horizontal (settings 2-3-4-5); and (3) orbiting-rotating (settings 6-7).

Protrusive. When adjusting the protrusive path, an adjustment of one side of the articulator will have a reciprocal influence on the horizontal stylus on the opposite side of the instrument. Therefore the location of both horizontal styli should be given consideration when adjusting the protrusive paths.

Horizontal. The vertical styli tracings reflect the translations and rotations of the mandible in the horizontal plane. All vertical styli are fixed relative to each other, and an adjustment of any one stylus has a reciprocal effect on the other three. It is important that settings 2, 3, 4, and 5 be done in that sequence.

Orbiting-rotating. The setting of the stylus to the orbiting path has a reciprocal influence on the position of the opposite horizontal styli relative to the rotating line. Therefore the location of both horizontal styli should be given consideration when adjusting the orbiting condylar path (setting 6) and the opposing rotating condylar path (setting 7).

CHECKBITE PROCEDURE

The checkbite procedure is employed to register the relation of the mandibular dental structures of the patient to the maxillary structures by means of an interocclusal or checkbite record. The checkbite record is subsequently used to accurately locate the mandibular cast in the articulation at the recorded position. Checkbite records can be used to register centric and eccentric mandibular positions at any vertical dimension (Chapter 29).

The maxillary cast is transferred to the articulator by registering the relation of the maxillary structures of the patient to the initial references with a face bow. Subsequently this record is used to accurately locate the maxillary cast in the articulator for mounting. The mandibular cast is transferred to the articulator by occluding it with the maxillary cast, checkbite procedure, or a combination of the two.

In the transfer of the mandibular cast to the articulator, if the mandibular casts can be occluded accurately in the most intercusped position, the most accurate way to transfer the mandibular cast to the articulator is by occluding it with the maxillary cast. However, if deflective contacts exist, these must either be removed by grinding so the cast can be accurately oriented in the desired most intercusped position or the centric relation record must be taken at an increased vertical dimension by checkbite procedure.

A combination of occluding casts and checkbite registration is employed when there is an absence of deflective contacts but there is insufficient interocclusal contacts to establish stability or accurate orientation of casts to each other. This condition is frequently established after partial mouth-tooth preparation and equilibration of the unprepared teeth.

There are many satisfactory recording agents such as waxes and bite registration pastes, and many technics with which these agents can be employed to advantage in checkbite registration. However, there is no universal method that proves optimum in all situations. Therefore, the dentist must be knowledgeable in the anatomy of the related structures, neuromuscle physiology, and in the physical properties of dental materials that determine checkbite accuracy. This will enable him to effect a method of choice as varying situations present themselves.

It is not within the scope of this chapter to present an exhaustive discourse on checkbite procedure. However, one recommended procedure that affects basic principle of checkbite technic is presented. Variations of this technic can be employed as circumstances dictate. The following basic principles should always be employed in any checkbite technic.

1. The checkbite record should be obtained as close to the vertical dimension at which the restoration is to be constructed as possible.
2. The dentist should always manipulate the patient's mandible in obtaining the checkbite. The patient must not be instructed or allowed to bite or close down in such a manner as to cause flexion of the mandible or movement of teeth in obtaining the record.
3. The recording medium interposed between the teeth should be of a dead soft consistency as the mandible is brought to the desired position so as to prevent deflection of the mandible or mobile teeth, or the programming of muscle function.

Technic

The following technic can be used to register the mandibular position at the correct vertical dimension or at an increased vertical dimension. It can be used to register centric or eccentric positions. Described will be the registration of the centric relation position of the mandible at the minimal increase of vertical dimension, which will result in lack of posterior tooth contact.

Fabricate an occlusal program by softening a small piece of base plate wax in a water bath to a soft consistency and adapt it over several teeth in the anterior segment of the mouth. Manipulate the mandible into centric relation and gently guide the patient in terminal hinge closure lightly tapping the soft wax. Establish a broad simultaneous contact of several mandibular teeth with the wax. The wax is then removed from the mouth and chilled in tap water. The thickness of wax used should be the minimum to effect posterior distocclusion.

A small amount of denture adhesive cream is applied to the wax (occlusal programmer) in the area that adapts to the lingual surfaces of the maxillary anterior teeth. The occlusal programmer is repositioned in the mouth by reindexing it to the maxillary teeth. This occlusal programmer thus establishes a predetermined stop to vertical closure with the condyles in centric relation and with an absence of contacting deflective inclines by group functioning of teeth in the anterior segment of the mouth where the occluding pressures are the least. The occlusal programmer reprograms muscle function so as to eliminate resistance to terminal hinge closure previously programmed by deflective contacts, and the dentist can now more easily manipulate the mandible in repeated terminal hinge closure in accomplishing the checkbite record. Similar occlusal programmers can be fabricated in eccentric position to facilitate obtaining eccentric checkbite records.

Suitable checkbite recording medium is placed on the mandibular posterior teeth area and the mandible is guided in terminal hinge closure. The checkbite recording medium is allowed to harden without the patient executing a biting pressure. Deep fissures, grooves, and undercuts on the teeth and cavity preparations are blocked out by wiping petroleum jelly over the teeth with the index finger before a zinc oxide–eugenol paste material is used for checkbite registration.

Occlusal programmers can be constructed to index the mandible in protrusive, rigid lateral, and left lateral mandibular positions to facilitate obtaining of checkbite records of these mandibular positions.

Maximum accuracy can be ensured if the fossa condylar settings are adjusted to the patient's temporomandibular joint characteristic prior to the time the mandibular cast is transferred to the articulator. This procedure should always be followed when casts on which restorations are to be constructed are transferred to the articulator. If the temporomandibular joint characteristics are unknown when the mandibular cast is transferred to the articulator, the anteroposterior angle of the eminentia should be set to 25 to 30° and the progressive side shift adjustments are set to 5 to 10°. All other adjustments are set to zero. The mediolateral orientation of the bows of the articulator should be maintained by the inner walls of the fossa and not the centric latch. A heavy elastic can be used to ensure positive seating of the condyles in their respective fossae.

The articulator is inverted and the mandibular cast is accurately oriented to the mandibular cast by means of the centric relation checkbite record. The mandibular cast is secured to the mounting plate with dental stone.

Eccentirc checkbite technic

The anteroposterior angle of the eminentia and the progressive side shift adjustment of the articulator can be set to eccentric check bites.

Protrusive adjustment. The incisal pin assembly is removed from the articulator. Set the progressive side shift adjustment to its maximum setting and set all other adjustments to zero including the angle of the eminentia. Place the protrusive checkbite record (not the occlusal programmer) on the mandibular cast. Relate the maxillary bow of the articulator to the mandibular by carefully seating the maxillary cast in the checkbite record. Stabilize the casts in the checkbite record by lightly pressing on the top of the articulator. Note that the condylar elements are displaced away from the posterior, medial, and superior walls of the fossa. Increase the anteroposterior angle of the eminentia until the superior wall of the fossa contacts the condylar element. Lock the fossa in this position and repeat on opposite side.

Progressive side shift adjustment. Place the lateral checkbite record on the mandibular cast. Relate the maxillary bow of the articulator to the mandibular bow by carefully seating the maxillary cast in the checkbite record. Stabilize the casts in the checkbite, applying slight pressure to the top of the articulator. Note that the medial fossa wall does not contact the condylar element. Decrease the progressive side shift adjustment from its maximum setting until the medial fossa wall contacts the condylar element. Lock the medial fossa wall in this position and repeat on the opposite side.

SUGGESTED READINGS

Granger, E. R.: Establishment of occlusion: the articulator and the patient, Dent. Clin. N. Amer., p. 527, Nov., 1962.

Granger, E. R.: Practical procedures in oral rehabilitation, Philadelphia, 1962, J. B. Lippincott Co.

McCollum, B. B.: A research report; basic text for the postgraduate course in gnathology, South Pasadena, California, 1955, The Scientific Press.

Posselt, U.: The physiology of occlusion, Philadelphia, 1962, F. A. Davis Co.

Ramfjord, S. P., and Ash, M.: Occlusion and rehabilitation, Philadelphia, 1966, W. B. Saunders Co.

GENERAL REFERENCES

Arstad, T.: Capsular ligaments of the temporomandibular joint and the retrusion facets of the dentition in relationship to mandibular movements, Am. Equilibration Soc. Compend. **4**:24, 1960 (abst.).

Atwood, D. A.: A critique of research of the posterior limit of the mandibular position, J. Prosth. Dent. **20**:21, 1968.

Atwood, D. A.: A critique of research of the rest position of the mandible, J. Prosth. Dent. **16**: 848, 1966.

Aull, A. E.: Condylar determinants of occlusal patterns, J. Prosth. Dent. **15**:826-846, 1965.

Avery, J. K., and Rapp, R.: Investigation of the mechanism of neural impulse transmission in human teeth, Oral Surg. **12**:190, 1959.

Baer, P. N.: Analysis of physiologic rest position, centric relation, centric occlusion, J. Periodont. **27**:181, 1956.

Ballard, C. F.: Consideration of the physiological background of mandibular posture and movement, Tr. Brit. Soc. Study Orthodont., pp. 117, 126, 1955.

Baraban, D. J.: Establishing centric relation and vertical dimension in occlusal rehabilitation, J. Prosth. Dent. **12**:1157, 1962.

Beck, H. O.: Jaw registrations and articulators, J.A.D.A. **73**:863, 1966.

Beck, H. O., and Morrison, W. E.: Method for reproduction of movements of the mandible; research progress report, J. Prosth. Dent. **12**: 873, 1962.

Bell, D. H.: Sagittal balance of the mandible, J.A.D.A. **64**:486-495, 1962.

Bennett, G. T.: The kinematic geometry of the small movements of the mandible, Brit. D. J. **45**:228, 1924.

Bennett, N. G.: Contribution to the study of the movements of the mandible, J. Prosth. Dent. **8**:41, 1958.

Bergman, S. A.: Importance of temporomandibular joint roentgenograms in mouth rehabilitation, New York D. J. **20**:103, 1954.

Berman, M. H.: Accurate interocclusal records, J. Prosth. Dent. **10**:620, 1960.

Berry, D. C.: Constancy of the rest position of the mandible, D. Pract. & D. Rec. **10**:129, 1960.

Berry, H. M., Jr., and Hoffmann, F. A.: Cineradiographic observations of temporomandibular joint function, J. Prosth. Dent. **9**:21, 1959.

Beyron, H. L.: Characteristics of functionally optimal occlusion and principles of occlusal rehabilitation, J.A.D.A. **48**:648, 1954.

Bolender, C. L.: Significance of vertical dimension in prosthetic dentistry, J. Prosth. Dent. **6**: 177, 1956.

Boos, R. H.: Maxillomandibular relations, occlusion, and the temporomandibular joint, Dent. Clin. N. Amer., pp. 19-35, March, 1962.

Boos, R. H.: Vertical, centric and functional dimensions recorded by gnathodynamics, J.A.D.A. **59**:682, 1959.

Borgh, O., and Posselt, U.: Hinge axis registration: experiments on the articulator, Odont. Revy. **7**:214, 1956; Dent. **8**:35, 1958.

Boucher, C. O.: Maxillomandibular relations and records, Tr. Am. D. Soc. Europe **68**:8, 1962 (abst.).

Boucher, C. O.: Occlusion in prosthodontics, J. Prosth. Dent. **3**:633-656, 1953.

Boucher, L. J.: Limiting factors in posterior movements of mandibular condyles, J. Prosth. Dent. **11**:23-25, 1961.

Boucher, L. J.: Anatomy of the temporomandibular joint as it pertains to centric relation, J. Prosth. Dent. **12**:464 (disc. pp. 473-475), 1962.

Boucher, L. J., and Jacoby, J.: Posterior border movements of the human mandible, J. Prosth. Dent. **11**:836, 1961.

Boyd, J. B., Jr.: Relationship between occlusion, occlusal equilibration and crown and bridgework and partial denture prosthesis, Alum. Bull. Indiana Univ. School Dent., pp. 4-7, 36-38, Aug., 1959.

Brodie, A. G.: The three arcs of mandibular movement as they affect wear of the teeth, Lecture presented before the University of Illinois Orthodontic Alumni Meeting, Chicago, March, 1968.

Brotman, D. N.: Hinge axis, J. Prosth. Dent. **10**: 436, 631, 636, 1960.

Chestner, S. B.: Considerations in the prescription of occlusal rehabilitation, J.A.D.A. **55**:790, 1957.

Christensen, F. T.: Effect of incisal guidance on cusp angulation in prosthetic occlusion, J. Prosth. Dent. **11**:48, 1961.

Christiansen, R. L.: Rationale of the face bow in maxillary cast mounting, J. Prosth. Dent. **9**: 388, 1959.

Cohen, R.: More on the Bennett movement, J. Prosth. Dent. **9**:788, 1959.

Cohen, R.: Hinge axis and its practical application in the determination of centric relation, J. Prosth. Dent. **10**:248, 1960.

Cohn, L. A.: Integrating treatment procedures in occluso-rehabilitation, J. Prosth. Dent. **7**:511, 1957.

Cohn, L. A.: Two techniques for interocclusal records, J. Prosth. Dent. **13**:438, 1963.

Cooper, H., Jr.: Bridge construction; functional occlusion in bridgework, J. Michigan D. A. **40**:296, 1958.

Courtade, G. L.: Foreword to symposium on occlusal rehabilitation, Dent. Clin. N. Amer., pp. 575-576, Nov., 1963.

D'Amico, A.: The canine teeth—normal functional relation of the natural teeth of man, J. South. California D. A. **26**:1, 49, 127, 175, 194, 239, 1958.

D'Amico, A.: Application of the concept of the functional relation of the canine teeth, J. South. California D. A. **27**:39, 1959.

D'Amico, A.: Functional occlusion of the natural teeth of man, J. Prosth. Dent. **11**:899, 1961.

Decker, J. C.: Traumatic deafness as result of retrusion of condyles of mandible, Ann. Otol. **34**: 519, 1925.

Derksen, A. A., and Van Haeringen, W.: Protrusive movement in articulators, J. Dent. Res. **37**:127, 1958.

DiSalvo, N. A.: Neuromuscular mechanisms involved in mandibular movement and posture, Am. J. Orthodontics **47**:330, 1961.

Dixon, A. D.: Structure and functional significance of the intra-articular disc of the human temporomandibular joint, Oral Surg. **15**:48, 1962.

Duncan, E. T., and Williams, S. T.: Evaluation of rest position as a guide in prosthetic treatment, J. Prosth. Dent. **10**:643, 1960.

Edwards, L. F.: Some anatomic facts and fancies relative to the masticatory apparatus, J. Prosth. Dent. **5**:825, 1955.

el-Aramany, M. A., and others: Evaluation of the needle point tracing as a method for determining centric relation, J. Prosth. Dent. **15**: 1043, 1965.

Foster, T. D.: Use of the face-bow in making permanent study casts, J. Prosth. Dent. **9**:717, 1959.

Fountain, H. W.: Seating the condyles for centric relation records, J. Prosth. Dent. **11**:1050, 1961.

Franks, A. S. T.: Observations on the rest position of the mandible, J. Dent. Res. **39**:1098, 1960.

Freese, A. S.: Myofascial trigger mechanism in temporomandibular joint and allied disturbances, Oral Surg. **14**:933, 1961.

Garnick, J., and Ramfjord, S. P.: Rest position; an electromyographic and clinical investigation, J. Prosth. Dent. **12**:895, 1962.

Gehl, D. H.: Vertical dimension, jaw relation records and occlusion, Dent. Clin. N. Amer., pp. 321-332, July, 1960.

Glickman, I.: Occlusion and the periodontium, J. Dent. Res. **46**:53, 1967.

Goodfriend, D. J.: Practical analysis of occlusal procedures, J. Prosth. Dent. **16**:557-571, 1966.

Gottsegen, R.: Centric relation; the periodontist's viewpoint, J. Prosth. Dent. **16**:1034-1038, 1966.

Graf, H., and Zander, H. A.: Tooth contact patterns in mastication, J. Prosth. Dent. **13**:1055-1066, 1963.

Granger, E. R.: Functional relations of the stomatognathic system, J.A.D.A. **48**:638, 1954.

Granger, E. R.: Functional concepts of dentistry, Illinois D. J. **25**:226, 1956.

Granger, E. R.: Prosthetic relations of the temporomandibular joint, North-West Dent. **38**: 117, 1959.

Granger, E. R.: Clinical significance of the hinge axis mounting, Dent. Clin. N. Amer., p. 205, March, 1959.

Granger, E. R.: Method of recording functional relations, J. South. California D. A. **27**:381, 1959.

Granger, E. R.: Temporomandibular joint in prosthodontics, J. Prosth. Dent. **10**:239, 1960.

Griffin, C. J., and Sharpe, C. J.: Distribution of elastic tissue in the human temporomandibular meniscus especially in respect to "compression" areas, Australian D. J. **7**:72, 1962.

Guichet, N. F.: Procedures for occlusal treatment, Anaheim, California, 1969, Denar Co.

Gysi, A.: Practical application of research results in denture construction (mandibular movements), George Wood Clapp, Collaborator, J.A.D.A. **16**:199, 1929.

Hankey, G. T., and Nash, D. F. E.: Temporomandibular disorders, the result of trauma, malocclusion and muscular imbalance, Am. Equilibration Soc. Compend. **4**:86, 1960.

Hickey, J. C., Allison, M. L., Woelfel, J. B., Boucher, C. O., and Stacy, R. W.: Mandibular movements in three dimensions, J. Prosth. Dent. **13**:72-92, 1963.

Huffman, R. W., Regenos, J. W., and Taylor, R. R.: Principles of occlusion, laboratory and clinical teaching manual (Ohio State University), Columbus, 1969, H. and R. Press.

Hughes, G. A., and Regli, C. P.: What is centric relation, J. Prosth. Dent. **11**:16-22, 1961.

Hurst, W. W.: Vertical dimension and its correlation with lip length and interocclusal distance, J.A.D.A. **64**:496, 1962.

Isaacson, D.: Clinical study of the Bennett movement, J. Prosth. Dent. **8**:64, 1958.

Jacobsen, A. M.: Function analysis of temporomandibular joint disturbances, J. South. California D. A. **30**:35, 1962.

Jankelson, B.: Physiology of human dental occlusion, J.A.D.A. **50**:671, 1955.

Jankelson, B.: Considerations of occlusion in fixed partial dentures, Dent. Clin. N. Amer., p. 187, March, 1959.

Jankelson, B.: Dental occlusion and the temporomandibular joint, Dent. Clin. N. Amer., pp. 51-62, March, 1962.

Jankelson, B.: A technique for obtaining optimum functional relationship for the natural dentition, Dent. Clin. N. Amer., pp. 131-141, March, 1960.

Jarabak, J. R.: Electromyographic analysis of muscular and temporomandibular joint disturbances due to imbalance in occlusion, Angle Orthodontist **26**:170, 1956.

Jerge, C. R.: The neurologic mechanism underlying cyclic jaw movements, J. Prosth. Dent. **14**:667-681, 1964.

Jerge, C. R.: Temporomandibular joints and centric relation, Pennsylvania D. J. **61**:5, 12, 1957.

Kapur, K. K., and Yurkstas, A. A.: Evaluation of centric relation records obtained by various techniques, J. Prosth. Dent. **7**:770, 1957.

Kawamura, Y.: Neuromuscular mechanisms of jaw and tongue movement, J.A.D.A. **62**:545, 1961.

Kazis, H., and Kazis, A. J.: Complete mouth rehabilitation, New York J. Dent. **28**:199, 1958.

Kazis, H., and Kazis, A. J.: Complete mouth rehabilitation through fixed partial denture prosthodontics, J. Prosth. Dent. **10**:296-303, 1960.

Kingery, R. H.: Maxillomandibular relationship of centric relation, J. Prosth. Dent. **9**:922, 1959.

Koski, K.: Axis of the opening movement of the mandible, J. Prosth. Dent. **12**:888, 1962.

Krajicek, D. D., and others: Clinical and electromyographic study of mandibular rest position, J. Prosth. Dent. **11**:826, 1961.

Kurth, L. E.: Methods of obtaining vertical dimension and centric relation; a practical evaluation of various methods, J.A.D.A. **59**:669, 1959.

Kurth, L. E.: From mouth to articulator; static jaw relations, J.A.D.A. **64**:517, 1962.

Kyes, F. M.: Temporomandibular joint disorders, J.A.D.A. **59**:1137, 1959.

Lauritzen, A. G., Bodner, G. H.: Variations in location of arbitrary and true hinge axis points, J. South. California D. A. **29**:10, 1961; J. Prosth. Dent. **11**:224, 1961.

Lauritzen, A. G., and Wolford, L. W.: Hinge axis location on an experimental basis, J. South. California D. A. **29**:354, 1961; J. Prosth. Dent. **11**:1059, 1961.

La Vere, A. M.: Lateral interocclusal positional records, J. Prosth. Dent. **19**:350, 1968.

Leff, A.: Gnathodynamics of four mandibular positions, J. Prosth. Dent. **16**:844, 1966.

Lieb, D. E.: Generated path in fixed denture prosthesis, Minneapolis Dist. D. J. **46**:25, 1962.

Lindblom, G.: Anatomy and function of the temporomandibular joint, Acta Odont. Scandinav. **17**(supp. 28):7, 1960.

Linkow, L. I.: Oral rehabilitation technique utilizing copper band impressions, J. Prosth. Dent. **11**:716, 1961.

Lipke, D., and Posselt, U.: Functional anatomy of the temporomandibular joint, Am. Equilibration Soc. Compend. **4**:73, 1960.

Lipke, D. P.: Hinge axis and its value, Bull. Greater Milwaukee D. A. **25**:197, 1959.

Logan, L. R.: Electromyographic investigation of the occlusal position of the mandible as determined by a hinge axis method, J. South. California D. A. **30**:133, 1962.

Lucia, V. O.: Centric relation—theory and practice, J. Prosth. Dent. **10**:849, 1960.

Lucia, V. O.: Gnathological concept of articulation, Dent. Clin. N. Amer., pp. 183-197, March, 1962.

McCollum, B. B.: Mandibular hinge axis and a method of locating it, J. Prosth. Dent. **10**:428, 1960.

MacQueen, D.: Is an early cuspid rise essential to periodontal health?, J. West. Soc. Periodont. **6**:76, 1958.

Mann, A. W., and Pankey, L. D.: Oral rehabilitation: part I, use of the P-M instrument in treatment planning and in restoring the lower posterior teeth; part II, reconstruction of the upper teeth using a functional generated path technique, J. Prosth. Dent. **10**:135-162, 1960.

Marevskaya, A. P.: Development of proprioceptive reflexes in the muscles of mastication, D. Abst. **4**:30, 1959.

Mazur, B.: Construction of plastic registration trays, J. Prosth. Dent. **16**:904, 1966.

Messerman, T.: A means for studying mandibular movements, J. Prosth. Dent. **17**:36-43, 1967.

Meyer, F. S.: Generated path technique in reconstruction dentistry, II: fixed partial dentures, J. Prosth. Dent. **9**:432, 1959.

Moller, E.: The chewing apparatus; an electromyographic study of the action of the muscles of mastication and its correlation to facial morphology, Acta Physiol. Scandinav. **69**: (Suppl.) 280-281, 1966.

Morgan, D. H.: Diagnosis of temporomandibular joint problems, J. S. Calif. Dent. Ass. **33**:523, 1965.

Moulton, G. H.: Centric occlusion and the freeway space, J. Prosth. Dent. **7**:209, 1957.

Moulton, G. H.: Importance of centric occlusion in diagnosis and treatment planning, J. Prosth. Dent. **10**:921, 1960.

Moyers, R. E.: Some physiologic considerations of centric and other jaw relations, J. Prosth. Dent. **6**:183, 1956.

Murphy, W. M.: Rest position of the mandible, J. Prosth. Dent. **17**:329. 1967.

Nevakari, K.: Analysis of the mandibular movement from rest to occlusal position; a roentgenographic-cephalometric investigation, Acta Odont. Scandinav. **14**(supp. 19):9, 1956.

Niswonger, M. E.: The rest position of the mandible and centric relation, J.A.D.A. **21**:1572, 1934.

Nuttall, E. B.: The principles of obtaining occlusion in occlusal rehabilitation, J. Prosth. Dent. **13**:699, 1963.

Osborne, J.: Mandibular-maxillary relationships in oral rehabilitation, Int. Dent. J. **16**:398-405, 1966.

Oursland, L. E., and Carlson, R. D.: Study of the horizontal axis of rotation of the mandible, J. South. California D. A. **26**:212, 1958.

Parsons, M. T., and Boucher, L. J.: The bilaminar zone of the meniscus, J. Dent. Res. **45**: 59-61, 1966.

Perry, H. T.: The temporomandibular joint, Amer. J. Orthodont. **52**:399-400, 1966.

Phillips, R. W.: Report of the Committee on Scientific Investigation of the American Academy of Restorative Dentistry, J. Prosth. Dent. **19**:416, 1968.

Posselt, U.: Hinge opening axis of the mandible, Acta Odont. Scandinav. **14**:49, 1956.

Posselt, U.: Movement areas of the mandible, J. Prosth. Dent. **7**:375-385, 1957.

Posselt, U.: Under what circumstances should the mandible be placed in terminal hinge position in occlusal adjustment or restorative procedures?, J. West Soc. Periodont. **5**:5, 1957.

Posselt, U.: An analyzer for mandibular positions, J. Prosth. Dent. **7**:368, 1957.

Posselt, U.: Range of movement of the mandible, J.A.D.A. **56**:10, 1958.

Posselt, U., and Addiego, B. J.: Gnatho-thesiometric study of various mandibular positions in individuals with normal and abnormal function of the temporomandibular joints, Odont. Revy **9**:1, 1958.

Posselt, U., and Nevstedt, P.: Registration of the condyle path inclination by intraoral wax records—its practical value, J. Prosth. Dent. **11**:43, 1961.

Posselt, U., and others: The split cast technique, Odont. Revy **13**:270, 1962.

Posselt, U., and Franzen, G.: Registration of the condyle path inclination by intraoral wax records; variations in three instruments, J. Prosth. Dent. **10**:441, 1960 (reprint).

Posselt, U., and Thilander, B.: Influence of the innervation of the temporomandibular joint capsule on mandibular border movements, Acta Odont. Scandinav. **23**:601-613, 1965.

Ptack, H.: Temporomandibular joint and its importance to the prosthodontist, J. Canad. D. A. **26**:341, 1960.

Pyott, J. E., and Schaeffer, A.: Centric relation and vertical dimension by cephalometric roentgenograms, J. Prosth. Dent. **4**:35, 1954.

Ramfjord, S. P.: Bruxism, a clinical and electromyographic study, J.A.D.A. **62**:21, 1961.

Ramfjord, S. P.: The significance of recent research on occlusion for the teaching and practice of dentistry, J. Prosth. Dent. **16**:96-105, 1966.

Ricketts, R. M.: Details of occlusion, Pacific Palisades, California, 1966, Dome, Inc.

Ricketts, R. M.: Occlusion—the medium of dentistry, J. Prosth. Dent. **21**:39, 1969.

Rivalut, M. A., and Tabet, G. A.: Factors determining the movements and positions of the mandible, Internat. D. J. **11**:217, 1961.

Roberts, M.: Comparison of the rest vertical dimension of the face as determined clinically and electromyographically, Am. J. Orthodontics **45**:872, 1959.

Ross, J. H.: Dentist's responsibilities in temporomandibular joint disturbances, J. Florida D. Soc. **32**:17, 1961.

Saizar, P.: Retrusive movement of the mandible, Actualities Odontostomat. **16**:187, 1962.

Sandquist, U.: Some remarks on the background to certain proprioceptive muscle reflexes with special regard to their occurrence in the jaw muscles, Acta Odont. Scandinav. **18**:331, 1960.

Schei, O., and others: Tooth mobility and alveolar bone resorption as a function of occlusal stress and oral hygiene, Acta Odont. Scandinav. **17**:61, 1959.

Schier, M. B. A.: Temporomandibular joint roentgenography; controlled erect technics, J.A.D.A. **65**:456, 1962.

Schuyler, C. H.: Considerations of occlusion in fixed partial dentures, Dent. Clin. N. Amer., pp. 175-185, March, 1959.

Schweitzer, J. M.: Conservative approach to oral rehabilitation, J. Prosth. Dent. **11**:119, 1961.

Schweitzer, J. M.: Masticatory function in man; mandibular repositioning, J. Prosth. Dent. **12**:262, 1962.

Shanahan, T. E. J., and Leff, A.: Mandibular and articulator movements: part VIII, physiologic and mechanical concepts of occlusion, J. Prosth. Dent. **16**:62-72, 1966.

Sheppard, I.: Effect of hinge axis clutches on condyle position, J. Prosth. Dent. **8**:260, 1958.

Sheppard, I. M.: Bracing position, centric occlusion, and centric relation, J. Prosth. Dent. **9**:11, 1959.

Sheppard, I. M.: Closing masticatory strokes, J. Prosth. Dent. **9**:946, 1959.

Sheppard, I. M.: Anteroposterior and posteroanterior movements of the mandible and condylar centricity during function, J. Prosth. Dent. **12**:86, 1962.

Shore, N. A.: Symptomatology of temporomandibular joint dysfunction, J. New Jersey D. Soc. **31**:10, 1959.

Shore, N. A.: Treatment of temporomandibular joint dysfunction, J. Prosth. Dent. **10**:366, 1960.

Shore, N. A.: Interpretations of temporomandibular joint roentgenograms, Am. Equilibration Soc. Compend. **4**:152, 1960.

Shpuntoff, H., and Shpuntoff, W.: Study of physiologic rest position and centric position by electromyography, J. Prosth. Dent. **6**:621, 1956.

Sicher, H.: Changing concepts of the supporting dental structures, Oral Surg. **12**:31, 1959.

Sicher, H.: Temporomandibular articulation; concepts and misconceptions, Oral Surg. **20**:281, 1962.

Stallard, H.: Physiology of chewing, J. Dist. Columbia D. Soc. **34**:9, 1959.

Stallard, H., and Stuart, C. E.: Eliminating tooth guidance in natural dentitions, J. Prosth. Dent. **11**:474, 1961.

Stansbery, C. J.: Functional position checkbite technique, J.A.D.A. **16**:421, 1929.

Storey, A. T.: Physiology of a changing vertical dimension, J. Prosth. Dent. **12**:912, 1962.

Stuart, C. E.: Why dental restoration should have cusps, J. South California D. A. **27**:198, 1959.

Stuart, C. E., and Stallard, H.: Diagnosis and treatment of occlusal relations of the teeth, Texas D. J. **75**:430, 1957.

Swenson, H. M.: Complete mouth reconstruction or destruction?, J.A.D.A. **65**:345, 1962.

Thilander, B.: Innervation of the temporo-mandibular joint capsule in man; an anatomic investigation and a neurophysiologic study of the perception of mandibular position, Tr. Roy. Schools Dent. Stockholm & Umea, no. 7, pp. 9-67, 1961.

Trapozzano, V. R., and Lazzari, J. B.: Study of hinge axis determination, J. Prosth. Dent. **11**:858, 1961.

Trapozzano, V. R., and Lazzari, J. B.: The physiology of the terminal rotation position of the condyles in the temporomandibular joint, J. Prosth. Dent. **17**:122-133, 1967.

Uccellani, E. L.: Use of a muscle relaxant as an aid in obtaining centric registration, J. Prosth. Dent. **10**:92, 1960.

Vaughan, H. C.: Occlusion and the mandibular

articulation, Dent. Clin. N. Amer. pp. 37-50, March, 1962.

Weinberg, L. A.: Physiologic objectives of reconstruction techniques, J. Prosth. Dent. **10:** 711, 1960.

Weinberg, L. A.: Evaluation of the face-bow mounting, J. Prosth. Dent. **11**:32, 1961.

Weinberg, L. A.: An evaluation of basic articulators and their concepts, J. Prosth. Dent. **13:** 622, 1963.

Weinberg, L. A.: An evaluation of basic articulators and their concepts: part II, arbitrary, positional, semiadjustable articulators, J. Prosth. Dent. **13**:645, 1963.

Wester, L. H.: Occlusion in the fixed bridge, Texas D. J. **76**:172, 1958.

Wing, G.: Temporomandibular joint and general dental practice, Australian D. J. **6**:94, 1961.

Woelfel, J. B., Hickey, J. C., Stacy, R. W., and Rinear, L.: Electromyographic analysis of jaw movements, J. Prosth. Dent. **10**:688-697, 1960.

Zimring, M. J.: Gnathology; an introduction, D. Students' Mag., **46**(2)131-187, 1967.

Zola, A.: Morphologic limiting factors in the temporomandibular joint, J. Prosth. Dent. **13:** 732-740, 1963.

Zola, A., and Rothschild, E. A.: Condyle positions in unimpeded jaw movements, J. Prosth. Dent. **11**:873, 1961.

Chapter 38

Use of acrylic resins in crowns and fixed partial dentures; early use of synthetic resins

The use of synthetic resins in dentistry is not new, but their application to the construction of crowns and bridges is of comparatively recent date. A search of the dental literature, however, discloses that as early as 1938 an article by Selbach[1] was published in which construction of crowns made of synthetic resins is described. The resins employed were made available in four colors, namely, yellow, white, light gray, and dark gray.

EARLY USE OF SYNTHETIC RESINS FOR CROWNS

Synthetic resins for crowns were first demonstrated and used in this country in May, 1940, by Wilson.[2] A search of the dental literature discloses an article by Weder[3] published in Europe in January, 1940, describing and illustrating in detail the use of a synthetic resinous plastic material for the construction of individual crowns.

Because the early resins used for this purpose were not suitable nor specifically designed for use in small dental restorations, the results were not entirely satisfactory. Also, many failures were due to the fact that the polymer particles that were used in crowns and fixed partial dentures were of too large a mesh, resulting in a product that was coarse and granular in appearance. During the intervening years, manufacturers have developed acrylic resins specially suited for making small restorations.

Not only has a fineness of particle size been developed but also hues have been made available that make it possible for the dentist to match the color of the natural teeth with the same degree of exactness as it is possible to do with the fired porcelain restorations.

Since the acrylic veneer crown has become generally used, it is well at this time to consider those factors which are essential to the successful use of this material. The acrylic resins are not a panacea—they have their limitations as well as their advantages. The acrylic resin crown is not intended to supplant the glazed porcelain veneer crown, but it should be used where indicated and not where contraindicated.

TYPES OF SYNTHETIC RESINS

The dental synthetic resins fall into one of the following types: phenolic, urea, polystyrene, cellulose, vinyl, the methyl methacrylate, and many types of copolymers. These resins and their copolymers appear to be well suited for the smaller types of restorations.

The methyl methacrylate synthetic resins belong to the thermal plastic group as distinguished from those that are thermal setting, such as the phenol formaldehyde types. There is also the autopolymerizing or self-curing group.

DESIRABLE PHYSICAL PROPERTIES OF RESINS

A synthetic resin, to be suitable for dental purposes, should have (1) toughness (impact strength), (2) flexural strength, (3) tensile strength, (4) permanency, (5) a low cold flow, (6) high resistance to water and solvents, (7) a minimum of dimensional change, (8) high relative hardness, (9) moldability, and, finally (10) adaptability to a simple technic employing inexpensive equipment. While there is no single type of synthetic resin that possesses all of these desirable qualities to the optimum degree, the acrylic resins possess these qualities to a degree to make them the material of choice for many dental purposes.

MONOMER AND POLYMER

The acrylic resins for crowns and bridges are generally available in the powder and liquid form. The powder, or polymer, is the polymerized form of the liquid monomer. In use, the powder and liquid are mixed in the approximate proportions of 3 to 1 by volume, or 65 to 35 parts by weight, polymer to monomer. This mixture, when permitted to stand in a closed jar, gradually changes to a doughy consistency. The change or the process by which the liquid monomer is converted into the solid polymer is known as polymerization, which is hastened by the application of heat, ultraviolet light, or oxidizing agents. The method which employs heat is generally used by dentists in the processing or polymerization of the resin. In a mixture of monomer and polymer, it is important that not too much of the liquid monomer be used, but only enough so that all the polymer particles are wetted. The greater the amount of monomer used, the greater will be the total shrinkage of the object molded; in fact, if monomer alone were used, the volumetric shrinkage of an object would be approximately 21 percent. Moreover, since the monomer is a clear liquid, it polymerizes into a clear, transparent polymer; hence, excessive use of the monomer may modify the color of the processed resin.

The physical properties of acrylic resin, which are of special interest to the dentist, relate to (1) dimensional changes, (2) water imbibition or adsorption, (3) color permanency, (4) flexural strength, (5) relative hardness, and (6) cold flow.

Methods of mixing monomer and polymer

Several methods can be used to mix the monomer and the polymer and place the mixture in the mold or tooth.

First method. In the first method, the one most generally used for small restoration, the liquid and the powder in proper proportions are placed in a jar and thoroughly mixed for several minutes with a glass rod. The cover is then screwed tightly on the jar, where the mixture is permitted to remain for a given length of time, whereupon it reaches a soft, doughlike consistency. In this state, it is suitable for packing in the mold. If a sufficient amount of the monomer has been used, the surface of every particle of the polymer has been penetrated by the monomer. The depth of penetration or dispersion of the monomer in the polymer depends on both the amount of liquid used and the time allowed for its penetration into the particles. When packed in a mold and subjected to heat and pressure, the monomer polymerizes and the entire mixture then becomes one solid mass. If an insufficient amount of monomer is used, and if insufficient pressure and heat are applied, it is probable that some of the polymer particles will not be molecularly welded into one solid piece. Hence, care must be exercised that: (1) the proper proportions of powder and liquid are used; (2) a sufficient length of time be allowed for the polymer particles to be thoroughly wetted; (3) the mass be mixed thoroughly, so that a uniform distribution of the coloring ingredients shall be obtained and all the gross and microscopic air spaces be eliminated within the mass.

Second method. There is a second method of mixing monomer and polymer for the construction of crowns and bridges. In this method, a small amount of the powder is first placed on a glass slab. To this, monomer is added drop by drop from a medicine dropper in an amount sufficient to saturate the polymer. The saturated mass, which has a granular appearance, is immediately taken up with the tip of a spatula, and placed in the mold. While in this granular state, the mass is vibrated and settled into place. More is added until the crown or bridge is filled to its proper form. When two or more colors are employed, a separate pile is made of each powder, saturated with monomer, and each is applied where indicated.

If there is an excess of the liquid, it may be absorbed by adding dry powder to the small pile. While this method seems to have certain advantages, it cannot be used with all of the acrylics on the market today. It is primarily intended for those acrylic powders, the grain size of which is 100 mesh or finer. This method is not suitable for those powders which are coarser, because the finished prosthesis would have a definite granular appearance.

Third method. The third method of mixing monomer and polymer may be called the dry pack technic. The polymer is sprinkled dry into the crown mold. First the gingival color is applied, then the incisal, also in dry powder form. When a sufficient amount has been used to develop the contour of the restoration, monomer is added drop by drop from a medicine dropper, until the mass is saturated. The metal flask containing the mold is now vibrated or tapped on the workbench, so that the moistened particles of the mass gravitate to the deepest portions of the mold. Sufficient monomer is added to slightly oversaturate the mass. The excess liquid is absorbed by sprinkling on additional dry powder. This process of alternately adding powder and liquid is continued until the proper contour is developed. Here again there exists the danger that the coloring ingredients settle to the lower portion of the mold, resulting in poor color distribution.

Fourth method. A fourth method, sometimes used to veneer cast metal crowns, combines the polymer moistened with a special monomer and applied in small increments to the metal (Pyroplast). It is cured directly, exposed to 275° F. for 8 minutes after each laminated application. The metal is first covered with an opaque layer and cured for 8 minutes. Then the gingival and the incisal colors are applied and blended, followed by curing each lamination. A special type of curing oven is used, which controls the desired temperature and correct distance at which the restoration is maintained. When fully processed, the veneer is finished and polished in the customary manner.

Closure of flask

After the mold has been filled or, better still, slightly overfilled by one of the first three methods just described, a piece of moistened cellophane is placed over the lower half of the flask, covering the exposed acrylic resin. Trial closure is made. On separating the two halves of the flask, more material is added if needed. Then another trial closure is made, but at no time during the trial are the two halves of the flask brought into complete contact; a space of 1 mm. is maintained by means of shims, which are removed at the time that final closure of the flask is made before processing. Thereafter, the case may be processed by either the slowly rising high heat technic or the constant low heat technic. The following discussion does not apply to the autopolymerizing type of resins.

METHODS OF PROCESSING

High heat method of processing

First, the high heat or boiling water method will be considered. Certain phenomena have been observed during the processing of the acrylic resins particularly during the time that polymerization takes place. A study of the chart in Fig. 38-1 will help to explain them. This chart indicates the use of boiling water for the processing. It is apparent that there exists a definite time-temperature relationship in this procedure. Since resins react quickly to higher temperatures, it is advisable to start the processing of the crown or bridge at a relatively low temperature. The temperature reading on this chart begins at 30° C. or 86° F.

When the water has reached this temperature, the two halves of the flask are placed in a press and closed to within 1 mm. of complete closure. The flask held within the press is now submerged in the water, and heat is applied gradually so that there is an approximate temperature rise of 1° C., or 1.8° F., per minute. The dotted line *A*, also designated by *T1*, indicates the temperature of the water bath.

Processing temperature curves. It will be observed that in 10 minutes the temperature of the water will be 40° C. or 104° F.; in 20 minutes, 50° C. or 122° F., and so on. This is continued until the boiling point of water is reached, 100° C. or 212° F. It will be observed that the broken line *T1*, representing the temperature rise of the water and the flask, continues in a curved line, rising in proportion to the increase in temperature and lapse of time.

Immediately below is the line desig-

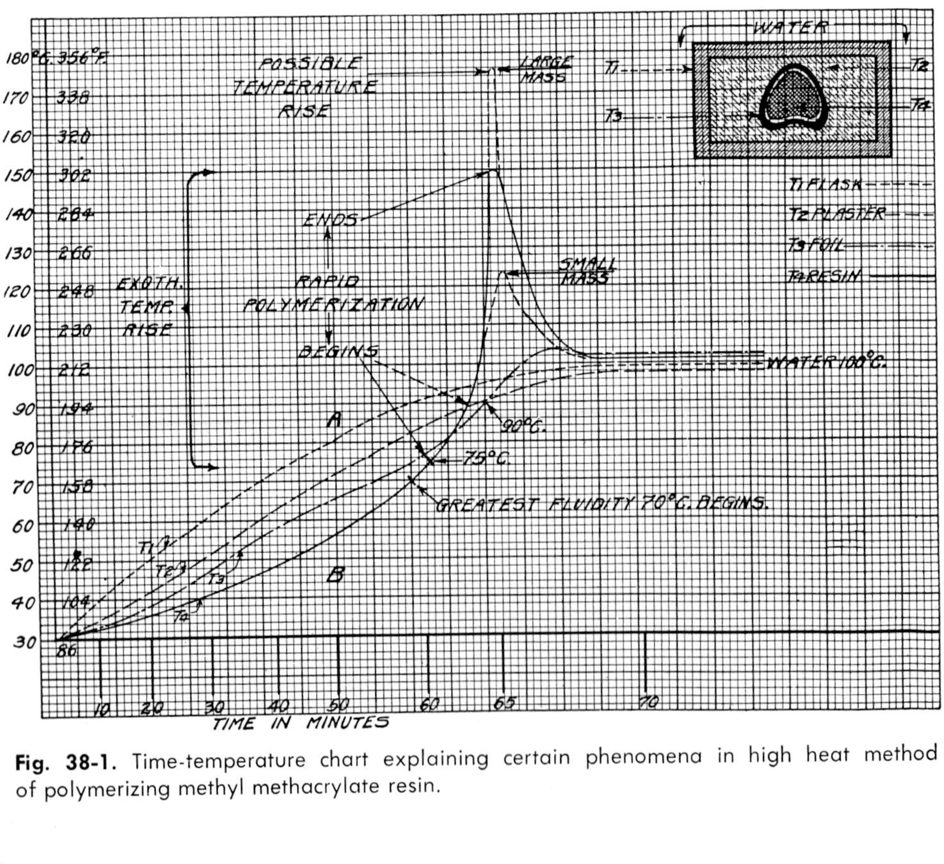

Fig. 38-1. Time-temperature chart explaining certain phenomena in high heat method of polymerizing methyl methacrylate resin.

nated as *T2*, representing the plaster investment material enclosed within the metal flask. This line also has a relatively proportional rise, but there is an initial lag because the investment is a relatively poor conductor of heat as compared to the metal flask, and, also, the investment is not in direct contact with the surrounding water.

The bottom, solid line *T4*, represents the resin enclosed within the tin-foiled, plaster-filled flask. It is observed that while the temperature of the resin mass also rises in proportion to the other curves during the first 40 or 50 minutes, there is a considerable initial lag in its relation to line *T1*, the temperature of the water.

In approximately 60 minutes, the temperature of the resin has risen to 70° C. (158° F.). This is the starting point of its greatest fluidity range, which extends approximately to 90° C. (194° F.). More will be said later regarding this fluidity range. Possibly a better term to explain the condition of the mass would be "plasticity," since the mixture does not revert to a fluid but merely becomes a softer mass.

Exothermic reaction—heat of reaction. During the next few minutes an interesting phenomenon manifests itself. Between 70 and 75° C. (158-168° F.), the resin temperature curve *T4* takes a sharp upturn, indicating an increase in temperature which is not due to externally transmitted heat. During the next few minutes, this temperature rise is very rapid, reaching its maximum at approximately 150° C. (302° F.). From this point it drops rapidly, and shortly the resin reaches the water temperature level of 100° C. (212° F.). This heat of reaction, also referred to as exothermic temperature rise, takes place during the time when the greatest amount and the most rapid polymerization occurs. According to Harold Vernon and to Willard Bartoe, chief physicist of Rhom and Haas Company, who assisted in the preparation of this chart, approximately 95 percent of the polymerization occurs during this short interval of time. As the volume of the polymerized mass is increased, the peak of the exothermic curve may rise to 175° C. (379° F.), or higher.

Where tin foil is used as a lining agent in the mold, the line *T3* indicates the temperature of the tin foil. It will be observed that where the acrylic line *T4* bends upward, it crosses *T3* at about 80° C. (176° F.). This causes the higher temperature of the acrylic resin to raise the temperature of the tin foil above 100° C. (212° F.), but only for a short time, for it quickly returns to the boiling point of water at the same time that the polymerized acrylic does. The temperature of the flask, investment, foil, and acrylic resin, at any given point, may be determined on the chart by dropping a vertical line. Such a line *A-B* at the 50-minute point indicates that when the flask is 80° C. (176° F.), the investment is 72° C. (161° F.), the tin foil 66° C. (150° F.), and the acrylic resin 56° C. (132° F.).

The data shown in the chart prompt the question, "When does polymerization begin and when is it completed?" It is known that only a slight degree of polymerization occurs before 75° C. (167° F.) is reached. At 75° C. (167° F.) polymerization develops rapidly, and in approximately 10 minutes, 95 percent of it is completed. The total time elpased from room temperature, 30° C. (86° F.), to this stage of polymerization is approximately 70 minutes. For safety's sake, it is recommended that an additional 30 to 60 minutes be allowed in boiling water in order to complete the polymerization, depending on the volume of resin in the mold.

When to close flask. The question may be raised, "Is complete closure of the two halves of the flask advisable before applying heat; if not, what is the temperature best suited for complete closure of the flask?" It is known that a thermal expansion of the acrylic resin occurs in the range

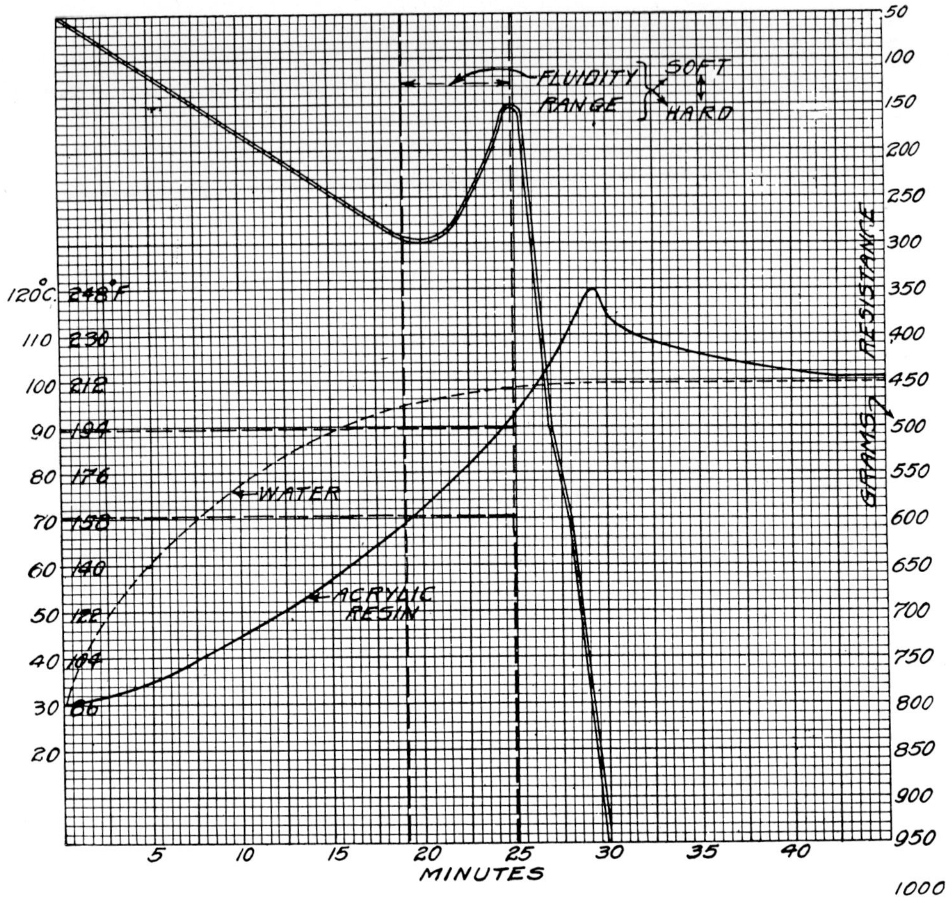

Fig. 38-2. Chart indicates why complete closure of flask should be made during certain temperature ranges.

extending from the initial temperature of 30° C. (86° F.), to 70° C. (158° F.); also, that an excess of material in the mold is recommended during this time-temperature interval. The complete closure of the flask should be made when the acrylic material is between 70 and 90° C. (158 to 194° F.), when the acrylic mass assumes its greatest state of plasticity. It is preferable to make the closure nearer 70° C. (158° F.) rather than the 90° C. (194° F.) temperature.

Plasticity curve. The chart in Fig. 38-2 shows the plasticity curve of the acrylic material during processing. It indicates in grams the resistance of the material to displacement under a load. Of the two lower curves, commencing at 30° C. (86° F.), the bottom dotted-line curve represents the reaction of the acrylic resin, and the middle broken-line curve represents the temperature rise of the heating medium, water. The upper double-line curve indicates the increased resistance of the acrylic material to displacement as the temperature of the acrylic resin is raised. This increase in resistance to displacement is characterized first by a gradual hardening of the mass, in this instance during the first twenty minutes or until the acrylic resin reaches the threshold of the plasticity range at a temperature of 70° C. (158° F.).

It will be observed that, at this point,

the downward path of the curve stops at 300 grams resistance, then reverses itself during the next 8 minutes, indicating a reduced resistance to displacement, or a gradual softening of the acrylic material until it reaches 90° C. (194° F.), or a point of resistance of 150 grams. The curve then drops sharply so that within 5 minutes it reaches a resistance of nearly 1,000 grams. It may be noticed that this approaches the crest of the exothermic curve; this may help to explain why complete closure of the flask is recommended during the short interval of time when the temperature of the acrylic material lies in the 70 to 90° C. (158 to 194° F.) range.

Elastic memory—skeletal molecular framework. During range of greatest plasticity and period of polymerization, a skeletal framework of molecules, or so-called elastic memory, is created; this is determined by the shape of the mold in which the restoration is processed. This skeletal molecular structure is permanent and is characteristic of each individual restoration. Any effort or technic that subsequently disturbs or displaces this molecular structure will set up internal stresses, which ultimately result in a distortion and misfit of the appliance, because the stressed molecular structure is constantly striving to resume its normal, original form.

Linear shrinkage of acrylic resin. It is impossible to eliminate entirely the shrinkage that occurs during the processing of acrylic resins. Linear shrinkage may vary from 0.47 to 0.56 percent, or an average of 0.53 percent, as shown by Sweeney,[4] at the Bureau of Standards. The use of the injector type of flask to force additional material into the hot mold while the enclosed polymerized resin is still soft, in an effort to eliminate this shrinkage, introduces stresses within the prosthesis. Shrinkage occurs only after polymerization of the resin has taken place; hence, any displacement of the polymerized resin by forcing additional material into the mold will result in setting up stresses. These are later released at mouth temperature resulting in a variation in the fit of the prosthesis.

When shrinkage occurs, it is not uniform throughout the molded object, due to variations in its size, shape, and cross-section areas.

Porosity. One of the annoying problems associated with acrylic resins is that of porosity. Porosity usually occurs in thick specimens containing a large volume of material, but it is sometimes a defect present in the less bulky restorations also.

As shown in the time-temperature curve (Fig. 38-1), when the acrylic resins reach the 70 to 90° C. (158 to 194° F.) range, the temperature rises precipitously within a short period of time, i.e., in a few minutes. When a large amount of acrylic resin is involved, polymerization, even though rapid, starts from the outer surface and progresses inwardly. When the temperature on the outer surface exceeds 100.3° C. and some free monomer remains within the center of the mass, it is possible for the monomer to be volatilized, and the gas so formed is trapped within the polymerized mass. It has been found that as the volume of the acrylic resin increases, the time of processing should be lengthened and continued at a lower temperature.

During the initial stages of polymerization, or before complete dispersion of the monomer and polymer has taken place, high temperatures may also cause the monomer to be volatilized and produce bubbles.

In order to control and reduce the excessive exothermic rise during the polymerization of acrylic resins, several time-temperature schedules have been recommended.

Low heat method of processing

A second method of processing has been suggested, in which the temperature of the water is brought to 160 to 165° F. and kept at this temperature range for a relatively long period of time. Recommendations* have been made which offer three posible methods[5]:

Method 1. (1) Immerse flask in room temperature water. (2) Adjust heat so that water will boil in from 1 to 3 hours (depending upon bulk of resin). (3) Boil 15 minutes.

Method 2. (1) Immerse flask in water at 160° F. constant temperature, and hold for 1½ hours. (2) Increase to boiling temperature and boil 30 minutes.

Method 3. (1) Immerse flask in water at 160° F. constant temperature. (2) Hold for 9 hours.

By the low, constant temperature method, polymerization occurs and the exothermic curve is flattened out; thus the possibility of gas and bubble formation is reduced.

Autopolymerization method (self-curing)

The autopolymerizing or self-curing types of resins have been developed that do not depend on heat to initiate the process of their polymerization. Extensive research has been done to determine the best methods for their use, and also to compare their physical properties with those processed by methods employing heat.

This method, used more in operative than in prosthetic dentistry, is the brush technic.[6, 7] The method is sometimes used to replace broken facings when it is impossible to do so with porcelain. To employ this method, self-curing resin powder and monomer are placed in separate dappen dishes. A fine-pointed camel or sable brush is moistened in the monomer, then touched to the dry powder. By capillary attraction a bead of wet powder attaches itself to the brush tip. This is then carried to the cavity and placed where desired. After 20 to 30 seconds when initial set has occurred, another bead is added. This procedure is continued until the mass is built up to the desired contour, whereupon it is covered with cocoa butter and permitted to polymerize for 15 to 20 minutes. At the expiration of this time it is trimmed to final contour with special burs and disks, after which it is ready for its final polish then, or at a later sitting.

This type of resin is self-curing and is activated by a catalyst to induce polymerization. The catalysts are of the benzoyl peroxide or of the paratoluene sulfinic acid types.

DISADVANTAGES OF POROSITY

Porosity has several definite disadvantages. (1) It weakens the structure in its resistance to forces. (2) The tiny bubbles produce a dispersion of light, which changes or modifies the color of the acrylic resin material. In clear acrylic material, this produces a milky or cloudy appearance in the finished prosthesis similar to that caused by exposure of the resin to water during processing. (3) The pores offer lodging places for bacteria and debris. (4) Pores are irritating to soft tissues.

DIMENSIONAL CHANGES DUE TO MOISTURE

When an acrylic appliance has been processed, there is still further opportunity for dimensional change after it is placed in the mouth. Although some acrylic resins have a water absorption factor of less than 0.5 percent by weight, others, on immersion in water, may show an absorption of almost 3 percent. The amount of water which an acrylic resin absorbs is quite important clinically. The work done at the Bureau of Standards[4] (Fig. 38-3) shows that acrylic resin dentures stabilized at a constant relative humidity of 32 percent, when placed in water, expanded approximately 0.8 percent within a period of 27 days. It was further noted that acrylic dentures which expanded on immersion in

*Developed by Harold Vernon, Vernon-Benshoff Co.

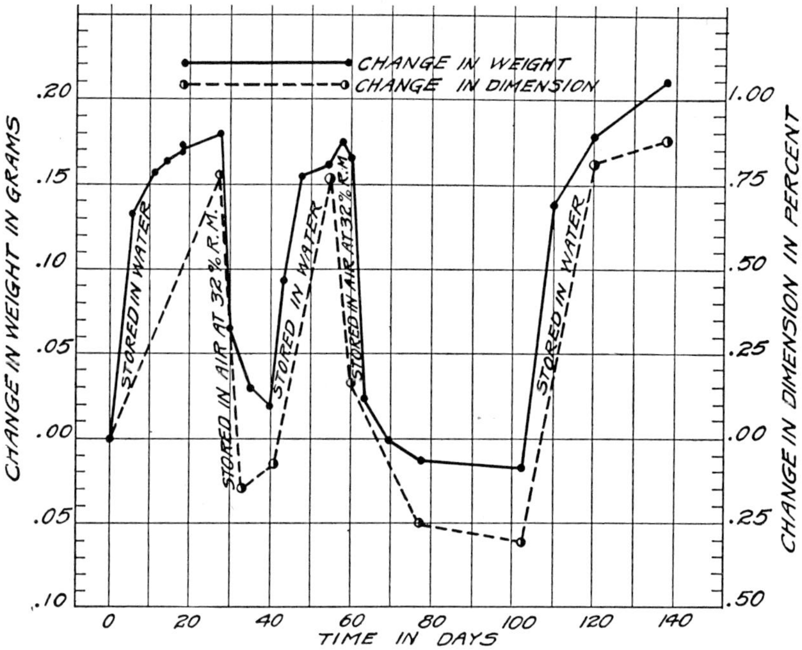

Fig. 38-3. Effect of water on acrylic resin denture at 37° C. (Courtesy U. S. Bureau of Standards; from Sweeney, W. T.: J. A. D. A. **26:**1963, 1939.)

water shrank when they were removed and exposed to the air to dry, and frequently shrank to less than their original dimensions. Slight dimensional changes occurring in complete dentures may be tolerated and compensated for by the resilient mucosa. They do not present the same degree of difficulties and dangers present in complete veneer crowns when the prostheses are in direct contact with hard and unyielding tooth tissue. Even a small fractional dimensional change of a cemented crown, from a dry to a saturated condition, may be sufficient to cause the failure of the restoration at the marginal cement joint. This reaction of the resin to moisture suggests that crowns made of acrylic resins should be immersed in water until they reach "saturation expansion," after which they are dried before being cemented.

No doubt a technic may be developed wherein the shrinkage incident to the processing of the material can be balanced by the subsequent expansion due to water absorption together with the use of a stone die material having a sufficient hygroscopic expansion.

BIOLOGIC COMPATIBILITY OF ACRYLIC RESINS

Clinically, the acrylic restorations have proved themselves to be biologically compatible if the tooth has been properly prepared, and if the restoration itself conforms to the same physiologic and mechanical requirement of the standard types of gold and porcelain restorations. Apparently, the absorption of water by the acrylic material does not react harmfully on the contiguous soft tissues. One of the objectionable features noted is a slight tendency of the material to become stained. This, however, may be the result of improper oral hygiene.

The acrylic resins are not resistant to abrasion when they are opposed by ground porcelain surfaces or by natural teeth whose surfaces are not smooth and rounded. Our observation has been that an acrylic tooth in contact with another acrylic prosthesis, in the presence of saliva, does not undergo any mechanical abrasion but it does flow.

COLD FLOW OF RESINS

The behavior of an acrylic resin in the mouth and under applied force has a decided influence upon its application and upon the design of the prosthesis in which it is used. The suitability of the acrylic resin for use in crowns and bridges has been questioned on the basis of its hardness, i.e., whether there is sufficient resistance of the material to penetration, abrasion, or cold flow.

The work of Peyton and Mann[8] indicated that even though an elastic recovery follows the removal of the load from the resin, this recovery is not complete, inasmuch as a permanent distortion remains. This finding of Peyton is based upon the application of a static load of 3,550 pounds per square inch, applied for 7 days continuously. It would be interesting to know what, if any, would be the permanent distortion of this material if loads comparable to the forces of occlusion were applied intermittently over a similar period of time. The question is raised whether such permanent deformation is cumulative under these conditions.

Clinical experience indicates that the acrylic resins possess the necessary toughness or resistance to impact force, provided there exists a sufficient bulk of material, and that no shearing planes are effective.

No attempt is made here to discuss the chemistry or detailed physical properties of the various types of synthetic resins, since this information may be found in texts on this subject.[9] It must be remembered that the profession is dealing with a comparatively new material applied to new uses. That the synthetic resins have their limitations is readily admitted by those studying their physical properties and clinical applications. The correct approach is not an effort to replace all other dental materials with it, but to determine by scientific study and clinical observation its rightful uses and limitations in dental practice.

INDICATIONS FOR ACRYLIC CROWNS

One of the prime indications for the use of the acrylic veneer crown is in very young patients.[9] There are instances, for example, in which the upper anterior central incisor has been fractured, or in which proximal decay has reached a point requiring the placement of a complete coronal restoration. In such patients the pulp chamber is usually large and the pulp would be endangered if a typical shoulder-type preparation were made for such a young patient in order to place a fired porcelain veneer crown. It is much better in such circumstances to use an acrylic veneer crown, which does not require the removal of all of the enamel nor the preparation of a gingival shoulder in the dentin. An acrylic crown would in this instance be the restoration of choice.

Occasionally, it is found that in close-bite patients the acrylic veneer is preferable to the porcelain veneer crown. In those mouths in which the teeth are of the opalescent dentin type, the so-called dentinogenesis imperfecta, it has been found that the acrylic veneer crown has served much better than the glazed porcelain type.

Where the bonded, porcelain veneer crown has failed over a cast gold core in combination with a bridge, it has been found that the acrylic type is less likely to fracture than one made of porcelain.

The second indication for acrylic resins in crowns is found in their use as a veneer for the cast gold crown. This type of veneer crown may be used in individual restorations or in crowns used as bridge retainers. Although the ground-in porcelain-facing type of crown may be used in the majority of cases, there are times when the acrylic veneer possesses certain advantages over the fired porcelain veneer.

Experience has shown that should a patient wear through the gold incisal protection, a porcelain veneer will snap out of the casting, whereas one made of acrylic veneer is elastic and flows under stress and will not break out of the casting. There are other conditions of unusual contour or occlusal relationship that have been more effectively met by the use of acrylic rather than glazed porcelain crowns.

Because the acrylic resins have a greater resilience than glazed porcelain, it is found that they are better able to absorb shock; for this reason acrylic crowns can be used successfully in very thin layers where porcelain could not be used (for example, in some adolescents). Consequently, in those instances in which a temporary protection is desired for the tooth of a child, and a shoulderless type of crown is indicated, it should be made of acrylic resin rather than of glazed porcelain.

Where temporary, corrective, or esthetic veneers are desired for public entertainers, these also may be made of synthetic resins.

ACRYLIC RESIN VENEER CROWNS: THE EFFECT OF TOOTH PREPARATION ON CROWN FABRICATION AND FUTURE PERIODONTAL HEALTH*

Acrylic resin veneers (or any of the tooth colored veneering materials) are placed on cast metal crowns for esthetic purposes only. Many veneered crowns that meet the requirements of fit and occlusion fail as restorations because they are not acceptable to the periodontium. They are not acceptable because they are oversized and improperly contoured, particularly on the veneered surface. As a general rule, unless the tooth is malposed, periodontally involved, or in contact with the clasp of a removable partial denture, the closer a veneered metal crown duplicates the size

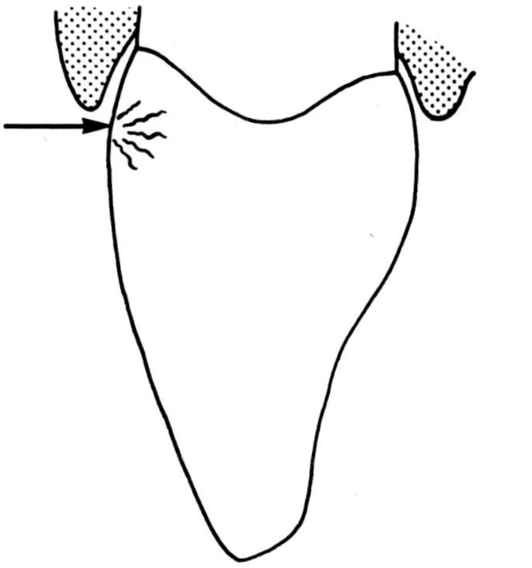

Fig. 38-4. Arrow on outline of upper central incisor indicates region of cervical finishing line on surface to be veneered. Preparation of this part of surface of tooth is critical to success of acrylic resin veneer crown. (Courtesy Dr. A. C. Long.)

and shape of the original tooth, the more acceptable it is to the periodontium. Improper tooth selection and inadequate reduction of the tooth surfaces to be veneered seem the most likely causes of oversized and overcontoured veneered metal crowns. All veneering materials require a certain thickness to esthetically mask the underlying metal, and the space for whatever thickness is necessary must be obtained during tooth preparation if overcontouring the veneer is to be avoided. While any tooth can be reduced enough to assure the necessary space, not all teeth can be successfully reduced because the end result with some teeth will be permanent pulp damage or exposure or insufficient tooth structure remaining to support the restoration. Therefore, not all teeth are suitable or can be successfully prepared for veneered crowns.[10]

To ensure adequate space for acrylic resin veneers on teeth that can be successfully reduced, two areas are most critical during tooth reduction; both are on the veneered surface or surfaces. First is the cervical finishing line which must be

*Summary by Alfred C. Long, Associate Professor of Dentistry, Ohio State University School of Dentistry.

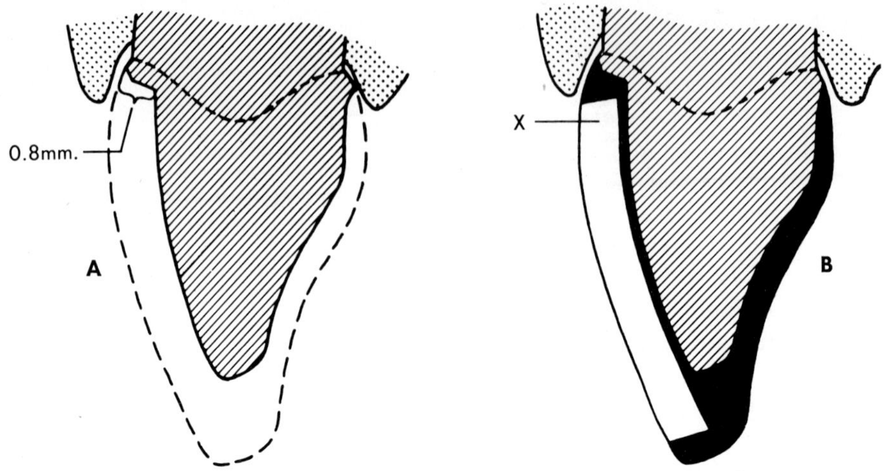

Fig. 38-5. Properly prepared tooth. **A,** Dotted line indicates contour of original tooth. Cervical finishing line on surfaces to be veneered must be a shoulder, at least 0.8 mm. wide. **B,** Acrylic resin veneer crown on tooth; 0.8 mm. shoulder permits acrylic resin veneer to extend apically to free margin of gingival tissues and to be thick enough at **X** to effectively mask underlying metal without being overcontoured. (Courtesy Dr. A. C. Long.)

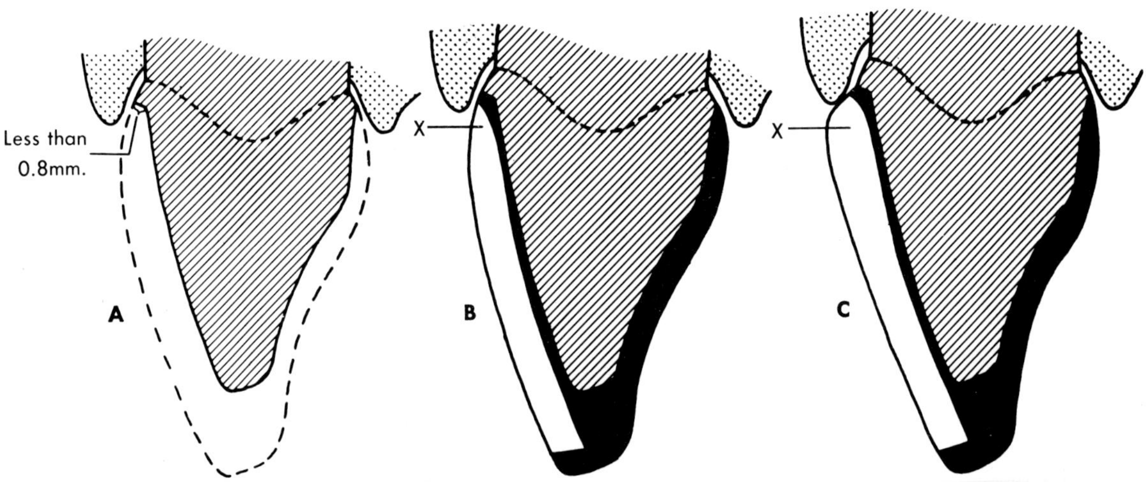

Fig. 38-6. Improperly prepared tooth. **A,** Cervical shoulder on this preparation is less than 0.8 mm. wide. **B,** Inadequate shoulder width permits acrylic resin veneer to extend apically to free margin of gingival tissues, but veneer is too thin at **X** to effectively mask underlying metal. **C,** Veneer on this crown is overcontoured at **X;** cannot mask metal. Resultant restoration does not duplicate size and shape of original tooth, as shown by dotted line in **A.** (Courtesy Dr. A. C. Long.)

a shoulder *at least* 0.8 mm. wide if the veneer is to extend apically to the free margin of the gingival tissues and also be thick enough in that area to mask the underlying metal without overcontouring (Figs. 38-4 to 38-6). If a wider shoulder can be successfully prepared, by all means do so. The shoulder must also extend onto the proximal surfaces if the veneer is to extend on to these surfaces (Figs. 38-7 to 38-9). The second critical area is the incisal or occlusal third of the veneered sur-

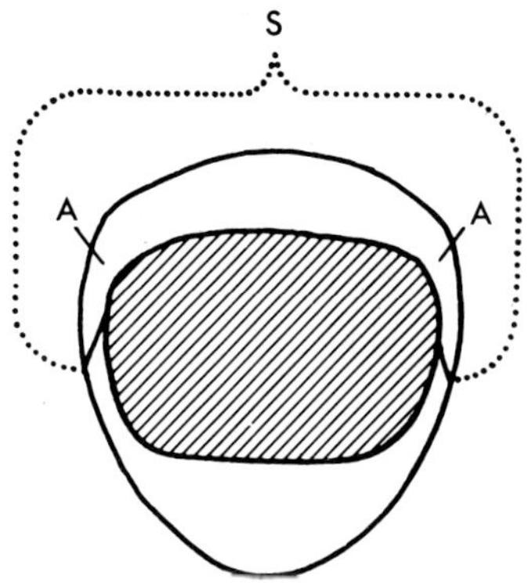

Fig. 38-7. Cross section through improperly prepared central incisor shown at level of proximal shoulder, **S.** Shoulder narrows or disappears as it approaches and extends onto proximal surfaces, **A.** (Courtesy Dr. A. C. Long.)

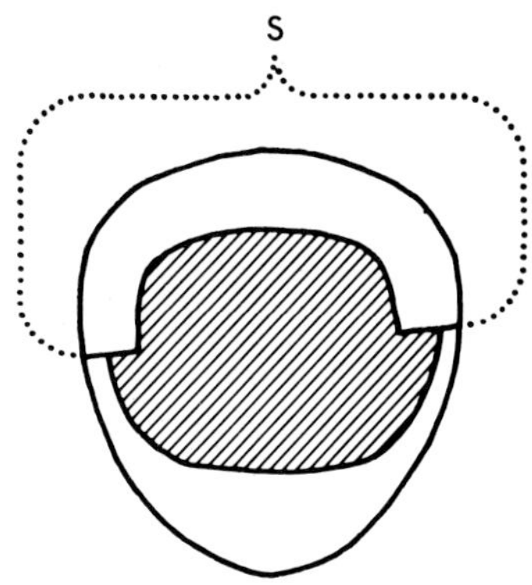

Fig. 38-8. Cross section through properly prepared central incisor shown at level of proximal shoulder, **S.** Entire shoulder must have adequate width to ensure veneer thickness. (Courtesy Dr. A. C. Long.)

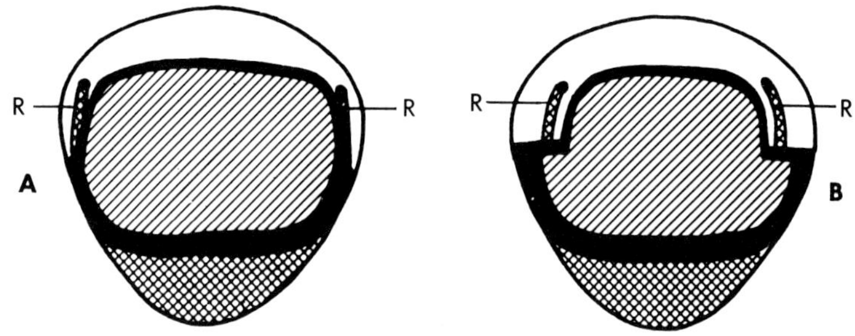

Fig. 38-9. Cross sections through two prepared upper central incisors and their acrylic resin veneered crowns shown at level of retentive loops, **R. A,** Inadequate proximal shoulder preparation has made proper positioning of retentive loops impossible. It is unlikely that loops in this position give adequate retention to veneer, and it is likely that veneer will not effectively mask them. **B,** Adequate proximal shoulder preparation permits proper positioning of retentive loops, **R.** (Courtesy Dr. A. C. Long.)

face. Most surfaces to be veneered have some vertical convexity and should have a similar convexity after preparation if the veneer is to have adequate thickness in these areas while duplicating original tooth size and shape in the restoration (Figs. 25-2, 25 3, 38-10, and 38-11). Too often, the prepared tooth surface from the shoulder to the incisal or occlusal is flat, while the original surface had some convexity. This practice usually results in inadequate veneer thickness at the incisal or occlusal third of the veneer (Figs. 38-12 and 38-13). When preparing posterior teeth, intercuspal distance can be used as a guide (Fig. 38-14). After preparation the distance between corresponding buccal and lingual cusps should be the same as or less than it was before preparation (Figs. 38-15 and 38-16).

The principles of tooth preparation for clasped veneered crowns are the same as for crowns that are not to be clasped. However, it is necessary to remember that the shape and size of a crown to be clasped usually differ to some degree from those of the original tooth. The difference and the degree are determined by the design of the removable partial denture and by its path of insertion (Fig. 38-17). Only

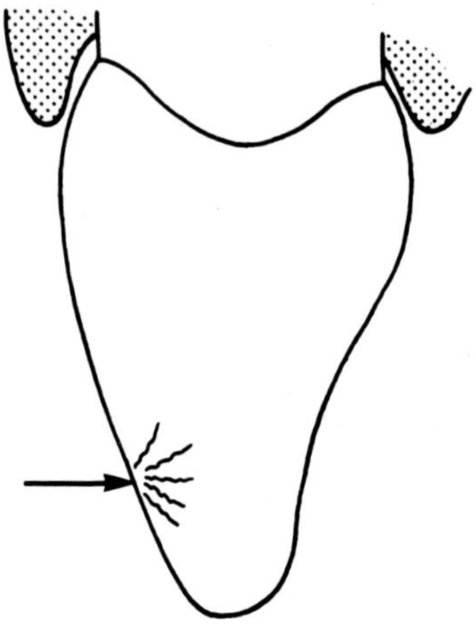

Fig. 38-10. Arrow indicates other critical part of preparation of labial surface of tooth to be veneered. Adequate tooth reduction in incisal third of labial surface is vital to success of acrylic resin veneer crown. (Courtesy Dr. A. C. Long.)

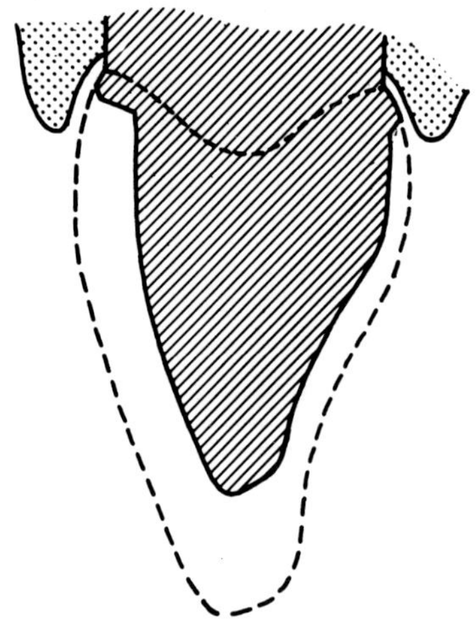

Fig. 38-11. Properly prepared tooth. Natural undercuts must be removed during preparation, but original tooth form or convexity, as shown by dotted line, is simulated in contour of preparation. (Courtesy Dr. A. C. Long.)

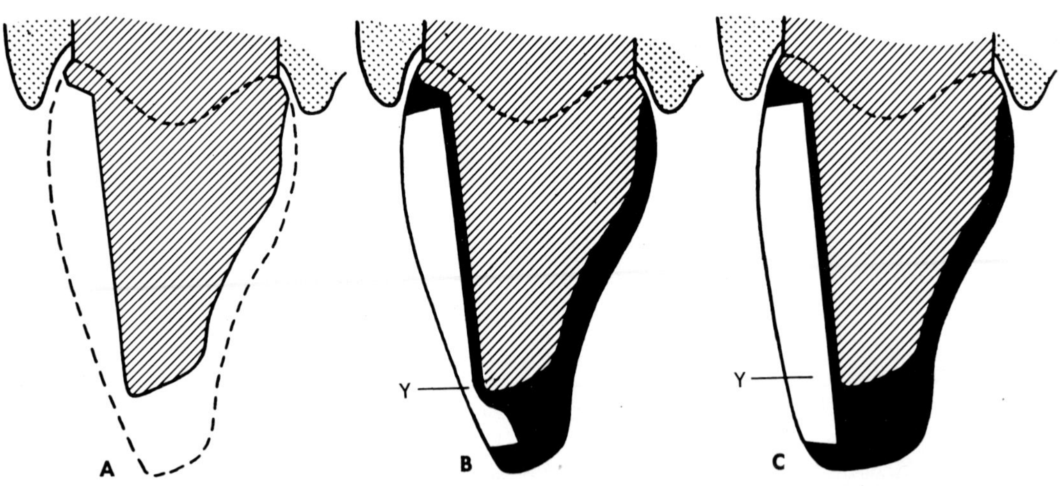

Fig. 38-12. Effect of inadequate preparation. **A,** Labial surface of preparation is too straight from shoulder to incisal edge. Adequate cervical shoulder has been prepared, but labial surface does not simulate form of original tooth. **B,** This error in preparation results in veneer being too thin at **Y** to effectively mask underlying metal. **C,** Alternative is overcontouring of veneer at **Y.** Resultant restoration does not duplicate size and shape of original tooth. (Courtesy Dr. A. C. Long.)

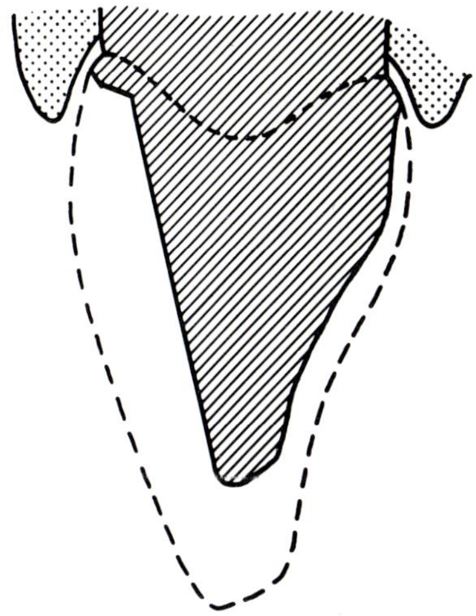

Fig. 38-13. Improperly prepared tooth. Flat labial surface in this preparation poses no problem in obtaining adequate veneer thickness at any point, but overreduction of middle and cervical thirds has weakened retention and resistance form and may have injured or exposed pulp. (Courtesy Dr. A. C. Long.)

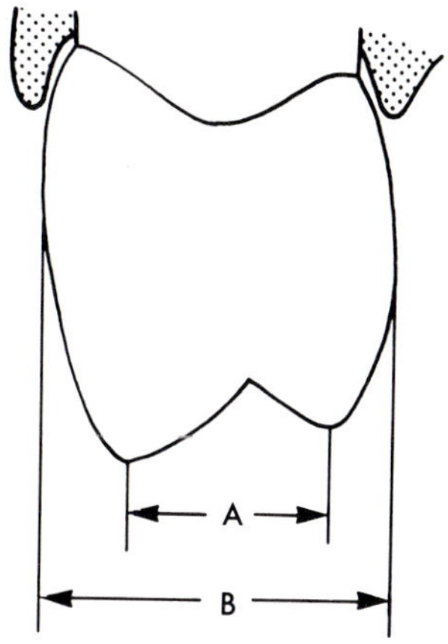

Fig. 38-14. Distance between cusp tips is less than overall width of posterior teeth. **A,** Buccolingual intercuspal measurement; **B,** greatest buccolingual crown measurement. **A** is one-half to two-thirds of **B** on approximately 80 percent of all posterior teeth. (Courtesy Dr. A. C. Long.)

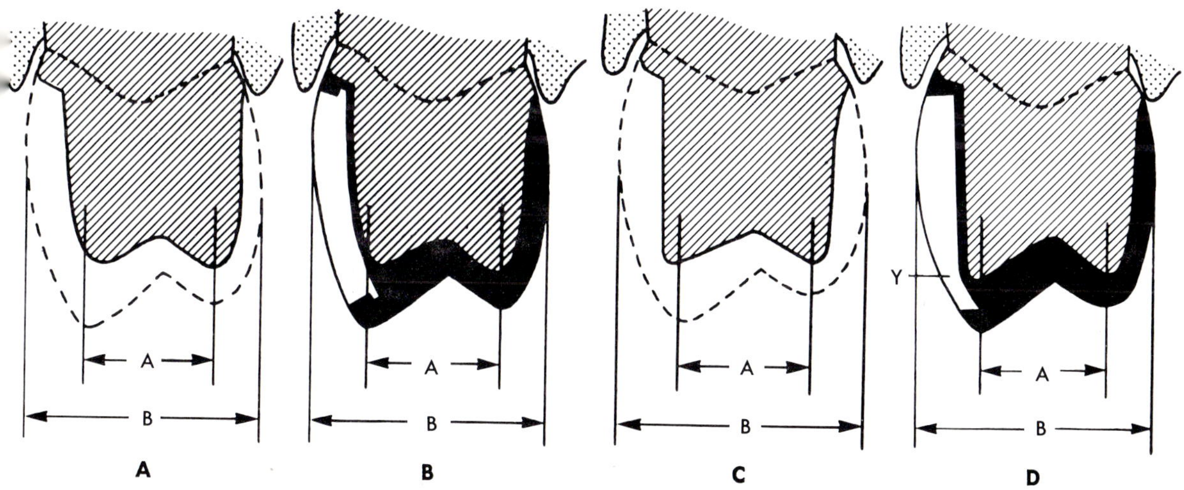

Fig. 38-15. Comparison of effects of properly and improperly prepared teeth. **A,** Properly prepared tooth (**A,** original buccolingual intercuspal distance; **B,** greatest original buccolingual crown width). Note that curvature of surface to be veneered closely follows original curvature of tooth (dotted line), and that intercuspal measurement of preparation is less than intercuspal measurement before preparation at **A. B,** Properly prepared tooth is covered by acrylic resin veneer crown that has adequate veneer thickness throughout. Note that dimensions at **A** and **B** have been duplicated in restoration. **C,** Improperly prepared tooth. Note that surface to be veneered is flat and that intercuspal measurement on preparation is greater than it was originally at **A. D,** Improperly prepared tooth is covered by acrylic resin veneer crown that does not have adequate veneer thickness at **Y,** because distances (**A** and **B**) are duplicated in restoration. (Courtesy Dr. A. C. Long.)

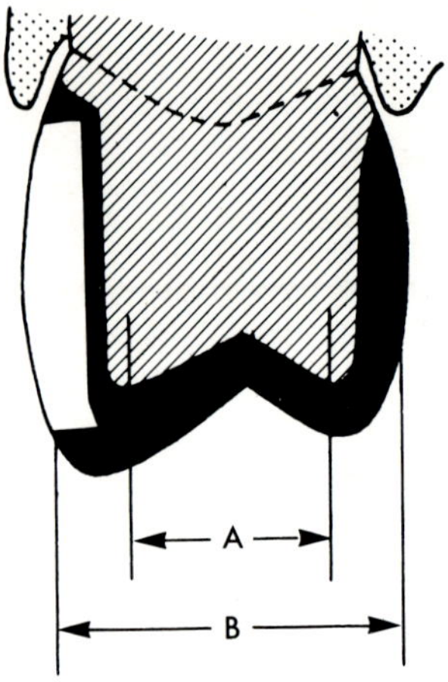

Fig. 38-16

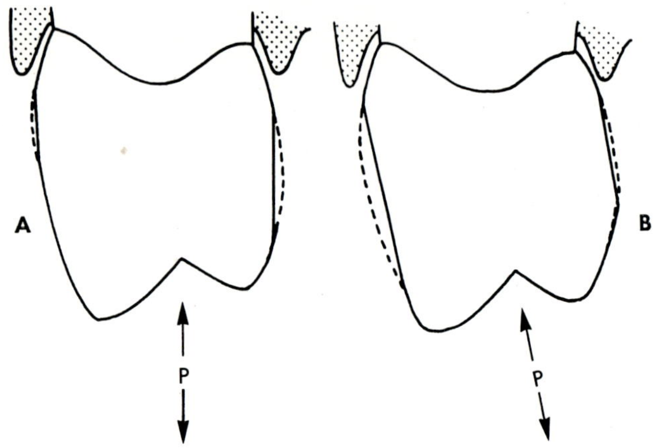

Fig. 38-17

Fig. 38-16. Improperly prepared tooth. **A,** Original buccolingual intercuspal distance; **B,** greatest original buccolingual crown width. Note general overcontouring of restoration necessary to obtain adequate thickness of resin veneer and metal thicknes and increased size of occlusal table; both changes resulted because insufficient tooth structure was removed from occlusal third of vertical walls of tooth and because intercuspal distance after preparation was greater than it was originally, **A.** (Courtesy Dr. A. C. Long.)

Fig. 38-17. Potential crown outlines are changed on identical tooth contours when indicated path of insertion, **P,** of removable partial denture is changed. **A,** Potential crown outline, as determined by path of insertion, **P,** varies only slightly from original tooth outline. **B,** Potential crown outline, as determined by path of insertion, **P,** varies considerably from original tooth outline, particularly on surface to be veneered. Dotted lines show original tooth outline in **A** and in **B.** (Courtesy Dr. A. C. Long.)

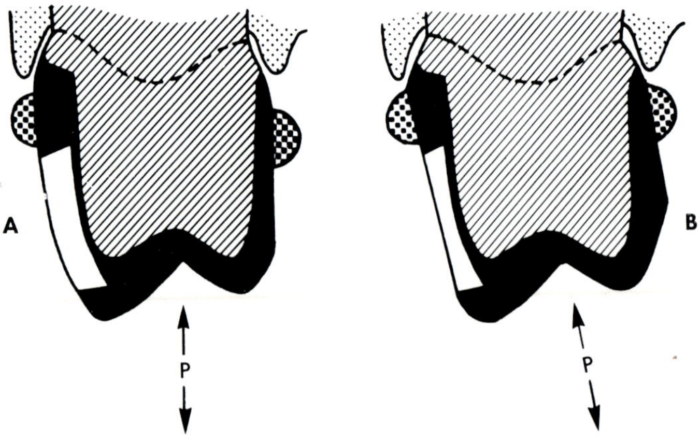

Fig. 38-18. Effect of changing path of insertion of removable partial denture on form of crown. Tooth has been properly prepared for veneer crown that is not to be clasped, but it has been restored with veneer crowns that are designed for clasping. Path of insertion, **P,** of removable partial denture is different on two drawings. **A,** Preparation is acceptable for this clasped crown since shape and size of this crown, as determined by path of insertion, **P,** still permit adequate veneer thickness. **B,** Identical preparation is not acceptable for this crown, since shape and size of this crown, as determined by different path of insertion, **P,** do not permit adequate veneer thickness. (Courtesy Dr. A. C. Long.)

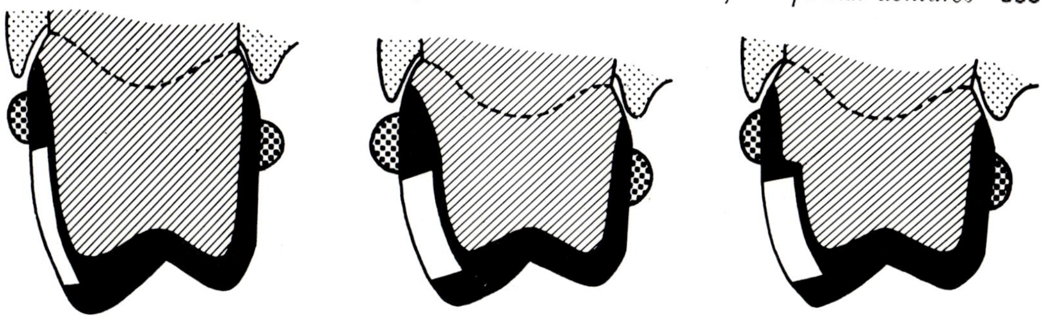

Fig. 38-19. Chamfer-type preparations are covered by acrylic resin veneer crowns that are retainers for clasps. **Left,** Retention and resistance forms have been maintained, but veneer thickness is inadequate. **Center,** There is adequate veneer thickness, but convergence of buccal and lingual walls of preparation toward occlusal surface has weakened retention and resistance forms. **Right,** Retention and resistance forms have been maintained, and there is adequate veneer thickness because of modification in preparation of buccal surface of tooth (note combination shoulder and chamfer on buccal surface of preparation). (Courtesy Dr. A. C. Long.)

when these factors become known, after a preliminary survey of the diagnostic cast, is it possible to estimate the amount and location of tooth reduction necessary to ensure adequate veneer thickness. Tooth reduction sufficient for a veneered crown that is not to be clasped, *may* or *may not* be sufficient for one that is to be clasped (Figs. 38-18 and 38-19).

Veneered crowns closely resembling original tooth shape and size cannot be used on every tooth since some teeth cannot be successfully prepared, and since a change from original tooth shape and size is indicated for some veneered crowns. However, many oversized, overcontoured, veneered crowns, which neither look like teeth nor are in harmony with the periodontium, could have been avoided if the critical areas of the preparation had been altered.

Repair of crowns utilizing synthetic resins

Acrylic resins may be used with satisfaction to replace a fractured, detached dowel type of crown. When such a fracture occurs and it is not deemed advisable to remove the dowel from the canal, the remaining portion is removed from the root face and a crown is contoured in ivory-colored wax, after which it is removed from the protruding portion of the dowel and prepared for investment in a crown flask.

A half-inch length of wire of the same diameter as the dowel remaining in the tooth is inserted into the opening in the base of the wax crown. After the crown has been processed and removed from the investment a pair of flat-nosed pliers is heated slightly. With this the wire extending from the base of the crown is grasped, and with a slight rotary motion it is withdrawn from the crown, leaving an opening that will fit the dowel extension still remaining in the natural tooth. The acrylic crown is then finished, polished, and cemented directly over the dowel.

Repair of facings

The acrylic resins have also proved very valuable in replacing fractured porcelain facings on pontics and crowns; these may be either of the long-pin-facing type or of the patented replaceable types. If the acrylic resins serve no other purpose than that of serving as a satisfactory material for repairing fractures, they deserve a place among dental materials. The fourth method, previously mentioned, of applying and curing the resin by open exposure to 275° F. is useful in repairing restorations not permanently attached to the teeth.

DISADVANTAGES OF ACRYLIC CROWNS

Opposed to the advantages mentioned above are certain disadvantages in the use of synthetic resins for crowns and bridges. Under certain conditions of pressure, the resins exhibit qualities of flow that may have serious end results. In individual restorations it has been observed that in the course of time well-rounded and well-placed contact areas frequently lose their convexities and become flat surfaces.

The property of flow in resins, while advantageous under certain conditions, as in the case of an acrylic veneer facing, may prove harmful if the flow of the material in a crown is sufficient to break the mechanical union at the gingival margins. Likewise, unless an acrylic crown has been saturated to its maximum expansion before being cemented, it will absorb an additional amount of water in the mouth, causing a dimensional change and breaking the existing union. Therefore, great caution must be used in the clinical application of this material. Just what the relationship is between the hardness of the synthetic resins and the amount of wear that restorations made of these materials undego is still being investigated. Whether actual attrition takes place or whether the loss of cusp height is the result of the displacement of the material due to flow should be determined by further investigation.

EARLY USE OF SYNTHETIC RESINS IN FIXED PARTIAL DENTURES

The first recorded use of synthetic resins for the construction of bridges is found in the literature as early as 1931; these were constructed by Geier[11] in Europe at that time. Due to the fact that the resins were not as highly developed as they are today nor available in the desired hues, the use of synthetic resin bridges did not make much progress until a more suitable type of acrylic resin was presented to the profession by the manufacturers in this country. The development of the acrylic bridge and its increased use parallels that of the acrylic veneer crown.

INDICATIONS FOR ACRYLIC FIXED PARTIAL DENTURES

Acrylic bridges are indicated in those places where esthetics are desirable. In the past, the fired porcelain bridge, reinforced with a metal truss, was the restoration of choice. This type of prosthesis, however, is very exacting in its technic and, usually, it is relatively expensive. The acrylic bridge meets the requirements of esthetics and at the same time it is economical to construct. Moreover, whereas the fired porcelain bridge requires manipulative skill above that possessed by the average dentist, the acrylic resin bridge is relatively simple to construct. Also, the acrylic bridge may be used at times where even the fired porcelain bridge is contraindicated. Its main advantage and use today is as a temporary structure while the permanent structure is being fabricated. It is also useful as a splint in periodontal treatment.

Advantages of acrylic fixed restorations

The advantages of the synthetic resin type of bridge[12] are the following.

"(1) It is esthetic to a high degree. The observation has been made and the nature of the material is such that it harmonizes and blends with the natural teeth better than any material at our disposal today. (2) The technic of constructing an acrylic bridge is relatively simple as compared to that required for making a glazed porcelain bridge which is reinforced with an iridioplatinum truss. (3) The time required for its construction is less than that necessary for other types of bridges, particularly the glazed porcelain bridge. (4) It is relatively inexpensive to make. (5) Reports in the literature, and clinical evidence, seem to substantiate the belief that the acrylic resin is biologically compatible to the oral tissues. (6) Properly processed methyl methacrylate is impermeable to bacteria, although the resin does not inhibit the growth of bacteria.

(7) The acrylic bridge is relatively durable. (8) It possesses a high impact strength. (9) It is light in weight. (10) It is easy to finish and polish. (11) Additional material may be added to it without remaking the entire structure. (12) If manufactured facings or crowns of acrylic resin are used, the color and contour of the bridge may be predetermined before the completion of the entire bridge."*

Disadvantages of acrylic fixed partial dentures

There have been noted, however, certain limitations and disadvantages:

(1) The acrylic resin is likely to be porous if it is not properly manipulated and processed. (2) If the restoration is placed under continuous pressure or submitted to intermittent pressure, it flows. This results in the loss of the contour, as well as its proximal contact areas. (3) Restorations made of acrylic resin have sometimes discolored in the mouth. While many explanations have been offered for this discoloration, the fact remains that occasionally it still occurs. (4) In the event of the failure of a pontic, it is almost inevitable that the entire restoration must be removed in order to make the repair. (5) It abrades easily. (6) There is the annoyance for those people who chew gum habitually of having the chewing gum stick to the restoration.[12]

In considering the above advantages and disadvantages it is evident that the acrylic bridge is not a panacea and that its use should be the exception rather than the general rule. The standard type of bridge using the porcelain facing with the cast gold occlusal portion is still the restoration of choice in the majority of cases.

Types of acrylic fixed partial dentures

Three types of bridges may be constructed in which the acrylic resins are employed. The first type of acrylic bridge is made entirely of the acrylic resin. Its primary use today is that of a temporary restoration. No metal is used either in the retainers or in the pontics of the restoration. Such a bridge is indicated in the anterior region of the mouth and is usually limited to a short span restoration. Because no metal is used, the two retainers are usually acrylic veneer crowns also.

The second type of acrylic restoration is that which employs metal retainers in the abutment teeth. These may be complete or partial cast veneer crowns or intracoronal inlays. The pontics are constructed in a manner similar to the regular type of fixed bridge except that instead of using a long pin porcelain facing, the porcelain part is replaced with acrylic resin. Special preparation and design of the gold portion of the pontic must be made in order to afford sufficient mechanical retention and protection against displacement of the resin. This type of acrylic bridge has proved quite satisfactory to date.

The third type of acrylic restoration is one in which the pontic is constructed entirely of acrylic resin but it is supported by an internal metal truss. With this type of bridge the standard cast retainers may be used or the ferrule type of castings may be made to go over the abutment teeth; these subsequently are covered entirely with the acrylic resin.

Types of abutment preparations

The preparation of teeth for three-quarter retainers and complete shoulder crowns has been fully described in previous chapters, and no further discussion of these is undertaken here. The metal, reinforcing truss, however, needs further consideration.

Use of metal trusses. The metal truss gives rigidity to the bridge, and at the same time it furnishes the necessary supporting strength to the acrylic pontic to withstand the forces of mastication. Therefore, the metal part must be made of an

*From Salisbury, G. B.: Modern trends in dental acrylics, D. Digest **51**:196, 1945.

alloy which possesses the necessary strength with minimum bulk. Pure gold and pure platinum are not suitable for this purpose; either type C or clasp metal gold alloys (type D) or one of the chrome cobalt types may be employed.

In order to obtain the maximum strength from a given amount of metal in the truss, various shapes and designs, similar to those considered in Chapter 35, have been developed for this purpose.

Types of metal trusses. Earlier, pieces of round wire extending from one retainer to the other were used; later, square wire was used. It was found, however, that wire alone did not afford the necessary amount of resistance to torsional or pressure forces.

The next development was the use of the T- and the Y-shaped metal bars, the same type as was used for fired porcelain bridges advocated by Swann (Chapter 34). While this shape of the truss bar was an improvement over the round or square bar, it still did not furnish the required amount of support for the resin.

Many other types of trusses were subsequently developed, some using cross pieces of heavy wrought wire placed at the center of each pontic; others resorted to a cast metal structure.

The advantage of the cast type of truss over the wrought-wire type lies in the fact that the extent and shape of the truss may be easily shaped in wax to meet any existing conditions irrespective of tissue irregularity or contour. Also the truss may be so positioned and shaped that it gives a saucerlike support to the pontic against the forces of compression and tension. A cast truss may also be reinforced and made thicker in those areas where greater forces will be exerted on the bridge.

Purpose of metal trusses. The question has been raised whether the incorporation of a metal within an acrylic restoration creates cleavage planes and areas of highly localized stress within the resin. To what degree these exist has not been definitely established; however, the characteristic properties of flow and elasticity that the acrylic resins exhibit are a definite handicap to their use in bridge restorations. A properly designed metal truss in an acrylic bridge has enabled it to withstand the forces of mastication to a limited degree.

A metal truss is always attached to the metal retainers in the abutment teeth. As previously stated, these may be either the complete cast crowns, the three-quarter crowns, or intracoronal retainers. At times the ferrule or thimble types of retainers are used, usually with the shoulder type of tooth preparation; these are covered entirely with the resin in the finished bridge.

Use of opaque resin. Where metal structures are used in conjunction with acrylic resins, it is necessary to cover the metal with an opaque resin to prevent the color of the metal from showing through in the finished bridge.

CONCLUSION

In conclusion it can be said that because the dental profession has a better understanding of the limitations as well as the advantages of this type of material in bridge prosthesis, the acrylic bridges as constructed today and the conditions under which they are used make it possible for the acrylic restorations to serve satisfactorily for longer periods of time under certain selected conditions.

SELECTED REFERENCES

1. Selbach, F. W.: Crowns and bridges of artificial resin, Zahnärztl. Rundschau. **26**:1, 1091, 1938.
2. Wilson, W. E.: Casting of plastic inlays and crowns, D. Digest **46**:202, 1940.
3. Weder, K.: Crowns, dowel teeth and bridges made of synthetic resins, Zahnärztl. Rundschau. **49**:3, 1940.
4. Sweeney, W. T.: Denture base material: acrylic resin, J.A.D.A. **26**:1963, 1939.
5. Vernonite Workbench: Low-heat technic pro-

cessing, Pittsburgh, Pa., 1945, Vernon-Benshoff Co., vol. 2, p. 1; vol. 4, p. 1.
6. Peyton, F. A.: Self-curing resins for direct inlay, J. Michigan D. Soc. **32**:32, 1950.
7. Nealon, F. H.: Acrylic restorations: operative non-pressure procedure, New York J. Dent. **22**:201, 1952.
8. Peyton, F. A., and Mann, W. R.: Acrylic and acrylic-styrene resins: their properties in relation to their uses as restorative materials, J.A.D.A. **29**:1852, 1942.
9. Tylman, S. D., and Peyton, F. A.: Acrylic and other synthetic resins used in dentistry, Philadelphia, 1946, J. B. Lippincott Co.
10. Long, A. C.: Acrylic resin veneer crowns: the effect of tooth preparation on crown fabrication and future periodontal health, J. Prosth. Dent. **14**:370, 1968.
11. Geier, W.: Experiences with Hekodent and Rockodenta-colloid as crown and bridge material in patients, Deutsche Zahnärztl. Wchnschr. **13**:191, 1931.
12. Salisbury, G. B.: Modern trends in dental acrylics, D. Digest **51**:196, 1945.

GENERAL REFERENCES

Adams, C.: Properties and uses of cold curing acrylic in prosthetics, Iowa D. J. **42**:20, 1956.

Alvares, L. C., and others: Radiopacity of acrylic resins, Oral Surg. **22**:318-324, 1966.

American Dental Association Specification No. 13 for Self-Curing Repair Resins (first revision approved December, 1958, effective Jan. 1, 1959), J.A.D.A. **58**:136, 1959.

Atkinson, H. F., and others: Pressure changes in polymerizing polymethyl methacrylate, J. Dent. Res. **44**:1040, 1965.

Buonocore, M. G.: Report on a resin composition capable of bonding to human dentin surfaces, J. D. Res. **35**:846, 1956.

Bowen, R. L.: Use of epoxy resins in restorative materials, J. D. Res. **35**:360, 1956.

Bergman, B. O.: Test denture for masticatory studies, D. Abst. **6**:678, 1961.

Bergman, B. O.: Studies on the permeability of acrylic facing material in gold crowns, a laboratory investigation using Na^{22}, Acta Odont. Scandinav. **19**:297, 1961.

Blatterfein, L.: Planning and contouring of acrylic resin veneer crowns for partial denture clasping, J. Prosth. Dent. **6**:386, 1956.

Brown, R. E.: Full gold-acrylic veneer crown, Roy. Canad. D. Corps Quart. **1**:11, 1960.

Caul, H. J., and Sweeney, W. T.: Relationship between residual monomer and some properties of self-curing dental resins, J.A.D.A. **53**:60, 1956.

Cornell, J. A., and Powers, C. M.: Effect of varying peroxide and polymer on the rate and degree of polymerization of polymethyl methacrylate slurries, J. D. Res. **38**:606, 1959.

Cornell, J. A., Stone, K., and Ellis, S.: Tensile strengths of modified methyl methacrylates and various rates of loading, J. D. Res. **34**:740, 1955 (abst.).

Cornell, J. A., and others: Method of comparative wear resistance of various materials used for artificial teeth, J.A.D.A. **54**:608, 1957.

Crone, F. L., and Bloch, P.: Penetration of C^{14}-labelled methyl-metacrylate into the dentine, Acta Odont. Scandinav. **16**:247, 1958.

Ehrlich, A.: Erosion of acrylic resin restorations, J.A.D.A. **59**:543, 1959.

Fiasconaro, J. E., and Sherman, H.: Sealing properties of acrylics, New York D. J. **18**:189, 1952.

Fitz Roy, D. C., Swartz, M. L., and Phillips, R. W.: Physical properties of selected dental resins, part II, J. Prosth. Dent. **13**:1108, 1963.

Frankel, H. J.: Uses of autopolymerizing acrylic resins in fixed partial prosthesis, J. Prosth. Dent. **8**:1003, 1958.

Franks, A. S. T.: Clinical appraisal of acrylic tooth wear, D. Pract. & D. Rec. **12**:149, 1962.

Goodfriend, D. J.: Practical analysis of occlusal procedures, J. Prosth. Dent. **16**:557-571, 1966.

Hall, R. W.: Retention for cast gold acrylic veneer crowns, Roy. Canad. D. Corps Quart. **1**:15, 1960.

Hedegard, B.: Cold polymerizing resins: a clinical and histological study, Acta Odont. Scandinav. **13**(supp. 17):13, 1955.

Hedegard, B.: Evaluation of materials for anterior bridges with special reference to acrylic resins, Internat. D. J. **12**:33, 1962.

Hirsch, L., and Weinreb, M. M.: Marginal fit of direct acrylic restorations, J.A.D.A. **56**:13, 1958.

Issa, H.: Marginal leakage in crowns with acrylic resin facings, J. Prosth. Dent. **19**:281, 1968.

Kafalias, M. C., Swartz, M. L., and Phillips, R. W.: Physical properties of selected dental resins, part I, J. Prosth. Dent. **13**:1087, 1963.

Klaffenback, A. O.: Anterior fixed bridge prosthesis including acrylic resins, J. South. California D. A. **13**:19, 1940.

Klaffenbach, A. O.: Anterior fixed bridge prosthesis including acrylic resins, J.A.D.A. **34**:670, 1947.

Kramer, I. R. H.: Development of characteristic changes in the dental pulp following the use of resins containing methacrylic acid, J. D. Res. **34**:782, 1955 (abst.).

Kramer, I. R. H.: Reaction of the pulp to self polymerizing resins, Brit. D. J. **101**:378, 1956.

Krikos, A.: Self-curing resins in constructing patterns for small castings, J. Prosth. Dent. **20**: 235-238, 1968.

Lamstein, A., and Blechman, H.: Marginal seepage around acrylic resin veneers in gold crowns, J. Prosth. Dent. **6**:706, 1956.

Langeland, K.: Pulp reactions to resin cements, Acta Odont. Scandinav. **13**:239, 1956.

Langeland, K.: Pulp reactions to resin cements, D. Abst. **2**:660, 1957.

Lastra, M. J.: Comparative study of acrylic and porcelain jacket crowns, D. Abst. **2**:76, 1957.

McCune, R. J., Phillips, R. W., and Swartz, M. L.: A study of a new resin veneering material, J. South. California D. A. **36**(12): 496, 1968.

McLean, J. W.: Some physical properties of a new cross-linked plastic filling material, Brit. D. J. **110**:375, 1961.

Manning, J. E.: Guide to use of acrylic resin filling materials, Internat. D. J. **8**:48, 1958.

Martins, E. A., and others: Properties of custom-made plastic teeth formed by different techniques, J. Prosth. Dent. **12**:1059, 1962.

Miller, T. H.: Allergies to acrylic resins, Iowa D. Bull. **40**:285, 1954.

Muller, O., and Maeglin, B.: Histological changes in the pulp of teeth filled with self polymerizing resins, Internat. D. J. **4**:167, 1953.

Myerson, R. L.: Use of porcelain and plastic teeth in opposing complete dentures, J. Prosth. Dent. **7**:625, 1957.

Myerson, R. L.: Effect of cross-linking on mechanical damping and stiffness of methacrylates, I.A.D.R. **40**:89, 1962 (abst.).

Nealon, F. H.: Acrylic restorations; operative non-pressure procedure, J. Prosth. Dent. **2**:512-518, 1959.

Ohashi, M.: Observations on the generating mechanism of internal porosity in polymerization of methyl methacrylic resin for dental use. J. Nihon Univ. School Dent. **4**:1, 1961.

Peyton, F. A., and others: Restorative dental materials, St. Louis, 1960, The C. V. Mosby Co.

Peyton, F. A.: Various developments in dental plastics, Minneapolis Dist. D. J. **38**:69, 1954.

Peyton, F. A., and Craig, R. G.: Current evaluation of plastics in crown and bridge prosthesis. J. Prosth. Dent. **13**:743, 1963.

Phillips, R. W.: Newer restorative resins, J. Indiana D. A. **42**:151-152, 1967.

Pine, B.: Pontics for gold-acrylic resin fixed partial dentures, J. Prosth. Dent. **12**:347, 1962.

Roche, H. A. P.: Assessment of the values of porcelain versus methylmethacrylate in jacket crown and bridgework, Brit. D. J. **87**:23, 1949.

Rose, E. E., Lal, J., and Green, R.: Effects of peroxide, amine and hydroquinone in varying concentrations on the polymerization rate of polymethyl methacrylate slurries, J.A.D.A. **56**: 375, 1958.

Rose, E. E., Lal, J., Green, R., and Cornell, J. A.: Direct filling resin materials; coefficient of thermal expansion and water sorption of polymethyl methacrylate, J. Dent. Res. **34**:589-596, 1955.

Ryge, G., and Foley, D. E.: Effect of dry heat processing on the physical properties of acrylic crowns, J.A.D.A. **66**:672, 1963.

Sausen, R. E., Armstrong, W. D., and Simon, W. J.: Penetration of radiocalcium at margins of acrylic restorations made by compression and noncompression technics, J.A.D.A. **47**:636, 1953.

Schwartz, N. L.: Processing acrylic resin veneers using sectional cores, J. Prosth. Dent. **10**:330, 1960.

Selberg, A.: Acrylic veneers and bridgework, J. Tennessee D. A. **29**:28, 1949.

Seltzer, S.: Penetration of microorganisms between the tooth and direct resin fillings, J.A.D.A. **51**:560, 1955.

Sim, J.: Allergic reaction to denture base material, J. Canad. D. A. **24**:292, 1958.

Skinner, E. W., and Jones, P. M.: Dimensional stability of self curing denture base acrylic resins, J.A.D.A. **51**:426, 1955.

Slack, F. A.: Notes on dentures, jackets, crowns and bridges, J.A.D.A. **32**:1112, 1945.

Slack, F. A., Jr.: Experiments in directional polymerization, D. Digest **63**:356, 1957.

Slack, F. A., Jr., Sweeney, W. T., McParland, P. V., and Miller, I. F.: Use of acrylics for crowns, bridges and inlays, Pennsylvania D. J. **12**:115, 1945.

Soremark, R., and Bergman, B.: Studies on the permeability of acrylic facing material in gold crowns; a laboratory investigation using Na^{22}, Acta Odont. Scandinav. **19**:297, 1961.

Terry, I. A., and Harrington, J. H.: Abrasion tests on acrylics, J.A.D.A. **65**:377, 1962.

Vernon, H. M.: Glossary of terms used in plastic arts, J. Prosth. Dent. **8**:1055, 1958.

Vieira, D. F., and Phillips, R. W.: Influence of certain variables on the abrasion of acrylic resin veneering materials, J. Prosth. Dent. **12**: 720, 1962.

Waerhaug, J., and Loe, H.: Tissue reaction to selfcuring acrylic resin implants, D. Pract. & D. Rec. **8**: 234, 1958.

Waerhaug, J., and Zander, H. A.: Reaction of gingival tissues to self-curing acrylic restorations, J.A.D.A., **54**:760, 1957.

Yamamoto, T.: Self-curing acrylic pattern used in indirect technic for casting full crowns, D. Abst. **7**:515, 1962.

Chapter 39

Fundamental mechanics of fixed dental restorations; relation of mechanical forces to biologic reactions*

Symbols used:

F	Force
P	Load
R	Resultant of force system; also reaction of a beam
M	Moment of a force; bending moment in a beam
x, y, and z	Unknown distances; indeterminate distances
S	A unit stress
S_x or S_z	Unit stresses at extremities of x and z
da	A very small or differential area
A	A cross-sectional area
S_s	A unit stress in shear
S_p	Unit stress at the proportional limit; yield strength of a material
E	Modulus of elasticity of material
K	Modulus of resilience of material
T	Torque; toughness of material
ε	Gr. letter epsilon used to denote unit elongation of material under stress
e	Total elongation of material under stress; also eccentricity
V	Total shear on a beam section
M_R, M_L	Bending moments at right and left
×	Sign for multiplication
dx or dz	Differential increments of indeterminate distances
NA	Neutral axis of a beam
c	Distance from neutral axis of a beam to outer fiber
Σ	Gr. letter sigma used to denote summation
cg	Center of gravity of a force system or of an area
I	Axial moment of inertia of a beam section
$\frac{I}{c}$	Section modulus of a beam
J	Polar moment of inertia of a torsion member
θ	Gr. letter theta used to denote an angle or angular rotation of a beam section
ϕ	Gr. letter phi also used to designate an angle
i and di	Used for intercepts, swept out by tangents to the elastic curve of a beam
f and y	Deflections of a beam
kL	Fractional parts of the span length of a beam
/ or —	Each indicates a sign for division; thus $bd^3/12$ indicates $\frac{bd^3}{12}$

*Text by R. C. Brumfield, C. E.: Formerly Associate Professor of Civil Engineering, Cooper Institute, New York, New York.

INTRODUCTION

Consideration of forces and materials should be an inevitable accompaniment to the planning and construction of a dental bridge. The primary purpose of the dental bridge is to receive the forces of occlusion and to transmit them through the abutments to the bony structure of the maxilla or the mandible. These forces arise from the facial muscles that are attached to the mandible and may be of considerable magnitude. The forces of mastication react upon the bridge, which transmits them, and produce effects within it that tend to destroy it, if the effects are large enough. A bridge that is properly proportioned to withstand these effects will retain its original form and give satisfactory service as a restorative device for carrying loads arising from mastication. If the bridge is not properly proportioned, it may be subject to permanent distortion or to actual rupture, thus interrupting its service and giving rise to patient dissatisfaction.

Since consideration of force and its relationship to the dental bridge is of vital importance to the service of the bridge, it becomes necessary to know what constitutes a force and to consider methods of dealing quantitatively with it and its effects upon the bridge that carries it.

FORCE

A force may be defined as any influence which, when exerted upon a body, tends to set the body into motion or to alter its state of motion, if such motion previously existed.

Examples of force are numerous. The force of gravity is a most familiar one. It is universal and tends to pull all objects toward the center of the earth. It is this force that must be combatted by most of our bodily exertions and by the devices of the rocketeer in launching satellites. Forces range from those too small to be comprehended to the irresistible ones of nature that bring about our earthshaking catastrophies.

The definition of a force, in terms of its effect upon a body, is not sufficient to permit it to be dealt with in the quantitative fashion necessary in considering its effects upon the dental bridge. Consideration will show that any force is completely defined only by evaluating three of its characteristics, which are entirely independent of each other. These independent characteristics are (1) the line of action of the force, (2) the direction of action of the force along this line, and (3) the intensity of the force (its value in pounds, kilograms, ounces, or grams).

It should be noted that each of these three characteristics is entirely independent of the other two. The line of action of a force may be changed but its direction and intensity remain unaltered. Also the direction of a force along a line may be reversed though the line and intensity remain unaltered. Again, intensity depends neither upon the line of action nor upon the direction along that line.

In order to visualize the force and its effects, it is convenient to represent it graphically. A straight line carrying an arrow does this quite satisfactorily as shown in Fig. 39-1. In this illustration the straight line itself represents the line of action of the force, the arrow placed on the line shows the direction of action along this line, and the length of the line (to some appropriate scale) may be made to represent the intensity of the force. This simple method of representation is quite useful in visualizing the force as well as in dealing quantitatively with its effects.

For convenience in discussion, forces are often classified from different standpoints. It is desirable to mention a few in connection with the dental bridge and the effects of forces of mastication upon it. Forces are said to be either coplanar or noncoplanar. When a number of lines are drawn to represent forces, such as those

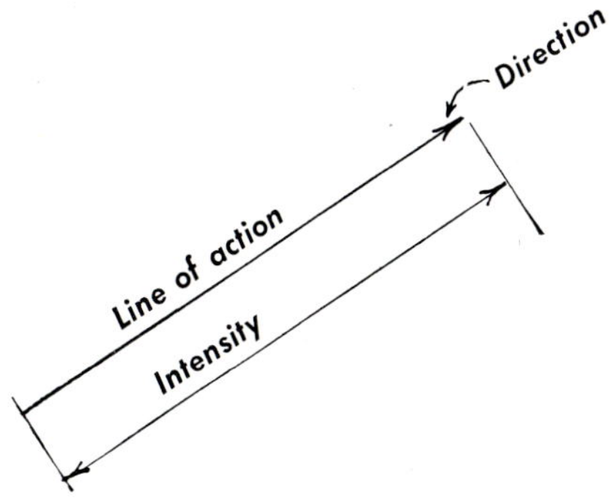

Fig. 39-1. Graphic representation of force.

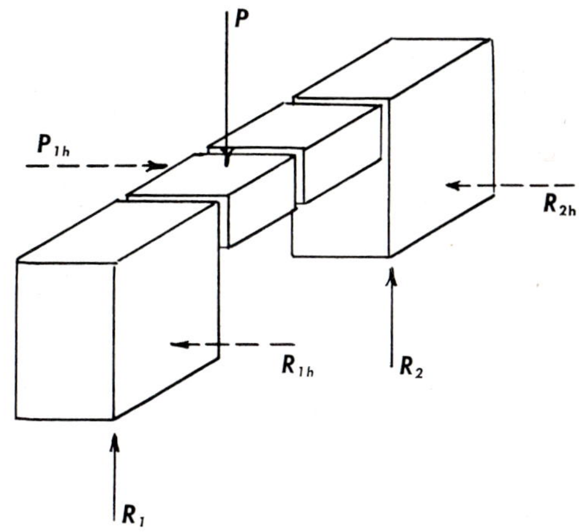

Fig. 39-2. Coplanar and noncoplanar forces.

shown in Fig. 39-1, and if these all lie in one plane, such a system of forces is said to be coplanar. An example of such a system is the forces acting upon the small dental bridge shown in Fig. 39-2 (full lines). Here an applied load, *P*, acts near the center of the bridge, and two forces of reaction, R_1 and R_2, act at the two abutments in the opposite direction. These three forces all lie in the plane of the axis of the bridge and its abutments and hence are coplanar. If to this system is added a lateral force P_{1h}, caused by the transverse motion of the mandible in mastication, this new force lies in a plane approximately perpendicular to the plane of the previously mentioned forces, as do the reactional forces R_{1h} and R_{2h}, caused by the lateral force. The combination of the two sets of forces is said to constitute a noncoplanar system of forces, since not all lie in the same plane. Such noncoplanar systems may become much more complicated than the one shown.

Forces may be classified also according to the impact effects that they produce upon the body to which they are applied. For instance, a book may lie quietly upon a table. The table and the book are both at rest. The force that the book exerts upon the table is simply its weight, as measured by its gravitational attraction. This force is said to be a *static* force. The book, upon being placed on the table, may have been dropped. In this case, when the book made contact with the table, it exerted against the table not only its weight but also an additional force caused by the check in velocity which the table produced. As a consequence, it momentarily exerted against the table more force than the static force previously mentioned; just as a hammer, when striking an anvil, momentarily exerts more force than it would if lying quietly upon the anvil. Thus the momentary effect of the falling book is greater than its static effect. Therefore, the table deforms more under this effect than it would if the book had been laid quietly upon it. However, at the peak of this excessive deformation it comes to rest, at which time the book can exert only its weight upon the table. The table, being deformed in excess of that which the weight alone could produce or can maintain, springs back and produces an excess deformation in the opposite direction. This process is repeated rapidly, causing vibrations in the table, until the excess energy of the falling book is dissipated through heat and the book and the table come to rest. In this final condition, the book again exerts static force against the table.

A force that exerts an influence upon an object, by virtue of its striking velocity as well as that resulting from its weight, is called an *impact force.* When striking velocities are high, impact effects upon a body may be very much greater than the static effects of the same force. Impact forces have a very wide range of effects, varying in intensity from those that in certain cases may theoretically approach infinity to very low effects that approach in value those of the static load.

If the book had been brought just in contact with the table but allowed to bear no weight upon it, and if then its weight had been released in zero time (assuming that this was possible), the book would have exerted its full gravitational force against the table during the deformation of the table. This is a very low form of impact load, called a *sudden load.* Theoretically, the sudden load momentarily exerts twice the pressure that the same load would exert after the receiving structure has vibrated to the deformation of a static load.

The moving mandible in the human mouth produces something of the effect of an impact load upon the occlusal surfaces. It is desirable to consider this effect in planning structures to carry the forces of occlusion.

RESOLUTION AND COMPOSITION OF FORCES

It has been stated that a force is an influence that moves or tends to move a body. If more than one force is exerted upon a body at the same time, it is a basic principle that the effect produced by one may be considered independently of that produced by each of the others. Such independent effects may later be combined to produce a composite effect. When a gun is fired, the explosion forces the bullet to travel in the line of the gun barrel and out through the muzzle. However, as soon as it leaves the muzzle, it begins to fall toward the earth—the action of gravity. Its composite line of travel is a curve, concave downward. The bullet strikes the earth's surface at the point at which this curve intersects that surface. The point of striking would be the same if the bullet had been allowed to travel in a straight line to a point directly over its striking point and had then been allowed to fall vertically to the earth.

With the principle in mind that each force produces an independent effect, consider Fig. 39-3. Here a body, *A*, is acted upon by two intersecting forces, F_1 and F_2. If each could produce its own effect independently, F_1, being the greater force, would move the body to p_1 in the same length of time that F_2 moved it to p_2. Actually the movements take place simultaneously in differential amounts, as indicated by the little triangle in the center of the diagonal of the rhombus, whose sides are parallel to the forces. The result is that movement occurs along the diagonal. The location of *A* at any particular instant will be found upon the diagonal. Since movements are proportional to intensities, it is evident that a similar procedure may be used for finding either movements or intensities of the forces that cause movement.

From this it is evident that if a system of coplanar intersecting forces acting upon a body is laid off successively to scale, each with its proper line of action, direction, and intensity, as shown in Fig. 39-4, the single force that would produce the same result upon the body, as regards its tendency to move, is represented completely and to scale by the line joining the ends of the first and last forces laid off. Thus the force labeled *R* is this force. It is called the *resultant* of the force system. It is axiomatic that if two forces are equal and have the same line of action but act in opposite directions along that line, each neutralizes the other and no motion is produced upon a body on which they may act. Thus, if the force at the right is added, exactly equal and opposite to *R*, the effect

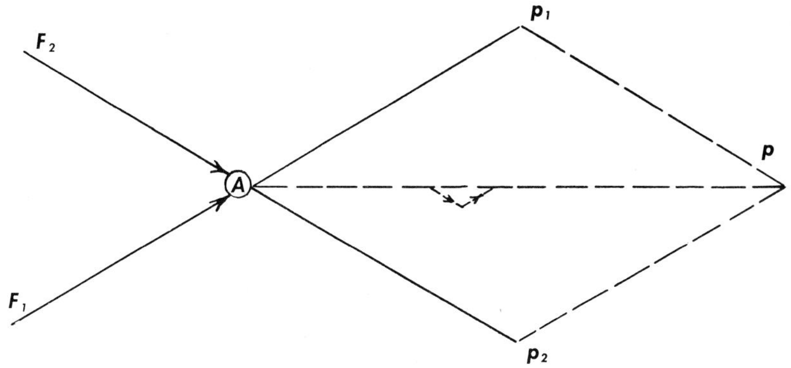

Fig. 39-3. Independent effects of forces.

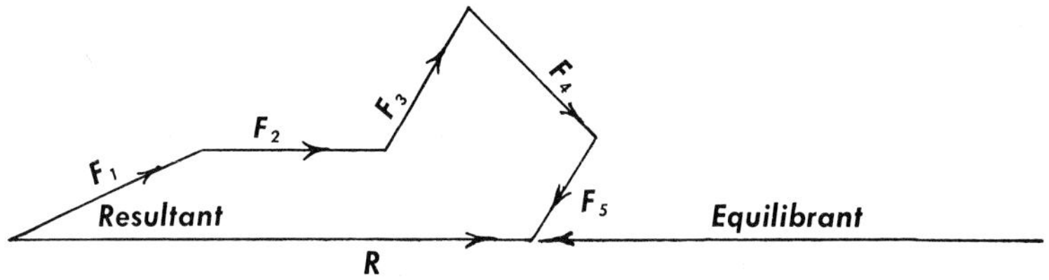

Fig. 39-4. Force system—resultant and equilibrant.

of the whole force system is neutralized. This force, equal and opposite to the resultant, is called the *equilibrant* of the force system. The equilibrant is exactly equal to the resultant in intensity, has the same line of action, but acts in an opposite direction to the resultant.

This process is called the composition of forces. Any system of coplanar forces that intersects at a common point may have its resultant determined exactly as shown in Fig. 39-4. The line joining the unattached ends of the first and last forces laid out is equal in intensity, according to scale, to either the resultant of the forces or to its equilibrant. The direction of action of the resultant is indicated by an arrow pointed in such a way as to indicate flow around the polygon, in a direction opposite to the flow indicated by the component forces. The direction of the equilibrant is opposite to this.

Resultants may also be found analytically rather than graphically. It is often necessary to find the resultant of two intersecting forces at right angles to each other. In such cases the polygon formed by the two forces and the resultant will be a right triangle, in which the hypotenuse is the resultant. Here the forces and their resultant partake of the same characteristics as the three sides of the triangle. The hypotenuse squared is then equal to the sum of the squares of the two legs. Consider two right-angled forces equal, respectively, to 3 and 4; the resultant then is equal to the square root of the sum of the squares of 3 and 4:

$$R = \sqrt{3^2 + 4^2} = 5 \qquad \text{(Eq. a)}$$

(See Fig. 39-4.)

Intersecting noncoplanar forces may be reduced to a single resultant by a similar although more complicated process. Such systems of forces will have little pertinence to the present discussion.

THE COUPLE AND FORCE TRANSFER

A system consisting of two equal forces having parallel lines of action but acting in opposite directions along those lines is called a couple. Such a system is shown

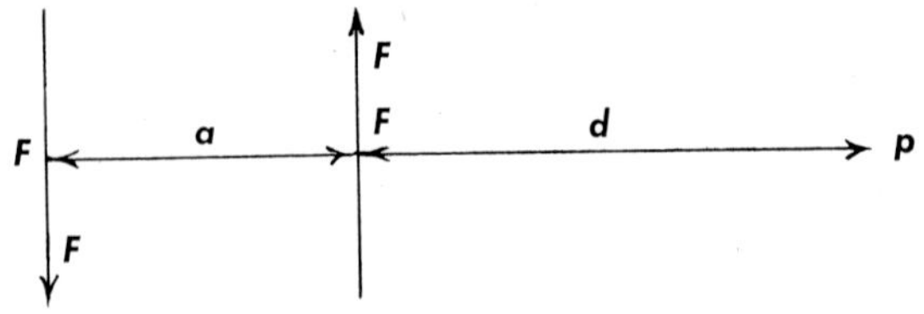

Fig. 39-5. Couple.

in Fig. 39-5. The distance between the forces is *a*, which may have any value. If *a* becomes zero, each of the forces becomes the equilibrant of the other. In this extreme case the couple could have no influence upon any body on which it might be placed.

From the foregoing statement it is evident that a couple may produce only rotation of a body to which it is applied, but not translation. There are many examples of the use and effects of a couple, such as the action of an automobile engine in producing torque to drive the car or the effect of a crank used to turn a wheel. In practical cases, couples occur more frequently associated with another force than they occur alone. In fact, by adding a couple a force may be transferred laterally to a new line of action parallel to its original line.

In Fig. 39-6, let it be required to transfer the line of action of the force *F* (at the left) to a point *p* at *a* distance to the right of its present line of action. At *p* add two forces parallel to *F*, with each equal in intensity to *F* but acting in opposite directions to each other. These two new forces cannot affect the equilibrium of the system, since each is the equilibrant of the other. However, if the added force at *p*, which acts in a direction opposite to that of *F*, is considered together with *F*, it is seen that these two constitute a couple, with moment *Fa*. The second force that was added is equal to *F* and acts in the same direction. Therefore, the force has been transferred a distance *a* to the right by adding a couple of moment *Fa*. This is a very useful procedure in dealing with beams, as will be seen in discussing curved anterior bridges.

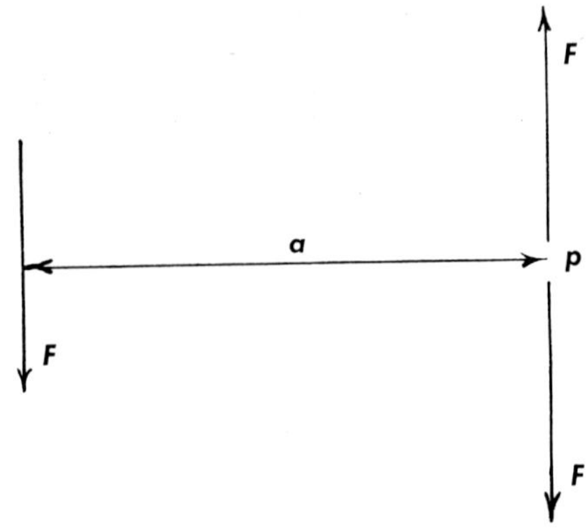

Fig. 39-6. Force transfer by adding couple.

MOMENT OF A FORCE—CENTER OF GRAVITY OF PARALLEL FORCES

Any force has a moment (tendency to rotate) about any point in space, except points on its own line of action. This moment is measured by the product of the force and the perpendicular distance of the point of rotation from the line of action of the force. If intensity is expressed in pounds and the distance in inches, the moment is said to be in inch pounds. The intensity may be in kilograms and the distance in centimeters, in which case the moment would be centimeter kilograms.

Moments of forces have signs arbitrarily given to them. Moments in a clockwise direction receive opposite signs to those in a counterclockwise direction. It is thus seen that the sign depends upon the viewpoint of the observer. If the viewpoint changes, allowance must be made. Consider the couple shown in Fig. 39-5. Let it be required to find the moment of this couple about the point *p*, at a distance *d* to the right of the right-hand force of the couple. The two forces of the couple act in opposite directions and their moments about *p* will have opposite signs. Also the moment of the couple is made up of the sum of the moments of its parts.

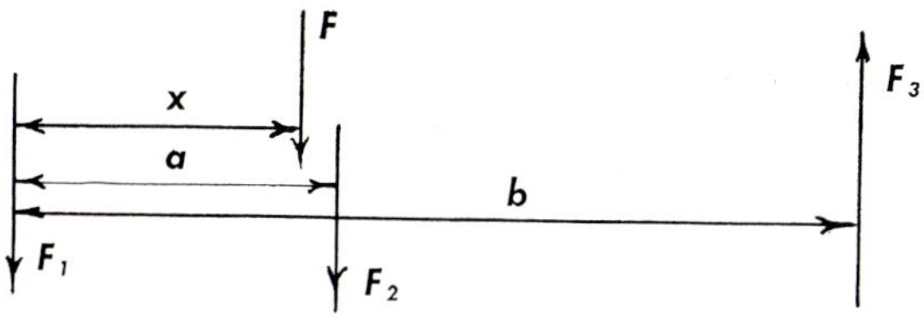

Fig. 39-7. Center of gravity of coplanar, parallel forces.

The moment of the couple is then expressed by the equation:

$$M = -F(a + d) + Fd = -Fa \qquad \text{(Eq. a)}$$

(See Fig. 39-7.)

From this equation it follows that the moment of a couple about any point in its own plane is a constant and is equal to the product of one of the forces that constitute the couple and the distance between the two forces of the couple. It should be noted that if the point p had been selected to the left of the couple or at any point between the forces, the result would have been thc same. In this example the minus sign was selected to represent counterclockwise turning.

It is often desirable to find the location of the center of gravity of coplanar forces for the purpose of locating the point about which there is no tendency of the system to rotate.

Fig. 39-7 shows such a system of forces consisting of F_1, F_2, and F_3. F_2 is *a* distance to the right of F_1, and F_3 is *b* distance to the right of F_1. The resultant of this system of forces would be a force *F, equal to their algebraic sum. F* is shown at x distance to the right of F_1. If F is the resultant, it should have the same moment about any point in its own plane as does the summation of moments of the separate forces of the system. Taking moments about F_1 for simplicity:

$$Fx = F_2a - F_3b, \text{ or } x = \frac{F_2a - F_3b}{F} \qquad \text{(Eq. a)}$$

(See Fig. 39-7.)

If the forces and lever arms are given specific values, the distance x to F may be found numerically. Since F has no moment about any point on its own line of action, it follows that, about this line, the sum of the moments of the component forces is zero.

It should be noted that any center of movements can be selected, A point on the line of action of F_1 was selected to make the leverage of F_1 zero and so eliminate it from the equation. The value of x is unknown until Eq. a is solved. Some assumption must be made as to the location of the center of gravity. If x should be negative as a result of the solution, it simply signifies that the wrong assumption was made and that the leverage x should have been located on the opposite side of the point of moments.

THE LAWS OF STATIC EQUILIBRIUM

The laws of static equilibrium refer to a body at rest, under the influence of a system of forces. They are axiomatic and require no proof. Since by postulation the body is at rest, it has no movement of either translation in any direction or of rotation. Also, since force, by definition, produces movement, it must further be granted that the summation of all components of forces acting upon the body in any given direction must be equal to zero. Otherwise there would be an unbalanced force in that direction and movement would result, violating the primary assumption of a body at rest. Likewise, since rotation is movement produced by a couple, it must also be assumed that there is no unbalanced couple resulting from combining the rotating effects of the forces on the body. Otherwise our primary assumption would again be violated. It should be remembered that no force can have a component at right angles to itself.

From these considerations the following conclusions result. They may be stated as the three laws of equilibrium for coplanar forces acting upon a body.

1. **The summation of all the vertical external forces acting upon a body at rest must be zero.**
2. **The summation of all horizontal external forces acting upon a body at rest must be zero.**
3. **The summation of the moments about any point in space of all external forces acting upon a body at rest must be zero.**

These are very important laws. They constitute the principles involved in determining the equilibrants of force systems acting upon a body at rest. They also are used in evaluating the forces set up within a body, called stresses, when the body is subject to external force. It is by these laws that reactions at the abutment teeth are determined when the dental bridge is subjected to occlusal load. In cases in which no horizontal components of force act, the second law drops from use, and only two laws remain.

When the system of force in noncoplanar, a fourth law becomes operative. In such cases the second law becomes two laws since horizontal forces may have components in either of two right-angled horizontal directions. The summation of the components in each of these two horizontal directions must then become zero, thus creating a fourth law. The terms vertical and horizontal as used here denote only directions at right angles to each other. Such selected directions need not be parallel to vertical or horizontal directions, with reference to the earth's surface.

As an example of the use of these laws, let it be required to find the reactions at the abutments of the bridge shown in Fig. 39-2 caused by the vertical force *P*. Let the span length be *L*, and let the occlusal load *P* be at distance *b* from the center of the right abutment, that is, from the right reaction R_2, and *a* distance from R_1. By applying the first law of equilibrium as stated, the following equation may be written:

$$R_1 + R_2 = P \qquad \text{(Eq. a)}$$

(See Fig. 39-2.)

Applying the third law and writing moments about the line of action of the right reaction, we have the following:

$$R_1L - Pb = O \qquad \text{(Eq. b)}$$

(See Fig. 39-2.)

or

$$R_1 = \frac{Pb}{L} \qquad \text{(Eq. c)}$$

(See Fig. 39-2.)

Putting this value of R_1 back into Eq. a, we have the following for R_2:

$$R_2 = P\,\frac{L - b}{L} = \frac{Pa}{L} \qquad \text{(Eq. d)}$$

(See Fig. 39-2.)

Specific values of *P*, *a*, *b*, and *L* may be assigned and numerical values obtained for the reactions. Let *P* be 100 lb., *L* be 1.125 in., *a* be 0.625 in., and *b* be 0.5 in. Inserting these in Eq. c:

$$R_1 = \frac{100 \times 0.625}{1.125} = 55.6 \text{ lb.} \qquad \text{(Eq. e)}$$

(See Fig. 39-2.)

From Eq. d:

$$R_2 = \frac{100 \times 0.5}{1.125} = 44.4 \text{ lb.} \qquad \text{(Eq. f)}$$

(See Fig. 39-2.)

Checking these results, using Eq. a:

$$R_1 + R_2 = 55.6 + 44.4 = 100 \text{ lb.} \qquad \text{(Eq. g)}$$

(See Fig. 39-2.)

APPLICATIONS OF LAWS OF EQUILIBRIUM ON POSTERIOR BICUSPID

The laws of static equilibrium are most important to the consideration of forces applied to the dental structure, either natural or artificial. It seems fitting to illustrate some of these applications in order to emphasize this fact.

Fig. 39-8, *A*, shows the lower bicuspid, ⌈5, in conventional perspective. The longitudinal axis of rotation is shown passing through the center of the lower tip of this tooth and the center of gravity of the right-tooth section, which section contains the midpoint of the line connecting the centers of gravity of the mesial and distal areas of contact of the same tooth. This section might perhaps be called the section of contact areas.

The axis of this tooth is also shown as the line of intersection of two right-angled planes. One of these planes, marked mesiodistal, should, under ideal anatomy, contain or be parallel to the line joining centers of the two contact areas of the tooth and may be called the mesiodistal plane of forces. The other, at right angles to the mesiodistal plane of forces, containing the longitudinal axis of the tooth, is called the buccolingual plane of forces. To these two right-angled planes may be added a third plane of force perpendicular to them and to the axis of the tooth at the P_R point. This plane would contain any horizontal, rotational component of a force applied to the tooth that would tend to rotate it about its longitudinal axis. (This plane however, is not shown in Fig. 39-8.)

The effect of any external force applied to the tooth, through the processes of analysis, eventually will be assigned to one of these three planes. No component so assigned may have any influence in either of the other planes, since a force cannot have a component at right angles to itself.

A point, marked P_R, is shown on the longitudinal axis of the tooth. It is about this point that the tooth is assumed to rotate when subjected to transverse torque. This point has never been definitely located and in fact may vary to some extent in location under varying types of loading. The writer has placed this rotational center near the midpoint of the length of the axis contained between the lower tip of the root and the cervical plane, even though some dental authorities feel it should lie at about the lower third region.

There is a compelling reason for locating it higher. When a transverse force comes upon the tooth, it tries to rotate it in the fundus, causing the lower end of the root to put pressure on one wall of the socket (below the point of rotation) and the upper portion of the root to put pressure on the opposite wall (above the point of rotation). This movement induces opposing forces in the bone of the fundus. The movement continues until the total force induced on one wall, when combined with the total-equal-and-opposite-force induced on the opposite wall, compose a couple equal to the applied couple. It is this couple, induced in the fundus, that tends to rotate the tooth in a direction opposite to that caused by the applied couple. At the time equilibrium results and rotation ceases, the induced couple becomes equal to the applied couple, as required by the third law of equilibrium.

The equality of the two sets of forces (above and below the center of rotation) results from the second law of equilibrium. If the two sets of forces are to be equal, those below the center of rotation must be considerably greater, in unit intensity, than those above this point because the area over which those below the point of rotation are distributed, is much smaller, (due to the taper of the root) than that over which the forces above the point of rotation are distributed. Moving the point of rotation downward would increase the unit intensities of pressures below the point of rotation.

It is also true the bone of the fundus diverges upward opposite to the taper of the tooth apically. The bone of the fundus also needs protection. Nature tends always to accomplish its purposes by the most efficient method possible. These are

A

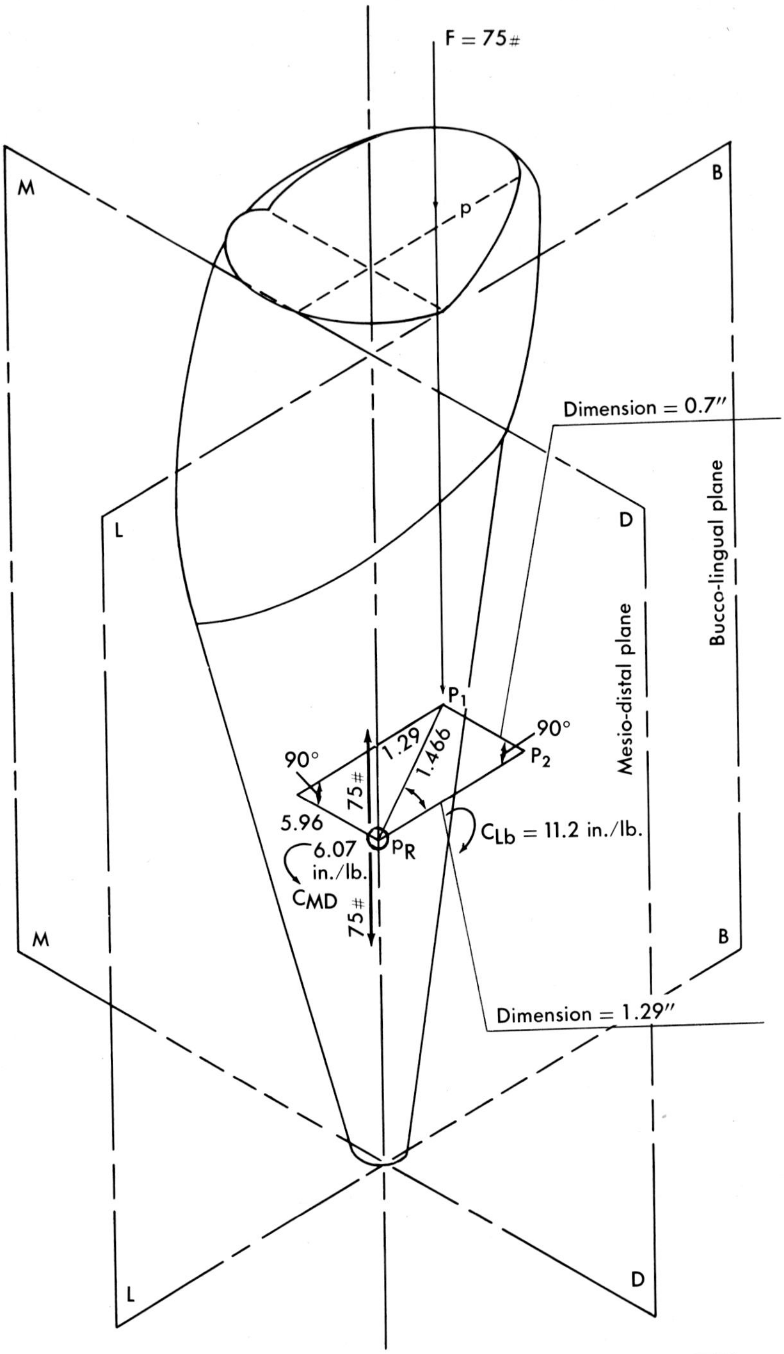

Fig. 39-8. A, Load, **F,** applied eccentrically to occlusal surface of cuspid |5; steps necessary for allocation of its separate effects in producing centric loads on root structure; torsional effects in mesiodistal plane, as well as in buccolingual plane. **B,** Probable resisting stresses on tooth root caused by axial load. **C,** Probable induced stresses on tooth root caused by application to tooth in bi-plane of clockwise torque. **D,** Possible distribution of resisting stresses caused by applied torque around periphery of tooth root.

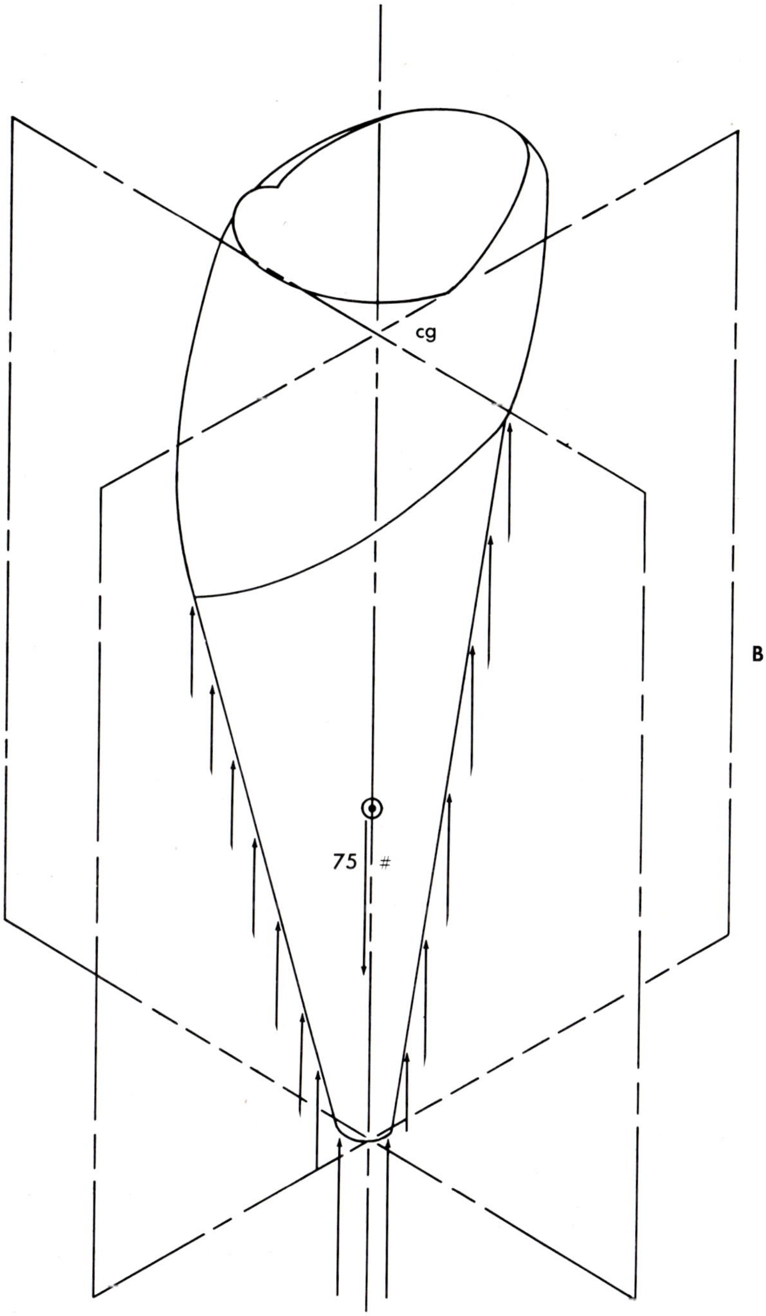

Fig. 39-8, cont'd. For legend see opposite page.

Continued.

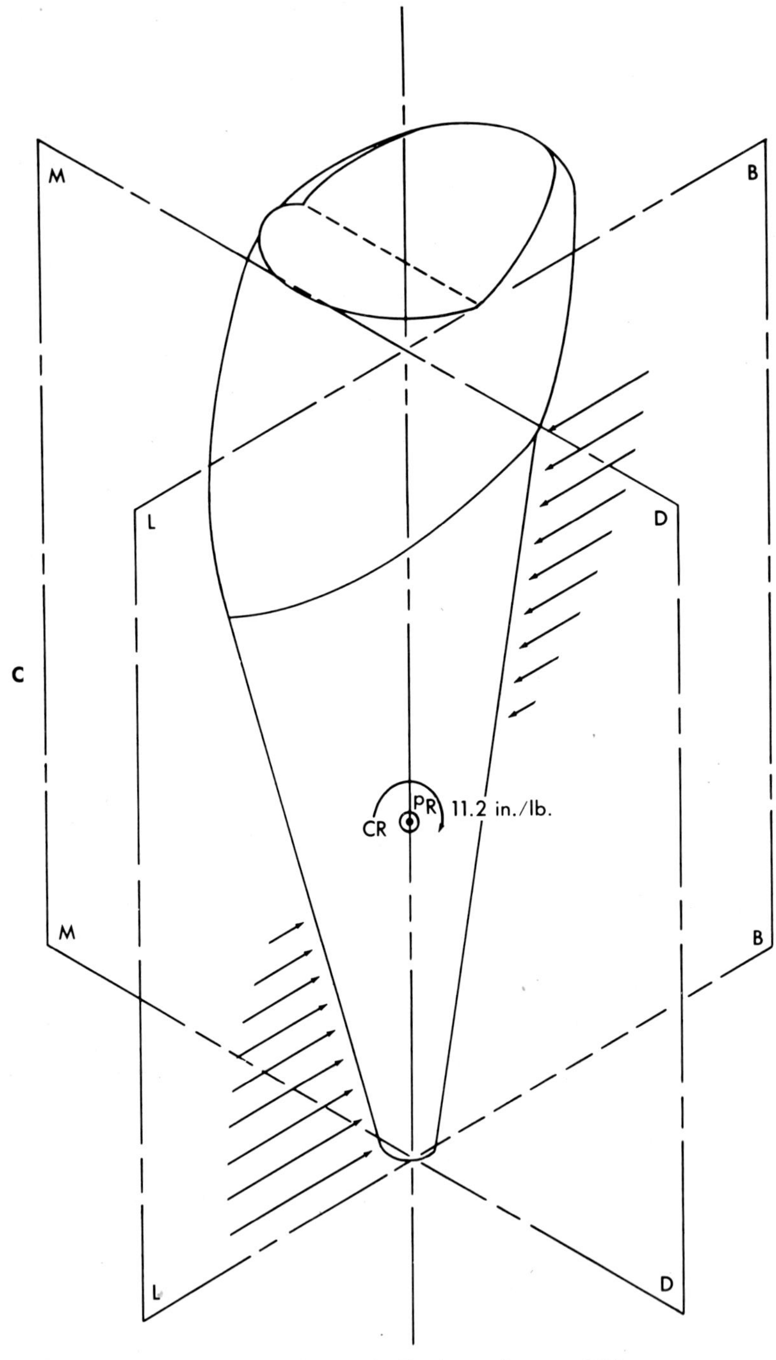

Fig. 39-8, cont'd. For legend see p. 868.

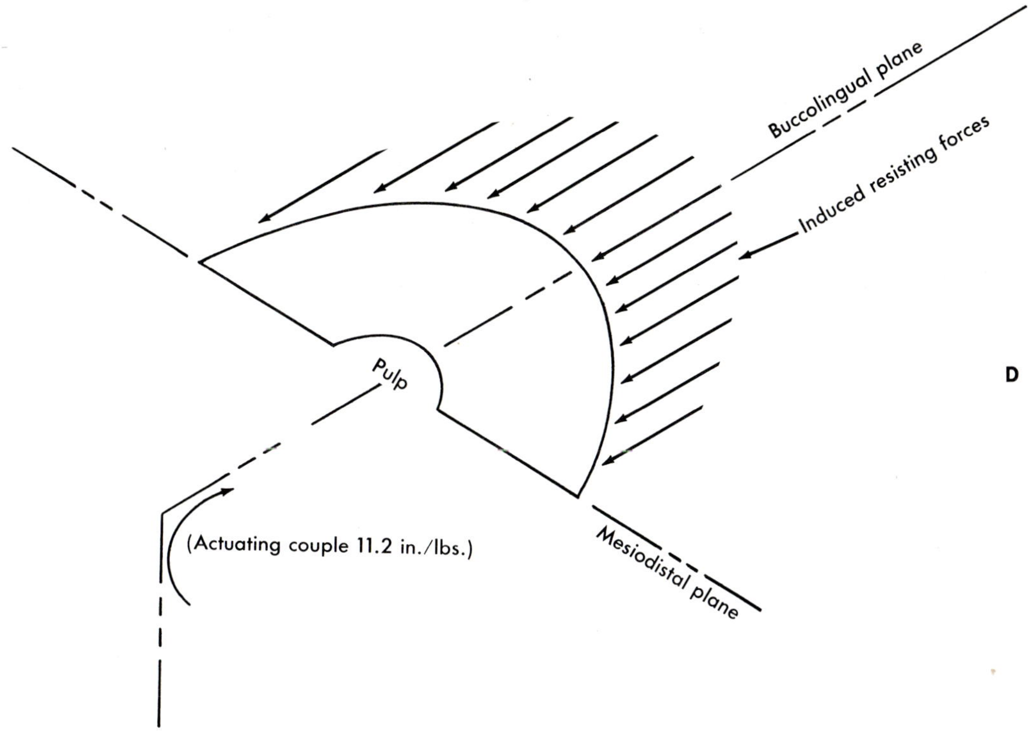

Fig. 39-8 cont'd. For legend see p. 868.

some of the reasons why the point of rotation has been raised. Experimentation should throw further light on this matter.

Application of an eccentric occlusal load to the tooth

Fig. 39-8 shows an eccentric occlusal load of 75 lbs. applied approximately parallel to the axis of tooth ⌈5 and perpendicular to the occlusal plane. The line of action of this force 'F' is produced to the point p_1, where it intersects the plane, normal to the tooth axis, through the point of rotation, p_R, of the tooth. The line p_1p_R is shown. The perpendicular distance of point P_1, to the left of the buccolingual plane is shown as 0.7 inch, as scaled from the drawing. The distance from the mesiodistal plane is shown as 1.29 inches obtained in the same way.

It is a peculiarity of the conventional perspective type of drawing that only distances parallel to the major axes of the drawing are shown in their true values. Other distances are distorted. The only distances shown that are of correct value are 0.7 inch and 1.29 inches, for the scaled eccentricities of the point of load application P_1. The length p_1p_R has been foreshortened. The triangle $p_1p_2p_R$ is shown as a right triangle. Even though the angle at p_2 has been distorted, its true value is ninety degrees. This being so, the true value of distance p_1p_R, the hypothenuse, is equal to the square root of the sum of the squares of the two distances 0.7 and 1.29, which do show in true lengths. Then:

$$p_1p_R = \sqrt{0.70^2 - 1.29^2} = 1.466 \text{ inches}$$

The true distance of the eccentric force 'F' from the axis being 1.466 inches and the value of F, from the table of design loads for various teeth being 75 lbs. for the tooth under consideration (Table 40-1), the value of the total torque tending to rotate the tooth, due to eccentric load, is the product of 75 and 1.466. The two added, equal, and opposite forces are shown just to the left of the tooth axis, on the upper and lower sides of point P_R. Of the two added forces, the upper one together with the original eccentric force makes an applied couple. The downward force, acting along the axis, is the original eccentric force, which has now been transformed into an axial force by adding the couple.

The value of the couple is now (to the scale of the drawing):

$$C = 75 \times 1.466 = 110 \text{ inch/lb.}$$

This 110 inch/lb., however, is obtained on the assumption that the tooth has been drawn to natural size. If it be assumed that the natural buccolingual width of the tooth is three-eighths of an inch and compare this with that shown on the drawing, we find the true enlargement of the drawing is 8.67 times. The value of the couple obtained above is then 8.67 times too great; its true value is 110/8.67 or 12.7 inch/lb.

This couple is, however, applied in a plane, making an angle with the buccolingual plane of forces whose cosine is 1.29/1.466 or 0.880. The angle, then, is 28 degrees/20 minutes. The couple, of value 12.7 inch/lb. is now resolved into components which lie respectively in the buccolingual and mesiodistal planes of force.

$$C_{BL} = 12.7 \times .880 = 11.2 \text{ inch/lb.}$$

$$C_{MD} = 12.7 \times 0.7/1.466 = 6.07 \text{ inch/lb.}$$

The effects of the eccentric occlusal load, placed on this tooth, have now been completely allocated into an applied load of 75 lbs., acting along the axis of the tooth; a counterclockwise couple of 6.07 inch/lb., in the mesiodistal plane of force; and an 11.2 inch/lb. clockwise couple acting in the buccolingual plane of force; these three are separate effects of the original eccentric load on the tooth. They have been produced by the musculature of the face and are external forces.

Induced forces in the fundus

For a complete wrap-up of the effect of the eccentric load we must now consider the separate effects of the various components of the eccentric load, in inducing forces in the tooth and its fundus that oppose and stabilize the tendencies, of these various components, in causing movements.

The axial load effect

In order to avoid confusion, the concentric load applied along the axis of the tooth, will first be considered alone. The effects of this force, in inducing stresses, are shown in Fig. 39-8, *B*. These induced forces, act in an upward direction over the root surfaces of the tooth. Not everything is known about these induced stabilizing forces, but the laws of equilibrium and the laws of symmetry give valuable bits of information about them.

(1) The first law of equilibrium states that their total sum must be 75 lbs.

(2) The laws of symmetry tell us that the upward forces on surfaces, which are approximately symmetrical, on the two sides of the tooth root, must be equal in intensity.

(3) Downward movement of the tooth produced these forces. They are divided into two groups, those on the tapered sides of the tooth root and those across the bottom or blunt point of the root. Those along the tapered sides of the root are produced by action of the fibers of the peridontal membrane. It is reasonable to believe that the intensity of forces across the bottom should be greater than those along the tapered sides, because they make more nearly 90 degree contact with the tooth root surfaces, with which they come into contact.

(4) The laws of equilibrium do not assure us that there are no lateral forces perpendicular to the axis of the tooth. The second law of equilibrium, however, does assure us that if such exist, they are equal and opposite on the two sides of the root.

(5) The third law of equilibrium says the line of action of the resultant, of all these induced upward forces, must lie along the tooth axis, to insure that there is no tendency to rotate the tooth in any direction.

Resisting forces due to a couple

The resisting forces shown in Fig. 39-8, *C*, are the sole result, in this plane, of the influence of the 11.2 in./lb. couple. They are indicated on the root surfaces, above the center of rotation on the right and below this point on the left. Rotation of the tooth about P_R will tend to be clockwise because the couple acts in a clockwise direction. The laws of equilibrium and other considerations show the following facts about these induced stabilizing forces.

(1) The resisting forces (or rather the resultants of those induced around the semi-peripheries of root sections) lie in, or parallel to, the plane BL because the applied couple lies in this plane.

(2) The sum of the induced leftward resisting forces above the center of rotation must equal the sum of the rightward forces below P_R as required by the second law of equilibrium.

(3) We do not know whether or not the induced forces acting against the root walls vary by a straight line law from zero, at p_R, to a maximum at the extremities of the root, because of lack of experimental work on this point. The variation has therefore been shown as a curve of unknown character.

(4) We do know that the sums of those above p_R and those below p_R are equal. We also know these two sets of equal and opposite forces times the unknown vertical distance between their two centers of gravity constitute a couple, and that this couple of resisting forces is exactly equal to and opposite in direction to the applied couple of 11.2 inch/lb., as required by the laws of equilibrium.

The peripheral stresses shown in Fig. 39-8, *D*, are induced by the actuating couple of 11.2 inch/lb., applied in the buccolingual plane. These intensities should be maximum at the intersection of the buccolingual plane with the tooth periphery and taper off to zero (by an unknown law) at each of the intersections of the mesiodistal plane with the same periphery. Fig. 39-8, *B*, simply indicates the resultants of all the variable induced forces, on a given periphery, as if they all acted in the buccolingual plane.

These conclusions are the principal ones which follow from the laws of equilibrium and other considerations, due to the couple of 11.2 inch/lb. applied to tooth |5. The forces produced by the couple would of course be combined with those caused by the axial load.

There is another couple of 6.07 inch/lb., which lies in the MD plane and is counterclockwise in direction. The effects of this couple in inducing pressures against the walls of the tooth root are similar to those shown for the BL plane, except that they lie in the MD plane at right angles to the BL plane.

These analyses and conclusions serve to illustrate the extreme importance of the laws of static equilibrium in considering the really complicated matter of analyzing the effects of force when applied to a tooth in the human mouth.

EFFECTS OF FORCE UPON MATERIAL

Determination of the effect of force when applied to material is primarily the result of observation. When a rubber band is loaded, it stretches; when a load is laid across a spline of wood, the spline bends; an automobile tire flattens under the weight of the car. Starting with these examples in which deformation as a result of loading is obvious to the naked eye, the curiosity of the observer is aroused as to whether or not deformation results in all cases in which load is applied to material. If load is applied along the axis of a straight, steel bar, does the bar elongate or deform otherwise? If a housefly alights upon a railroad rail, does the rail bend?

As more and more sensitive measuring devices have been devolped, the answer to these questions is that material does deform when load is applied to it. Though very sensitive devices now exist which will measure to one millionth of an inch and even smaller, it is still impossible to measure infinitely small quantities. However, investigators confidently extrapolate and state a general law as follows: *When force is applied to any material, deformation of that material results.*

Now if deformation of material results when force is applied to it, why then does not this deformation continue indefinitely as the force continues to be applied? Observation shows that deformation does cease in most structural materials after a certain amount has taken place. In other materials, such as pitches and tars, or in metals at high temperatures, deformation continues indefinitely (though not at a uniform rate) until rupture eventually occurs.

The answer to these queries must be concerned with force. Since force is the cause of movement, it is logical to look for a counteracting force to cause movement to cease. This counterforce is called stress. It is postulated to be induced within the material and to oppose the deformation caused by the applied force.

The following is a definition for stress: *Stress is that internal, induced force which results from deformation caused in a material by an external, applied load.* Stress tends to oppose such deformation.

Consider the bar shown in Fig. 39-9. This bar is loaded with a load P and its equilibrant acting in the opposite direction. The original length of the bar was L. Under the influence of load it elongates an amount e. The bar decreases in diameter, also according to a law, which will not be discussed here. It has been postulated that there is an internal induced force, called stress, which opposes the elongation of the bar and eventually causes elongation to cease. Let it be required to evaluate this induced stress.

For this purpose, use will be made of the laws of static equilibrium. Let it be assumed that the bar is cut into two pieces at the section *b-b*. Consider the upper portion of this bar as shown on the right in Fig. 39-9. Since the force P is still applied to the upper portion of the bar and since this portion of the bar was in equilibrium before the section was cut, it must be assumed that the portion taken away exerted a total force equal to P on the lower end of the upper portion, in order to satisfy the first law of equilibrium, as previously stated. The total force (replaced now as an external load) is indicated at the lower end of the portion shown on the right in Fig. 39-9. It is equal to a summation of the individual stresses acting on very small areas, *da*, over the whole section of the bar.

Then from the first law of equilibrium, we know that

$$P = \Sigma S \; da \qquad \text{(Eq. a)}$$

(See Fig. 39-9.)

We do not know, however, that the individual unit stresses on each of the individual areas, *da*, are all equal. In fact, it is true that they are not, as indicated by the varying lengths of the force arrows

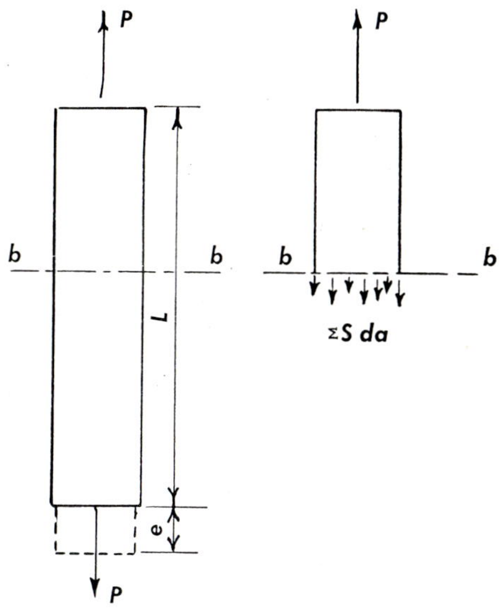

Fig. 39-9. Bar under tensile load.

shown on the cut section. These differential areas might logically be those of the individual crystalline grains of metal that make up the section. It is reasonable to assume that these individual unit stresses are not all equal. If the directions of both the load and the replaced stresses were reversed, the case would have some analogy to that of a man standing on a pile of gravel. In this case it is not probable that each particle of the gravel would bear an equal portion of the man's weight. Nevertheless, it is necessary, for practical purposes, to arrive at a usable unit stress on each potrion of the bar. The *assumption* is therefore made that the average unit stress acts on each unit of area of the bar. Under this assumption, the S of Eq. a becomes a constant and the summation of *da* becomes the whole area of the bar. Eq. a then becomes

$$P = S\,A \quad \text{or} \quad S = \frac{P}{A} \qquad \text{(Eq. b)}$$

(See Fig. 39-9.)

This equation yields a statistical average for the unit stress on each square unit of area of the cross section of the bar. Justification for this result is found in the fact that the equation has been used in the design of engineering structures for a great many years with satisfactory results. However, the assumption is not true for practical purposes when stresses are the result of intermittent loads applied an enormous number of times. This occurs in the case of rapidly reciprocating parts of machines. In such special cases allowances must be made.

TYPES OF STRESS

There are three, and only three, types of stress induced in a material by applied loads.

1. *Tensile stress* is the internal induced force that opposes elongation of a material in a direction parallel to the direction of the *stress*.
2. *Compressive stress* is the internal induced force that opposes shortening of the material in a direction parallel to the direction of the *stress*.
3. *Shearing stress* is the internal induced force that opposes the sliding of one plane of the material on the adjacent plane in a direction parallel to the *stress*.

The stress shown on the right in Fig. 39-9 is an example of tensile stress as defined. This figure also serves to illustrate compressive stress, if the directions of the applied load and the induced stresses were reversed.

One of the common occurrences of shearing stress is the stress induced in a circular bar subjected to a twist. Such a bar is shown in Fig. 39-10. Here a circular bar has a counterclockwise torque, *T*, applied at its left end. The right end of the bar is assumed to be firmly held as in a vise. As the torque *T* is applied, the left end of the bar moves in a circular motion with respect to the right end. This motion may be visualized by thinking of the bar as made up of a great number of extremely thin washers whose centers lie on the axis

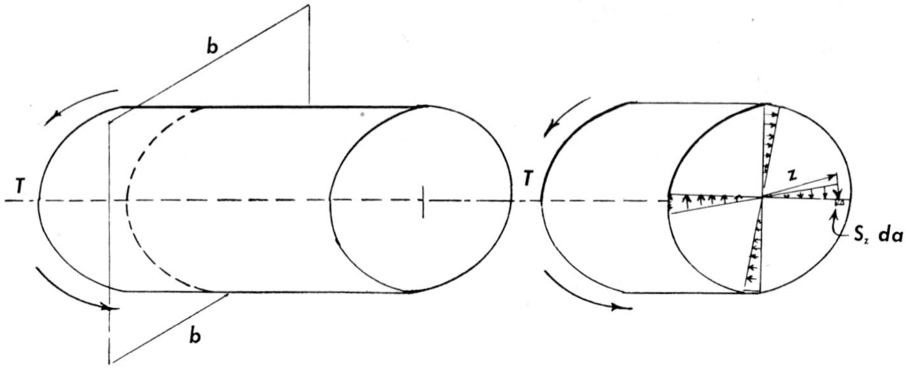

Fig. 39-10. Shearing stress.

of the bar. The movement consists of these washers sliding in a circular path, each upon the adjacent one. The outer peripheries, of course, slide most, and sliding at the center is zero. Since there is this variable movement, the stress at the outside of the bar will be greatest because movement there is greatest. If, now, a section is cut at *b-b* and the left end of the bar is considered as a separate free body, subject to the laws of equilibrium, stresses may be replaced on the cut end of the bar to restore equilibrium, as was done for the tensile bar of Fig. 39-9.

These stresses are shown on the right in Fig. 39-10. The applied torque at the left end tends to cause counterclockwise rotation. The replaced stresses at the right end oppose this and cause clockwise rotation. Since there are no unbalanced vertical or horizontal forces, the applied force being a couple and the induced stresses being couples, it follows from the third law of equilibrium that

$$T = \Sigma S_z \text{ da} \qquad \text{(Eq. a)}$$
(See Fig. 39-10.)

where S_z varies as a straight line (experimental determination) from zero at the center of the bar to a maximum of S_s at the outer surface. Methods of evaluating S_s will be developed. This is only one example of shearing stress. Many others occur. Shearing stress becomes important in short deep beams. All stresses in material may be resolved into tensile, compressive, or shearing stress.

The discussion up to this point has dealt with total stress on a section. It is normally desired to deal with the maximum stress on any square unit of the section. The unit ordinarily used in the English system is the square inch, and the unit of force is the pound. Accordingly, unit stresses are usually expressed in pounds per square inch. They may also be readily expressed in kilograms per square millimeter or otherwise. The unit of area upon which the unit stress acts is measured ordinarily at right angles to the stress in cases of tensile or compressive stress and parallel to the stress in case of shearing stress. There will be further reference to methods of determining unit stresses in beams and in torsion bars. A method of determining the unit stress in an axially loaded tensile or compression bar has been included in the discussion of effects of force upon material.

PHYSICAL PROPERTIES OF MATERIALS

It has been shown that materials deform under the influence of forces applied to them. It has been further stated that the type of deformation varies with the material and also with the temperature of the material. Nothing has been said of the laws followed in the progress of the de-

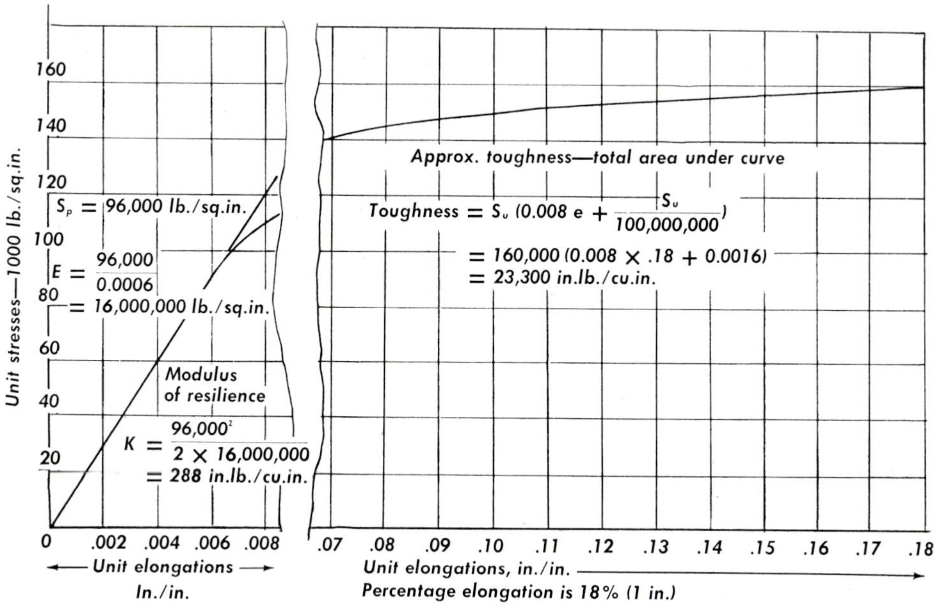

Fig. 39-11. Load-deformation curve, dental gold wire. (Courtesy J. F. Jelenko Co.)

formation of the material when the load is applied. It is necessary to know these laws in order to make use of the material for constructing dental bridges and other structures. This necessity arises from the fact that, within the material of the structure, applied load induces stresses, that are independent of the material and depend only upon the form of the structure and the intensity and placement of the load.

Although there is a beginning of some theoretical basis for predicting the strength of material from the character of its crystalline and atomic structures, this basis is so tentative at present and so hedged about with practical considerations not included in the prediction that results do not bear much relationship to facts. As a consequence, the ability of a material to withstand induced stresses must be determined by actual test. For metals from which dental bridges are constructed, the test used is a tensile test, in which an axial, tensile load is applied to a straight cast bar of the metal and deformations are recorded for each increment of applied load throughout the test. Measurements of deformation are made by means of sensitive measuring devices, which record deformations as small as 0.0001 inch or smaller.

A typical record of such a test is shown, plotted graphically, in Fig. 39-11. Loads are plotted on the vertical ordinates in units of 1000 lb./sq. in. Unit deformations are plotted along the horizontal axis in units of inches of elongation per linear inch of test bar.

It will be noted from this curve that the first law of deformation is as follows: *Deformations are proportional to applied loads up to a certain unit stress called the proportional limit.*

At the proportional limit, unit deformation was comparatively small, being between six and seven thousandths of an inch per inch. It should be stated further that if the load had been released at any unit stress below the proportional limit, the corresponding unit deformations would have disappeared and the bar would have returned to its unstressed length.

After the induced stresses passed the proportional limit of the material, deformation no longer continued to be proportional to the applied load but began to progress at a much faster pace. The type of deformation that took place before the proportional limit stress was attained is called *elastic* deformation, because it is all recoverable when the load is removed. The type that began after the proportional limit is called *plastic* deformation. Plastic deformation is not all recoverable when the load is removed. During removal of the load in the plastic stage, the return curve follows a course somewhat parallel to the elastic curve. When the entire load is taken away, there remains a *permanent* deformation of the material, called *permanent set.*

The next significant unit stress is the ultimate strength, marked S_u on the curve. *Ultimate strength* is the greatest unit stress that may be induced in the material in a test to complete rupture. It should be noted that the unit stress at the maximum load is computed from the original, unstressed area of the bar and not from the reduced cross section. This rule also applies to all stresses computed during the test. Such a stress is called *engineering unit stress.* For most purposes it serves just as well as the true physical unit stress and offers much more convenience in practice.

After the bar is broken, the ruptured ends are carefully fitted together. The percentage by which a gauge length, marked on the bar in its original, unstressed condition, has increased in length up to the time of rupture is called the *percentage of elongation.*

Modulus of elasticity is found by dividing the unit stress, at any point up to the proportional limit, by its corresponding unit *elongation* (for tension) or *strain.* For the curve in Fig. 39-11 the modulus of elasticity is found by dividing the unit stress of 96,000 lb./sq. in., near the proportional limit, by its corresponding unit strain of 0.006 in./in., giving a modulus of elasticity of 16,000,000 lb./sq.in. To make it reasonable to think of modulus of elasticity in terms of a unit stress, modulus of elasticity may be defined as that unit stress which (if the material could withstand such a stress) would exist in a tensile bar, when sufficient load had been applied to double its original length. It will be seen that this definition is compatible with the first one given, for if the length is doubled, the unit stress is divided by unity, and modulus and unit stress become identical. The fact that material will not withstand such stresses does not invalidate the usefulness of the concept.

Modulus of resilience is defined as the work or energy required to stress a cubic inch of the material (in one direction only) from zero up to the proportional limit of the material. Work is defined as the product of force and distance through which it moves. The average force acting upon a cubic inch of the material during stressing to the proportional limit is one half the proportional limit unit stress. The distance through which the force travels is (for the bar shown in Fig. 39-11) 0.006 in. The modulus of resilience then is $0.006 \times S_p/2$. However, by definition of modulus of elasticity, in this case $0.006 = S_p/E$, where E represents modulus of elasticity. Letting K stand for modulus of resilience, and making the substitution, we have the following:

$$K = Sp^2/2E \qquad \text{(Eq. a)}$$

(See Fig. 39-11.)

K is expressed in terms of energy and usually as inch pounds per cubic inch of material.

In a similar manner *toughness* is the total work or energy expended in stressing a cubic inch of a material (in one direction only) from zero up to the breaking point. Toughness is strictly equal to the total area under the unit stress–unit strain curve as shown in Fig. 39-11. Again it is expressed in inch pounds per cubic inch. Toughness for dental gold may be approximated, with good accuracy, by the following semi-empirical equation:

$$T = S_u \left(0.008\ e + \frac{S_u}{100{,}000{,}000}\right) \qquad \text{(Eq. b)}$$

(See Fig. 39-11.)

In this equation, *T* stands for *toughness* in inch pounds per cubic inch, *e* for *percentage of elongation,* and S_u for ultimate strength. For the test piece plotted on the curve, the *toughness* is computed as 23,300 in.lb./cu.in.

STRUCTURAL SIGNIFICANCE OF PHYSICAL PROPERTIES

It was shown previously that material will not return to its original form when stressed beyond its proportional limit. This being true, it is obvious that a dental bridge built from the material cannot retain its original form and fit if the material of the bridge becomes stressed beyond its proportional limit. It is apparent that a bridge that does not retain its original form is no longer useful in the mouth. Therefore, *proportional limit* of material measures, according to laws to be developed, the maximum load that can be placed upon the structure in service and still have the structure retain its usefulness. Of two bridges of identical form, the one made from the material of higher proportional limit can be expected to sustain the higher load. Thus, it is seen that proportional limit has its great significance as a measure of maximum permissible load on the bridge. This is not to say that permissible loads on the bridge induce proportional limit stresses in the material.

It is desirable that the bridge not be loaded to exceed the proportional limit stress of its material. It is also desirable, if unforeseen circumstances should cause momentary stresses beyond the proportional limit, that rupture does not occur, because of such circumstance. *Ultimate strength* is a rough measure of the load required to cause rupture and, as such, becomes important in measuring *inelastic strength* of the bridge under static loads.

Impact loads are those that induce stresses as a result of their weight as well as their velocity at contact. In mastication, when the individual unexpectedly bites on an object such as a bone fragment, an impact load is produced upon the bridge. Such a load produces much of its effect because of its velocity energy. The ability of the material to withstand this momentary effect and still have stresses remain within the proportional limit is measured by the *modulus of resilience.* If stresses are induced beyond the proportional limit, the ability of the material to withstand them and avoid rupture is measured by its *toughness.*

It will be noted that for the material shown the toughness is many times the modulus of resilience. Thus toughness represents a cushion for absorbing shocks that may cause momentary streses beyond the proportional limit. Ductile materials, having high percentages of elongation, have high toughnesses. The toughness of brittle materials is much lower. Since percentage of elongation is an important factor in determining toughness, it is desirable to retain *percentage of elongation* as high, as is consistent with other requirements.

Modulus of elasticity was defined (p. 1132) as the ratio of unit stress within the proportional limit to its corresponding unit strain. It was shown to be a unit stress ordinarily expressed in terms of pounds per square inch. This definition may be set down in an equation as follows:

$$E = \frac{S}{\varepsilon} \quad \text{or} \quad \varepsilon = \frac{S}{E} \qquad \text{(Eq. c)}$$

(See Fig. 39-11.)

In this equation, the Greek letter epsilon stands for the unit elongation, which corresponds to a unit stress, S, within the proportional limit, while *E* stands for modulus of elasticity. Since the total elongation of such a test bar, as shown in

Fig. 39-9, is made up of the sum of the values of ε for each linear inch and since in this case the unit elongations in each inch are the same, then it follows that

$$e = L\,\varepsilon \quad \text{or} \quad e = L\,\frac{S}{E} \qquad \text{(Eq. d)}$$

(See Fig. 39-11.)

Thus Eq. a makes it possible to determine the elongation of a bar at any given unit tensile stress. Suppose a bar is 10 in. long and is stressed to 12,000 lb./sq.in. Its modulus of elasticity is 12,000,000 lb./sq.in. Let it be required to determine its elongation under this stress. Substituting:

$$e = 10 \times \frac{12{,}000 \times 10}{12{,}000{,}000} = 0.01 \text{ in.} \qquad \text{(Eq. e)}$$

(See Fig. 39-11.)

Thus it is seen that modulus of elasticity is an inverse measure of deformation of structure under load. Since beams bend under load, modulus of elasticity becomes one of the characteristics of the material in the determination of how much the beams bend. A high modulus means a stiff material and a low modulus a limber one.

Other physical properties exist, such as melting range and hardness. These do not relate closely to structural matters and will not be discussed here.

BEAMS—DEFINITIONS

A *beam* is any bar whose curvature changes under load. This is a broad definition but a correct one. Under this definition a ring or a hook supporting a load would be a beam. In dental work, only beams that are approximately straight in their unstressed condition will be considered. Most dental bridges fall into this class. Such beams have supports, and in the case of dental bridges these are the abutment teeth.

A point of *support* of a beam is that point at which is placed one of the induced equilibrants to the applied loads. The equilibrants to the applied loads, which are induced at the supports, are called *reactions.* The length of the beam between two supports is called the *span length.* Beams are divided into classes according to the methods used in supporting them and the consequent methods that must be used in determining the reactions at the supports. The classes that will be mentioned here are cantilever beam, simple beam, restrained beam, and continuous beam. Supports for beams are divided into three classes: free supports, restrained supports, and fixed supports.

For purposes of mathematical discussion, a *cantilever beam* is a beam that is supported by only one fixed support at one of its ends. A *simple beam* is a straight beam that has two, and only two, free supports, one at either end. A *restrained beam* is one that has two or more supports, at least one of which permits some freedom of rotation to the beam at the point of support but not as much as would be the case if the support was a free support. A *continuous beam* is one that continues over three or more supports—those supports not at the beam ends being usually free supports.

A *free support* is one that does not permit translation of the beam perpendicular to its axis and is presumed to offer no restraint to any tendency of the beam to rotate at the support. A knife edge is usually considered a typical example of such a support. A *restrained support* is one that permits no motion perpendicular to the beam axis but does permit some rotation at the support, although not as much as in the case of a freely supported beam. A *fixed support* is one that permits no motion, either of translation or of rotation at the support. A bar clamped in a vise is often taken as a typical example of this type support. A dental bridge soldered to a crown of an abutment tooth is considered a typical restrained support. The tooth rotates to some extent in its alveolar socket, but it may also offer some restraint at the point of support. This rotation is in the plane of the beam and the abutment as opposed to rotation around its longitudinal axis.

It will be realized that these definitions are idealized for purposes of mathematical discussion. Even a knife edge or a pin through the beam at the point of support will offer some small restraint to rotation, since friction always exists. Also, a bar clamped in a vise will rotate a small amount because of the deformation of both the bar and the vise. Vertical movement, though small at support points, must take place, since the material of the supports deforms under loads. Nevertheless, these exceptions are sufficiently negligible to make the definitions valuable for purposes of discussion.

BEAM REACTIONS—THE LAWS OF STATIC EQUILIBRIUM

On p. 865 the reactions for a simple beam were determined through the use of the laws of static equilibrium. It will now be profitable to consider the possibilities and limitations of these laws when used for this purpose.

It will be remembered from the previous discussion on force that a force is determined by three independent characteristics, each of which can be altered without affecting the other two. Each of these characteristics requires a separate mathematical equation for the complete determination of the force. A simple beam, supported at its two ends as shown in Fig. 39-12, has a reaction at each of its two ends. The three characteristics of each of these two forces constitute six unknowns, and the laws of equilibrium supply only three equations for their determination. Thus it follows that, in the most general case, the reactions of a beam on more than one support may not be fully determined by the laws of equilibrium. However, in the case of the simple beam, if the loading

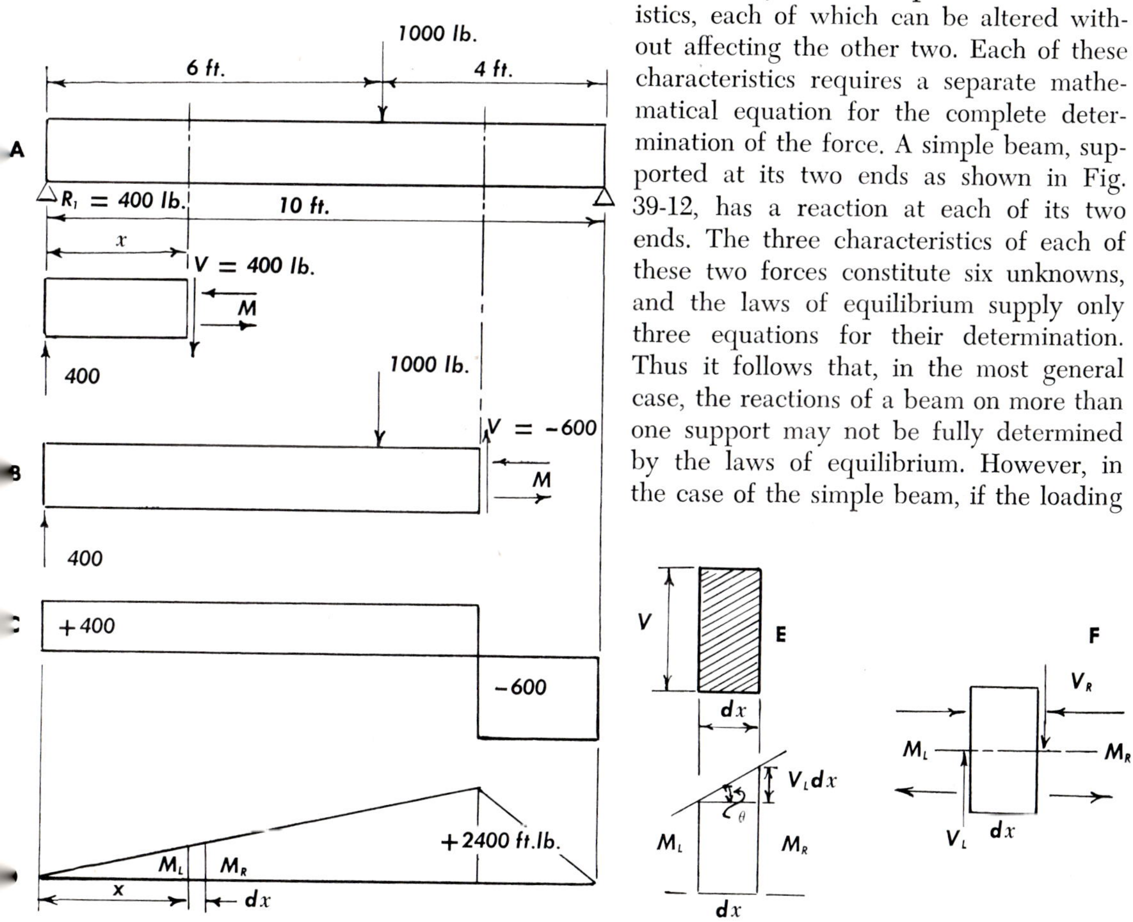

Fig. 39-12. **A** to **D**, Shear and bending moment diagrams. **E** and **F**, Interrelationships between shear and bending moment.

be assumed perpendicular to the beam and in the plane of its axis, then the direction of the reactions may also be assumed in the plane of the beam and perpendicular to the axis. Thus the two lines of action of the two unknown reactions are determined. Also, each of the reactions may be assumed to act in a direction opposite to the loads, which eliminates two more of the six unknowns. This leaves only the magnitudes of the two reactions. The laws of equilibrium supply equations for them. In all other cases, except the portion of a cantilever beam projecting from the support, the reactions are not capable of being completely determined by the laws of equilibrium.

SHEAR AND BENDING MOMENT IN A BEAM

In Fig. 39-12, let the span length be 10 ft. and the distance of the 1000 lb. load from the left and right supports, respectively, be 6 ft. and 4 ft. Then from Eq. c (Fig. 39-2) and Eq. d (Fig. 39-2):

$$R_1 = \frac{1000 \times 4}{10} = 400 \text{ lb.}$$

and

$$R_2 = \frac{1000 \times 6}{10} = 600 \text{ lb.}$$

As a check:

$$R_1 + R_2 = 400 + 600 = 1000 \text{ lb.}$$

as should be the case in order to satisfy the laws of equilibrium which say the sum of vertical forces must be zero.

At any point to the left of the load, and at x distance from the left reaction, let a section x-x be imagined cut across the beam. Now consider the equilibrium of the left portion of the beam. This portion still has the left reaction of 400 lb. acting upon it (Fig. 39-12, *A*). In order to satisfy the laws of equilibrium, an equal and opposite downward force of 400 lb. must be applied to the cut section as shown. This is known as the shear on the section. This shear, combined with the left reaction, forms a couple with a turning moment of 400 (x). In order to satisfy the law of equilibrium that requires that the moment of external forces must be zero, a counteracting couple, M, must be applied to the cut section as shown. This is called the bending moment on the section. Both V and M are total stresses on the section.

Again, consider a section to the right of the load, as shown in Fig. 39-12, *B*. Now the shear must be 600 lb., acting upward on the cut section, to satisfy the laws of equilibrium. The bending moment must be 400 (x) – 1000 $(x - 6)$. Thus the shear changed sign as the load was passed and the bending moment began to diminish.

From these illustrations we may define the shear and the bending moment at any section of a beam as follows:

The total *shear* on any section of a beam is equal to the algebraic sum of all the external, normal forces acting on the beam to one side of the section. For horizontal beams, if this sum is upward to the left of the section, the shear is arbitrarily said to have a *positive sign*. The reverse is true on the right of the section.

Bending moment at any section of a beam is the algebraic sum of the moments about the section of all external forces to one side of the section. For horizontal beams, clockwise moments of forces to the left of the section are said to be *positive*. The reverse is true of forces on the right of the section.

Shear and bending moment in a beam are extremely important; from them the maximum induced stresses in the beam are computed. By the use of their diagrams it is possible to determine the elastic deformation of the beam under load, as well as to find the angular rotations of the beam at its supports. It is then desirable to investigate their interrelationships.

The shear diagram for the whole beam is shown in Fig. 39-12, *C*, and the bending moment diagram in Fig. 39-12, *D*.

INTERRELATIONSHIPS BETWEEN SHEAR AND BENDING MOMENT

In Fig. 39-12, *E*, is shown a portion of the bending moment diagram from *A*, for two sections at a differential distance, *dx* apart. These sections are indicated on the bending moment diagram of *D*, with bending moments M_L and M_R at the left and right ends of the portion of beam. This portion has been indicated in *E*, together with the corresponding portion of the shear diagram directly above it.

The portion of the beam, included in the length *dx* is shown *F*. On the cut section to the left of this portion has been replaced the bending moment M_L and the shear V_L, and at the right end, the bending moment M_R and the shear V_R, as shown. These internal stresses now become external forces, since the sections have been cut and the necessary stresses replaced to restore equilibrium for this portion, considered as a free body.

The free body of Fig. 39-12, *F*, must satisfy the laws of equilibrium, since it was at rest in the beam. Therefore:

$$M_R = M_L + V_L \ d \qquad \text{(Eq. a)}$$
(See Fig. 39-12.)

and

$$V_L = V_R \qquad \text{(Eq. b)}$$
(See Fig. 39-12.)

Eq. a satisfies the law which says the moments of all external forces acting upon the free body must be zero. It will be noted that V_R does not enter the equation, since moments are being taken about the right-hand end and its moment arm is zero. If there had been an intervening applied load, it would have been included. Eq. b is from the law that states that the sum of the vertical forces must be zero.

In Fig. 39-12, *E*, the difference between M_L and M_R is indicated by a dimensional arrow. Eq. a shows that the actual difference between these two bending moments is $V_L \ dx$. Now the inclination of the bending moment diagram, with the horizontal, is indicated on the figure as an angle, designated by the Greek letter Θ. The tangent of the angle Θ is obviously the following:

$$+ \text{an } \Theta = \frac{M_R - M_L}{dx} = V_L \qquad \text{(Eq. c)}$$
(See Fig. 39-12.)

If this expression is multipled by *dx*, there results the difference between the bending moments to the right and left of the portion. But this has already been proved to be $V_L \ dx$ by Eq. a. Therefore, it may be concluded that:

1. *The shear at any section of a beam is equal to the tangent of the angle of inclination of the bending moment diagram at the same section. Or, as often stated, the shear is the slope of the bending moment diagram.*

Since, mathematically, any curve attains a maximum (or minimum) value when its tangent or slope becomes zero, it follows that:

2. *Maximum (or minimum) bending moment in any beam occurs at any section where the shear diagram passes through zero.*

In connection with Fig. 39-12, *E*, it has been shown that the increment of the bending moment for the length *dx* has the value $V_L \ dx$. It will be seen that $V_L \ dx$ is the area of the differential portion of the shear diagram shown directly above the bending moment portion. If a longer section were to be considered, the differences between the bending moments to the left and right would be the sum of the separate values of $V_L \ dx$ for the distance. It therefore follows that:

3. *The increment of the bending moment between any two sections of a beam is numerically equal to the net area of the shear diagram lying between the same two sections.*

The term *net area* is used to indicate that positive and negative areas are to be added algebraically. In Fig. 39-12, *C* and *D*, it will be noted that the bending moment begins to decrease as soon as the shear passes through zero at the load. Negative area of the shear diagram on the right also begins to subtract from the positive area on the left as the load is passed. As a corollary to principle 3, it may then be stated:

4. *The net area of the shear diagram for any complete beam is equal to zero.*

Or

5. *The net area of the shear diagram for any beam is equal to zero between any two points of zero bending moment on the same beam.*

The first of these statements applies to beams with fixed ends if the portion of the beam within the clamp may be considered. This is usually not feasible.

Finally, the law expressed in Eq. a may be stated as a principle:

6. *The bending moment at any section of a beam is equal to the bending moment at any section to the left, plus the shear at that section (just to the right if a load occurs there), times the distance between sections, minus the moments of intervening loads about the section in question.*

STRESSES IN A BEAM DUE TO BENDING MOMENT

In Fig. 39-13 is shown a portion of a beam that is assumed to be subject to bending caused by loads not shown. On the side of the beam, two straight lines were drawn parallel to each other before bending occurred. After bending, these lines were still straight but now were converging toward the top of the beam and diverging toward the bottom, as indicated by the dashed lines. The distance between them decreased at the top and increased at the bottom. At a point near the center, the distance remained constant.

Since, within the proportional limit, deformation is proportional to stress, and since the lines came closer at the top and diverged at the bottom, it may be concluded that tensile stress exists at the bottom, that compressive stress exists at the top, and that at a point near the center, where the distance remained constant,

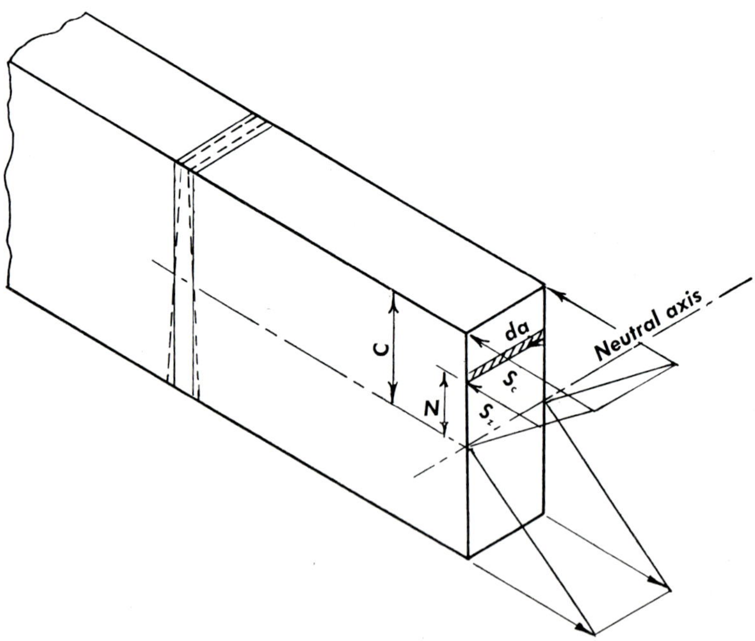

Fig. 39-13. Stresses caused by bending.

there was neither tension nor compression. The line across the section of the beam, where neither tension nor compression exists, is known as the *neutral axis.*

These tensile and compressive stresses are indicated at the right of Fig. 39-13, replaced on the cut section. Since the lines remained straight during bending, and since stress is proportional to strain or deformation, it may be concluded that the stresses increased from zero at the neutral axis, in a straight line ratio, to a maximum value of S at the outer surface of the beam, as indicated.

If it be assumed that the bending is induced by loads (in the plane of the drawing), perpendicular to the axis of the beam, then the induced tensile and compressive forces replaced on the cut section are the only horizontal forces acting on the portion of the beam shown. As a result, according to the laws of equilibrium, the sum of the tensile unit stresses times the areas over which they act must be equal to the sum of the compressive unit stresses times the areas over which they act.

Let the unit stress, induced at a distance z from the neutral axis, be designated S_z, and the unit stress induced at the outer fiber or surface be called S_c. S_z acts over an infinitely small or differential strip of the beam designated *da.* Both above and below S_z, the value of S_z changes. To satisfy the law of equilibrium, the following equation must maintain:

$$\Sigma S_z \, da = 0 \qquad \text{(Eq. a)}$$

(See Fig. 39-13.)

But it has been established that S_z varies from its minimum value of zero at the neutral axis to its maximum of S at the outer fiber, according to a straight line ratio. Therefore:

$$\frac{S_z}{z} = \frac{S}{c} \text{ or } S_z = S\frac{z}{c} \qquad \text{(Eq. b)}$$

(See Fig. 39-13.)

where c is the distance from the neutral axis to the outer surface. Substituting into Eq. a the value of S_z given by Eq. b, there results:

$$\frac{S}{c}\Sigma z da = 0 \qquad \text{(Eq. c)}$$

(See Fig. 39-13.)

Eq. c is a very important one. It enables us to locate the neutral axis of any beam subject to bending stresses within the proportional limit. Since the quantity S/c is a constant, being the induced unit stress at one unit out from the neutral axis, it does not participate in the summation. Then Eq. c states that the summation of the moments of the differential areas of the cross section of a beam, about the neutral axis, is equal to zero. But this is the exact requirement for locating the center of gravity of an area. Therefore, it may be concluded that: *The neutral axis of any straight beam, at stresses within the proportional limit, lies at the gravity axis of the cross section of the beam. This axis is perpendicular to the plane of loading.*

To find the neutral axis of any beam it is necessary only to locate the gravity axis of the cross section, perpendicular to the plane of loading. (Of course, gravity axis of an area is strictly a misnomer, since area has no weight. The term is used for an area since the mathematical equation for locating the center of gravity of a mass in a thin sheet would be identical.)

The gravity axis of any beam of symmetrical cross section will, of course, lie at the beam's center. This will apply to such sections as a circle, a rectangle, etc. Methods will later be developed for locating the gravity axis for such irregular sections as those found in the metal portions of a pontic.

Referring to Fig. 39-13 and remembering that the bending moment M, produced on any section by the external loads, must be equal to the opposing moment, produced by the induced bending stresses, it is possible to evaluate induced stresses by equating these two moments. The unit stress S_z, acting over the differential area *da,* with a leverage of *z* about the neutral axis, produces a moment $S_z\ da(z)$. Then

$$\Sigma S_z\ da(z) = M \qquad \text{(Eq. d)}$$
(See Fig. 39-13.)

But it has been shown that S_z is equal to $\frac{S}{c}$ z. Making this substitution:

$$\frac{S}{c}\ \Sigma z^2\ da = M \qquad \text{(Eq. e)}$$
(See Fig. 39-13.)

The quantity S/c is a constant. The summation of the products $z^2\ da$ for the whole cross section is called the moment of inertia of the cross section, about the neutral axis, and is designated by the letter *I.* Making this substitution:

$$S = \frac{Mc}{I} \qquad \text{(Eq. f)}$$
(See Fig. 39-13.)

Eq. f (Fig. 39-13) gives the stress in any beam, originally straight, that is subject to a bending moment, *M,* in terms of the moment of inertia of the cross section about the neutral axis and the distance from the neutral axis to the point where the unit stress is being computed. Since we are ordinarily interested in the greatest unit stress induced in the beam, the *c* used is the distance from the neutral axis to the most remote fiber.

STRESSES IN A CIRCULAR BAR SUBJECT TO TORQUE

In a manner exactly similar to that shown for the formula Eq. f (Fig. 39-13) in the discussion of stresses in a beam due to bending moment, it may be shown that the stresses induced in a circular bar subject to torsion are induced in quite an analogous manner.

In Fig. 39-10 is shown a torsion bar, with a torque, *T,* applied to its left end. On the cut section at the right is shown the induced unit stresses replaced on the cut section. These stresses vary as a straight line from zero, at the center of the bar, to a maximum value of S_s, at the outer surface. The fact that the variation is according to a straight line results from experimental determinations.

Let S_z be the induced unit stress at any point *z* distance from the center. This stress acts over a differential area, *da.* Now, from the laws of equilibrium, the summation of the actuating torque *T* and the opposing torques resulting from the induced stresses must be zero. Therefore:

$$T = \Sigma S_z\ da\ (z) \qquad \text{(Eq. g)}$$
(See Fig. 39-13.)

where *z* is the leverage of the total stress $S_z\ da$, about the center or pole of the circle. But, as was the case in Eq. f (Fig. 39-13) for beams, S_z equals $S_s\ z/c$, where *c* is the radius of the circle. Making this substitution in Eq. a:

$$T = \frac{S_s \Sigma_z{}^2\ da}{c} \quad \text{or} \quad T = \frac{S_s J}{c} \qquad \text{(Eq. h)}$$
(See Fig. 39-13.)

where $\Sigma z^2\ da$ is equal to *J,* which is called the polar moment of inertia of the cross section of the circle. Polar moment of inertia is equal to the summation of the differential areas times the squares of their distances from the center of the circle, or the "pole."

Eq. h (Fig. 39-13) applies only to circles. It gives grossly erroneous results when used with other shapes, such as a rectangle. It is, of course, valid only within the proportional limit of the material.

MOMENTS, CENTERS OF GRAVITY, AND MOMENTS OF INERTIA OF AREAS

In Fig. 39-14 is shown an area, *A,* of irregular perimeter. Let it be required to find the distance *c* from its gravity axis *o-o* to any parallel axis *y-y.* Let *x* be the distance from the gravity axis *o-o* to any differential area *da* of the area *A. x* is considered positive when it lies above *o-o* and negative when below. The moment of the

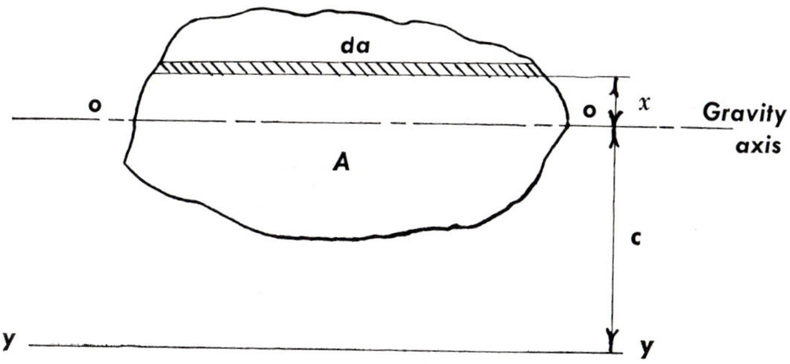

Fig. 39-14. Moment of area—moment of inertia.

area *A*, about *y-y*, is equal to the following:

$$m_{y-y} = \Sigma da\ (c + x) = c\Sigma da + \Sigma xda$$

(Eq. a)
(See Fig. 39-14.)

But $c\Sigma da$ is equal to *cA*, and by definition of center of gravity, $\Sigma\ x\ da$ must be equal to zero. Therefore:

$$cA = m_{y-y} \quad \text{or} \quad c = \frac{m_{y-y}}{A}$$

(Eq. b)
(See Fig. 39-14.)

Thus, in order to find the gravity axis of an area, in any given direction, it is only necessary to find the moment of the area about any parallel axis and to divide this moment by the total area. The result is the distance from the known axis to the gravity axis.

Again, take moments of inertia of the total area *A* about the axis *y-y*. This is given by the equation

$$I_{y-y} = \Sigma da(c + x)^2 = \Sigma da(c^2 + 2cx + x^2)$$

(Eq. c)
(See Fig. 39-14.)

or

$$I_{y-y} = c^2A + 2c\Sigma\ x\ da + \Sigma\ da\ x^2$$

(Eq. d)
(See Fig. 39-14.)

But the middle term of the right-hand member of Eq. d (Fig. 39-14) is zero by definition of center of gravity. The right-hand member is by definition the moment of inertia of the area about its own gravity axis *o-o*. Making these substitutions, Eq. d becomes

$$I_{y-y} = I_{o-o} + A\ c^2$$

(Eq. e)
(See Fig. 39-14.)

The law expressed in Eq e may be stated as follows: *The moment of inertia of any area about any axis is equal to its moment of inertia about its gravity axis parallel to the axis in question, plus the area, times the distance squared, between axes.*

The is an important principle. In the case of an irregular area, the gravity axis is not known in advance. Its gravity axis and moment of inertia about that axis may be found at one operation by taking first and second moments of the parts of the area, about any convenient axis parallel to the direction of the axis desired, and using the results thus found in Eq. b and Eq. e.

As an example of the use of Eq. b and Eq. e, let it be required to find the gravity axis, perpendicular to the long side, and the moment of inertia about that axis of the 3 by 12 inch rectangle shown in Fig. 39-15. Of course, the gravity axis of the rectangle is known in advance through symmetry. The moment of inertia of the rectangle about its gravity axis is known from calculus to be $b\ d^3/12$. In this expression, *b* is parallel to the axis about which moment of inertia is to be taken and *d* is perpendicular to that axis.

Divide the rectangle into twelve strips, parallel to the short side as shown. Each

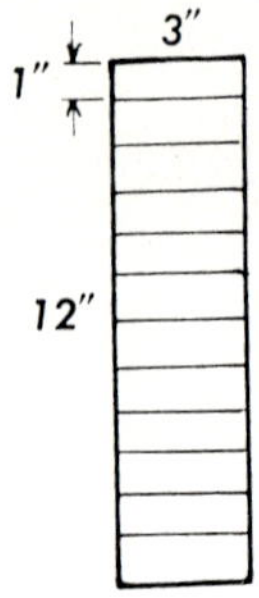

	Leverage	Area	First moment	Second moment
	0.5	3	1.5	0.75
	1.5	3	4.5	6.75
	2.5	3	7.5	18.75
	3.5	3	10.5	36.75
	4.5	3	13.5	60.75
	5.5	3	16.5	90.75
	6.5	3	19.5	126.9
	7.5	3	22.5	169.
	8.5	3	25.5	217.
	9.5	3	28.5	271.
	10.5	3	31.5	331.
	11.5	3	34.5	397.
Totals		36	216	1726.4

From Eq. 7: $c = \dfrac{216}{36} = 6.0$ in.

From Eq. 8: $I_{o\text{-}o} = 1726 - 36 \times 6^2 = 1726 - 1296 = 430$ in.^{4}

Fig. 39-15. Tabular determination of **c** and $\mathbf{I_{0\text{-}0}}$.

strip is one unit high and three units wide. The distance of the center of each strip from the top of the rectangle (the axis y-y here selected for moments) is indicated at the right of each rectangle in the illustration. The area of each strip is 3, as shown in column 2 of the tabular material. If 3 for each strip is multiplied by the indicated moment arms for the strips, the product, shown in column 3, is obtained. Thus 3 times 1.5 gives 4.5. When the figure in column 3 is again multiplied by the moment arm of its strip, the second moments of column 4 are obtained. Thus the figure 13.5 of column 3 is multipled by 4.5 to give the 60.75 of column 4.

When columns 2, 3, and 4 are each added, the total area of the rectangle is seen to be 36, as it should; the sum of the first moments of the strips is seen to be 216, and the sum of the second moments of the area is 1726.4.

From Eq. b (Fig. 39-14), distance c from the top of the rectangle to its center of gravity is computed by dividing 216 by 36, which gives the number 6, as it should from symmetry.

Attention is called to Eq. e. Here it was shown that $I_{y\text{-}y}$ was equal to the moment of inertia of the area about its own gravity axis, plus the area times the square of the distance between axes. Column 4 of the table of Fig. 39-15 gives only the area times the square of the distance between axes. The moment of inertia of each strip about its own gravity axis (as called for in Eq. e) does not appear. Suppose the last are ignored for these narrow strips. Let an examination be made of the error so produced.

It has been stated that the moment of inertia of a rectangle about its gravity axis is equal to b $d^3/12$. For one of these narrow strips this would be $(3 \times 1^3)/12$ or 0.25. A glance at column 4 will show that if 0.25 is added to each of the figures, the total of 1726.4 will be increased by only 3. Therefore, it may be concluded that the portion $I_{o\text{-}o}$ of Eq. e may be neglected when the strips, as here, are taken narrow enough. Then for the rectangle of Fig. 39-15:

$$I_{o\text{-}o} = 1726 - 36 \times 6^2 = 1726 - 1296 = 430 \text{ in.}^4$$

The figure for moment of inertia of the rectangle may be checked by using the formula b $d^3/12$, from which it is found that $I_{o\text{-}o}$ is 432 in.^{4}. Thus it is seen that the tabular method of determining moment of inertia and center of gravity is quite accurate (error less than 0.5%) if width of strips is taken small enough. This

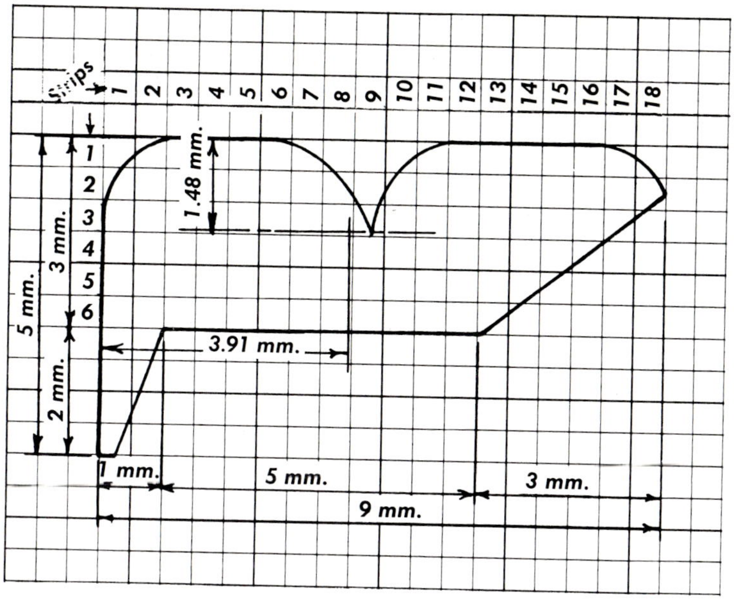

Fig. 39-16. Moment of inertia and center of gravity for typical section of dental bridge pontic. (Courtesy J. F. Jelenko Co.)

Table 39-1 (see also Figs. 39-15 and 39-16)

(1) Strip no.	*(2) Areas (sq. mm.)*	*(3) Moment arm (mm.)*	*(4) First moment (mm.³)*	*(5) Second moment (mm.⁴)*
1	3.1	0.25	0.77	0.19
2	4.0	0.75	3.00	2.25
3	4.1	1.25	5.13	6.41
4	3.75	1.75	6.56	11.50
5	3.45	2.25	7.76	17.50
6	3.15	2.75	8.65	23.60
Totals	21.55		31.87	61.45

tabular method must be resorted to for sections whose peripheries do not follow any regular geometric pattern. This is almost always the case for sections of beams applicable in dental bridges.

As a second example of the use of Eq. b and Eq. e, let it be required to determine the gravity axis parallel to the occlusal plane and the moment of inertia about this axis for the section of the metal portion of a bridge pontic, as shown in Fig. 39-16. This section was made from actual measurements of such a pontic. It has been plotted on cross-sectioned paper to such a scale that 0.5 mm. is equal to the side of one of the squares of the paper, as shown. The stop on the lingual side of the pontic will be ignored, since it does not extend the full length of the bridge.

Here the bridge section has been divided into six strips, each 0.5 mm. in depth. These are numbered at the left. The areas of the strips may be estimated quite closely from the squares of the paper included in each.

Estimates for the areas of strips affected by the carvings will not be serious, since if moments are taken about the occlusal surface, the leverage will be small. The estimates for the area of each of the strips are shown in Table 39-1.

Computing the distance from the occlusal surface to the gravity axis according to Eq. b (Fig. 39-14):

$$c = \frac{31.87}{21.55} = 1.48 \text{ mm.}$$

Computing the moment of inertia from Eq. e and ignoring the moments of inertia of the strips about the gravity axis of each:

$$I_{o-o} = 61.45 - 21.55 \times 1.48^2 = 61.45 - 47.2 = 14.25 \text{ mm.}^4$$

Center of gravity

In Table 39-1 was computed the distance *c* from the occlusal plane to the gravity axis, parallel to that plane. This axis only partially locates the center of gravity of the cross section. The center of gravity lies on that axis, but its exact location is still indeterminate. In order to locate the exact center of gravity, it is necessary to determine another gravity axis, making an angle with the one previously determined. Then the true center of gravity will lie at the intersection of the two axes.

Table 39-2 is used to determine a second gravity axis at right angles to the first one determined. Moments are taken about a line representing the lingual side of the metallic portion of the pontic. One-half millimeter strip widths are retained because they were used in the first determination (Fig. 39-15). The computations are exactly similar to those used for determining the axis parallel to the occlusal plane. Second moments are not included because they are not pertinent to gravity axis determination.

Proceeding exactly as previously:

$$x = \frac{84.95}{21.69} = 3.91 \text{ mm.}$$

This vertical axis is shown together with the horizontal axis previously determined in Fig. 39-16. Their intersection is the center of gravity of the cross-sectional area. The center of gravity of the cross section of the metallic portion of the pontic has significance for the constructor of the bridge. The centers of gravity of contiguous pontics and that of the soldered joint between them should all coincide when the bridge is assembled. Knowledge of the locations of these centers of gravity is of assistance to the judgment of the technician in making this proper assembly. With this idea in mind, the straightness of the longitudinal axis of the bridge may be much better controlled.

Table 39-2. Gravity axis parallel to lingual side of pontic (see also Fig. 39-17)

(1) Strip no.	(2) Areas (mm.^{2})	(3) Moment arms (mm.)	(4) First moments (mm.^{3})
1	1.3	0.25	0.33
2	1.5	0.75	1.12
3	1.5	1.25	1.87
4	1.5	1.75	2.62
5	1.5	2.25	3.36
6	1.5	2.75	4.12
7	1.4	3.25	4.15
8	1.25	3.75	4.68
9	0.92	4.25	3.91
10	1.2	4.75	5.70
11	1.4	5.25	7.34
12	1.5	5.75	8.62
13	1.4	6.25	8.73
14	1.2	6.75	8.10
15	1.02	7.25	7.40
16	0.8	7.75	6.20
17	0.6	8.25	4.95
18	0.2	8.75	1.75
Totals	21.69		84.95

A quick and reasonably accurate method of graphically locating the center of gravity of the section is indicated in Fig. 39-17. Take an accurate cutout of a scale drawing of the metallic part of the pontic section. Make two pinholes at different points on the cutout. Enlarge these slightly so that the cutout rotates freely on the pin. From the pin suspend a thread, with weight

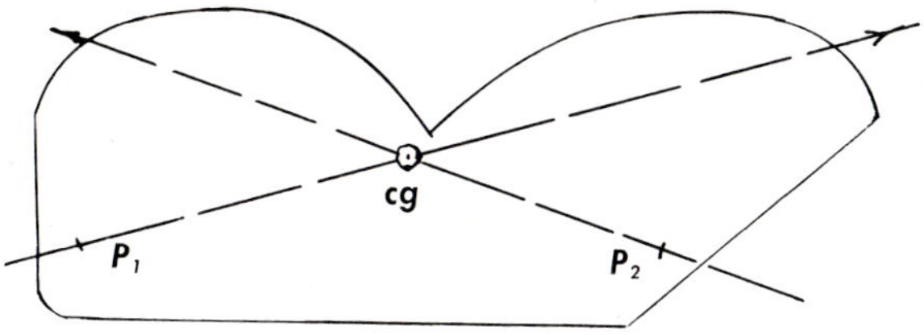

Fig. 39-17. Center of gravity of pontic section.

attached. When cutout and weight hang freely and at rest, mark the line which the thread makes on the cutout. This is one gravity axis. Hang the assembly from the second pinhole and repeat. The intersection of the two axes is the center of gravity of the section. Fig. 39-17 shows this type of determination for the center of gravity of the metallic portion of the pontic section shown in Fig. 39-16. It will be noted that the center of gravity, so determined, compares very favorably with that determined by tabular computation.

SECTION MODULUS—COMPUTING STRESSES IN A BRIDGE

Referring to Eq. f (Fig. 39-13) in the discussion on stresses in a beam due to bending moment, it is shown here that the unit stress induced in a beam at any section is equal to the bending moment at that section, divided by the fraction I/c. This fraction is called the *section modulus* of the beam. The maximum induced unit stress, in any beam at its outer fiber, times the section modulus of the beam is equal to the bending moment applied at the section. Ordinarily, we are interested only in the greatest induced unit stress. Therefore, the greatest distance *c* from the neutral axis to the outer surface is to be used in determining the section modulus. For the beam of Fig. 39-16, the depth is 3 mm. The distance from the occlusal surface to the neutral axis is 1.48 mm. Therefore, the distance from the neutral axis to the lower surface is 1.52 mm. From this and the value previously computed for $I_{o\text{-}o}$, the section modulus is

$$\frac{I}{c} = \frac{14.25}{1.52} = 9.38 \text{ mm.}^3$$

The dentist is accustomed to the use of a millimeter scale for taking measurements in the mouth. However, almost universally the physical properties of materials used for bridges are given in terms of the English system of measurement. It is therefore necessary to reduce the section modulus from mm.^{3} to in.^{3} This is done by multiplying by the cube of the factor of 0.03937 used for reducing millimeters to inches. This cube is 0.0000609. The section modulus is then, in terms of inches:

$$\frac{I}{c} = 9.38 \times 0.0000609 = 0.000571 \text{ in.}^3$$

The bridge from which the pontic section (Fig. 39-16) was taken is shown in Fig. 39-18. Let an occlusal load of 100 lb. be assumed to be applied at a distance of 8 mm. from the left support. From Eq. c in the discussion on the laws of static equilibrium:

$$R_L = \frac{100 \times 12}{20} = 60 \text{ lb.}$$

$$M = 60 \times 8 = 480 \text{ mm. lb.} = 18.85 \text{ in. lb.}$$

From Eq. f (Fig. 39-13) in the discussion on stresses in a beam due to bending moment using the value of I/c previously computed:

$$S = \frac{18.85}{0.000571} = 33{,}000 \text{ lb./sq.in.}$$

It will be seen that the operation illustrated in Fig. 39-16 and in Table 39-1 represents a considerable amount of detailed work. Data are given in Chapter 40 that are designed to shorten this work.

As a second example of the determination of stress, let it be required to find the greatest bending moment in inch pounds that the section of Fig. 39-18 will sustain. Assume the allowable unit stress in the material is 21,000 lb./sq.in. and use the approximate I/c computed above:

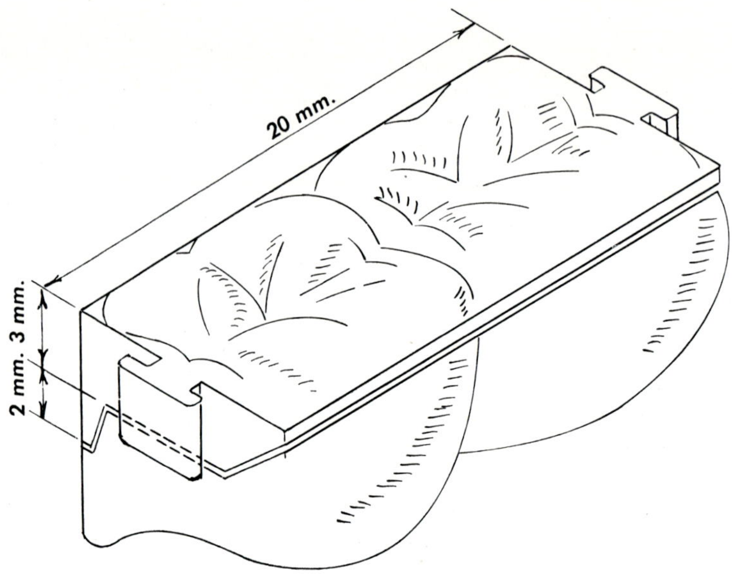

Fig. 39-18. Typical dental bridge—freely supported. (Courtesy J. F. Jelenko Co.)

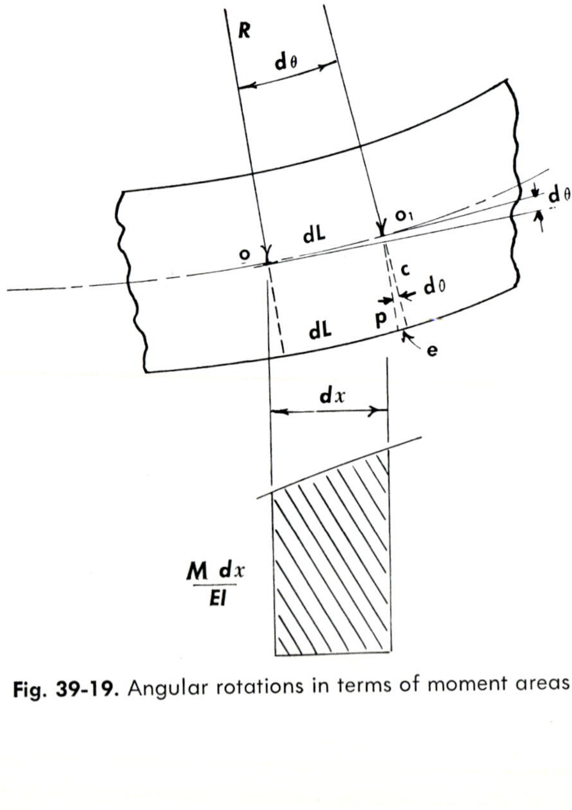

Fig. 39-19. Angular rotations in terms of moment areas.

$$\frac{I}{c} = 0.000571 \text{ inches cubed}$$

$$M = 21{,}000 \times 0.000571 = 12.0 \text{ in.lb. of bending moment}$$

If the load that produced it be assumed at the center of the span:

$$\frac{PL}{4} = 12.0 \text{ in.lb. } P = 12.0 \frac{4}{20 \times 0.0394} = 61 \text{ lb.}$$

The use of Eq. h (Fig. 39-13) in the discussion on stresses in a circular bar subject to torque is exactly similar to that shown for the flexure formula. The value of the polar moment of inertia for a circle is $\frac{\pi d^4}{32}$ or $\frac{\pi r^4}{2}$. The value of the section modulus is $\frac{\pi d^3}{16}$ or $\frac{\pi r^3}{2}$. When the applied torque in inch pounds is known, the induced unit stresses at the surface of the circle may be found by substituting in Eq. h the torque and the values given for the section modulus. It should be kept in mind that Eq. h is valid for circular sections only.

ANGULAR ROTATIONS OF BEAM SECTIONS IN TERMS OF MOMENT AREAS

In Fig. 39-19 is shown a short length of beam (originally straight) bent into a curve by forces not shown. The trace of the intersection of the neutral plane of the beam with facing elevation is indicated by the dash-dot line. Any short length, *dL,* of the beam at the neutral axis may be considered to substantially coincide with a circle of unknown radius *R,* since the length *dL* may be considered as infinitely short. The radius of this circle is said to be radius of curvature of the beam at the point where *dL* is taken.

Draw radii of curvature of the beam at points *o* and o_1 on the axis at the neutral plane. The points *o* and o_1 are *dL* distance apart. These radii meet at some point above the beam, which is the momentary center of curvature. These converging radii make a very small angle with each other, labeled $d\theta$. At point o_1, *dL* distance to the right of *o,* draw a line parallel to the left-hand radius. Also draw a line *c* by extending the right-hand radius. These two lines cut off a distance *e* on the lower fiber of the beam. The distance *e* is the elongation of the lower fiber of the beam, in the length *dL,* caused by the tension induced by bending. This is true because the original length of the fiber was *dL.* This length did not change at the neutral plane, since no bending stresses exist there. The dashed line o_1p is parallel to the left-hand radius. Therefore, these two lines cut off the original length on the lower fiber, as shown. Its elongation is then *e* by identity. Also, if deflections are small, *dL* will be substantially equal to *dx,* as shown in Fig. 39-19, for the width of the corresponding portion of the bending moment diagram shown immediately below.

Now

$$R\, d\theta = dL = dx \qquad \text{(Eq. a)}$$

(See Fig. 39-19.)

and

$$c\, d\theta = e, \text{ or } d\theta = \frac{e}{c} \qquad \text{(Eq. b)}$$

(See Fig. 39-19.)

Substituting this value of $d\theta$ in Eq. a, there results:

$$\frac{Re}{c} = dx \qquad \text{(Eq. c)}$$

(See Fig. 39-19.)

And, in turn, from Eq. f (Fig. 39-13) in the discussion on stresses in a beam due to bending moment:

$$S = \frac{Mc}{I}$$

where S is the unit stress, due to bending, at the fiber c distance from the neutral axis. It is this unit stress that opposes the elongation *e* in this fiber. From Eq. d (Fig. 39-11) in the discussion on structural significance of physical properties:

$$e = \frac{S}{E}\, dx = \frac{Mc}{EI}\, dx \qquad \text{(Eq. d)}$$

(See Fig. 39-19.)

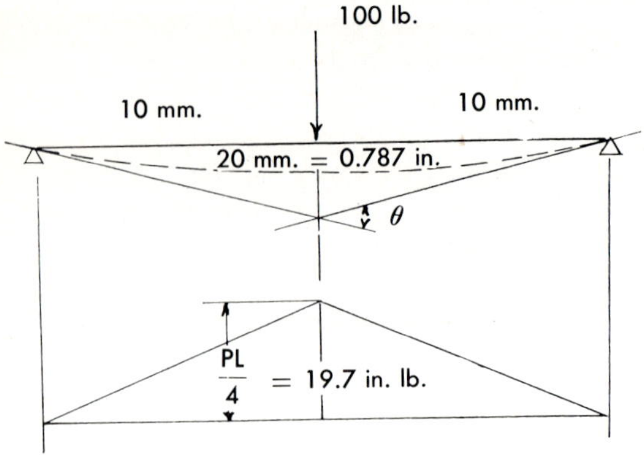

Fig. 39-20. Angular rotations.

Substituting this value of *e* back into Eq. c, we have:

$$\frac{R\ M}{EIc}\ c\ dx = dx \text{ or } MR = EI$$

(Eq. e)
(See Fig. 39-19.)

Eq. e is important. It shows that the product of the bending moment and the radius of curvature are always a positive constant, that is, EI. If the bending moment is small, the radius of curvature is large; if the bending moment is zero, the radius of curvature becomes infinite, that is, we have a straight beam; if the bending moment is constant for a considerable distance along the beam, the radius of curvature is also constant, that is, the beam is bent into the arc of a circle; if the bending moment is positive, the radius of curvature is also positive in order that the product may be positive; if the bending moment is negative, the radius of curvature must also be negative, that is, extend from the beam in the direction opposite to that considered positive, in order that the product may remain positive.

Substituting the value of *e* shown in Eq. d, back into Eq. b, there results:

$$d\theta = \frac{Mc\ dx}{EI}\ \frac{1}{c} = \frac{M\ dx}{EI}$$

(Eq. f)
(See Fig. 39-19.)

Eq. f shows that the very small or differential angle between the radii of curvature drawn a differential distance apart is equal to area of the M/EI diagram for the beam, within the length *dx*. This is shown in Fig. 39-19 as a cross-hatched area. That the right-hand member of Eq. f is this area is seen by the fact that the height of the rectangle (differential trapezoid) is M/EI, and the width is *dx*.

If tangents to the elastic curve of the beam are drawn at the extremities of each of the radii, the angle between these tangents is also equal to dθ, since the sides of the new angle are, respectively, perpendicular to the radii. Now, if two tangents are drawn to the elastic curve at any two points of a beam, the angle between these two tangents is obviously made up of the sum of the differential angles (as indicated in Fig. 39-19) for the lengths d*x* lying between the points of tangency. This is evidently the area of the M/EI diagram lying between the points of tangency. Therefore, it may be stated: *If two tangents are drawn to any two points on the elastic curve of a beam, the angle these tangents make with each other is expressed in radians and is equal to the net area of the M/EI diagram lying between the two points of tangency.*

In Fig. 39-20 is shown the span of Fig. 39-18 loaded with 100 lb. placed at its center. The elastic curve is indicated by the dashed line, and the *M/EI* diagram is shown below with its bending moment at the span center, $\frac{PL}{4}$. Tangents are drawn to the elastic curve at each of the supports. These tangents intersect at the center of the beam (because of symmetry) and make an angle θ with each other. Let it be required to find this angle if the modulus of elasticity of the material of the beam is 14,000,000 lb./sq.in.

In the discussion on moments, center of gravity, and moments of inertia of areas

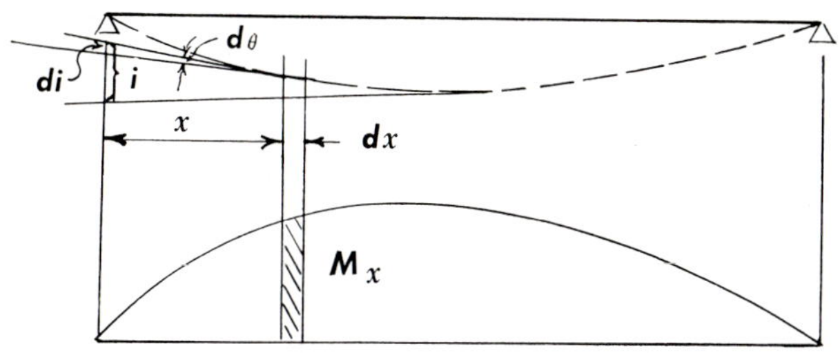

Fig. 39-21. Beam deflections in terms of moment areas.

it was shown that the moment of inertia for the cross section of this beam was 14.25 mm.[4] Let it be assumed that this value is constant for the span (not entirely true for a dental bridge). The moment of inertia then reduces to $14.25 \times 0.03937^4 = 0.0000341$ in.[4] when transferred into the English system.

According to the principle stated, the angle θ is equal to the entire area of the M/EI diagram for the beam. Then:

$$\theta = \frac{19.7 \times 0.787}{2 \times 14{,}000{,}000 \times 0.0000341} = 0.0162 \text{ radian}$$

A radian is 57.3 degrees. Therefore:

$$\theta = 57.3 \times 0.0162 = 0.93 \text{ degree}$$

This is a very small angle and, of course, is equal to double the angle of rotation at each support, for this particular case, these angles being equal because of symmetry.

DEFLECTIONS OF BEAMS IN TERMS OF MOMENT AREAS

In Fig. 39-21 is shown a beam that is bent, although causes are not shown. Its elastic curve is indicated by the dashed line. A bending moment diagram is shown below the beam. Two tangents to the elastic curve have been drawn at a differential distance apart and x distance from the left support. These tangents make an angle $d\theta$ with each other. This angle $d\theta$ is shown, according to the previous discussion on angular rotations of beam sections in terms of moment areas, to be equal to $M_x\,dx/EI$.

These two tangent lines cut off an intercept, *di,* on a line normal to the unstressed position of the beam and passing through the left support. If the tangents were horizontal, this intercept would be exactly equal to $x\,d\theta$, the differential arc of a circle of radius x. It has been shown in the discussion on angular rotations of beam sections in terms of moment areas that the rotations of these tangents is quite small. If rotations remain small, it may be assumed, without sensible error, that di is equal to $x\,d\theta$. But in Eq. f (Fig. 39-19) it was shown that $d\theta$ is equal to $\frac{Mdx}{EI}$. Therefore:

$$di = x\,d\theta = \frac{M \times dx}{EI} \qquad \text{(Eq. a)}$$

(See Fig. 39-21.)

Expressed in words, Eq. a states: *If two tangents are drawn at any two points on the elastic curve of a beam, these tangents cut off an intercept on any line perpendicular to the unstressed position of the beam, which is equal to the moment of that part of the M/EI diagram lying between the two points of tangency about the line where the intercept is taken.*

As an example of the use of this principle, consider the cantilever beam shown in Fig. 39-22. A single load P is applied at the free end. The bending moment diagram is shown below with a bending moment of $-PL$ at the clamp. The variation of the bending moment from the free end to the clamp is according to a straight line.

Draw tangents to the elastic curve at the

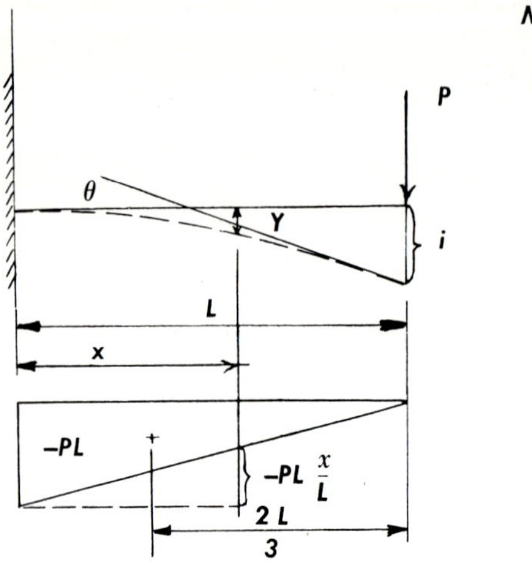

Fig. 39-22. Cantilever beam deflection in terms of moment areas.

free end and at the clamp. These intersect to form the angle Θ. The tangent at the left end retains the unstressed position of the beam, since no rotation is permitted at the fixed end. The angle Θ has been shown to be equal to the area of the triangular $\frac{M}{EI}$ diagram.

The intercept *i*, on a normal line to the unstressed position of the beam, drawn at *P*, will, according to the stated principle, be equal to the moment of the triangular bending moment diagram about the right end, divided by EI. The center of gravity of a triangle lies at two thirds the distance from the apex to the base, as shown. Then:

$$i = -\frac{PL}{EI}\frac{L}{2}\frac{2L}{3} = -\frac{PL^3}{3\ EI}$$

(Eq. a)
(See Fig. 39-22.)

The deflection of the cantilever could readily have been determined at any point, intermediate between the fixed and free ends, by taking moments of the trapezoidal portion of the bending moment diagram lying between the fixed support and the point in question, about a normal line through this point, and dividing by EI. Thus at *x* distance from the fixed support,

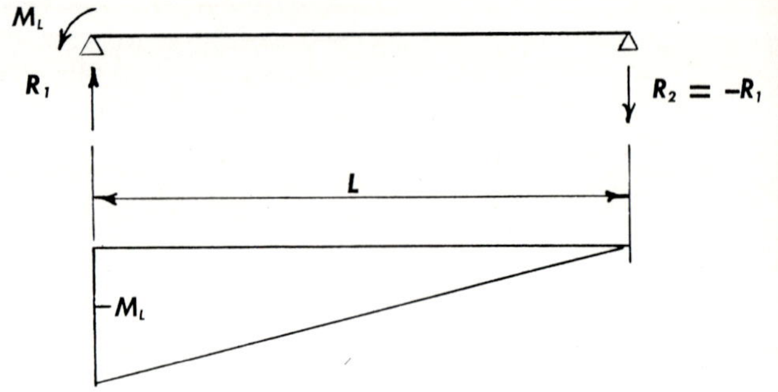

Fig. 39-23. Couple on simple beam.

the trapezoidal area of the bending moment diagram is made up of the rectangle whose height is *–PL* and whose base is *x*, minus the triangle whose base at *x* (vertical ordinate) is $-PL\frac{x}{L}$ and whose apex is at the fixed support. Taking moments of these two parts about a normal line through *x*, there results:

$$EI\ y = -\frac{PL\ x^2}{2} - (-PL)\frac{x}{L}\frac{x}{2}\frac{x}{3}$$

$$EI\ y = -\frac{PL\ x^2}{2} + \frac{P\ x^3}{6} \qquad \text{(Eq. b)}$$

(See Fig. 39-22.)

It will be noted that the right-hand member of this equation becomes $-PL^3/3$, when *x* is equal to *L*. This checks the value found in Eq. a.

BENDING MOMENT FROM A COUPLE APPLIED AT THE END OF A BEAM

In Fig. 39-23 is shown a simple span of length *L*. Let a counterclockwise couple of value M_L be applied at the left support, as shown. It has been demonstrated that a couple has the same moment about any point in its plane (see Fig. 39-6). Its moment about the right support will then be M_L. This moment is resisted by the induced reaction, at the left, times the span length *L*. Thus:

$$R_1\ L = M_L \quad \text{or} \quad R_1 = \frac{M_L}{L} \qquad \text{(Eq. a)}$$

(See Fig. 39-23.)

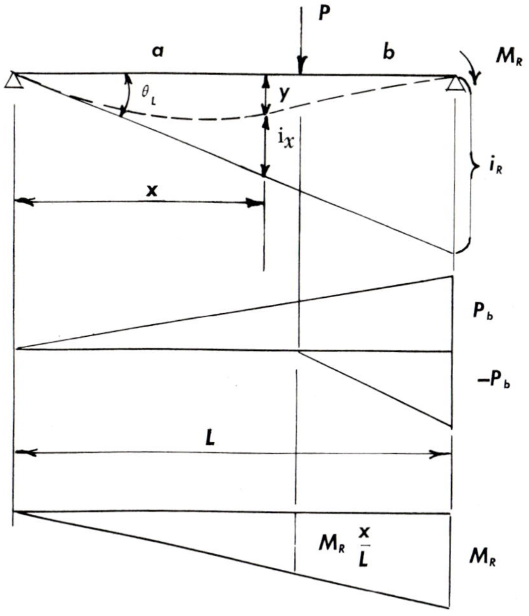

Fig. 39-24. Deflections of any span of any beam.

The bending moment diagram produced by this couple and its induced reaction at the left end will obviously be the triangle with the base M_L at the left end and its vertex at the right end. This bending moment is shown as negative because M_L is counterclockwise on the left.

If a second couple is applied at the right end, it will produce a second triangle of bending moment with a base M_R at the end and apex at the left. The composite bending moment diagram, due to the two couples, is found by adding their ordinates at various points along the length of the beam.

DEFLECTIONS OF ANY SPAN OF ANY BEAM

Fig. 39-24 shows a beam of span length, *L,* loaded with a single load, *P,* at *b* distance from the right support and *a* distance from the left support. A clockwise couple, M_R, is applied at the right support. A possible elastic curve for this loading is indicated by the dashed line.

At any distance x (x being less than a) from the left support, the deflection is given by the equation:

$$y = \Theta_L x - i_x \qquad \text{(Eq. a)}$$

(See Fig. 39-24.)

where i_x is the intercept between tangents drawn to the elastic curve at the left support and at the right extremity of x. But Θ_L is equal to i_R divided by L.

For the loading shown:

$$\text{LEI } \Theta_L = \text{Pb} \frac{L}{2}\frac{L}{3} - \text{Pb} \frac{b}{2}\frac{b}{3} - M_R \frac{L}{2}\frac{L}{3}$$

or

$$\text{LEI } \Theta_L = \frac{\text{P b}}{6} (L^2 - b^2) - \frac{M_R}{6} L^2 \qquad \text{(Eq. b)}$$

(See Fig. 39-24.)

or

$$\text{EI } \Theta_L = \frac{\text{P b}}{6L} (L^2 - b^2) - \frac{M_R L}{6} \qquad \text{(Eq. c)}$$

(See Fig. 39-24.)

In a similar manner:

$$\text{EI } i_x = \text{Pb} \frac{x \;\; x \;\; x}{L \;\; 2 \;\; 3} - M_R$$

$$\frac{x \;\; x \;\; x}{L \;\; 2 \;\; 3} = \frac{\text{Pb}}{6L} x^3 - \frac{M_R}{6L} x^3 \qquad \text{(Eq. d)}$$

(See Fig. 39-24.)

These values of Θ_L and i_x may be substituted back into Eq. a and a specific equation obtained for the elastic curve of the left portion of the beam shown in Fig. 39-24. Making these substitutions:

$$\text{EI } y = \frac{\text{Pb}}{6L} [(L^2 - b^2)x - x^3] - \frac{M_R}{6L} (L^2 x - x^3) \qquad \text{(Eq. e)}$$

(See Fig. 39-24.)

Eq. e applies only to the portion of the beam lying to the left of the load. If the equation of the curve to the right of the load is required, a new equation must be written for this portion.

The accuracy of the equation may be tested by assuming that M_R becomes zero and that b is equal to L/2, thus placing the load at the span center. Then, if x also is placed equal to L/2, the deflection under the load becomes $\frac{PL^3}{48EI}$ as it should.

A convenient concept for remembering the principles demonstrated in this discussion may be had by considering the $\frac{M}{EI}$ diagram as a load on a simple span, the original loading that produced the diagram having been removed. If the three $\frac{EI}{M}$ triangles that made up the bending moment diagram for the original loading had been considered as a load on the simple span of length L (negative moment areas being considered as upward load), then the left reaction due to this auxiliary loading would have been obtained exactly as Θ_L was obtained, that is, by writing moments about the right support and dividing by L. The angle Θ_L then becomes, under this concept, the left reaction for the auxiliary loading. When Θ_L is multiplied by x, it becomes the bending moment at the right extremity of x due to the left reaction. (See Eq. a [Fig. 39-24]).

In turn, i_x is found by taking moments about the right extremity of x of all the parts of the $\frac{M}{EI}$ moment diagram lying within x. Combining these two steps, it will be seen that the procedures for evaluating $(\Theta_L x - i_x)$ are identical with those for writing the bending moment at the right extremity of x, the $\frac{M}{EI}$ moment areas considered as a load on the simple span. Consequently, the following general law may be stated: *In order to write the equation of the elastic curve of any span under any loading consider the original loading removed and the span as a simple beam. On this simple span, place the M/EI diagram, produced by the original loading, and consider it as an auxiliary load. Write the bending moment equations for the various parts of the span for this new loading. These bending moment equations are the equations of the elastic curve of the beam, produced by the original loading.*

The above principle is applicable to any span of any beam. It does not apply to cantilever beams. Elastic curve equations have certain limitations. These are inherent in assumptions made in derivations of various formulas basic to elastic curve derivations. It is important that these be stated in order that equations are not misused.

1. Induced stresses within the material of the beam must be within the proportional limit of the material.
2. The material of the beam must have substantially the same modulus of elasticity in compression as in tension.
3. The beam must have been straight in its unstressed condition.
4. Deflections of the beam must be relatively small. Equations give increasingly inaccurate results as the beam becomes more limber.
5. Free supports allow no motion of translation normal to the beam but allow perfect freedom of rotation.
6. Fixed supports allow neither translation nor rotation at the support.

DEFLECTIONS OF BEAMS DUE TO BENDING IN TERMS OF MAXIMUM ALLOWABLE UNIT STRESS

The simple beam, with a concentrated load at its center, may be used as a concrete example for the discussion of this case (Fig. 39-20). Here the maximum bending moment in the beam is under the load. Its value is $\frac{P\ L}{4}$. The maximum deflection of the beam (also under the load) is $\frac{P\ L^3}{48\ EI}$ (see Fig. 39-24). The greatest unit stress in this beam is given by the formula $S = \frac{M\ c}{I}$ (see Eq. f [Fig. 39-

14]). The equation for the deflection of the beam may be rewritten as follows:

$$f = \frac{1}{12}\,\frac{PL}{4}\,\frac{c}{I}\,\frac{L^2}{Ec} = \frac{1}{12}\,\frac{SL^2}{Ec}$$

Similarly the deflection of a cantilever beam (with a concentrated load at its free end, is shown to be $\frac{PL^3}{3\,EI}$. The maximum bending moment (PL) and therefore the maximum unit stress is located at the fixed support. The deflection at the free end is shown to be:

$$f = \frac{PL^3}{3\,EI} = \frac{1}{3}\,\frac{PLc}{I}\,\frac{L^2}{Ec} = \frac{1}{3}\,\frac{SL^2}{Ec}$$

This operation could be repeated for many beam types and results would be of a similar nature. A general law may then be written, but only for relatively straight beams.

> For a beam, stressed to a given unit stress within the proportional limit of its material (usually its maximum allowable unit stress), its deflection varies directly as the square of its length times the allowable unit stress in its material and inversely as the modulus of elasticity of its material times some fraction of its depth, all multiplied by a constant, which depends upon the type of its load, the load placing, as well as the type of beam and cross section.

$$f = k\frac{S\,L^2}{E\,c}$$

STATICALLY INDETERMINATE BEAMS

A beam is said to be statically indeterminate when its reactions at the supports and its shear and bending moment diagrams cannot be completely evaluated by use of the laws of static equilibrium. It was previously stated that only the simple span met this requirement. Other beams (except cantilevers as regards the portion projecting from the clamp) are indeterminate.

In order to obtain reactions, shears, and bending moments for indeterminate beams, laws other than those of equilibrium must be brought into use. One of the important uses of the laws of elastic deformation of beams lies in the aid they supply in the determination of reactions, shears, and bending moments for indeterminate beams.

In Fig. 39-24, let it be assumed that the bending moment M_R was induced at the right support, because this support was fixed. Under this assumption, there is, of course, no rotation, and the tangent to the elastic curve over the support remains horizontal. Consequently, the intercept at the left support, between that tangent and one drawn at the left support, becomes zero. (See discussion on deflections of beams in terms of moment areas, Fig. 39-21.) In this case, since M_R is an unknown bending moment, it will receive a positive sign. If this is a wrong assumption, the sign obtained will be opposite and therefore correct. Writing for the intercept at the left end:

$$Pb\,\frac{L}{2}\,\frac{2L}{3} - Pb\,\frac{b}{2}\left(L - \frac{b}{3}\right) + M_R\,\frac{L}{2}\,\frac{2L}{3} = 0 \qquad \text{(Eq. f)}$$

(See Fig. 39-24.)

Solving this equation for M_R:

$$M_R = -\frac{P\,ab}{2\,L^2}\,(L + a) \qquad \text{(Eq. g)}$$

(See Fig. 39-24.)

If the load is placed at the span center, then *a* and *b* each become L/2 and M_R is (–3 PL/16) as it should be.

The left reaction may now be obtained from the definition of bending moment:

$$M_R = R_1L - Pb$$

or

$$R_1 = \frac{M_R + Pb}{L}$$

From which, substituting for M_R:

$$R_1 = \frac{Pb}{L}\left(1 - \frac{a(L + a)}{2\,L^2}\right) \qquad \text{(Eq. h)}$$

(See Fig. 39-24.)

The value of R_1 may be found from Eq. c, in cases in which the load lies at the span center, by letting *b* and *a* each become L/2. In this case, R^1 becomes 5P/16, as it should.

The values of R_1 and M_R each being known, the composite shear and bending moment diagrams may be drawn in the usual manner.

THE THEOREM OF THREE MOMENTS

Beams of multiple spans often occur, though not in a true sense in dentistry. However, a common method of solving for the bending moments at the supports of such beams also applies to single span beams with fixed ends and is included here for that reason.

In Fig. 39-25 is shown any two continuous spans of any continuous beam. This beam extends indefinitely to the right and left of the two spans shown. The spans are numbered 1 and 2 and the supports 1, 2, and 3, as shown. Let the unknown bending moments at the three supports be labeled M_1, M_2, and M_3 and the span lengths L_1 and L_2. Let a load, P_1, be placed in span 1, at a distance k_1L_1 from support 1. Let P_2 be placed in the right-hand span, at a distance k_2L_2 from support 3. The symbols k_1 and k_2 stand for fractions less than unity which, when multiplied by the respective values of L, give the required distances.

As previously stated, since the values of M_1, M_2, and M_3 are unknown, it will be proper to give them positive signs, and if their signs should really be negative, results will come out opposite to the assumption and be correct. The simple beam effects of the loads P_1 and P_2, in producing bending moments, are shown separately from the triangular moment areas produced by the bending moments at the supports.

The character of the elastic curve of the beam is, of course, unknown. A possible one is indicated by the dashed lines. A tangent line is drawn to this curve over the center support. This tangent makes angle Θ_{2L} in the left-hand span and Θ_{2R} in the right-hand span with the unstressed position of the beam. It is obvious that the two angles are equal but opposite in

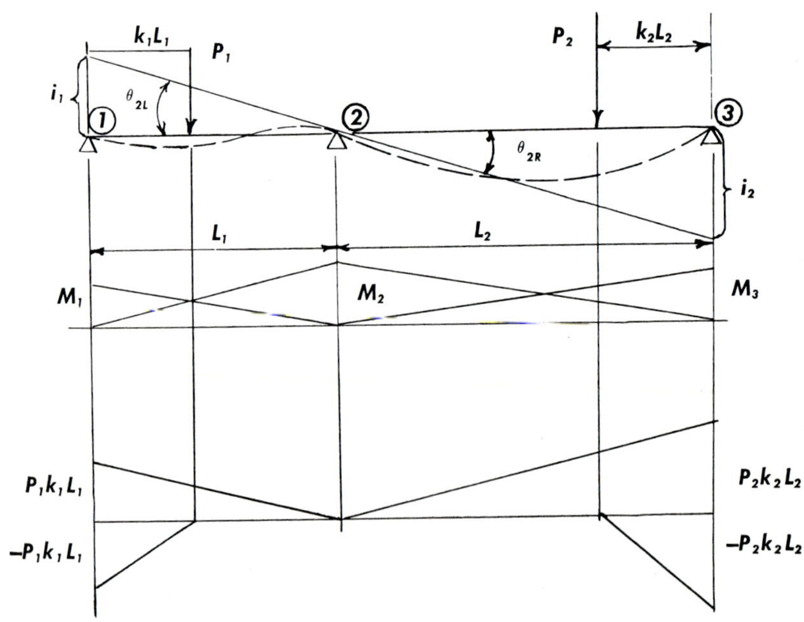

Fig. 39-25. Two spans of continuous beam.

sign, one being above the unstressed position and the other below. These angles are equal to the intercepts i_1 divided by L_1 for the left-hand span and i_2 divided by L_2 for the right-hand span. The intercepts i_1 and i_2 may be found by taking moments of the bending moment areas in span 1, about support 1, and span 2, about support 3; thus:

$$L_1 \, EI \, \theta_{2L} = M_1 \frac{L_1}{2} \frac{L_1}{3} + M_2 \frac{L_1}{2} \frac{2L_1}{3} + P_1k_1L_1 \frac{L_1}{2} \frac{L_1}{3} - P_1k_1L_1 \frac{k_1L_1}{2} \frac{k_1L_1}{3}$$

or

$$EI \, \theta_{2L} = \frac{M_1L_1}{6} + \frac{2\,M_2L_1}{6} + \frac{P_1L_1^2}{6} (k_1 - k_1^3)$$

(Eq. a)
(See Fig. 39-25.)

In a similar manner, taking moments in span 2, about support 3:

$$EI \, \theta_{2R} = \frac{2\,M_2L_2}{6} + \frac{M_3L_2}{6} + \frac{P_2L_2^2}{6} (k_2 - k_2^3)$$

(Eq. b)
(See Fig. 39-25.)

Equating Eq. a to the negative of Eq. b, there results:

$$M_1L_1 + 2\,M_2\,(L_1 + L_2) + M_3L_2 = - P_1L_1^2\,(k_1 - k_1^3) - P_2L_2^2\,(k_2 - k_2^3)$$

(Eq. c)
(See Fig. 39-25.)

Eq. c is the familiar theorem of three moments. It is applicable to any two contiguous spans of any continuous beam, which does not violate the limitations stated in the discussion on deflections of any span of any beam. It is also applicable to single spans with fixed supports.

Consider the span shown in Fig. 39-24 with a fixed support at the right end. A fixed support differs in definition from a free support only in that it permits no motion of rotation. The fixed support may be replaced by two free supports a differential distance apart, as shown in Fig. 39-26. Thus the fixed ended beam of a single span has been replaced by a beam of two spans, one of which has only a differential length which may be considered zero. The two free supports, at a differential distance apart, allow no vertical movement at support points. If the vertical position of two points on a line, at differential distance apart, is fixed, it is obvious that the direction of the tangent line is also fixed. Therefore, the two free supports, for mathematical purposes, replace the single fixed support. That no material would withstand the infinite stresses at the support, if such a concept were put into practical operation, makes no difference at all for mathematical purposes.

For the case shown in Fig. 39-26, the value of k is 0.5 and the load is at the span center. The bending moments at supports 1 and 3 are zero, these being the ends of the beam supported by free supports. There are no loads in the right-hand span, so that all terms involving P_2 drop out. Substituting directly in Eq. c.

$$O + 2\,M_2L + O = -PL^2 \left(\frac{1}{2} - \frac{1}{8}\right)$$

(Eq. a)
(See Fig. 39-27.)

From which:

$$M_2 = -3\,PL/16$$

Now consider the beam fixed at both ends, as shown in Fig. 39-27. This beam simulates a dental bridge, soldered to complete crowns of the abutment teeth, one at either end. A single load of 100 lb. is placed at the quarter point of the 1 inch span. It is required to find the bending moments at the fixed supports and to draw

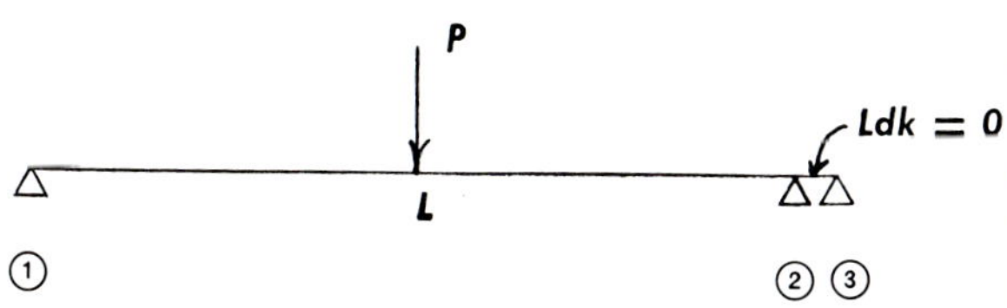

Fig. 39-26. Beam, right end fixed, considered as two spans.

the shear and bending moment diagrams for the fixed span.

Just below this span is shown the fixed supports replaced by two freely supported auxiliary spans of zero length. The four supports are marked 1, 2, 3, and 4. These numbers, as subscripts, also designate the bending moments at these supports. The bending moments at supports 1 and 4 are zero, the free supports being at beam ends. The span length is 1 in., and the load is placed 0.25 in. from support 2 and 0.75 in. from support 3.

The theorem of three moments may be applied first to the left-hand pair of spans and then to the right-hand pair, thus giving two equations by which to solve for the two unknown bending moments. It should be remembered that in the derivation, kL is measured in each of the spans from the outer support and not from the common support of the two spans.

Applying the theorem to the left-hand pair of spans:

$$O + 2M_2\,(1 + O) + M_3\,(1) = -100 \times 1^2\left(\frac{3}{4} - \frac{27}{64}\right)$$

(Eq. a)
(See Fig. 39-27.)

$$2M_2 + M_3 = -32.8$$

Applying the theorem to the right-hand pair of spans:

$$M2\,(1) + 2M_3\,(1 + O) + O = -100 \times 1^2\left(\frac{1}{4} - \frac{1}{64}\right)$$

(Eq. b)
(See Fig. 39-27.)

$$M_2 + 2M_3 = -23.44$$

The simultaneous solution of Eq. e and Eq. d gives:

$$M_2 = -14.05 \text{ in.lb.}$$

$$M_3 = -4.7 \text{ in.lb.}$$

(It should be noted that in Eq. b the value of k became 1/4 instead of 3/4 used in Eq. a, since support 2 now becomes the outer support of the two spans under consideration.)

Using the sixth interrelationship between shear and bending moment (see discussion on interrelationships between shear and bending moment, Fig. 39-12), the shears at the supports and the positive bending moment at the load may now be computed.

$$M_3 = M_2 + V_{2R} \times 1 - 100 \times 0.75$$

Substituting and solving:

$$V_{2R} = +\ 84.35 \text{ lb.}$$

(Eq. c)
(See Fig. 39-27.)

and

$$M_2 = M_3 - V_{3L} \times 1 - 100 \times 0.25$$

$$V_{3L} = -15.65 \text{ lb.}$$

(Eq. d)
(See Fig. 39-27.)

which is a check on V_{2R}, for the arithmetic sum of V_{2R} and V_{3L} is equal to 100, as it should be.

Finally M_P, the bending moment under the load may be computed:

$$M_P = M_2 + V_{2R} \times 0.25 = -14.05 + 84.35 \times 0.25 = +7.04 \text{ in.lb.}$$

(Eq. e)
(See Fig. 39-27.)

From these values the composite shear and bending moment diagrams are drawn as shown in Fig. 39-27.

It is worth noting that the bending moment diagram which would have existed if the span was a simple beam has been depressed as a result of placing the fixed supports at the ends. Thus, the bending moment under the load, which would have been +18.75 in.lb. for a simple beam, has now been reduced to +7.04 in.lb. The bending moment at the left support, which for the simple beam would be zero, has become –14.05 in.lb. This distribution, with the decrease in greatest bending moment, would be highly desirable, if it could always be depended upon. However, with the type supports available for dental bridges, results are quite undependable, as will be seen in the next discussion.

SETTLEMENTS OF SUPPORTS—INDETERMINATE BEAMS

It has been stated that the bending moments, in the case of indeterminate beams, are found by the aid of the laws of fluxure. The limitations of these laws have been discussed (see Figs. 39-12 and 39-13). One of the limitations found there is that the supports of the beam must permit no motion of translation normal to the beam axis. In other words, the supports of the beam must be stable.

In dealing with practical beams we know that the supports cannot be entirely stable. Materials of the supporting structure deform under load, thus giving somc movement. It then becomes of interest to examine and see by what rate a vertical movement of the support would affect computed bending moments.

In Fig. 39-28 is shown a beam with a fixed support at the left end and a free support at the right end. A single load, *P*, is placed at *b* distance from the right end. The span length is *L*. Let it be assumed that the right support settles and amount *f* and let it be required to find the bending moment at the fixed support, taking this settlement into account.

The settlement *f* is given a negative sign, since it obviously would increase the negative bending moment at the fixed support. The bending moment diagrams for the beam are shown on Fig. 39-28.

If tangents are drawn to the elastic curve of the beam at the fixed end and at the right support, they would cut off an intercept equal to *f* on a normal line through the right support. Taking moments of the bending moment areas about the right support:

$$M_L \frac{L}{2}\frac{2L}{3} + Pb\frac{L}{2}\frac{L}{3} - Pb\frac{b}{2}\frac{b}{3} = -EI\,f$$

from which

$$M_L = -\frac{3\,EI\,f}{L^2} - \frac{P\,b}{2L^2}(L^2 - b^2)$$

(Eq. a)
(See Fig. 39-28.)

Eq. a gives the bending moment required. It will be seen that the right-hand member of this equation is made up of two terms. The last of these two terms is the bending moment at the left support, if no settlement is assumed. This may be seen by letting *b* become L/2,

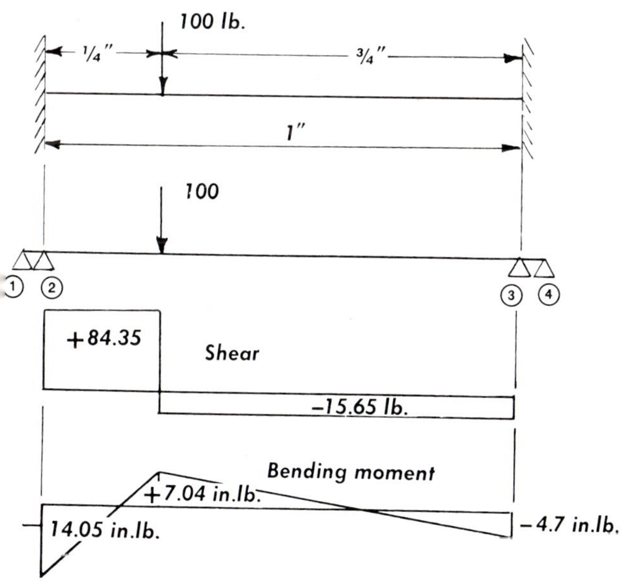

Fig. 39-27

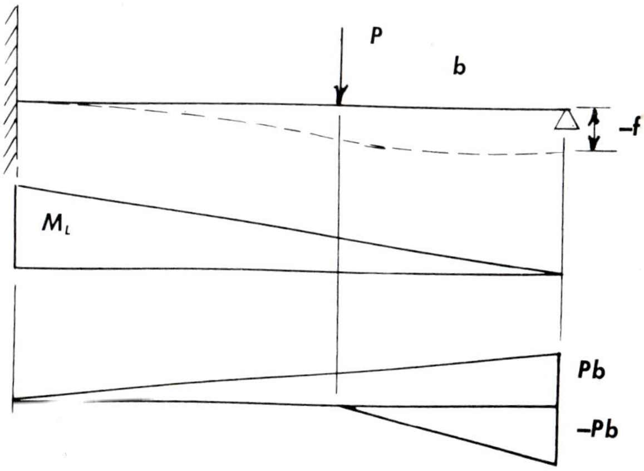

Fig. 39-28

Fig. 39-27. Indeterminate beam fixed at both ends.
Fig. 39-28. Settlement of supports, indeterminate beams.

in which the term becomes $(-3PL/16)$. This is the bending moment obtained in the same beam with the load at the center (see Fig. 39-24). The term $(-3\ EI\ f/L^2)$ must then be the effect of the settlement of supports on the bending moment at the fixed end. In this expression, the modulus of elasticity is a multiplier of *f*. The modulus of elasticity being very large, it becomes clear that change in bending moment is quite rapid as settlement progresses. Caution is indicated in permitting any settlement at all, if dependence is to be placed on reliability of computations.

It will be worthwhile to investigate support settlement for the dental bridge as shown in Figs. 39-16 and 39-18. Let it be assumed that the left support, of the 20 mm. span, is fixed and the right end freely supported. Let it be further assumed that the right end settles 0.01 in. If the bridge is of gold, the modulus of elasticity will be about 14,000,000 lb./sq.in. In the discussion on moments of inertia of areas, the moment of inertia of the cross section was computed to be 14.25 mm.^{4}, which is 0.0000341 in.^{4}. The 20 mm. span length reduces to 0.79 in. Using these figures in the term for effect of settlement of the support:

$$\frac{3\ EI\ (-f)}{L^2} =$$

$$\frac{3 \times 14{,}000{,}000 \times 341 \times 1 \times 10{,}000}{10{,}000{,}000 \times 100 \times 79^2} = -23 \text{ in.lb.}$$

(Eq. b)
(See Fig. 39-28.)

Thus the bending moment at the fixed support would be increased by 23 in.lb. over that which would exist if no settlement took place.

We shall now determine what proportion this is of the allowable bending moment on the section of this beam. Assume that the material of the bridge may be safely loaded up to 20,000 lb./sq.in. The value of I/c was 0.000571 in.^{3}. Substituting these figures in Eq. f (Fig. 39-13) of the discussion on stresses in a beam due to bending moment:

$$M = \frac{S\ I}{c} = \frac{20{,}000 \times 571}{1{,}000{,}000} = 11.4 \text{ in.lb.}$$

(Eq. c)
(See Fig. 39-28.)

Thus the settlement of the support of this beam by 0.01 in. would theoretically cause a moment to be induced at the fixed support which is double the allowable bending moment—a situation not permissible. A settlement of only one tenth of this amount, 0.001 in., would induce a bending moment of 2.3 in.lb., about 25% of the allowable.

The conclusion, then, is obvious that if supports are not stable, beams with fixed ends cannot be depended upon to have stresses close to those computed for them. A similar conclusion does not apply to the simple beam, where supports may settle great amounts, without substantially invalidating results.

BEAMS OF THE ANTERIOR BRIDGE TYPE

A curved restoration is constructed to fit the anatomy when edentulous areas occur in the anterior portion of the mouth. Such restorations are anchored to cuspids or first bicuspids and often tied back to adjacent teeth. They are sometimes partially mucosa-supported. The supporting curved metal of the bridge is not, strictly speaking, a beam but is a combination of beam and torsion member. From a structural standpoint, the worst feature of such a bridge is the heavy rotational effect upon the abutments or the uplift exerted upon teeth posterior to the abutment to which the bridge may be tied, as well as the torsion induced in the metal of the bridge span whose section does not effectively carry torsion.

These combination beams and torsion members are strictly indeterminate beams and not readily solved by the methods previously given. The irregular, noncircular sections may not be solved by means of the torsion formula (Fig. 39-10). However, when the load is placed at the center, symmetry results. Under this special condition, a solution may be had which will give stresses that are perhaps as great as any that may exist for any placing of the load. This solution will illustrate the problem involved.

Fig. 39-29, *A*, shows the plan view of such a curved anterior bridge. The illustration is drawn to scale, with the load placed at the center line and perpendicular to the occlusal plane. The bridge is assumed to be soldered to crowns on the abutments. These abutments are symmetrically placed in the mouth. In this instance, abutments are not tied back to teeth in a posterior direction. The axis *A-A* extends from center to center of abutments. Load *P* is normal to the occlusal plane at the bridge center. From Table 40-1, the biting force on the central tooth, by which the load is produced, will be assumed to be 40 lb. The bridge is assumed to be cut free from its supports and is considered as a free body. The load has an eccentricity of *e*, which in this case is assumed to be 0.3 in., with respect to the axis of abutments, *A-A*. The width between abutments is 2b and is assumed to be 1.5 in. If the moment of *P* is taken about the axis *A-A*, the laws of equilibrium require that shears be applied at the two cut sections at *A* and *A*, whose sum is equal to *P*. The laws of symmetry say also that these shears must equal each other, that is, each is $\frac{P}{2}$. The laws of equilibrium also require that equal couples be

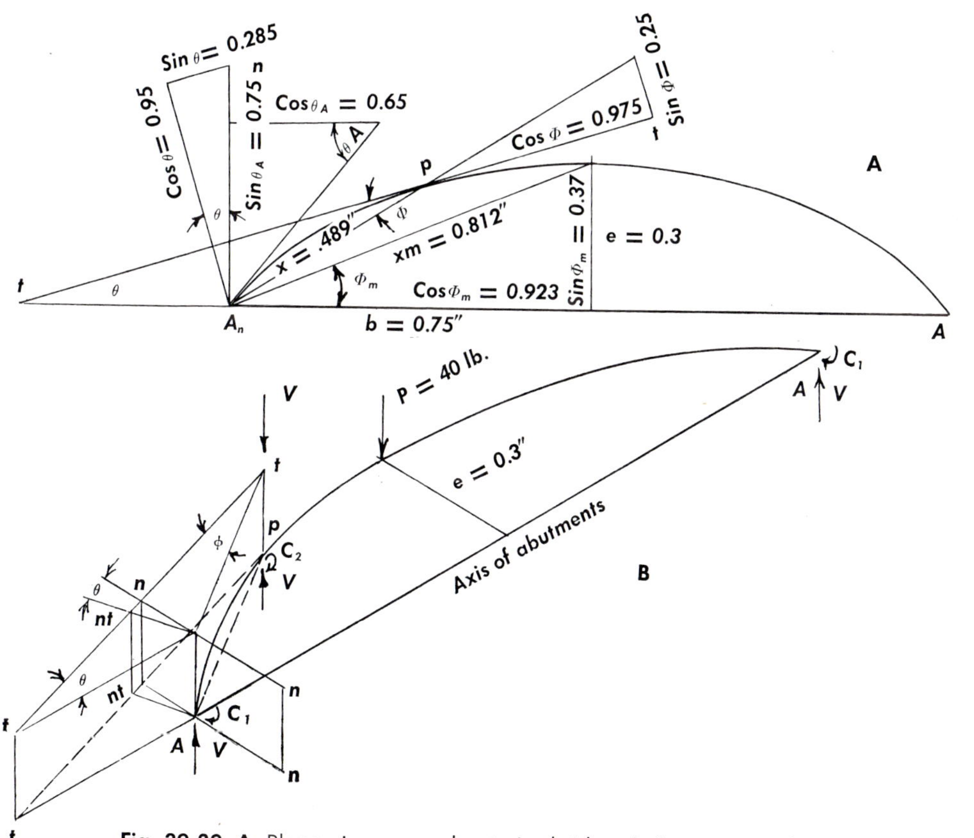

Fig. 39-29. A, Plane view, curved anterior bridge. **B,** Perspective of **A.**

applied at each of supports *A*, acting in planes perpendicular to *A-A*, such that Pe is equal to the sum of these two couples. Designate each as C_1.

At any point *p* on the curved axis of the bridge draw a plane tangent to the bridge axis and perpendicular to the occlusal plane. The trace of this plane on the occlusal plane is shown at *t-t* in Fig. 39-29, *A*, and the plane is shown in perspective in *B*. This plane intersects the plane which includes the axis *A-A* and is perpendicular to the occlusal plane, at an angle Θ, in the vertical line *t-t* (Fig. 39-29, *B*). The plane *n-n-n* is perpendicular to the occlusal plane and also to axis *A-A*. The plane *nt-nt-A* is perpendicular to the tangent plane *p-t-t*, passes through *A*, and is perpendicular to the occlusal plane. Planes *n-n-n* and *nt-nt-A* make an angle Θ with each other. Last, the plane *A-p-t* is perpendicular to the occlusal plane, passes through *A*, and makes an angle ø with the plane *t-t-t*. Now place two equal and opposite forces at *p* as shown, each equal to *V*. The point *p* is *x* distance from *A*. That one of these two forces which acts downward, acting together with the upward shear at *A*, constitutes a couple *Vx*, acting clockwise at *p*. The other upward force at *p* becomes a direct shear on the bridge section at *p*. Let the couple *Vx*, acting in the plane *t-p-A*, be designated C_2. Now the couple C_1, acting in the plane *n-n-n*, and the couple C_2, acting in the plane *t-p-A*, each have a component, one of which produces a torsion and the other a bending moment on the bridge section at *p*.

$$C_1 = -\frac{Pe}{2}$$

and

$$C_2 = Vx = \frac{Px}{2}$$

The sign of the couple C_1 is made arbitrarily negative because it produces counterclockise bending moment on the right-hand portion of the bridge as divided at *p*, and C_2 is designated as positive because it produces clockwise bending. Resolving couples and adding:

$$M_p = C_1 \sin \Theta + C_2 \cos \phi \quad \text{(Eq. a)}$$

(See Fig. 39-29.)

$$M_p = -\frac{Pe}{2} \sin \Theta + \frac{Px}{2} \cos \phi$$

or

$$M_p = \frac{P}{2} (x \cos \phi - e \sin \Theta)$$

(Eq. b)

(See Fig. 39-29.)

where M_p is the bending moment on the bridge section at *p*.

Similarly let T_p represent the torque at *p*. Then:

$$T_p = C_1 \cos \Theta + C_2 \sin \phi = -\frac{Pe}{2} \cos \Theta + \frac{Px}{2} \sin \phi$$

(Eq. c)

(See Fig. 39-29.)

$$T_p = \frac{P}{2} (x \sin ø - e \cos \Theta)$$

(Eq. d)

(See Fig. 39-29.)

It will of course be recognized that Θ, ø, and *x* are variables that change with the location of the point *p*.

At the left support, the couple C_2 becomes zero because the value of *x* becomes zero.

Then, Eq. b reduces to

$$M_A = -\frac{Pe}{2} \sin \Theta \quad \text{(Eq. e)}$$

(See Fig. 39-29.)

and Eq. d to

$$T_A = -\frac{Pe}{2} \cos \Theta \quad \text{(Eq. f)}$$

(See Fig. 39-29.)

At the span center (the load P), the value of Θ becomes zero, that is, the tangent plane is parallel to the abutment axis plane, and they theoretically meet at infinity. In this case the arm *x* becomes x_m, or 0.812 in., and the value of the sine ø becomes e/x_m and the cosine becomes b/x_m. Eq. b reduces to

$$M_P = \frac{P}{2} x_m \cos \phi = \frac{Pb}{2} \quad \text{(Eq. g)}$$

(See Fig. 39-29.)

and

$$T_p = \frac{P}{2} (x_m \sin \phi - e) = 0 \quad \text{(Eq. h)}$$

(See Fig. 39-29.)

It would be possible, where the bridge curvature followed a regular geometric pattern, to interrelate the values of Θ and ϕ. Since dental bridges seldom follow such a pattern, it is more practical to draw the bridge to scale and to scale off the various values. The sines and cosines of ϕ and Θ may be found by setting off the distance unity to any scale on one leg of the angle, completing the right triangle, and scaling off the values of sine and cosine, to the same scale, on these legs: values of x may be scaled directly from Fig. 39-29, *A*.

At the support A for the bridge shown on Fig. 39-29, *A* (remember *P* is 40 lb.):

From Eq. e:

$$M_A = -\frac{40 \times 0.3}{2} \times 0.75 = -4.5 \text{ in.lb.}$$

From Eq. f:

$$T_A = -\frac{40 \times 0.3}{2} \times 0.65 = -3.9 \text{ in.lb.}$$

At the point *p:*

From Eq. b:

$$M_p = \frac{40}{2}(0.489 \times 0.975 - 0.3 \times 0.285) = 7.56 \text{ in.lb.}$$

From Eq. d:

$$T_p = \frac{40}{2}(0.489 \times 0.25 - 0.3 \times 0.95) = +3.25 \text{ in.lb.}$$

At the middle of the span (load *P*):

From Eq. g:

$$M_P = 20 \times 0.75 = 15.0 \text{ in.lb.}$$

From Eq. h:

$$T_p = 0.0$$

It will be noted from the foregoing that the negative bending moment is greatest at the abutment, becomes positive at the point *p*, and reaches its greatest positive value under the load at mid-point of the bridge. On the other hand, the torque is greatest at the abutment and tapers off to zero at the middle of the span, under the load.

The analysis given here is valid for conditions of symmetry as previously noted. Lack of symmetry would invalidate the calculations made. A tendency of one abutment to rotate more than the other could produce such asymmetry. No attempt will be made to discuss asymmetric conditions. Such a discussion would involve the types of distortion taking place in the nonuniform and irregular sections of the dental bridge. The problem, as outlined, serves to show the nature of the factors involved and gives some quantitative idea of the moments and torques induced. These are perhaps nearly as great as would occur under any conditions.

This analysis was made without assuming any tie-backs for the abutment teeth. Whether or not there are such tie-backs does not in any way affect the analysis given of the curved portion of the bridge that extends between abutments. Equations are still valid for this portion under any conditions of tying the abutment. This portion of the bridge is in much the same situation as the free end of a cantilever beam projecting from the support. The analysis of this free end does not in any way depend upon the method used for clamping the fixed end.

Tied-back abutments

It will be noted from the foregoing that the turning moments at the abutment *A* (4.5 in.lb. in bending and 3.9 in.lb. in torsion) are large. Orthodontists are accustomed to rotate a tooth with only a fraction of these moments. The necessity is then obvious for taking measures to prevent a forward or a rotational move-

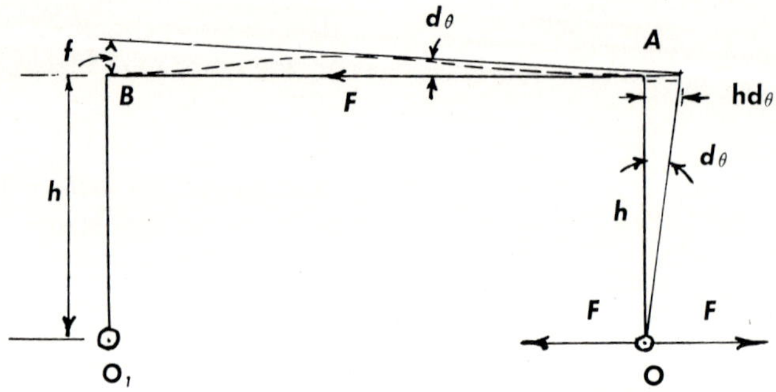

Fig. 39-30. Tied-back abutment, anterior bridge.

ment and the extraction of the abutments. This is often done with tie-backs to a more posterior tooth.

Fig. 39-30 shows a skeleton drawing of a tied-back abutment arrangement. The line *AO* represents the longitudinal axis of the abutment tooth. *O* is its point of rotation in the fundus. The vertical height *AO* is represented by *h*. The line BO_1 represents the longitudinal axis of the posterior tooth to which the tie-back is made. *BA* is the axis of the tie-back bar which is presumed to coincide, at *A*, with the axis of the curved anterior bridge, attached to the abutment at *A*.

As the bending moment M_A at the abutment (Eq. e) in the curved anterior bridge is applied, the abutment rotates forward though a small angle $d\theta$, as shown. One result of this forward movement is a tendency to elongate the tie-back bar *BA*. This induces a tensile force *F* within the tie-back and in turn causes a forward rotation of lesser amount than $d\theta$ in the posterior anchor tooth BO_1. Apply at *O*, two equal and opposite forces, *F*, as shown. One of these forces acting in an anterior direction, when considered with *F*, produces a counterclockwise couple, *Fh*, which opposes the forward rotation of the abutment, produced by M_A. The remaining force *F* applied at *O* induces a fairly uniformly distributed compressive force in the fundus.

If the tie-back bar *AB* has some kind of so-called stressbreaker that does not permit it to transmit moment, then the force *F* is the only one involved. The moment *Fh* must be equal to the bending moment M_A. The distance *h* may be reasonably assumed to be in the neighborhood of 3/8 inch.

Then

$$0.375\ F = M_A = 4.5$$
$$F = 12.0\ \text{lb. approximately}$$

This 12 lb. force is a considerable pull to put upon the tie-back tooth. It is obvious that if the tie-back bar *BA* extends over more than one tooth, the load will be distributed and less forward force will be placed upon any one tooth.

No uplifting force has been shown so far. Certainly there is none on the abutment, for the shear here is directly downward. If there is no stressbreaker in the tie-back bar *BA* then it will become of the nature of a fixed-ended beam, with supports on different levels (see discussion on settlement of supports—indeterminate beams, Fig. 39-24). The tie-back tooth will then be subject to the uplift due to the shear at *B*, as suggested by the dashed line elastic curve for bar *BA* in Fig. 39-30. It is futile to try to evaluate quantitatively this shear, since there are a number of imponderables. It is sufficient to note that it will be greater if *BA* is short and heavy and lesser if it is longer and lighter. The cross-sectional area of *BA* need not be excessive, since it only carries 12 lb. of tensile load. Nevertheless, if it is too light, the elongation of *BA* caused by the induced stress will be greater and the angle of rotation of the abutment will increase.

One other point will be made. The bending moments and torques of Eq. b and Eq. d resulted from the occlusal load placed at the span center, assumed to be 40 lb. If this load can be reduced, all dependent quantities will grow smaller and there is less damage to abutments. The effective manner of reducing the load *P* is to introduce some mucosa support. The load is then partly transmitted directly into the mucosa and does not become available for inducing moments and shears in the beam sections. This diminution is not capable of exact evaluation, but it is certainly on the side of safety and becomes larger if there is undue rotation of the abutment.

Functions of θ and ϕ (Eq. b and Eq. d) depend upon an accurately drawn curvature of the anterior bridge axis and upon accurate tangents. Care should be exercised in placing a correct curve upon paper, to represent the anterior bridge (Fig. 39-29, *A*).

GENERAL REFERENCES

Brumfield, R. C.: Load capacities of posterior dental bridges, J. Prosth. Dent. **4**:530-547, 1954.

Burgess, J. K.: Coordinating the mechanics of bridge construction with the biologic requirements of the periodontal structures, J.A.D.A. **14**:1494, 1927.

Craig, R. G., and others: Experimental stress analysis of dental restorations, part I, two-dimensional photoelastic stress analysis of inlays, J. Prosth. Dent. **17**:277, 1967.

Craig, R. G., and Peyton, F. A.: Measurement of strains in fixed bridges with electronic strain gauges, J. Dent. Res. **46**:615, 1967.

Craig, R. G., and Peyton, F. A.: Measurement of stresses in fixed-bridge restorations using a brittle coating technique, J. Dent. Res. **44**: 756, 1967.

DeForest, A. V., Ellis, G., and Stern, F. B., Jr.: Brittle coating for quantitative strain measurements, J. Appl. Mech. **64**:184-188, 1942.

Evans, R. G., and Lissner, H. R.: "Stresscoat" deformation studies of the femur under static vertical loading, Anat. Res. **100**:159, 1948.

Hollenger, H. H.: Photography in the photoelastic stress analysis of restorations, Dent. Radiog. Photog. **31**:31, 1958.

Huang, H. K., and Ledley, R. S.: Numerical experiments with a linear force-displacement tooth model, J. Dent. Res. **48**:32, 1969.

Johnson, E. W., and others: Stress pattern variations in operatively prepared human teeth, studied by three-dimensional photoelasticity, J. Dent. Res. **47**:548-558, 1968.

Ledley, R. S., and Huang, H. K.: Linear model of tooth displacement by applied forces, J. Dent. Res. **46**:427, 1968.

Mahler, D. B., and Terkla, L. G.: Analysis of stress in dental structures, Dent. Clin. N. Amer., pp. 796-797, Nov., 1958.

Mahler, D. B., and Peyton, F. A.: Photoelasticity as a research technique for analysing stresses in dental structures, J. Dent. Res. **34**:831-838, 1955.

Noonan, M. A.: The use of photoelasticity in a study of cavity preparations, J. Dent. Child. **16**:24-28, 1949.

Reed, R. R.: Application of mechanical laws to bridge construction, North-West Dent. **21**:191, 1942.

Roucoules, L.: Fixed prosthetic appliances: basic principles and architectural laws, Rev. Franc. Odontostomat. **13**:1537-1563, 1966.

Short, H.: Relation magnitudes of stress on abutment teeth with different retainers, J. Prosth. Dent. **21**:267, 1969.

Chapter 40

Structural investigation and design of dental restorations (bridges); relationship of structural design to biologic acceptance*

FUNDAMENTAL CONSIDERATIONS

The word design is a familiar one to the dental practitioner. He has long been accustomed to speak of the design of his structures. In the design of the dental bridge he has taken many factors into account, such as esthetics, physiologic function, feasibility of construction, prophylaxis, and structural adequacy. In carrying out the steps of design procedure, his attitude has been that of an artist rather than that of a scientist. The distinction between the two types of approach is largely one of basic training. The artist's approach to a problem is often an intuitive one. He arrives at conclusions not by conscious reasoning but through subconscious preferences resulting from long-acquired skills and manual dexterities for which basic rules have never been written. The scientific approach is more likely to be one based on written rules and conscious rationalizing from known facts to a resulting conclusion.

This comparison in methods of approach should not disparage either. Most sciences have had their beginnings as an art. The tendency has been to move from the artistic viewpoint toward the more scientific method as underlying principles have been developed and consciously recorded. In most sciences, also, some art will always linger. The highly trained artist will often produce results equal to those obtained by the more scientific method. However, written rules and codified methods of procedure tend to make the results obtained by the less-skilled person more nearly in line with those obtained by his co-worker of much longer training and experience.

Thus, the material presented here, far from deprecating the value of judgment, is designed to aid it by writing down some of the basic procedures for arriving at a rational conclusion on one phase only of the design of dental bridges, namely, that of structural adequacy. When there is a conflict among the many factors that enter into the design of the bridge, the decision as to which will be sacrificed for the other will always be the responsibility of the practitioner. In making this decision, the realization will be ever present that lack of structural adequacy may cause the failure of all other purposes of his bridge. It is hoped that the rules and principles

*Text by R. C. Brumfield, C. E.; Formerly Associate Professor of Civil Engineering, Cooper Institute, New York, New York.

embodied in this chapter may enable the dentist to more readily reconcile such conflicts and so to produce serviceable restorations that otherwise might not have been possible.

FACTORS RELATED TO LOAD-CARRYING CAPACITY

There are three factors that are of determinative influence on the load-carrying capacity of the dental bridge or, for that matter, on any structure that carries loads:

1. The loads that are to come upon the bridge, both as to intensity and as to character (static, impact, concentrated)
2. The form and shape of the structure that receives the loads; the load placing and the consequent stresses induced within the structure
3. The ability of the material from which the structure is built to withstand the stresses induced within it

These three factors are not related to each other. In the case of the dental bridge, the loads that come upon it are entirely a matter of experimentation with occlusal forces. They are not dependent upon the structure itself nor upon its material. These loads arise primarily from the biting force of the various teeth, which stem in turn from the musculature of the individual. A tabular listing of the biting forces on the various teeth in the mouth, from measurements made at the University of Illinois, is shown in Table 40-1, together with recommended loads for each tooth, to be used as design criteria (S.D.T.).

Although the loads given in Table 40-1 are recommended for use as design criteria, it is recognized that the practitioner may wish to exercise judgment in certain cases and use some load other than the recommended one. In using judgment, it should be kept in mind that the measured loads on artificial teeth are usually less than the corresponding loads on natural teeth and that heavily muscled individuals are likely to exert greater biting forces than the average, whereas lightly muscled persons will exert lesser biting forces. The type and condition of the supporting periodontal tissues and bone likewise influence the biting forces exerted.

The second factor related to load-carrying capacity has to do with stresses induced within the material of the bridge by the applied loads. These stresses, although they depend upon the loads applied, also depend upon the form of the structure and the placing of the loads upon it. The value of the load may remain constant, but if the form of structure is changed or the placing of the load is altered, the induced stresses may be greatly

Table 40-1. Biting forces of human teeth and recommended design loads (From Measurements Made at the University of Illinois Dental School)

	Biting force (pounds)					
	Uppers			*Lowers*		
Tooth no., mesiodistally	*Natural denture*	*Restoration*	*Design loads*	*Natural denture*	*Restoration*	*Design loads*
1	47	43	50	40	40	40
2	28	30	35	48	31	50
3	52	48	55	81	57	80
4	70	73	75	75	65	75
5	68	67	70	68	69	75
6	82	66	75	89	82	90
7	82	75	75	73	70	75
8	38	20	40	62	49	70

altered. Thus, stresses may be altered even though the load remains constant.

Ability of materials to withstand induced stresses is wholly unrelated to either the applied loads or the form of the structure. The character of the material of the structure does not enter into computations for induced stresses so long as these are within the proportional limit of the material. On the contrary, ability of material to withstand stress is a matter of experimentation for each material. If a weak material is used to build a structure, its load-carrying capacity will be small and the parts of the structure must be correspondingly heavier. A greater load-carrying capacity may be had by substituting a stronger material in a structure of the same form. Conversely, the same load-carrying capacity may be maintained and at the same time a more lightly proportioned structure may be built by using a stronger material. In Chapter 39, pp. 874 to 879, are listed some of the possibilities and limitations of materials commonly used to construct dental bridges. In Table 40-2 are listed pertinent physical properties of some dental gold alloys that dental practitioners have been accustomed to use in constructing dental bridges. When adequate strength is difficult to obtain, the stronger materials commonly used for partial dentures must be substituted for the type C inlay golds. Data for some partial denture alloys are therefore included in Table 40-2.

BEAM TYPES REPRESENTED AMONG DENTAL BRIDGES

A number of dental bridge types are in general use or have been employed at one time or another. *The discussion of these beam types will be from a strictly structural standpoint.* In some cases this will differ from the usual dental viewpoint. To the dentist, a fixed bridge is one that may not be readily removed from the mouth because of a soldered connection to a cemented crown at one end or both. Structurally, a fixed bridge is one whose supports allow no motion of either translation or rotation at the support points. From a structural standpoint, dental bridges may be classified as follows:

1. A bridge freely supported at each of the two ends
2. A bridge freely supported at one end and soldered and cemented at the other
3. A bridge supported by precision connectors at each end
4. A bridge soldered to a cemented crown on an abutment tooth at each end
5. A bridge (or bridges) tied across a common abutment (pier) tooth that intervenes between adjacent, edentulous areas
6. A bridge partially abutment-supported and partially mucosa-supported
7. A bridge in the anterior part of the mouth, with curved axis, subject to bending as well as to torsion

The first type listed unquestionably falls into the class of simple beams. An example of this type is the Nesbitt, which is not used as much as formerly. This type (usually a single tooth replacement) is supported by occlusal rests on two abutment teeth and held in approximate position by clasps. It often has a saddle support. It should be analyzed in quite the same manner as the bridge illustrated in Figs. 39-16 and 39-18.

Type 2, which is freely supported at one end and soldered and cemented at the other, appears to fall in the classification of beams fixed at one end and freely supported at the other. The discussion of this beam type will be found in Chapter 39. In this discussion bending moments were computed and complete shear and bending moment diagrams drawn. However, the conclusion should not be reached that this bridge is to be considered a fixed and freely supported beam without first con-

Table 40-2. Properties of alloys used in bridge construction

A.D.A. Spec. No. 5

	Type	Gold and platinum group metals (per-cent minimum)	Brinell no. quenched Min.	Brinell no. quenched Max.	Min. hardened	Elongation 2" gauge length (percent minimum) Quen.	Elongation 2" gauge length (percent minimum) Hard.	Tensile hard-ened (lb./sq. in. minimum)	Fusion tem-perature—°F. minimum
Detailed require-ments for dental inlay casting golds	I	83	40	75	—	18	—	—	1700
	II	78	70	100	—	12	—	—	1650
	III	78	90	140	—	12	—	—	1650
	IV	75	130	—	200	10	2	90,000	1599

Physical properties of typical cast gold alloys

Casting alloys			Solders recommended	Casting temp. (°F.)	Brinell hardness*	U.T.S. (lb./sq. in.)	Percent elongation (2 in.)	Yield strength (lb./sq. in.)	Melting range (°F.)
For hard inlays, fixed, removable, and partial dentures	Jelenko no. 7	Type IV, Extra hard	650 Color Blend	1890	Q. 135 H. 240	71,000 112,500	35 7	40,000 71,500	1690 to 1720
	Sturdicast	Type IV, Extra hard	615 585	1780	Q. 135 H. 225	70,000 128,000	34 3	43,500 97,500	1630 to 1660
	Jel-4	Type IV, Extra hard	650 615	1870	Q. 150 H. 215	66,000 111,000	35 4	43,000 87,500	1635 to 1675
	Super White, platinum color	Type IV, Extra hard	Alboro H.F.	2090	Q. 130 H. 215	65,000 105,000	16 5	37,500 67,500	1840 to 1870
	Palloro, platinum color	Type IV, Extra hard	Alboro H.F.	2070	Q. 175 H. 231	90,000 139,500	13 3	65,500 89,000	1715 to 1860
	Firmilay	Type III, hard	650 Color Blend	1890	Q. 110 H. 165	63,000 77,000	39 19	30,000 40,000	1710 to 1760
For inlays, crowns, and fixed prostheses	Durocast	Type III, hard	708 650	1860	Q. 118 H. 200	66,000 87,000	34 20	37,500 45,000	1710 to 1755
	Bridge White, platinum color	Type III, hard	Alboro H.F.	2170	Q. 116 H. 190	58,000 85,000	16 13	33,500 43,500	1885 to 1970
	Carmilay	Type III, hard	650 615	1870	Q. 103 H. 175	59,000 86,100	34 11	29,500 52,000	1675 to 1770
For M.O.D. and other individual inlays	Modulay	Type II, medium hard	708 650	1880	Q. 92	58,000	38	27,000	1695 to 1760
For one- and two-surface inlays	Special Inlay	Type I, soft	708 650	1860	Q. 73	50,000	35	15,000	1730 to 1760
For parallel pin work	Ponto Gold		650	1925	Q. 175 H. 265	82,000 133,000	23 3	67,000 111,000	1650 to 1680
For fusing porcelain to gold			Ceramco	2300	165 after firing	63,000	3	47,500	2100 to 2150

*Q, quenched, or softened; H, hardened.

sidering the discussion on settlement of supports. It was shown that if the support settled as little as 0.001 in., computed results at the fixed end were altered by a large percentage. The periodontal membrane does permit vertical movement of the abutment and probably as much as the amount stated. As was shown, economies for this type of beam consist in reducing the greatest bending moment near the center of a beam of the simple type and adding bending moments of lesser amount near the fixed end. Since probable abutment movement does not permit these economies to be depended upon, they obviously may not be realized.

It is therefore safer procedure in designing this beam type to consider it a simple beam, of a span length extending from the center of the free support to the center of the fixed abutment. Also be sure to maintain the section to the soldered connection in order to care for any negative bending moment that may be induced there. It should be remembered that the bending moments of simple beams are not appreciably affected by support settlements.

The third type of dental bridge is supported by precision connectors at each of its ends. This type should be considered as a simple beam of span length from center to center of connectors. It is true that these connectors would seem to lend some degree of fixity to the supports. However, mechanical devices of this type are not rigid in the sense contemplated in the definition of a fixed support. When uncertainty exists, it is safe procedure to consider the span as a simple beam, for in this type bending moments near the center are always greater than they would be in any restrained beam of the same dimensions. As previously stated, sections required near midspan should be maintained also at beam ends to care for any restraining moments that may exist there.

The fourth type of bridge is soldered to a cemented crown at either end of the bridge. This would seem to ideally simulate the fixed-ended beam type. Certainly the soldered joints form rigid connections between the bridge and the abutment crowns.

A little consideration will show that if the supports are rigidly attached to the beam, as they are with the soldered joint, then instead of a beam there exists a two-legged bent, as shown in Fig. 40-1, *A*. The vertical legs of this bent represent the abutment teeth. The height is from the center of gravity of the attachment of the bridge to the crown to the center of rotation of the abutment. The bottoms of these legs are represented as pinned, since the tooth may rotate. If the vertical legs were allowed no lateral movement at the bottom, then the elastic curve and the accompanying type elastic deformation pattern for the bent would be as shown by the dashed and full lines. However, just as the periodontal membrane permits some vertical movement to the abutment, so also may some lateral movement occur, as shown in Fig. 40-1, *B*. If this movement

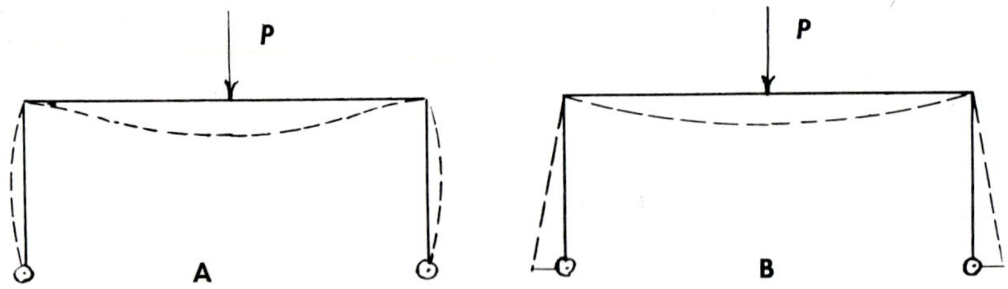

Fig. 40-1. Bridge soldered to crown at either end simulates two-legged bent type of beam.

is sufficient, the case would be just as if the lower end were on frictionless rollers, and the lateral movement would relieve all bending moments shown at the junction of horizontal and vertical members in *A*. Under these conditions the bridge would consist of a simple beam supported on struts (the abutments), as shown in *B*.

It will be of value to make a brief investigation in order to determine approximately how much lateral movement of the abutment would be required to relieve the induced bending moments at the junction of the bridge and the abutment. In Fig. 39-20 it was shown that the angle of rotation at the support of a specific beam of the dental bridge type was 0.0162/2, or 0.0081 radian. Assume that the vertical leg of the bent (abutment) is 0.375 in. long. Then the lateral movement required to relieve the bending moment at the junction of the bridge and the abutment would be approximately three-thousandths of an inch (0.003 inch).

$$\frac{3 \times 0.0081}{8} = 0.003 \text{ in.}$$

Although data do not exist to show whether or not the abutment may move enough laterally to relieve entirely the induced restraining moment at the support, it is certain that some movement does take place and that there is some relief. Since any movement makes computed results uncertain, and since the greatest bending moment for a given load will exist in a simple beam, it would seem wise to treat this case also as a simple beam, carrying the heavier section near the middle on to the supports in order to care for any residual restraining moment induced there.

Bridges of type 5 are tied together across a common abutment (pier) tooth that intervenes between two edentulous areas. At first glance these would seem to fall into the classification of continuous beams. Such beams were discussed previously. However, induced bending moments in these beams were shown in the discussion to be very sensitive to settlement of supports. Since this is true and since any of the supports may settle, it is better to consider each span of such a beam as a simple beam, separate from the one to which it may be tied, and to look upon any continuity that may exist as an added margin of safety in that it will reduce bending moment concentrations near span centers.

Type 6, the partially mucosa-supported bridge, is used when abutments are less than satisfactory or when there are spans and low clearance between the mucosa and occlusal plane. In this case the mucosa supports an unknown part of the load, which may be designated P_u. The remainder, P_c, is taken by the abutments and may be considered as a concentrated load. According to a previously stated principle, each of these loads may be considered to produce its own independent effect. The effect of P_u will be considered as though the load were applied at or near the center from above, its reactions constituting a uniformly distributed load over the mucosa for the full length of the saddle. This is shown in Fig. 40-2. Here the shear and bending moment diagrams produced by P_u are shown above and those by P_c are shown below.

It is obvious that the induced bending moment produced by the load P_u is only half as great as that produced by P_c, if these loads are considered equal in intensity. Thus mucosa support reduces the bending moment in the bridge near the span center. It also reduces the part of the load "carried by the abutments" by the amount P_u. If a reasonable decision as to the relative intensities of P_c and P_u can be had, the design may be carried out in the usual manner by adding the separate bending effects near the center caused by each type of load.

The curved type (type 7) anterior bridge has been discussed separately (Fig. 39-29). No further discussion is required

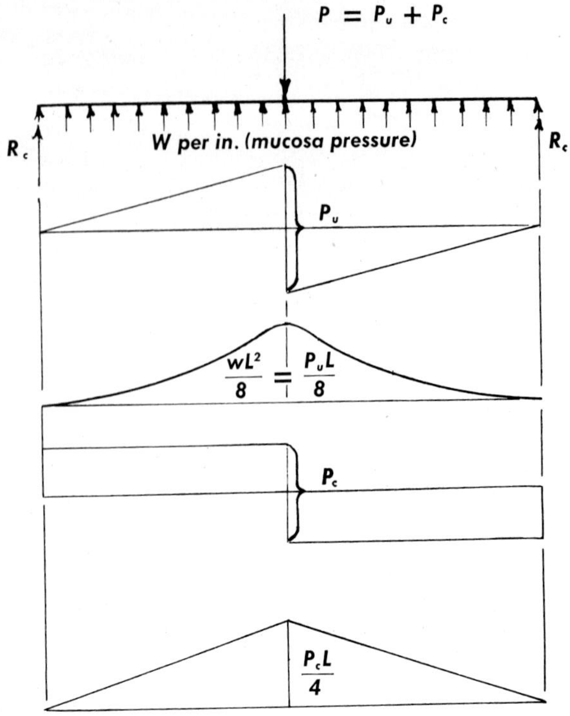

Fig. 40-2. Shears and bending moments in partially mucosa-supported bridge.

here. Its investigation and approximate design will be considered further in a subsequent discussion.

In summary it may be said that all dental bridge types, with the exception of type 7, should be analyzed as though the separate spans were those of simple beams. This practice results from lack of stability of supports and other considerations. The procedure is followed because it represents the safe course to pursue.

COMPARATIVE LOAD-CARRYING CHARACTERISTICS OF BEAM SECTIONS

For a discussion of the methods that were developed for computing the section characteristics of beams in order to determine the maximum stresses induced in them due to bending and the allowable loads they are capable of carrying (Fig. 40-3). However, the tabular computations shown there for beams of irregular peripheries are cumbersome in daily practice. In Table 40-3 those computations have been made and the results incorporated in tabular form for typical bridge pontic sections in order that normal computations may be facilitated.

Table 40-3 shows three beam sections of standard shape with peripheries of geometric form. Column 1 shows the type of section; columns 2 and 3 show the over-all dimension parallel to the vertical and the horizontal dimensions, respectively; column 4 shows the product obtained from multiplying the horizontal dimension by the square of the vertical dimension; column 5 gives the section modulus of the section; and column 6 gives a constant obtained by dividing the section modulus by the breadth-depth product shown in column 4. Column 7 shows the area of the section and column 8 the constant obtained by dividing the area by the product of the first powers of the breadth and the depth.

The results in column 6 of Table 40-3 show that for the beam sections dealt with, the section modulus is always some constant (as listed) times the product of the horizontal dimension of the beam and the square of the vertical dimension. For the purpose of this discussion, the direction named *horizontal* may be taken as that perpendicular to the direction of the applied load, and that called *vertical* as the over-all dimension parallel to the applied load. Any number of beam sections might have been listed and the result would have been similar. This establishes a law: *The section modulus of any beam section is equal to some constant times the product of the over-all breadth of the beam section and the square of its depth.*

In a similar manner, the results shown in column 8 establish the law that: *The cross-sectional area of any beam section is equal to some constant times the product of the over-all breadth of the section and the over-all depth.*

It will be noted from the above laws that the size of the beam section does not in any way affect the constant. It would

Table 40-3. Section characteristics in terms of over-all beam dimensions

(1) Section	*(2)* Depth	*(3)* Breadth	*(4)* $b\ d^2$ (in.^{3})	*(5)* Section modulus	*(6)* Constant (k)	*(7)* Area (in.^{2})	*(8)* Area constant (k_1)
Circle	d	d	$d\ d^2$	$\pi\ d^3/36$	0.088	$\pi\ d^2/4$	0.786
Triangle	d	b	$b\ d^2$	$b\ d^2/24$	0.042	$b\ d/2$	0.500
Rectangle	d	b	$b\ d^2$	$b\ d^2/6$	0.167	$b\ d$	1.000

be the same if the section were microscopic in dimensions or if the over-all dimensions were miles in extent.

These laws also hold for the irregular sections of dental bridge pontics in exactly the same manner. The only difference in the case of the bridge section is that since the periphery of the pontic is not of a geometric pattern, the law is not so apparent. However, if computations of section characteristics are made for usual pontic sections, it will be found that, so long as section variations are proportionately made, as they would be by photographic enlargements, the laws apply for different sizes of a given pontic section. The section modulus characteristic of any one of these could be found by multiplying the modulus constant of the original section by the product of the breadth and the square of the depth of the enlarged section. In a similar manner, the area of the enlarged section could be found by multiplying the area constant of the original section by the product of the breadth and depth of the enlarged section.

These computations have been made for three typical bridge pontic sections as shown in Table 40-4. Characteristics of each of these sections have been computed for eight or nine variations in depth and proportional variations in width. All dimensions are given in millimeters—the unit normally used for dental measurements. Columns 5 and 7, however, show the section modulus and the area in terms of inches, because tables of physical properties are printed in those terms. The lower three listings are for soldered joints for use with corresponding pontic sections. Column 1 shows a sketch of each pontic section and the center of gravity of each in terms of the fractional parts of depth and breadth. Center of gravity is useful in assembling the bridge, for the centers of gravity of adjacent pontics should coincide in order that the bridge axis be straight after assembly.

The section modulus listed in column 5 is a direct measure of the strength of the bridge section in which the pontic may be placed. It will be noted that the range of strengths (measured by section modulus) varies as much as from ten to fifteen times the lowest strength listed in Table V for each section. It will also be noted that the strength of the soldered joint for any particular section (which must of necessity be about 3 mm. less in depth than the pontic section) will show strengths that are often less than half of that of the corresponding pontic. This shows that the soldered joint is likely to be the controlling or critical point in the bridge if it occurs near the center.

The modulus constant of column 4 and the area constant of column 6 are shown in case it is desired to compute section moduli or section areas for dimensions of pontics similar to those shown at the left but differing in dimensions from any listed in Table 40-4. To compute the section modulus of column 5 it is necessary only to multiply the section constant of column 4 by the breadth (in mm.) of the section and the square of the depth (in mm.) and to multiply this result in turn by the cube of the number 0.03937, to re-

Table 40-4. Section characteristics of dental pontic sections*

Section (fractional dimensions)	*Location in mouth*	*Variations in dimensions (mm.)* b	*Variations in dimensions (mm.)* d	*Modulus constant*	*Section modulus (in.³)*	*Area constant*	*Section area (sq. in.)*
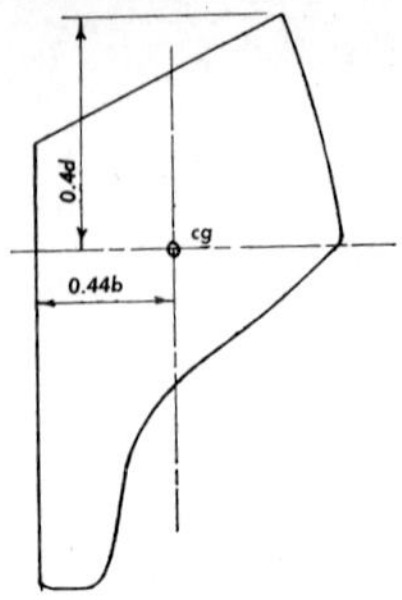	Lingual Lateral incisor	3.3	6		0.000442		0.070
		3.9	7		0.000710		0.0245
		4.5	8		0.000107		0.0309
		5.0	9		0.00151		0.0387
		5.5	10		0.00205		0.0462
		6.1	11		0.00275		0.0577
		6.7	12	0.061	0.0036	0.555	0.0690
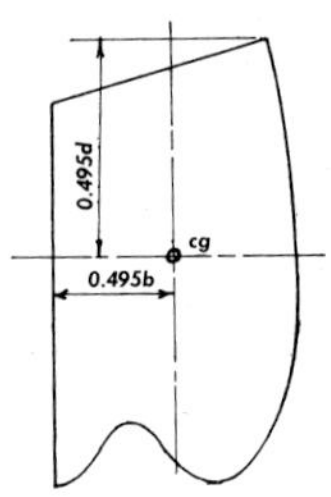	Lingual Bicuspid No. 4	3.0	5		0.000526		0.0207
		3.5	6		0.000885		0.0290
		4.1	7		0.00141		0.0399
		4.7	8		0.00211		0.0519
		5.3	9		0.00301		0.0659
		5.9	10		0.00414		0.0814
		6.5	11		0.00552		0.0988
		7.1	12		0.00716		0.1160
		8.0	13.5	0.115	0.0102	0.890	0.1490
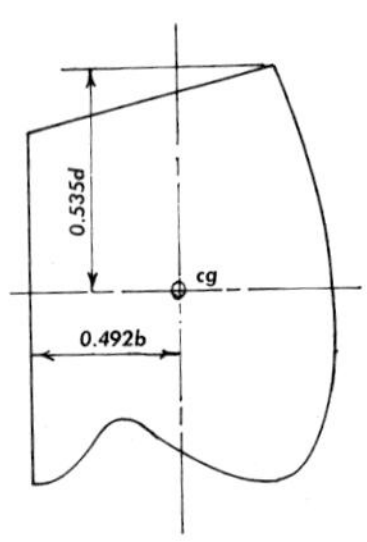	Lingual Molar No. 6	3.8	5		0.000523		0.0230
		4.6	6		0.000913		0.0335
		5.4	7		0.00146		0.0460
		6.1	8		0.00215		0.0592
		6.9	9		0.00308		0.0755
		7.7	10		0.00424		0.0935
		8.5	11		0.00481		0.1135
		9.2	12		0.00730		0.1340
		10.0	13	0.0904	0.00931	0.782	0.1580
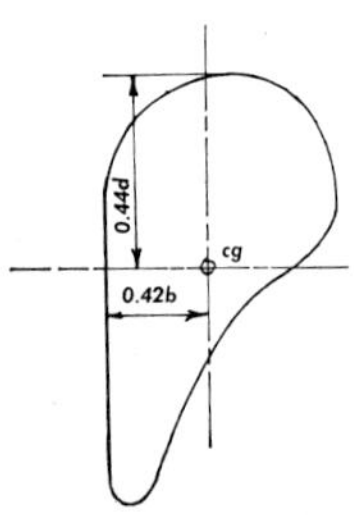	Lingual Soldered joint 3-2	1.69	3		0.0000376		0.0049
		2.25	4		0.000089		0.0087
		2.8	5		0.000173		0.0120
		3.4	6		0.000302		0.0196
		4.0	7		0.000484		0.0269
		4.5	8		0.000711		0.0346
		5.1	9		0.00102		0.0441
		5.7	10	0.0405	0.00141	0.622	0.0548
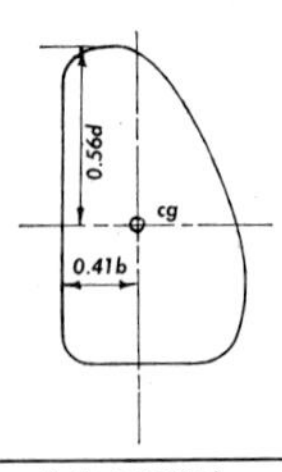	Lingual Soldered joint 5-4	1.8	3		0.000107		0.00745
		2.4	4		0.000254		0.0119
		3.0	5		0.000495		0.0166
		3.6	6		0.00086		0.0268
		4.2	7		0.00136		0.0365
		4.8	8		0.00204		0.0475
		5.4	9		0.00289		0.0603
		6.0	10		0.00396		0.0744
		6.6	11		0.00526		0.0900
		7.2	12	0.108	0.00684	0.890	0.1070

*Square of 0.03937 = 0.00155; cube of 0.03937 = 0.0000610, approximately.

Table 40-4. Section characteristics of dental pontic sections—cont'd

Section (fractional dimensions)	*Location in mouth*	*Variations in dimensions (mm.)*		*Modulus constant*	*Section modulus ($in.^3$)*	*Area constant*	*Section area (sq.in.)*
		b	*d*				
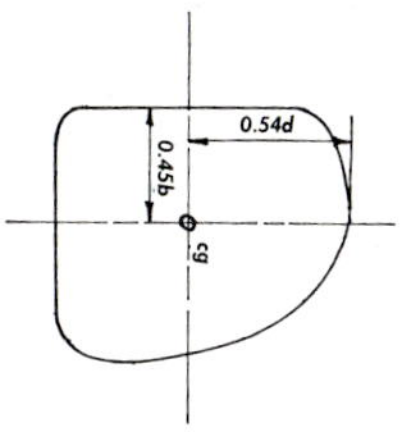	Lingual Soldered joint 7-6	2.7	3		0.000170		0.0108
		3.4	4		0.000384		0.0182
		4.0	4.7		0.000620		0.0251
		4.3	5		0.000752		0.0284
		5.1	6		0.00128		0.0408
		6.0	7		0.00206		0.0560
		6.8	8		0.00306		0.0725
		7.7	9		0.00436		0.0925
		8.5	10		0.00596		0.1135
		9.4	11		0.00797		0.1380
		10.0	12	0.115	0.0101	0.860	0.1600

duce millimeters to inches. Areas may be found in a similar manner by multiplying the constant of column 6 by the breadth times the depth and multiplying this in turn by the square of the reduction factor 0.03937. Neither of these operations should be required frequently, since it is believed that Table 40-4 covers the normal range of variance. It should be satisfactory to consider pontics 7 and 8 like pontic 6 shown and pontic 5 like pontic 4. Anterior pontics will be considered like pontic 1.

INVESTIGATION OF THE DENTAL BRIDGE

A two-pontic bridge, somewhat stylized, is shown in Fig. 40-3. The over-all span of the bridge from center of abutment 4 to center of abutment 7 is shown as 1.15 in. The metal portion of each pontic is not distinguished from the porcelain or acrylic resin, but the assembled pontic is indicated. However, the metal will be used only in computations for strength (data being taken from Table 40-4). The depths of pontics as well as buccolingual dimensions are shown in millimeters, this being the unit of measurement normally used. The mesiodistal dimensions are shown in inches because these dimensions will be involved in bending moment computations. Tooth numbers, representing the abutments as well as the pontics, are shown in Fig. 40-3. It is required to investigate this bridge for adequate strength, assuming that metal portions and soldered joints are constructed about as shown in Table 40-4.

Load at center of span

The span center falls well on the pontic replacing tooth 6. From Table 40-1 the design load on this lower tooth is 90 lb. The bending moment produced by this load at span center is

$$M = \frac{P\ L}{4} = \frac{90 \times 1.15}{4} = 26 \text{ in.lb.}$$

The total depth of pontic 6 is shown in Fig. 40-3 to be 8.2 mm. Let it be assumed that the metal portion of the pontic has a depth of 7 mm. and a width to correspond as shown in Table 40-4. From this table the section modulus for this depth is 0.00146. Then

$$S = \frac{Mc}{I} = \frac{26}{0.00146} = 17{,}800 \text{ lb./sq.in.}$$

This would not be satisfactory if the alloy from which the bridge was constructed was the University of Illinois alloy, type C, in its soft condition. However, apply-

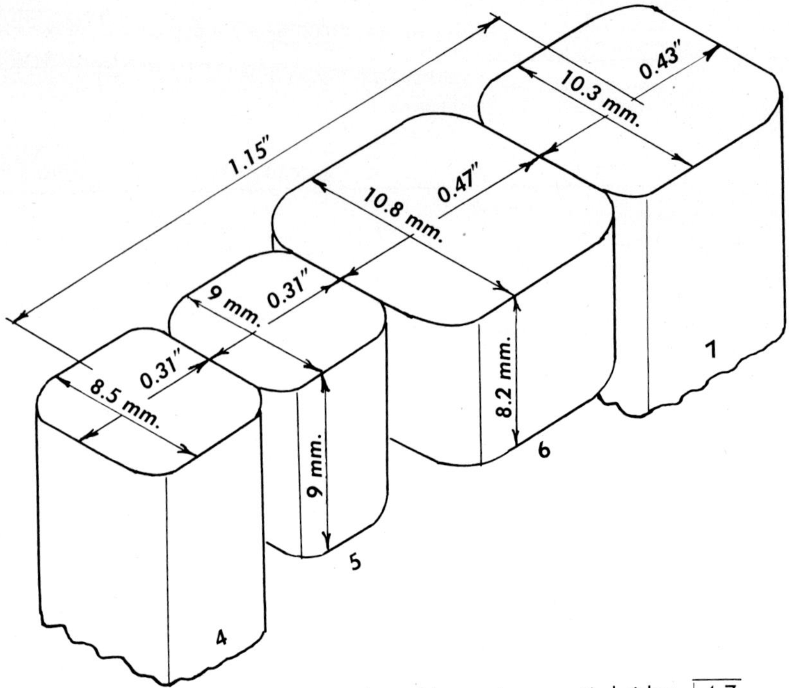

Fig. 40-3. Problem in investigation of lower two-pontic bridge, $\overline{|4\text{-}7}$.

ing a factor of safety of 2 to the yield strength, in the heat-hardened condition, the allowable unit stress would be 57,000/2, which is 28,500 lb./sq.in., and the bridge would be satisfatory at the center span.

Soldered joint 5-6

The soldered joint 5-6 is nearest to span center and a point of weakness, since the joint must be less in dimension than adjacent pontics. Use the design load for pontic 5, which from Table 40-1 is 75 lb. The joint is located at 0.465 in. from the left support and 0.685 in. from the right support. The bending moment then is

$$M_{5\text{-}6} = \frac{Pab}{L} = \frac{75 \times 0.465 \times 0.685}{1.15} = 20.7 \text{ in.lb.}$$

Now the depth of joint 5-6 must be less than either the depth of pontic 5 or that of pontic 6. From Fig. 40-3 let it be assumed that this depth is 5.5 mm. Now from Table 40-4 assume the joint is like that of joint 7-6. Then interpolating the section modulus:

$$I/c = \frac{0.000752 + 0.00128}{2} = 0.001016 \text{ in.}^3$$

and

$$S = \frac{20.7}{0.001016} = 20{,}400 \text{ lb./sq.in.}$$

It will be noted that the unit stress at this joint is considerably higher than the stress at span center, despite the fact that the joint is located 10% off center. This stress is higher than would be allowable for solder, unless great care was exercised to fully heat-harden the joint. It may be permissible in view of the fact that the joint is thin, and failure may not occur without a distortion which also involves surrounding materials of the stronger pontics. For this reason allowable unit stresses in solders may be raised 25 per-cent.

Punching shear—joint 4-5

Joint 4-5 is near enough to the support that danger of high unit stress as a result of bending need not be feared. However, the design load for pontic 5 may be applied at joint 4-5 and the resulting shear at the soldered joint required to be investigated. This shear will be the left reaction when the load is at 4-5. The design load for pontic 5 is 75 lb. Then:

$$R_4 = \frac{75 \times 1.0}{1.15} = 65 \text{ lb.}$$

From Table 40-3 the area of joint 4-5 for a depth of 5.5 mm. is

$$A = \frac{0.0166 + 0.0268}{2} = 0.0217 \text{ sq.in.}$$

Then the punching shear at this joint is

$$S_s = \frac{65}{0.0217} = 3000 \text{ lb./sq.in.}$$

SOME CONSIDERATIONS IN DESIGNING A DENTAL BRIDGE

The design of the dental bridge will be considered from a strictly structural standpoint. The investigation of an existing bridge does not involve these considerations. A structure under investigation already exists, and its stresses are fixed by the conditions under which it was built. Therefore, none of the factors that might have a bearing on defects that may develop in the investigation is capable of change.

However, in designing a structure all viewpoints may be taken into account. The critical loading and its placing may be coordinated with structural form, which may be altered to best meet requirements, and the best available material may be selected to withstand induced stresses. The critical loading selected for the structure stems primarily from the data given in Table 40-1, which show the biting forces (as measured by researchers at the University of Illinois) on both the natural teeth and restorations of the natural teeth. Biting forces on restorations are often not quite as large as those on natural teeth. There is also included a column of recommended biting forces for each of the teeth, which are to be used as critical loads in designing the bridge. These should prove satisfactory in the majority of cases.

The question arises as to whether or not each pontic of the restoration should be loaded with its design load in making the load placing for the design. It is believed that this is not necessary and that it places an improbable burden on the bridge. It is suggested rather that the maximum biting forces listed in Table 40-1 are the unusual forces that come upon the bridge: e.g., when the wearer unexpectedly bites down upon a bone splinter or other hard object. In such cases the load would come upon one pontic only and not upon all pontics in the bridge. It is therefore recommended that for each bridge the design load be selected for a single pontic and that this be allowed to be placed in positions where it will be possible to induce greatest stresses at critical points on the bridge span.

In each case a careful examination should be made of abutment teeth to determine their adequacy for carrying the reactions from the proposed bridge. This examination should include a roentgenograph of each abutment to determine whether the root structure is complete and sound, whether the tooth is seriously tilted toward the edentulous area, and whether the surrounding tissues are healthy. Abutments must carry more than their normal biting loads, since they convey the reactions of the bridge to the periodontium and bony structures of the maxilla or mandible. Such overloads indicate that these abutments should begin their service in as sound and healthy a condition as possible. Determination should also be made as to whether or not the bridge is to be soldered to a crown on the abutment or whether it is to be freely supported by the abutment. In connection with this it should be remembered that the freely supported bridge is usually of shorter span than the one soldered to the crown, because the free supports ordinarily do not lie at the abutment center. Fixed-ended bridges require slightly greater strength, because of the longer span. In the case of the freely supported bridge, special consideration must sometimes be given to the manner of supporting the bridge in order to avoid tipping the abutment (see discussion on transferring bridge reaction to abutment, Chapter 10).

In selecting pontics for the bridge, the mesiodistal dimension of the pontic will be varied to suit the necessities of filling the edentulous area in which the bridge is to be placed. Such variation will not affect the bending strength of the pontic section. The depth (occlusogingival) of the pontic should be kept as large as is compatible with the particular case under study. It should be remembered that in determining strength, *depth* is the more important of the two dimensions of the pontic. After the maximum permissible depth is determined, the width (buccolingual or linguolabial) should be kept in about the proportion to the depth as given in Table 40-4. If a greater width should be determined upon, the figures for section modulus and area given in Table 40-4 for the depth selected will be safe to use. If lesser widths are used, these figures should be reduced.

Design of the dental bridge differs in one important particular from the design of ordinary engineering structures. In engineering design, one very important consideration, secondary only to safety, is that the design represent economy of material, because it is desired to keep the cost low. The possibility of saving material in dental bridge design has a negligible effect on total cost and therefore is not regarded as important. Structural strength is paramount.

The range of properties of gold alloys available for making dental bridges is given in Table 40-2. The best alloy must be selected for constructing the bridge. In making this decision, adequate strength of the bridge is the first consideration, but ease in working, tarnish, cost, and other factors should also be considered. A discussion of the significance of physical properties of gold alloys is given in Chapter 31. It was stated that allowable working stress of the alloy was based upon its proportional limit, or yield strength. Working stress cannot, however, be equal to the proportional limit. To obtain working stress, the unit stress at the proportional limit is divided by a factor, called factor of safety. Factor of safety is also applied to ultimate strength, a custom formed before adequate measuring devices permitted the determination of proportional limit.

The necessity for the use of a factor of safety arises because there is a lack of information on a number of data that affect the use of the structure. The exact magnitudes of the loads that are to come upon the bridge, as well as their character (static impact), are uncertain. These things depend upon the wearer of the bridge and are beyond the control of the designer. Again, the exact proportional limit of the material depends upon heat handling. Under present conditions of practice, this is inclined to be uncertain. All these and other factors require that a margin of unused strength of material be left to cover uncertainties. It is recommended that a factor of safety of 2 be applied to the proportional limit of material. Thus, if the proportional limit of the material be 40,000 lb./sq.in., the working stress would be 20,000 lb./sq.in. This is in line with good engineering practice.

Solder should be selected for the joints of the bridge just as carefully as the material is selected for the pontics. Again, strength is of paramount importance. Soldered joints, by the nature of the contoured bridge, are of less area than the pontics. Depths of joints are as much as 3 mm. less than those of the pontics which they join. A glance at joint strengths shown in Table 40-4 (section moduli) will show that such a decrease of depth may lower strength considerably. Two guiding principles follow: the solder should have as great a strength as possible, when bending moments are large, and *joints should be located as far as possible from the center of the bridge span.* The last is not always possible. It is also obvious that care should be exercised to obtain the full area of solder contemplated in the design.

Manufacturers have not been accustomed to publishing the strengths of their solders. Table 40-2 lists some solder strengths for the varying finenesses for the solders of one manufacturer. It is probable that these are fairly representative. The stronger solders lie in finenesses from 585 to 615. None of these strengths is as great as those for the best partial denture casting golds. In critical situations, consideration may well be given to making cast joints (instead of soldered joints) near bridge centers in order to take advantage of the greater strength of the high-strength casting golds. There is one redeeming feature in connection with soldered joints. Such joints are thin (perhaps 0.01 in. thick in a well-soldered joint). It is desirable that this thickness maintain for the full depth of the joint. If so, the thin joint will be stronger than it would otherwise be, because of the small thickness, since distortion must take place before rupture may ensue. In distorting, the thin joint involves some of the stronger material of the adjacent pontics and thus its strength is enhanced. Properly made thin joints may be allowed as much as 25% more working stress than is indicated by the factor of safety applied to the proportional limit. Heat-hardening possibilities of solders should also be examined, as well as the compatibility of the hardening process with that required for the material of the pontics. (See Tables 31-1 to 31-4.)

STEPS IN THE STRUCTURAL DESIGN OF A DENTAL BRIDGE

1. Examine the abutment teeth and determine their adequacy for carrying the reactions of the proposed bridge. Upon their soundness, stability, degree of tilt toward the edentulous area, and other factors will rest the decision as to whether a tooth-borne bridge is to be used or whether it is to be partially mucosa supported.

2. Using the model, lay a straight edge across the occlusal surface of the two abutment teeth, or if opposing teeth protrude into the area, use their occlusal plane. Measure the distance from this plane (whichever is chosen) to the mucosa. This distance will be the potential total depth of the pontics of the proposed bridge. It should be divided into two parts: (a) the minimum thickness of porcelain or acrylic resin, which is to be used to cover the lower surface of the metal of the pontic, and (b) the remaining space to be occupied by the metal portion of the pontic. The acrylic resin or porcelain portion should always be kept at a minimum in order to allow a maximum depth for the metal of the pontic. It is this metal that carries all the bending moment induced by the load on the bridge. Since depth is the more important dimension of the cross section, it should be as large as is obtainable. An acrylic resin or porcelain depth of 1 mm. should be sufficient. Although it is true that the acrylic resin or porcelain portion of the pontic may carry some bending, at best it will be small. Because of uncertainties of cement joints and other factors, it should not be depended upon.

3. Determine the type of end conditions that are to be used; that is, soldered to crowns on abutments at one or both ends or freely supported by a rest or by precision connectors.

4. Measure the span length of the bridge in inches. If the bridge is to be fixed-ended (soldered to crowns) measure from center to center of abutments. If it is to be fixed at one end and freely supported at the other, measure from the center of the abutment at the fixed end to the center of the seat of the free support at the other. When the bridge is to

be freely supported at each end, measure from center to center of support seats.

5. Select from Table 40-1 the design load to be used in determining the induced stresses in the bridge. It is recommended that the load selected to be the largest design load of Table 40-1 that is listed for any tooth to be replaced in the edentulous area.

6. Determine the widths (mesiodistal) of pontics to be used in the area. Buccolingual widths should be maintained. If it is necessary to shorten mesiodistal widths because of drifting of abutments, this will not greatly affect the strength.

7. Make a sketch of the bridge, with pontics in place such as that shown in Fig. 40-3. Mark the distance from the center of each support to the critical placings of load. Remember that joints are likely to be critical locations, even though they do not lie at or near span centers.

8. From Table 40-4 select the pontic type as that shown for each particular tooth in the replacement. The pontic depth will be that determined in step 2. When the depth has been determined, select from Table 40-4 the section modulus and area constant for each pontic and each joint. Use the buccolingual pontic widths shown in Table 40-4 or larger widths.

9. Place the critical load at the span center and at other previously selected positions. Determine the bending moment under the load for each placing from the expression $M = P\,ab/L$. In the expression, a and b are the distances, in each placing, from the load to the respective supports.

10. Read from the manufacturer's chart the proportional limits of the material or materials to be used. Divide this by the factor of safety of 2 and establish the working stress of the material.

11. From the bending moments computed in step 9 and the equation $S = Mc/I$, compute the maximum stress in the bridge caused by bending. Compare this with the selected working stress of step 10. If the computed stress is within the allowable stress, the bridge represents safe design from a structural standpoint. If the computed stress is above the allowable stress, methods must be considered to improve the strength of the bridge. If these fail, consideration must be given as to whether or not the bridge will be abandoned as a restoration or whether it shall be placed with full knowledge that failure is a possibility.

To improve strength, the first thing to be considered is the increase of depth of the pontic or, of less effectiveness, the increase in the buccolingual width. Since space between the occlusal plane and the mucosa is fixed, increase in depth may be possible only by sacrificing some of the acrylic resin or porcelain of the pontic at the ridge portion.

A second method of increasing strength is to select a material of higher proportional limit. Thus, if a type C inlay gold was first considered, it may be desirable to go to a partial denture type D gold alloy, with higher proportional limit. In this connection, careful heat handling should be considered to give the highest possible proportional limit.

Third, neither of these alternatives may be sufficient, especially if the span is long. In such a case, consideration should be given to a bridge that is partially mucosa supported. If all these devices fail, it is possible that consideration of a bridge as a restoration type should be abandoned. If existing circumstances make it mandatory to place a bridge, it should be done with full realization on the part of the patient that it is structurally inadequate and subject to possible failure, should the full design load come upon it.

DESIGN OF A TWO-PONTIC BRIDGE

In Fig. 40-4, are shown two teeth and an edentulous area. The teeth have been approved in root structure and soundness of supporting tissues as suitable for abut-

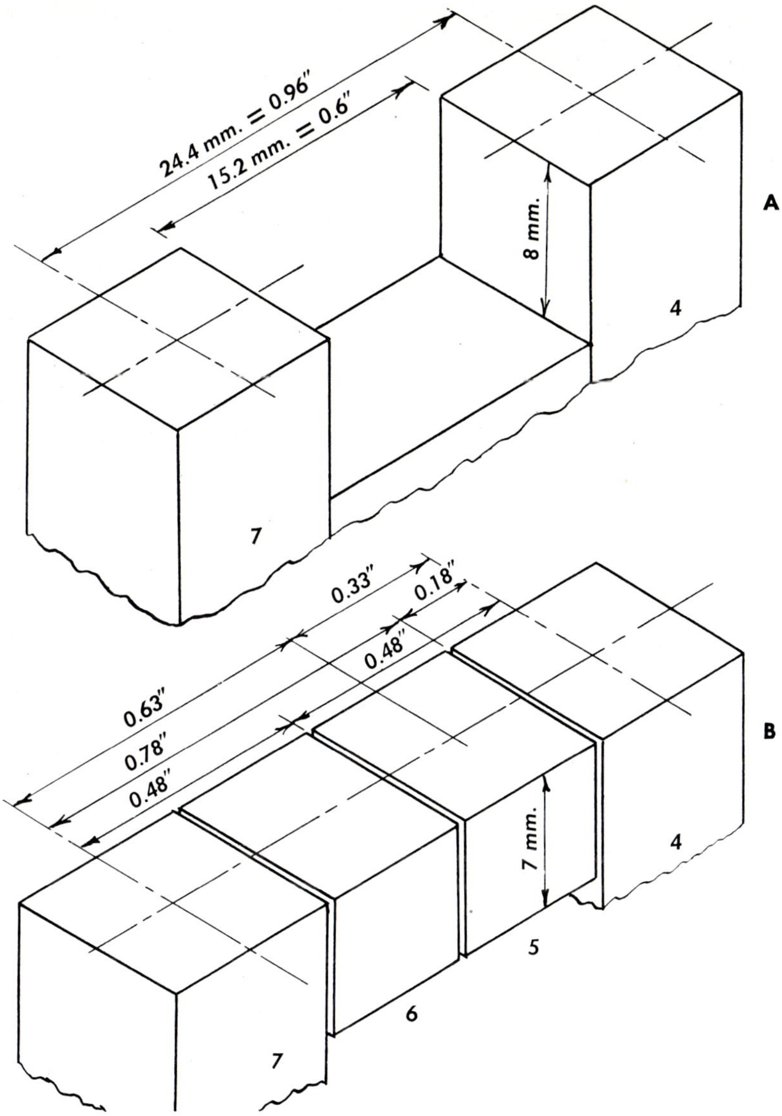

Fig. 40-4. A, Abutments $\overline{7}|$ and $\overline{4}|$ and edentulous areas $\overline{6}|$ and $\overline{5}|$. **B,** Pontics $\overline{6}|$ and $\overline{5}|$ in place and span dimensions.

ments. The edentulous area is to be bridged. It has been established that the opposing teeth do not protrude into this area. A straight edge has been laid across the two abutments, and the distance from this line to the mucosa has been determined as 8 mm. The clear distance between abutments has been measured as 15.2 mm. or 0.6 in. The distance from center to center of abutments has been recorded as 0.96 in. Two pontics have been selected to fill the gap, each 0.3 in., mesiodistally. Their widths buccolingually will be taken as those of Table 40-4 for the 7 mm. effective depth determined upon. A design and investigation will be made for the bridge.

The depth to the mucosa being 8 mm., it will be assumed that 1 mm. is sufficient for the porcelain or acrylic resin gingival platform of the pontic. The effective depth of the metal is then 7 mm. The tooth numbers of the abutments and pontics are marked on Fig. 40-4, *B*. It will be assumed that the pontics are like those of tooth $\overline{6}|$, and the soldered joints are like those of joint 7-6 and 5-4.

From Table 40-1, the largest critical load for either of the pontics is 75 lb. for tooth $\overline{6}|$. Place this load at the soldered joint at span center. Then:

$$M_c = \frac{75 \times 0.96}{4} = 18 \text{ in.lb.}$$

From Table 40-4, for the soldered joint $\overline{6\text{-}7}|$ (table depth as 4 mm.):

$$\frac{I}{c} = 0.000384$$

$$A = 0.0182$$

Substituting:

$$S = \frac{M\ c}{I} = \frac{18}{0.000384} = 46{,}900 \text{ lb./sq.in.}$$

The stress in the two adjacent pontics at the joint is much lower. From Table 40-4, for pontics $\overline{5}|$ and $\overline{6}|$:

$$\frac{I}{c} = 0.00146 \text{ for the 7 mm. depth.}$$

$$S = \frac{18}{0.00146} = 12{,}300 \text{ lb./sq.in.}$$

Punching shear at joint $\overline{5\text{-}4}|$

From Fig. 40-4, *B*, the reaction when the load of 75 lb. is placed at joint $\overline{5\text{-}4}|$ becomes the shear on the joint.

$$R_4 = \frac{75 \times 0.78}{0.96} = 61 \text{ lb.}$$

From Table 40-3, the area of the $\overline{5\text{-}4}|$ joint for the 4 mm. depth is 0.0119 sq.in. Then the punching shear is

$$S_s = \frac{61}{0.0119} = 5{,}100 \text{ lb./sq.in.}$$

A glance at Fig. 40-4 will show that the only part of the bridge that is stressed dangerously high is the soldered joint $\overline{5\text{-}6}|$ at the span center. Since greater depth for this joint is difficult to obtain because of the limited space between the occlusal and the mucosa, and since the stress indicated is high for a solder, it is recommended that the pontics be cast as a unit from a good grade of partial denture gold with a proportional limit, when heat hardened, of as much as 75,000 lb./sq.in. This will make the working stress of the joint 37,500 lb./sq.in. When this is increased by 25 percent, in consideration of the thinness of the joint, the allowable stress becomes 47,000 lb./sq.in. This procedure will render the joint safe. It does require, however, that care be taken that the two pontics cast as a unit be carefully heat hardened to develop the required strength.

Another possibility for this joint lies in increasing the buccolingual width of the adjacent pontics and consequently of the soldered joint by 2 mm. If this is possible, the strength of the joint may be materially improved. From Table 40-4, the section modulus of the joint as previously used is 0.000384. The dimensions that produced this modulus were d= 4 mm. and b = 3.4 mm. The depth cannot be increased. If the width can be increased to 6 mm., the section modulus becomes

$$\frac{I}{c} = \frac{0.000384 \times 6}{3.4} = 0.000675 \text{ in.}^3$$

NOTE: The procedure in the above equation is an approximation and does not give an exact result.

When this new modulus is used

$$S = \frac{18}{0.000675} = 26{,}600 \text{ lb./sq.in.}$$

This stress is possible for a fully heat-hardened joint soldered with a properly selected solder and represents an alternative procedure.

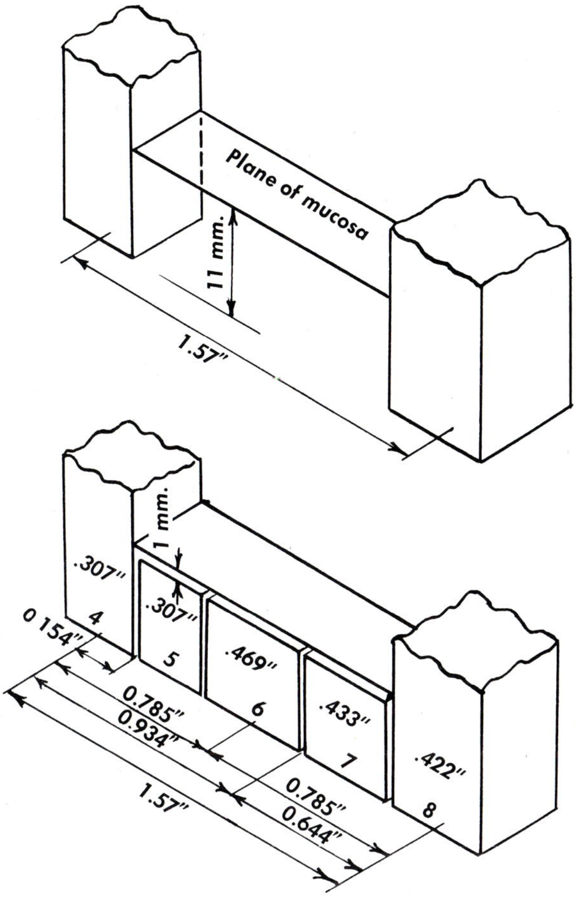

Fig. 40-5. Design of three-pontic |5-|6-|7 upper bridge extending from abutment teeth |4 to |8.

DESIGN OF A THREE-PONTIC UPPER BRIDGE

Fig. 40-5, *B*, shows a schematic drawing of a three-pontic upper bridge, whose abutments, which have been approved, are existing teeth |4 and |8. The clearance between the occlusal plane (or the level of the opposing teeth whichever may control) and the mucosa is 11 mm. Allowing 1 mm. for acrylic resin or porcelain gingival cover of the metal of the pontic, the effective depth of the metal then becomes 10 mm. The mesiodistal widths of the abutments and the respective pontics are also given. Many dentists would make the pontics of equal widths, but the variation shown conforms more nearly to the natural dentures. Span dimensions and dimensions from supports to critical soldered joints are shown. From Table 40-1, the critical load will be taken as 75 lb., as recommended. Take moments first at joint |6-|7. This joint will be assumed to have an effective depth of 7 mm., that is, 3 mm. less than those of the pontics that it joins. From Table 40-4, for joint |6-|7, the section modulus is 0.00206 in.³. The bending moment is

$$M\ |6\text{-}|7 = \frac{75 \times 0.644 \times 0.934}{1.57} = 28.5 \text{ in. lb.}$$

Then

$$S = \frac{28.5}{0.00206} = 13{,}850 \text{ lb./sq.in.}$$

This stress is satisfactory for the soldered joint. The strength of pontic |6 will be investigated at the span center. From Table 40-4, the section modulus of pontic |6 for an effective depth of 10 mm. is 0.00424 in.³. The bending moment at span center is

$$M_c = \frac{75 \times 1.57}{4} = 29.4 \text{ in.lb.}$$

The stress then is

$$S_6 = \frac{29.4}{0.00424} = 6{,}950 \text{ lb./sq.in.}$$

This is a satisfactory stress for any type C gold or better.

The punching shear will be computed at joint |4-|5. The shear at this joint is the reaction at abutment |4, when the load is placed at the joint.

$$R_4 = \frac{75(1.57 - 0.154)}{1.57} = 67.5 \text{ lb.}$$

From Table 40-4, the area of the joint of effective depth 7 mm. is

$$A\ |4\text{-}|5 = 0.0365 \text{ sq.in.}$$

$$S_s = \frac{67.5}{0.0365} = 1{,}850 \text{ lb./sq.in.}$$

The punching shear is entirely satisfactory.

It is noted that the stresses for this bridge are well within the allowable stresses and quite safe. This is a desirable condition. However, it may be of value to see how much the effective depth of the bridge might be lessened and still be within the safe stress. Let the working strength of the solder be assumed to be 18,000 lb./sq.in. Then, assuming the strength of the joint will be the controlling one:

$$\frac{I}{c} = \frac{28.5}{18{,}000} = 0.00158 \text{ in.}^3$$

Interpolating between the section moduli for depths of 7 and 6 mm., we find that the depth of the joint might be 6.37 mm. Adding 3 mm., we find the depth of the pontic might be 9.37 mm., which is not much different from that used in the design.

DESIGN OF AN ANTERIOR BRIDGE

The gravity axis of the bridge is represented by the line drawing shown in Fig. 40-6. (For details see Fig. 39-29.) The points *A* and *A* represent the centers of symmetrically placed abutment teeth, 3| and |3. Their distance, center to center, is 1.4 in. The bridge at its mesial point is 0.25 in. from the axis of abutments, giving an eccentricity of 0.25 in. The design load of 40 lb. is placed at the mesial point, perpendicular to the occlusal plane (not shown in Fig. 40-6). It is required to compute (1) the stresses induced by bending at the center, where bending is greatest, and (2) the bending and torsional or shearing stresses at the point of attachment to the abutments. Also the tie-back to more posterior teeth will be considered. Fig. 40-6 should be consulted in conjunction with Fig. 39-29.

It will be assumed that the effective depths of the pontics, as measured from the occlusal plane to the mucosa, may be 10 mm. This will make a 7 mm. effective depth of the soldered connections, according to the rule previously followed.

Moments at the left support

From Eq. e (Fig. 39-29) and Eq. f (Fig. 39-29):

$$M_A = -\frac{P\ e}{2} \sin \Theta_A = -\frac{40 \times 0.25}{2} \times 0.75 = -3.75 \text{ in.lb.}$$

and

$$T_A = -\frac{P\ e}{2} \text{Cos } \Theta_A = -\frac{40 \times 0.25}{2} \times 0.65 = -3.25 \text{ in.lb.}$$

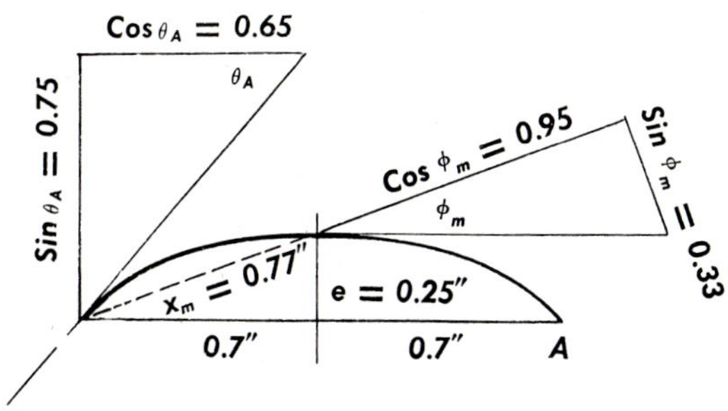

Fig. 40-6. Line diagram of upper anterior bridge, cuspid to cuspid 3|3. (See also Fig. 39-29.)

At the mesial point (span center)

See Eq. g (Fig. 39-29).

$$M_c = \frac{P}{2} b = \frac{40}{2} \times 0.7 = 14.0 \text{ in.lb.}$$

The greatest bending moment occurs at the mesial point and this is at the soldered joint 1|1. This soldered joint has previously been stated to have an effective depth of 7 mm. From Table 40-4 (assuming the joint is like that of 3-2|):

$$\frac{I}{c} = 0.000484 \text{ in.}^3$$

At the center line:

$$S = \frac{14.0}{0.000484} = 29{,}000 \text{ lb./sq.in.}$$

This is high for any ordinary solder. As was recommended for a previously solved bridge, it is concluded that pontics 1| and |1 of the bridge be cast as a unit from a good grade of partial denture gold and that this cast joint, together with the two pontics, be heat hardened.

The torque at the center is zero; therefore, there is no shearing stress here.

At point A (connection to the abutments): 3-2|, |2-3

The torque here has been computed to be 3.25 in.lb. and the bending moment, 3.75 in.lb. Because of the bending moment, the stress is as follows (assume soldered joint like that at 1|1):

$$S_A = \frac{3.75}{0.000484} = 7{,}750 \text{ lb./sq.in.}$$

There is no accurate formula for computing the shearing stress caused by torsion in an irregular cross section (as the section of an anterior dental bridge). However, the following empirical equation, used for rectangles, will give a rough approximation:

$$S_s = \frac{T}{d\,b^2}\left(3 + 1.8\,\frac{b}{d}\right)$$

In Eq. 17, *b* and *d* are the breadth and depth of the section, as shown in Table 40-4. Using this formula, the shearing stress caused by torsion at *A* approximates

$$S_s = \frac{3.25}{7 \times 4^2\,(0.0394^3)}\left(3 + 1.8 \times \frac{4}{7}\right)$$

$$= 1920 \text{ lb./sq.in.}$$

This shearing stress is safe, and if the precaution suggested for the 1|1 joint is observed, it may be concluded that the part of the bridge between abutments is structurally safe.

The question suggests itself as to whether or not the above computed shearing stress induced by torsion should be combined with the stress induced by bending, previously computed. Theoretically, this should be done. However, the shearing stress in a rectangle to which the preceding applies is concentrated near the middle at the extremities of the short side. The extremities of the long side are not highly stressed in shear. On the other hand, the greatest stresses induced by bending are at these extremities. This fact makes it unnecessary to combine the two.

An examination of the abutments and tie-backs is desirable. The overturning moment at *A* is

$$\frac{Pe}{2} = \frac{40 \times 0.25}{2} = 5 \text{ in.lb.}$$

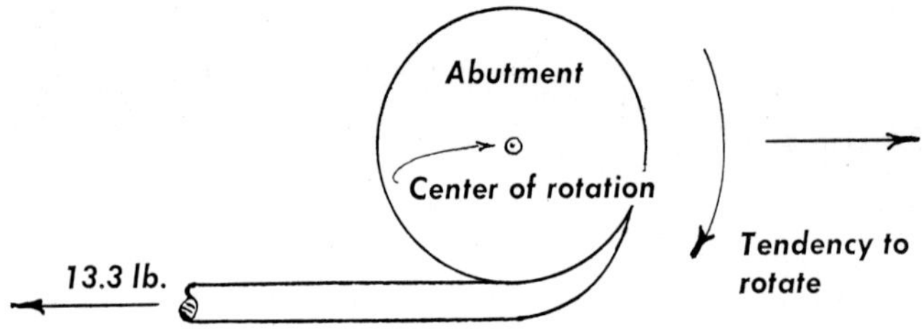

Fig. 40-7. Tendency to rotate abutment using only lingual tie-backs.

If it is assumed that the distance, from the center of gravity of the point of attachment of the bridge to the abutment to the center of rotation of the abutment tooth in the fundus, is 3/8 in., then the pull or tension in the tie-back will be due to the

$$F = \frac{Pe}{2} \times \frac{8}{3} = \frac{40 \times 0.25}{2} \times \frac{8}{3} = 13.3 \text{ lb.}$$

critical occlusal load of 40 lb.

This tie-back, in addition to holding the forward pull of the bridge resulting from occlusion, must also check the tendency of the bridge to rotate the abutment labially, the result of torsion in the bridge. Perhaps, also, it must take some forward thrust in occlusion, since the bridge pontic (particularly in the case of the upper teeth) is not set at right angles to the occlusal plane and takes some bending, if no stressbreaker is provided. The allowable stress in tension then should be set low. Let it be assumed that this allowable stress is 10,000 lb./sq.in. Then:

$$13.3 = 10{,}000 \text{ A}$$

or

$$\text{A} = 0.00133 \text{ sq.in.}$$

d (the diameter of a circular section to hold this) would be:

$$d = \sqrt{0.00133/.7854} = 0.041 \text{ in.}$$

Thus a bar of the area of an 18-gauge wire would be satisfactory for the tie-back. If the bar is made heavier, it would of course be satisfactory from a strength standpoint. The heavier the bar the more uplift it will exert on the secondary anchor tooth, if no stressbreaker is provided. It is therefore desirable that this bar not be too heavy. (See Fig. 39-30.)

One additional point needs to be discussed. Fig. 40-7 is a diagram of the abutment and the tie-back bar, with its pull of 13.3 lb. If the tie-back is placed only upon the lingual side, which is desirable from an esthetics standpoint, then a clockwise rotation of the abutment is indicated. If the tie-back bar is soldered both to a crown on the abutment and to the secondary anchor tooth, 4|, |4, this tendency to rotate (direction of rotation dependent on attachment) is shared by both teeth, which will minimize its effect on either tooth. However, it would be better if tie-backs were used on both the lingual and labial sides to avoid such tendency. If a wire is used on both lingual and labial sides, it may be smaller (half the area of the 18-gauge wire suggested).

TRANSFERRING THE BRIDGE REACTION TO THE ABUTMENT

The manner of transferring the bridge reaction into the abutment tooth is often important. The brief analysis given here is more pertinent to one or more abutments receiving reactions from freely supported bridges, although the tendencies noted take place in all abutments.

Fig. 40-8 shows a single-rooted lower bicuspid abutment tooth. There is an assumed center of rotation of this tooth marked at *o*. In practice, the tooth may have an indeterminate number of inclina-

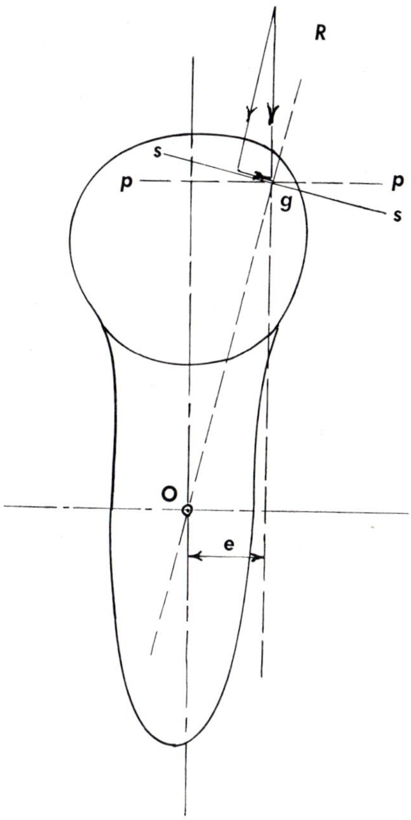

Fig. 40-8. Bridge reaction transfer into abutments.

tions toward the edentulous area. It is usually inclined toward it. It is here shown with its axis vertical. If the reaction could be applied to the abutment, directly along its longitudinal axis, and if the axis were normal to the occlusal plane, there would be no problem. The seat would always be perpendicular to the axis, or horizontal.

Because of mechanical difficulties, it is not always practicable to apply the reaction in line with the longitudinal axis. On the contrary, it is most often applied at some point between the proximal contact of the bridge and the abutment axis. Such a reaction is indicated in Fig. 40-8, as *R*, applied at *e* distance from the axis. If the reaction is vertical, it then has a tendency to rotate the abutment in a clockwise direction. This tendency is overcome in various ways. It may be easily overcome, when the bridge is a freely supported one, by attention to the angulation of the keyway seat upon which the key of the bridge rests.

Let the plane *p-p* in Fig. 40-8 represent the elevation of the center of this seat. The line of action of the bridge reaction, *R*, intersects this plane at *g*. From the center of rotation, *o*, draw the line *og*. The plane *s-g-s*, perpendicular to this line, represents very closely the proper inclination of the bridge seat on the abutment.

This may be proved as follows. Resolve the reaction *R* into components. The larger one is parallel to the line *og* and passes through the center of rotation, *o*. The smaller one is parallel to the seat *s-s* and acts in that plane. Since the large component passes through *o*, a very small clockwise rotation of the tooth gives it a small leverage which is sufficient to produce a counterclockwise tendency to rotation that is equal to the clockwise tendency produced by the small component parallel to *s-s*. Equilibrium results and rotation ceases. This is easily demonstrated by a model. Teeth so prepared are quite stable.

When a removable bridge has an abutment at either end and the seats are not carefully prepared, the abutments usually tend to rotate toward the edentulous area. In so doing they come into contact with the bridge, and the thrust each exerts toward the edentulous area tends to neutralize the other, so that little actual rotation results. When a bridge is soldered to both terminal abutment crowns, bending moments induced at the points of connection are neutralized by counteracting couples in the root structure.

GENERAL REFERENCE (See also p. 909.)

Tylman, S. D.: Relationship of the structural design of dental bridges to their supporting tissues, Int. Dent. J. 13:303, 1963.

Chapter 41

Gothic arch tracings with Hanau adjustable articulator H2-XPR and face bow: separable registration trays and stone checkbites

When malocclusion and mandibular malrelationships are accompanied by other subjective symptoms, it is advisable to make a comprehensive study of the existing conditions. To restore the oral environment with restorations that are also biologically acceptable, a prerequisite is a method to be used in mounting both the study and the working casts in an adjustable articulator using a hinge axis face bow. Casts so mounted are related to each other in the instrument as the dentition and arches are in the mouth, also in relation to the temporomandibular articulation. This relation is correct in centric and in functional positions of the mandible.

In previous chapters consideration was given to the functionally generated path method—a technic capable of giving satisfactory results with the simpler types of restorations that do not involve extensive restorative procedures or corrections. In Chapter 29, a procedure was discussed that employs interocclusal wax records; it also utilizes an adjustable articulator and a hinge axis face bow. In Chapter 37, procedures were also presented using a gnathologic instrument of recent development, likewise a face bow and pantograph for obtaining and recording the positions and movements of the mandible. This procedure utilizes styli and recording plates to indicate graphically the positions and movements of the mandible for transfer to and setting of the articulator.

A fourth method of recording functional relations of the mandible also utilizes the adjustable articulator and hinge axis face bow. However, instead of using the interocclusal records or the stylus type of pantograph recorder, this procedure utilizes cast aluminum registration trays (clutches) with stone checkbites, and gothic arch tracings. These are then used to transfer the casts to the articulator, which is adjusted to the gothic arch tracings and stone checkbites.

The first step, therefore, is to determine the hinge movement of the mandible. Later the slant which the condyle and meniscus travel along the posteroinferior border of the articular eminence is recorded. Actually, the temporomandibular joint consists of not one but of two joints, one rotating, the other sliding. The two movements may occur separately but usually take place simultaneously.

The mandible cannot be held long in a static position without the musculature becoming fatigued; the mandible habitually returns to its postural position which is determined by a neuromuscular mechanism which restores the muscles to their physiologic, tonic length. In this state of muscle equilibrium the mandible can be held a long time without fatigue. In this postural position, there normally exists from 2 to 4 mm. of interocclusal space between the anterior maxillary and mandibular teeth.

To obtain correct registrations of the movements of the mandible and to transfer them to an articulator for functional analysis and oral rehabilitation, it is first necessary to place the condyles functionally and terminally in their glenoid fossae in order to determine their axes of vertical rotation.

Although the axis running through the vertical rotation centers of the condyles remains constant with reference to the two condyles, the position of the axis in its spatial relation to the glenoid fossae varies. The position of the condylar axis differs when the mandible is in a postural or so-called rest position, from the one which the mandible occupies in its physiologically retruded, terminal, functional position.

In functional vertical closure, the condyles move upward and posteriorly in their glenoid fossae, being limited in the amount of their movement by their anatomy, muscles, and capsular ligaments. They are *not positioned in their most retruded position or in the deepest part of the fossae* in normal functional occlusion. This view is confirmed by Sicher.[1]

Therefore, it is not recommended to apply external force to the mandible in an effort to position the condyles in their *physiologically retruded functional position.* An acceptable method is given later to locate and register the axis of vertical condylar rotation designated as the functional hinge axis.

To try and locate these axes by placing fingers on the side of the face near the tragus is largely guesswork. A more precise method of locating these centers of rotation utilizes a metal registration tray rigidly attached to the mandibular teeth (Figs. 41-29, 41-30, and 41-45). By means of a stud, the registration tray is attached to a hinge bow having an adjustable stylus opposite each condyle. As the functionally retruded mandible is gently opened and closed with a pure hinge rotation, each stylus is adjusted vertically and anteroposteriorly until each stylus rotates on a point. This is done on both sides of the face. These points which establish the axes of vertical rotation of the condyles are then marked permanently on the skin on both sides of the face (Figs. 41-38 and 41-42). A third point, on a plane with the infraorbital notch, is determined and marked permanently on the right side of the nose. This latter point, with the two others which mark the hinge axis, establishes the "axis-orbital plane" (Figs. 41-44 and 41-76).

By utilizing this plane of reference, study casts as well as working cases may at any time be correctly orientated on the articulator by means of the face bow and the axis orbital indicator. The relation of the upper model to the axis is the same in the articulator as it is in the patient. All subsequent registrations are made with reference to this established plane; likewise, the validity of all subsequent registrations is determined by the accuracy of this step.

The starting point for such registrations on the patient is the centric relation of the mandible to the cranium in the articular fossae. This must relate the mandible to the maxillae in its *physiologically retruded functional terminal position* in the articular fossae. This is the most important registration, for all other records are worthless if the centric relation registration is incorrect; all eccentric positions of the mandible are oriented with reference to it.

The determination of the correct centric relation of the mandible is subjective on the part of the dentist and depends on the understanding, judgment, and skill of the individual dentist. The finest mechanical instruments will not correct false registrations; articulators accept what the dentist imposes on them.

The purposes of recording functional relation have been summed up by Contino and Stallard[2] as follows: (1) to determine the dimensional relationship of teeth and jaws to the cams and to the axes of the joint movements on a patient; (2) to determine and locate the centric axis position of the opening and closing action of the mandible; (3) to establish the slant and curve of the condyle path; (4) to set and direct the amount and direction of the Bennett path; (5) to transfer these recordings to the articulator to reproduce the movement that the patient makes.

There are many types of articulators available,[3] ranging from the simple and less expensive ones to those more comprehensive in the scope of their recordings[4] and, therefore, more expensive. From among the several types, we shall discuss the Hanau adjustable type articulator, model H2-XPR, since this type is more generally used by students and the general practitioner.[5]

TECHNIC OF USING GOTHIC ARCH TRACINGS WITH THE HANAU ADJUSTABLE ARTICULATOR, MODEL H2-XPR; THE ADJUSTABLE FACE BOW AND SEPARABLE REGISTRATION TRAYS (CLUTCHES)

This method is primarily indicated for the partially edentulous patient. For this technic, the following items of equipment are utilized: (1) two sectional aluminum registration trays with detachable stems (Fig. 41-1); (2) Hanau H2-XPR articulator (Fig. 41-2); (3) hinge axis face bow (Fig. 41-3); (4) transfer board (Fig. 41-4); and (5) two sets of upper and lower stone casts of patient's mouth.

To construct registration trays of cast aluminum for taking registrations, it is first necessary to mount the casts on the articulator. This initial, *temporary mounting* of the casts may be done by the method customarily employed, namely, the condyle areas are palpated with the fingers and marked on the skin with a pencil, after which the infraorbital notch level is located and marked on the right side of the nose. A bite fork is covered on both sides with a layer of impression compound to a thickness of ⅛ inch (Fig. 41-5).

With an alcohol torch the compound is softened, then carried to the mouth; the stem of the fork extends anteriorly. The compound bite should extend posteriorly to the second molar area. The compound and fork are carried against the upper teeth while the patient is instructed to close lightly until the cusps of the lower teeth make an imprint in the lower surface of the compound. *The teeth must not penetrate the compound to the metal.* Only the cusps of the upper and lower teeth should make imprints in the compound. The compound bite is then chilled and removed from the mouth. The accuracy of the cuspal imprints may be verified by seating the stone casts into the imprints. If a more accurate registration is desirable, some zinc oxide–eugenol impression cement is placed over the cuspal indentations in the compound, and it is returned to the mouth, after which the jaw is again closed lightly (Fig. 41-6).

When the cement has set, the patient is instructed to hold the bite firmly between the teeth (Fig. 41-7). The face bow is slipped over the bite-fork stem and the condylar-pointers are adjusted so they lie opposite the condylar marks on the skin on either side of the face and the orbital pointer placed next to the mark on the right side of the nose (Fig. 41-8). The condylar and infraorbital locknuts are

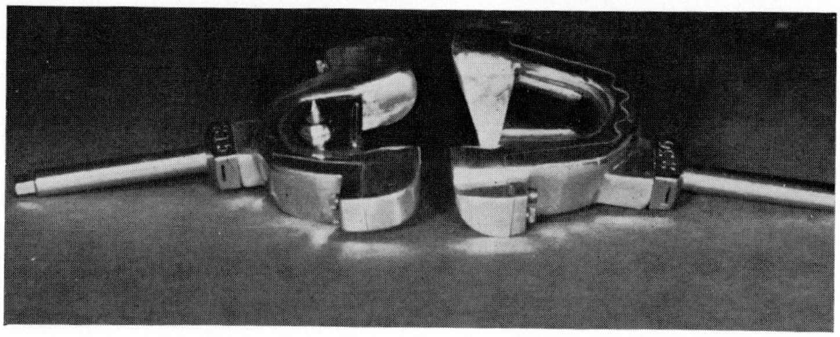

Fig. 41-1. Upper and lower cast aluminum registration trays with detachable stems.

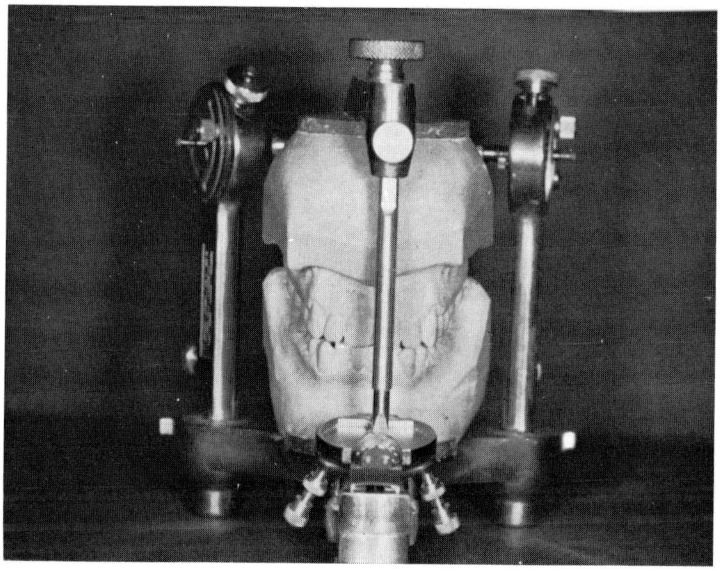

Fig. 41-2. Arbitrary mounting of upper and lower casts on Hanau articulator, H2-XPR.

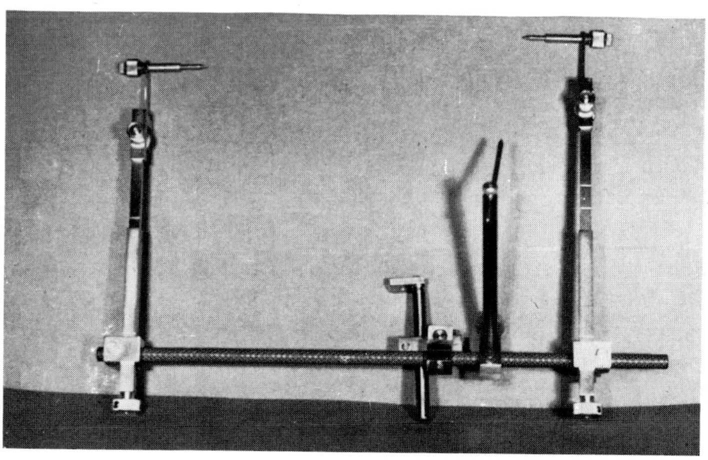

Fig. 41-3. Hanau adjustable face bow with infraorbital pin and detachable tray stem.

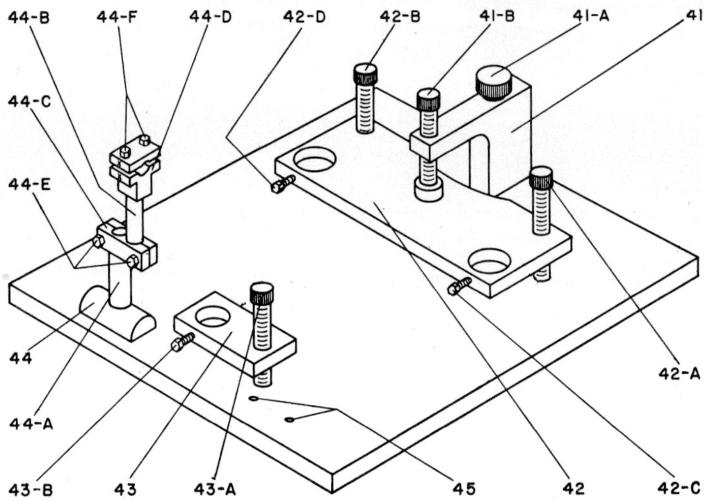

Fig. 41-4. Transfer board. **41,** Locking clamp with lock screws, **41-B. 42,** Rear articulator support with elevating screws, **42-A** and **42-B,** and leg screws, **42-C** and **42-D. 43,** Front articulator support with elevating screws, **43-A,** and leg screw, **43-B. 44,** Face bow support, complete assembly with supporting studs, **44-A** and **44-B,** clamps, **44-C** and **44-D,** and lock screws, **44-E** and **44-F. 45,** Two holes in board permit mounting face bow support, **44,** opposite to position shown here. (Courtesy Hanau Engineering Co., Inc.)

Fig. 41-5

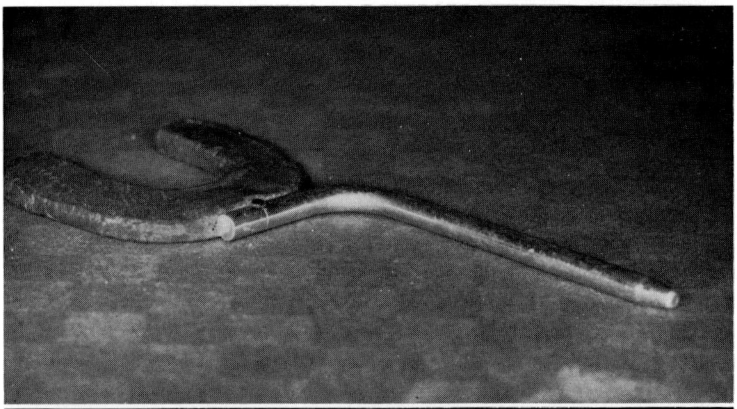

Fig. 41-6

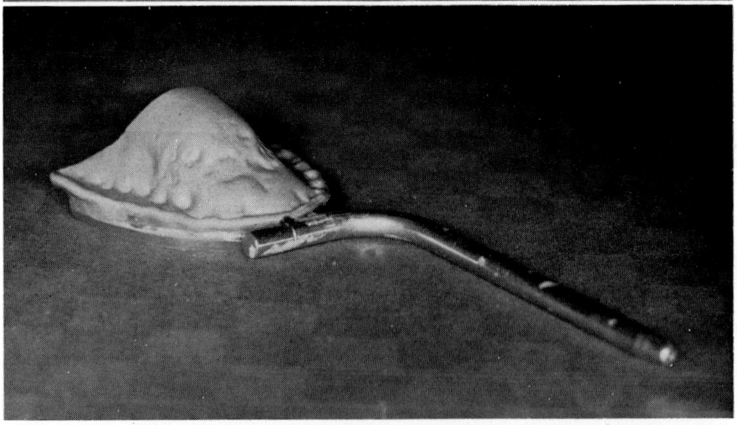

Fig. 41-5. Bite fork with modeling compound.
Fig. 41-6. Bite fork with zinc oxide–eugenol cement bite registration.

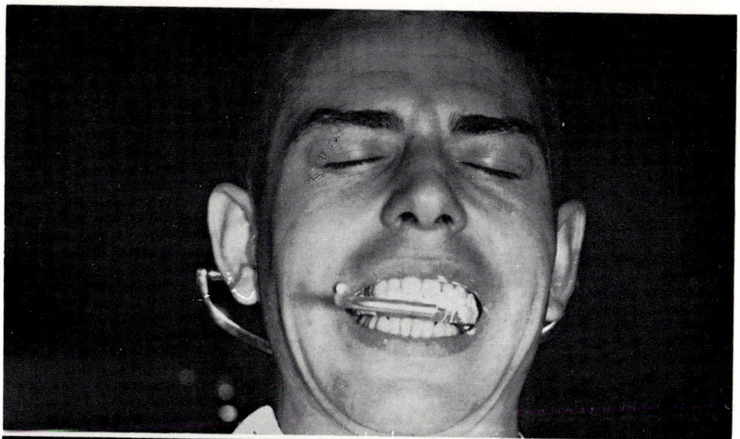

Fig. 41-7

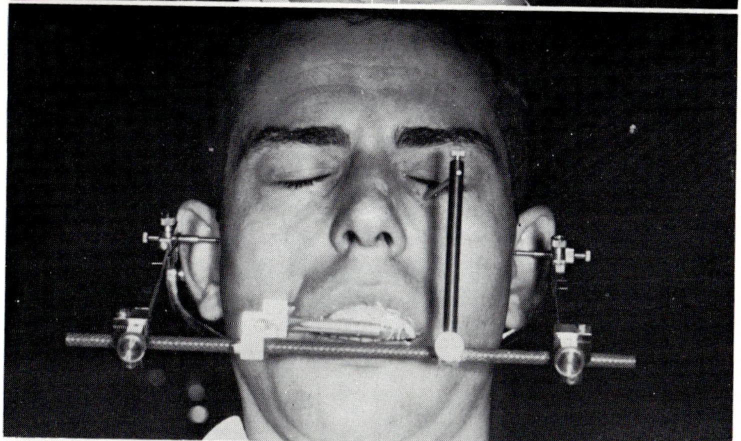

Fig. 41-8

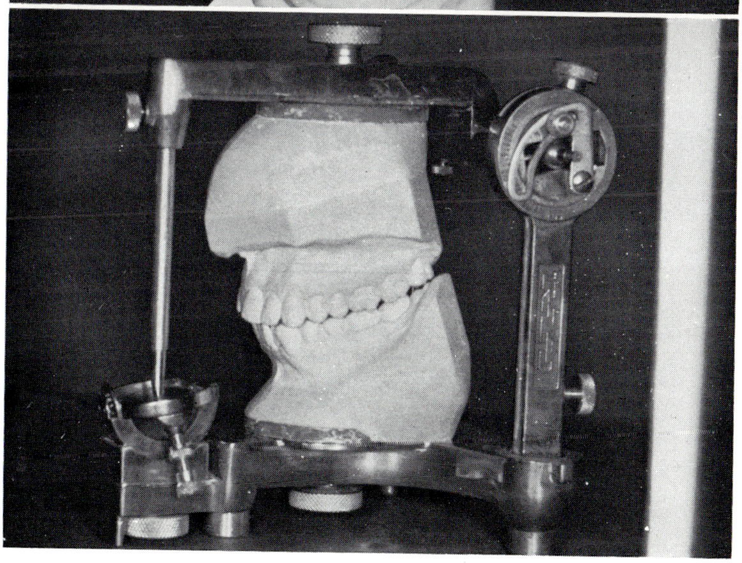

Fig. 41-9

Fig. 41-7. Patient holding bite fork in place with mandibular teeth.
Fig. 41-8. Locating and attaching infraorbital pointer to face bow.
Fig. 41-9. Casts mounted in articulator using arbitrary locations of hinge axis and centric wax bite.

tightened, also the toggle-clamp fastening the bite-fork stem to the face bow. With the face bow securely locked to the bite fork it is carried to the transfer board and clamped tightly in clamp 44-D (Fig. 41-4).

The articulator is then placed on the transfer board and adjusted as closely as possible to (1) the condylar pointers and (2) the infraorbital plane pointer attached to the face bow. The upper cast is now seated in the zinc oxide–compound bite and attached to the upper bow of the articulator.

The centric wax bite customarily used is then used to mount the lower cast to the lower frame of the articulator (Fig. 41-9).

The *arbitrary mounting of the casts,* just described, is done for one purpose only, namely, to facilitate the construction of the cast aluminum trays and to align the tray stems in their proper vertical and horizontal relationship to each other and to the trays. *This mounting, it must be stressed again, is an arbitrary one used only to construct the trays;* after the aluminum trays have been constructed, the casts will be removed from the articulator.

Registration trays (clutches)*

Although cast aluminum registration trays may be purchased with detachable tray stems as shown in Fig. 41-10, better results are obtained if individual trays are made for each cast. Some recommend the use of registration trays made of acrylic resin (Fig. 41-11) or of double thickness base-plate; however, for the most reliable and accurate results, the cast aluminum registration tray has proved most satisfactory. As later described, the metal tray is divided into labial and lingual sections, which are assembled by means of screws.

There are several methods of making the individual trays, and the following method is the one generally used by many dentists.

*The term registration tray is preferred to the term clutch; the former designates the use and purpose of the instrument.

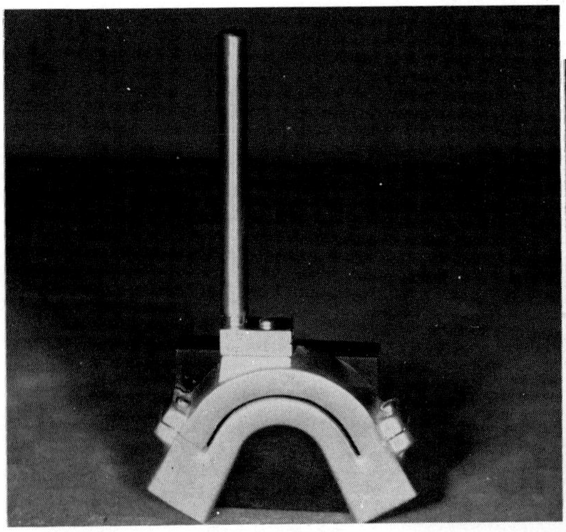

Fig. 41-10

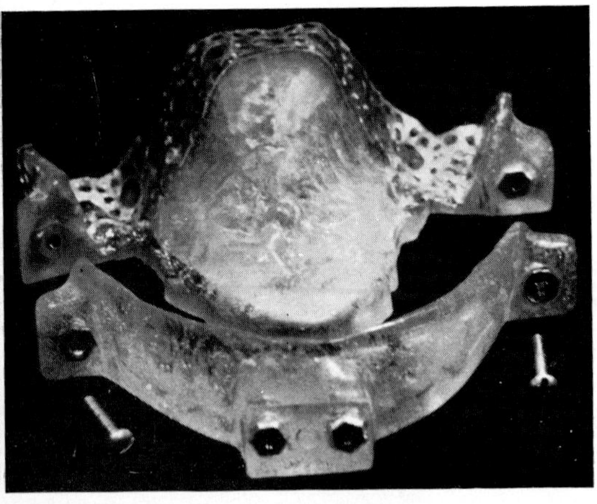

Fig. 41-11

Fig. 41-10. Manufactured Hanau aluminum separable registration tray with detachable stem. (Courtesy Hanau Engineering Co., Inc.)
Fig. 41-11. Custom-made reinforced acrylic resin registration tray for upper arch. (Courtesy Dr. B. Mazur.)

To make trays for the cast, the casts with mounting plates are first removed from the articulator by unscrewing their mounting plate screws. Wax is adapted to the models to fill in all undercuts. The wax should cover the buccal and labial surfaces of the models from 2 mm. below the buccal and labial edges of the teeth, down over the undercuts, with one layer of Tenax wax on the thinnest portion (Fig. 41-12). The lingual surfaces are covered in a similar manner (Fig. 41-13), also the palatal area. Then the entire occlusal surface of the model and gingival area is covered with one thickness of 0.003 inch tin foil. This is burnished smooth and should present no undercuts (Fig. 41-14).

A film of cocoa butter is applied over the tin foil to allow the next application of wax to separate freely from the tin foil. One layer of Tenax wax is then applied over the tin foil. It should extend ½ inch below the incisal and occlusal surfaces on the buccal, labial, and lingual surfaces of the lower cast. On the upper cast it should cover the entire palate and extend ½ inch below the occlusal surface on the labial and buccal surfaces but in no case should encroach onto the tissue reflections. Strips ½ inch wide are then placed over the

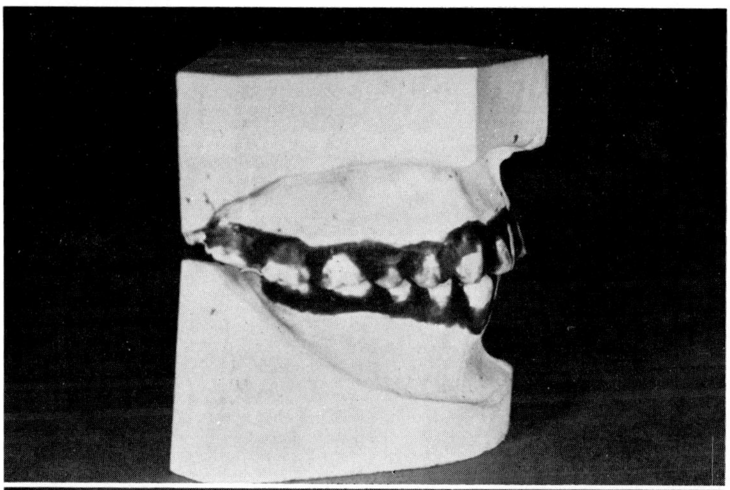

Fig. 41-12

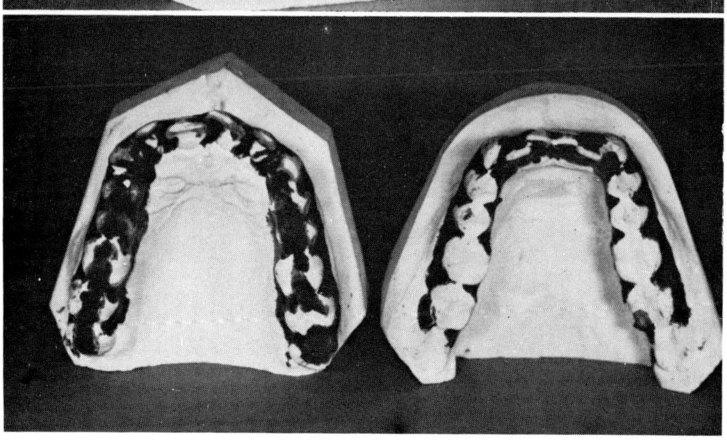

Fig. 41-13

Fig. 41-12. Undercuts removed from casts prior to waxing registration trays.
Fig. 41-13. Undercuts on lingual surfaces also eliminated with wax prior to waxing registration trays.

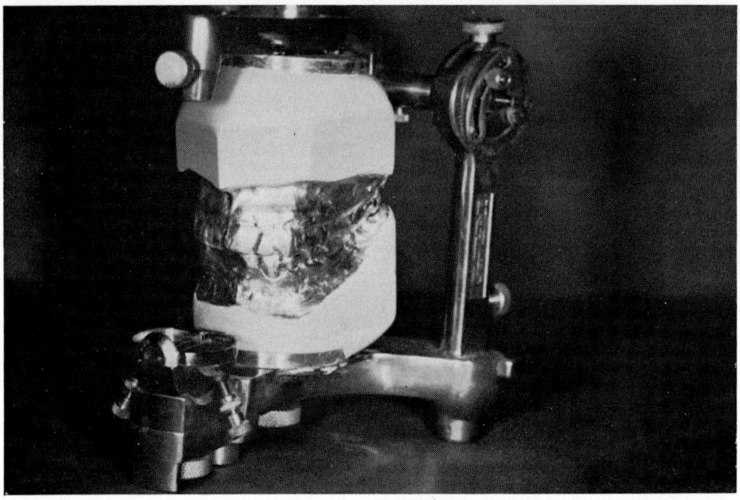

Fig. 41-14. Teeth covered with tin foil.

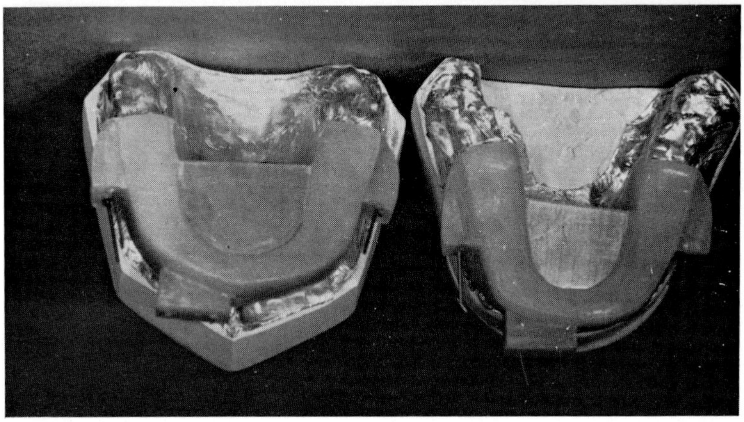

Fig. 41-15. Registration trays waxed.

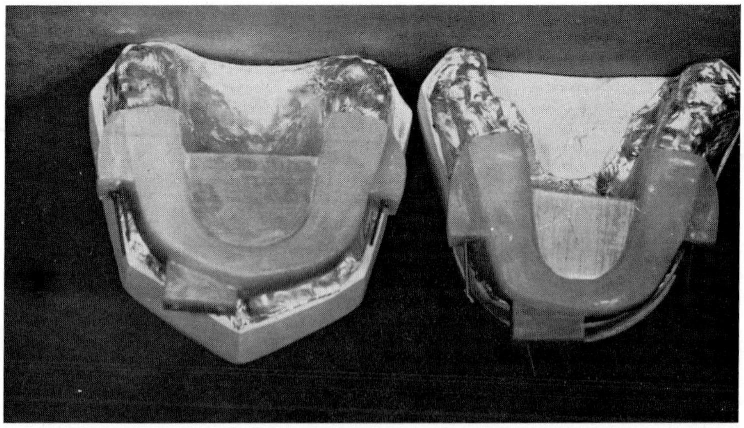

Fig. 41-16. German-silver plates cast into upper and lower waxed registration trays.

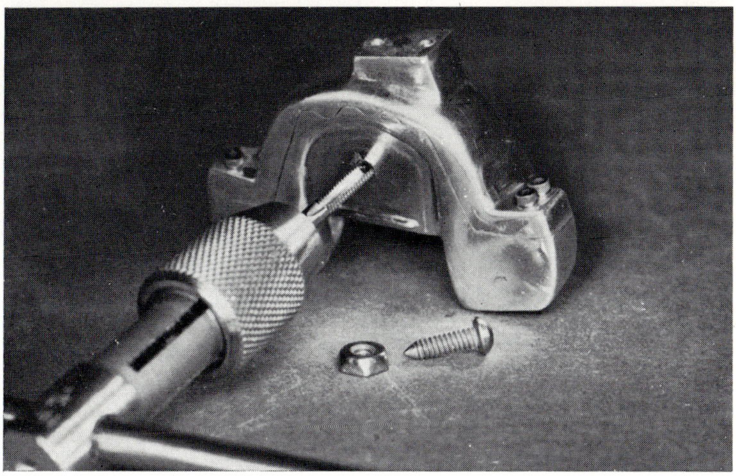

Fig. 41-17. 6-32 screw and hole tapped in German-silver plate to accommodate screw used as center-bearing screw.

labial, buccal, and lingual surfaces, but not extending onto the occlusal. This is luted to the underlying layer of wax. There is now a covering of one layer of wax over the occlusal surfaces and two layers over the rest of the areas (Fig. 41-15).

One-quarter inch square blocks of Tenax wax, ½ inch long, are placed on the buccal surface opposite the mesial cusps of the first molars. These blocks are placed vertically and will later be drilled, tapped, and sawed on the casting, to allow removal of the cemented trays from the mouth.

The lower registration tray. German-silver plate, or brass (Fig. 41-16, *right*), ¹⁄₁₆ inch thick, is sawed out to fit the inner curvature of the lower anterior teeth. It should be about 1½ inches wide at its maximum width and semicircular in shape. At the center of the plate and near its anterior curved edge, a hole is drilled with a No. 36 drill or a No. 6 round bur; this hole is tapped with a 6-32 tap (Fig. 41-17). A 6-32 screw sharpened to a rounded point and a locknut are now placed in the tapped hole, which will serve as the center-bearing screw. The plate is then waxed in behind the lower anterior teeth, kept parallel to the plane of occlusion and about ⅛ inch below the plane of occlusion. The center-bearing screw should be centered between the two arms of the arches.

The upper registration tray. A semicircular plate of ¹⁄₁₆ inch German-silver or brass is cut to fit behind and close to the upper anterior teeth (Fig. 41-16, *left*). It should be about 1 inch anteroposteriorly and about 1 inch in width. The plate should be bent to present a slight concavity into the upper tray. The bend will give some vertical shift in the lateral movement of the mandible to aid the clearance of the trays in those movements. When placing the curved plate lingual to the upper anterior teeth in the upper tray, the posterior edge of the plate should be depressed to give opening to the trays in the protrusive movement. As the plate is placed in the upper wax, it should be about ⅛ inch below the incisal edge of the anterior teeth and slope to about ¼ inch depth below the plane of occlusion at its posterior edge.

The models and wax are returned to the articulator, and the center-bearing-screw contact with the upper German-silver or brass plate is checked: first, to see that

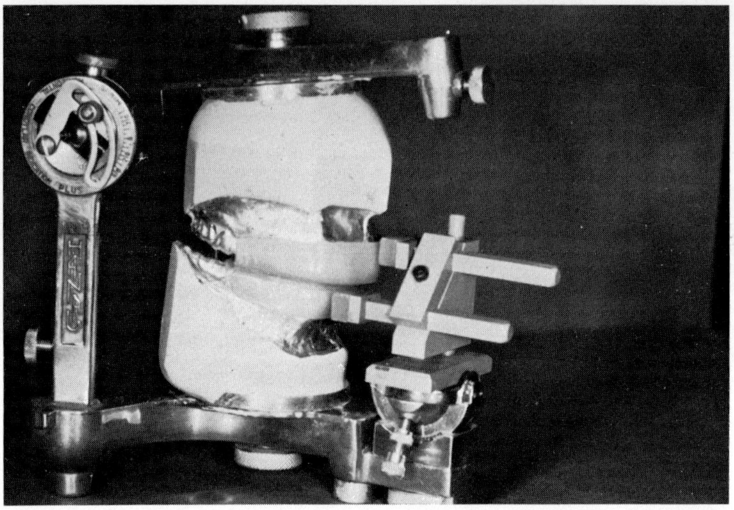

Fig. 41-18. Waxed registration trays on casts with stud alignment for proper placement of separable studs in finished aluminum castings.

A

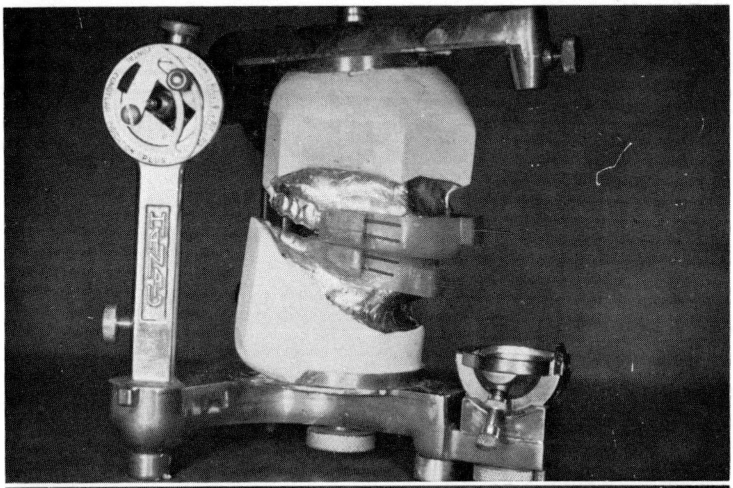

B

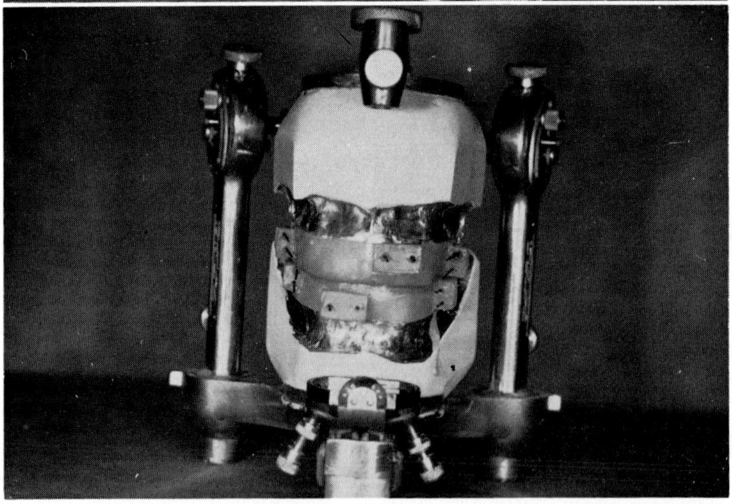

Fig. 41-19. Pencil leads placed on buccal and labial aspects of waxed trays; holes are later enlarged and tapped in cast trays.

the screw is centered in the deepest portion of the bend in the opposing plate in centric closure; second, that the wax forms of the trays do not touch in centric, lateral, and protrusive positions. In other words, the only bearing between the two models is through the center-bearing screw.

The separable-stud alignment-jig (Fig. 41-18) is then placed in front of the casts on the articulator. Wax is applied to the tray pattern so that the studs will be placed (1) equally above and below the incisal edge and (2) at right angles to the hinge axis in both vertical and horizontal planes. Wax is placed anteriorly between the jig-stud-plate and the waxed tray. The wax addition is then luted down smoothly to the tray pattern.

Warm the end of each stud and press it into the wax block. Close the articulator and set the studs so that they are approximately parallel and separated vertically about ½ inch, and horizontally about 1 inch. Chill the wax pattern. Warm the tip of the stud with a small flame, until it drops off the wax pattern from its own weight. Separate the end of the stud, which will be attached to the tray. Apply a thin coat of petrolatum. Replace it on the pattern. Medium hard pencil leads are used in Okler style mechanical pencils to form the holes for later threading. Insert a heated broken explorer into the wax through the screw hole of the stud. Hold a piece of pencil lead in the flame until it is red hot, then insert in the pattern, carrying it all the way through. Do the same with both holes. In a similar fashion insert leads in the tapered side blocks, parallel to the buccal surface and far enough apart to permit room for the screw heads (Fig. 41-19).

A reinforcing ridge of wax ⅛ inch by ⅛ inch is then laid on both patterns bilaterally, extending from the anterior separable-stud-attachment-block to the posterior screw-block, placed at the mesial of the first molar; this reinforcing ridge is smoothly luted to the pattern.

The patterns can then be removed from the casts and the borders trimmed to eliminate as much material from the edges as is consistent with adequate strength. The corners around the second molar areas are also trimmed off to avoid contact with the muscles when in the mouth.

Investing and casting registration trays

The patterns are then placed on the models again to check for fit. They are chilled, removed, and placed occlusal side up on the bench. Three sprues are then made for each tray of double thickness Tenax wax ⅜ inch wide. One is placed at the anterior-most portion of each tray and one at each heel. The three are waxed together at a convenient intersection depending upon the type of casting flask used (Fig. 41-20, *A*).

The next step is to invest the pattern making sure to allow a sufficient capacity in the crucible for the considerable amount of aluminum necessary for the casting (Figs. 41-20, *B*, and 41-21).

Upon setting of the investment material, the wax is dissipated, first, by boiling out in water and, second, by heating in an oven for sufficient time and temperature of about 1100 to 1200° F., to burn out all wax residue completely. The flasks are then allowed to cool to about 500° F. or until they can be picked up in the hands. The aluminum will cast best in a cooled mold. Do not overheat the aluminum.

After casting and thoroughly cooling, the castings can be removed from the mold. The sprues are sawed off and a wire brush finish given to the trays (Fig. 41-22). With soft solder, attach to each nickel-silver plate short sections of 14-gauge brass or German-silver rods as indexes for the checkbites. Place these where they will not interfere with the movements of the center-bearing screw point. Holes are drilled in the trays for anterior attach-

A

B

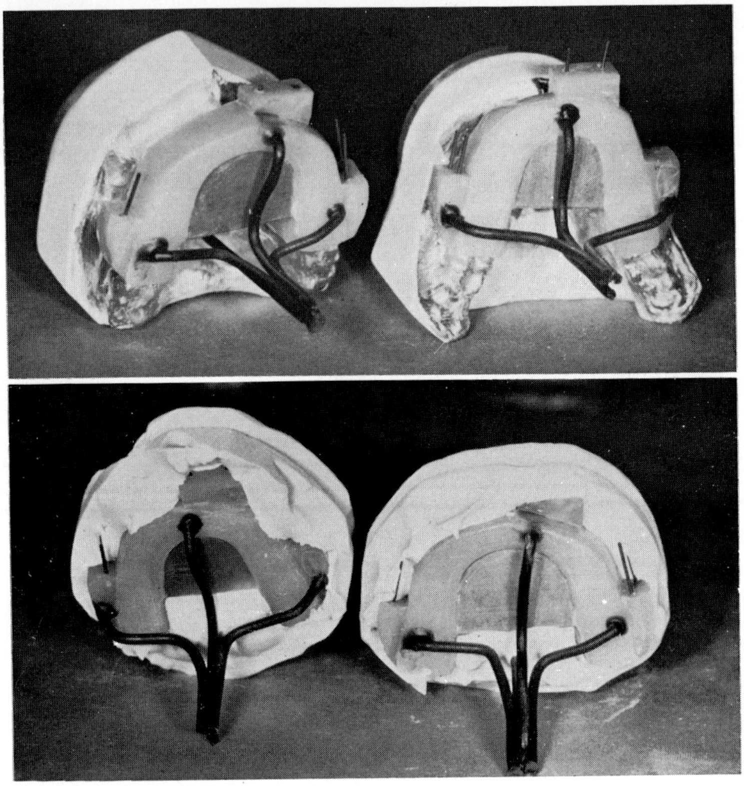

Fig. 41-20. Waxed registration trays sprued with casting investment poured against tissue surfaces of trays prior to investing in flask.

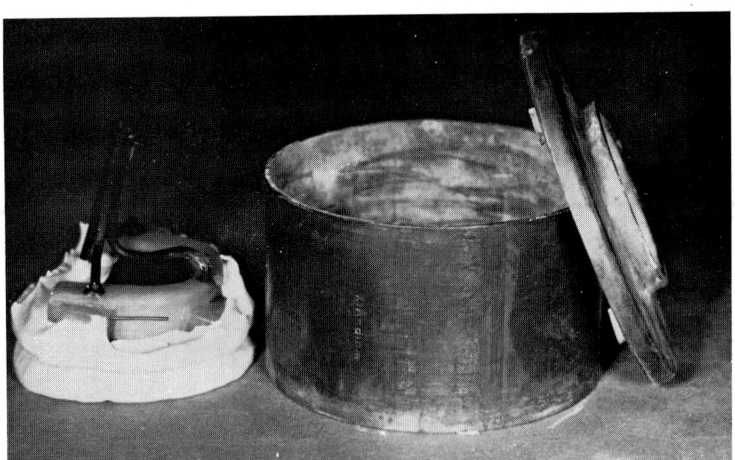

Fig. 41-21. Sprued, waxed tray ready to be invested in casting ring and crucible forming top.

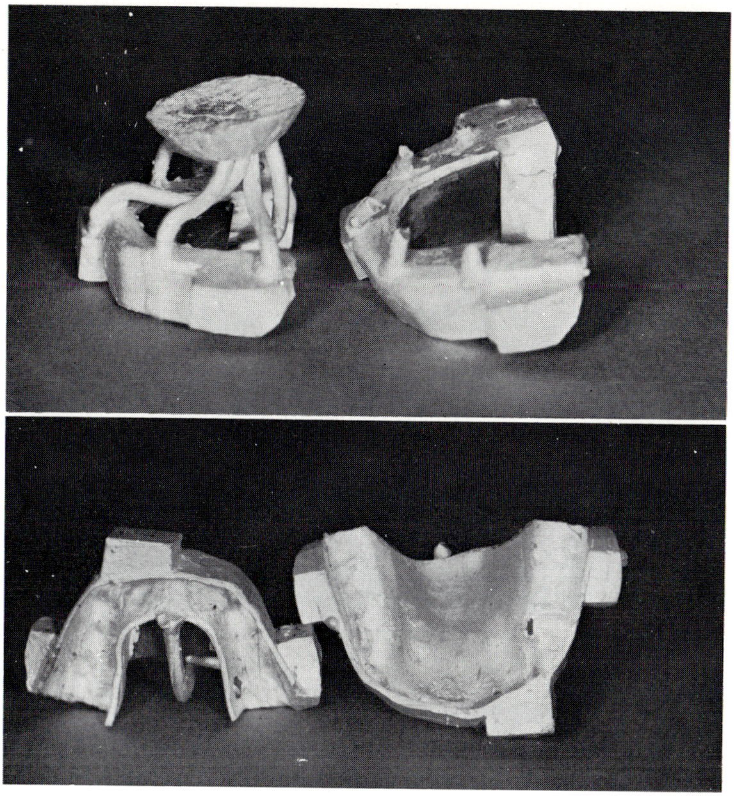

A

B

Fig. 41-22. External and internal surfaces of cast aluminum registration trays before and after sprues are cut off.

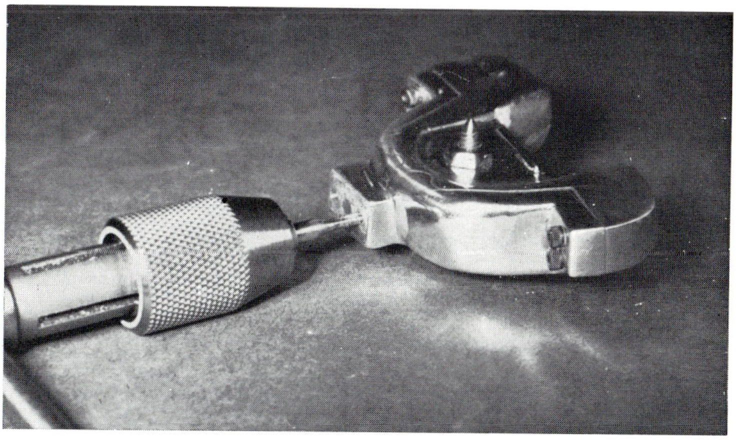

Fig. 41-23. Drilling out lead points and tapping holes with 2-56 tap.

ment of the separable-stud-plates (Fig. 41-23). Drill out the pencil leads with a No. 44 drill, creating pilot holes. These are then enlarged with a No. 48 drill. The hole is now tapped with a 2-56 tap (Fig. 41-24). The separable-stud-plates (Fig. 41-25) can then be attached to the trays (Figs. 41-26 and 41-27). Turpentine, carbon tetrachloride, or lard oil are excellent lubricants for drilling and tapping aluminum. The studs are then screwed to the plates on the trays, which provide a convenient handle for succeeding operations. Next, drill two holes in each of the side blocks at the first molar location, one hole above and one

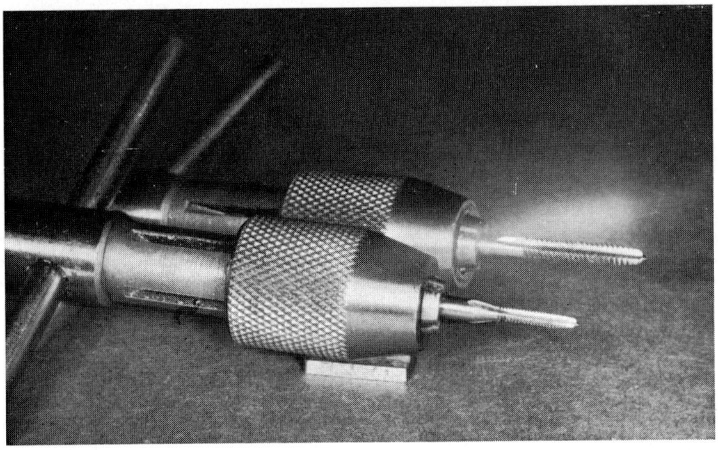

Fig. 41-24. Taps for 2-56 screw and for 6-32 screw for center-bearing screw.

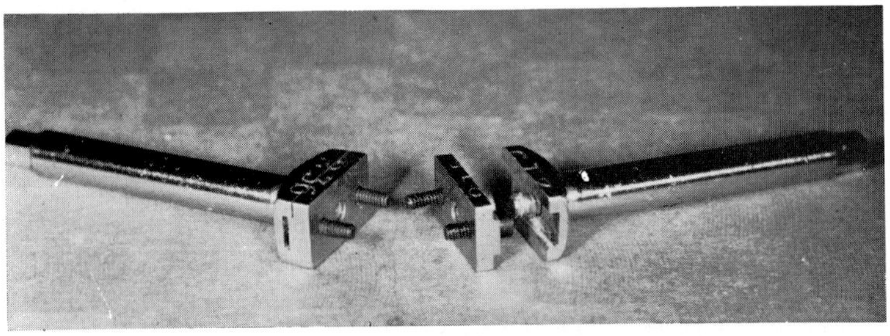

Fig. 41-25. Detachable tray stem and separable stem plates.

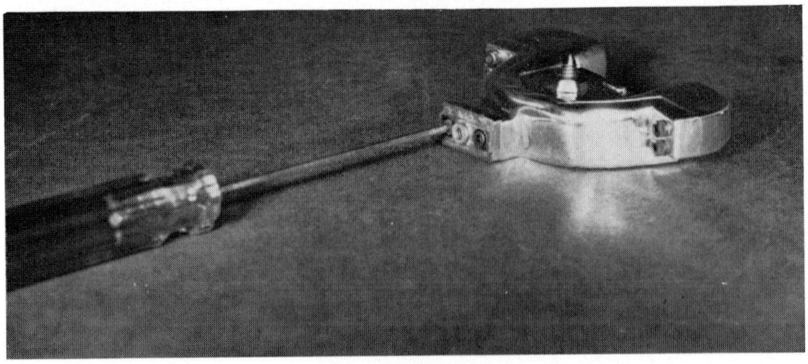

Fig. 41-26. Attaching stem plate to aluminum tray.

below the ⅛ inch by ⅛ inch reinforcing ribs; drill out the pencil leads with a No. 44 drill to establish pilot holes. Next the pilot holes are enlarged with a No. 48 drill; the holes are then tapped with a 2-56 tap.

With a fine jeweler's saw cut buccolingually and vertically through the buccal blocks at their centers, leaving about ⅛ inch on each side of the cut (Fig. 41-28). Proceed with the cut vertically over the buccal cusps of the bicuspids and over the incisal edges of the anterior teeth until the anterior portion of the trays is separated from the posterior portion (Fig. 41-29). A saw-tooth shaped cut can be made over the central and lateral incisors which will provide better locking of the two parts of the trays. The anterior portion of the tray, at the first molar block, is then drilled with a No. 50 drill to remove the threads. No. 2-56 screws are then placed in the first molar blocks. A screwdriver slot is cut on the outside of each molar block in the saw-cut line between the two screws to allow for a pry-slot in removing the anterior portion of the tray from the teeth. The trays are now complete (Fig. 41-30) and ready for trial on the mounted casts.

Without removing the tin foil and wax from the cast, place the trays on them and raise the center-bearing screw so that no contact exists in centric, lateral, and protrusive positions of the casts, except on

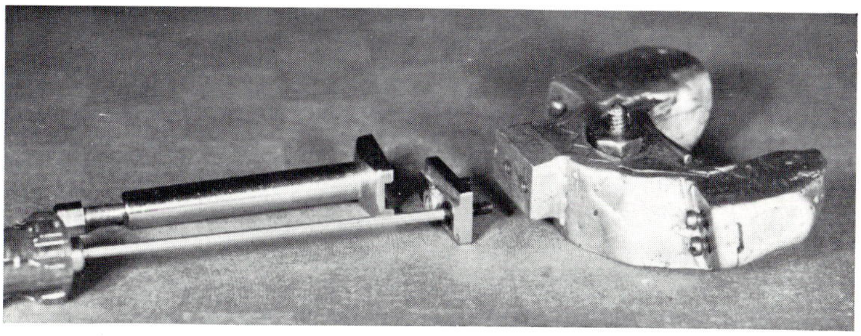

Fig. 41-27. Separable stud ready to be inserted and screwed to stem plate, which is rigidly attached to tray.

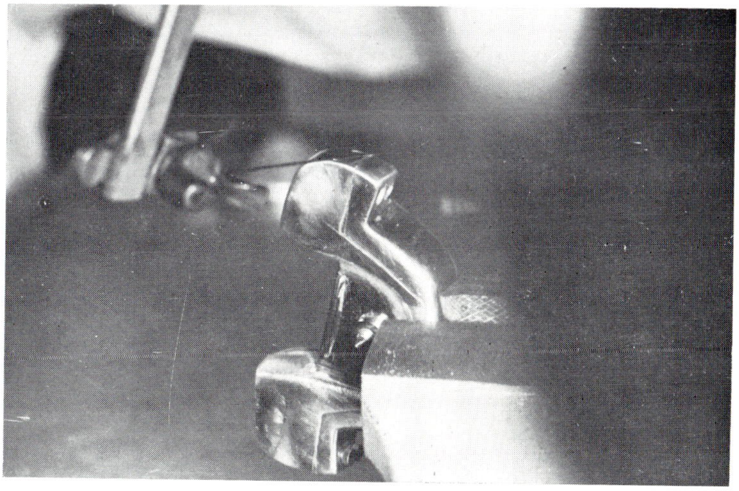

Fig. 41-28. Aluminum tray held rigidly in vise; with jeweler's saw, cut is made through buccal blocks and extended through occlusal surface of tray. This leaves a separable anterior section of tray.

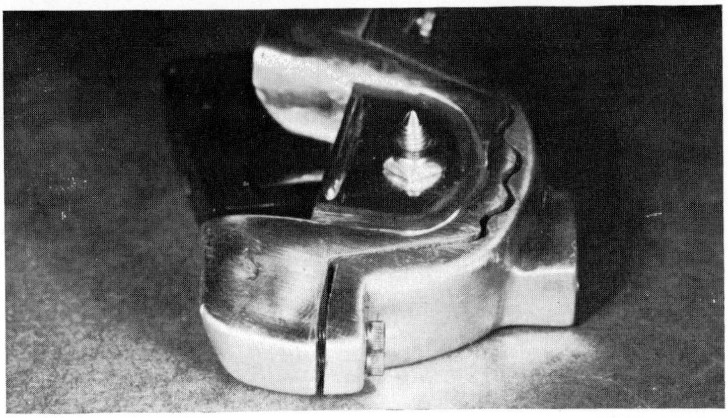

Fig. 41-29. Two portions of tray are reunited with 2-56 screws.

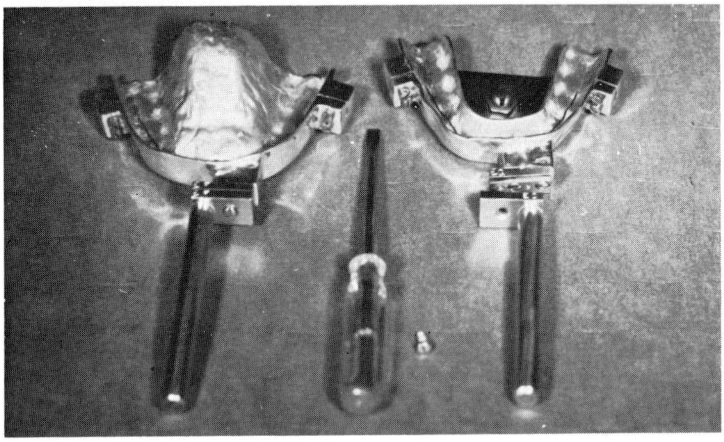

Fig. 41-30. Upper **(left)** and lower **(right)** registration trays; upper has its separable stem attached to tray; lower is detached.

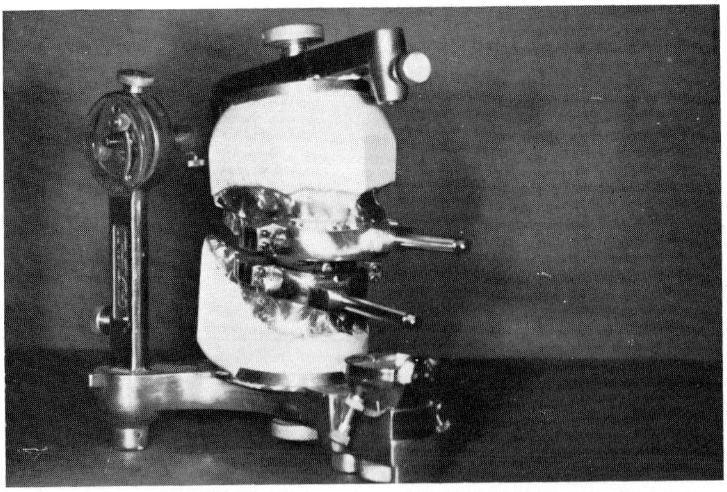

Fig. 41-31. Finished registration trays with separable stems attached and placed on mounted casts to verify parallelism and to adjust center-bearing pin.

the screw. To bring the trays as close as possible together, some grinding may be done on the posterior occlusal surfaces as long as adequate metal is left to firmly support the lingual portion of the trays from the buccal and labial sections (Fig. 41-31).

To save time later at the chair, the face bow arms may be preadjusted on the articulator beforehand. This, however, is optional.

Placing the recording apparatus on the patient

With the patient in the chair, the trays are now tried in the mouth to make certain that the only contact between the jaws is on the center-bearing screw. No part of the trays should touch in any position of the mandible. The two sections of the aluminum trays should be securely screwed together (Fig. 41-31) and attached to the stems with screws. The trays are now removed from the mouth and dried. All the teeth in the lower and upper arches are dried and a mix of zinc oxide–eugenol cement is made to cement the trays to the teeth. Only a sufficient amount of the zinc oxide-eugenol cement should be used to envelop the teeth to their cervical margins. It is not necessary to carry the cement over the vault or onto the soft tissues. If severe undercuts are present, as in the case of fixed bridges, they should be blocked out with soft wax.

The zinc oxide–eugenol cement is placed in the trays; both trays are then placed in the mouth and the patient is asked to close at the same time on the center-bearing pin. The precaution must be taken to prevent the heels of the trays from rising or dropping in the posterior regions; this can be avoided by interposing cotton rolls or by maintaining finger pressure against the upper and lower heels of the trays (Fig. 41-32). However, the center-bearing pin must be in continuous contact with the German-silver plate in the upper tray. Care must be taken to avoid having the excess cement flow over the screw heads uniting the two sections of the trays; nor should the cement be allowed to flow over the anterior stud-plates attached anteriorly.

When the cement has set, the doweled male stems of the separable stud are now united with the stud-plate attached to the trays by tightening the two screws. If the preliminary mounting of the casts on the articulator and the waxing of the separable studs were done correctly, the tray stems should be parallel as they were on the articulator.

Next, the upper bar is attached to the upper tray stem by means of a tray clamp. The bar is centered over the stem *close to*

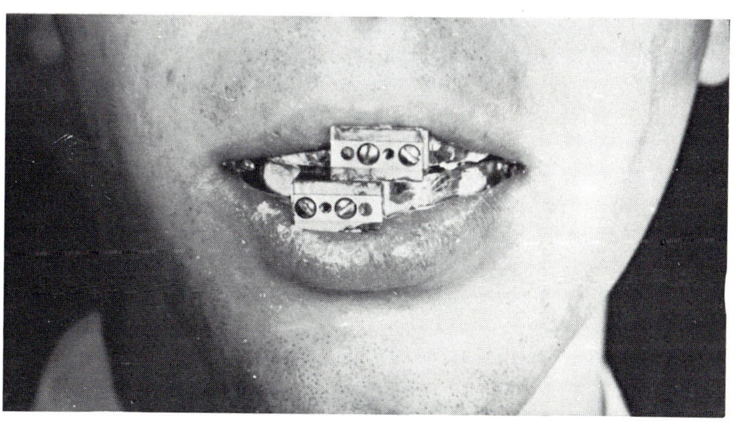

Fig. 41-32. Upper and lower registration trays cemented to upper and lower arches.

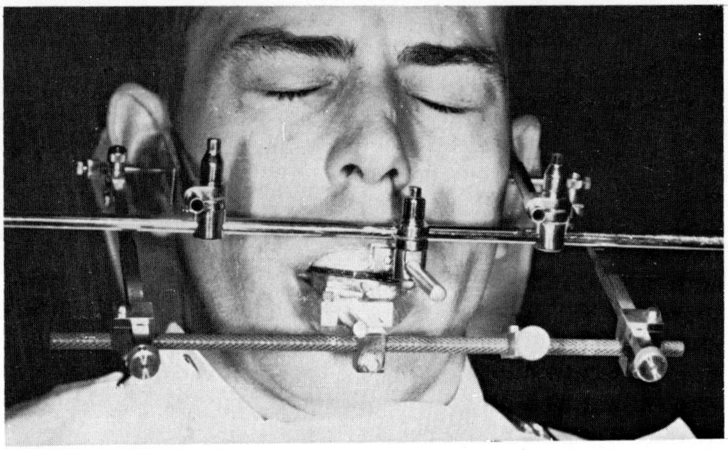

Fig. 41-33. Upper bar with condyle flags attached to upper cemented tray; adjustable face bow attached to lower cemented tray.

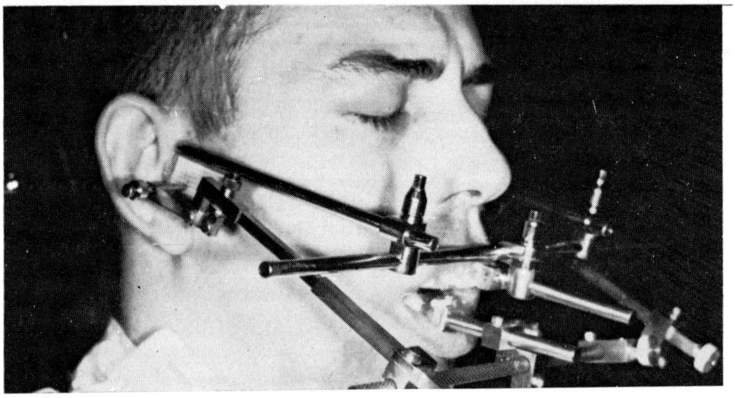

Fig. 41-34. Hinge axis flags attached to upper bar.

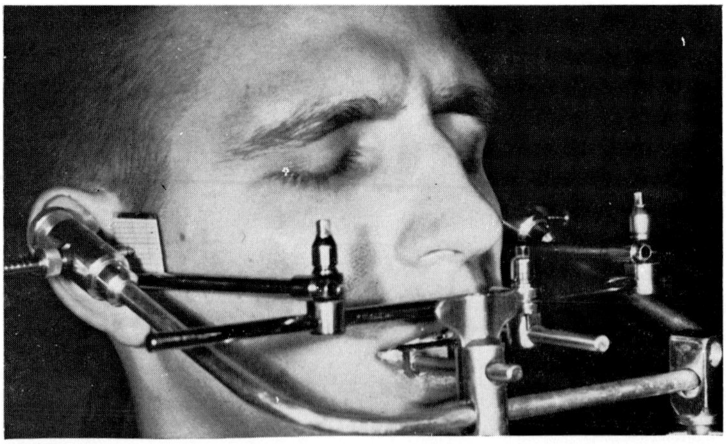

Fig. 41-35. Using more simple, student type of face bow with hinge axis flags attached to upper bar.

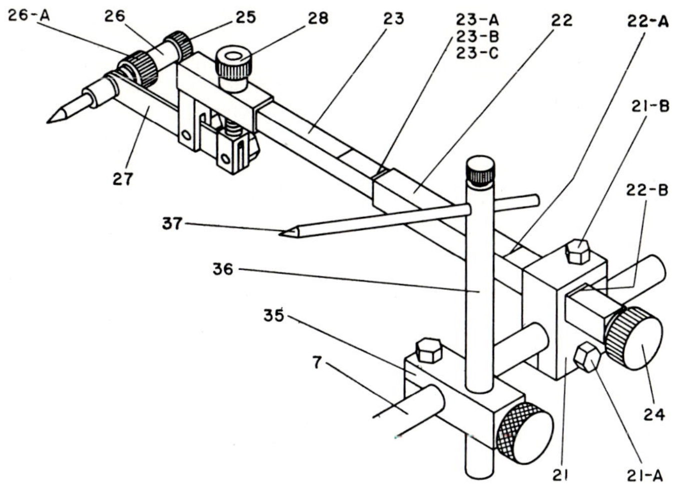

Fig. 41-36. Face bow arms. **7,** Transverse bar of face bow. **21,** Face bow arm clamp with lock screw, **21-A** and **21-B. 22,** Square tubular segment of face bow arm; indicator lines, **22-A** and **22-B. 23,** Square sliding segment of face bow arm; indicator lines, **23-A, 23-B,** and **23-C. 24,** Knob for adjusting **23. 25,** Condylar pointer. **26,** Condylar pointer sleeves with locknut, **26-A. 27,** Condylar pointer adjusting lever. **28,** Condylar pointer adjusting knob. **35,** Orbital pointer clamp. **36,** Orbital pointer holder. **37,** Orbital pointer. (Courtesy Hanau Engineering Co., Inc.)

the lips and is placed parallel to the hinge axis, both horizontally and vertically (Fig. 41-33). The right and left hinge axis flags are attached to the upper front bar, placing the vertical flags in the region of the condylar axes (Fig. 41-34). The flags do not touch the skin but are brought to within $\frac{1}{16}$ inch of the face. The outer surface of the flag is covered with a piece of 1 mm. crosshatched paper. These stationary flags are used as a background for locating the hinge axes of the condyles. Some prefer to apply a piece of adhesive tape to the skin in the condylar area as a background for this purpose. This is not as satisfactory, since the adhesive tape and skin may move with the opening and closing movements of the mandible. Fig. 41-35 shows the same procedure, but using the simpler and less expensive type of Hanau adjustable face bow.

Next, the transverse bar of the hinge axis face bow is slipped over the lower tray stem and securely attached with a tray clamp (Figs. 41-33 and 41-34). This attachment should be near the center of the face bow bar. The bar should be placed parallel with the patient's eyes on the calculated hinge axis, and positioned anteroposteriorly so that later when the face bow arms are attached and adjusted there will be a distance from the transverse bar to the condylar pointers of about 6 inches.

Face bow arms*

The face bow arm assemblies are now preadjusted before they are attached permanently to the transverse bar of the face bow (Fig. 41-36). The manufacturer suggests that the following preliminary settings be made in order to permit a maximum range of adjustments of the movable components in any required direction: (1) the condylar pointers, *25,* are screwed all the way into their sleeves, *26;* (2) the sleeves are then set so that the groove on each sleeve registers at the

*Discussion adapted and quoted in part from *Hanau Axis Face Bow Technic in Conjunction With Hanau Articulator Model H2-XPR,* Hanau Engineering Co., Inc.

pointer adjusting lever, *27*, and locked with locknut, *26-A*. The adjusting levers, *27*, are positioned parallel to the square telescoping arms of the face bow by turning adjusting knob, *28*, in the required direction. Lock screw, *21-B*, of clamp, *21*, is loosened, and either of the two indicator lines, *22-A* and *22-B*, of the square tubular segment, *22*, of the face bow arm is registered with the appropriate edge of the clamp, *21*. By turning adjusting knob, *24*, in the required direction, the square sliding segments, *23*, are positioned so that the second (middle) of the three indicator lines, *23-A*, *23-B*, and *23-C*, register with the edges of the square tubular segments, *22*.

It must be borne in mind that these adjustments are only preliminary settings and that any major adjustment required later to bring the condylar pointers over the general condyle area on the patient's face will be accomplished by loosening lock screw, *21-B*, and moving square tubular segment, *22*, in or out. For the purpose of these preliminary settings, the condyle head is digitally located and identified by a temporary mark on the skin as was previously done.

The preadjusted face bow arms are now placed on the transverse bar, *7*, of the face bow one at a time. The condylar pointers are suitably oriented to the previously determined condyle area of the patient, and the lock screws, *21-A* and *21-B* of clamp, *21*, are finally and securely tightened. The condylar pointers should be very close to, but not touching, the patient's skin or flags. In-and-out movement of the condylar pointers is accomplished only with sleeves, *26*, and not the threaded condylar pointers, *25*, which are left undisturbed at this stage and provide a positive position index. To facilitate the nonbinding movement of the sleeve, the condylar sleeve should be rotated while it is simultaneously sliding in and out.

Locating the hinge axis using the Hanau hinge axis face bow. The Hanau hinge axis face bow consists of the following parts: transverse bar; a right and a left, calibrated, face bow arm; two face bow arm clamps with lock screws; one orbital pointer clamp; one tray clamp with lock screws; one orbital pointer; one orbital pointer holder (Fig. 41-37).

In order to locate the hinge axis it is necessary first to assemble the hinge axis face bow.

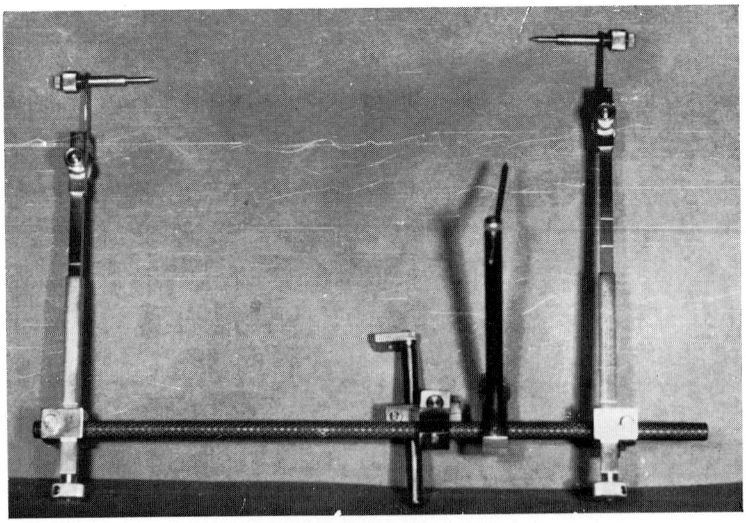

Fig. 41-37. Hanau hinge axis face bow.

The manufacturer of the Hanau axis face bow recommends the following sequence of procedure in the assemblage: (1) With tray stem clamp, *6* (Fig. 41-45), loosened at *6-A*, *6-B*, and *6-C*, insert the tray stem into its clamp and tentatively tighten the three lock screws, keeping the transverse bar, *7*, *as close to the lips as permissible.* Next, any necessary adjustments are now made so that the transverse bar is parallel with the patient's eyes, and its ends extend equally on either side of the face. Securely, but not excessively, tighten clamp lock screws *6-A*, *6-B*, and *6-C*, to ensure against the slightest mechanical movement at any point in the assembly. The tightening of the screws should not be excessive.

The right and left face bow arm assemblies (Fig. 41-36) are now preadjusted before they are attached to the transverse bar of the face bow. The following preliminary settings are suggested by the manufacturer to permit maximum range of adjustment of the movable components in any required direction: (1) the condylar pointers, *25*, are screwed all the way into their sleeves, *26;* (2) the sleeves are then set so that the groove on each sleeve registers at the pointer adjusting lever, *27*, and locked with locknuts, *26-A*.

The adjusting levers, *27*, are positioned parallel to the square telescoping arms of the face bow by turning adjusting knobs, *28*, in the required direction. Lock screw, *21-B*, of clamp, *21*, is loosened, and either of the two indicator lines, *22-A* and *22-B*, of the square tubular segment, *22*, of the face bow arm is registered with the appropriate edge of clamp, *21*.

By turning adjusting knob, *24*, in the required direction, the square sliding segments are positioned so that the second (middle) of the three indicator lines, *23-A*, *23-B*, and *23-C*, registers with the edges of the square tubular segments, *22*.

It must be borne in mind that *these are only preliminary settings,* and that any major adjustment required later to bring the condylar pointers over the general condyle areas on the patient's face will be accomplished by loosening screw, *21-B*, and moving square tubular segment, *22*, in or out. For these preliminary settings, the condyle head can be digitally located and identified by a temporary mark placed on the skin.

The preadjusted face bow arms are now placed on the transverse bar, *7*, of the face bow one at a time. The condylar pointers are suitably oriented to the previously arbitrarily determined condyle areas of the patient, and the lock screws, *21-A* and *21-B*, of clamp, *21*, are finally and securely tightened. The condylar pointers should be very close to, but not touching, the crosshatched paper on the vertical flags attached to the upper transverse bar locked to the cemented upper tray (Fig. 41-38). In-and-out movement of the condylar pointers is accomplished only with sleeves, *26*—not the threaded condylar pointers, *25*, which undisturbed at this stage, provide a positive index. To facilitate nonbinding movement of the sleeve, the condylar sleeve may be rotated while simultaneously sliding in and out.

The patient is instructed to open and close within a limited range. The condylar pointers, *25*, will be observed to move in arcs when not in line with the exact hinge axis. NOTE: *Every precaution must be taken to prevent incorporation of a protrusive component in the opening and closing movements of the mandible.* To simplify the procedure, *observe the direction of movement of the condylar pointers only on the closing stroke of the mandible* (Fig. 41-39).

By observing the type and position of movement of the condylar pointers, the necessary adjustment of the pointers may be made in the correct direction. Anterior-posterior adjustment of the condylar pointers is made by turning adjusting knobs, *24;* adjustment of the pointers above and

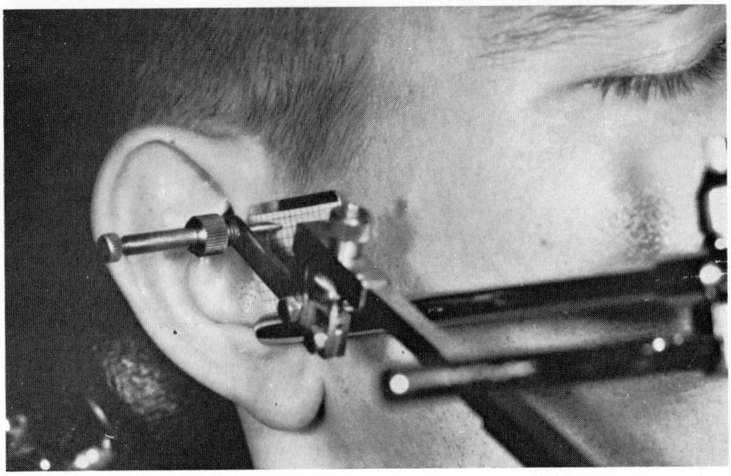

Fig. 41-38. Locating condylar pins of face bow close to vertical flags attached to upper cross bar.

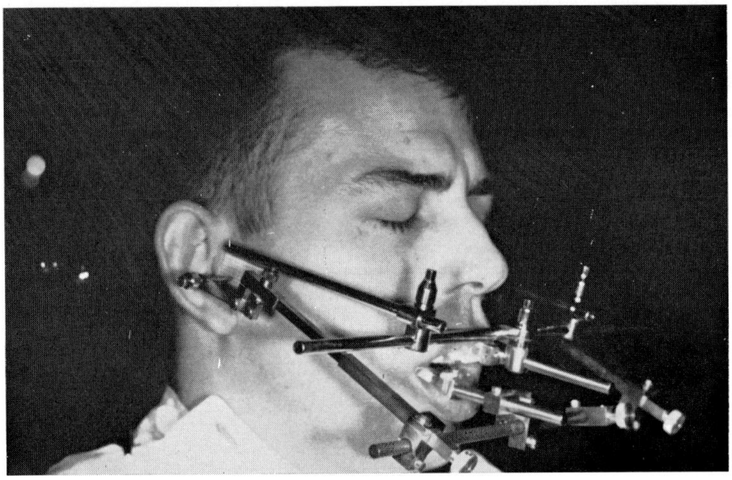

Fig. 41-39. Condylar pin of face bow shows whether or not it moves in arc or on hinge axis point.

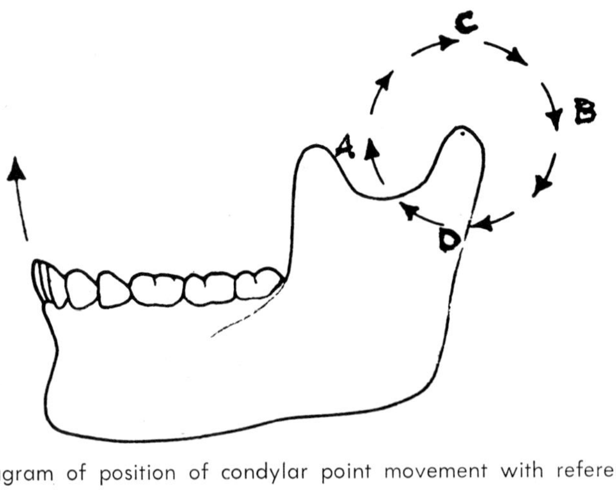

Fig. 41-40. Diagram of position of condylar point movement with reference to position of hinge axis.

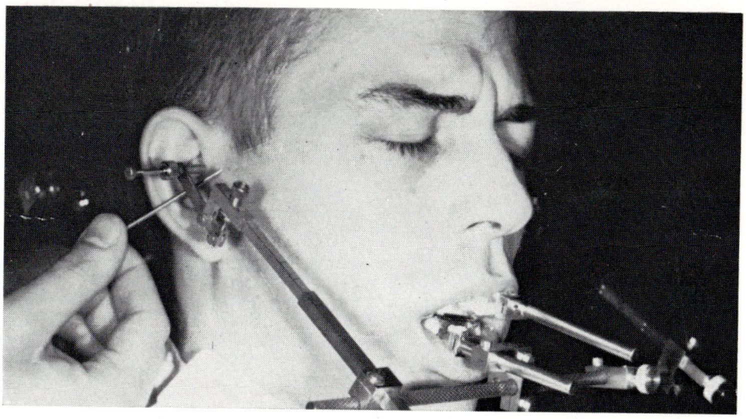

Fig. 41-41. With vertical flags removed, condylar pointer, wetted with indelible pencil, is touched against skin to indicate position of hinge axis; this is done on both sides.

below the hinge axis is made by turning adjusting knobs, *28*.

When, on closing, the pointer moves in the same direction as the closing jaw, then the face bow pointer is anterior to the hinge axis; therefore, it must be moved backward (Fig. 41-40).

When, on closing, the pointer moves in the opposite direction of the closing jaw, the face bow pointer is posterior to the hinge axis and must be moved anteriorly.

When, on closing, the pointer moves toward the back of the head, the face bow pointer is above the hinge axis and therefore it must be moved downward.

When, on closing, the pointer moves forward toward the chin, the face bow pointer is below the hinge axis and therefore it must be raised.

It will be noted that, the farther away the pointers are from the true hinge axis, the longer will be the stroke of the pointer. The closer the hinge axis, the shorter will be the stroke. When both pointers are opposite the hinge axis, they will be seen not to move in relation to the cross-hatched markings on the flags but will be observed to hinge or rotate on a point.

During the registrations and the adjustment of the condylar pointer, it is not necessary to have the patient open more than half an inch. Some recommend a gentle pressure on the chin directed backward during the opening and closing of the mandible. Instead of applying the pressure, it is recommended that, during the closing, the patient elevate and retract his tongue, bringing the tip up and back during the closing movement. The mandible is thus brought into a *physiologically retruded, functional terminal position,* and it is in this position that we wish to locate the hinge axis of the mandible. If abnormal pressure is used, there is danger of forcing the mandible into a strained, retruded, posterior position beyond its true centric relation. It is also advisable to have the patient's head tilted back during this procedure.

After the hinge axis has been located on each side of the face and marked with indelible pencil, the two flags and the clamps attaching them to the upper front bar are loosened and removed (Fig. 41-41). The patient is instructed to sit erectly in the chair without the use of the headrest.

Locknut, *26-A* (Fig. 41-36), is now loosened, the condylar pointer-sleeve, *26,* is slightly withdrawn and the tip of the condylar pointer is touched with wet indelible pencil. The condylar pointer and sleeve are gently pushed medially until

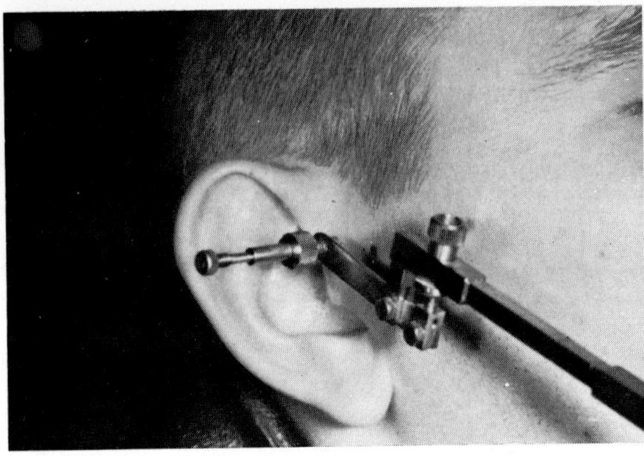

Fig. 41-42

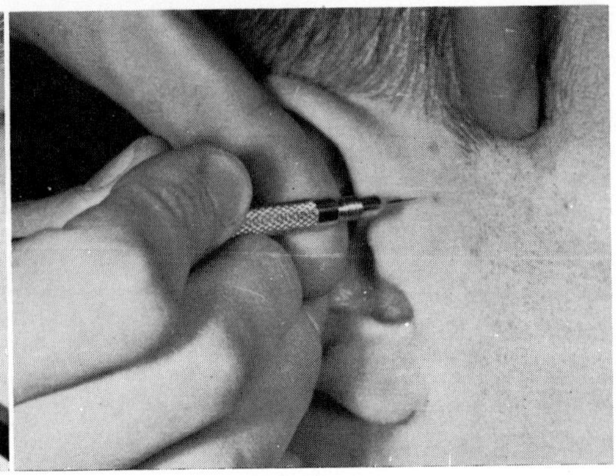

Fig. 41-43

Fig. 41-42. Position of hinge axis marked on skin.
Fig. 41-43. Permanent hinge axis reference point tattooed on skin.

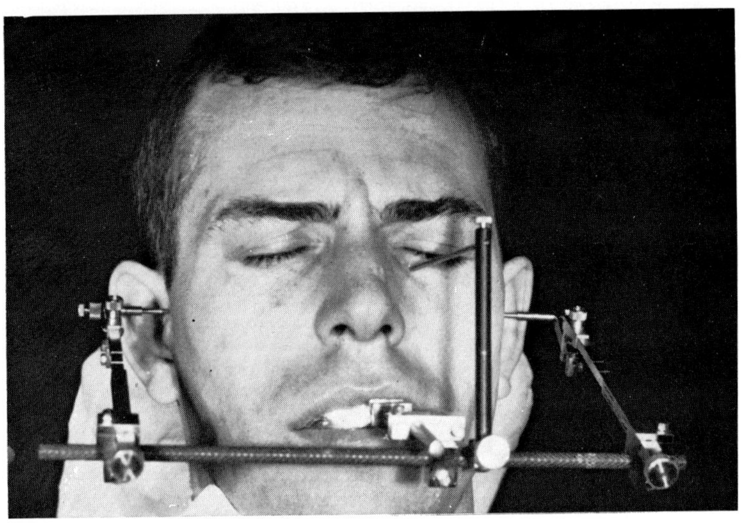

Fig. 41-44. Infraorbital reference point located and marked on skin.

the indelible ink touches the skin; this marks the axis opening on one side of the face (Fig. 41-42). The same procedure is repeated on the opposite side. If permanent marks are desired, they are obtained by tattooing on the skin (Fig. 41-43). A third reference point is established by placing a mark on the right side of the nose in line with the infraorbital border; this also may be tattooed (Fig. 41-44). This establishes the hinge axis-orbital plane.

The first objective of the adjustable hinge axis face bow having been attained, namely, the location and marking of the hinge axes, it may now be removed from the *lower tray stem.* A convenient and safe method for the removal of the calibrated arms of the face bow is to loosen the locknuts, *21-A* (Fig. 41-36). Locknut, *6-A,* is then loosened in clamp, *6* (Fig. 41-45), and the remainder of the face bow may be slipped off the lower tray stem. Tray stem, *5,* with plate is removed from

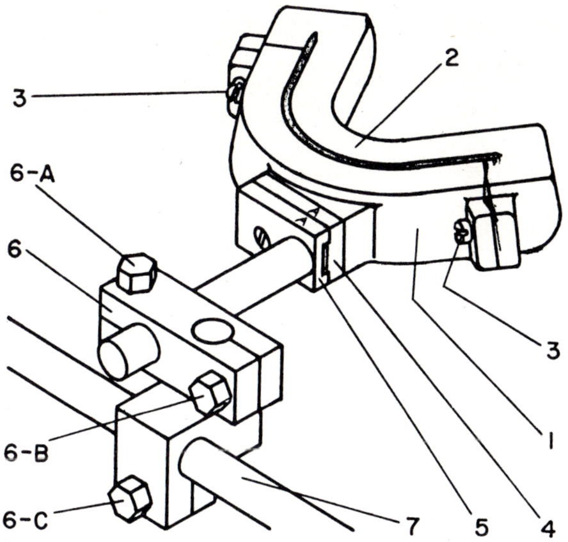

Fig. 41-45. Registration tray, stem, and clamp assembly. **1,** Labial tray section. **2,** Lingual tray section. **3,** Screws assemble tray sections, **1** and **2** (screws No. 2-56 × 3/8 inch fillister head, brass). **4,** Tray plate attached with two screws (No. 2-56 × 3/16 inch fillister head, brass). **5,** Tray stem assembled to **4** with screw (No. 2-56 × 3/16 inch fillister head, brass). **6,** Tray clamp with lock screws, **6-A, 6-B,** and **6-C. 7,** Transverse bar of face bow. (Courtesy Hanau Engineering Co., Inc.)

the tray (Fig. 41-45). All extraoral recording apparatus has now been removed from the patient, leaving only the two aluminum trays still cemented to their respective upper and lower arches.

The patient is now asked to sit erect in the chair without using the headrest. All subsequent registrations are made with the patient in an upright position without the use of the headrest.

The patient is now conditioned to raise the mandible from an open position to a centric closure. No surfaces of the trays should touch; contact is made only between the center-bearing pin in the lower tray and the nickel-silver plate in the upper. From centric position the patient is then directed to go into protrusive position, then the right and the left lateral positions of the mandible. The paths which the center-bearing pin follows from centric to protrusive, to right, and to left lateral positions are marked on the upper nickel-silver plate (Fig. 41-46). Extreme care must be taken that first the true centric relation position has been established and then marked on the plate.

Points are now marked 1/4 inch away from the centric position on the three lines radiating from centric position (Fig. 41-47). With a No. 6 round bur, a slight depression is made in the nickel-silver plate at the four points: centric, protrusive, right, and left lateral. The depressions are very slight, approximately 0.2 to 0.3 mm. in depth, just sufficient to permit the center-bearing pin to locate and maintain the four respective positions of the mandible.

Again, it must be emphasized that the only contacts made between the upper and lower trays are those made between the center-bearing pin and the nickel-silver plate.

The next step is to record the centric, protrusive, right, and left lateral positions of the mandible by means of stone checkbites. The opposing surfaces of the upper and lower trays, also their buccal surfaces, are lubricated with petrolatum (Fig. 41-

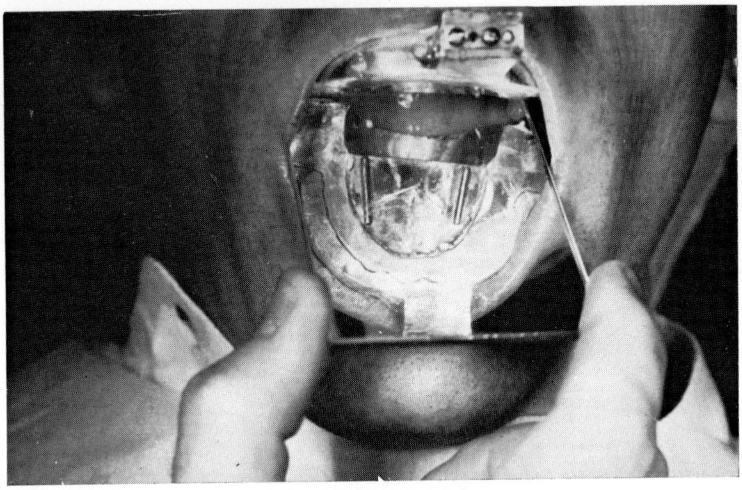

Fig. 41-46. Palatal view of upper tray showing protrusive, right and left lateral, and centric positions of center-bearing pin.

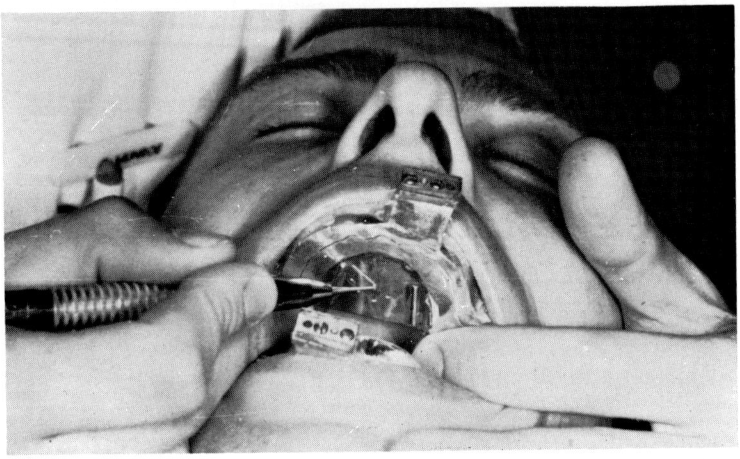

Fig. 41-47. Four positions marked with No. 6 round bur in German-silver plate.

48). A small piece of soft wax is placed over the tapped screw opening of the anterior tray stem plates (Fig. 41-45, *4-A*).

With the patient sitting in an upright position, the mandible is brought into centric relation, with the point of the center-bearing pin resting in the slight depression previously made in the plate. The patient is instructed to maintain this position while rapid-setting stone is injected between the two trays and allowed to set (Fig. 41-49). When hard, the stone checkbite is marked *C* and set aside (Fig. 41-50).

The mandible is now placed in the protrusive position so that the center-bearing point rests in the protrusive depression in the plate. Rapid stone is again injected between the two trays and when set it is removed, marked *P*, and set aside (Fig. 41-51).

After each registration the patient returns to centric position, since all the eccentric movements start from and return to centric relation.

The mandible is next carried in a left lateral direction until the center-bearing pin rests in the left lateral depression in

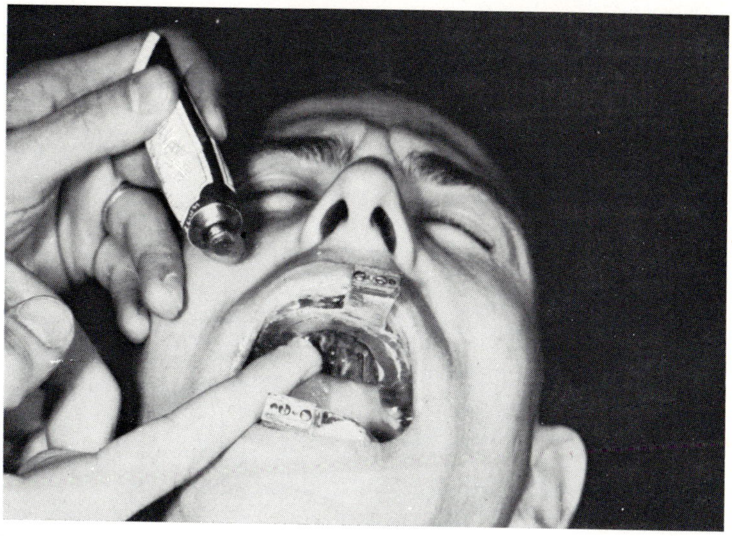

Fig. 41-48. Lubricating registration trays prior to taking stone checkbites.

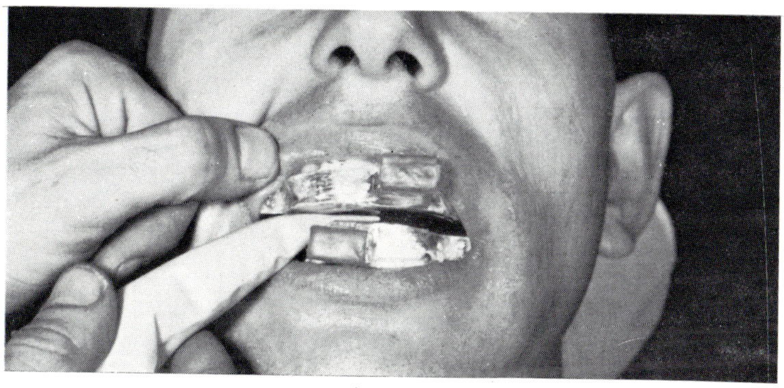

Fig. 41-49. Injecting rapid-setting stone between upper and lower registration trays in centric relation position.

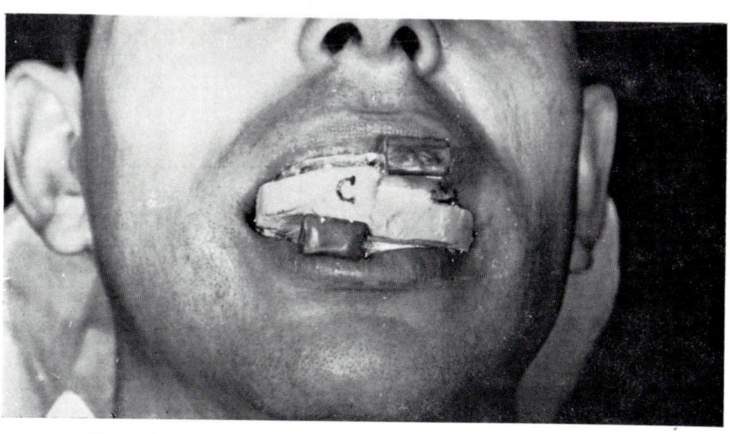

Fig. 41-50. Stone checkbite registering centric relation.

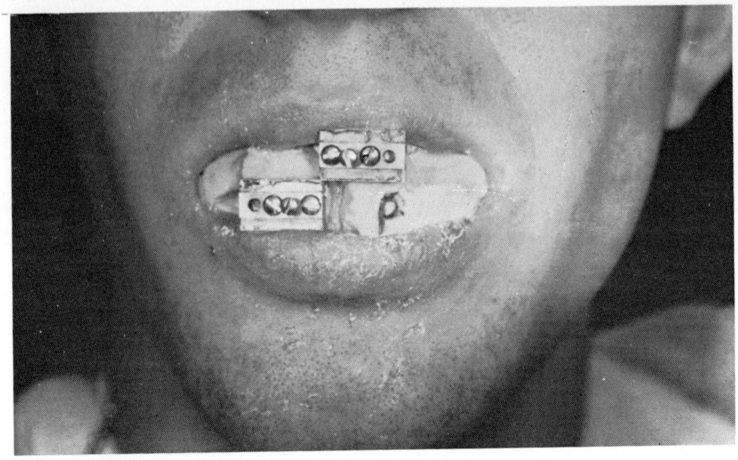

Fig. 41-51. Stone checkbite registering protrusive relation of maxilla to mandible.

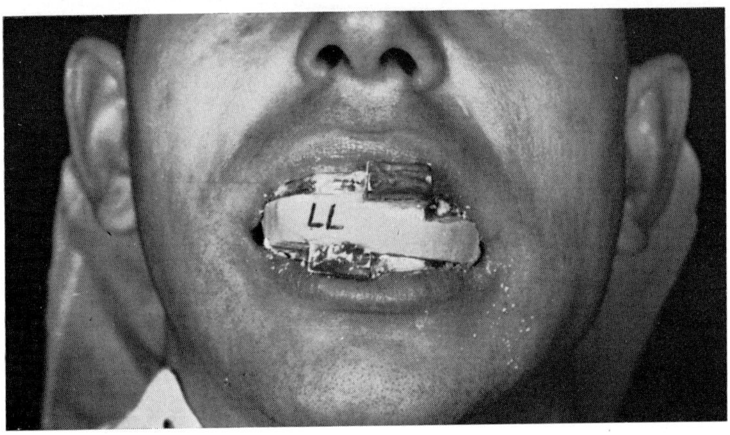

Fig. 41-52. Stone checkbite registering left lateral relation.

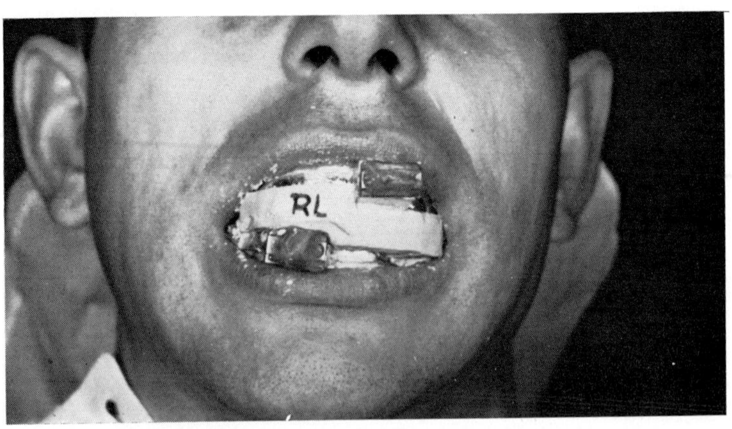

Fig. 41-53. Stone checkbite registering right lateral relation.

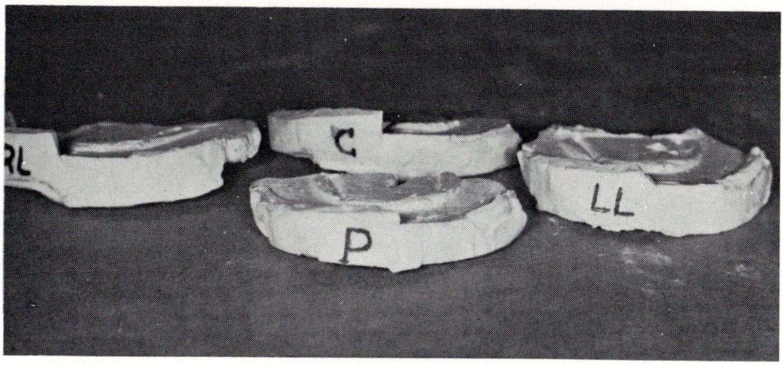

Fig. 41-54. Stone checkbites indicating four relations of mandible to maxilla.

the plate. Again quick-setting stone is injected between the two trays, allowed to set, and removed. *LL* is placed on the stone checkbite (Fig. 41-52).

Again the procedure is repeated by having the mandible move from centric into the right lateral position at which point rapid-setting stone is injected; when set the stone checkbite is removed and marked *RL* (Fig. 41-53). We now have four stone checkbites (Fig. 41-47).

Tray stem, *5* (Fig. 41-45), is now reattached to the upper tray, which is still in the mouth. The transverse bar is reattached at its midpoint to the stem by means of the tray clamp, *6* (Fig. 41-45). The orbital pointer clamp, *35* (Fig. 41-36), is placed on the transverse bar just to the right of the tray clamp, *6* (Fig. 41-45), and fastened securely. The orbital pointer holder, *36*, with the orbital pointer, *37*, is prepared and laid aside for later insertion in the orbital pointer clamp, *35* (Fig. 41-36).

The two calibrated side arms, *22*, which were previously used to locate the hinge axis, are replaced on the transverse bar. They may be preadjusted as previously described, placing the condylar pointers as near to the hinge axis markings on the side of the face, previously placed. Minute adjustments are made as required, to position the condylar pointers opposite the condyle axes markings on the skin. The points of the condylar pointers must be exactly opposite to the tattoo marks and in contact with the skin. The condylar pointers and the side arms are then locked securely to the transverse bar. The orbital pointer with the holder, *37, 36* (Fig. 41-36), is inserted into its clamp, *35*, and is adjusted to contact the infraorbital point previously marked. A final check is made that all clamps and locknuts are securely tightened and that the condylar and orbital pointers coincide with the markings previously made (Fig. 41-55).

To prevent interference with the incisal pin of the articulator during subsequent transfer of the face bow, be sure that the face bow arms are adjusted so that the distance from the transverse bar to the condylar pointer is about 6 inches. Set clamp, *21*, approximately at the end of the square segment of the arm, *22*, or at the first indicator line; set the sliding segment, *23*, of arms to middle indicator lines, *23-B* (Fig. 41-36).

To remove the assembled face bow from the tray the following steps are observed: (1) the threaded, condylar pointers, *25* (Fig. 41-36), are unscrewed from their sleeves and removed to eliminate the possibility of scratching the patient's face; (2) remove the screw which attaches the tray stem plate, *5*, to the tray plate, *4* (Fig. 41-45). By inserting a small flat instrument between the tray stem plates, *the face bow with its attached tray stem* is now disengaged from the

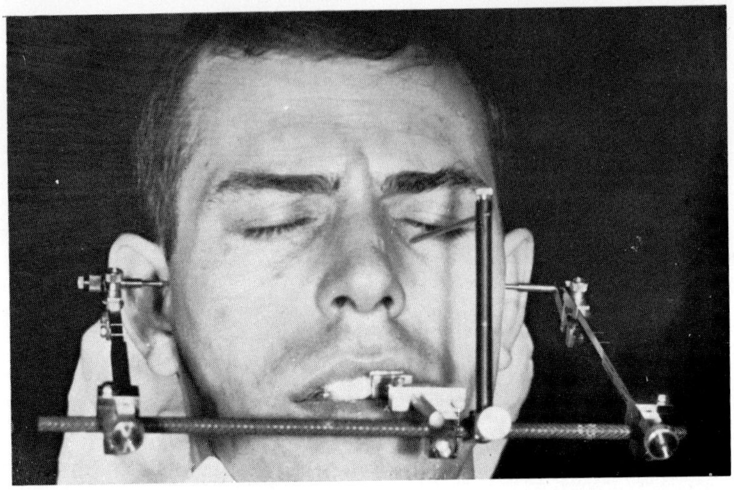

Fig. 41-55. Face bow repositioned and attached to cemented upper tray using hinge axis and infraorbital markings as orientation points.

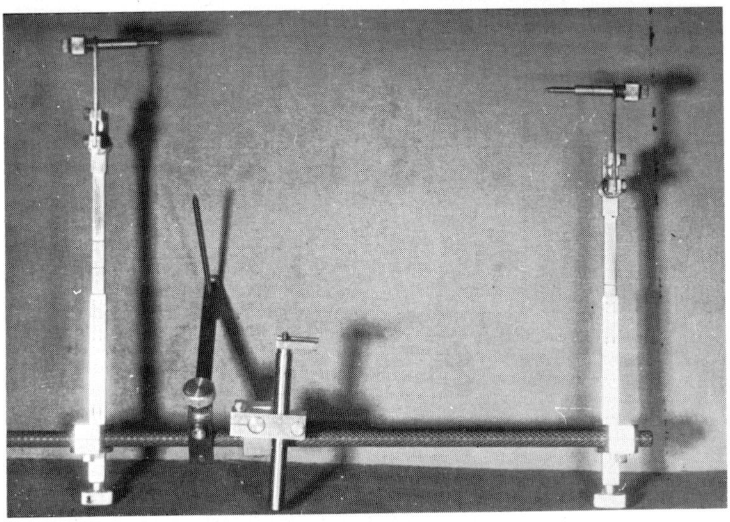

Fig. 41-56. Face bow, with detachable upper tray stem attached, is separated from upper tray, which is left in mouth temporarily. Condylar and infraorbital pins are securely locked in face bow.

tray and removed from the patient (Fig. 41-56). This is laid aside for subsequent reattachment to the tray.

Buccal tray screws, *3* (Fig. 41-45), are now loosened (Fig. 41-57), and the labial and palatal portions of the tray are removed separately from the mouth (Fig. 41-58). The sections are reassembled with the screws (Fig. 41-45, *3*, and Fig. 41-59).

The upper and lower reassembled trays are now filled with stone to a height ¼ inch above their peripheries, and the stone is allowed to set (Fig. 41-60).

When the stone has hardened in the upper tray, it is reattached with screws to the tray stem plate, *5* (Fig. 41-45), which was left locked in the face bow when it was removed from the patient (Fig. 41-61). The upper stone-filled tray again bears the same relationship to the hinge axis and orbital markings that the tray did in the mouth (Fig. 41-62).

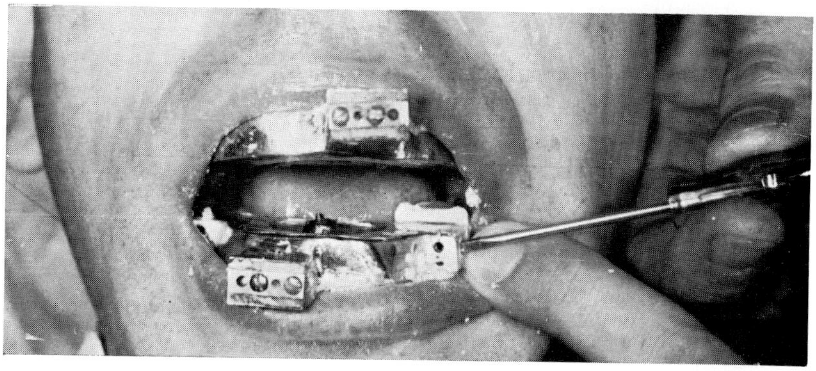

Fig. 41-57. Detaching anterior segment of lower registration tray.

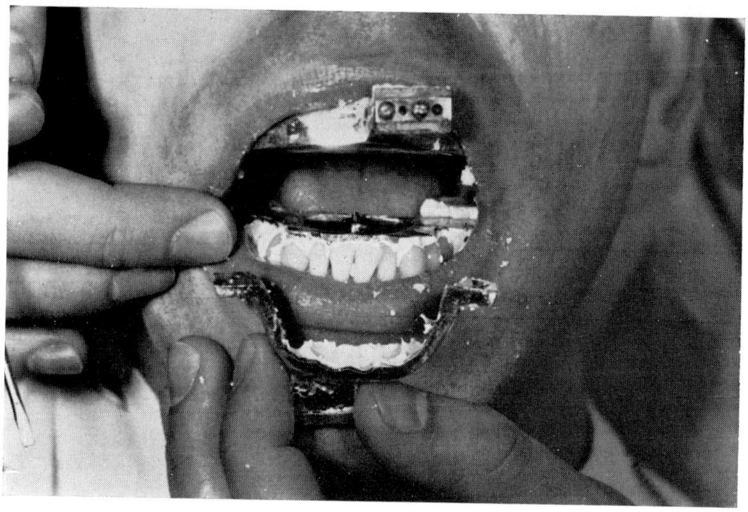

Fig. 41-58. Anterior segment of lower registration tray removed.

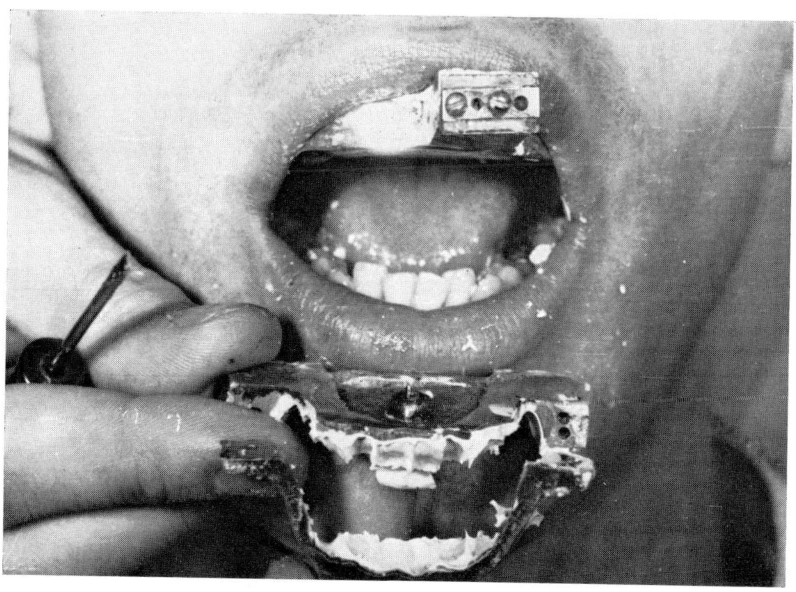

Fig. 41-59. Anterior and buccal segments are removed from mandibular arch.

A

B

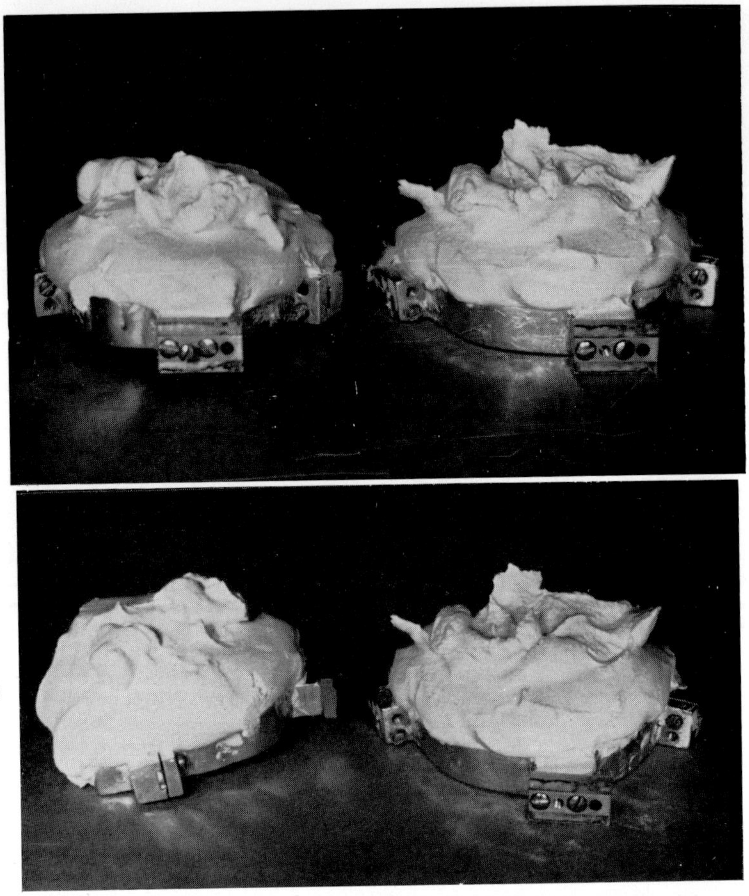

Fig. 41-60. Upper and lower reassembled registration trays filled with stone.

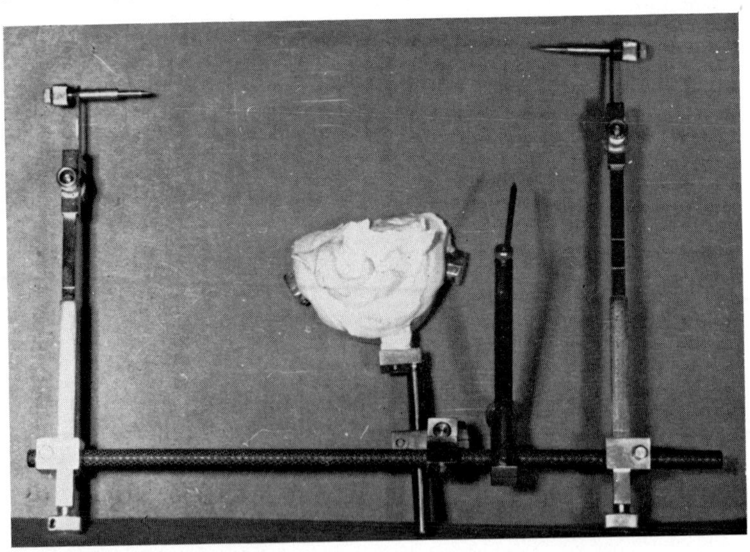

Fig. 41-61. Upper tray filled with stone is reattached to tray stem plate, which was left locked in face bow when removed from patient (Fig. 41-55).

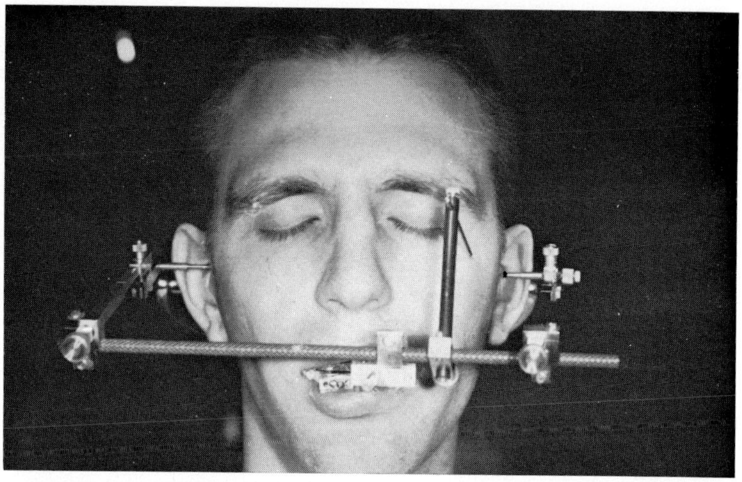

Fig. 41-62. Face bow as originally attached to upper tray in patient's mouth (Fig. 41-55).

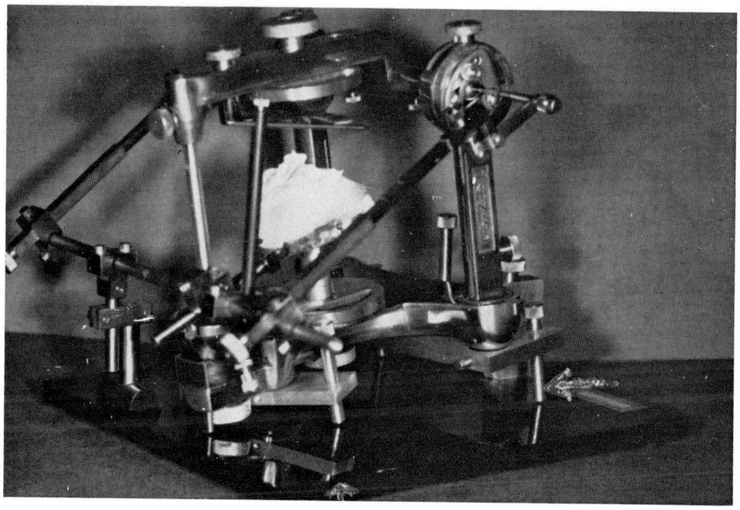

Fig. 41-63. Articulator positioned on transfer board and face bow with poured, attached tray locked to face bow support of transfer board.

Setting the Hanau H2-XPR adjustable articulator to the face bow and stone checkbite registrations

The front and rear articulator supports, *43, 42* (Fig. 41-4), are securely attached to the legs of the articulator with lock screws, *43-B, 2-C,* and *42-D.* With elevating screws, *43-A, 42-A,* and *42-B,* raise the articulator so that its three legs are about ½ inch above the surface of the transfer board (Fig. 41-63). The upper member of the articulator is latched in centric, and *the instrument is tentatively positioned on the transfer board.* Locking clamp, *41,* is temporarily removed from the transfer board by disengaging lock screw, *41-A* (Fig. 41-4).

The face bow assembly is locked to the face bow support, *44* (Fig. 41-4), of the transfer board (Fig. 41-64), following which the *articulator is oriented to the face bow registration using the orbital, 37, and condyle pointers, 25, as guides* (Fig. 41-65). When model H2-XPR articu-

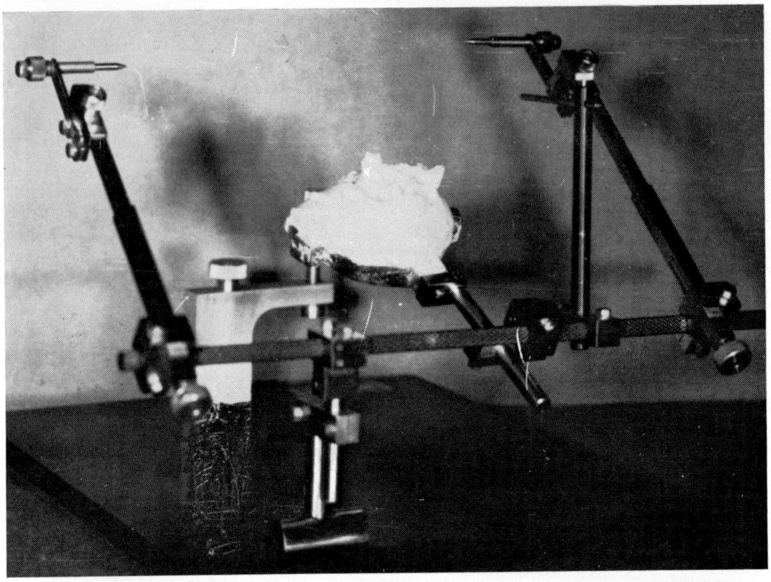

Fig. 41-64. Face bow locked to transfer board support.

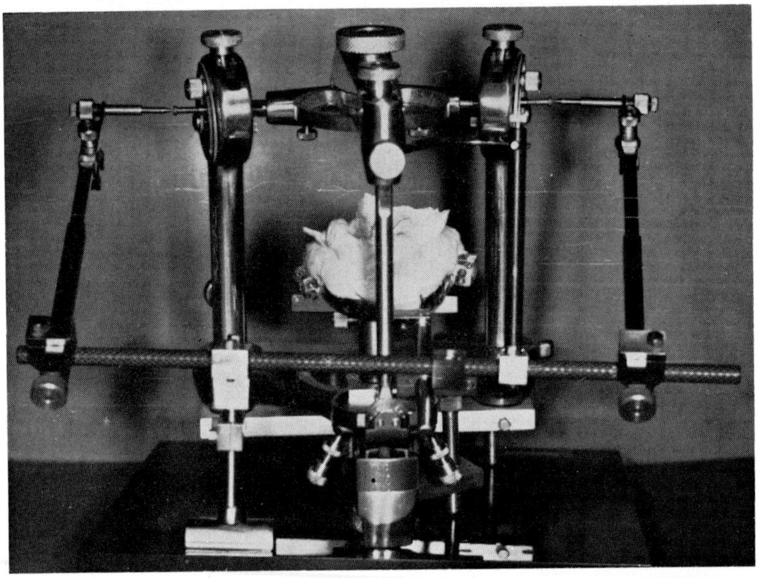

Fig. 41-65. Orienting articulator to condylar hinge axis and infraorbital pins.

lator is used, the centric stop in the "condylar assembly" must be set at zero (Fig. 41-66).

The locked condylar pointers of the face bow are placed opposite and slightly above the centers of the extendible condylar shafts of the articulator (Fig. 41-67). These extendible shafts must be brought out equally to meet the face bow condylar pointers (Fig. 41-68). Position the orbital pointer by raising or lowering the face bow on the upright support of the mounting board, until the orbital pointer is level with the orbital plane indicator which is attached to the upper bow of the articulator (Fig. 41-68, *B*).

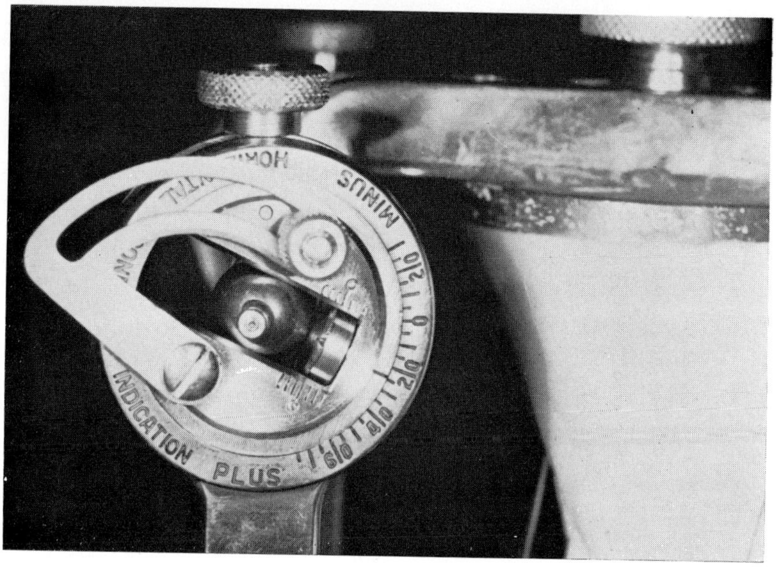

Fig. 41-66. Condylar assembly of new H2-XPR Hanau articulator.

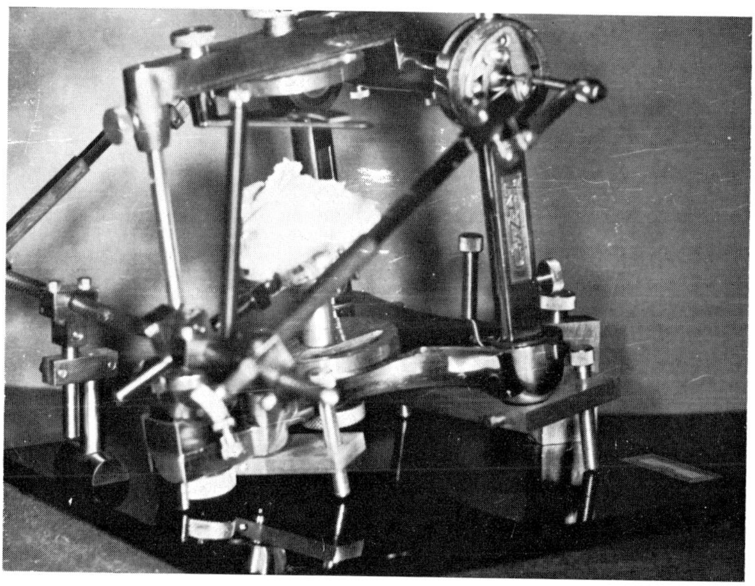

Fig. 41-67. Lateral view showing adjustment of extendible condylar rods of articulator to meet exactly the points of the condylar pins of face bow.

The articulator is now moved around on the transfer board, raised and lowered by means of the elevating screws in the articulator support, *42, 43* (Fig. 41-4), until an exact vertical alignment is obtained of each condylar pointer point with the center of each extendible condylar shaft of the articulator (Fig. 41-69). The orbital pointer is also adjusted to the height of the infraorbital swivel plane of the articulator.

When perfect vertical and horizontal alignment between the extendible shafts and condyle pointers has been attained, the articulator is locked in the transfer board as follows: Locking clamp, *41* (Fig.

A

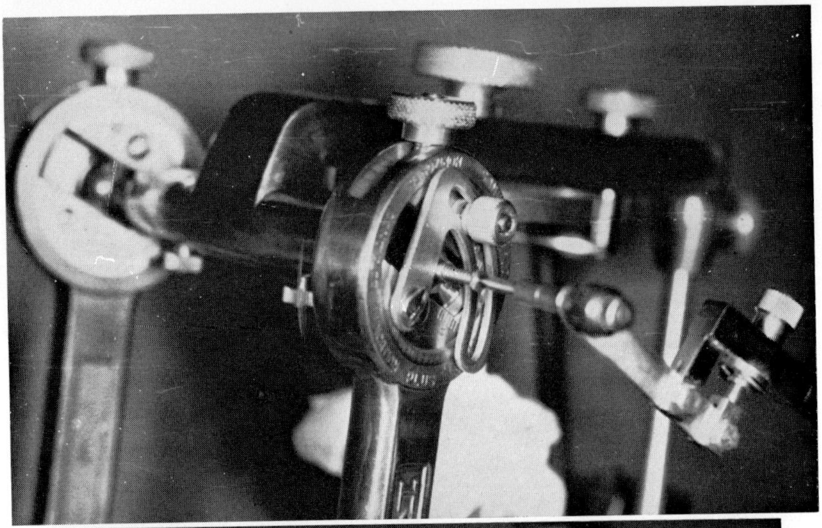

B

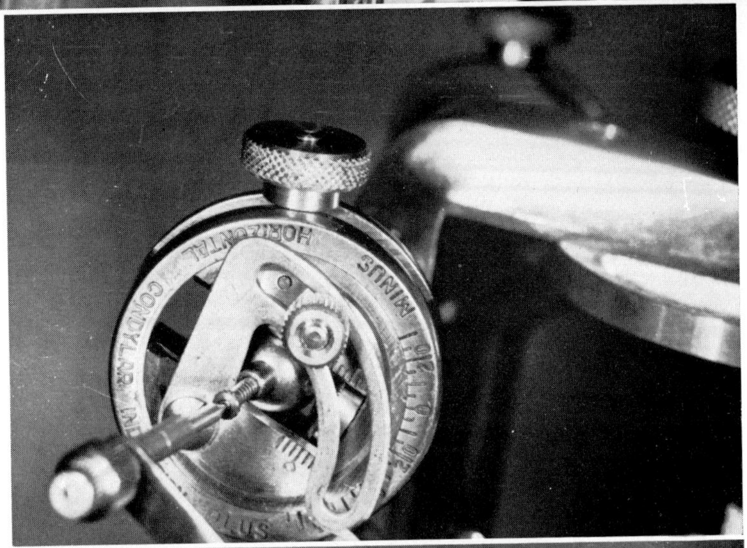

C

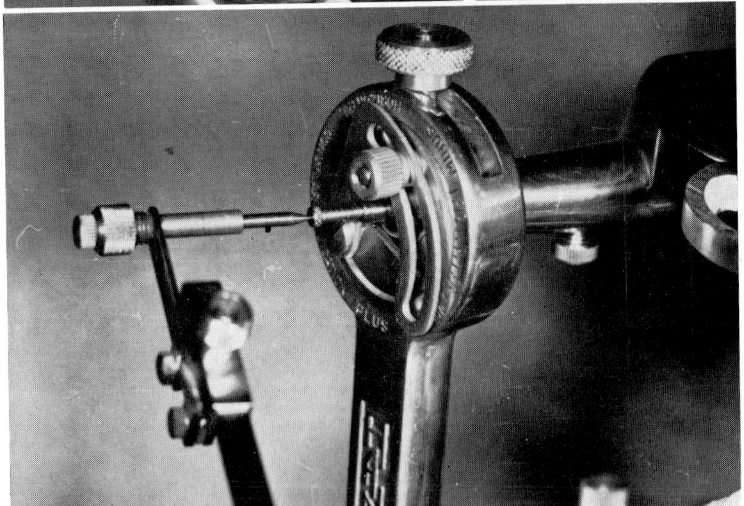

Fig. 41-68. A to **C,** Close-up views of precise placement of condylar rod points in centers of extendible condylar rods of articulator.

41-4), is carefully replaced on the transfer board with lock screw, *41-A*, engaging any of the three holes in the board that will permit lock screw, *41-B*, to contact the rear support, *42*. Lock screw, *41-B*, is raised sufficiently to allow lock screw, *41-A*, to draw clamp, *41*, down to the surface of the board. Lock screw, *41-B*, is then tightened against the rear support, *42*, and the articulator is thus locked in place. Make certain that any minute change in the alignment of the pointers has not resulted from accidental movement of the articulator during this phase of the procedure.

The upper stone-filled tray is supported beneath by two wood wedges or by a cast support (Figs. 41-70 and 41-71), so as not to disturb the tray from its locked position in the face bow. The stone-filled tray is attached with stone to the upper mounting plate of the articulator, after which the incisal pin is set and tightened securely (Fig. 41-72).

When the stone has set, the screws attaching the tray stem plate and face bow to the upper tray are now removed, and the face bow with tray stem is disengaged from the articulator and removed from the face bow support, *44* (Fig. 41-4). This leaves the stone-filled upper tray attached to the upper mounting plate of the articulator. The articulator may now be removed from the transfer board.

The reassembled lower tray filled with stone is now oriented to the upper tray in centric relation. This is done by interposing the *centric*, stone checkbite between the two trays, keeping the surfaces of both trays in perfect contact with both surfaces of the stone checkbite. This relation is maintained by luting the stone checkbite and the trays with wax or by any other dependable means (Fig. 41-72, *A*). The lower, stone-filled tray is then attached with stone to the lower mounting plate of the articulator (Fig. 41-72, *B*).

The two mounted trays are separated from the *C* stone checkbite, and the *protrusive* stone checkbite is interposed between the trays, again bringing their sur-

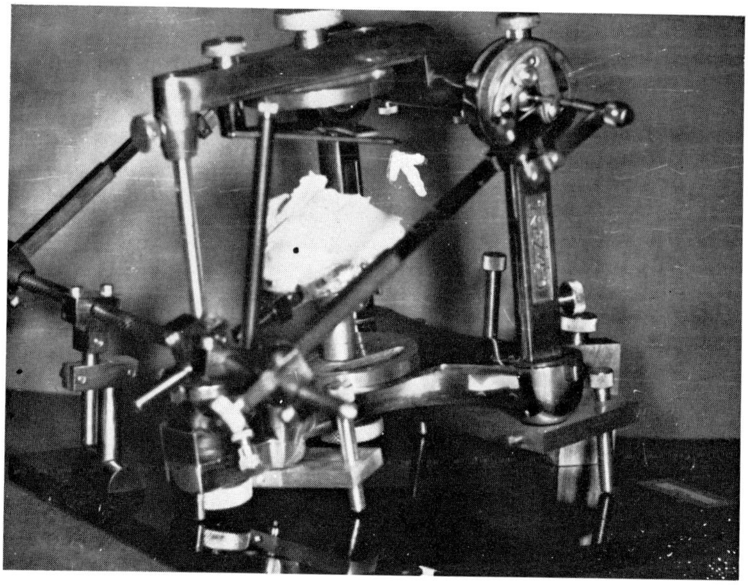

Fig. 41-69. Vertical plane of face bow is determined by position of infraorbital pointer related to swivel plane of articulator (arrow).

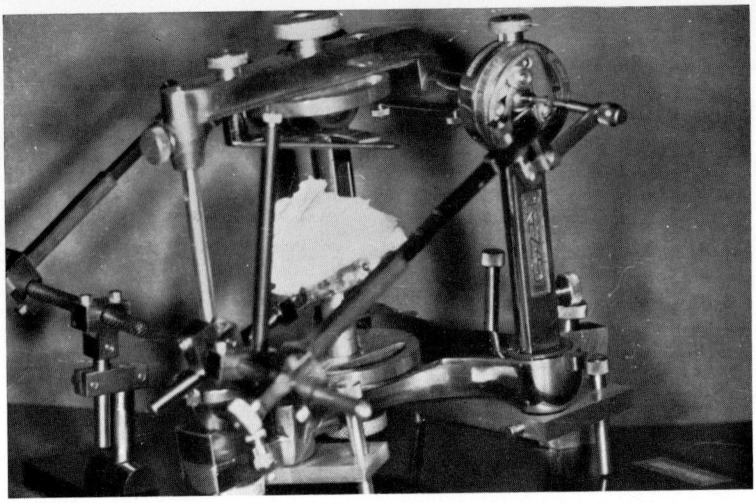

Fig. 41-70. Articulator adjusted to registrations in face bow; stone-filled upper tray ready to be attached to upper mounting ring of articulator.

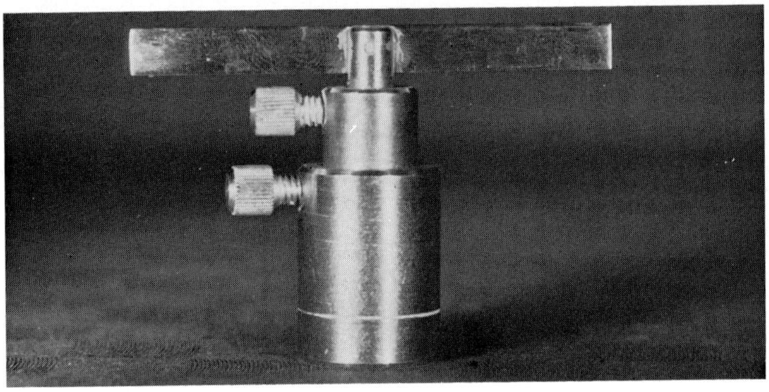

Fig. 41-71. Support used for stabilizing stone-filled tray during attachment to upper mounting ring of articulator.

A

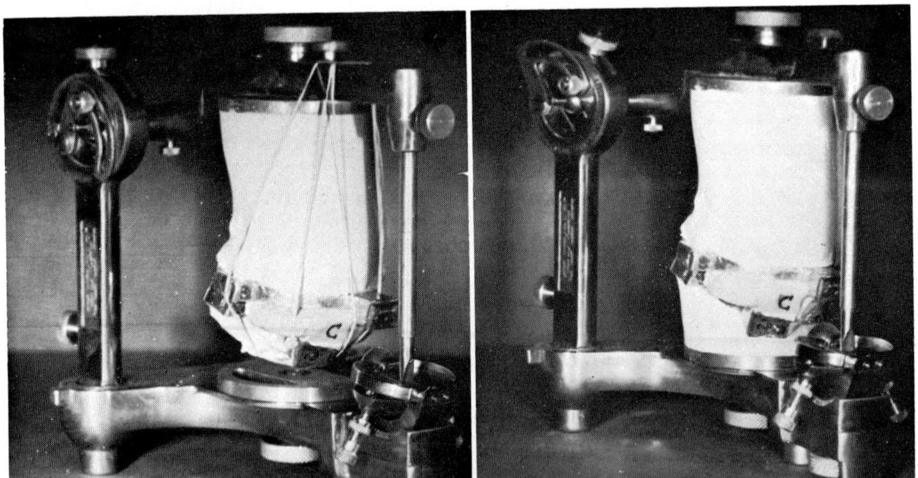

B

Fig. 41-72. A, Upper stone-filled tray attached with stone to upper mounting ring; centric stone checkbite interposed between lower and upper registration trays. **B,** Lower stone-filled tray attached to lower mounting ring with centric stone checkbite interposed; mandibular tray in centric relation to maxillary tray.

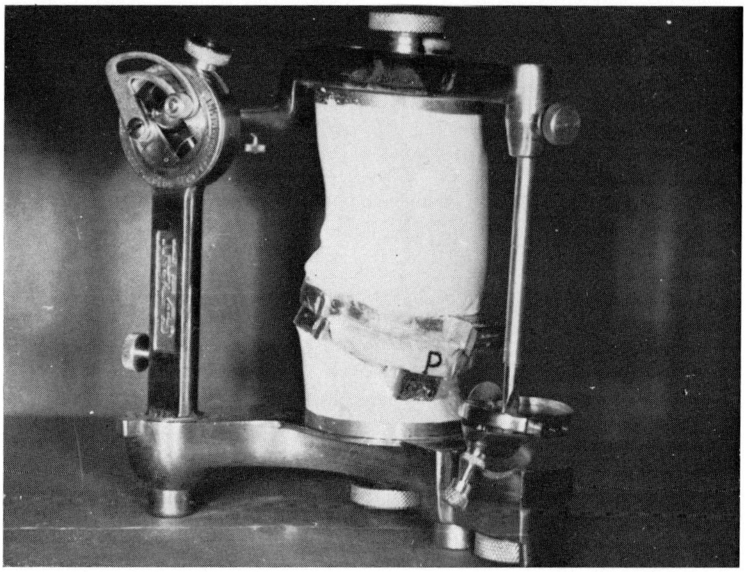

Fig. 41-73. Protrusive stone checkbite interposed between two mounted trays to record condyle path registration.

faces into complete contact with the *P* checkbite (Fig. 41-73). With the two trays held firmly in this relationship, the left and the right condylar guides are set so that there is no rocking or spaces evident between the stone checkbite and the surfaces of the trays.

The protrusive checkbite is replaced with the *right lateral checkbite,* and the condylar post is adjusted to the right lateral Bennett position; also any incisal plane interference is adjusted (Fig. 41-74, *A*).

The right lateral stone checkbite is replaced with the *left lateral checkbite,* and the other condylar post is adjusted to the left lateral Bennett position; also any incisal plane interference is adjusted (Fig. 41-74, *B*).

The articulator has now been adjusted to the four positions of the mandible in its centric, protrusive, right and left lateral relations. All locknuts of the articulator are tightened securely, and the upper and lower stone-filled trays and mounting rings are removed from the articulator; these are replaced with new mounting rings.

Clean out the stone from the upper tray and reassemble its two sections; attach its tray stem. Place 4 mm. to 5 mm. of wax on the underneath surface of the tray carrying the wax from first molar to first molar areas. Mix zinc oxide–eugenol cement and place a layer 4 mm. thick *inside* the occlusal trough of the tray. Bring the tray lightly up against the occlusal surfaces of the upper teeth and *hold until the cement hardens;* only the occlusal and cuspal imprints are needed in this impression. *After* the zinc oxide–eugenol cement has hardened have the patient bite uniformly into the outer occlusal layer of wax and hold the jaw immobile (Fig. 41-75). The only purpose of the wax bite is to stabilize the tray and impression during the subsequent steps.

The face bow is now reassembled as previously described and the tray clamp, *6* (Fig. 41-45), slipped over the tray stem. The condyle pointers are aligned exactly with the condylar axes marks and the orbital pointer with the orbital plane mark on the skin; all clamps and lock screws are then tightened securely (Fig. 41-76).

A

B

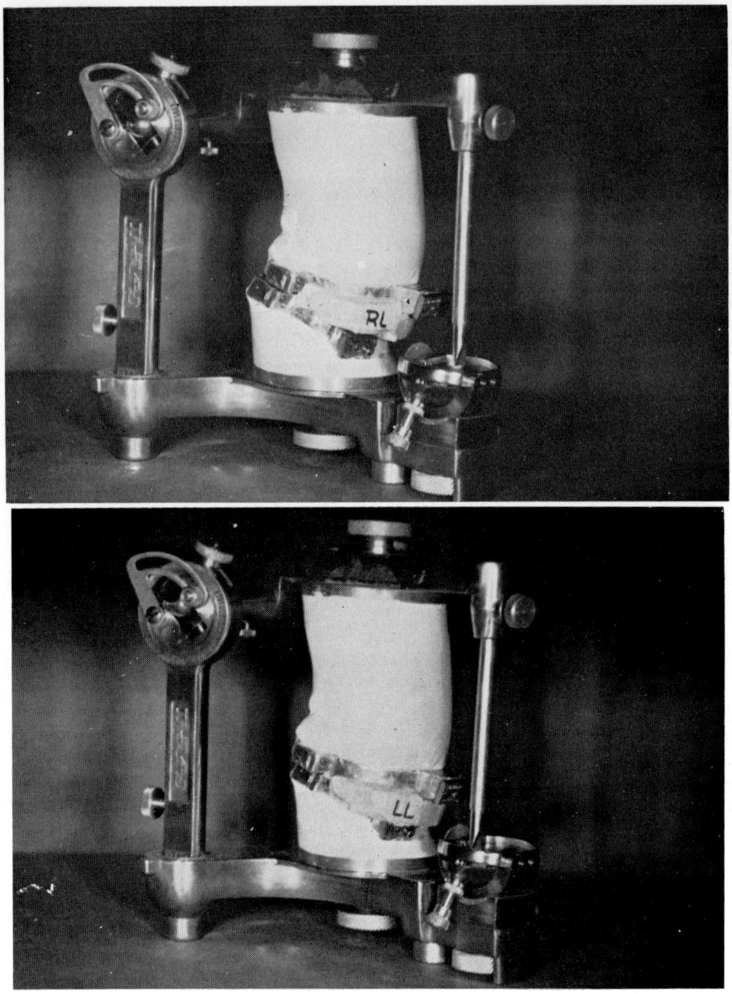

Fig. 41-74. Right and left stone checkbites are interposed for adjusting upright posts of articulator to Bennett right and left paths.

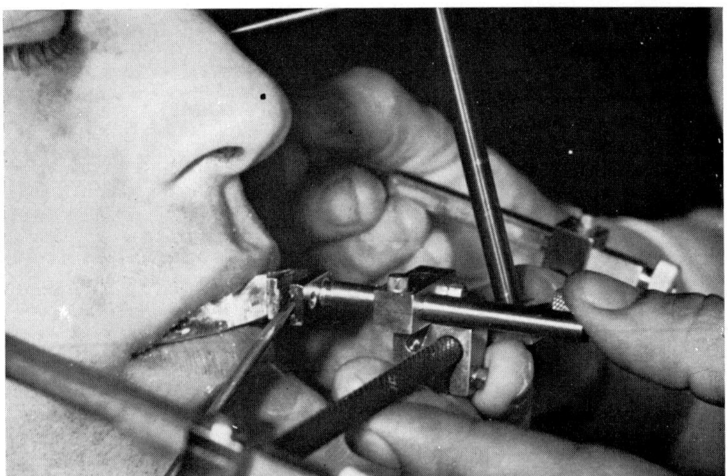

Fig. 41-75. Patient biting against wax attached to undersurface of upper registration tray to hold it in position while face bow is attached to stem of tray lined with zinc oxide-eugenol cement.

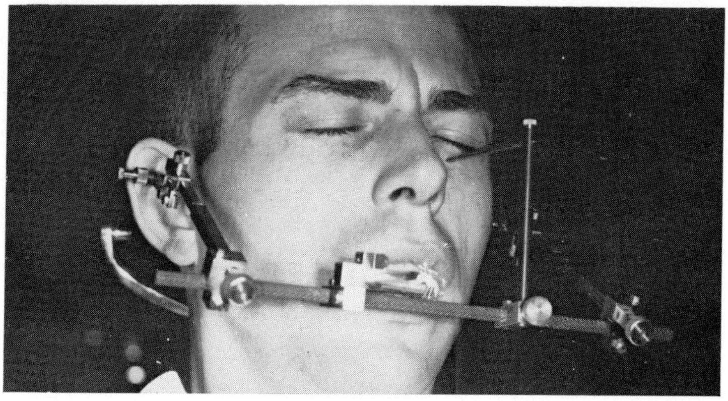

Fig. 41-76. Infraorbital pointer locked to face bow oriented to three reference points.

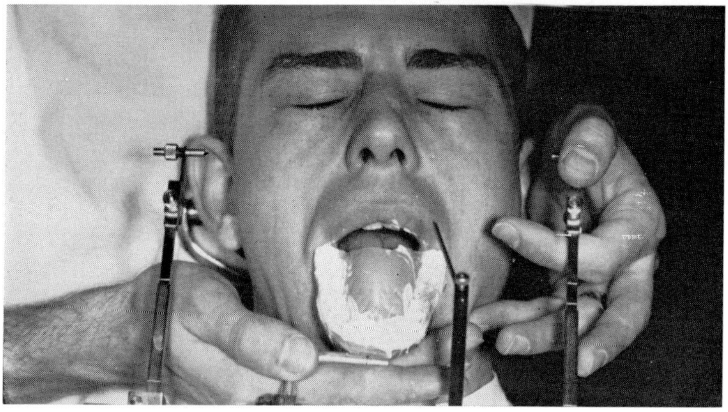

Fig. 41-77. Completely locked assembly of face bow and tray with zinc oxide-eugenol occlusal imprints, removed from patient's mouth.

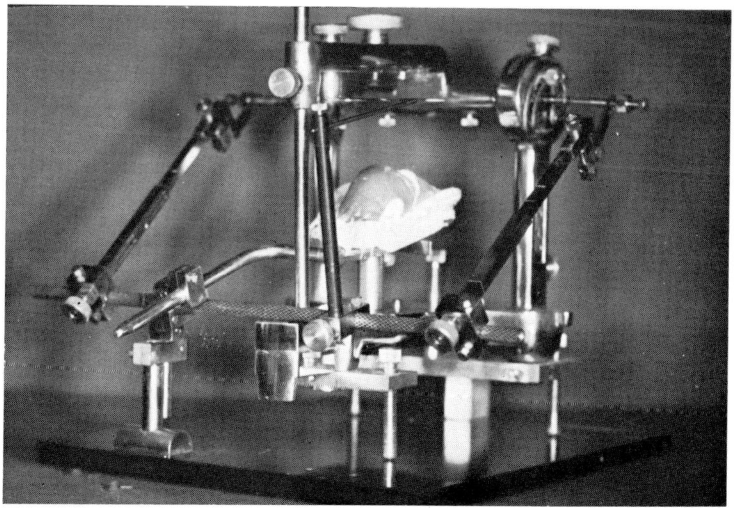

Fig. 41-78. Assembly shown in Fig. 41-77 is locked to face bow support of transfer board. Articulator is oriented to condylar pins and infraorbital pointer of face bow. Articulator is locked to transfer board.

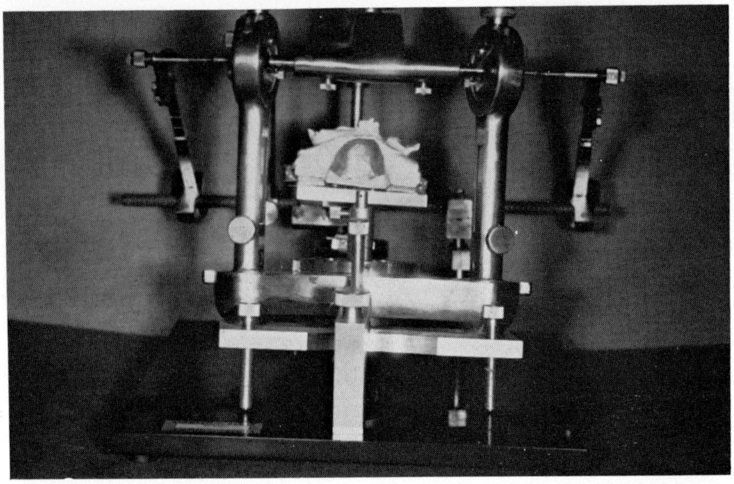

Fig. 41-79. Rear view of Fig. 41-78; articulator locked to transfer board and tray supported underneath.

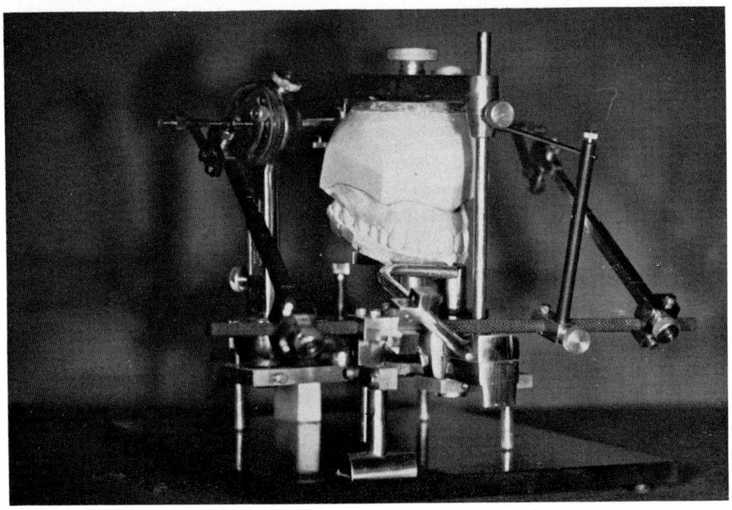

Fig. 41-80. New stone cast is seated in cusp indentations in zinc oxide–eugenol cement in upper tray and attached to mounting ring of upper bow of articulator.

The patient is instructed to open carefully from the wax bite; the upper tray with its zinc oxide–eugenol occlusal imprints, and still locked to the face bow assembly, is depressed and detached from the teeth. Only imprints of the cusp tips and occlusal surfaces of the teeth should be seen in the zinc oxide–eugenol cement (Fig. 41-77).

The articulator, which previously was adjusted to the various registrations with the stone checkbites, is again reoriented on the transfer board to the face bow assembly and locked to the face bow support, *44* (Fig. 41-4), as was previously done (Fig. 41-78). The tray impression is supported beneath by means of the cast support (Fig. 41-79). A new, accurate upper stone cast is seated in the zinc oxide–eugenol occlusal imprints. Any interferences in the cement are cut away if necessary so the cast is positioned perfectly. The cast is now attached to the upper mounting plate of the articulator with stone (Fig. 41-80).

Next, the mandibular cast must be

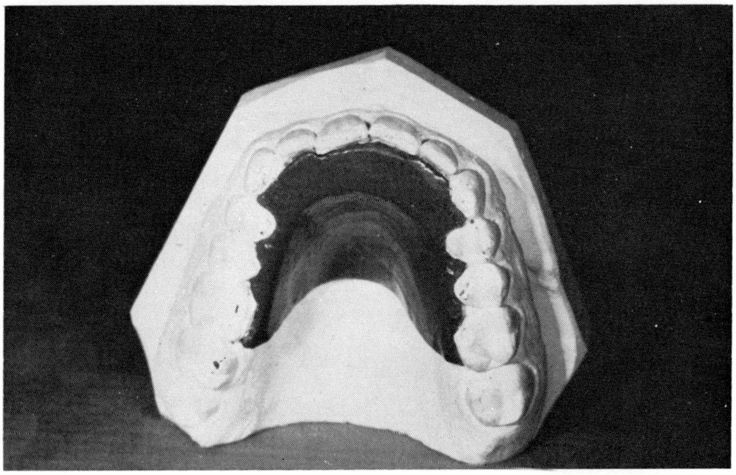

Fig. 41-81. Modeling compound bite plane shaped over tin-foiled palate surface of upper cast.

placed in centric relation to the maxillary cast mounted on the articulator. This may be done by several methods: (1) using the centric wax bite which is customarily employed; (2) the Ash metal, wax, and zinc oxide–eugenol technic; or (3) the modeling compound zinc oxide–eugenol centric registration with buccal and labial stone indexes.

MODELING COMPOUND ZINC OXIDE–EUGENOL METHOD OF OBTAINING CENTRIC RELATION REGISTRATION

After the articulator which has been adjusted to the various registrations obtained by means of the face bow and the stone checkbites, the customary procedure employs the centric wax-bite technic for relating the mandibular to the maxillary cast in centric relation. Such methods require the patient to bite into a relatively resistant substance, which induces the mandible to close in a noncentric relationship. There is the additional danger in such technics of having the dentist force the condyles abnormally into a posterior position in the fossae beyond the desired functionally retruded, terminal position.

The following technic avoids these shortcomings and is readily mastered by the average student and patient.

First, 0.003-inch tin foil is swaged over the palatal surface of the upper cast, including the palatal surfaces of the teeth. A ⅛-inch layer of heated modeling compound is adapted to the tin foil and extended posteriorly from second molar to second molar; it covers the palatal surface. A flat incisal plane is built up, level with the upper incisal edges extending from cuspid to cuspid; it is ½ inch wide labiolingually (Fig. 41-81).

The occluded position of the mandible is first determined. Where an overbite exists, a pencil line is marked on the labial surfaces of the lower incisors, indicating the position of the upper incisal edges when the mandible is in occlusion (Fig. 41-82, *A*, *c*).

Another line, *b*, parallel to and 2 mm. *above the first one*, is placed on the labial surfaces of the lower incisors.

The flat modeling compound plane is now trimmed down or built up, so that the lower incisors touch it when the jaw is in a position of rest (Fig. 41-83).

The tin-foiled, compound bite plane is now removed from the maxillary stone cast and thoroughly chilled.

With an alcohol torch the flat incisal

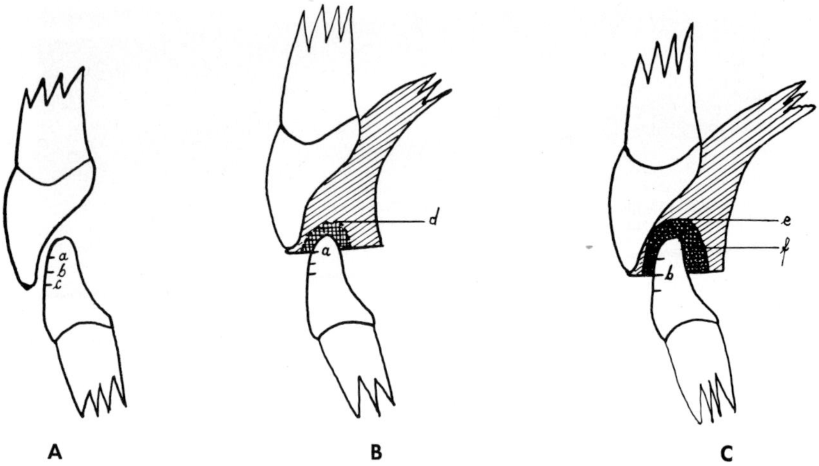

Fig. 41-82. Diagrammatic illustrations of steps shown in Figs. 41-83 to 41-87 in treatment of patient having normal incisal relationship.

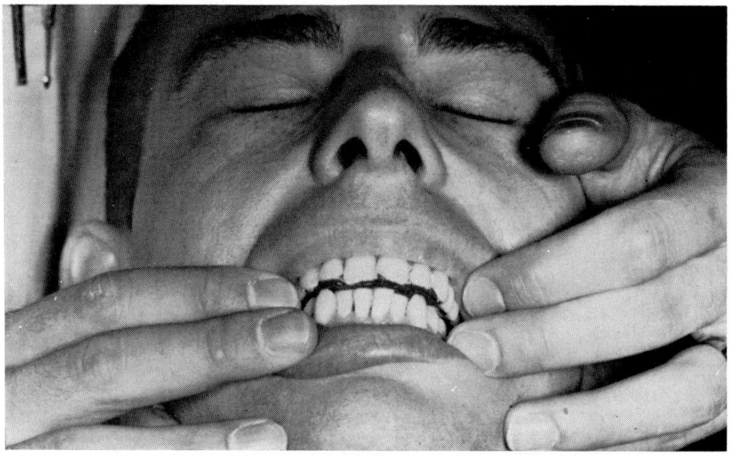

Fig. 41-83. Lower incisors touching modeling compound plane when jaw is in rest position.

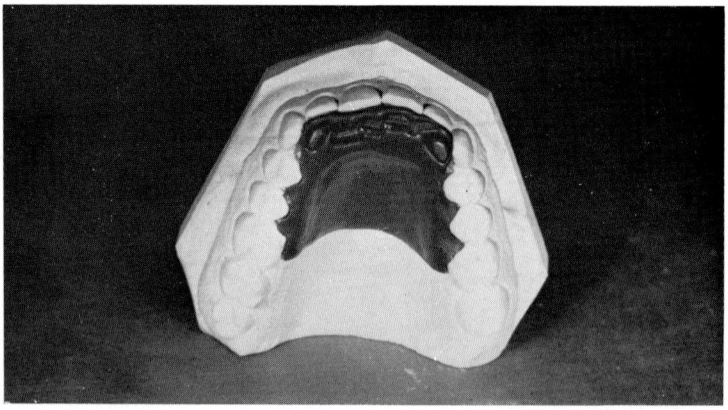

Fig. 41-84. Compound index with lower incisor indentations in flat plane.

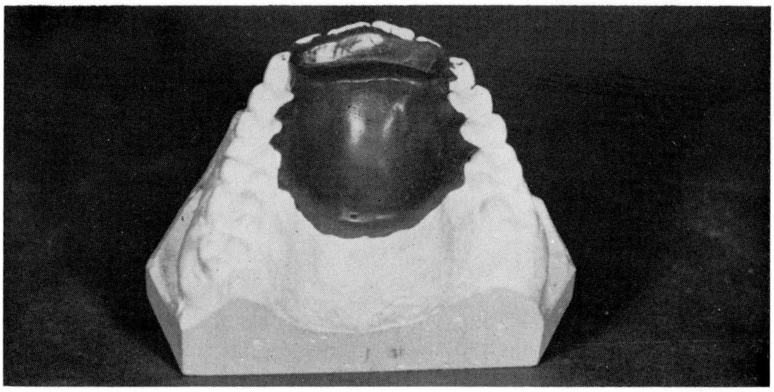

Fig. 41-85. Trench 5 mm. wide and 5 mm. deep cut out along line of indentations made by lower incisal edges.

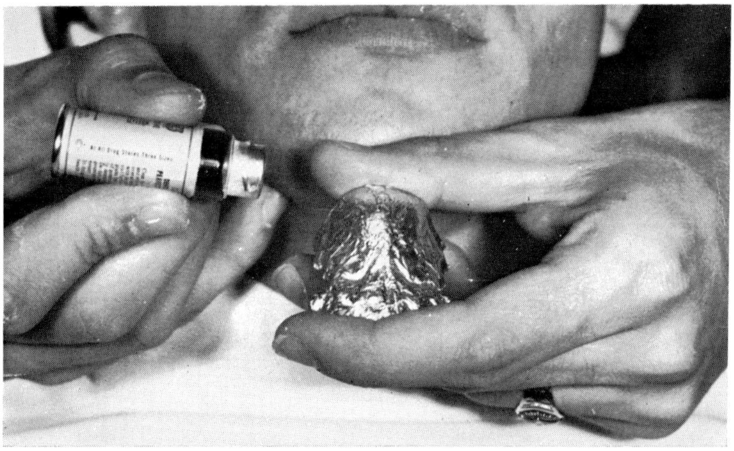

Fig. 41-86. Adhesive powder applied to palatal surface of compound bite plane and zinc oxide-eugenol cement placed in incisal trench.

plane is heated to a depth of 1 mm.

Quickly it is reinserted in the mouth and the patient is instructed to close lightly, only touching the softened surface of the compound (Figs. 41-82, *B, a,* and 41-84). *During closure the patient brings the tip of the tongue up and back, touching the palate posteriorly.* This conditions the patient to position the condyles in their *physiologically retruded, functional terminal positions* in the glenoid fossae.

The compound bite plane is removed from the mouth and chilled thoroughly (Fig. 41-84). It is replaced and the correctness of the vertical closure is verified.

If the closure is correct, the compound bite plane is again removed and chilled. A channel 5 mm. wide and 5 mm. deep (Fig. 41-82, *C*), is now cut out from bicuspid to bicuspid following the curve of the lower incisor imprints. This will eliminate the lower incisal imprints previously made in the compound plane (Fig. 41-85).

The channel is filled with zinc oxide–eugenol cement, and the tissue side of the tin foil is sprinkled with adhesive powder; the compound bite plane is then returned to the mouth (Fig. 41-86).

With the tongue raised so that the tip

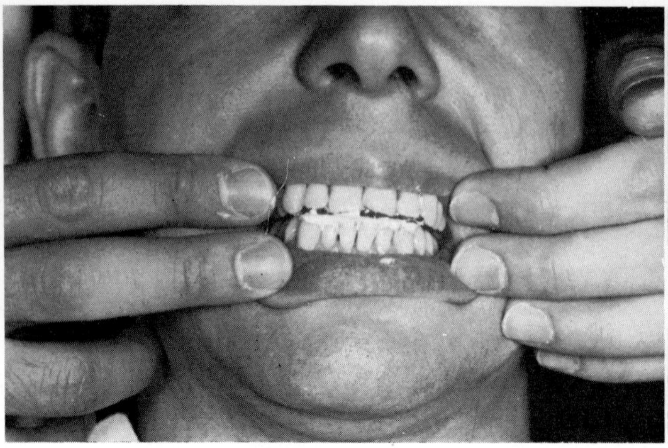

Fig. 41-87

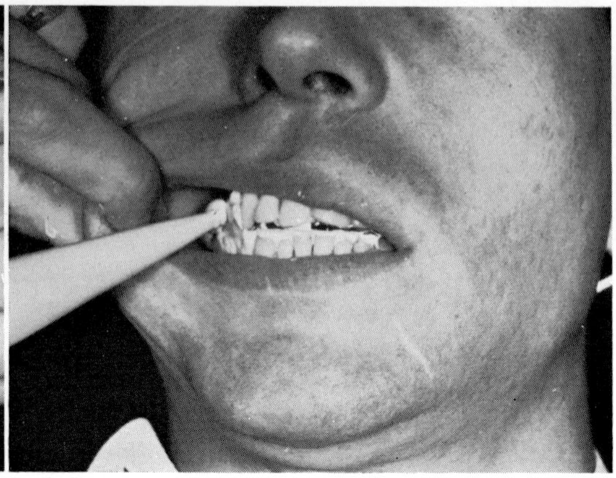

Fig. 41-88

Fig. 41-87. Mandible raised so that lower incisors "float" into zinc oxide–eugenol cement.
Fig. 41-88. Injecting quick-setting stone into buccal vestibules to "freeze" position of mandible in its terminal, centric relation position. Modeling compound plane is in position during this procedure.

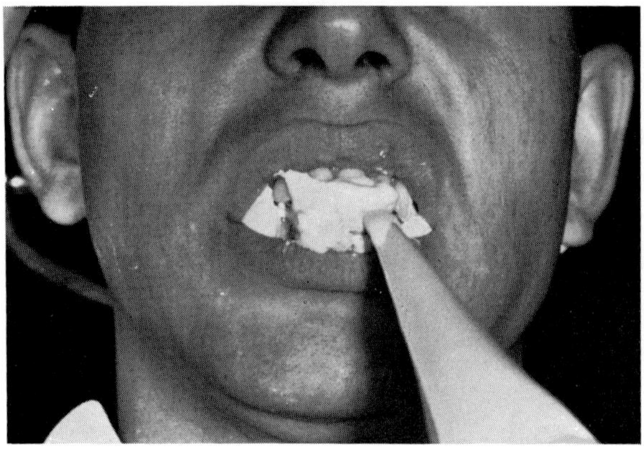

Fig. 41-89

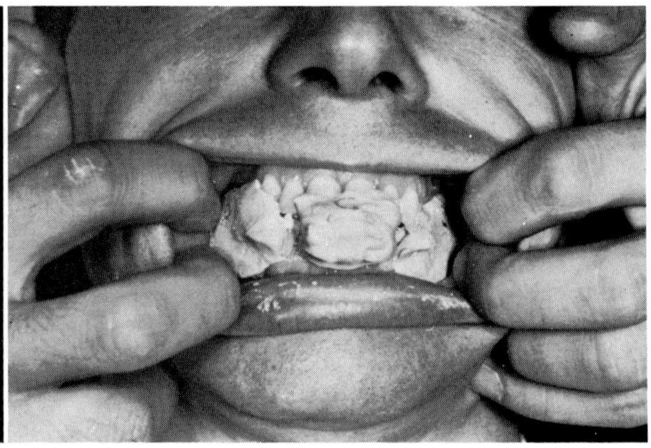

Fig. 41-90

Fig. 41-89. Injection quick-setting stone anteriorly against labial surfaces of incisors.
Fig. 41-90. Three stone cores or indexes registering mandible in its centric relation to glenoid fossae.

touches the posterior border of the modeling compound bite plane during closure, the patient raises the mandible until the middle pencil line on the mandibular incisors (Fig. 41-82, *C, b*) is even with the upper incisal edges. This gives a closure 2 mm. short of complete occlusal contact (Fig. 41-82, *A, c*), but lying in the path of centric relation closure. The mandibular incisors and cuspids have been *floated* into the zinc oxide–eugenol cement without encountering any solid resistant material or interference. The condyles also are in their physiologically retruded, functional terminal positions in the glenoid fossae.

Do not have the lower incisors at any time come in contact with the compound plane. The patient holds this vertical, functionally retruded, terminal position un-

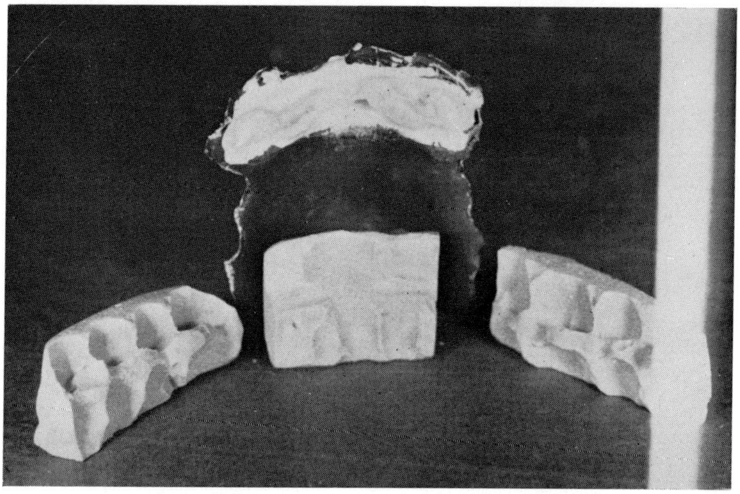

Fig. 41-91. Stone cores are trimmed to cervical lines of enamel of all teeth. Incisal imprints are seen in zinc oxide–eugenol cement of compound bite plane.

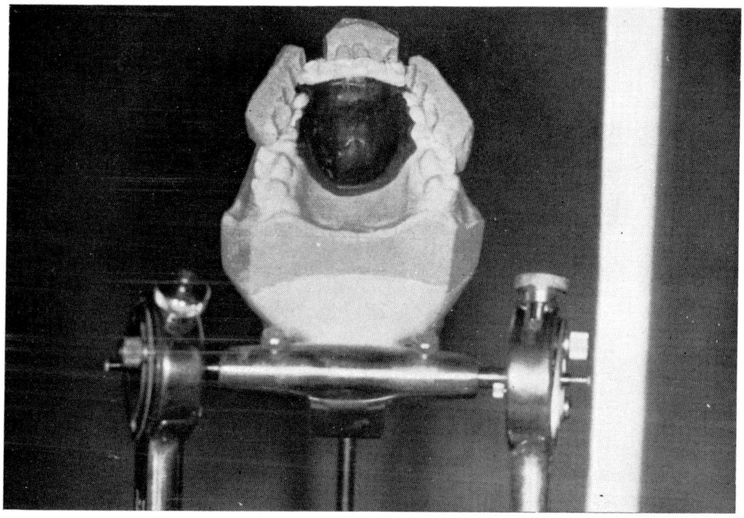

Fig. 41-92. Maxillary cast is fitted accurately to each core individually; same procedure is done with mandibular cast, individually.

til the zinc oxide–eugenol cement hardens completely (Fig. 41-87).

When it has set, some quick-setting stone is immediately injected into the left and right buccal vestibules, against the buccal surfaces of the upper and lower bicuspids and molars (Fig. 41-88); the same is done against the anterior surfaces of the incisors (Fig. 41-89). The stone cores are allowed to set completely (Fig. 41-90).

When hardened, the three cores are removed, as well as the compound bite plane with its incisal imprints in the zinc oxide–eugenol cement (Fig. 41-91). The three stone cores are trimmed so that only the impressions of the buccal and the labial enamel surfaces of the teeth are retained; the gum tissue areas are cut away to the cervical margins of the teeth.

Each core area is now fitted individually to its specific quadrant, tooth area on

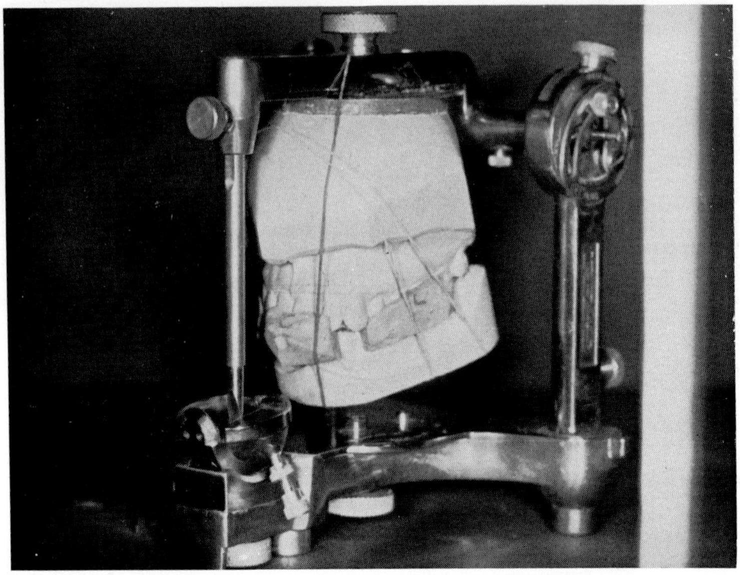

Fig. 41-93. Upper and lower casts related to each other with cores are held together with sticky wax or other means, and lower cast is attached with stone to lower ring of articulator.

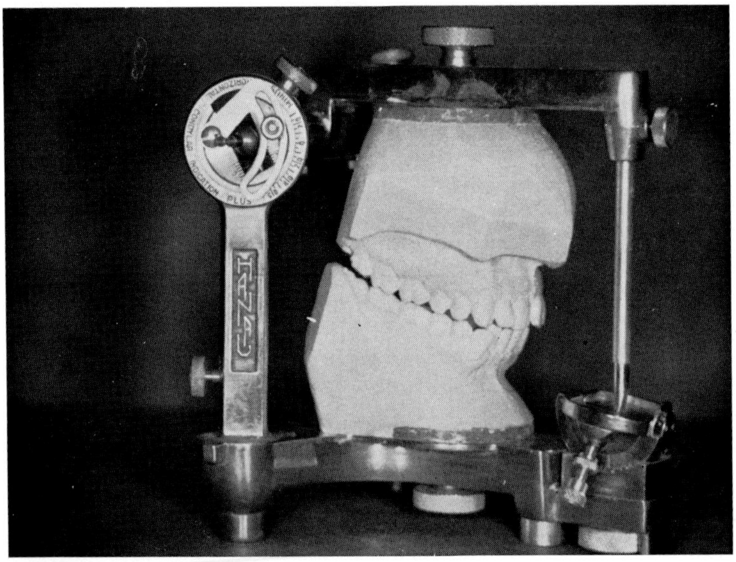

Fig. 41-94. Casts mounted to each other on articulator previously adjusted to centric, protrusive, and two lateral positions of mandible.

the casts, first to the upper, then to the lower (Fig. 41-92). By means of the three stone cores and the compound zinc oxide–eugenol bite index, the mandibular cast is related to the upper cast in centric relation without the teeth coming in contact with each other. The two casts fitted into the stone cores are held together with wax or by other suitable means (Fig. 41-93); the maxillary cast, having been previously mounted to the articulator, the lower cast is now attached to the lower

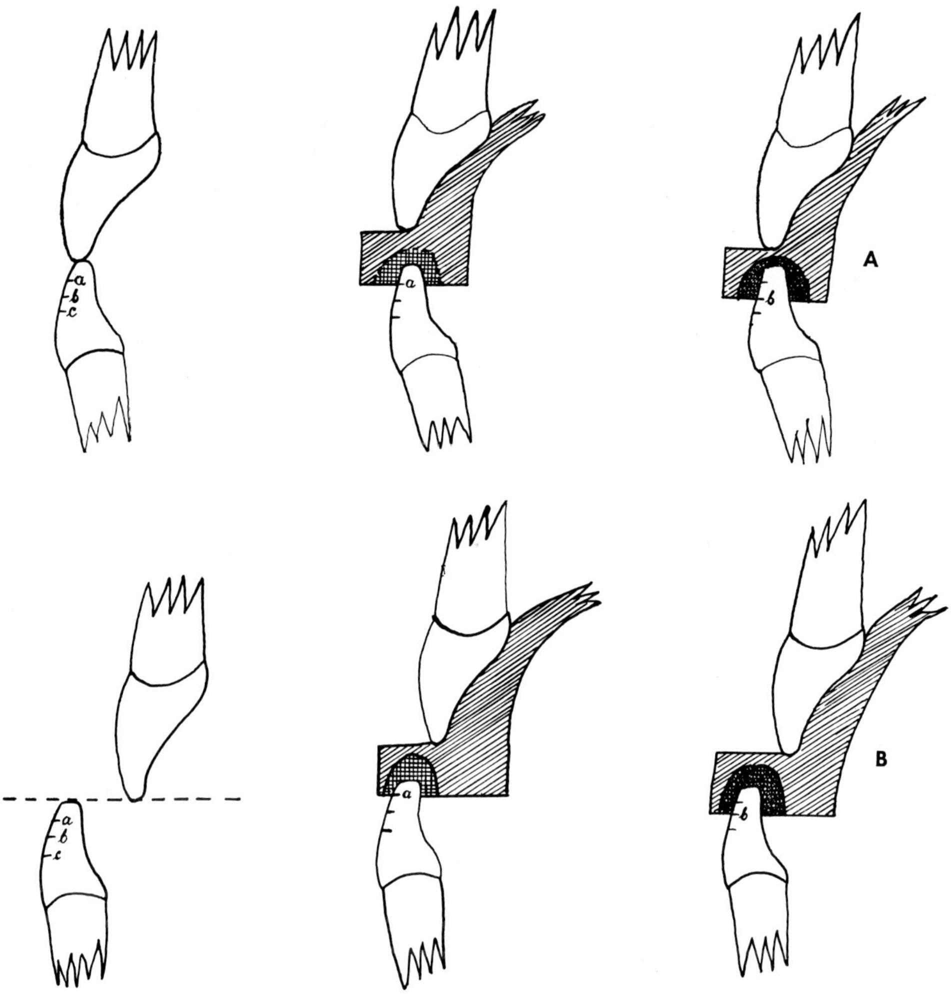

Fig. 41-95. Use of compound bite plane with zinc oxide–eugenol cement in end-to-end, **A,** and prognathous, **B,** types of relationships.

mounting plate of the articulator with stone.

When the stone has set, the three stone cores and the compound zinc oxide–eugenol bite plane are removed. The mandibular cast has now been related to the maxillary in centric relation, and in a functionally retruded position in the glenoid fossae (Fig. 41-94).

In those patients having an end-to-end bite or a prognathous jaw relationship, the technic may also be used by modifying the shape of the modeling compound bite plane (Fig. 41-95, *A* and *B*).

Because the articulator was previously adjusted to centric, protrusive, and right and left lateral positions of the mandible, the locknut of the incisal pin may now be loosened and the two casts be slowly brought together to make initial occlusal or incisal contact.

When this is done, the following determinations may be made:

1. How much vertical distance is available in reconstruction if a vertical increase is decided upon
2. The amount of existing interocclusal space when the jaw is at rest

3. The teeth which make initial occlusal contact
4. Additional closure which occurs after initial occlusal contact is made
5. The direction in which the mandible moves from initial to final occlusion, whether laterally or anteroposteriorly
6. Any other malrelations of the teeth and arches associated with temporomandibular joint dysfunctions
7. Correlation of roentgenographic, pathologic, and physiologic data with stomatognathic findings
8. The amount and type of occlusal equilibration required, if any
9. The most acceptable plan of restorative treatment compatible with the registrations of (1) the mandibular movements in the glenoid fossae and (2) the occlusal interrelations of the teeth during function
10. Any changes which may take place in the stomatognathic system in the future

Analyzing positions of condylar spheres

To determine the direction and the amount in which the mandible moves laterally and anteroposteriorly from initial to final occlusion, the condylar-element-assembly has been modified as shown in Figs. 41-96 and 41-97. The manufacturer's description and instructions for the adjustment and use of this assembly are given as follows:

The articulator is in correct "zero" centric position when on each side, the notch No. 7 marked 0 on the periphery of the centric stop No. 4 coincides with the indicating line No. 6 on the condylar element, and the flat underedge of the stop is aligned with 0 of the protrusive-retrusive calibration No. 3. Each full turn of the centric stop, gauged by the notch, is 1 mm. Each line on the top surface of the stop indicates 0.25 mm. The stops are individually calibrated and therefore are not interchangeable.

The shoulders on the condylar shaft must contact the flat on the spheres No.

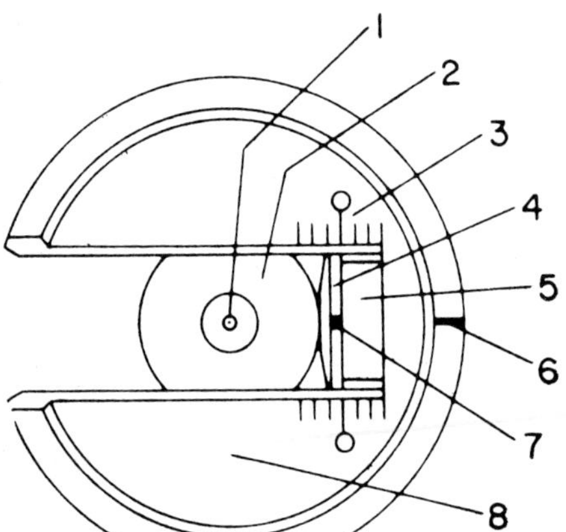

Fig. 41-96

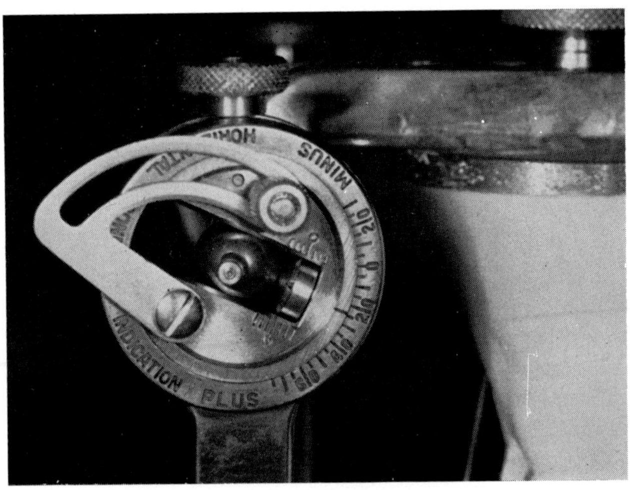

Fig. 41-97

Fig. 41-96. **1,** Extendible condylar shaft. **2,** Condylar sphere. **3,** Protrusive-retrusive calibration. **4,** Centric stop. **5,** Spacer. **6,** Indicating line. **7,** Notch and flat undersurface. **8,** Condylar element, complete assembly. (Courtesy Hanau Engineering Co., Inc.)

Fig. 41-97. Improved condylar element on the Hanau H2-XPR articulator, showing newly added spacer, stop, and condyle path calibrations. (Courtesy Hanau Engineering Co., Inc.)

2 when these rest upon the centric stops without binding or excessive side-to-side play of the shaft; the flat of the incisal pin exactly coincides with the width of the center groove of the incisal guide. All adjustments are secured by tightening the thumbscrews.

A spacer No. 5 (Fig. 41-98, *B*) is fitted under the centric stop No. 4 for convenient setting and retention of the condylar spheres No. 2 at "zero" centric position. This spacer, until removed, also limits adjustment of the condylar spheres to "anatomical protrusive"; removal of the spacer permits adjustment to "anatomical retrusive." (NOTE: These spacers and their stops are individually fitted, and therefore are not interchangeable.)

IMPORTANT: When the spacer No. 5 is in position and engages the flat undersurface of the centric stop No. 4, the condylar spheres No. 2 are within "zero" centric range. If necessary, the notch No. 7 is realigned to exactly coincide with indicating line No. 6, and while carefully held in that position, the thumbscrew on the inner surface of the condylar element is securely tightened.

Repositioning condylar spheres. When it is necessary to reposition the condylar spheres in the condylar slots, either protrusively or retrusively, the following adjustments are made.

Anatomic protrusive. Posterior to articulator "zero" centric (after protrusive and lateral guidances have been adjusted):

Loosen thumbscrews on inside face of condylar elements. Adjust centric stops No. 4 posteriorly, the required number of fraction of millimeters. Now loosen thumbscrews in the underpart of the upper member and equally extend both shafts by turning counterclockwise until the shoulders on condylar shaft again contact the flat on the condylar spheres No. 2 when these rest upon the centric stops without binding or side-to-side play of shaft; the flat of incisal pin centers the groove of the guide. Lock adjustments by tightening thumbscrews.

Anatomic retrusive. Anterior to articulator "zero" centric after protrusive and lateral guidances have been adjusted:

Remove the spacers No. 5 from under the centric stops No. 4 (Fig. 41-98, *A*);

A

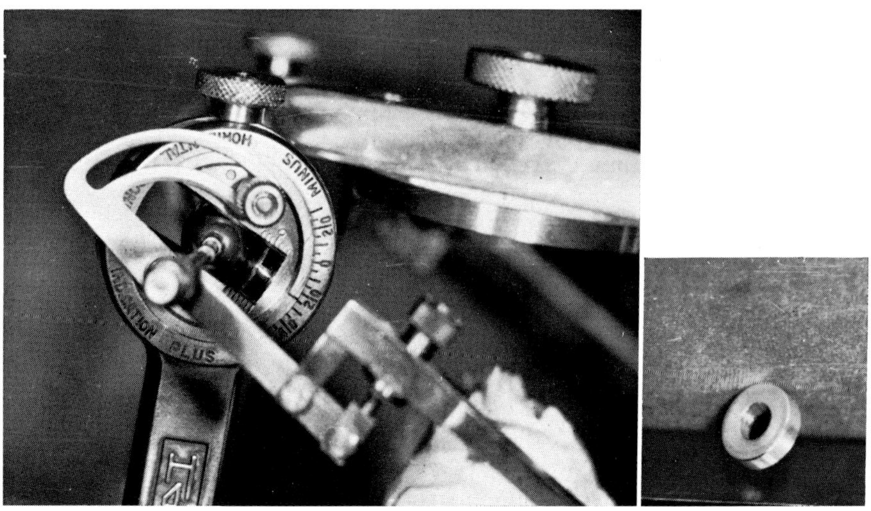

B

Fig. 41-98. A, Condylar assembly with spacer removed. **B,** Spacer. (Courtesy Hanau Engineering Co., Inc.)

replace the stops to position of "zero" centric.

Proceed as above described, except adjust centric stops anteriorly and reduce length of shaft by turning its ends clockwise.

It will frequently be possible to set both condylar posts to zero on calibrations at their base, thus eliminating the necessity for changing the shaft length.

SELECTED REFERENCES

1. Sicher, H.: Movements and positions of the mandible, Illinois D. J. **25**:220, 1956.
2. Contino, R. M., and Stallard, H.: Instruments essential for obtaining data needed in making a functional diagnosis of the human mouth, J. Prosth. Dent. **7**:66, 1957.
3. Stuart, C. E.: Gnathological instruments, Ventura, California, 1956.
4. Denar Model D4 Articulator and Pantograph, Anaheim, California, Denar Co.
5. Hanau axis face bow technic in conjunction with Hanau articulator model H2-XPR, Buffalo, N. Y., Hanau Engineering Co., Inc.

GENERAL REFERENCES

Refer to pp. 831-836.

Index

F